From-the-Editor Columns

Published in *The American Journal of Cardiology* 1982–2015

by

WILLIAM C. ROBERTS, MD
Editor in Chief

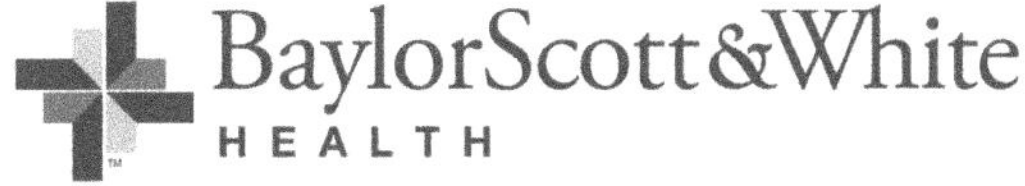

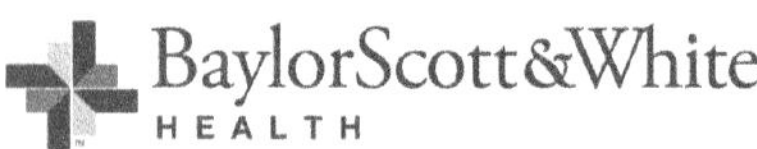

Baylor Scott & White Health
3500 Gaston Avenue, Dallas, TX 75246
1-800-4BAYLOR
http://baylorscottandwhite.com/

ISBN: 978-0-9845237-6-4

Table of Contents

Preface

When I became editor of *The American Journal of Cardiology* in June 1982, I thought that it might be useful for the readers and authors to have some idea of the thoughts of the new editor. The result was the initiation of the *From the Editor* columns beginning in July 1982. During the first 1.5 years, the publisher placed these columns among the advertising pages with an "A" page number, which excluded them from indexing and binding. In 1984, these columns began appearing in the regular editorial pages of the journal. During the first 5 years, the columns appeared in each issue, and during that time there were 15 issues a year. We now publish 24 issues a year, and these *From the Editor* columns appear about 5 times yearly. Through the years, some colleagues have suggested to me that the columns—or at least some of them—be collected in a single volume. This book is a result.

I have been honored to serve and to continue to serve as *The American Journal of Cardiology's* editor in chief, and that position has allowed the smooth publication of these columns, only a few of which have gone through the strenuous manuscript review process. My hope is that a few readers will find some of these 221 columns interesting, and all possibly a useful record.

—*William C. Roberts, MD*

Preventive Cardiology

An Agent with Lipid-Lowering, Antihypertensive, Positive Inotropic, Negative Chronotropic, Vasodilating, Diuretic, Anorexigenic, Weight-Reducing, Cathartic, Hypoglycemic, Tranquilizing, Hypnotic and Antidepressive Qualities

About 20 million Americans are runners or joggers. The difference between the two is the speed of the pace, with the divider being about 8 minutes/mile. About 70% of U.S. runners or joggers log in <10 miles/week and 4%, >40 miles/week. The champion marathoners usually run 100 to 120 miles/week. The winner of the 1983 New York marathon had a 4.9-minute/mile pace for the 26.22 miles and the 327th finisher and a 5.9-minute/mile pace. I started running 4 years ago and now average 13 miles/week. I usually enjoy the run and afterwards I always feel better—both mentally and physically. It's virtually the only exercise I do now. I like it because of its efficiency, its lack of dependence on another person (a tennis partner, for example) or on a particular place (golf course, for example) or time. One can run day or night, rain or shine and anywhere. I've run in most major cities in the U.S. and some abroad, and when I think back on those trips, it's usually what I saw during the runs that I remember the most. I think and plan during a run. I rethink my priorities. Many ideas for research projects and "From-the-Editor" columns have come during runs.

But what is the real value of running? I believe that running is a recapturing of some of our individual independence lost to the automobile and other industrial inventions of the 20th century. Paul Dudley White said that coronary heart disease came with the automobile. Running is getting out of the car and moving with one's own horsepower.

There is no question that running is healthful. It *decreases* the resting heart rate, resting blood pressure, body fat, appetite, low-density lipoprotein cholesterol (the bad one) and triglyceride levels, and *increases* mental health and tolerance to stress, resistance to infections, soundness of sleep, fibrinolytic (clot-dissolving) capability, high-density lipoprotein cholesterol (the good one), cardiac, pulmonary, bowel and thyroid glandular function, and the strength of ligaments, tendons, skeletal muscles and bones. Running, then, is a pretty good "medicine" without the use of drugs, or scalpels or psychiatrists.

A great benefit of running is that it makes one health-responsible. Few runners smoke, and those who do smoke less than before. Runners are diet-conscious. On a recent plane trip I sat next to a woman who, I learned, ran about 20 miles/week. When noticing that she did not eat her pie with the meal, I inquired as to why not. She answered that "It was 4 miles" (400 calories = 4 miles). It takes nearly 32 minutes to run those 4 miles and <3 minutes to eat those 400 calories! The trade-off for the runner is simply not worth it. The more the body weight the harder the running. Fish is digested more easily than is red meat and good gastrointestinal function is important to a runner. Running provides a calmer disposition and few regular runners need psychiatrists.

Individual responsibility for health has taken a giant step forward in the U.S. in the last 2 decades. The U.S. population is healthier today than 20 years ago. The death rate from coronary heart disease is decreasing in the U.S., and the U.S. is the only country in the Western world where this is so. Renewed interest in exercise almost surely has played a role in this improvement in health.

A major stimulant for the emphasis on self-responsibility for health came from Dr. George Sheehan, who writes a

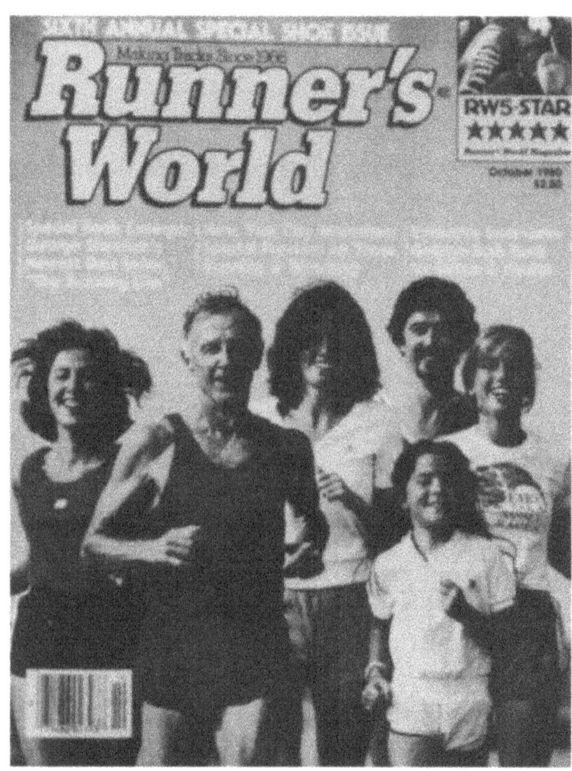

Cover of *Runner's World* magazine showing Dr. Sheehan running with several of his 12 children. (Reprinted with permission from *Runner's World.*)

piece on the importance of exercise in this issue (see page 260). George Sheehan was born 65 years ago in Brooklyn, New York. He went to Manhattan College on a track scholarship, was a member of a championship cross-country team, and was runner-up to the U.S. champion miler in 1940. He graduated from Long Island College of Medicine and in 1949 began private practice of internal medicine and cardiology in Red Bank, New Jersey. At the same time, his family was enlarging and eventually numbered 12 children.

In 1963 he broke a bone in his hand and could not play tennis, and thus, at age 44, his second running career began. Since then he has missed training on the road only when ill or injured. He runs about 30 miles/week—10 on Tuesday, 10 on Thursday, and a race every Sunday. He calls himself a "mainline jogger" who gets withdrawal symptoms if he goes more than 48 hours without running. At age 50, he was the world record holder for milers aged 50 years or older, with a time of 4 minutes, 47 seconds. He has run dozens of marathons, and at age 61 ran his fastest one (3 hours, 1 minute). That means he averaged 7 minutes for each of the 26.22 miles. In recent years, he has run the 6-mile race in 37 minutes. He has, of course, the runner's physique (weight in pounds = twice height in inches) and mystique.

The renewal of running brought out Sheehan's pen. In 1968, he started and has continued a weekly column titled "The Innocent Bystander" in his local newspaper, the *Red Bank Daily Register.* In 1970, he started a monthly medical advice column in the magazine *Runners World,* which has nearly a half million subscribers, and in 1972, he became its medical editor. Since 1974, he also has written a monthly column in *The Physician and Sports Medicine* entitled, "Running Wild." In addition, he has written books.

Running not only brought out the writer in Sheehan, but also brought out the philosopher. He started going to the public library rather than the medical library. Someone remarked that James F. Fixx writes on how to run and George Sheehan on *why* we run. Sheehan found his philosophy in his many philosophical friends; they include Emerson, Thoreau, Ortega, Santayana, William James, certain Greek philosophers, and Goethe, and he introduced them to many readers for the first time. Sheehan shows that athletes do not need to retire by age 40. He is an inspiration to me and I suspect to many others. He has demonstrated that a single cardiologist can improve the health of the entire country by setting an example of healthfulness rather than serving entirely as an advisor for healthfulness.

William C. Roberts

William C. Roberts, MD
Editor-in-Chief

Reducing the Blood Cholesterol Level Reduces the Risk of Heart Attack

During this century, many human and nonhuman studies have demonstrated clearly that the higher the blood total cholesterol (TC) level, the greater the chance of developing atherosclerotic coronary heart disease (CAD). However, the proof that lowering the blood TC lowered the risk of developing symptomatic or fatal CAD has been lacking. But no more; the proof is in. If the plasma TC level is lowered in persons with initially high levels (>265 ml/dl), the risk of developing fatal CAD or nonfatal acute myocardial infarction (AMI) also is lowered. The evidence is unequivocal. For each 1% that the plasma TC is lowered, the risk of developing fatal CAD or nonfatal AMI is lowered by about 2%.

The long-awaited data come from the National Heart, Lung, and Blood Institute's Lipid Research Clinics Coronary Primary Prevention Trial (LRC-CPPT), the results of which were reported in the January 20, 1984, JAMA (pages 351–374). This study, surely to be a classic, was 10 years in the making and cost $150 million. It was carried out in 12 clinics in North America and involved 3,806 men, at entry aged 35 to 59 years, with fasting plasma TC levels >265 mg/dl and no clinical evidence of CAD. To get the 3,806 men, 436,679 had to be screened. The participants were randomized into 2 groups: 1,900 who received 24 g of placebo (P) each day plus a moderate (400 mg of cholesterol) lowfat diet and 1,906 who received the same diet plus 24 g of cholestyramine (C) resin each day. The design was double-blind and 100% of the participants were followed for 7 years, some for 10 years. The baseline characteristics of both the P and C groups were virtually identical: mean plasma TC = 292 mg/dl; mean low-density lipoprotein (LDL) cholesterol = 219 mg/dl; mean high-density lipoprotein cholesterol = 44 mg/dl; percent currently smoking cigarettes (37% and 39%); mean systemic blood pressure (120/78 mm Hg) (patients with systemic hypertension were excluded); and age (mean = 48 years). The magnitude of the trial is mind-boggling. The 3,806 men who entered the trial had 193,000 clinic visits, 341,000 blood tests and 72,000 ECGs; 1,055,000 clinic data forms were filled out. Each participant took up to 24 g of P or C each day and most adhered to the specified diet during the entire 7-year period. The clinic appointments were every 2 months and each was preceded by a 12-hour fast. The participants never had knowledge of their blood lipid levels, and no guarantee of benefit from participation in the trial.

The cholesterol-lowering effects in the participants were as follows: Between the initial baseline level and time 0, when both treatment groups were on diet alone, a 3.5% decrease in TC and a 4.0% decrease in LDL cholesterol occurred in both groups. In year 1, with the introduction of drug therapy, an additional 14% decrease in TC and a 21% decrease in LDL cholesterol occurred in the C group. The cholesterol differences between the 2 groups became highly significant in year 1. Although the gap between the C and P groups narrowed as the study continued, the differences in cholesterol levels at the end of 7 years were statistically significant. The average differences between the C and P groups were 8.5% in TC and 12.6% in LDL cholesterol. In the C group, the overall reduction of TC was 13.4% and of LDL cholesterol, 20.3%. The overall differences in cholesterol levels between the 2 groups would probably have been better had there been a more optimal adherence to therapy. By the end of year 7, the number of medication packets consumed daily was down to 3.6 (from 6) in the C group and to 4.4 in the P group, and 27% of the participants were consuming no C or P.

The difference in the study's primary end point—the number of definite CAD deaths and/or nonfatal AMIs—was significantly different ($p < 0.05$) between the 2 groups: 187 definite CAD deaths or nonfatal AMIs in the P group and 155 in the C group, a 19% reduction in risk. This figure reflected a 24% reduction in definite CAD deaths and a 19% reduction in definite nonfatal AMIs. By the end of 7 years, 8.6% of the P group and 7.0% of the C group had had a primary end point event, a 19% reduction. The risk of developing 3 other "softer" CAD end points also was significantly reduced: 20% for developing angina pectoris (235 vs 287), 25% for developing a positive exercise ECG (260 vs 345) and 21% for having aortocoronary bypass surgery (93 vs 112. A clear relation also was observed between the amount of reduction in both TC and LDL cholesterol levels and the amount of decrease in CAD risk.

Although the LRC-CPPT study included only men aged 35 to 59 years with plasma TC >265 mg/dl, the conclusion of the study, i.e., that decreasing both TC and LDL cholesterol levels reduces the risk of developing CAD, are readily applicable to women and to younger persons with both similar and less elevated cholesterol levels. Irrespective of the manner in which the blood TC and LDL cholesterol levels are lowered—whether by diet alone, diet plus lipid-lowering drugs or lipid-lowering drugs alone—the important factor is to lower the TC and LDL cholesterol levels. The lower these levels, the lower the risk of developing CAD and vice versa. The high plasma TC levels on entry of the participants in the LRC-CPPT study occur in only 5% of Americans aged 35 to 59 years, and levels <150 mg/dl, below which symptomatic or fatal CAD is almost nonexistent, also occur in only 5% of Americans in this age group. The average plasma TC of all Americans aged 35 to 59 years now is down to 211 mg/dl, but the average of male victims of AMI is only about 225 mg/dl. Thus, our levels must continue to decrease. The results of this landmark study provide support for lay persons in assuming greater responsibility for the health of their systemic arteries by controlling their intake of saturated fat and for physicians to actively work toward lowering the blood TC and LDL cholesterol levels when elevated in their patients. In my view, simple maintenance of an ideal or near-ideal body weight is most helpful in this regard, for in adults this nearly always requires limiting the intake of high-cholesterol containing foods, which are usually high in calories.

Although this study involved men without clinical evidence of CAD at entry, the study's conclusion also appears applicable to patients with symptomatic CAD. The lowering of the TC and LDL cholesterol levels in patients with angina pectoris and healed myocardial infarction may well slow the progression of the atherosclerotic process.

To Bob Levy who initiated the study, to Basil Rifkind who carried it through. and to the staff of the 12 clinics, congratulations for producing this long-needed information. To the 3,806 participants who each consumed up to 61.32 kg (135 lbs) of the unpleasant-tasting powdered medicines or placebos during the 2,555 days of the study, and, especially to the 1,906 participants who received the placebo and, consequently no benefit from it, our hearty thanks.

William C. Roberts

William C. Roberts, MD
Editor-in-Chief

Extreme Hypercholesterolemia = Malignant Atherosclerosis

In adults with plasma total cholesterol (TC) levels <150 mg/dl, atherosclerotic plaques large enough to narrow arterial lumens rarely develop and symptomatic or fatal organ ischemia rarely occurs. Most such adults live in underdeveloped countries or in the Eastern world or both. In contrast, in adults with plasma TC levels >150 mg/dl, atherosclerotic plaques large enough to narrow arterial lumens often develop and symptomatic or fatal ischemia of 1 or more body organs is frequent; most of these adults live in developed or Western world countries.

In the USA, the average plasma TC level of persons 20 years of age is about 160 mg/dl, but thereafter the level progressively increases.[1] The increase, however, is not as high today as it was a decade ago.[2] The average plasma TC of adults older than 40 years in the USA is down to 210 mg/dl, from about 225 mg/dl a decade ago.[2] The average plasma TC of persons in coronary care units with acute myocardial infarction is about 225 mg/dl.[3] All these figures, however, are considered "normal" in most laboratories in the USA. In the Clinical Chemistry Laboratory of the Clinical Center (i.e., the Hospital) of the National Institutes of Health, the "normal" range for serum TC is stated to be 163 to 263 mg/dl. The upper limit in some laboratories is 300 mg/dl. For laboratories, particularly those of prominent research institutions, to present values of this level as normal prevents attempts of physicians and of patients to make efforts to lower the plasma TC to levels where signs and symptoms of organ ischemia do not occur, and that level, for practical purposes, is <150 mg/dl. I consider any plasma TC level >150 mg/dl to be elevated.

If the upper limit of the normal plasma TC level is considered to be 250 or 300 mg/dl, hypercholesterolemia does not fall out as a greater risk factor for development of symptomatic or fatal cardiovascular atherosclerosis than does systemic hypertension or cigarette smoking. In areas of the world, however, where the frequency of systemic hypertension and cigarette smoking is high but the level of plasma TC is low, i.e., <150 mg/dl, the occurrence of symptomatic or fatal coronary heart disease is virtually nonexistent. About 15 years ago, I visited Kampala, Uganda, and examined many aortas, coronary arteries and circles of Willis at necropsy. Other than a few small yellow dots or streaks that produced virtually no luminal narrowing, these arteries were free of atherosclerotic plaques. Yet, the frequency of systemic hypertension in this central African population was extremely high—indeed, hypertension was their most common cardiovascular condition—and a high percentage of the hearts were heavier than normal, presumably the result of the systemic hypertension. I was also impressed with the high frequency of cigarette smoking among the population. In Central Africa, many adults have plasma TC levels of about 100 mg/dl, a value >100% less than the average plasma TC level in adult Americans. In my view, evidence is lacking to implicate either systemic hypertension or cigarette smoking as an accelerator of atherosclerosis in the absence of hypercholesterolemia if the normal plasma TC level is defined as a level <150 mg/dl; if the TC level, however, is >150 mg/dl, as is the situation in 95% of adults over 40 years of age in the USA, both systemic hypertension and cigarette smoking are highly atherogenic.

In contrast to the levels in Central Africa, where symptomatic and fatal coronary heart disease is virtually nonexistent, only 5% of Americans older than 40 years have plasma TC levels <150 mg/dl. Thus, to perform studies on meaningful numbers of adults over 40 years of age in the USA with plasma TC levels <150 mg/dl (ideal normal value) and compare findings to those with levels 160 to 260 mg/dl (usual values) is virtually impossible. In contrast to the 5% of middle-aged and older adult Americans with plasma TC levels <150 mg/dl, 5% of American adults older than 40 years have plasma TC levels >265 mg/dl, and about 1 in a million have plasma TC levels >600 mg/dl and normal plasma triglyceride levels.

Elsewhere in this issue (page 20), Sprecher and associates describe certain clinical and morphologic cardiovascular findings in a group of patients with extremely elevated plasma TC levels. Of the 16 patients, all but 2 before therapy had plasma TC levels >400 mg/dl and normal and near-normal plasma triglyceride levels; most had TC levels >600 mg/dl and the average was 729 ± 58 mg/dl. Additionally, 90% of the TC was composed of low-density lipoprotein, the water-soluble, extremely atherogenic component of the TC, and little high-density lipoprotein, the good cholesterol, was present. The consequence of this devastating hypercholesterolemia was what might be called "malignant atherosclerosis." Without therapy to lower the plasma TC level dramatically, coronary heart disease is usually fatal by the teenage years in these unfortunate persons with homozygous familial (both mother and father had type II hyperlipoproteinemia) hypercholesterolemia.

Of the 16 patients, 4 had died from coronary heart disease at a mean age of 12 years; 3 others, aged 5, 10 and 38 years, had symptoms of myocardial ischemia, and 9 at the time of initial study were still free of symptomatic coronary heart disease, but their mean age was only 9 ± 1 years. Of the 4 patients who had died (mean age 12 years), the extent of the atherosclerotic plaquing was severe and, at the same time, unusual. In the usual adult with severe atherosclerosis, the atherosclerotic process virtually always spares the ascending aorta (except for a few plaques in or about the sinotubular junction), the process is most extensive in the abdominal portion of aorta, and it is present, but less extensive, in the arch and descending thoracic aorta. In the 4 necropsy patients described by Sprecher et al, the ascending aorta in each was extensively and diffusely involved by atherosclerotic plaques, the extent being greater than that in the abdominal aorta; the reverse of the usual. Furthermore, the atherosclerotic process actually involved the aortic valve cusps, which became thickened by lipid and fibrous tissue and calcific deposits, and in 2 of the 4 patients aortic valve stenosis was a consequence. Additionally, the ostia of the coronary arteries were extremely narrowed by the atherosclerotic plaques, an unusual occurrence in adults without extreme hypercholesterolemia (unassociated with hypertriglyceridemia) or aortitis. The coronary arteries and other arteries arising from the aorta were extensively involved by atherosclerotic plaques in 3 of the 4 patients. In 1 patient, however, the arteries arising from the aorta were virtually spared of atherosclerotic plaques; the ostia of the coronary arteries, however, were so narrowed by the aortic atherosclerotic plaques that severe generalized myocardial ischemia resulted (ischemic cardiomyopathy).

The 4 necropsy patients described above had plasma TC levels before therapy of 588 to 1164 mg/dl (mean 870). The extreme degree of atherosclerotic plaquing in them demonstrates the devastating effect of extreme hypercholesterolemia. These patients and those with lower TC levels show that the risk of the plasma TC is proportional to its level. The higher the level, the greater the risk and vice versa. The recent Lipid Research Clinic study[4] of patients with plasma TC levels >265 mg/dl (patients with homozygous familial hypercholesterolemia were excluded) clearly shows that lowering plasma TC lowers the risk of heart attack. To believe that lowering the TC level is not important in 1984 in preventing coronary heart disease is simply not to be familiar with the facts. The problem arises in the definition chosen for hypercholesterolemia. The usual definition of normal in the USA is, of course, an *average* and for the adults over 40 years of age it is usually stated to be 160 to 300 mg/dl (mean 211). These levels are highly atherogenic and the consequence is near-epidemic symptomatic and fatal atherosclerosis. The nonatherogenic populations living on planet Earth have plasma TC levels <150 mg/dl; it is this level, in my view, that should be considered normal, for it is below 150 mg/dl where, for practical purposes, persons do not have to worry about the development of atherosclerosis and its consequences.

William C. Roberts

William C. Roberts, MD
Editor-in-Chief

References

1. Lipid Research Clinics Population Studies Data Book. Vol. I. The Prevalence Study. U.S. Dept. Health and Human Services, Public Health Service, National Institutes of Health (NIH Publ. No. 80-1527), July 1980:136.
2. **Beaglehole R, LeRosa JC, Heiss GE, Davis CE, Rifkind BM, Muesing RM, Williams OD.** Secular changes in blood cholesterol and their contribution to the decline in coronary mortality. *In* Proceedings of the Conference on the Decline in Coronary Heart Disease Mortality, U.S. Dept. Health, Education, and Welfare, Public Health Service, National Institutes of Health (NIH Publ. No. 79-1610), May 1979:282–295.
3. **Gore JM, Goldberg RJ, Matsumoto AS, Castelli WP, McNamara PM, Dalen JE.** Validity of serum cholesterol levels obtained within 24 hours of acute myocardial infarction. Am J Cardiol 1984;54: accepted for publication (Sept. 1984).
4. Lipid Research Clinics Program. The Lipid Research Clinics Coronary Prevention Trial Results. I. Reduction in incidence of coronary heart disease. II. The relation of reduction in incidence of coronary heart disease to cholesterol lowering. JAMA 1984;251:351–374.

Cardiac Rupture, Abdominal Aneurysmal Rupture and Dissecting Aortic Rupture: A Preventive Trio

Today, 5 March 1985, I visited an impressive local hospital for a cardiovascular conference. I was 5 minutes late; about 60 persons were waiting (5 × 60 = 5 hours of human time wasted). A table in the front of the conference room contained 3 hearts. I started with A86-28. A thick-walled, nondilated, nonscarred left ventricle with a transmural acute myocardial infarct in the posterolateral wall. On the epicardial surface was a 1-cm-long left ventricular rupture site. The 61-year-old woman had been well, except for systemic hypertension, until 7 days earlier when the substernal chest pain began and within 4 hours streptokinase had been injected intravenously. The next day the serum creatinine kinase level was nearly 1,400 with 10% MB fraction. The next 6 days were uneventful: no shock, no congestive heart failure, no arrhythmias. On day 7 she was found in bed dead; 450 ml of blood was present in the pericardial sac. The subepicardial fat was so extensive that the heart floated in water. All 3 major epicardial coronary arteries were narrowed >75% in cross-sectional area by plaque. She had been well for all 61 years and chest pain occurred and disappeared quickly 7 days before death. Weight was too much: 149 pounds on the 62-inch frame. Cardiac rupture occurs in about 10% of patients with fatal acute myocardial infarction. Rupture of the free wall, ventricular septum or papillary muscle appears to be increasing as fewer arrhythmias are fatal in the coronary care units. Why are ruptured hearts so heavily covered with adipose tissue? Does a skinny person ever rupture the left ventricular wall during acute myocardial infarction? I thought no.

The next case was A86-29. An 8-cm-diameter aneurysm of the abdominal aorta was present and it had ruptured. This 73-year-old man also had had systemic hypertension. Computed tomography had shown the abdominal aortic aneurysm also to be 8 cm in diameter and its lumen was about 30% filled with thrombus. The abdominal aortic aneurysm was to be resected after the carcinoma of the lung had been treated by rads and chemotherapy. But the aneurysm ruptured at home. Necropsy also disclosed severe coronary narrowing by atherosclerotic plaques. Most persons with abdominal aortic aneurysm die from coronary artery disease, not from complications of the aortic aneurysm. This man was different.

The next heart (A86-30) had blood within the wall of the swollen ascending aorta, around the pulmonary trunk and around both left and right main pulmonary arteries. These findings meant dissection of the aorta. She, a 73-year-old woman, had been well all her life except for systemic hypertension until 2 days earlier when back pain, followed by abdominal pain, suddenly appeared. Radiograph showed the ascending aorta to be bigger than normal. Suddenly it was over. The outer partition of the false channel of the ascending aorta ruptured, first into the aortic adventitia, which shares a common adventitia with the pulmonary trunk. Blood entering the aortic adventitia rapidly spread to the adventitia of the pulmonary trunk and then into the adventitia of both right and left main pulmonary arteries. The adventitial hemorrhage into the wall of the left main pulmonary artery caused severe cross-sectional area narrowing of the lumen of this artery, i.e., peripheral pulmonic stenosis. The aortic dissection stopped shortly after origin of the innominate artery because severe atherosclerosis of the aortic arch had caused atrophy and fibrosis of the underlying aortic media. The left ventricular wall was thickened but free of scars and its cavity was of normal size. (The dilated left ventricle is not capable of generating a hypertensive pressure, which is essential for aortic dissection to occur.)

Thus, 3 ruptures: one of the left ventricular free wall, one of an abdominal aortic fusiform aneurysm and one of the outer wall of the false channel of a dissected ascending aorta. All 3 patients had had systemic hypertension with hypertrophied hearts. Left ventricular rupture during acute myocardial infarction, abdominal aortic aneurysm and aortic dissection rarely occur in the absence of earlier systemic hypertension.[1–4] Of course, atherosclerosis was crucial in causing the coronary narrowing in case 1, in allowing the abdominal aortic aneurysmal formation in case 2, and in preventing progression of the dissection further than the ascending aorta in case 3, but it too is preventable by getting the plasma or serum total cholesterol level below 150 mg/dl. The best treatment for cardiac rupture and abdominal aortic aneurysm begins with proper eating in early life, and the proper treatment of aortic dissection begins with prevention of systemic hypertension at any time in life.

I hope the 5-minute wait will be forgiven and the benefit of blood pressure–lowering and lipid-lowering preventive therapies will be long remembered.

William C. Roberts

William C. Roberts, MD
Editor in Chief

1. Roberts WC. *The hypertensive diseases. Evidence that systemic hypertension is a greater risk factor to the development of other cardiovascular diseases than previously suspected. Am J Med 1975;59:523–532.*

2. Roberts WC. *The aorta: its acquired diseases and their consequences as viewed from a morphologic perspective. In: Lindsay J Jr, Hurst JW, eds. The Aorta. New York: Grune & Stratton, 1979:51–117.*

3. Roberts WC. *Aortic dissection: anatomy, consequences, and causes. Am Heart J 1981;101:195–214.*

4. Roberts WC, Ronan JA Jr, Harvey WP. *Rupture of the left ventricular free wall (LVFW) or the ventricular septum (VS) secondary to acute myocardial infarction (AMI): an occurrence virtually limited to the first transmural AMI in the hypertensive individual (abstr). Am J Cardiol 1975;35:166.*

In One Day in the USA

In 1984, the book *In One Day* by Tom Parker was published by Houghton Mifflin (Boston). In its 94 pages are 365 entries describing what 236 million Americans do in each 24-hour period.

Every day in the USA, 10,000 persons are born, 5,500 die, and the population increases over 5,000 (the result of births and immigration minus deaths and emigration). Each day, 30 become 100 years of age and 5,500 become 65 years of age. Americans spend $800 million daily on personal health care, an average of $3.50 per person. Two million visit a doctor's office, 100,000 are admitted to a hospital and stay an average of just over 7 days (shorter now), 67,000 have an operation (circumcision in 4,100, tonsillectomy in 1,250, appendectomy in 850 and coronary artery bypass in 500). About 4,125 gallons (4 quarts, 3.785 liters) of blood are donated and used. About 3 million depend on someone else to help them in going to the toilet, and 827,000 need help getting out of bed. About 137,000 stay home from work because of a cold which also keeps 164,000 children from school. About 4,100 have a heart attack; 1,500 die. Heart disease of some sort kills 2,700 despite the consumption of 52 million aspirin tablets. Cancer is discovered in 2,200 persons and 1,000 die from it. Americans scrub their teeth with 550,000 pounds of toothpaste, spend $12,000 on dental floss, but, nevertheless, 1 million persons see dentists who fill 500,000 cavities using 80 pounds of gold.

Our daily oral intake includes some of the following: About 815 billion *calories* of food are consumed, roughly 200 billion more than we need to maintain a moderate level of activity. (That's enough extra calories to feed everyone in Mexico, a country in 1984 of 80 million people). Nearly 100,000 *cattle* are herded into slaughter houses and they leave 60 million pounds of red meat and nearly 4 million square feet of hide. About 250,000 *hogs* are butchered and 17,700 *lambs* and *sheep*. More than 4 million pounds (454 g) of bacon are eaten. About 1.5 million pounds of lard (hog fat) and 47 million hot dogs (smoked sausage of beef or beef and pork) are eaten daily. McDonald's restaurants serve the equivalent of 2,250 head of cattle. The fishing industry processes 33 million pounds of *fish* and *shellfish*, 22 million pounds (67%) of which is used for human food; the remainder is fed to nonhuman animals or used to make chemicals and paint. We eat 1.7 million pounds of canned tuna (enough to make nearly 16 million tuna-salad sandwiches), 190,000 of sardines, 247,000 of fish sticks and 250,000 pounds of lobster. We eat 600 pounds of beef, however, for every 1 pound of live lobster.

Dairy cows in the USA produce 47 million gallons of milk daily, 19 of which are used as *liquid milk*, and the rest as *cheese*, *yogurt* and other dairy products. We eat 12.5 million pounds of cheese, including 85,000 pounds of blue cheese, 700 pounds of cream cheese, 650,000 pounds of Swiss and 5.8 million pounds of cheddar cheese. Cottage cheese alone makes up >2.5 million pounds or 312,000 gallons of the daily diet. Americans eat 170 million *eggs* and 12 million *chickens*.

We also eat >200 million pounds of fresh fruit and vegetables, including 550,000 bushels (22 million pounds) of *apples*, half of which are eaten fresh; 400,000 bushels of *bananas* and 23,500 bushels of fresh *lemons*. We eat 1.2 million bushels (35 liters) of *potatoes;* 1.0 million of *tomatoes;* 100,000 of *broccoli;* 90,000 of fresh *carrots*; 88,000 of *green peppers* and >100,000 bushels of shelled or roasted *peanuts*. We also eat 1.5 million pounds of *cauliflower*, 17 million of *lettuce*, 2.8 million of *cucumbers*, 72 million of *wheat flour* and 220,000,000 million pounds of *salt*. Also, 400,000 gallons of canned *corn* and 6.5 million gallons of popcorn are consumed daily.

Americans eat 50 million pounds of *sugar*, an average of 21 teaspoons apiece for all 236 million persons; 3 million gallons of *ice cream* and *ice milk;* and 10 million pounds of *candy*, including 5.8 million pounds of chocolate candy and 56,000 gallons of *honey*. The average American eats 1 teaspoon of *artificial colors, flavors* and *preservatives*, or almost 4 pounds a year. Americans eat 1.3 million *TV dinners* daily, warm up 2 million pound of *frozen entrees* and "nationality" dishes, and 75 acres (43,560 square feet) of *pizza*. We spend $300 million eating out and drink $64 million worth at the bar.

We use 450 billion gallons of water in our homes, factories and farms; we drink 115 million gallons of *water*, 23 million of *soft drinks*, 17 million of *coffee*, 6 million of *tea*, 3 million of *orange juice*, 15.7 million of *beer and ale* and 1.5 million gallons of *hard liquor* (enough to get 26 million persons thoroughly drunk).

Americans smoke 85 million packs of *cigarettes*. If 1 cigarette deducts 5.5 minutes of life from the smoker, collectively, Americans shorten their lives by 18,000 years every day. We fill 85,000 bushels with cigarette butts. Four thousand children and teenagers take up smoking each day.

We take 30 million *sleeping pills*. Smugglers fly 150 planeloads of illegal drugs into the USA, or 1 shipment every 10 minutes, and earn 123 million dollars selling the illegal drugs. Americans smoke 85,000 pounds of *marijuana* and snort 325 pounds of *cocaine;* everyday 5,000 people try cocaine for the first time. Americans inject themselves with 25 pounds of heroin. Americans swipe 100,000 doses of narcotics, stimulants and depressants from pharmacies, drug manufacturers, hospitals and doctors' offices.

We also dispose of considerable quantities of solid and liquid matter. Each day, we use 6.8 billion gallons of water to flush our toilets, filter 10 billion gallons of liquids with our kidneys and produce 88 million gallons of urine. We produce 88 million gallons of moisture by breathing and sweating, and give off enough heat with our bodies to boil 140 million gallons of water (It would take 12 million gallons of gasoline to boil the same amount). Our public sewers drain off enough organic waste to make 6.0 million pounds of nitrogen plant food, an amount equivalent to 54 million pounds of commercial fertilizer. Collectively, we pass >9 million cubic feet of gas, enough to inflate a balloon 250 feet in diameter.

The hearts of Americans pump collectively >400 billion gallons of blood, equivalent to 8 million kilowatt-hours of energy, enough to run 150 locomotives for 24 hours.

William C. Roberts

William C. Roberts, MD
Editor in Chief

Fast Foods and Quick Plaques

In 1955, in Des Plaines, Illinois, the first McDonald's restaurant opened its doors. By 1960 there were 250 McDonald's in the USA and by 1986 there were more than 9,000 McDonald's worldwide. In late 1985, 1 McDonald's went up every 15 hours around the world. Other fast-food restaurant chains followed so that by the end of 1986 about 60,000 units were present worldwide (Table I). Fast-food restaurants are located everywhere including shopping malls, airports, bus and train terminals, zoos, military bases, college campuses, museums, Mississippi River boats, and *hospitals*! Burger King hauls its Whoppers to your door or playground. It's been converting $110,000 recreational vehicles into mobile restaurants ("burger wagons"). The 50 top fast-food restaurant chains sold about $50 billion in food and drink in 1986. Fast-food sales jumped 40% between 1977 and 1984. Americans in 1986 spent an average of over $200 per person in fast-food restaurants. One half of all monies spent in restaurants in the USA today is spent in the fast-food restaurants. Twenty percent of Americans eat their lunch every day in a fast-food restaurant; 13%, their supper, and 5%, their breakfast. They move in and out of the restaurant rapidly. The seating is hard, uncushioned, immobile. After shifting in the seat once or twice, the typical customer is on his/her way.

The above information comes from the book *Fast-Food-Guide* by Michael F. Jacobson, PhD (Executive Director, Center for Science in the Public Interest, Washington, DC), and Sara Fritschner, a food writer (Workman Publishing, New York, 1986, 225 pp, $4.95). The book examines the foods and drinks served by the 15 top fast-food chains with charts (Tables II, III and IV) showing the caloric, fat, sodium and sugar content of their foods. It is astounding to see what some of the most popular products contain. If one squeezed real hard either a Burger King Double Beef Whopper with Cheese or a Wendy's Triple Cheeseburger, about 15 teaspoons of saturated fat, more than a quarter of a cup of fat, would ooze out; both contain about 1,000 calories and 1,200 and 1,850 mg of sodium, respectively (Table II). Add to that Hardee's French Fries, large, and 5 more teaspoons of saturated fat, 306 g of sodium, and more than 400 calories are consumed. Most chains cook the french fries in beef fat and 1 chain (Taco Bell), in coconut oil. And, of course, some liquid drink is needed with the burger and fries. The Dairy Queen Chocolate Shake, large, 21 fluid ounces, provides 6 more teaspoons of fat, 360 mg of sodium, 29 teaspoons of sugar, and 970 calories (Table IV). Wendy's Triple Cheeseburger, Hardee's French Fries and Dairy Queen's Shake total nearly 2,500 calories and over 2,500 mg of sodium. The ketchup for the burger and fries contains more sugar than ice cream (29% vs 23%).

It wasn't easy for Jacobson and Fritschner to obtain the information on the accompanying tables. Two of the 15 companies would not release any "nutritional" information and others were "slow" to do so. The result of this reluctance to provide ingredient information is that the consumers of the fast-food products have little concept of what is in the foods or drinks. Jacobsen spent 1 long weekend on the fast-food track visiting a dozen different restaurants and ordering a variety of foods. He asked the clerks what were the *ingredients* in the foods. Some clerks were uncooperative. Some brought out the bulk containers that had the ingredient labels on them, and some asked what the word "ingredient" meant.

The present and preceding generations were the first to "grow up" on fast foods, which are tasty, convenient and predictable, but obviously not nutritious. These restaurants are particularly attractive to the younger generation. The chains appeal to the children and the children hook their parents. The fast-food chains spend millions in marketing to attract the kids. Ronald McDonald is better known to children than any figure other than Santa Claus. Taco Bell provides Huggletts stuffed animals. Others provide Star Wars and Star Trek, Care Bears, Masters of the Universe, Fast Macs—the themes change with the times. Hardee's provide a recorded Gremlins Story. Fast-food restaurants with playgrounds have higher sales than restaurants without. Roy Rogers established the Buckaroo Club for children under 10.

TABLE I The Biggest Franchised Restaurant Chains

Company	1985 Sales ($ millions)	Restaurants
1. McDonald's	11,000	8,901
2. Burger King	3,990	4,225
3. Kentucky Fried Chicken	3,100	6,396
4. Wendy's	2,700	3,459
5. Hardee's	2,200	2,411
6. Pizza Hut	2,100	4,912
7. Dairy Queen	1,572	4,822
8. Taco Bell	1,140	2,173
9. Big Boy	1,135	870
10. Domino's Pizza	1,097	2,816
11. Arby's	814	1,545
12. Church's	739	1,647
13. Ponderosa	681	641
14. Long John Silver's	637	1,359
15. Jack in the Box	612	822
16. Dunkin' Donuts	577	1,447
17. Shoney's	576	488
18. Roy Rogers	507	540
19. Sizzler	443	465
20. Baskin-Robbins	423	3,305
21. Bonanza	421	542
22. Western Sizzlin'	420	500
23. Popeye's	355	540
Total	$37,239 billion	54,826 units

*Excerpted with permission from Restaurant Business, March 20, 1986. Figures include overseas outlets.

TABLE II Fast Food: Hamburgers, Cheeseburgers

Company/Product	Calories	Fat (tsp)	Sodium (mg)	Gloom
D'Lites Jr. D'Lite	200	2	210	9
Wendy's Kid's Meal Hamburger	200	2	265	11
D'Lites ¼ lb. D'Lite Burger	280	3	240	14
McDonald's Hamburger	263	3	506	16
Burger King Hamburger	275	3	509	17
Wendy's Hamburger, Multi-Grain Bun	340	4	290	20
Wendy's Hamburger, White Bun	350	4	410	22
Hardee's Hamburger	276	3	589	22
Jack in the Box Cheeseburger	323	3	749	22
Burger King Whopper Jr.	322	4	486	22
McDonald's Cheeseburger	318	4	743	23
D'Lites Double D'Lite	450	5	290	24
Carl's Jr. Old Time Star	450	5	625	26
Dairy Queen Single with Cheese	410	5	790	28
McDonald's Quarter Pounder	427	5	718	31
Roy Rogers Hamburger	456	6	495	34
Burger King Double Cheeseburger	478	6	827	35
Jack in the Box Mushroom Burger	477	6	906	36
Hardee's Big Deluxe	503	7	903	38
Burger King Bacon Double Cheeseburger	510	7	728	38
Carl's Jr. Famous Star	530	7	705	40
Wendy's Double Hamburger, White Bun	560	8	575	40
Hardee's Bacon Cheeseburger	556	7	888	42
McDonald's Quarter Pounder with Cheese	525	7	1,220	43
McDonald's Big Mac	570	8	979	45
Dairy Queen Double with Cheese	650	8	980	46
Burger King Whopper	626	9	842	47
Wendy's Double Cheeseburger, White Bun	630	9	835	48
Jack in the Box Ham & Swiss Burger	638	9	1,330	51
Dairy Queen Triple Hamburger	710	10	690	51
Jack in the Box Jumbo Jack with Cheese	630	8	1,665	52
McDonald's McD.L.T.	680	10	1,030	54
Burger King Whopper with Cheese	709	10	1,126	56
Roy Rogers RR Bar Burger	611	9	1,826	57
Jack in the Box Bacon Cheeseburger Supreme	724	10	1,307	59
Carl's Jr. Super Star	780	11	785	59
Burger King Double Beef Whopper	887	13	922	66
Burger King Double Beef Whopper with Cheese	970	15	1,206	76
Wendy's Triple Cheeseburger	1,040	15	1,848	85

Befriend your arteries by choosing small burger and skipping the "special sauces." Cheeseburgers provide some calcium, but skim milk, yogurt, and green vegetables are much better, lower-calorie sources.

TABLE III Fast Food: French Fries

Company/Product	Calories	Fat (tsp)	Sodium (mg)	Gloom
Arby's French Fries	211	2	30	9
Dairy Queen Fries, regular	200	2	115	11
McDonald's Fries, regular	220	3	109	13
D'Lites French Fries, regular	260	3	100	14
Long John Silver's Fryes	247	3	6	14
Kentucky Fried Chicken Kentucky Fries	268	3	81	15
Church's French Fries	256	3	—	15
Jack in the Box French Fries, regular	221	3	164	15
Arthur Treacher's Chips	276	3	39	15
Hardee's French Fries, regular	239	3	180	15
Wendy's French Fries, regular	280	3	95	16
Roy Rogers French Fries	268	3	165	16
D'Lites French Fries, large	320	3	120	17
Burger King French Fries, regular	227	3	160	17
Dairy Queen French Fries, large	320	4	185	21
Carl's Jr. French Fries, regular	250	3	460	21
Roy Rogers French Fries, large	357	4	221	22
Hardee's French Fries, large	406	5	306	27

Although they're deep-fried and salted, french fries are not quite as bad as their reputation would have them. A small serving should be more than enough, and ask the clerk to hold the salt. Kudos to Long John Silver's for making salt-free "Fryes" its standard.

TABLE IV Fast Food: Shakes, Malts

Company/Product	Calories	Fat (tsp)	Sodium (mg)	Sugar (tsp)	Gloom
Jack in the Box Strawberry Shake, 11 fl. oz.	320	2	240	9	13
McDonald's Vanilla Shake, 10.2 fl. oz.	352	2	201	10	15
McDonald's Strawberry Shake, 10.2 fl. oz.	362	2	207	10	15
Arby's Vanilla Shake, 8.8 fl. oz.	295	2	245	8	16
Burger King Vanilla Shake, 10 fl. oz.	321	2	205	9	16
Roy Rogers Vanilla Shake, 10.8 fl. oz.	306	2	282	9	17
Hardee's Milkshake, 11 fl. oz.	391	2	241	11	17
Carl's Jr. Shakes, large	490	2	350	14	17
McDonald's Chocolate Shake, 10.2 fl. oz.	383	2	300	11	17
Burger King Chocolate Shake, 10 fl. oz.	374	3	225	9	18
Dairy Queen Chocolate Malt, small, 10 fl. oz.	520	3	180	12	21
Dairy Queen Chocolate Malt, regular, 14 fl. oz.	760	4	260	18	29
Dairy Queen Chocolate Shake, large, 21 fl. oz.	990	6	360	29	43

Typical shakes contain about as much sugar as a can of cola, as much fat as a glass of milk, and as many calories as a cola and milk combined. They are good sources of calcium. Not a bad choice for a combined beverage and dessert, you can also make it better by sharing one with a friend (or, in the case of Carl's Jr. and Dairy Queen's large shakes and malts, 2 or 3 friends.

Our cardiovascular health is most dependent on what goes into our mouths. There is nothing wrong with the idea of eating fast but the food can be far more nutritious than it is presently. As William Castelli has stated, the Golden Arches of McDonald's are the entrances into the Pearly Gates.

William C. Roberts

William C. Roberts, MD
Editor in Chief

Stone Agers in the Atomic Age: Lessons from the Paleolithic Life-Style for Modern Man

The archeological record of the Stone Age or Paleolithic period consists of unfleshed, time-cleansed, grinning skulls with emptied eyes, a few finer bones, some loose teeth, jaws, broken hips, the remains of meals, habitation floors or workplaces, hard-stone tools and a few man-made images of animals and strange signs and symbols. From these studies and from those of the few remaining groups of preliterate people, who are still living in many ways like our Stone Age ancestors, anthropologists have learned much about our early predecessors. The April 1988 issue of *The American Journal of Medicine* contained an article entitled "Stone Agers in the Fast Lane: Chronic Degenerative Diseases in Evolutionary Perspective" by S. Boyd Eaton, Melvin Konner and Marjorie Shostak. The authors present evidence that the genetic makeup of humanity has changed little during the past 10,000 years, but during the same period, our culture has been transformed to the point that there now is a mismatch between our ancient, genetically controlled biology and certain important life-style factors like nutrition, exercise and exposure to noxious substances like alcohol and tobacco. The mismatch between our genetic makeup and the myriad of life-style changes—especially great since the Industrial Revolution began about 200 years ago—promotes chronic degenerative diseases (atherosclerosis, essential hypertension, diabetes mellitus, obesity and certain cancers [lung, breast, colon]) that together cause 75% of all deaths in Western nations, but that were rare or nonexistent among preagricultural hunter-gatherers.

The 3 authors of the "Stone Agers" article are eminently qualified to discuss the subject. *Boyd Eaton*, born in 1938, a radiologist at a private hospital in Atlanta, Georgia, has had a lifelong interest in anthropology and paleontology and is adjunct associate professor of anthropology at Emory University. His book, *The Paleolithic Prescription*, coauthored with Marjorie Shostak and Melvin Konner, will be published by Harper & Row this month; it describes diets, exercise, child care and relations between men and women from an evolutionary perspective. *Melvin Konner*, born in 1946, received a Doctor of Philosophy degree from Harvard University in anthropology and was a departmental faculty member for 6 years thereafter. He spent 2 years in Botswana living in grass huts on the sand with the !Kung San, or Bushman, hunter-gatherers of the Kalahari Desert. His first book was *The Tangled Wing: Biological Constraints on the Human Spirit* (New York: Harper & Row, 1982:543). This book received wide acclaim; it was selected for the Science Book-of-the-Month Club, as an alternate for the regular Book-of-the-Month Club and it was nominated for the National Book Award. In 1981 Konner entered the Harvard Medical School and received his medical degree in 1985. Some observations on his medical school experiences (almost entirely those of the third year) were published in the widely acclaimed book entitled *Becoming a Doctor: A Journey of Initiation in Medical School* (New York: Elizabeth Sifton Books, Viking, 1987:390). This book received rave reviews in the *New York Times Book Review* of July 26, 1987, and in the January 14, 1988, *New England Journal of Medicine*. Presently, Konner is the Samuel Candler Dobbs Professor of Anthropology at Emory; he also has an appointment in Emory's Psychiatry Department; he is a contributing editor of *The Sciences*, for which he writes a regular column "On Human Nature" and he is a regular contributor to the column called "Body and Mind" in the *New York Times Sunday Magazine*. *Marjorie Shostak*, born in 1945, is married to Melvin Konner, the mother of 3 children, adjunct assistant professor of anthropology at Emory and the author of the widely heralded book entitled *Nisa: The Life and Words of a !Kung Woman* (Boston: Harvard University Press, 1981:380 [Vintage 1983]), which is considered a classic in the field of anthropology. Shostak is fluent is the !Kung language (she was with her husband for 2 years in Botswana), a sought-after speaker and an award-winning photographer.

Some observations from "Stone Agers in the Fast Lane."

Lack of genetic change: The gene pool has changed little since anatomically modern humans, *Homo sapiens sapiens*, became widespread about 35,000 years ago. From a genetic standpoint, current humans are still late Paleolithic preagricultural hunter-gatherers. We have Stone Age bodies in an Atomic Age. Our genetic makeup was selected, over geologic eras, ultimately to fit the life-style of Paleolithic humans.

Enormous environmental change: The increasing industrialized affluence of the last 200 years has affected health both beneficially and adversely. Improved housing, sanitation and medical care have ameliorated the impact of infection and trauma, the chief causes of death from the Paleolithic era until 1900. The result is that average life expectancy is now approximately double what it was for preagricultural humans. Concomitantly, the past century has accelerated the biologic estrangement that has increasingly differentiated humans from other mammals for over 2 million years. In today's Western nations, we have little need for exercise, consume foods quite different from those available to other mammals and expose ourselves to such harmful agents as alcohol and tobacco. We have crossed an epidemiologic boundary and entered a watershed in which disorders such as atherosclerosis, systemic hypertension, obesity, diabetes mellitus and certain cancers have become common in contrast to their rarity or near nonexistence among remaining preagricultural humans.

The late Paleolithic life-style: The period, 35,000 to 20,000 years ago, is the last time period during which the collective human gene interacted with bioenvironmental circumstances typical of those for which it had been originally selected. Thus, the diet, exercise patterns and social adaptions of that time have continuing relevance today.

Nutrition: The dietary requirements of all Stone Age persons were met exclusively by uncultivated vegetables and wild game. The amount of protein was great, probably 33% of calories, compared with the current American diet, which derives 12% of its calories from protein. Because game animals are lean, Paleolithic humans ate much less fat than Americans and Europeans do today. Stone Agers ate more polyunsaturated than saturated fat. Their cholesterol intake equaled or exceeded that now common in industrialized nations. Stone Agers ate much more dietary fiber than do most Americans. They obtained far more potassium than sodium from their food (as do all other mammals). Because they had no domesticated animals, they had no dairy foods; despite this, their calcium intake far exceeded that consumed today.

Physical exercise: The hunter-gatherer way of life generated high levels of physical and aerobic fitness. Strength and stamina were characteristic of both sexes at all ages. The hunter-gatherers were stronger and more muscular than succeeding agriculturalists.

Alcohol: Alcoholic beverages were infrequently consumed and those available, all products of natural fermentation, were far less potent than that of present day distilled liquors. Solitary, addictive drinking did not occur.

Tobacco: Tobacco was practically unavailable until agriculture appeared in the Americas about 5,000 years ago. Pipes and cigars were the only methods used for smoking until about 1850 when cigarettes first appeared. The major impact of tobacco abuse is a post-cigarette phenomenon of this century.

Effects of changes in life-style on disease prevalence: The 3 chief killers of the Stone Agers were childbirth and diseases of infancy, infection (particularly parasitism) and trauma. The effects of life-style changes on our present "diseases of civilization" were thoroughly discussed by Eaton and associates:

Obesity: Stone Agers were lean, and leanness today in the Western world is nearly the exception. Most food today is calorically concentrated in comparison to the wild game and uncultivated fruits and vegetables that constituted the Paleolithic diets. In eating a given volume, enough to create a feeling of fullness, Paleolithic humans consumed fewer calories than those consumed in a similar volume in the Western world today. Most beverages consumed today provide a significant caloric load. Paleolithic humans, in contrast, drank water. Energy expenditure, i.e., calories burned, by modern man is much less than by the Stone Agers.

Atherosclerosis: Present day preliterate societies have little or no coronary artery disease. Like our Paleolithic ancestors, they rarely use tobacco, are normotensive, have low blood cholesterol levels and live lives characterized by considerable physical exertion. The adverse changes that occur in atherosclerotic risk factors when persons from societies with little such disease become Westernized recapitulate the patterns observed for other diseases of civilization. The present day remaining hunter-gatherers and the other remaining preliterates (rudimentary horticulturists, simple agriculturists and pastoralists) consume diets low in total fat with more polyunsaturated than saturated fatty acids (a higher polyunsaturated than saturated fat ratio), but with an amount of cholesterol similar to that in the current American diet (600 mg). Because the fibrinolytic activity of blood and platelet aggregation are enhanced by physical activity but decreased by cigarette smoking, obesity and hypercholesterolemia, the preliterate peoples also have more such activity and less platelet aggregation than do average Westerners.

Systemic hypertension: There are still several cultures on earth whose members do not have essential hypertension and their blood pressure does not rise with age. When persons living in these remaining preliterate cultures, however, adopt a Western life-style, either by migration or acculturation, they first develop a tendency for their blood pressure to rise with age and then an increasing tendency to develop hypertension. The diets of these normotensive preliterates are low in sodium, high in potassium, high in calcium and low to absent in alcohol.

Diabetes mellitus: Obesity and maturity-onset diabetes are among the first disorders to appear when unacculturated persons undergo economic development. The overall prevalence of noninsulin-dependent diabetes among adults in industrialized countries ranges from 3 to 10%, but among unacculturated native populations it is zero to 2%. The most powerful risk factor to diabetes is obesity, and excessive weight gain is virtually absent in preliterate societies. Obese persons have reduced numbers of cellular insulin receptors, a relative tissue resistance to insulin and higher blood insulin levels than those of lean persons. Conversely, high-level physical fitness, characteristic of aboriginal persons, is associated with an increased number of insulin receptors and better insulin binding, both of which enhance the body's sensitivity to insulin. Diets containing ample amounts of non-nutrient fiber and complex carbohydrates lower both fasting and postprandial blood glucose levels, and these types of diets are the rule among technologically primitive societies but the exception in Western nations.

Thus, the message from Eaton and associates is this: we need to eat and exercise like the Stone Agers. If we do, our health will improve substantially, and our medical bills will decrease substantially.

William C. Roberts

William C. Roberts, MD
Editor in Chief

The Friedewald-Levy-Fredrickson Formula for Calculating Low-Density Lipoprotein Cholesterol, the Basis for Lipid-Lowering Therapy

The recently published report of an Expert Panel of the National Cholesterol Education Program provides new guidelines for the treatment of elevated blood cholesterol in adults aged 20 years and older.[1] The report recommends that all adults having a nonfasting or fasting serum total cholesterol >240 mg/dl (>5.2 mmol/liter) should have "lipoprotein analysis" and that persons with levels from 200 to 239 mg/dl also should have lipoprotein analysis if they have clinical evidence of myocardial ischemia or if they have 2 coronary artery disease risk factors (male sex, family history of premature coronary artery disease [acute myocardial infarction or sudden coronary death[2] before 55 years of age in a parent or sibling], cigarette smoker [>10 cigarettes a day]), systemic hypertension [not defined], serum high-density lipoprotein [HDL] cholesterol <35 mg/dl, diabetes mellitus, history of cerebrovascular or peripheral arterial disease and severe obesity [≥30% overweight]). Because nearly 3 of every 4 patients with clinical evidence of myocardial ischemia are men and nearly half of them are either cigarette smokers or have systemic arterial pressures >140/90 mm Hg or both, for practical purposes, all men with serum total cholesterol levels >200 mg/dl need lipoprotein analysis. The panel recommended that both dietary and drug treatment decisions be based on the low-density lipoprotein (LDL) cholesterol, not on the total cholesterol level. The desirable serum LDL cholesterol level was considered to be <130 mg/dl. Dietary treatment was recommended for persons with LDL cholesterol ≥130 mg/dl if evidence of myocardial ischemia was present or if 2 coronary risk factors were present or if LDL cholesterol was ≥160 mg/dl without evidence of myocardial ischemia or 2 risk factors. Drug treatment in addition to diet was recommended for persons with serum LDL cholesterol ≥160 mg/dl if evidence of myocardial ischemia or 2 risk factors were present and ≥190 mg/dl if evidence of myocardial ischemia were absent and either only 1 or no risk factors were present.

In contrast to the serum total cholesterol, which is measured directly and which is similar in both nonfasting and fasting bloods, the LDL cholesterol is a calculated value from 3 determinations, 2 of which, the blood triglyceride and the HDL cholesterol, require fasting (about 12 hours) samples for accuracy. A method to calculate the blood LDL cholesterol was reported by Friedewald, Levy and Fredrickson[3] in 1972. Their formula is based on the fact that TC = LDL + HDL + VLDL, where TC = total cholesterol, LDL = LDL cholesterol, HDL = HDL cholesterol and VLDL = very low-density lipoprotein cholesterol. The LDL cholesterol, therefore, is derived from the following: LDL = TC − HDL − VLDL.

VLDL cholesterol usually is not measured directly, but is derived by dividing the serum or plasma triglyceride (TG) by 5. Thus, the serum or plasma LDL cholesterol can be determined by measuring the serum or plasma total cholesterol, the HDL cholesterol and the triglyceride, so that the clinically useful Friedewald-Levy-Fredrickson formula for calculating the LDL cholesterol is the following:

$$\text{LDL} = \text{TC} - \text{HDL} - \text{TG}/5.$$

This formula loses its accuracy, however, when the plasma or serum triglyceride level is considerably elevated. Friedewald et al[3] reported that the calculated LDL cholesterol was most accurate when the blood triglyceride level was <400 mg/dl. A 1986 report[4] suggested that dividing the triglyceride level by 6 rather than 5 provided a more accurate calculated LDL cholesterol.

There are differences in the cholesterol and triglyceride levels in serum and plasma. To convert serum values to plasma, multiply by 0.97; to convert plasma values to serum multiply by 1.03.[1] The total, HDL and LDL blood cholesterol values in the report of the National Cholesterol Education Program are from serum. Although most laboratories use serum for measuring blood lipids, the Lipid Research Clinics Primary Prevention Trial used plasma mixed with the anticoagulant ethylene-diamine-tetraacetic acid (EDTA).

To assure comparative blood lipid values, it is important that the blood be drawn the same way each time. Levy[5] recommended that blood be drawn into a syringe after the patient has sat for 5 minutes and after the tourniquet has been released. If 1 sample is taken with the patient lying down and the tourniquet unreleased while blood fills the syringe and the sample on the next visit is drawn while the patient is seated and after the tourniquet has been released, the cholesterol values may differ by as much as 10 to 15%. This difference might be translated into a total cholesterol value of 210 mg/dl rather than 190 mg/dl or vice versa. According to the Expert Panel recommendations[1] a person having an initial serum total cholesterol of 190 mg/dl need not have it repeated for another 5 years, whereas the person with a value of 210 mg/dl might return for the full lipoprotein analysis.

We have entered the cholesterol era and we must do it right.

William C. Roberts, MD
Editor in Chief

1. The Expert Panel. *Report of the National Cholesterol Education Program Expert Panel on Detection, Evaluation, and Treatment of High Blood Cholesterol in Adults. Arch Intern Med 1988;148:36–69.*

2. Roberts WC. *Sudden cardiac death: definitions and causes. Am J Cardiol 1986;57:1410–1413.*

3. Friedewald WT, Levy RI, Fredrickson DS. *Estimation of the concentration of low-density lipoprotein cholesterol in plasma, without use of the preparative ultracentrifuge. Clin Chem 1972;18:499–502.*

4. DeLong DM, DeLong ER, Wood PD, Lippel K, Rifkind BM. *A comparison of methods for the estimation of plasma low- and very low-density lipoprotein cholesterol: the Lipid Research Clinics prevalence study. JAMA 1986;256:2372–2377.*

5. Levy RI. *Cholesterol screening—when, why, and how? Cholesterol and Coronary Disease . . . Reducing the Risk (official newsletter) 1986;1:1-4.*

Factors Linking Cholesterol to Atherosclerotic Plaques

Although the relation between cholesterol and atherosclerosis has been discussed for nearly 80 years, only in recent years has sufficient evidence accumulated to indicate without reasonable doubt that cholesterol plays a major role in the development of atherosclerotic plaques, and, therefore, symptomatic and fatal atherosclerotic coronary artery disease. This piece reviews the various factors linking cholesterol to atherosclerosis:

(1) *Feeding high-cholesterol diets to certain nonhuman animals produces atherosclerotic plaques similar to those occurring in humans.* The initial connection between cholesterol and atherosclerotic plaques began in 1912 when Anitschkow reported finding atherosclerotic plaques, similar to those occurring in humans, in rabbits after feeding them diets high in cholesterol.[1,2] (This was the same year that James Herrick first reported that acute myocardial infarction could be diagnosed clinically and that it was not always immediately fatal.[3]) Subsequently, atherosclerotic plaques were produced also in other nonhuman animals (guinea pig, dog and chicken) by feeding them high-cholesterol diets.[2] Anitschkow from his experiments laid down the dictum that increased cholesterol in the blood was the exciting cause of atherosclerosis.[1]

(2) *Cholesterol is found in both experimentally induced atherosclerotic plaques in nonhuman animals and in plaques in humans.* It has been known for nearly 80 years that cholesterol is a major component of atherosclerotic lesions. Three main types of lipid accumulate in atherosclerotic lesions: free sterols (almost exclusively cholesterol), cholesterol esters (mainly cholesteryl linoleate, oleate and palmitate) and phospholipids (mainly phosphatidylcholine and sphingomyelines).[4] All 3 lipids are insoluble in water.[4] These lipids make up about 95% of the total lipids in both normal intima and in atheromatous plaques.[4] The lipids present in small amounts include triacylglycerols, fatty acids and lysophospholipids.[4] Cholesterol esters are nearly absent in newborn intima but they are a major part of atherosclerotic plaques.[4] Triglycerides are lowest in newborn intima and they never become a major component of plaques, although they rise to 6% in the gruel-like material of plaques.[4]

(3) *Atherosclerotic plaques large enough to produce clinical problems occur only in persons having serum or plasma total cholesterol levels >150 mg/dl for long periods of time.* Most native African, Latin American and Oriental populations have a low frequency of coronary atherosclerosis.[5] Their diets are low in saturated fat, cholesterol and animal protein. Most adults in these populations have serum total cholesterol levels <150 mg/dl. In 1969 I had the opportunity to spend a week at the Mulago Hospital in Kampala, Uganda, and during the visit examined at necropsy the hearts, portions of aorta and many circles of Willis of numerous adults. Although many hearts were hypertrophied because of systemic hypertension—the most common cardiovascular condition in central Africa at the time—I rarely encountered an atherosclerotic plaque and the few seen were so small that they were of no functional significance. I learned that the serum total cholesterol levels in adults in Kampala usually were <150 mg/dl. To my knowledge, I have not observed fatal atherosclerotic vascular disease in the USA in anyone with a serum total cholesterol level <150 mg/dl for many years. In the USA, however, only 5% of the population >40 years of age has a serum or plasma total cholesterol level <150 mg/dl.[6] I consider the ideal serum or plasma total cholesterol level to be <150 mg/dl because those persons with these levels over decades do not develop atherosclerotic plaques large enough to cause organ ischemia or infarction.

Nathan Pritikin, PhD, who died in February 1985 at 69 years of age, followed during his last 30 years of life the Pritikin high complex carbohydrate, low fat, low cholesterol diet and his serum total cholesterol progressively decreased from 280 to 94 mg/dl.[7] Specifically, at age 39 (December 1955) his serum total cholesterol was 280 mg/dl; by age 42 (February 1958) it was 210; by July 1958, it was 162; by September 1958, 122; by December 1963, 102; and in November 1984, 94 mg/dl. Pritikin led a vigorous life, running several miles weekly, until lymphocytic lymphoma appeared about a year before death. At necropsy, his coronary arteries and aorta were free of atherosclerotic plaque.[7]

(4) *The higher the blood total cholesterol level the greater the chance of having symptomatic and fatal atherosclerotic disease.* Although the Framingham,[8] the "Seven Countries"[5] and the Israeli[9] studies have demonstrated that persons with higher serum total cholesterol levels have higher incidences of atherosclerotic disease than persons of similar age and sex with lower levels, the best study in my view demonstrating the relation between serum total cholesterol level and symptomatic or fatal atherosclerotic disease is the Multiple Risk Factor Intervention Trial (MRFIT).[10] The reason is that MRFIT involved >350,000 persons whereas the 7-country study involved just over 12,000 men from each of 7 nations and

TABLE I Deciles of Serum Total Cholesterol (TC) and Six-Year Coronary Artery Disease (CAD) Mortality in 356,222 Primary Screenees (All Men Aged 35 to 37 Years in 1973 to 1975) of the Multiple Risk Factor Intervention Trial*

Decile	Serum TC (mg/dl) Range	Mean	CAD Mortality (Rate/1,000)	Relative Risk
1	≤167	153	3.2	1.0
2	168–181	175	3.3	1.1
3	182–192	187	4.1	1.3
4	193–202	198	4.2	1.3
5	203–212	208	5.4	1.7
6	213–220	216	5.8	1.8
7	221–231	226	6.9	2.2
8	232–244	238	7.4	2.3
9	245–263	253	9.1	2.9
10	≥264	290	13.1	4.1

* Modified from Stamler et al.[10]

the Framingham study, 5,127 persons. As shown in Table I, the 356,222 persons without clinical evidence of coronary artery disease sampled in the MRFIT study were divided into deciles on the basis of their serum total cholesterol levels. The 6-year coronary-artery-disease mortality rate per 1,000 persons increased as the serum total cholesterol level increased. This study shows dramatically that the serum total cholesterol level is a quantity and that the greater the quantity the greater the risk of symptomatic and fatal coronary artery disease.

Persons with enormously elevated (6 to 10 times normal) low-density lipoprotein (LDL) cholesterol levels usually die from consequences of atherosclerosis in the first 2 decades of life.[11,12] These individuals have familial hypercholesterolemia of the homozygote variety. They inherit 2 mutant genes at the LDL receptor locus, 1 from each parent, and about 1 in 1,000,000 persons have this abnormality. The heterozygote variety of familial hyper-

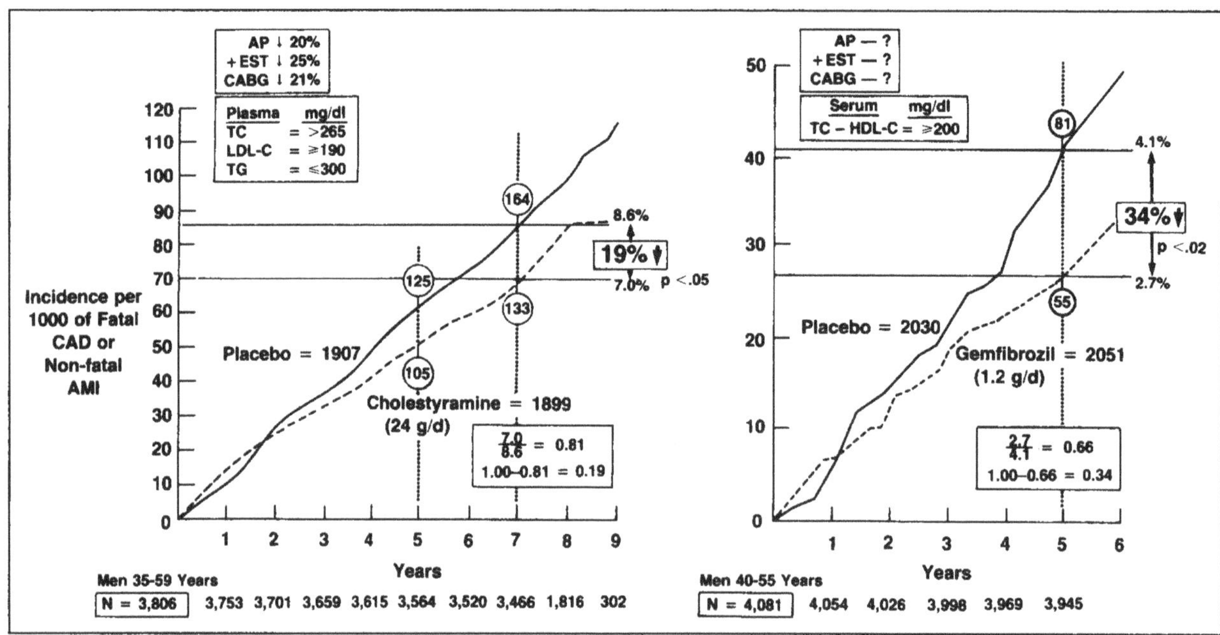

FIGURE 1. Life-table cumulative incidences of fatal coronary artery disease (CAD) and nonfatal acute myocardial infarction (AMI) in the treatment and placebo groups of the Lipid Research Clinics–Coronary Primary Prevention Trial (*left*) published in January 1984[16,17] and the Helsinki Heart Study (*right*) published in November 1987.[19] Both studies showed significant decreases in incidence of fatal CAD or nonfatal AMI in the groups treated with cholestyramine or gemfibrozil. All patients in the Lipid Research Clinics trial were followed for 7 years and at that point 133 (7.0%) of the 1,899 patients treated with cholestyramine and 164 (8.6%) of the 1,907 subjects not receiving cholestyramine had died or had nonfatal AMI. The difference in the 7.0% and 8.6% frequency of "hard" endpoints at 7 years represented a 19% reduction. In contrast, in the Helsinki Heart Study all patients and subjects were analyzed after 5 years and at that point 55 (2.7%) of the 2,051 patients in the gemfibrozil group and 81 (4.1%) of the 2,030 subjects in the placebo group had died or had had nonfatal AMI. The difference in the 2.7% and 4.1% frequency of hard endpoints at 5 years represented a 34% reduction. At 5 years in the Lipid Research Clinics study the frequency of hard endpoints was 5.5% (105 of 1,899 patients) in the cholestyramine group and 6.6% in the placebo group (125 of 1,907 subjects), a difference of 8.4% (not significant).

The reason(s) the incidence of hard endpoints in the gemfibrozil study is much less than in the Lipid Research Clinics study is not certain, but it may be related to the fact that the average decrease in both plasma total and LDL cholesterol levels in the placebo group in the Lipid Research Clinics study was about 8% for each. In contrast, the serum total and LDL cholesterol levels in the placebo group in the gemfibrozil study were not reduced at all; indeed, they rose slightly but insignificantly. The average decrease in the plasma total and LDL cholesterol levels in the placebo group of the Lipid Research Clinics study actually was about the same as the decreases in these 2 serum lipids in the gemfibrozil treatment group of the Helsinki Heart Study.

In the publications of the Lipid Research Clinics study[16,17] the number of subjects in the placebo group was listed as 1,906, not 1,907, and the number of patients in the drug treatment group as 1,900, not 1,899. After the publication appeared, however, the investigators learned that 1 patient in the cholestyramine group should have been in the placebo group, but since this patient did not have a fatal coronary event or a nonfatal AMI, the incidence percentage did not change. AP = angina pectoris; CABG = coronary artery bypass grafting; EST = exercise stress test; g/d = grams/day; HDL-C = high-density lipoprotein cholesterol; LDL-C = low-density lipoprotein cholesterol; TC = total cholesterol; TG = triglyceride.

cholesterolemia has a 2-fold increase in blood LDL levels and these individuals often have fatal heart attacks in their 30s and 40s. About 1 in every 500 persons among most ethnic groups throughout the world has familial hypercholesterolemia of the heterozygote variety. Both the homozygote and the heterozygote varieties of familial hypercholesterolemia provide strong evidence that persons with severe elevations of serum LDL and total cholesterol levels have both symptomatic and fatal coronary artery disease at much earlier ages than do persons with lower levels.

(5) *The higher the serum total and LDL cholesterol levels, the greater the extent of the atherosclerotic plaques.* The International Atherosclerosis Project quantified the extent of coronary and aortic atherosclerotic plaques at necropsy in 23,207 persons in 14 countries.[13] The extent of the atherosclerotic plaques differed markedly among populations, and the mean serum total cholesterol level correlated positively with the severity of the atherosclerotic plaques. The severity of the atherosclerotic plaques also correlated positively with the percent of dietary calories from fat. The extent of atherosclerotic plaques in aorta correlates directly with LDL cholesterol levels in the serum.[14]

(6) *Lowering the blood total cholesterol and LDL cholesterol levels decreases the chances of fatal or nonfatal atherosclerotic disease.* Two studies, the Lipid Research Clinics-Coronary Primary Prevention Trial (LRC-CPPT) (cholestyramine)[15-17] and the Helsinki Primary Prevention Trial (gemfibrozil),[18,19] both provided evidence that lowering the blood total and LDL cholesterol levels reduces the frequency of fatal and nonfatal coronary artery disease (Figure 1). Both studies were randomized, double-blind, placebo-controlled, multicenter, primary prevention trials analyzed by the intention-to-treat method.

The LRC trial results, published in January 1984,[16,17] included 3,806 men aged 35 to 59 years (mean 48) at entry with plasma total cholesterol levels ≥265 mg/dl and LDL cholesterol levels ≥190 mg/dl (≥175 mg/dl after dieting); half the subjects received the bile acid sequestrant cholestyramine 24 g a day and the other half an equivalent amount of placebo. All subjects were followed a minimum of 7 years and up to 10 years (mean 7.4). The cholestyramine group (1,899 men) had average total and LDL cholesterol reductions at the end of the first year of 18% (292 → 239 mg/dl) and 28% (216 → 159 mg/dl), respectively, and by the end of the seventh year of 12% (292 → 257 mg/dl) and 19% (216 → 175 mg/dl), respectively. In contrast, the placebo group (1,907 men), also on a cholesterol-lowering diet, had average total and LDL cholesterol reductions at the end of the first year of 6% (292 → 275 mg/dl) and 8% (216 → 199 mg/dl), respectively, and by the end of the seventh year of 5% (292 → 277 mg/dl) and 9% (216 → 198 mg/dl), respectively. The primary endpoints—fatal coronary artery disease or nonfatal acute myocardial infarction—were reduced 19%, which is the difference in the cumulative 7-year incidence of the primary endpoint which was 7.0% in the cholestyramine group (133 of 1,899 men) and 8.6% (164 of 1,907 men) in the placebo group (Figure 1), or the difference in the cumulative rate of cardiac endpoints at 7 years of 70/1,000 in the cholestyramine group and 86/1,000 in the placebo group (Figure 1). In addition, other cardiovascular events also decreased in the cholestyramine group compared with the placebo group: *positive exercise test results* fell 25% (260 [14.9%] vs 345 [19.8%]); *angina pectoris* fell 18% (235 [12.4%] vs 287 [15.1%]); and need for *coronary artery bypass grafting* fell 17% (93 [4.9%] vs 122 [5.9%]).

The Helsinki gemfibrozil trial results, published in November 1987,[19] included 4,081 men aged 40 to 55 years (mean 47) at entry with serum non-high-density lipoprotein (HDL) cholesterol, i.e., total cholesterol minus HDL cholesterol, >200 mg/dl. The mean serum total cholesterol for the 4,081 men was 290 mg/dl and the mean HDL cholesterol was 48 mg/dl. Half of the subjects received gemfibrozil 1.2 g a day and the other half an equivalent amount of placebo. All subjects were followed a minimum of 5 years. The gemfibrozil group had average total and calculated LDL cholesterol reductions during both the first 2 years and during the last 3 years of study of 9% (270 → 245 mg/dl) and 9% (189 → 173 mg/dl), respectively. The HDL cholesterol rose during both the first 2 years and the last 3 years of study by 9% (47 → 52 mg/dl). In contrast, the placebo group, also on a cholesterol-lowering diet, had no change in either serum total (270 → 273 mg/dl) or LDL cholesterol (48 → 47 mg/dl) during the entire 5 years of the trial. The primary endpoints—fatal coronary artery disease or nonfatal acute myocardial infarction—were reduced 34%, which is the difference between the 2.7% incidence of primary endpoints in the gemfibrozil group (56 in 2,051 men) and the 4.1% incidence in the placebo group (84 in 2,030 men), or, the difference in the cumulative rate of cardiac endpoints at 5 years of 27/1,000 in the gemfibrozil group and 41/1,000 in the placebo group (Figure 1).

Thus, both the LRC and Helsinki primary prevention trials demonstrate that lowering the blood total and LDL cholesterol levels reduces the incidence of fatal and nonfatal coronary artery disease.

(7) *Atherosclerotic plaques regress when high blood cholesterol levels are lowered.* Many experimental studies in nonhuman animals have shown that atherosclerotic plaques regress when blood lipid levels fall after atherogenic diets are eliminated.[20-22] Two major studies in humans demonstrate that lipid lowering both retards the rate of progression of angiographically demonstrated coronary arterial narrowing or causes reduction in size of atherosclerotic plaques as evidenced by increased luminal diameters.

The first major study in this regard was the National Heart, Lung, and Blood Institute Type II Coronary Intervention Study conducted by Brensike and associates.[23,24] This double-blind study evaluated in 116 patients the effects of cholestyramine (24 g/day) (59 patients) or placebo (57 patients) on the progression of coronary arterial narrowing assessed by 2 angiograms done 5 years apart. The patients had elevated (>upper tenth percentile of the distribution of the general population) blood LDL cholesterol after 1 month of therapy with a low-cholesterol, low-fat diet and angiographic and clinical evidence of coronary artery disease (previous acute myocardial infarction, angina pectoris, positive exercise stress test result or calcific deposits by fluoroscopy in ≥1 coronary artery). At the time of study, most patients were asymptomatic or only mildly limited by symptoms of myocardial ischemia despite medical therapy. The cholestyramine-treated group (74% adherence to therapy) had a 17% (310 → 256 mg/dl) decrease in total cholesterol levels from baseline after diet 5 years later, and a 26% reduction (242 → 178 mg/dl) in LDL cholesterol. In contrast, the placebo group had a 1% decrease (293 → 289 mg/dl) in total cholesterol levels in the 5 years and a 5% decrease (229 → 219 mg/dl) in LDL cholesterol levels.

Angiographic definite or probable increase in coronary arterial narrowing occurred in 32% of the cholestyramine group (19 of 59 patients) and in 49% (28 of 57 patients) of the placebo group (p 0.05). Angiographic definite or probable regression without any evidence of angiographic progression occurred in 4 (7%) of 59 cholestyramine-treated patients and in 4 (7%) of 57 placebo-treated patients, but the regression part of the analysis is less likely than progression because 22 (37%) of the 59 cholestyramine-treated patients and 22 (39%) of the 57 placebo-treated patients had none of the major epicardial coronary arteries narrowed as much as 50% in diameter at the baseline angiogram.

The Cholesterol-Lowering Atherosclerosis Study (CLAS) reported by Blankenhorn et al[25] in June 1987 is a better study than the Type II Coronary Intervention Study. CLAS was a randomized, placebo-controlled angiographic trial testing combined colestipol (30 g daily) and niacin (3 to 12 g daily) therapy in 162 nonsmoking men aged 40 to 59 years (mean 54) who had had coronary artery bypass grafting at least 3 months (but up to 7 years) before entering the study. The colestipol–niacin-treated group (80 patients) achieved a 26% reduction in blood total cholesterol (246 → 180 mg/dl), a 43% decrease in LDL cholesterol (171 → 97 mg/dl) and a 37% increase in HDL cholesterol (45 → 61 mg/dl) at the end of 2 years when the second coronary angiogram was done. In contrast, the placebo group (82 patients) at the end of 2 years had a 4% decrease in blood total cholesterol (243 → 232 mg/dl), a 5% decrease in LDL cholesterol (169 → 160 mg/dl) and no change in HDL cholesterol (44 mg/dl). Compared with the initial coronary angiogram, the second one 2 years later showed a significant reduction in the percent of patients with new narrowings or new closures (18 of 80 drug-treated patients [23%] vs 31 of 82 placebo patients [38%], p 0.03) in the native coronary arteries, and also a decrease in the percent of patients with new narrowings or new closures in bypass conduits (18 of 80 drug-treated patients [23%] vs 33 of 82 placebo patients [40%], p 0.03). Lessening of coronary narrowing, i.e., atherosclerotic regression, occurred in 16% of the colestipol–niacin-treated group and in 2% of the placebo-treated group (p = 0.002). An important feature of this study was the significant effect of cholesterol lowering on the "global change in coronary score" in the patients with lower baseline total cholesterol levels compared to those with higher baseline levels. The global change in the drug-treated group was over twice that in the placebo group in the 78 patients with blood total cholesterol levels 185 to 240 mg/dl (mean 216) and in the 84 patients with total cholesterol levels 241 to 350 mg/dl (mean 270) at baseline.

The data from the CLAS study suggest that it is never too late to attempt to reduce the total and LDL cholesterol levels, and that persons with lower initial levels may benefit from the reduction almost as much as those with higher initial levels. The latter finding is important because the other studies, namely the Lipid Research Clinics Study, the Helsinki Heart Study and the Type II Coronary Intervention trial included only patients with very high blood total cholesterol levels, essentially only subjects in the upper fifth percentile, i.e., blood total cholesterol >265 mg/dl.

In summary, 7 factors provide evidence that elevation of the blood total (specifically the LDL) cholesterol level is the cause of atherosclerosis. Of the 7 factors, the last 4 were confirmed during the present decade. There no longer is any controversy about cholesterol's role in atherosclerosis. In my view, physicians should provide a clear and united voice to the public regarding the dangers of elevation of the blood LDL cholesterol level. Every person needs to know his/her serum or plasma total cholesterol level and if it is elevated every attempt should be made to lower it. Atherosclerotic cardiovascular disease is responsible for 50% of the deaths in the Western world. In the USA alone 5.5 to 7.5 million persons have symptoms of myocardial ischemia. The most effective means of improving the health of the largest percent of Americans is for each to lower his/her LDL cholesterol level. The cost of medical care almost surely will diminish as the blood LDL cholesterol level falls.

William C. Roberts, MD
Editor in Chief

1. Anitschkow NN. *Lesions of organs under lipoid infiltration. Proc Med Soc Petersburg 1912;80:1.*
2. Anitschkow NN. *A history of experimentation on arterial atherosclerosis in animals. In: Blumenthal HT, ed. Cowdry's Arteriosclerosis. A Survey of the Problem, second edition. Springfield, Illinois: Charles C. Thomas, 1967:21–44.*
3. Herrick JB. *Clinical features of sudden obstruction of the coronary arteries. JAMA 1912;59:2015–2019.*
4. Small DM. *Progression and regression of atheriosclerotic lesions. Insights from lipid physical biochemistry. Arteriosclerosis 1988;8:103–129.*
5. Keys A, ed. *Coronary heart disease in seven countries. Circulation 1970; 41;42(suppl I):I-1–I-211.*
6. The Lipid Research Clinics Population Studies Data Book, vol. 1, The Prevalence Study. *Aggregate Distributions of Lipids, Lipoproteins and selected variables in 11 North American Populations. NIH Publication No. 80-1527, July 1980:1–136.*
7. Hubbard JD, Inkeles S, Barnard RJ. *Nathan Pritikin's heart. N Engl J Med 1985;313:52.*
8. Castelli WP. *The epidemiology of coronary heart disease. The Framingham study. Am J Med 1984;76:4–12.*

9. Brunner D, Weisbort J, Meshulam N, Schwartz S, Gross J, Saltz-Rennert H, Altman S, Loebl K. *Relation of serum total cholesterol and high-density lipoprotein cholesterol percentage to the incidence of definite coronary events: twenty-year follow-up of the Donolo-Tel Aviv prospective coronary artery disease study. Am J Cardiol 1987;59:1271–1276.*

10. Stamler J, Wentworth D, Neaton JD, for the MRFIT Research Group. *Is relationship between serum cholesterol and risk of premature death from coronary heart disease continuous and graded? Findings in 356,222 primary screenees of the Multiple Risk Factor Intervention Trial (MRFIT). JAMA 1986;256: 2823–2828.*

11. Brown MS, Goldstein JL. *A receptor-mediated pathway for cholesterol homeostasis. Science 1986;232:34–47.*

12. Goldstein JL, Brown MS. *Regulation of low-density lipoprotein receptors: implications for pathogenesis and therapy of hypercholesterolemia and atherosclerosis. Circulation 1987;76:504–507.*

13. McGill HC Jr, ed. *The Geographic Pathology of Atherosclerosis. Baltimore: Williams & Wilkins, 1968:193.*

14. Newman WP, Freedman DS, Voors AW, Gard PD, Srinivasan SR, Cresanta JL, Williamson GD, Webber LS, Berenson GS. *Relation of serum lipoprotein levels and systolic blood pressure to early atherosclerosis: The Bogalusa Heart Study. N Engl J Med 1986;314:138–144.*

15. The Coronary Primary Prevention Trial: design and implementation. *The Lipid Research Clinics Program. J Chronic Dis 1979;32:609–631.*

16. The Lipid Research Clinics Coronary Primary Prevention Trial results. *I. Reduction in incidence of coronary heart disease. Lipid Research Clinics program. JAMA 1984;251:351–364.*

17. The Lipid Research Clinics Coronary Primary Prevention Trial results. *II. The relationship of reduction in incidence of coronary heart disease to cholesterol lowering. Lipid Research Clinics Program. JAMA 1984;251:365–374.*

18. Manttari M, Elo O, Frick MH, Haapa K, Heinonen OP, Heinsalmi P, Helo P, Huttunen JK, Kaitaniemi P, Koskinen P, Manninen V, Maenpaa H, Malkonen M, Norola S, Pasternack A, Pikkarainen J, Roma M, Sjoblom T, Nikkila EA. *The Helsinki Heart Study: basic design and randomization procedure. Eur Heart J 1987;8(suppl 1):1–29.*

19. Frick MH, Elo O, Haapa K, Heinonen OP, Heinsalmi P, Helo P, Huttunen JK, Kaitaniemi P, Koskinen P, Manninen V, Maenpaa H, Malkonen M, Manttari M, Norola S, Pasternack A, Pikkarainen J, Romo M, Sjoblom T, Nikkila EA. *Helsinki Heart Study: primary-prevention trial with gemfibrozil in middle-aged men with dyslipidemia. Safety of treatment, changes in risk factors, and incidence of coronary heart disease. N Engl J Med 1987;317:1237–1245.*

20. Armstrong ML, Megan MB. *Lipid depletion in atheromatous coronary arteries in rhesus monkeys after regression diets. Circ Res 1972;30:675–680.*

21. Schettler G, Strange E, Wissler RW, eds. *Atherosclerosis—Is It Reversible? Berlin: Springer-Verlag;1978:104.*

22. Clarkson TB, Bond MG, Bullock BC, McLaughlin KJ, Sawyer JK. *A study of atherosclerosis regression in macaca mulatta. Exp Mol Pathol 1984;41:96–118.*

23. Brensike JF, Kelsey SF, Passamani ER, Fisher MR, Richardson JM, Loh IK, Stone NJ, Aldrich RF, Battaglini JW, Moriarty DJ, Marianthopoulos MB, Detre KM, Epstein SE, Levy RI. *NHLBI Type II Coronary Intervention Study: design, methods and baseline characteristics. Controlled Clin Trials 1982;3:91–111.*

24. Brensike JF, Levy RI, Kelsey SF, Passamani ER, Richardson JM, Loh IK, Stone NJ, Aldrich RF, Battaglini JW, Moriarty DJ, Fisher MR, Friedman L, Friedwald W, Detre KM, Epstein SE. *Effects of therapy with cholestyramine on progression of coronary arteriosclerosis: results of the NHLBI Type II Coronary Intervention Study. Circulation 1984;69:313–324.*

25. Blankenhorn DH, Nessim SA, Johnson RL, Sanmarco ME, Azen SP, Cashin-Hemphill L. *Beneficial effects of combined colestipol-niacin therapy on coronary atherosclerosis and coronary venous bypass grafts. JAMA 1987;257: 3233–3240.*

Atherosclerotic Risk Factors—Are There Ten or Is There Only One?

In the January 1988 publication of the National Cholesterol Education Program on Detection, Evaluation and Treatment of High Blood Cholesterol in Adults, the expert panel listed 10 risk factors, hereafter termed "atherosclerotic risk factors," which were predictive of coronary arterial atherosclerotic events.[1] The 10 atherosclerotic risk factors were the following:

1. *Serum (or plasma) total cholesterol >200 mg/dl (>5.2 mmol/liter) and low density lipoprotein (LDL)-cholesterol >130 mg/dl (>3.4 mmol/liter).*
2. *Definite clinical evidence of coronary artery disease* (either myocardial infarction or ischemia [angina pectoris]).
3. *Male sex.*
4. *History of either myocardial infarction or sudden death before 55 years of age in a parent or sibling.*
5. *Cigarette smoking* (>10 cigarettes a day).
6. *Systemic hypertension* (undefined).
7. *High density lipoprotein (HDL)-cholesterol* <35 mg/dl.
8. *Diabetes mellitus.*
9. *Cerebrovascular or peripheral vascular disease* (by history).
10. *Severe obesity* (>30% overweight).

This piece examines each of these 10 risk factors to ask if each is an independent atherosclerotic risk factor or if it is not.

Serum (or plasma) total cholesterol or low density lipoprotein-cholesterol level: In my view, the only absolute, unequivocal, independent atherosclerotic risk factor is an elevated serum total or LDL-cholesterol level. What constitutes an *elevated* level is debatable. If an elevated level is that minimal level above which atherosclerotic events occur, then that level in my view would be 150 mg/dl (3.9 mmol/liter). If it is the level where the risk of atherosclerotic events is substantially increased compared to lower levels, then that level would be 200 mg/dl. Irrespective of which level is chosen, the higher the level the greater the risk of an atherosclerotic event. From study of >350,000 men, Stamler et al[2] have clearly demonstrated that the higher the serum total cholesterol level, the greater the risk of an atherosclerotic event. The Framingham study, involving approximately 5,000 residents of that Massachusetts community, also has shown that the higher the total and LDL-cholesterol levels and the lower the HDL-cholesterol level, the greater the risk of having an atherosclerotic event.[3] International epidemiologic studies also have shown that populations having serum total cholesterol levels <150 mg/dl for decades have a virtual absence of atherosclerotic events.[4] A certain critical serum total cholesterol level is necessary before an atherosclerotic event can occur and this critical level appears to be approximately 150 mg/dl. As the level increases above this value, the risk of an atherosclerotic event increases roughly proportional to the level. Thus, the only absolute prerequisite for a fatal or nonfatal atherosclerotic event is a serum total cholesterol level >150 mg/dl.

Male sex: Fatal and nonfatal atherosclerotic events are more common in men than women by a ratio of 2:1.[5] At least half of the atherosclerotic events in men occur before their sixtieth birthday, whereas atherosclerotic events in women are relatively infrequent before their sixtieth year.[5] After age 70, atherosclerotic events in women are as frequent as in men, but by age 70, over 75% of men destined to have a fatal atherosclerotic event have already had it. The average age of death in men in the USA from atherosclerotic coronary artery disease is 60, whereas the average age of women is 68.[5] Men have higher total and LDL serum cholesterol levels earlier in life than do women, but later in life women have higher levels than do men.[6] Neither men nor women, however, have atherosclerotic events unless the total cholesterol level is >150 mg/dl, and the higher the level the greater the chance of an event and the earlier the event occurs irrespective of sex. Thus, it is the person's blood cholesterol level, not the sex, that determines whether an atherosclerotic event occurs. Male sex, in my view, cannot be viewed as an independent atherosclerotic risk factor.

Family history: When atherosclerotic events occur in persons <55 years of age, it generally means (1) that the affected individuals have serum total cholesterol levels considerably higher than persons of similar age and sex without atherosclerotic events, and (2) that the affected individuals have total cholesterol levels much higher than those found in older individuals with atherosclerotic events. In persons with untreated familial hypercholesterolemia of the heterozygous type, the serum total cholesterol level is usually 300 to 400 mg/dl, and these individuals usually have atherosclerotic events when they are 31 to 55 years of age. In untreated individuals with familial hypercholesterolemia of the homozygous variety, the serum total cholesterol is usually >800 mg/dl and these individuals usually have atherosclerotic events before they are 20 years of age. Thus, individuals having atherosclerotic events before age 55 generally have higher total cholesterol levels than do individuals having atherosclerotic events later in life, and the genetic forms of hyperlipidemia are in these younger groups. A young age of an atherosclerotic event simply denotes very high serum total cholesterol levels and it is the cholesterol level, not the patient's age or the presence of atherosclerotic events in other family members, that is the villain.

Cigarette smoking: Although it is incompatible with good health, cigarette smoking, in my view, does not, in and of itself, produce atherosclerotic plaques. In populations where serum total cholesterol levels are <150 mg/dl, atherosclerotic events are rare even when cigarette smoking is widespread. In Japan, cigarette smoking is common, but atherosclerotic events are relatively uncommon. The average serum total cholesterol in adults in Japan is about 160 mg/dl, not a level associated with a high frequency of atherosclerotic events. Many Japanese adults have serum total cholesterol levels <150 mg/dl. In populations where the average serum total cholesterol in adults is >200 mg/dl—such as the USA—smoking cigarettes appears to accelerate atherosclerosis. In the USA, only 5% of the population >40 years of age have serum total cholesterol <150 mg/dl.[6] Therefore, in 95% of the USA population, cigarette smoking does appear to be associated with an increased frequency of atherosclerotic events, but this acceleration appears to be a cholesterol-dependent phenomenon. Thus, cigarette smoking is not an independent atherosclerotic risk factor.

Systemic hypertension: In nonhuman experimental animals given atherogenic diets (high fat-high cholesterol), those previously made hypertensive develop more atherosclerotic plaques than do the normotensive animals.[7] Hypertensive persons with total and LDL-cholesterol levels similar to those in normotensive persons have a higher frequency of atherosclerotic events compared to normotensive subjects.[7] These 2 facts have supported the contention that systemic hypertension is an atherosclerotic risk factor. Most studies describing benefits of antihypertensive therapy have not demonstrated a reduction in coronary or peripheral atherosclerotic events by such therapy. There is no evidence that systemic hypertension accelerates atherosclerosis if the serum total cholesterol level is <150 mg/dl.

In the late 1960s I spent a week in Kampala, Uganda, where I examined several hundred hearts. Many of them were severely hypertrophied without ventricular cavity dilatation or associated valvular disease. I learned that systemic hypertension was by far the most common cardiovascular condition in adults in Uganda. Yet, examination of hundreds of coronary arteries in these hypertrophied adult hearts disclosed virtually no atherosclerotic plaques. I also learned that most adults in Kampala at the time had serum total cholesterol levels ranging from 90 to 140 mg/dl. Thus, despite the high frequency of systemic hypertension, there was a low frequency of atherosclerosis. It appears that systemic hypertension also is a cholesterol-dependent risk factor in that the serum total cholesterol must be >150 mg/dl before hypertension has the ability to accelerate atherosclerosis and, therefore, hypertension is not an independent atherosclerotic risk factor.

In persons with serum total cholesterol levels >150 mg/dl, elevation of the pulmonary arterial pressure clearly causes the development of atherosclerotic plaques in the major pulmonary arteries. Whether these plaques develop in the extrapulmonary pulmonary arteries in patients with severe chronic elevation of pulmonary arterial pressures associated with low serum total cholesterol levels is unclear to me.

Although the evidence is lacking, in my view, implicating systemic hypertension as a direct atherosclerotic risk factor, it clearly is the major risk factor for development of stroke and aortic dissection.[7] These 2 lesions are not atherosclerotic dependent. The prime effect of hypertension is on the media of arteries causing this arterial layer to tear, dissect or rupture. Atherosclerosis is an intimal process and only indirectly is the media affected.

Diabetes mellitus: Juvenile diabetic patients clearly have more atherosclerotic plaques and a higher frequency of atherosclerotic events than do nondiabetics of similar age and sex.[8] But the juvenile diabetics have higher serum total and LDL-cholesterol levels than do their nondiabetic counterparts.[8] Likewise, adult-onset diabetics have more atherosclerosis and a higher frequency of atherosclerotic events than do nondiabetics of similar age and sex. Moreover, the adult-onset diabetics have higher serum total and LDL-cholesterol levels than do their nondiabetic counterparts. Thus, diabetes mellitus appears to be an atherosclerotic risk factor because these individuals have higher total and LDL-cholesterol levels than do their nondiabetic counterparts. There is no evidence that diabetics who have serum total cholesterol levels <150 mg/dl have an increased frequency of atherosclerotic events compared to nondiabetic counterparts with similar cholesterol levels. Indeed, there is no evidence that diabetics with low serum total cholesterol levels have atherosclerosis of any significance. Thus, diabetes mellitus also appears to be a cholesterol-dependent risk factor.

Severe obesity: In general, obese persons have higher total and LDL-cholesterol levels than do nonobese persons of similar age and sex. This fact is, of course, not surprising because obese persons eat more fat than do nonobese persons. Usually about a third of the fat eaten is of the saturated variety and most of the saturated fat once absorbed is converted into cholesterol. Although few exist to study, I am not aware that obese adults with serum total cholesterol levels <150 mg/dl have any risk to development of atherosclerotic events. Thus, obesity is a cholesterol-dependent risk factor, not an independent risk factor.

Low levels of serum high density lipoprotein-cholesterol: In adults in the USA the mean plasma HDL level in men is 45 mg/dl and in women it is 55 mg/dl.[6] Data, especially from Framingham, Massachusetts, have shown that high levels of HDL are associated with decreased risk and that low levels, with increased risk of atherosclerotic events.[3,9] Although there are some doubters about the beneficial effects of high HDL levels and the harmful effects of low HDL levels, the evidence is convincing, in my view, that high HDL is good and low HDL is bad. But what is the risk of a serum HDL level of 20 mg/dl if the LDL-cholesterol is only 100 mg/dl and the serum total cholesterol is <150 mg/dl? The answer is no risk. Is an HDL of 100 mg/dl protective when the LDL is 200 mg/dl? The answer is no. Whether the HDL-cholesterol is an independent risk factor, i.e., independent of the LDL-cholesterol level, is, in my view, not yet clear. I believe it best to view a low HDL-cholesterol as an additive atherosclerotic risk factor if the LDL-cholesterol is elevated, but not as an additive atherosclerotic risk factor if the LDL-cholesterol is low. Whichever is proper, the HDL-cholesterol is a type of cholesterol, and, therefore, consistent with the thesis that the blood cholesterol is the only direct atherosclerotic risk factor.

Definite clinical evidence of coronary artery disease: An atherosclerotic risk factor is a predictor of an atherosclerotic event, not necessarily in a single individual, but certainly in groups of individuals. Therefore, if an atherosclerotic risk factor is a predictor of an atherosclerotic event, how can the atherosclerotic event itself be an atherosclerotic risk factor? On the other hand, the presence of one atherosclerotic event is highly predictive of another atherosclerotic event. The person most prone to an atherosclerotic event is the person who has already had an atherosclerotic event. I believe it inappropriate, however, to include an atherosclerotic event as an atherosclerotic risk factor. By doing so, no distinction is made between primary and secondary prevention.

History of peripheral or cerebrovascular disease: Most peripheral vascular events are atherosclerotic events and many cerebrovascular events are atherosclerotic events. Therefore, the same aforementioned argument concerning a definite coronary event is applicable here. An atherosclerotic event is best not considered to be synonymous with an atherosclerotic risk factor (predictor).

In summary, in my view there are not 10 atherosclerotic risk factors, there is only 1—and that is an elevated (>150 mg/dl) serum total cholesterol level and specifically an elevated serum LDL-cholesterol level. A low (<35 mg/dl) HDL-cholesterol level in the presence of an elevated LDL-cholesterol level probably should be viewed as an additive atherosclerotic risk factor. Male sex, family history of coronary events before age 55 in a parent or sibling, cigarette smoking, systemic hypertension, diabetes mellitus, and severe obesity are best viewed as cholesterol-dependent atherosclerotic risk factors and not in themselves atherogenic in the absence of a serum total cholesterol level >150 mg/dl. Atherosclerotic events (coronary, cerebrovascular and peripheral), although predictive of future atherosclerotic events, are not by definition true atherosclerotic risk factors and they should not be viewed as such. Nevertheless, all of the aforementioned cholesterol-dependent atherosclerotic risk factors take effect when the serum total cholesterol level is >150 mg/dl, and because 95% of Americans >40 years of age have total cholesterol levels >150 mg/dl, these indirect risk factors need to be dealt with and managed accordingly.

William C. Roberts

William Clifford Roberts, MD
Editor in Chief

1. The Expert Panel. Report of the National Cholesterol Education Program Expert Panel on detection, evaluation, and treatment of high blood cholesterol in adults. *Arch Intern Med 1988;148:36–69.*

2. Stamler J, Wentworth D, Neation JD, for the MRFIT Research Group. Is relationship between serum cholesterol and risk of premature death from coronary heart disease continuous and graded? Findings in 356,222 primary screenees of the Multiple Risk Factor Intervention Trial (MRFIT). *JAMA 1986;256:2823–2828.*

3. Castelli WP, Garrison RJ, Wilson PWF, Abbott RD, Kalousdian S, Kannel WB. Incidence of coronary heart disease and lipoprotein cholesterol levels: the Framingham study. *JAMA 1986;256:2835–2838.*

4. Keys A. Seven Countries: A Multivariate Analysis of Death and Coronary Heart Disease. *Cambridge, Massachusetts: Harvard University Press, 1980.*

5. Roberts WC, Potkin BN, Solus DE, Reddy SG. Modes of death, frequency of healed and acute myocardial infarcts, numbers of major epicardial coronary arteries severely narrowed by atherosclerotic plaque, and heart weight in fatal atherosclerotic coronary artery disease: analysis of 889 patients studied at necropsy. *JACC, in press.*

6. The Lipid Research Clinics Program Epidemiology Committee: Plasma lipid distributions in selected North American populations: the Lipid Research Clinics Program Prevalence Study. *Circulation 1979;60:427–439.*

7. Roberts WC. Frequency of systemic hypertension in various cardiovascular diseases. *Am J Cardiol 1987;60:1E–8E.*

8. Crall FV Jr, Roberts WC. The extramural and intramural coronary arteries in juvenile diabetes mellitus. Analysis of nine necropsy patients aged 19 to 38 years with onset of diabetes before age 15 years. *Am J Med 1978;64:221–230.*

9. Gordon T, Castelli WP, Hjortland MC, Kannel WB, Dawber TR. High density lipoprotein as a protective factor against coronary heart disease. *Am J Med 1977;62:707–714.*

Lipid-Lowering Therapy After an Atherosclerotic Event

When considering lipid-lowering therapy (diet ± drug) for a patient who has had an atherosclerotic event, the following facts might be considered:

1. Whatever the levels of the serum (or plasma) total and low density lipoprotein (LDL) cholesterol in the patient with an atherosclerotic event, they are too high for that particular patient.

2. The greatest risk factor for a subsequent atherosclerotic event is a previous atherosclerotic event.

3. The greatest danger period for a subsequent atherosclerotic event is the first 6 months after the previous atherosclerotic event.

4. The higher the serum total and LDL cholesterol levels, the greater the chance of a subsequent atherosclerotic event.

5. Portions of atherosclerotic plaques disappear ("reverse") when the total and LDL-cholesterol levels are lowered, and when portions of plaques disappear the arterial lumens widen and blood flow to the organ supplied increases.

6. The greater the percent drop in serum total and LDL-cholesterol levels, the greater the disappearance (reversibility) of portions of atherosclerotic plaques.

7. Diet therapy alone (percent of calories from fat reduced from 40% to 30%) usually lowers the serum total and LDL-cholesterol levels only about 10%, and a reduction of this magnitude probably causes little to no disappearance of portions of atherosclerotic plaques.

8. Most persons having atherosclerotic events have serum total cholesterol levels from 200 to 240 mg/dl (5.2 to 6.2 mmol/liter) and LDL cholesterol levels from 130 to 160 mg/dl (3.4 to 4.1 mmol/liter).

If the aforementioned 8 items are accepted as facts, is it appropriate to manage serum cholesterol levels in persons who have had atherosclerotic events in the same fashion as these levels are managed in persons who have not had atherosclerotic events? My answer is "no."

To better understand this answer it may be useful to summarize the therapeutic guidelines of the Adult Treatment Panel (29 members) of the National Cholesterol Education Program (slightly modified for simplicity), published in January 1988, for management of LDL-cholesterol levels in persons aged 20 to 74 years in the USA.[1] The Panel had 3 therapeutic recommendations:

1. If the serum LDL cholesterol was 130 to <160 mg/dl and if definite coronary artery disease or 2 other risk factors were present, a low-fat, low-cholesterol diet should be prescribed. The "other risk factors" were male sex, history of acute myocardial infarction or sudden coronary death before 55 years of age in a parent or sibling, cigarette smoking (>10 cigarettes a day), systemic hypertension (not defined), serum high density lipoprotein cholesterol <35 mg/dl (<0.9 mmol/liter), diabetes mellitus, history of cerebrovascular or peripheral arterial disease, and severe obesity (≥30% overweight).

2. If the serum LDL cholesterol was 160 to 190 mg/dl (4.1 to 4.9 mmol/liter) in the absence of definite evidence of coronary artery disease and without the presence of 2 other risk factors, diet therapy should be prescribed.

3. If the LDL cholesterol was >190 mg/dl in the absence of definite evidence of coronary artery disease or 2 other risk factors, a lipid-lowering diet should be started and if the goal of <190 mg/dl was not obtained by diet in 6 months, then lipid-lowering drug therapy should be added.

Thus, the therapeutic recommendations of the National Cholesterol Education Program[1] are based primarily on the serum LDL-cholesterol level and only secondarily on the presence of definite clinical evidence of coronary artery disease or other risk factors. The therapeutic recommendations are not greatly different for persons who have had definite coronary events (secondary prevention) and for those persons who have not (primary prevention). In my view, the occurrence of a coronary event (myocardial infarction, nonfatal cardiac arrest, angina pectoris associated with angiographically confirmed coronary arterial narrowing, and positive exercise test in the absence of symptoms of myocardial ischemia but in the presence of angiographically confirmed coronary arterial narrowing) should take precedence over the serum LDL-cholesterol levels, and lipid-lowering therapy should be approached quite differently in the person who has had a coronary event compared to the person who has not.

Of persons residing in the USA who have not had an atherosclerotic event—and coronary events are by far the most common of them—slightly less than 50% will have one eventually if our lipid-consuming habits are not altered. Furthermore, of persons who have had 1 atherosclerotic event and survived, the chances are >90% that another atherosclerotic event will occur, and the chances also are >90% that the mode of death will be another atherosclerotic event. The major focus of management of a person who has had 1 atherosclerotic event is the prevention of a subsequent atherosclerotic event (secondary prevention).

The best deterrent to the occurrence of a subsequent atherosclerotic event is the lowering of the serum total

TABLE I Maximal Recommended Daily Doses of "Lipid-Lowering" Drugs Presently Available in the USA and Their Average Effects on Serum Lipids

Drug	Daily Dose (g)	Daily Dose (mg)	Effects on Serum Lipids‖			
			TC	LDL	HDL	TG
Colestipol	30	30,000	↓18%	↓24%	↑6%	↑10%
Cholestyramine	24*	24,000	↓18%	↓24%	↑6%	↑10%
Nicotinic acid	3†,‡	3,000†,‡	↓20%	↓25%	↑10%	↓25%
Gemfibrozil	1.2†	1,200†	↓11%	↓12%	↑15%	↓40%
Probucol	1†,‡	1,000†,‡	↓10%	↓10%	↓23%	↓3%
Lovastatin	0.08§	80§	↓34%	↓42%	↑10%	↓25%

* Each gram of regular Questran contains 0.44 g of cholestyramine, and each gram of Questran light (nutrasweet) contains 0.86 g of cholestyramine.
† This dose also is the usual dose.
‡ This dose can be increased but side effects increase considerably.
§ About 70% of the nearly 1.0 million persons in the USA now receiving lovastatin take only 20 mg a day (1 tablet). This is the only drug of the 6 that is a once-a-day medicine when taken in 20- or 40-mg dosage.
‖ These average values were obtained from several studies.[2–19] The averages assume that the study subjects are also on a lipid-lowering diet.
HDL = high density lipoprotein; LDL = low density lipoprotein; TC = total cholesterol; TG = triglyceride.

and LDL-cholesterol levels below the levels that were present at the time of the earlier atherosclerotic event. Even if the serum total cholesterol level was <200 mg/dl and the LDL cholesterol <130 mg/dl at the time of the first atherosclerotic event, these levels are too high for that patient. (Levels above these values are recognized to be too high for all persons irrespective of whether or not they have had atherosclerotic events.) Thus, irrespective of the actual serum total and LDL-cholesterol levels at the time of or preceding an atherosclerotic event, the levels should be lower. If serum total and LDL-cholesterol levels are lowered, the chances of a subsequent atherosclerotic event are lowered; the chances of dissolving (reversing) portions of atherosclerotic plaques and of increasing organ perfusion are increased; and, consequently, the chances of longer survival are increased.

Because the initiation of low-fat, low-cholesterol diet therapy usually causes only modest lowering of serum total and LDL-cholesterol levels; because the chances of, and extent of, plaque reversibility appears to be roughly proportional to the extent of the lowering of the serum total and LDL-cholesterol levels; because the chances of a subsequent atherosclerotic event decrease roughly proportional to the drop in serum total and LDL-cholesterol levels; and because the greatest danger of an atherosclerotic event is during the first 6-month period after a previous atherosclerotic event, maximal lowering of serum total and LDL-cholesterol levels should occur as soon as possible after an atherosclerotic event. Maximal lowering is not best achieved by a 6-month trial of diet therapy. *It is best achieved by simultaneous initiation of both low-fat, low-cholesterol diet therapy and lipid-lowering drug therapy as soon as possible after the atherosclerotic event has occurred.* The goal is maximal reduction of both serum total and LDL cholesterol levels as soon as possible after the atherosclerotic event.

The drug or drugs chosen should be those that have the greatest capacity to lower the serum total and LDL-cholesterol levels (Table I). In persons who have not had atherosclerotic events, a 1% reduction in serum total cholesterol yields at least a 2% reduction in the frequency of fatal coronary artery disease or nonfatal acute myocardial infarction.[2,3] There is no reason to believe that this 2 for 1 principle is inapplicable to persons who have had atherosclerotic events. The combination of a 3-hydroxy-3-methyl glutaryl-coenzyme-A (HMG CoA) reductase inhibitor (e.g., lovastatin) and a bile-acid sequestrant (e.g., cholestyramine, colestipol) have the capability of lowering the serum LDL cholesterol by 50%,[4] and theoretically this degree of reduction before an atherosclerotic event could eliminate the possibility of an atherosclerotic event. For those persons who have had an atherosclerotic event, it is reasonable to believe that a 50% reduction in serum LDL cholesterol would substantially decrease the chances of a subsequent atherosclerotic event.

Opponents of the viewpoint that simultaneous lipid-lowering diet and drug therapy should be initiated soon after an atherosclerotic event irrespective of the actual serum total and LDL-cholesterol levels (assuming that secondary causes of hypercholesterolemia have been ruled out and that there are no contraindications to drug therapy) might argue that lipid-lowering drugs are expensive and that they have real or potential toxic effects. Yes, these drugs are expensive, but coronary artery disease is an expensive disease. It occurs because most of us eat expensive foods. Coronary angioplasty is an expensive procedure (each about $10,000) and about 200,000 were performed in the USA in 1988. Coronary bypass is an even more expensive procedure (each about $30,000) and about 250,000 of these operations were performed in the USA in 1988. Thirty percent of persons undergoing coronary angioplasty have restenosis at the angioplasty site within 6 months after the procedure. Although coronary bypass has proved to be highly beneficial, about 25% of persons having it increase both their serum cholesterol levels and their body weight during the first year after the procedure and both of these occurrences increase the chances of another atherosclerotic event.

In the USA an estimated 5.5 to 7.5 million persons have symptomatic myocardial ischemia, and, therefore, the lipid-lowering drug cost potentially could be very expensive. If 5.5 million Americans with symptomatic myocardial ischemia each were treated with a single 20-mg tablet of lovastatin daily, then the total cost would be $2.75 billion a year ($1.50/tablet and $550/person/year). For this cost the average reduction in serum total cholesterol would be 17%, in LDL cholesterol 20% and in serum triglycerides 20%, and the serum high density lipoprotein cholesterol would increase about 7%. A serum total cholesterol reduction of 17% should yield a sizable reduction in the frequency of subsequent coronary events. In contrast, the cost of performing 250,000 coronary bypasses each year presently is about $7.5 billion (nearly 3 times as much), and the cost of performing 200,000 coronary angioplasties each year presently is about $2.0 billion. The impact of treating several million persons who have had a coronary event with lipid-lowering drugs (+

lipid-lowering diet) might have an enormous impact on the nation's health.

Although 4 of the 6 drugs presently available (Table I) in the USA to lower the serum total and LDL-cholesterol levels do cause an alteration in hepatic enzymes in 1 to 2% of recipients, these alterations are completely reversible when the drug is discontinued, and these hepatic enzyme alterations may not occur on another trial of the same drug. Rhabdomyolysis occurs in about 1 in 5,000 persons who receive lovastatin and are not concomitantly receiving cyclosporine. The operative procedures (angioplasty and bypass) designed to increase myocardial blood flow also, of course, have their "toxic" effects including death. The greatest danger for a person who has had a coronary event, however, is not a toxic effect from a drug or a complication of a coronary procedure or operation, it is the occurrence of another coronary event. The prevention of another coronary event should be the major thrust of therapy for those who have had an earlier event.

In my view, virtually all persons who have had coronary events would benefit from combined diet and drug lipid-lowering therapy including persons who have had coronary angioplasty and bypass procedures. Several studies are now in progress to definitely answer the question of the usefulness of lipid-lowering drugs in persons who have had coronary events. Enough data already are available, however, to support the view to increase the use of lipid-lowering drugs irrespective of serum total and LDL-cholesterol levels in patients who have had atherosclerotic events.

William C. Roberts

William C. Roberts, MD
Editor in Chief

1. The Expert Panel. Report of the National Cholesterol Education Program Expert Panel on Detection, Evaluation, and Treatment of High Blood Cholesterol in Adults. *Arch Intern Med 1988;148:36–69.*

2. The Lipid Research Clinics Coronary Primary Prevention Trial results. I. Reduction in incidence of coronary heart disease. Lipid Research Clinics program. *JAMA 1984;251:351–364.*

3. The Lipid Research Clinics Coronary Primary Prevention Trial results. II. The relationship of reduction in incidence of coronary heart disease to cholesterol lowering. Lipid Research Clinics Program. *JAMA 1984;251:365–374.*

4. Grundy SM, Vega GL, Bilheimer DW. Influence of combined therapy with mevinolin and interruption of bile-acid reabsorption on low density lipoproteins in heterozygous familial hypercholesterolemia. *Ann Intern Med 1985;103:339–343.*

5. Frick MH, Elo O, Haapa K, Heinonen OP, Heinsalmi P, Helo P, Huttunen JK, Kaitaniemi P, Koskinen P, Manninen V, Mäenpää H, Mälkönen M, Mänttäri M, Norola S, Pasternack A, Pikkarainen J, Romo M, Sjöblom T, Nikkilä EA. Helsinki heart study: primary-prevention trial with gemfibrozil in middle-aged men with dyslipidemia. Safety of treatment, changes in risk factors, and incidence of coronary heart disease. *N Engl J Med 1987;317:1237–1245.*

6. Manninen V, Elo MO, Frick MH, Haapa K, Heinonen OP, Heinsalmi P, Helo P, Huttunen JK, Kaitaniemi P, Koskinen P, Mäenpää H, Mälkönen M, Mänttäri M, Norola S, Pasternack A, Pikkarainen J, Romo M, Sjöblom T, Nikkilä EA. Lipid alterations and decline in the incidence of coronary heart disease in the Helsinki heart study. *JAMA 1988;260:641–651.*

7. Atmeh RF, Stewart JM, Boag DE, Packard CJ, Lorimer AR, Shepherd J. The hypolipidemic action of probucol: a study of its effects on high and low density lipoproteins. *J Lipid Res 1983;24:588–595.*

8. Kesamiemi YA, Grundy SM. Influence of probucol on cholesterol and lipoprotein metabolism in man. *J Lipid Res 1984;25:780–790.*

9. Yamamoto A, Matsuzawa Y, Yokoyama S, Funahashi T, Yamamura T, Kishino B. Effects of probucol on xanthomata regression in familial hypercholesterolemia. *Am J Cardiol 1986;57:29–35.*

10. Kuo PT, Wilson AC, Kostis JB, Moreyra DE. Effects of combined probucol-colestipol treatment for familial hypercholesterolemia and coronary artery disease. *Am J Cardiol 1986;57:43H–48H.*

11. Sirtori CR, Sirtori M, Calabresi L, Franceschini G. Changes in high-density lipoprotein subfraction distribution and increased cholesteryl ester transfer after probucol. *Am J Cardiol 1988;62:73B–76B.*

12. The Coronary Drug Project Research group. Clofibrate and niacin in coronary heart disease. *JAMA 1975;231:360–381.*

13. Grundy SM, Mok HYI, Zech L, Berman M. Influence of nicotinic acid on metabolism of cholesterol and triglycerides in man. *J Lipid Res 1981;22:24–36.*

14. Havel RJ, Hunninghake DB, Illingworth DR, Lees RS, Stein EA, Tobert JA, Bacon SR, Bolognese JA, Frost PH, Lamkin GE, Lees AM, Leon AS, Gardner K, Johnson G, Mellies MJ, Rhymer PA, Tun P. Lovastatin (mevinolin) in the treatment of heterozygous familial hypercholesterolemia. A multicenter study. *Ann Intern Med 1987;107:609–615.*

15. Tikkanen MJ, Helve E, Jaattela A, Kaarsalo E, Lehtonen A, Malbecq W, Oksa H, Paakkonen P, Salmi J, Veharanta T, Viikari J, Aarynen M, and the Finnish Lovastatin Study Group. Comparison between lovastatin and gemfibrozil in the treatment of primary hypercholesterolemia: the Finnish multicenter study. *Am J Cardiol 1988;62:35J–43J.*

16. The Lovastatin Study Group III. A multicenter comparison of lovastatin and cholestyramine therapy for severe primary hypercholesterolemia. *JAMA 1988; 260:359–366.*

17. Grundy SM. Drug therapy in hyperlipidemia. *Cholesterol and Coronary Disease . . . Reducing the Risk 1987;1:1–8.*

18. Bilheimer DW. Therapeutic control of hyperlipidemia in the prevention of coronary atherosclerosis: a review of results from recent clinical trials. *Am J Cardiol 1988;62:1J–9J.*

19. Blum CB, Levy RI. Current therapy for hypercholesterolemia. *JAMA 1989;261:3582–3587.*

We Think We Are One, We Act As If We Are One, But We Are Not One

Natural carnivores live on meat. Natural herbivores live on vegetables, fruits and starches (rice, corn, potatoes, beans, pasta). Carnivores and herbivores are made differently (Table I). Carnivores have claws and sharp teeth for ripping meat apart; herbivores have hands (unless they have hoofs) for gathering food and flat teeth for grinding the vegetables, fruits and grains. Carnivores have short bowels and rapidly digest the flesh and rapidly excrete the putrefying animal products. The time required for food to travel through their intestinal tract is short. Herbivores have long intestines so that there is plenty of time to digest the nutrients in the plants, fruits and starches, and when these animals eat these foods their transient times also are relatively short despite the long intestinal tracts. Meat eaters pant to cool themselves and lap water; plant eaters, in contrast, sweat to cool and sip water. Carnivores synthesize their own vitamin C, which is virtually absent in meat and dairy products; herbivores obtain their vitamin C from plant foods in which it is abundant.

Although human beings eat meat we are not natural carnivores (Table I). We were intended to eat plants, fruits and starches! No matter how much fat carnivores eat, they do not develop atherosclerosis. It is virtually impossible, for example, to produce atherosclerosis in the dog even when 100 grams of cholesterol and 120 grams of butter fat are added to its meat ration.[1] (This amount of cholesterol is approximately 200 times the average amount that human beings in the USA eat each day!) In contrast, herbivores rapidly develop atherosclerosis if they are fed foods, namely fat and cholesterol, intended for natural carnivores. Adding only 2 grams of cholesterol daily for 2 months to a rabbit's chow, for example, produces striking fatty changes in its arteries.[1] And humans are like rabbits, natural herbivores, not like dogs or cats, natural carnivores.

Thus, although we think we are one and we act as if we are one, human beings are not natural carnivores. When we kill animals to eat them, they end up killing us because their flesh, which contains cholesterol and saturated fat, was never intended for human beings, who are natural herbivores.

TABLE I Differences in Carnivores and Herbivores

Characteristic	Carnivores	Herbivores
Appendages	Claws	Hands or hoofs
Teeth	Sharp	Flat
Intestines	Short	Long
Body cooling	Pant	Sweat
Drinking water	Lap it	Sip it
Vitamin C	Make it themselves	Obtained solely from diet

William C. Roberts

William Clifford Roberts, MD
Editor in Chief

1. Collens WS. Atherosclerotic disease: an anthropologic theory. *Medical Counterpoint.* December 1969;1:53–57.

The Best Antiarrhythmic Agent Will Be a Lipid-Lowering Agent

In September 1990 I attended a 2-day conference on Sudden Cardiac Death and heard a number of talks on malignant and potentially malignant ventricular arrhythmias. A variety of cardiac conditions, of course, have an increased propensity to develop ventricular arrhythmias. These include coronary artery disease, systemic hypertension, idiopathic dilated cardiomyopathy, hypertrophic cardiomyopathy, amyloidosis, sarcoidosis, mitral valve prolapse, some congenital cardiac anomalies, among others, and occasionally some malignant arrhythmias develop in the absence of "structural heart disease."Although they may be associated with several conditions, malignant ventricular arrhythmias most commonly (>75%) occur in association with severe coronary arterial narrowing from atherosclerosis. And the frequency of symptomatic and fatal myocardial ischemia increases as the amount of atherosclerotic plaque in our coronary arteries increases. And the amount of plaque increases as our total and low-density lipoprotein cholesterol levels in the serum increase and as the high-density lipoprotein cholesterol level decreases. If the percentage of calories from fat diminished in our diets from 40–42% to about 10%, our serum total cholesterol levels and the frequency of symptomatic and fatal myocardial ischemia would drop to rates where malignant ventricular arrhythmias would be "non-problems." Because reducing our percentage of calories from fat by 75% is unrealistic for most of us, the lipid-lowering drugs are needed.

In conjunction with low fat-low cholesterol diets, lipid-lowering agents slow, retard and reverse the atherosclerotic process, and, therefore, delay, retard and prevent the formation of atherosclerotic plaques by lowering our total and low-density lipoprotein serum levels, and by raising our high-density lipoprotein levels. The lower the total and low-density lipoprotein levels, the less the atherosclerotic plaque and the less the chance of developing malignant and potentially malignant arrhythmias.

I kept wondering during the sudden-cardiac-death conference how much the cardiac electrical experts knew or cared about cholesterol. I'll wager a bet with anyone that lipid-lowering agents eventually will prove to be the best antiarrhythmic agents.

William C. Roberts

William Clifford Roberts, MD

More on Fast Foods and Quick Plaques

Five of every 10 dollars spent on restaurant food in the USA is spent at a fast-food restaurant. Each person in the USA spends an average of $250 a year on fast foods. Over 160,000 fast-food restaurants are available in the USA and $70,000,000,000 (10 zeros) are spent at them each year. The fast-food restaurants outnumber the traditional restaurants in the USA. McDonald's, the largest of the fast-food chains, has over 11,000 outlets and a new one goes up somewhere in the world every 15 hours. McDonald's is the largest owner of commercial real estate in the world, and they employ over 500,000 persons. One of 5 persons in the USA visits a fast-food restaurant everyday, and 4 of 5, every month. More than half of the fast-food business is done at drive-through windows. Fast-food restaurants are located in hospitals, zoos, military bases, college campuses (including dormitories), museums, airports, naval ships and boats (Mississippi River), bus stations, amusement parks, private-office and state-government buildings, and department stores. Mobile (restaurants on wheels) fast-food restaurants visit neighborhoods, playgrounds, and beaches. Menus are being diversified. McDonald's now offers more than 40 items. The top 15 fast-food chains spent $1,217,000,000 on advertising in 1989, directing many of their ads to children. Survey after survey shows that parents let their

TABLE I Hamburgers and Cheeseburgers

Company/Product	Calories	Fat (tsp)	Sodium (mg)	Gloom
McDonald's Hamburger	255	2	490	16
Hardee's Hamburger	270	2	490	16
Burger King Hamburger	272	3	505	18
Jack in the Box Hamburger	267	3	556	18
McDonald's McLean Deluxe	320	2	670	18
McDonald's Cheeseburger	305	3	710	22
Hardee's Real Lean Deluxe	340	3	650	22
Burger King Cheeseburger	318	3	661	24
Burger King Burger Buddies	349	4	717	26
Burger King Hamburger Deluxe	344	4	496	27
Dairy Queen Single Hamburger with Cheese	365	4	800	29
McDonald's Quarter Pounder	410	5	650	31
Carl's Jr. Carl's Original Hamburger	460	5	810	31
Hardee's Big Twin	450	6	580	33
Dairy Queen Double Hamburger	460	6	630	37
Wendy's Double Hamburger	520	6	710	39
Jack in the Box Double Cheeseburger	467	6	842	40
Burger King Double Cheeseburger	483	6	851	40
McDonald's Big Mac	500	7	890	41
Hardee's Big Deluxe Burger	500	7	760	42
Hardee's Quarter-Pound Cheeseburger	500	7	1,060	42
McDonald's Quarter Pounder with Cheese	510	7	1,090	43
Burger King Bacon Double Cheeseburger	515	7	748	45
Wendy's Big Classic	570	7	1,085	48
Burger King Whopper	614	8	865	49
Jack in the Box Jumbo Jack	584	8	733	50
Hardee's Bacon Cheeseburger	610	9	1,030	54
Wendy's Big Classic with Cheese	640	9	1,345	56
Carl's Jr. Western Bacon Cheeseburger	730	9	1,490	59
Burger King Whopper with Cheese	706	10	1,177	61
Dairy Queen DQ Homestyle Ultimate Burger	700	11	1,110	63
Wendy's Double Big Classic	750	10	1,295	64
Burger King Double Whopper	844	12	933	72
Wendy's Double Big Classic with Cheese	820	12	1,555	72
Burger King Double Whopper with Cheese	935	14	1,245	83
Jack in the Box Ultimate Cheeseburger	942	16	1,176	88
Carl's Jr. Double Western Bacon Cheeseburger	1,030	14	1,810	91

Befriend your arteries by choosing small burgers and skipping the "special sauces." Cheeseburgers provide some calcium, but skim milk, yogurt, and green vegetables are much better, lower calorie sources.

The "Gloom" rating was designed by Jacobsen and Fritschner to give a quick summary of a food's or a meal's overall nutritional value. The formula for the Gloom rating provides 0.9 point/g of polyunsaturated oil; 1.1 point/g of highly saturated animal fat; 0.1 point/g of refined sugar or corn syrup; 1 point/20 mg of cholesterol; and 1 point/133 mg of sodium. This sum is then multiplied by a number ranging from 0.5 to 1.5 depending on the food's nutrient density, which is the ratio of nutrients/calorie (based on protein, calcium, iron, vitamin A, and vitamin C). For example, the multiplier would be 1 if a food contained 100% of the FDA of each of the 5 nutrients.

Reprinted with permission of the publisher.

TABLE II Roast Beef

Company/Product	Calories	Fat (tsp)	Sodium (mg)	Gloom
Dairy Queen BBQ Beef Sandwich	225	1	700	10
Arby's Junior Roast Beef	218	2	345	16
Subway Roast Beef Sandwich, 6 in.	375	3	839	16
Arby's French Dip (roast beef sandwich)	345	3	678	20
Hardee's Roast Beef Sandwich (RR)	350	3	732	20
Hardee's Roast Beef Sandwich, large (RR)	373	3	840	21
Hardee's Regular Roast Beef	310	3	930	22
Arby's Regular Roast Beef	353	3	588	23
Hardee's Roast Beef Sandwich with Cheese (RR)	403	3	954	27
Hardee's Big Roast Beef	360	3	1,150	28
Hardee's Roast Beef Sandwich with Cheese, large (RR)	427	4	1,062	28
Arby's French Dip 'N Swiss (roast beef sandwich)	425	4	1,078	32
Arby's Beef 'N Cheddar	451	5	955	33
Carl's Jr. Roast Beef Deluxe Sandwich	540	6	1,340	38
Arby's Super Roast Beef	529	6	798	38
Arby's Philly Beef'N Swiss	498	6	1,194	40
Arby's Giant Roast Beef	530	6	908	40
Arby's Bac 'N Cheddar Deluxe	532	7	1,672	52

Plain roast beef is lower in fat than most hamburger meat, but a sandwich, topped with bacon, cheese, or sauces, may be quite fatty. Hardee's sandwiches marked "(RR)" are available in the New York-Washington region; they are made from the very lean roast beef that has been used by Roy Rogers restaurants.

Reprinted with permission of the publisher.

children make restaurant choices. When children under age 17 years eat at a restaurant in the USA, 83% of the time it is at a fast-food chain.

The above information comes from the second edition of the *FAST-FOOD GUIDE* published in 1991 and written by Michael F. Jacobson, PhD, Executive Director, Center for Science in the Public Interest, and Sarah Fritschner, a nutritionist and the food editor of the Louisville *Courier-Journal*.[1] Like their first edition, which appeared in 1986[2] (and also reviewed in this column[3]), this new book details the amounts of calories, fat, sodium, sugar, and other "nutrients" in the foods and liquids sold by the 15 largest fast-food chains in the USA (Tables I to VII). When Jacobson and Fritschner wrote their 1986 book, virtually all fast-food chains were resistant to supplying them with the ingredients of the products sold. For their 1991 book, in contrast, most chains freely supplied them the ingredients of the products.

TABLE III Chicken and Turkey

Company/Product	Calories	Fat (tsp)	Sodium (mg)	Gloom
Carl's Jr. Charbroiler BBQ Chicken Sandwich	310	1	680	12
Arby's Light Roast Chicken Deluxe	253	1	874	13
Long John Silver's Chicken Plank, 1 piece	130	1	490	13
Jack in the Box Chicken Fajita Pita	292	2	703	14
KFC Original Recipe Drumstick	146	2	275	14
Hardee's Chicken Stix, 6 pieces	210	2	680	15
Burger King BK Broiler Chicken Sandwich	267	2	728	15
Dairy Queen Grilled Chicken Fillet Sandwich	300	2	800	16
Subway Turkey Sandwich, 6 in.	357	2	839	16
Wendy's Grilled Chicken Sandwich	320	2	715	16
Long John Silver's Baked Chicken Sandwich (no sauce)	320	2	900	17
KFC Original Recipe Wing	178	3	372	18
Burger King Chicken Tenders, 6 pieces	236	3	541	21
KFC Extra Tasty Crispy Drumstick	204	3	324	22
Hardee's Chicken Fillet	370	3	1,060	24
KFC Original Recipe Center Breast	283	3	672	25
Arby's Grilled Chicken Barbecue	378	3	1,059	25
Wendy's Chicken Sandwich, fried	430	4	725	25
KFC Original Recipe Side Breast	267	4	735	27
Arby's Turkey Deluxe	399	5	1,047	28
Jack in the Box Grilled Chicken Fillet	408	4	1,130	28
KFC Extra Tasty Crispy Wing	254	4	422	30
McDonald's McChicken	415	7	770	30
Wendy's Crispy Chicken Nuggets, 6 pieces	280	5	600	31
Dairy Queen Breaded Chicken Breast Fillet Sandwich	430	5	760	32
KFC Original Recipe Thigh	294	4	619	33
KFC Hot Wings, 6 pieces	376	5	677	40
Arby's Roast Chicken Club	513	7	1,423	43
KFC Colonel's Chicken Sandwich	482	6	1,060	45
KFC Extra Tasty Crispy Thigh	406	7	688	48
Arby's Chicken Cordon Bleu	658	8	1,824	60
Burger King Chicken Sandwich	685	9	1,417	61

Chicken starts out lean and wholesome, but once it is battered, breaded, fried, and smothered with a mayonnaise sauce, it will be loaded with fat and calories. Look for baked or broiled chicken, hold the sauces, and discard the grease-soaked breading.
Reprinted with permission of the publisher.

TABLE IV Fish

Company/Product	Calories	Fat (tsp)	Sodium (mg)	Gloom
Long John Silver's Shrimp, battered, 1 piece	60	1	180	7
Long John Silver's Fish, Homestyle, 1 piece	125	2	200	8
Wendy's Seafood Salad	110	2	455	9
Subway Tuna Sandwich, 6 in.	402	3	905	17
Long John Silver's Clams, breaded	240	3	410	19
Subway Seafood and Crab Sandwich, 6 in.	388	3	1,306	20
Long John Silver's Fish, battered, 1 piece	210	2	570	21
Dairy Queen Fish Fillet Sandwich	370	4	630	26
McDonald's Filet-O-Fish	370	6	930	32
Dairy Queen Fish Fillet Sandwich with Cheese	440	5	880	33
Burger King Ocean Catch Fish Filet	495	6	879	37
Wendy's Fish Fillet Sandwich	460	6	780	38
Hardee's Fisherman's Fillet	500	5	1,030	38
Jack in the Box Fish Supreme	510	6	1,040	41
Arby's Fish Fillet Sandwich	537	7	994	46
Carl's Jr. Carl's Catch Fish Sandwich	560	7	1,220	47

Most fresh fish is low in fat and quite healthful. But most fast-food fish is deep-fried and as fatty as many hamburgers. Seek broiled or baked fish, and season with lemon juice instead of butter and tartar sauce.
Reprinted with permission of the publisher.

TABLE V French Fries

Company/Product	Calories	Fat (tsp)	Sodium (mg)	Gloom
Long John Silver's Fryes (3 oz.)	170	2	55	7
Dairy Queen, small (2.5 oz.)	210	2	115	13
Hardee's, regular (2.5 oz.)	230	3	85	14
Jack in the Box, small (2.5 oz.)	219	3	121	14
McDonald's, small (2.4 oz.)	220	3	110	16
KFC (2.5 oz.)	244	3	139	16
Arby's, small (2.5 oz.)	246	3	114	18
Hardee's, large (4 oz.)	360	4	135	21
Wendy's, large (4.2 oz.)	312	4	189	22
Jack in the Box, regular (4 oz.)	351	4	194	22
McDonald's, medium (3.4 oz.)	320	4	150	23
Dairy Queen, large (4.5 oz.)	390	4	200	24
Jack in the Box, Jumbo (5 oz.)	396	5	219	24
Arby's Curly Fries (3.5 oz.)	337	4	167	27
Hardee's Crispy Curls (3 oz.)	300	4	840	27
Carl's Jr., regular (4.5 oz.)	420	5	200	29
McDonald's, large (4.3 oz.)	400	5	200	29
Arby's, medium (4 oz.)	394	5	182	29
Burger King, medium (4 oz.)	372	5	238	30
Hardee's, "Big Fry" (5.5 oz.)	500	5	180	30
Wendy's, Biggie (6 oz.)	449	5	271	32
Arby's Cheddar Fries (5 oz.)	399	5	443	35
Arby's, large (5 oz.)	492	6	228	37

Though they're deep-fried and salted, french fries are not quite as bad as their reputation would have them. But a small serving should be more than enough, and ask the clerk to hold the salt. Kudos to Long John Silver's for making salt-free "Fryes" its standard.
Reprinted with permission of the publisher.

TABLE VI Shakes and Malts

Company/Product	Calories	Fat (tsp)	Sodium (mg)	Sugar (tsp)	Gloom
McDonald's, Low-fat (average)	310	<1	193	9	7
Carl's Jr., regular	350	2	230	10	14
Jack in the Box (average)	323	2	247	10	15
Hardee's (average)	433	2	320	12	19
Arby's, Vanilla	330	3	281	7	20
Arby's, Jamocha	368	2	262	8	20
Arby's Chocolate	451	3	341	12	24
Dairy Queen Malt, regular	610	3	230	9	25
Burger King Chocolate, large	472	3	286	12	26
Dairy Queen Shake, regular	520	3	230	11	26
Dairy Queen Shake, large	600	4	260	13	30
Wendy's Frosty Dairy Dessert, medium	520	4	286	7	30
Arby's Snickers Polar Swirl	511	4	351	9	33
Wendy's Frosty Dairy Dessert, large	680	5	374	9	40
Arby's Peanut Butter Cup Polar Swirl	517	5	385	14	41
Dairy Queen Heath Blizzard, regular	820	8	410	14	58

Typical shakes contain about as much sugar (figures shown are estimates) as a can of cola, as much fat as a glass of milk, and as many calories as a cola and milk combined. However, they are all good sources of calcium. McDonald's was first to offer a low-fat shake. For some companies, the average of several flavors is shown.
Reprinted with permission of the publisher.

TABLE VII Salads

Company/Product	Calories	Fat (tsp.)	Sodium (mg)	Gloom
Arby's Side Salad	25	0	30	0
Wendy's Garden Salad	70	<1	60	1
Burger King Chunky Chicken Salad	142	1	443	6
McDonald's Chunky Chicken Salad	150	1	230	6
Wendy's Chef Salad	180	2	140	10
Subway Turkey Salad, small	167	2	479	10
Long John Silver's Seafood Salad	230	2	580	10
Subway Roast Beef Salad, small	185	2	479	11
McDonald's Chef Salad	170	3	400	12
Subway Tuna Salad, small	212	3	545	12
Burger King Chef Salad	178	2	568	13
Carl's Jr. Charbroiler Chicken Salad	200	2	300	15
Hardee's Garden Salad	210	3	270	15
Long John Silver's Ocean Chef Salad	250	2	1,340	17
Hardee's Chicken Fiesta Salad	280	3	640	19
Hardee's Chef Salad	240	3	930	20
Jack in the Box Chef Salad	325	4	900	25
Taco Bell Taco Salad, no shell	484	7	680	34
Wendy's Taco Salad	660	8	1,110	39
Taco Bell Taco Salad, with shell	905	14	910	68

Most salads, other than taco salads, are low in calories and fat. Be sure to ask for a low-calorie dressing or you risk ruining a good thing with several hundred additional calories.
Reprinted with permission of the publisher.

From 1986 to 1991, the 5-year period between the 2 editions of the 2 fast food books, most, but not all, of the fast-food chains decreased the calorie, fat and sodium contents of their foods. Several (McDonald's, Burger King, Hardee's, Arby's, Dairy Queen, Jack in the Box, and Wendy's) switched from beef fat to vegetable shortening for all frying, and 1 (Taco Bell) switched from coconut oil (92% saturated) to a less saturated vegetable shortening for all frying. McDonald's became the first chain to offer 1% low-fat milk and breakfast cereals. Frozen and non-fat yogurt was introduced by McDonald's and Baskin-Robbins. Wendy's dropped completely the Triple Cheeseburger from its menus. This hamburger/cheeseburger was number 1 for calories (1,040), fat (15 teaspoons), and sodium (1,848 mg) in 1986. Today's worst is Carl's Jr. Double Western Bacon Cheeseburger which contains 1,030 calories, 14 teaspoons of fat and 1,810 mg of sodium (Table I). Several (Arby's, Dunkin' Donuts, and Hardee's) either switched to cholesterol free or to a lower calorie mayonnaise. Despite these type changes, the saturated fat and cholesterol contents of the fast-food products remain far too high. Most changes, however, are in the right direction, and many others can be expected by the time the Jacobson/Fritschner third edition appears.

Congratulations to Jacobson and Fritschner for keeping the pressure on the fast-food suppliers to supply us with more healthy foods and liquids.

William C. Roberts

William Clifford Roberts, MD
Editor in Chief

1. Jacobson MF, Fritschner S. The Completely Revised and Updated Fast-Food Guide, Second Edition. New York: Workman Publishing, 1991:333.
2. Jacobson MF, Fritschner S. Fast Food Guide. New York: Workman Publishing, 1986:225.
3. Roberts WC. Fast foods and quick plaques. *Am J Cardiol* 1987;59:721–723.

Getting Cardiologists Interested in Lipids

Several surveys have shown that cardiologists rank only slightly above general internists, general practitioners and the general public in considering "cholesterol" of major importance for development of atherosclerosis.[1] It takes few fingers to name prominent cardiologists around the world who have become recognized as lipid experts or who have a major interest in lipids. Yet the data are in showing that cholesterol causes atherosclerosis![2–6] When high cholesterol levels are lowered clinical atherosclerotic events decrease, deaths from atherosclerotic events decrease, and the amounts of atherosclerotic plaque deposited in arteries decrease.[7–21] Although there are many exceptions, cardiologists in general have relatively little interest in cholesterol and its role in atherosclerosis. This piece examines why that might be the case:

1. *Cardiologists as a group are not completely convinced of the important role of cholesterol in atherosclerosis.* Most patients seen by cardiologists have serum total cholesterol levels >200 mg/dl (>5.2 mmol/liter), and there is not much difference in the cholesterol levels in those patients with and those without overt evidence of myocardial ischemia. Thus, the actual serum total cholesterol level is not very helpful in separating patients with from those without myocardial ischemia. Furthermore, nearly half the patients with angiographic evidence of significant coronary arterial narrowing have serum total cholesterol levels <200 mg/dl (<5.2 mmol/liter).[22,23] (Most of the latter group, however, have relatively low high-density lipoprotein cholesterol levels.) It is impossible to get excited about cholesterol if one is not convinced of its importance!

2. *Cardiologists view cholesterol management as unexciting.* Cholesterol management is long-term. Witnessed changes in outcome are rarely apparent. It is similar to the management of systemic hypertension. Cardiologists are certainly convinced of the importance of lowering elevated blood pressure, but as a group cardiologists are not interested in the management of systemic hypertension. The same goes for the management of hypercholesterolemia. Its management is relatively boring compared to the excitement of treating patients with chest pain, arrhythmias, overt congestive heart failure, heart block, etc. Cardiology focuses primarily on management of acute events, the management of which is exciting. Dramatic changes in outcome in response to therapies (drugs and procedures) are witnessed. Lowering of cholesterol or blood pressure levels do not, in contrast, produce overt changes in the patients' symptoms or appearances. Cardiologists also tend to be more excited by the acute lesions in coronary arteries than by the masses of plaque in the coronary arteries.

3. *Cardiologists avoid cholesterol management because they know that successful management requires expert knowledge of nutrition, of cholesterol-lowering drugs, and a change in their own lifestyles.* Cardiologists as a group are uncomfortable when nutrition is the topic. Cardiologists are not calorie counters or grocery-store shoppers. Housewives know more about calories, fats, and carbohydrates than do many cardiologists. Cardiologists as a group are not experts on lipid-lowering drugs. Cardiologists, in contrast, are comfortable with nitroglycerin, digitalis, β blockers, calcium antagonists, angiotensin-converting enzymes, antiarrhythmic agents, thrombolytic agents, aspirin, heparin, warfarin, and vasopressors, but not lipid-lowering and antioxidant agents. I am afraid that we all tend to dismiss as unimportant that which we do not understand well or are not interested in.

4. *Cardiologists are a bit confused by the recommendations of the lipid experts regarding whom to treat and whom not to treat with diet and lipid-lowering agents.* The recommendations do change. The first USA recommendations, however, appeared in January 1988,[24] and the second USA recommendations appeared in June 1993,[25] so the argument that the recommendations are "always changing" is not valid. The recommendations continue to intermix primary and secondary prevention, which I believe is inappropriate. I am convinced that patients who have had atherosclerotic events should be clearly separated from those who have not because management of the 2 is entirely different. I too believe that the recommendations can be simplified, but that subject is for another day.

5. *Cardiologists resent being excluded from important roles in the cholesterol-lowering world.* The adult-lipid-expert committee in the USA is composed almost entirely of persons whose subspecialty in medicine is endocrinology and metabolism.[24,25] Only one cardiologist is a member of the recent adult-lipid-expert panel in the USA.[25] I suspect that cardiologists as a group are a bit uncomfortable in a situation where they are not the dominant players. Leaders in the lipid world are not physicians whose training had focused on cardiology. Yet in the real world it is the cardiologists who see patients who have had atherosclerotic events. Lipidologists, i.e., non-cardiologists, see lipid disorders in patients who have not had atherosclerotic events. In other words, lipidologists dominate primary prevention, i.e., managing persons with lipid disorders before atherosclerotic events. Cardiologists, however, because they see persons who have or have had atherosclerotic events, are the dominant forces of secondary prevention. And in the USA alone an estimated 5.5 to 7.5 million persons have had one or more coronary atherosclerotic events. In my view, all of these patients should be on a low-fat, low-cholesterol diet, and, with few exceptions, on one or more lipid-lowering or antioxidant drugs. Cardiologists

simply have no choice but to become better informed about these diets and these drugs.

6. *Cardiologists view the lipid-lowering drugs as too expensive.* Compared to what? In the USA in 1992, about 18 billion dollars was spent on coronary bypass alone, and probably about half that much on coronary angioplasty procedures. The lipid-lowering drugs are cheap in comparison and cost-effective.[26] If every person in the USA with symptomatic myocardial ischemia was given a 20 mg tablet of lovastatin daily the cost would be approximately 3 billion a year and I suspect the benefit would be substantial.

7. *Cardiologists consider cholesterol-lowering drugs to have too many side effects with too high risk/benefit ratios.* The presently used lipid-lowering drugs are some of the safest of all drugs available. The EXCEL study showed the side effects of a 20 mg tablet of lovastatin daily to be no more than that of placebo![27,28] The bile acid resins have no systemic effects although the quantity of them required to provide good cholesterol lowering is high. Although enormously effective, the unpleasant side effects of niacin are considerable. Thus, compared to the toxic effects of atherosclerosis, the lipid-lowering drugs, in contrast, are essentially nontoxic.

8. *Cardiologists view cholesterol management as financially unrewarding.* Certainly in comparison to the financial rewards resulting from the various cardiologic procedures, lipid-lowering endeavors are time consuming, often discouraging, and financially of relatively little benefit. Additionally, some cardiologists consider lipid management the purview of their referring physicians.

Thus, because secondary prevention is in the hands of cardiologists and because cholesterol lowering has proven benefit after atherosclerotic events, cardiologists must increase their knowledge of and use of low-fat, low-cholesterol diets and lipid-lowering agents.

William C. Roberts

William Clifford Roberts, MD
Editor in Chief

1. Schucker B, Wittes JT, Cutler JA, Bailey K, Mackintosh DR, Gordon DJ, Haines CM, Mattson ME, Goor RS, Rifkind BM. Change in physician perspective on cholesterol and heart disease. Results from two national surveys. *JAMA* 1987; 258:3521–3531.

2. Dock W. Atherosclerosis. Why do we pretend the pathogenesis is mysterious? *Circulation* 1974;50:647–649.

3. Consensus Development Panel. Lowering blood cholesterol to prevent heart disease. *JAMA* 1985;253:2080–2086.

4. Roberts WC. Factors linking cholesterol to atherosclerotic plaques. *Am J Cardiol* 1988;62:495–499.

5. Roberts WC. Atherosclerotic risk factors—are there ten or is there only one? *Am J Cardiol* 1989;64:552–554.

6. Gotto AM Jr, LaRosa JC, Hunninghake D, Grundy SM, Wilson PW, Clarkson TB, Hay JW. The cholesterol facts. A summary of the evidence relating dietary fats, serum cholesterol, and coronary heart disease. A Joint Statement by the American Heart Association and the National Heart, Lung, and Blood Institute. *Circulation* 1990;81:1721–1733.

7. Lipid Research Clinics Program. The lipid research clinics coronary primary prevention trial results. I. Reduction in incidence of coronary heart disease. *JAMA* 1984; 251:351–364.

8. Lipid Research Clinics Program. The lipid research clinics coronary primary prevention trial results. II. The relationship of reduction in incidence of coronary heart disease to cholesterol lowering. *JAMA* 1984;251:365–374.

9. Stamler J, Wentworth D, Neaton JD. Is relationship between serum cholesterol and risk of premature death from coronary heart disease continuous and graded? Findings in 356 222 primary screenees of the multiple risk factor intervention trial (MRFIT). *JAMA* 1986;256 No. 20:2823–2828.

10. Frick MH, Elo O, Haapa K, Heinonen OP, Heinsalmi P, Helo P, Huttunen JK, Kaitaniemi P, Koskinen P, Manninen V, Maenpää H, Mälkonen M, Mänttäri M, Norola S, Pasternack A, Pikkarainen J, Romo M, S√joblom T, Nikkilä EA. Helsinki heart study: primary prevention trial with gemfibrozil in middle-aged men with dyslipidemia. Safety of treatment, changes in risk factors, and incidence of coronary heart disease. *N Engl J Med* 1987;317:1237–1245.

11. Blankenhorn DH, Nessim SA, Johnson RL, Sanmarco ME, Azen SP, Cashin-Hemphill L. Beneficial effects of combined colestipol-niacin therapy on coronary atherosclerosis and coronary venous bypass grafts. *JAMA* 1987;257:3233–3240.

12. Roberts WC. Lipid-lowering therapy after an atherosclerotic event. *Am J Cardiol* 1989;64:693–695.

13. Ornish D, Brown SE, Scherwitz LW, Billings JH, Armstrong WT, Ports TA, McLanahan SM, Kirkeeide RL, Brand RJ, Gould KL. Can lifestyle changes reverse coronary heart disease? The lifestyle heart trial. *Lancet* 1990;336:129–133.

14. Buchwald H, Varco RL, Matts JP, Long JM, Fitch LL, Campbell GS, Pearce MB, Yellin AE, Edmiston WA, Smink RD Jr, Sawin HS Jr, Campos CT, Hansen BJ, Tuna N, Karnegis JN, Sanmarco ME, Amplatz K, Castaneda-Zuniga WR, Hunter DW, Bissett JK, Weber FJ, Stevenson JW, Leon AS, Chalmers TC, POSCH Group. Effect of partial ileal bypass surgery on mortality and morbidity from coronary heart disease in patients with hypercholesterolemia. Report of the Program on the Surgical Control of the Hyperlipidemics (POSCH). *N Engl J Med* 1990;323:946–955.

15. Rossouw JE, Lewis B, Rifkind BM. The value of lowering cholesterol after myocardial infarction. *N Engl J Med* 1990;323:1112–1119.

16. Brown G, Albers JJ, Fisher LD, Schaefer SM, Lin J-T, Kaplan C, Zhao X-Q, Bisson BD, Fitzpatrick VF, Dodge HT. Regression of coronary artery disease as a result of intensive lipid-lowering therapy in men with high levels of apolipoprotein B. *N Engl J Med* 1990;323:1289–1339.

17. Kane JP, Malloy MJ, Ports TA, Phillips NR, Diehl JC, Havel RJ. Regression of coronary atherosclerosis during treatment of familial hypercholesterolemia with combined drug regimens. *JAMA* 1990;264:3007–3012.

18. Watts GF, Lewis B, Brunt JNH, Lewis ES, Coltart DJ, Smith LDR, Mann JI, Swan AV. Effects on coronary artery disease of lipid-lowering diet, or diet plus cholestyramine, in the St. Thomas' Atherosclerosis Regression Study (STARS). *Lancet* 1992;339:563–569.

19. LaRosa JC, Cleeman JI. Cholesterol lowering as a treatment for established coronary heart disease. *Circulation* 1992;85:1229–1235.

20. Manson JE, Tosteson H, Ridker PM, Satterfield S, Hebert P, O'Connor GT, Buring JE, Hennekens CH. The primary prevention of myocardial infarction. *N Engl J Med* 1992;326:1406–1416.

21. Brown BG, Zhao X-Q, Sacco DE, Albers JJ. Lipid lowering and plaque regression. New insights into prevention of plaque disruption and clinical events in coronary disease. *Circulation* 1993;87:1781–1791.

22. Miller M, Mead LA, Kwiterovich PO Jr, Pearson TA. Dyslipidemias with desirable plasma total cholesterol levels and angiographically demonstrated coronary artery disease. *Am J Cardiol* 1990;1–5.

23. Romm PA, Green CE, Reagan K, Rackley CE. Relation of serum lipoprotein cholesterol levels to presence and severity of angiographic coronary artery disease. *Am J Cardiol* 1991;67:479–483.

24. The Expert Panel. Report of the national cholesterol education program expert panel on detection, evaluation, and treatment of high blood cholesterol in adults. *Arch Intern Med* 1988;148:36–69.

25. Expert Panel on Detection, Evaluation, and Treatment of High Blood Cholesterol in Adults. Summary of the second report of the National Cholesterol Education Program (NCEP) expert panel on detection, evaluation, and treatment of high blood cholesterol in adults (Adult Treatment Panel II). *JAMA* 1993;269:3015–3023.

26. Reckless JPD. Cost-effectiveness of hypolipidaemic drugs. *Postgrad Med J* 1993;69:S30–S33.

27. Bradford RH, Shear CL, Chremos AN, Dujovne C, Franklin FA, Hesney M, Higgins J, Langendorfer A, Pool JL, Schnaper H, Stephenson WP. Expanded Clinical Evaluation of Lovastatin (EXCEL) study: design and patient characteristics of a double-blind, placebo-controlled study in patients with moderate hypercholesterolemia. *Am J Cardiol* 1990;66:44B–55B.

28. Bradford RH, Shear CL, Chremos AN, Dujovne C, Downton M, Franklin FA, Gould AL, Hesney M, Higgins J, Hurley DP, Langendorfer A, Nash DT, Pool JL, Schnaper H. Expanded Clinical Evaluation of Lovastatin (EXCEL) study results. I. Efficiency in modifying plasma lipoproteins and adverse event profile in 8245 patients with moderate hypercholesterolemia. *Arch Intern Med* 1991;151:43–49.

The Ineffectiveness of a Commonly Recommended Lipid-Lowering Diet in Significantly Lowering the Serum Total and Low-Density Lipoprotein Cholesterol Levels

It has long been recognized that long-term excessive intake of salt often leads to elevation of the systemic arterial pressure.[1] Adults in the USA consume an average of about 10 g of salt daily and an estimated 60 million adults in the USA have systemic arterial pressures >140/90 mm Hg. If the salt intake is decreased by 50% to 5 g daily, there is an insignificant change in the systemic arterial pressure.[1] If, however, the salt intake is decreased to <1 g daily, the blood pressure falls significantly.[2]

It has also long been recognized that long-term excessive intake of saturated fat and cholesterol often leads to severe atherosclerosis.[3,4] The average adult in the USA consumes nearly 140 g of fat daily, one third of which is of the saturated variety, approximately 0.4 g of cholesterol daily, and an estimated 40 million adults in the USA have serum total cholesterol levels >240 mg/dl (>6.2 mmol/liter).[5,6] The former translates into nearly 40% of total calories being derived from fat. A reduction in the percentage of calories from fat from near 40% to 30% with saturated fat <7% and cholesterol <200 mg/day (The National Cholesterol Education Program Step 2 diet[7,8]) results in an average reduction in both the serum total and low-density lipoprotein (LDL) cholesterol levels of only 5% (e.g., 240→228 mg/dl [6.2→5.9 mmol/liter])![9] Although a reduction in the calories from fat from 40% to 20% (The American Heart Association phase III diet) decreases the total and LDL cholesterol levels by an average of 20% (e.g., 240→192 mg/dl [6.2→5.0 mmol/liter]),[10] most adults in the USA are unwilling to reduce to this level their percentage of calories from fat. (The average percentage of calories from fat for the average adult in Japan is now 23%, although historically it has been about 10%.) A reduction to 10% of calories from fat, a level achieved for practical purposes only by a vegetarian-fruit diet, can lower the serum total cholesterol level to near 150 mg/dl (3.9 mmol/liter), a level where atherosclerotic plaques do not form, and where those present shrink in size.

Fortunately, for those of us unwilling to reduce our percentage of calories from fat to more desirable levels, the addition of a single 20 mg tablet daily of lovastatin (and probably also of simvastatin [10 mg] and pravastatin [20 mg]) will reduce both the serum total and LDL cholesterol levels by an average of 27% (e.g., 240→175 mg/dl [6.2→4.5 mmol/liter]) even if the percentage of calories from fat remains at nearly 40%![9] If the percentage of calories from fat is reduced from 40% to 30% and at the same time a 20 mg tablet of lovastatin is administered, both the serum total and LDL cholesterol levels are reduced an additional 5% on the average for a total 32% reduction (e.g., 240→163 mg/dl [6.2→4.2 mmol/liter]). And the side effects of a once-daily 20 mg tablet of lovastatin are the same as a similar dose of placebo.[11,12]

How should this heretofore mentioned information be used clinically? It should be applied now, in my view, to virtually all patients who already have had an atherosclerotic event (secondary prevention). Several studies, 5 published in 1990, have indicated that further luminal narrowing by atherosclerotic plaques can be delayed or even prevented, and that the frequency of subsequent atherosclerotic events can be decreased in patients who have had atherosclerotic events if their total and LDL cholesterol levels are substantially lowered indefinitely.[13–18] If the serum total cholesterol is lowered to about 150 mg/dl (3.9 mmol/liter), the atherosclerotic plaques will shrink with a resulting increase in luminal size and new plaques will not form. Furthermore, the vasoconstrictor substances released by platelets and other cells may lose their effect when the serum cholesterol levels are substantially lowered. In other words, atherosclerotic arteries that lose the fatty components of their plaques may revert physiologically to behave like normal arteries. Additionally, the frequency of plaque disruption may be decreased.[19]

The Expert Panel of the National Cholesterol Education Program issued guidelines for adults with hypercholesterolemia in 1987.[7,8] This group of experts recommended as the first step a diet low in saturated fat and cholesterol to be followed later, if needed, by lipid-lowering drug therapy. Although its effectiveness in some patients may be impressive, particularly when the serum triglyceride level is >300 mg/dl (3.4 mmol/liter), the 30%-of-calories-from-fat and 200 mg cholesterol diet used by Hunninghake and associates[9] on the average lowered the serum total and LDL cholesterol levels by only 5%, and there is no evidence that such a small reduction would either halt plaque progression or initiate plaque regression. In actuality, this 25% reduction in percentage of calories from fat simply leads to false hope on the part of both patient and physician and, indeed, to the frustration of each. The person who has had an atherosclerotic event needs to lower the serum total and

The Editor in Chief and his family have no stocks in any pharmaceutical company, and the Editor in Chief is not a consultant to any pharmaceutical company.

LDL cholesterol levels (and raise the serum high-density lipoprotein cholesterol) as much and as rapidly as possible to reduce the chance of a subsequent atherosclerotic event. Therefore, lipid-lowering drug therapy, in my view, should be initiated immediately after an atherosclerotic event, irrespective of the level of the serum total or LDL cholesterol, because whatever these levels are, they are too high for that particular patient.[20] At the same time, the change to a lower fat–lower cholesterol diet can begin, but unless the fat–cholesterol reduction is dramatic (about a 50% reduction in calories from fat), meaningful serum LDL cholesterol reductions will not be achieved in most patients. Diet, in other words, *after an atherosclerotic event* should be viewed as secondary rather than as primary lipid-lowering therapy, the reverse of what has been recommended by the Expert Panel of the National Cholesterol Education Program. In contrast, *before an atherosclerotic event*, a low fat–low cholesterol diet should be the primary lipid-lowering therapy, and lipid-lowering drug therapy should be viewed as secondary and only necessary when the reduced fat and cholesterol intake do not achieve meaningful reductions in the serum total and LDL cholesterol levels.

William C. Roberts

William Clifford Roberts, MD
Editor in Chief
Baylor University Medical Center
Dallas, Texas

1. Freis ED. Salt, volume and the prevention of hypertension. *Circulation* 1976;53:589-595.

2. Watkin DM, Fraeb HF, Hatch FT, Gutman AB. Effects of diet in essential hypertension. II. Results of unmodified Kempner rice diet in fifty hospitalized patients. *Am J Med* 1950;9:441-450.

3. Roberts WC. Factors linking cholesterol to atherosclerotic plaques. *Am J Cardiol* 1988;62:495-499.

4. Task Force on Cholesterol Issues, American Heart Association chaired by LaRosa JC. The Cholesterol Facts. A summary of the evidence relating dietary fats, serum cholesterol, and coronary heart disease. A joint statement of the American Heart Association and the National Heart, Lung, and Blood Institute. *Circulation* 1990; 81:1721-1733.

5. Johnson CL, Rifkind BM, Sempos CT, Carroll MD, Bachorik PS, Briefel RR, Gordon DJ, Burt VL, Brown CD, Lippel K, Cleeman JI. Declining serum total cholesterol levels among US adults. The National Health and Nutrition Examination Surveys. *JAMA* 1993;269:3002-3008.

6. Sempos CT, Cleeman JI, Carroll MD, Johnson CL, Bachorik PS, Gordon DJ, Burt VL, Briefel RR, Brown CD, Lippel K, Rifkind BM. Prevalence of high blood cholesterol among US adults. An update based on guidelines from the second report of the National Cholesterol Education Program Adult Treatment Panels. *JAMA* 1993;269:3009-3013.

7. Report of the National Cholesterol Education Program Expert Panel on detection, evaluation, and treatment of high blood cholesterol in adults. *Arch Intern Med* 1988;148:36-69.

8. Expert Panel on Detection, Evaluation, and Treatment of High Blood Cholesterol in Adults. Summary of the Second Report of the National Cholesterol Education Program (NCEP) Expert Panel on Detection, Evaluation, and Treatment of High Blood Cholesterol in Adults (Adult Treatment Panel II). *JAMA* 1993; 269:3015-3023.

9. Hunninghake DB, Stein EA, Dujovne CA, Harris WS, Feldman EB, Miller VT, Tolbert JA, Laskarzewski PM, Quiter E, Held J, Taylor AM, Hopper S, Leonard SB, Brewer BK. The efficacy of intensive dietary therapy alone or combined with lovastatin in outpatients with hypercholesterolemia. *N Engl J Med* 1993;328:1213-1219.

10. Grundy SM, Nix D, Whelan MF, Franklin L. Comparison of three cholesterol-lowering diets in normolipidemic men. *JAMA* 1986;256:2351-2355.

11. Bradford RH, Shear CL, Chremos AN, Dujovne C, Franklin FA, Hesney M, Higgins J, Langendörfer A, Pool JL, Schnaper H, Stephenson WP. Expanded clinical evaluation of lovastatin (EXCEL) study: design and patient characteristics of a double-blind, placebo-controlled study in patients with moderate hypercholesterolemia. *Am J Cardiol* 1990;66:44B-55B.

12. Bradford RH, Shear CL, Chremos AN, Dujovne C, Downton M, Franklin FA, Gould AL, Hesney M, Higgins J, Hurley DP, Langendörfer A, Nash DT, Pool JL, Schnaper H. Expanded Clinical Evaluation of Lovastatin (EXCEL) study results. I. Efficacy in modifying plasma lipoproteins and adverse event profile in 8245 patients with moderate hypercholesterolemia. *Arch Intern Med* 1991;151:43-49.

13. LaRosa JC, Cleeman JI. Cholesterol lowering as a treatment for established coronary heart disease. *Circulation* 1992;85:1229-1235.

14. Watts GF, Lewis B, Brunt JNH, Lewis ES, Coltart DJ, Smith LDR, Mann JI, Swan AV. Effects on coronary artery disease of lipid-lowering diet, or diet plus cholestyramine, in the St. Thomas' Atherosclerosis Regression Study (STARS). *Lancet* 1992;339:563-569.

15. Schuler G, Hambrecht R, Schlierf G, Niebauer J, Hauer K, Neumann J, Hoberg E, Drinkmann A, Bacher F, Grunze M, Kubler W. Regular physical exercise and low-fat diet. Effects on progression of coronary artery disease. *Circulation* 1992;86:1-11.

16. The Pravastatin Multinational Study Group for Cardiac Risk Patients. Effects of Pravastatin in patients with serum total cholesterol levels from 5.2 to 7.8 mmol/liter (200 to 300 mg/dl) plus two additional atherosclerotic risk factors. *Am J Cardiol* 1993;72:1031-1037.

17. Blankenhorn DH, Azen SP, Kramsch DM, Mack WJ, Cashin-Hemphill L, Hodis HN, DeBoer LWV, Mahrer PR, Masteller MJ, Vailas LI, Alaupovic P, Hirsh LJ, and the MARS Research Group. Coronary angiographic changes with lovastatin therapy. The Monitored Atherosclerosis Regression Study (MARS). *Ann Intern Med* 1993;119:969-976.

18. Haskell WL, Alderman EL, Fair JM, Maron DJ, Mackey SF, Superko HR, Williams PT, Johnstone IM, Champagne MA, Krauss RM, Farquhar JW. The effects of intensive multiple risk factor reduction on coronary atherosclerosis and clinical cardiac events in men and women with coronary artery disease: The Stanford Coronary Risk Intervention Project (SCRIP). *Circulation* 1994;89:000-000 (due March or April 1994).

19. Brown BG, Xue-Qiao X, Sacco DE, Albers JJ. Lipid lowering and plaque regression. New insights into prevention of plaque disruption and clinical events in coronary disease. *Circulation* 1993;87:1781-1791.

20. Roberts WC. Lipid-lowering therapy after an atherosclerotic event. *Am J Cardiol* 1989;64:693-695.

Calculating the Percentage of Calories from Fat and the Grams of Fat Consumed Daily to Maintain an Ideal Body Weight

Recently I was asked to review records of 60 patients who had had coronary arteriography, angioplasty or bypass to express an opinion regarding the appropriateness of and outcome of each procedure at a hospital that had started a cardiovascular program only a few months earlier. I noticed that nearly all patients had been placed at discharge on a diet consisting in part of 30% of calories from fat (the step I American Heart Association diet). Not long after the chart review I encountered one physician who had prescribed the 30%-of-calories-from-fat diet to nearly all of his patients. I asked him if he knew what percentage of calories in his own diet came from fat and how many grams of fat he consumed daily. He said that he had never calculated that percentage and furthermore he was not sure he knew how to do it. I then asked how many calories he consumed each day and how many he should consume to maintain an ideal body weight. He was not sure of that either. Now here is a physician who routinely prescribes a 30%-of-calories-from-fat diet to his patients and he is not aware of the percentage of calories from fat he consumes or should consume and he is not certain how to calculate the percentage of calories from fat. And this physician is not alone among physicians.

Most adults in the Western World need from 11 to 18 calories per pound per day to sustain an ideal weight: 11 for the near sedentary individual(+), 13 for the moderately active(++), 15 for the moderate exerciser or physical laborer(+++), and 18 for the extremely active exerciser or physical worker(++++) (Table I). Because I am 6 feet tall and like to weigh no more than 170 pounds and am moderately active(++), I need about 2300 calories daily: a 30%-of-calories-from-fat diet for me would be 690 calories from fat (2300 × 0.30); at 20% fat, 460 calories (2300 × 0.20) and at 10% fat, 230 calories (2300 × 0.10). It is easier and maybe more reasonable to calculate the grams of fat rather than the percentage of calories from fat in each of the various percent-of-calories-from-fat diets. Thus, the maximal grams of fat I should consume can readily be determined by dividing by 9 (the number of calories in 1 g of fat) the number of calories derived from fat were I

TABLE I Calories Needed Daily to Sustain Ideal Body Weight

Height (inches)	Ideal Body Weight (pounds)	Activity Level +	++	+++	++++
		Women			
59	95	1,045	1,235	1,425	1,710
60	100	1,100	1,300	1,500	1,800
61	105	1,155	1,365	1,575	1,890
62	110	1,210	1,430	1,650	1,980
63	115	1,265	1,495	1,725	2,070
64	120	1,320	1,560	1,800	2,160
65	125	1,375	1,625	1,875	2,250
66	130	1,430	1,690	1,950	2,340
67	135	1,485	1,755	2,025	2,430
68	140	1,540	1,820	2,100	2,520
69	145	1,595	1,885	2,175	2,610
70	150	1,650	1,950	2,250	2,700
71	155	1,705	2,015	2,325	2,790
72	160	1,760	2,080	2,400	2,880
		Men			
62	118	1,298	1,534	1,770	2,124
63	124	1,364	1,612	1,860	2,232
64	130	1,430	1,690	1,950	2,340
65	136	1,496	1,768	2,040	2,448
66	142	1,562	1,846	2,130	2,556
67	148	1,628	1,924	2,220	2,664
68	154	1,694	2,002	2,310	2,772
69	160	1,760	2,080	2,400	2,880
70	166	1,826	2,158	2,490	2,988
71	172	1,892	2,236	2,580	3,096
72	178	1,958	2,314	2,670	3,204
73	184	2,024	2,392	2,760	3,204
74	190	2,090	2,470	2,850	3,420
75	196	2,156	2,548	2,940	3,528
76	202	2,222	2,626	3,030	3,636

TABLE II Maximal Grams of Fat Allowed with Four Different Percent-of-Calories-from-Fat Diets

Daily Calorie Intake	Maximum Grams of Fat Allowed for Ideal Body Weight With Four Different Percent-of-Calories-From-Fat Diets: 15%	20%	25%	30%
1,200	20	27	33	40
1,300	22	29	36	43
1,400	23	31	39	47
1,500	25	33	42	50
1,600	26	36	44	53
1,700	28	38	47	57
1,800	30	40	50	60
1,900	31	42	53	63
2,000	33	44	56	67
2,100	35	47	58	70
2,200	36	49	61	73
2,300	38	51	64	77
2,400	40	53	67	80
2,500	41	56	69	83
2,600	43	58	72	87
2,700	45	60	75	90
2,800	46	62	77	93
2,900	48	64	80	96
3,000	50	67	83	100

to consume a 30% (690 ÷ 9 = 75 g), a 20% (460 ÷ 9 = 50 g) or a 10% (230 ÷ 9 = 25 g) calories-from-fat diet (Table II).

Total calories is the important factor from the standpoint of body weight, but fat calories or fat grams is the important item from the standpoint of atherosclerotic disease. If all of us consumed no more than 25 g (the average weight of a normal-sized thyroid gland in adult humans) of fat daily, none of us would have atherosclerosis of clinical significance, but unfortunately few of us are pure vegetarians, a near requirement to maintain a 25 g fat intake. At 50 g of fat daily (a little <2 ounces) our risk of significant atherosclerotic disease also is small. At 75 g it is greater. Incidentally, a deck of cards weighs 75 g and we should all try to make that size our maximal daily fat intake. If the quantity could be closer to 50 g of fat daily our arteries would be cleaner and then heart disease and excessive body weight would not be so prevalent. Unfortunately, most American adults consume >100 g of fat daily, many of us >140 g, and our body weights are increased, and our risk for developing significant atherosclerosis is enormous.

William C. Roberts

William Clifford Roberts, MD
Editor in Chief
Baylor University Medical Center
Dallas, Texas

Mexican Food: Oilé

They did it with the fast foods, then the Italian and Chinese restaurant foods, and now it's the Mexican restaurants' turn. Jayne Hurley and Stephen Schmidt of the Center For Science in the Public Interest, in their publication *Nutrition Action Healthletter* of July/August 1994, do a number on the Mexican restaurant cuisine. The study included the most popular dishes served at typical mid-priced table-service restaurants in Dallas, Texas, and in 3 other US cities, including Chi-Chi's, El Torito, El Chico, and also some smaller chains and independents.

The results of their analyses of typical Mexican appetizers, side dishes, and main dishes are summarized in Tables I and II. If we consider our maximal daily allowances of total fat to be 65 grams, saturated fat 20 grams, and sodium 2,400 milligrams, several of the main Mexican dishes, particularly when rice, refried pinto beans, sour cream, and guacamole are added, overshoot these daily values. A *chicken burrito* dinner (cheese-topped flour

TABLE I Calories, Fat, and Sodium in Typical Mexican Appetizers and Side Dishes

	Calories	Percent of Calories From Fat	Total Fat (g)	Saturated Fat (g)	Sodium (mg)
Mexican rice*	229	15	4	1	818
Refried pinto beans*	375	39	16	7	791
Tortilla chips†	645	47	34	6	679
Cheese quesadillas with sour cream, pico de Gallo, and guacamole	900	59	59	24	1,628
Beef & cheese nachos† with sour cream and guacamole	1,362	59	89	28	2,426
Cheese nachos	807	62	55	25	876

*3/4 cup.
†50 chips.
Adapted from *Nutrition Action Healthletter*, July/August 1994; ©1994 by the Center for Science in the Public Interest, Washington, D.C.

TABLE II Calories, Fat, and Sodium in Typical Mexican Main Dishes

	Calories	Percent of Calories From Fat	Total Fat (g)	Saturated Fat (g)	Sodium (mg)
Chicken fajitas*	839	26	24	5	1,526
(with B, R, SC & G)	(1,661)	(34)	(63)	(19)	(3,657)
Chicken burrito	724	36	29	8	1,736
(with B, R, SC & G)	(1,530)	(40)	(68)	(22)	(3,691)
Beef burrito	833	44	40	13	1,965
(with B, R, SC & G)	(1,639)	(44)	(79)	(28)	(3,921)
Crispy chicken taco	219	45	11	3	356
Soft chicken taco	208	49	11	4	545
Chicken enchilada	329	50	18	6	619
Beef chimichanga	802	52	47	13	1,680
(with B, R, SC & G)	(1,607)	(48)	(86)	(27)	(3,634)
Beef enchilada	324	53	19	4	636
Cheese enchilada	372	57	24	7	635
Taco salad (with SC & G)	1,099	58	71	20	1,847
Chile relleno	487	70	38	11	872

B = beans; G = guacamole; R = rice; SC = sour cream.
Adapted from *Nutrition Action Healthletter*, July/August 1994; ©1994 by the Center for Science in the Public Interest, Washington, D.C.

tortilla stuffed with chicken and refried beans) contained enough sodium for 1½ days. A *chile relleno* dinner (cheese-stuffed, deep-fried pepper, topped with cheese and red sauce) contained as much saturated fat as 27 slices of bacon. Two *crispy chicken tacos* (crisp corn tortillas stuffed with chicken, cheese, lettuce, and tomato) with refried beans and rice amounted to 1,042 calories, 36% of which came from fat; a total of 42 grams of fat, including 13 grams of saturated fat; and 2,320 milligrams of sodium. Two *soft chicken tacos* with refried beans and rice were just as bad: 1,022 calories, 38% of which came from fat; a total of 43 grams of fat, including 15 grams of the saturated variety; and 2,700 milligrams of sodium. Two *chicken enchiladas* (chicken and cheese in an oil-dipped corn tortilla) with beans and rice totaled 1,264 calories, 40% of which came from fat; a total of 57 grams of fat, 19 grams of which are saturated; plus 2,847 milligrams of sodium. Two *beef enchiladas* with beans and rice amounted to 1,253 calories, 42% of which came from fat; a total of 58 grams of fat, 16 grams being saturated; plus 2,880 milligrams of sodium.

The appetizers and side dishes were not much better. The *mexican rice* (¾ cup), sautéed in oil or shortening before being cooked in sodium-soaked chicken broth, is 15% fat, and *refried pinto beans* (¾ cup) contains nearly 40% more calories than the rice, and 39% of its 375 calories came from fat (Table I). The only dish the authors considered decent enough to recommend was *chicken fajitas*, but without the beans, sour cream, and guacamole. The authors also concluded that, unlike Chinese or Italian restaurant food, it's tough to make typical Mexican restaurant dishes less fatty and less salty. I think that I will avoid most Mexican restaurants in the future.

William C. Roberts

William Clifford Roberts, MD
Editor in Chief
Baylor University Medical Center
Dallas, Texas 75246

Retail Costs of the Statin Lipid-Lowering Drugs

Several physicians have mentioned to me that their patients cannot afford the lipid-lowering drugs. Their patients, however, seem able to afford the far more expensive procedures—angioplasty and bypass—which help relieve, at least temporarily, the acute consequences of severe narrowings in the coronary and peripheral arterial systems. If the 12-ounce steaks are eliminated or reduced drastically in size, there would be plenty of change left over to purchase any of the lipid-lowering agents that have been proven to decrease recurrences of atherosclerotic events and to decrease progression and cause some regression in persons who have already had atherosclerotic events. The lipid-lowering agents appear to be better than aspirin, β blockers, and other agents for decreasing subsequent atherosclerotic events in persons who have already had an event. The retail costs (the prices patients pay) of the 4 currently available statin drugs in one metropolitan area in the USA in 1 month of 1994 are listed in Table I. *Simvastatin* is roughly 4 times more potent than is *fluvastatin* and twice as potent as both *lovastatin* and *pravastatin*. Thus, equivalent doses would be simvastatin 10 mg = lovastatin 20 mg = pravastatin 20 mg = fluvastatin 40 mg, or simvastatin 20 mg = lovastatin 40 mg = pravastatin 40 mg = fluvastatin 80 mg.

William Clifford Roberts, MD
Editor in Chief
Baylor University Medical Center
Dallas, Texas 75246

TABLE I Retail Costs of Four 3-Hydroxy-3-Methylglutaryl Coenzyme A Reductase Inhibitors in the Dallas/Fort Worth, Texas Area–September 1994

Product (mg/day)	A	B	C	D	E	F	Mean Cost/Month	Cost (mg/day)	LDL (%↓)	Cost/Dose/Day for 1% LDL↓
Fluvastatin (20)	$36.39	$30.92	$31.69	$31.12	$32.89	$34.81	$32.97	$1.10	−18	$0.06
Lovastatin (10)	39.96	38.78	34.19	37.69	38.78	37.79	37.86	1.26	−19*	0.07
Pravastatin (10)	54.59	46.98	47.39	35.84	49.62	56.91	48.55	1.61	−20	0.08
Simvastatin (5)	49.79	46.68	48.19	46.29	46.98	48.86	47.79	1.59	−24*	0.07
Fluvastatin (40)	39.79	33.98	35.19	35.34	35.72	38.71	36.46	1.21	−24*	0.05
Lovastatin (20)	53.39	50.74	52.69	50.84	47.49	52.21	51.22	1.71	−24*	0.07
Pravastatin (20)	51.29	49.72	54.29	46.95	51.97	49.44	50.61	1.68	−25	0.07
Simvastatin (10)	50.29	48.92	50.19	48.21	49.68	51.23	49.75	1.65	−33*	0.05
Fluvastatin (80) (40 bid)	79.58	67.96	70.38	70.68	71.44	77.42	72.92	2.43	−34	0.07
Lovastatin (40)	93.79	94.68	99.49	91.24	82.69	89.71	91.93	3.06	−30*	0.10
Lovastatin (40) (20 bid)	118.18	98.79	107.89	97.53	94.27	106.99	103.94	3.46	−34*	0.10
Pravastatin (40)	99.49	82.84	84.29	86.89	88.54	81.11	87.19	2.91	−34*	0.09
Pravastatin (40) (20 bid)	102.58	97.78	108.58	93.68	103.94	102.99	101.59	3.38	—	—
Simvastatin (20)	99.59	85.98	97.59	87.77	84.49	86.39	90.29	3.01	−34*	0.09
Lovastatin (80) (40 bid)	181.18	185.97	178.99	194.09	188.76	189.99	186.51	6.22	−40*	0.16
Simvastatin (40)	101.29	91.62	102.29	92.43	91.97	93.25	95.47	3.18	−41*	0.08

*From Manufacturer's Product Insert.
bid = twice daily; LDL = low-density lipoprotein cholesterol; — = no information available; ↓ = reduction.
Columns A to F represent different pharmacies.

The Underused Miracle Drugs: The Statin Drugs Are to Atherosclerosis What Penicillin Was to Infectious Disease*

When penicillin appeared in World War II, it was immediately recognized as a miracle drug for certain infectious diseases. Physicians clamored for the new curative drug, but manufacture of it, at least initially, was slow. Enough could not be produced. Dr. Chester Keefer from Boston, Massachusetts, was the "Penicillin Czar" in World War II, and he determined the civilians who received the drug and those who did not.[1] Eventually, mass production techniques were developed and penicillin became available in ready supply. Today, penicillin is still considered a miracle drug.

In 1987 another miracle drug was approved, namely *lovastatin* (L). Subsequently, 3 other statin drugs have been approved, namely *pravastatin* (P), *simvastatin* (S), and *fluvastatin* (F), and in 1997 it is likely that a fifth statin drug will be approved, namely *atorvastatin*. These statin drugs are to atherosclerosis what penicillin was to infectious diseases. They have the capacity to prevent atherosclerosis, and they have the capacity to arrest the process, i.e., to prevent further plaque formation.

The preventing and arresting abilities of the statin drugs are unlikely to take effect at the lower doses, but they do have this capacity when used in higher doses or in combination with other lipid-lowering drugs. To repeat, these drugs not only possess the ability to decrease the risk of the first or subsequent atherosclerotic events, but they have the capacity to prevent events in the first place and to prevent subsequent events after the first one.

Other than efficacy, there appears to be little difference in the 4 currently available statin drugs. The equivalent doses in mg are as follows: S10 = L20 = P20 = F40; S20 = L40 = P40 = F80; S40 = L80 = P80 = F160. Pravastatin at 80 mg and fluvastatin at 160 mg/day are not presently approved by the Food and Drug Administration. Fluvastatin at 80 mg/day apparently will be approved shortly. A recent study has indicated that simvastatin at 5 mg/day is approximately equivalent to fluvastatin at 40 mg/day.[2] Atorvastatin appears to be about 50% more powerful than simvastatin. It apparently has the capacity to lower low-density lipoprotein (LDL) cholesterol by 60%, i.e., from 240 to 100 mg/dl, and it is unlikely that new plaques form when the LDL cholesterol is <100 mg/dl. Because of the relative safety of the statin drugs, simvastatin is currently being tested in human beings at doses of 80 mg/day and 160 mg/day.

In the USA, according to data from the Lipid Research Clinic Study[3] about 25% of the 160 million USA citizens over 20 years of age have plasma total cholesterol levels >240 mg/dl. The percentage of these 40 million Americans on lipid-lowering drug therapy is unclear, but it is estimated to be <5%. Furthermore, it is estimated that about 7 million living Americans have had nonfatal myocardial ischemic events and probably over a million others have claudication, transient ischemic attacks, abdominal aortic aneurysm, or other forms of atherosclerotic events, and it is estimated that <2 million of them are on 1 or more lipid-lowering drugs.

The Adult Treatment Panel II of the National Cholesterol Education Program has recommended that persons having coronary atherosclerotic events be placed on lipid-lowering drug therapy if the serum LDL cholesterol is >130 mg/dl with the goal of lowering that level to <100 mg/dl.[4] A recent survey by a pharmaceutical company has shown that <10% of persons placed on a lipid-lowering drug after a coronary atherosclerotic event actually lower the LDL cholesterol to <100 mg/dl at 6 months.

Additionally, approximately 50% of patients placed on a lipid-lowering drug quit taking the drug in 1 year and only 25% still take the drug 2 years after it was started. And these are life-long drugs unless the patient is willing to be a pure vegetarian!

Thus, we have available 4, and soon 5, drugs that have the capacity to prevent and the capacity to arrest atherosclerosis, but few patients who need them are on them. Furthermore, of the patients on them, few are taking doses sufficient to lower the

The editor has no stocks in any pharmaceutical or medical device company. He is on the speaking faculty, he thinks, of a large number of pharmaceutical companies.

* This piece also is included as part of an article entitled "Facts and ideas from anywhere" in the July 1996 issue of the *Baylor University Medical Center Proceedings*.

serum LDL cholesterol level to the point where plaques do not form, i.e., <100 mg/dl, and of those taking the drug, most (75%) quit taking the drug within 2 years.

All of this, of course, is good news for coronary angioplasty, coronary bypass, carotid endarterectomy, abdominal aortic resection, and peripheral vascular operative procedures, but it is bad news for patients and an embarrassment for physicians. It took 80 years after it was demonstrated that high cholesterol diets caused atherosclerosis in rabbits before a safe, efficacious, once-a-day drug became available which could actually prevent and/or arrest atherosclerosis. The challenge now is to use these miracle antiatherosclerotic drugs more frequently, to use them in sufficient doses to do their job, and to convince patients that these miracle drugs taken every day are the best antiatherosclerotic insurance they can purchase. The cost of 5 cigarettes readily pays for the drug each day. If the quantity of meat consumed was reduced in half, there would be plenty of money left over to purchase the miracle statin drugs.

William C. Roberts

William Clifford Roberts, MD
Editor in Chief
Baylor University Medical Center
Dallas, Texas 75256

1. Tompsett RR. Reminiscing about penicillin. *Baylor Univ Med Ctr Proceed* 1995 (April); 8:11–13.
2. Illingworth DR, Stein EA, Knopp RH, Hunninghake DB, Davidson MH, Dujovne CA, Miller VT, Tobert JA, Laskarzewski PM, Isaacsohn JL, Bacon SP, Tate AC. A randomized multicenter trial comparing the efficacy of simvastatin and fluvastatin. *J Cardiovasc Pharmacol Ther* 1996;1:23–30.
3. The Lipid Research Clinics Program Epidemiology Committee. Plasma lipid distributions in selected North American populations: the Lipid Research Clinics Program Prevalence Study. *Circulation* 1979;60:427–439.
4. Expert panel on detection, evaluation, and treatment of high blood cholesterol in adults. Summary of the Second Report of the National Cholesterol Education Program (NCEP) Expert Panel on Detection, Evaluation, and Treatment of High Blood Cholesterol in Adults (Adult Treatment Panel II). *JAMA* 1993; 269:3015–3023.

Tobacco

Hardly a newspaper or magazine these days is devoid of a piece on tobacco. Several states are suing tobacco companies to recoup huge medical costs resulting from consumption of tobacco. The federal government has just issued new regulations on tobacco. Two books on tobacco, each appearing this year, provide perspective on the industry and the ironies and paradoxes about this problem. One is entitled *Smokescreen: The Truth Behind the Tobacco Industry Coverup* by Philip J. Hilts, Addison-Wesley, 288 pp, $22. The other is *Ashes to Ashes, America's Hundred-Year Cigarette War, the Public Health, and the Unabashed Triumph of Philip Morris* by Richard Kluger, Knopf, 807 pp, $35.

Some observations; the downside:

(1) About 46 million Americans smoke cigarettes; each averages 25 cigarettes a day which means 70,000 nicotine "hits" a year.

(2) Tobacco kills about 420,000 Americans each year or about 1,160 Americans each day. That is the equivalent of 3 jumbo jet crashes 365 days a year. Worldwide, tobacco kills 3 million people each year or 6 people every minute. If current smoking patterns persist, when the young smokers of today reach adulthood, there will be 10 million deaths a year from tobacco or 1 every 3 seconds worldwide.

(3) Cigarette consumption in the USA is no longer decreasing. Although the percentage of Americans aged 18 and over who smoke is down to 25% (from 50% in the early 1970s), there has been essentially no decrease in numbers of cigarettes smoked in the USA since 1993. In 1995 it was 487 billion cigarettes, a 2 billion increase over 1994. (In 1981, 640 billion cigarettes were smoked in the USA.) Per capita consumption in 1995 was 2,515 cigarettes per American aged 18 years and older. The percentage of high school seniors who smoke is now 22%, the highest since 1979. (Most smokers of course take up the habit before age 18.)

(4) Tobacco is addictive. Tobacco fulfills the recognized definition of addiction: it controls the users behavior; its use is continued despite harm, and it causes the user to seek out the substance and puts that substance ahead of other priorities. Mark Twain said that "quitting smoking is one of the easiest things to do. He had done it a 1000 times." But quitting isn't easy as we all know. Only 75% percent of smokers, according to a recent Gallup poll (for SmithKline Beecham), say that they have tried to quit. But only 32% were smokefree for >3 months, 22% for 1 to 3 months, and 44% for <1 month.

(5) Although cigarette smoking is stable in the USA or increasing only slightly, in Europe, Asia, and the developing countries, it is increasing at astounding rates. In Europe the smoking sections of restaurants in the large cities are crammed with adults and teenagers, while the nonsmoking areas are small isolated corners of restaurants.

(6) The direct costs of cigarette smoking in the USA are estimated to be $50 billion a year.

(7) Cigarette butts litter our land. Of the nearly one-half trillion cigarettes smoked a year in the USA, 97% of them have cellulase acetate filters which have an after-smoke life of 5 to 7 years. These filter-tip cigarette butts now languish in every conceivable crammy, from cemetery statuary to bellies of whales. Several trillion are out there at any given time—in landfills, park trails, storm sewers, beaches, etc.

(8) Cigarettes are probably the most common cause of residential fires.

(9) Cigarette smokers have more nonfatal illnesses than do nonsmokers, and lost productivity is greater among smokers than nonsmokers.

(10) Federal subsidies to tobacco farmers increase the taxes to nonsmokers as well as smokers.

(11) The federal, state, and local governments subsidize the costs of treatment of illnesses produced by tobacco.

(12) Cigarette smoking is a major cause of miscarriages and underweight newborns.

(13) Tobacco makes for untruthfulness in both advertisers and politicians. This summer Philip Morris Europe ran full-page newspaper ads in major cities in Europe urging nonsmokers to be tolerant of smokers. The ads indicated that second-hand smoke was less dangerous than drinking 1 or 2 glasses of milk (1.62), or eating 1 biscuit (1.49), or drinking chlorinated water (1.38), or eating pepper (1.30). Second-hand smoke had a relative risk of 1.19. The tobacco industry has been a major contributor to congressional candidates and to both the Democratic and Republican parties. Dole, who had a terrible time ending his cigarette smoking habit 50 years ago, has recently stated, "There is a mixed view among scientists and doctors whether it is addictive or not. I'm not certain whether it's addictive. It is to some people." And this man is running for the presidency of the USA. Tobacco money alters the thought processes.

(14) Cigar smoking is also increasing rapidly. About $1 billion worth of cigars were sold in the USA in 1995, 98% to men and 2% to women. About 10 million persons in the USA smoke cigars, up from 100,000 a decade ago. It has become fashionable since the glossy, celebrity-studded *Cigar Aficionado* magazine appeared in 1992.

(15) Smokeless or spit tobacco sales also are increasing rapidly. About 40% of the nearly 700 major league baseball players use it. In Texas, 26% of

eighth graders have chewed spit tobacco. Nationally, about 1 million adolescents, including nearly 20% of all high school boys, use spit tobacco according to the U.S. Department of Health and Human Services, and chewing tobacco increases the frequency of cancers of the mouth and pharynx about 6 times compared to nonusers.

Although the downside for tobacco is much greater than the upside, here are some positives:

(1) The tobacco industry provides jobs for about 700,000 Americans in farming, manufacturing, and retailing. The numbers of lawyers and lobbyists supported by the industry is unclear but obviously large. There are 124,000 tobacco farms in the USA and they produce 1.6 billion pounds of tobacco, a 25% reduction compared to 1975. A total of 674 million acres grew tobacco in the USA in 1995. Farmers in North Carolina gross about $3,400 per acre of tobacco compared with $210 per acre of soybeans and $700 per acre of cotton.

(2) Tobacco provides about $21 billion a year in revenue from its agriculture and manufacturing. The tobacco crop itself in the USA is valued at $3 billion a year. Advertising expenditures in the USA exceed $6 billion a year. Fees for lawyers and lobbyists are in the multimillion dollar range.

(3) The tobacco industry provides about $13 billion to federal, state, and local governments in tax revenue. Cigarettes are the world's most heavily taxed consumer product! In the USA, the tax is 81.5 cents a pack (20 cigarettes), but in 20 other industrialized countries the taxes are even higher, sometimes 5 times higher.

(4) Tobacco reduces the expenditures on Medicare and Social Security as a result of the premature deaths of smoking victims. If every cigarette smoker quit today, there would be a crisis for Social Security and all pension plans that incorporate actuarial assumptions about millions of smokers dying before they can receive benefits they otherwise would collect.

(5) Tobacco is beneficial to the USA's balance of trade. (The tobacco industry, of course, is pushing cigarette sales in overseas markets to help make up for the loss of customers at home.)

(6) Because the tobacco companies have plenty of money, they are beginning to use it more to support some research endeavors unrelated to tobacco and also various charities.

(7) Smoking is banned in more and more sites in the USA including, most recently, prisons. The peer pressure to smoke is not as great as in years past.

(8) Some stores have discontinued selling tobacco products (Target for example).

(9) New regulations on tobacco. What are they? (a) declare nicotine an addictive drug, giving the Food and Drug Administration authority to control its sale and distribution; (b) require all tobacco advertising in magazines read by a significant number of teenagers to be in black and white and text only; (c) ban cigarette brand name sponsorship of sporting events, teams, and race cars, although corporate sponsorship could continue; (d) bar brand names on products such as hats and T-shirts; (e) prohibit single-cigarette sales, "kiddie packs," and other gimmicks; (f) require tobacco sales to occur in face-to-face transactions with photo identification showing proof of age for all sales unless they are by mail or from self-service displays in places where only adults are allowed; (g) require tobacco billboards to be in black and white and text only, and ban them within 1,000 feet of schools and playgrounds; and (h) bar cigarette vending machines from places where minors have access.

Will they work? Who knows? They will probably have little effect on the 46 million present cigarette smokers in the USA. But 3,000 teenagers take up smoking in the USA every day! It's these 1,095,000 new teenage smokers each year in the USA to whom these regulations are directed.

It is important that tobacco be ruled an addictive substance and controlled by the FDA. Here's why. The U.S. Supreme Court in May 1996 ruled that talk about a product, even one considered a vice, cannot be banned if the product is legal. The actual case occurred in 1956 when Rhode Island banned advertising on liquor prices. It took 40 years but the Supreme Court ruled that unconstitutional. The same would presumably occur with tobacco if it was not declared an addictive drug.

Cigarette smoking is the number 1 preventable cause of death in the USA. Humans were not made to smoke, chimneys were.

William C. Roberts

William Clifford Roberts, MD
Editor in Chief
Baylor University Medical Center
Dallas, Texas 75246

The Rule of 5 and the Rule of 7 In Lipid-Lowering by Statin Drugs

There are now 5 hydroxy-3-methylglutaryl-coenzyme A (HMG-CoA) reductase inhibitors. The first of these is *lovastatin* (Mevacor) which was introduced in the United States in 1987, and the latest one is *atorvastatin calcium* (Lipitor) which became available in the United States in February 1997. The relative efficacy of each of the 5 drugs is shown in Table I. The newest statin drug, atorvastatin, appears to be about twice as potent as *simvastatin* (Zocor), which in turn is about twice as potent as lovastatin and *pravastatin* (Pravachol); both of these are at least twice as potent as *fluvastatin* (Lescol). Rather than focusing on the relative efficacy of each of the statin drugs, it might be best to ask which drug at which dose lowers low-density lipoprotein (LDL) cholesterol 27%. Thereafter, a doubling of the dose of each statin drug lowers serum LDL cholesterol an additional 7%. This concept might be thought of as the rule of 7. Furthermore, it may be useful to remember which drug at which dose lowers the serum total cholesterol 22%. Thereafter, a doubling of the dose of each statin drug lowers the total cholesterol an additional 5%. This concept might be thought of as the rule of 5. Simvastatin at 10 mg/day, either lovastatin and pravastatin at 20 mg/day, and fluvastatin at 40 mg/day each lower LDL cholesterol approximately 27%, and each reduces serum total cholesterol approximately 22%. Atorvastatin is not available in the 5-mg dose. Nevertheless, 5 mg of atorvastatin appears to be roughly equivalent to 10 mg of simvastatin, 20 mg of either lovastatin or pravastatin, and 40 mg of fluvastatin. Eighty mg of atorvastatin and 160 mg of simvastatin (not yet approved) each lowers LDL cholesterol about 55% (and in some studies >60%) and each lowers total cholesterol approximately 42%. The high-density lipoprotein (HDL) cholesterol increase is not dose related; thus, both the lower and the higher doses of all of the statin drugs raise HDL cholesterol approximately 7%. Serum triglyceride lowering is dose related, but it is also related to the beginning triglyceride level. Thus, patients with higher initial triglyceride levels receive a greater reduction of these levels than those patients starting with lower levels.

HMG-CoA reductase inhibitors, like other lipid-lowering drugs, in some patients are associated with biochemical abnormalities of liver function. At the lower dosages shown in Table I, persistent elevations (>3 times the upper limit of normal occurring on ≥2 occasions in serum transaminases) are no more frequent than that occurring in placebo groups, namely 0.25% or 1 in 400 patients. With each doubling of the dose, the frequency of liver enzyme elevations >3 times the upper limit of normal also doubles. Thus, with simvastatin, for example, at 10 mg/day, liver enzyme elevation >3 times the upper limit of normal is 0.25%, and at a dose of 40 mg/day, 1%. At the highest available doses of atorvastatin and simvastatin, the frequency of abnormal enzyme elevations appears to level off at approximately 2%.

If the reductions in total and LDL cholesterol at the lower doses are remembered, the rule of 5 and the rule of 7 will be helpful in predicting further reductions in these cholesterol levels with an increase in the dosage of the statin drugs. By knowing these average cholesterol reductions, it is relatively easy to predict which

TABLE I Comparative Efficacy of the 5 Currently Available Statin Drugs

Statin Drug (mg)					Cholesterol Levels			
Atorvastatin (Lipitor)	Simvastatin (Zocor)	Lovastatin (Mevacor)	Pravastatin (Pravachol)	Fluvastatin (Lescol)	Total	LDL	HDL	LE ↑ >3 × ULN
5	10	20	20	40	22%↓	27%↓	↑	0.25%
10	20	40	40	80	27%↓	34%↓		0.50%
20	40	80			32%↓	41%↓	7%↑	1%
40	80*				37%↓	48%↓		2%
80	160*				42%↓	55%↓	↓	2%

*Approval for use at this dose level applied for to the Federal Drug Administration.
LE >3 × ULN = liver enzyme increase >3 times upper limit of normal.

dose of which statin is necessary to reach the goal for any particular patient. It is useful to calculate the necessary dose of any of the statin drugs to achieve the goal before placing a patient on the drug. If the serum LDL cholesterol before therapy is 145 mg/dl, 10 mg of simvastatin or 20 mg of lovastatin, or pravastatin or 40 mg of fluvastatin will, on average, reduce the LDL cholesterol to 106 mg/dl and higher doses will be needed to lower the level to <100 mg/dl. If the serum LDL cholesterol before therapy is 165 mg/dl, then 10 mg of atorvastatin, 20 mg of simvastatin, 40 mg of either pravastatin or lovastatin, and 80 mg of fluvastatin would be required to lower the level to 109 mg/dl and twice those doses to get the level to <100 mg/dl. The "starting dose," in other words, should be the one necessary to achieve goal, not the lowest available dose.

William C. Roberts

William Clifford Roberts, MD
Editor in Chief
Baylor University Medical Center
Dallas, Texas 75246

Floating in Fat: Fat Kids and Fat Adults

In June 1988, while visiting the University of Mississippi Medical Center in Jackson, I happened upon a book entitled *Choices for a Healthy Heart* by Joseph C. Piscatella and decided that this would be a good addition to my collection of books on nutrition and healthy living. I learned that Joe Piscatella, who had earlier written *Don't Eat Your Heart Out Cookbook* (1982, 1987, and 1994), was a highly successful businessman who in 1977 at age 32 developed angina pectoris and underwent coronary artery bypass surgery. Not long thereafter he became a student of atherosclerosis. Subsequently, *Controlling Your Fat Tooth* (1987), *The Fat Tooth Fat Gram Counter* (1993), *The Fat Tooth Restaurant* and *Fast Food Fat Gram Counter* (1993), and *Fat-Proof Your Child* (1997) appeared. Although Piscatella is not a physician, any physician would be proud to have authored any of these books. Of the writers of nutrition books, Joe Piscatella is one of the best. The following are some of his observations and practical recommendations from *Fat-Proof Your Child* (New York: Workman Publishing, 1997:494.), his most recent book:

1. *Overweightness in the USA.* About 60% of adults in the USA are overweight (that's nearly 100,000,000 folks) and nearly 30% of them are obese (≥20% above ideal weight for age, height, and gender). We have an epidemic of fatness in this country! As overweightness has increased in adults, so too has it in children and teenagers. Compared to 30 years ago, our kids are more sedentary, weigh more, have more body fat, and are less fit. An estimated 35% of children aged 6 to 17 years in the USA are overweight and 11% are extremely overweight (≥40% over ideal body weight). Since the 1960s, obesity has increased by 54% in children aged 6 to 11 and by 13% in those aged 12 to 17 years; extreme obesity has increased 98% in the age group 6 to 11 and 64% in the age group 12 to 17 years. On average, a 12-year-old today weighs 11.4 pounds more than a 12-year-old in 1973. Classroom desks made in the 1940s are now too small for today's grade school students. And overweight bodies lead to elevated cholesterol levels. About 35% of persons aged 2 to 19 years in the USA have serum total cholesterol levels >170 mg/dl (desirable <150 mg/dl).

The USA is a nation where slimness is seen as a virtue and overweightness, as a character flaw. Worth and weight seem to have an inverse relation. We feel bigger when we are smaller and smaller when we are bigger! An unhealthy obsession with weight is found everywhere. In 1972, 23% of women in the USA said they were dissatisfied with their overall appearance; by 1996, that figure had increased to 48%. Nine of 10 Americans think they weigh too much. One-half of American women are on a diet at any given time. About 80% of 10-year-old girls in the USA have a fear of fatness, and 40% of them—many of whom are of normal weight or even underweight—are trying to lose weight. Although girls are particularly prone to obsessing about the shape of their bodies, boys are not exempt. One study showed that 50% of 12- to 20-year-old males were dissatisfied with their weight and 33%, with their bodies' shapes.

2. *Physical consequences of overweightness.* Atherosclerosis, stroke, systemic hypertension, diabetes mellitus, certain cancers, gallbladder disease, arthritis, and gout are more common in adults who are overweight than in those at ideal weight. Overweight adults die from all causes at an earlier age than adults of normal weight. When suffering from the same disease, those overweight are sicker longer than those at normal weight. Overweight children and adults have more complications from surgery, and wound healing is slower than in those at ideal weight. Overweight girls are more prone to menstrual problems.

3. *Genetics of overweightness.* The chance of a child's being overweight is 15% if both parents are of average weight, 50% if one parent is overweight, and 80% if both parents are overweight. Members of the same family, however, tend to eat the same food. Although genetics can influence the metabolic rate, i.e., the speed at which calories are burned, so can exercise. Calories not burned are stored as fat. When 3,500 unused calories have been accumulated, body weight increases by 1 pound. Thus, because we use about 100 calories when we either walk or run 1 mile, we must walk or run 35 miles to lose 1 pound! Maintaining a proper balance between calories consumed and calories used, of course, prevents weight gain. Some people burn more calories than others when doing the same things: some people have high metabolic rates, burn calories at rapid rates, and they tend to be lean; other people have slow metabolic rates and they tend to be overweight.

Genetics may play a role in creating a set-point weight which is a predetermined weight that the body works to keep. Genetics also may determine, at least in part, the *number* of fat cells in the body. The average healthy baby at birth has 5 to 6 billion fat cells. Adults of normal weight have 30 to 40 billion fat cells, and obese adults have 80 to 120 billion fat cells. The more fat cells the heavier the body wants to be and the harder it is to keep weight down. The development of too many fat cells during childhood may signal the beginning of a lifelong weight problem. Fat cells shrink and swell according to the amount of fat inside them. The amount of fat in a cell can be reduced by restricting caloric intake, but the number of fat cells never diminishes.

Although genetics may play some role, obesity and poor fitness in American youngsters is a modern phenomenon and kids in most parts of the world are not as overweight as are American children and teens. Thus, for most overweight children, the problem is not genes, it's lifestyle. Exercise, for example, can boost metabolic rates by 20% to 30%. Although the set-point theory is a bit discouraging, implying we do not have much control over our weight, when a prudent diet is combined with physical activity, set-point can be favorably changed. Also, while the base number of fat cells may be genetically determined, that number is less important to weight control than their size and content, both of which are controlled by diet and exercise. Just as an overabundance of fat cells does not necessarily lead to obesity, as long as those fat cells are small, a scarcity of fat cells does not guarantee slimness because those fat cells present can become large. In the final analysis, the amount of fat contained in the cells determines body weight, and cell content is a product of lifestyle choices. Our gene pool is clearly not changing. It is the environment which is changing and that environment encourages overeating and underexercising. For every $1 spent for research to prevent and treat obesity, $100 is spent by the food industry to lull people into eating more fattening foods. We are being fattened up by the food industry and slimmed down by the diet and exercise industries! It's a fast fork not a slow metabolism that makes us fat. The Pima Indians in the USA are obese, whereas those in Mexico are thin. The genetics are the same, but their lifestyles are quite different.

4. *Parents' roles.* Toddlers and preschoolers rarely overeat. They tend to regulate how much food and drink they need. Left to their own devices, children are naturally active. Running and jumping are a way of life. Adults set kids on paths to overweightness and poor fitness. Children don't crawl to fast food restaurants, someone takes them there. Children don't turn on television sets initially, parents do. It is easier for parents to watch over children watching television rather than playing outdoors. It is easier to keep children at home than to take them to a recreation center to play ball. It is easier to hand children a bag of chips than to make a sandwich. The easy way for parents is an expensive way for children! The ability to regulate food intake found so naturally in babies and toddlers can be destroyed by well-meaning parents who use food as a bribe or a reward, treat certain foods as forbidden, or insist on clean plates regardless of hunger. Today's children also are bombarded with unhealthy messages, attitudes, and behaviors in the media.

Helping children without causing alarm or stress or sending the wrong message is a challenge. Berating children or teens about their weight or body shape can destroy self-esteem and be counterproductive. The goal of thinness needs to be replaced by the goal of fitness. If we want to influence the health and fitness of those we love, we must first take care of ourselves. Personal example is the best example. The attitudes and actions of parents about food and fitness have an enormous impact on children. Children do what parents do, not what parents say! Parents are the single most influential factor regarding how active and healthy a child will be. Health is more infectious than disease! Emphasis should not be on weight or appearance, but rather on changing the lifestyle habits that impact on weight and appearance. The proper prospective is not to produce a slim child but to foster healthy lifestyle habits that produce fitness and health for a lifetime. Criticizing children for being overweight and using restrictive diets or strict exercise regimens do not work, and indeed they may do more harm than good. Actions to control weight should be taken only to produce better health and fitness. Losing weight is a byproduct of that effort.

5. *Impediments to regular physical exercise.* The percentage of teenagers who exercised regularly in 1994 was 21%. Youngsters in the USA average <15 minutes of physical activity each day. Three of 4 children live a sedentary lifestyle! The average child rides about 22 miles a day in a car, bus, or other form of motorized transportation. As a result, kids sit down for a minimum of 10 hours a day, including the 6.5 hours sitting down in school, and sleep 8 to 10 hours of the remaining 14. Most of the day actually is spent sitting or lying down! Most kids reach their fitness peak, such as it is, at age 14 and it is downhill from there. Kids are starting off on sedentary lifestyles earlier than ever before. American kids as a result are in worse shape than ever before in history. Not only do boys and girls today weigh more than their same age counterparts in the past, two-thirds fail tests of endurance and strength. And the physically inactive child tends to become the physically inactive adult; the physically active tends to become the physically active adult. The challenge then is for parents to identify and remove the barriers that stand in the way of their kids' being more active. But 85% of families say their children are physically fit. Unless parents recognize the problem, the current patterns of inactivity among children are likely to continue.

The reason for the inactivity is mainly television, which kids watch 3 to 7 hours a day (20 to 35 a week). Computer games use time that used to be spent outdoors. Many kids now go to summer camp to learn how to use the latest computer programs rather than for physical activities. Kids now know more about bytes than batting averages! Kids now play baseball on a video game rather than on the ball field. More dense living also has decreased the amount of open spaces for play. And some parents worry about the safety of their kids' going to the park or playing on their own outside and the result is increased staying-home time. Often it is organized sports or nothing. Finally, many parents are simply out of time. With so many families (70%) having 2 working parents or a single parent, there is less time for 1 or both parents to be active with their children. And physical exercise during school time also is declining. Children in the fifth grade and above in the USA average only 3% of their school day in physical education or physical activity. In Japan, it's 18%. Even playing on a varsity team does not necessarily mean that a student is getting regular vigorous exercise. Football, basketball, baseball, softball, and volleyball are not considered aerobic because they do not require sustained hard exercise. Running, swimming, walking, jogging, aerobics, and bicycling are what count most because these exercises burn fat, enhance cardiopulmonary health, and produce fitness. Community programs too often emphasize competitive sports which usually mean that only select athletes benefit. Winning becomes all important. Such programs should instead enhance the goal of regular physical activity for *all* children and adolescents. Little league and other community organizations might best be judged by the number of children involved in sports and exercise, not on the won-lost record.

6. *Benefits of regular physical exercise.* Being physically active is a crucial lifestyle factor in losing weight, controlling weight, and in preventing cardiovascular disease. Body fat rarely stays off by dieting alone. About 9 of 10 adults who have gone on a weight-loss diet gain back the lost weight and usually more within 2 years. Low-fat eating habits work best in concert with physical activity. It takes exercise, so to speak, to squeeze the fat out of fat cells. The message for overweight kids is simply *become physically active.* Only when a child or teen is physically active will his/her body utilize stored fat as fuel. The physical activity must be on a regular basis. For children being outdoors is basic to increasing physical activity. Therefore, maximizing the time a child spends outside is crucial. The more time children spend outdoors, the more active they are. Simply being outdoors may be better than formal exercise programs. Childhood activity is often intermittent and sporadic and this is fine, because intermittent bursts of activity add up. The child's activity level should be linked with his/her developmental age. In general, fitness improves if a person exercises >3 days a week, is maintained by exercising 3 days a week, and lost when exercising <3 days a week. Regular exercise does the following:

It raises metabolism. Regular physical activity not only burns calories, but it also raises the body's metabolic rate such that after exercise (rest) the body needs more calories to function. Physically active kids burn excess calories literally while sleeping. Crash dieting, in contrast, can produce the opposite effect, namely reduce the metabolic rate because diet alone can deplete the lean body muscle.

It increases fat-burning muscle. Building up lean muscle through regular exercise increases the body's ability to burn calories and to utilize body fat as energy. Overweight people may need up to one-half fewer calories to maintain their weight than do people of normal weight. This is why of 2 people who eat the same amount of food, the fat person gets fatter and the lean person stays thin.

It increases cardiac health. Regularly exercising people have more energy, more endurance, and can do more physically with less strain on the heart than those who do not exercise regularly. Regular exercise also raises the serum high-density lipoprotein cholesterol level.

It enhances emotional health. Regular physical activity enhances emotional health, particularly in adolescents. Exercise helps to decrease stress, produce less anxiety and depression, and create greater self-image/self-esteem. Exercise indeed is nature's true tranquilizer! Exercise also helps to change stress-related eating habits. A calm, relaxed, nondistressed person is less likely to ''pig out'' on sweets and high fat foods. Physically active people eat more healthful foods and fewer high fat foods than do sedentary people. If exercise could be packaged into a pill it would be the single most widely prescribed and beneficial medicine in the nation!

In summary, adults need to be better role models for children. Children tend to eat what parents eat, and most parents in the USA eat unhealthy food regularly. Physically inactive parents tend to produce physically inactive youngsters. No factor so strongly motivates kids to exercise than regularly exercising parents. Unfortunately, nearly half of American adults are sedentary. Inactivity is especially marked among Blacks, Hispanics, low-income people, and the unemployed. Thus, many parents are actually negative role models for kids because of their own lifestyles. If we adults shape up, there is a better chance that kids will.

William C. Roberts

William Clifford Roberts, MD
Editor in Chief
Baylor Cardiovascular Institute
Baylor University Medical Center
Dallas, Texas 75246

Obtaining and Maintaining an Ideal Body Weight

Immediately following the 71st Scientific Session of the American Heart Association in November 1998, I flew to Tokyo. The 209 passengers were 90% Japanese returning home after the meeting. While observing the boarding process, I did not see a single Japanese passenger who was overweight!

In contrast, think what they saw in the USA, the heaviest nation in the world and yet a nation whose population is fixated on weight. A large percentage of our population is constantly dieting. Leanness is an obsession, but the minority of our population ≥20 years of age are lean. Indeed, 60% of adults in the USA are overweight and 30% are obese (>20% over ideal body weight). No nation in the history of the planet has witnessed overweightness to the extent as that in the USA. Only the Bible sells better in America than do diet books. The most common New Year's resolution in the USA is to lose weight. (Most are broken within 2 weeks.) Many men and women in the USA seem to have their plan for obtaining and maintaining an ideal body weight. Here's mine:

1. I weigh myself every morning upon arising. My number is 170 pounds (I am 72 inches tall), which means that if I am over that number I am particularly careful that day. I have good scales, like those found in physicians' offices, and, therefore, I believe the number. Weighing daily helps to prevent the sudden 5-pound gain. Having a weight number and not changing that number as the weight increases is crucial.
2. I usually eat a light breakfast, consisting, for example, of bran cereal with skim milk or a banana, both with a glass of grapefruit juice. Often on weekends I skip breakfast.
3. For lunch I usually have 3 vegetables.
4. I usually eat whatever I like at supper. If I have flesh, it is fish.
5. I rarely eat anything between meals. When we have these long "starvation periods" between meals, that's when we eat our anterior panniculus.
6. I make desserts on special occasions, such that I eat no more than about 1 dessert a week.
7. I drink water with most meals and avoid the high-caloric cokes. Stone-age men and women drank essentially only water. I drink coffee black and tea as it is served. The caloric cost (7 calories/g of alcohol) is taken into consideration.
8. I plan for festive occasions (or long, usually foreign, plane rides) so that I can eat heartily if I wish. If I'm going to a party or a Thanksgiving feast I eat very little preceding or immediately following the event. I try to count calories by the week, not by the day or by the meal. It's important to be able to "cheat" occasionally. Calories need to be budgeted by the week, just like money. In this way the particularly good meal can be fully enjoyed.
9. I virtually never eat at bedtime.

Vigorous exercise of course allows for a higher caloric intake, but exercise, unless it is frequent and not followed by a Big Mac, is a difficult way to lose pounds. One has to walk or run 35 miles to lose 1 pound! I try to avoid elevators and to walk rapidly around the hospital. Sometimes, I purposely park my automobile a distance from my destination so that I am required to walk.

Thus, weighing myself daily, limiting consumption of flesh and desserts, avoiding snacks, limiting intake of high-caloric liquids, walking rapidly and using stairs seems to work for me.

I welcome your methods and recommendations.

William C. Roberts

William Clifford Roberts, MD
Baylor University Medical Center
Dallas, Texas 75246

Shifting from Decreasing Risk to Actually Preventing and Arresting Atherosclerosis

A number of guidelines and task force recommendations have appeared in recent years, focusing on levels of serum or plasma low-density lipoprotein (LDL) cholesterol deserving of treatment with lipid-lowering diet and/or drugs either before or after an atherosclerotic event.[1–13] These guidelines and task force reports have focused on decreasing the risk of an atherosclerotic event. Pediatricians do not focus on decreasing the risk of mumps, measles, pertussis, or rheumatic fever. They focus on preventing these illnesses entirely. The same concept needs to be applied to atherosclerotic events.

What level of serum LDL cholesterol is needed to prevent the formation of atherosclerotic plaques either before or after an atherosclerotic event? Although it has been debated and is not entirely clear,[14,15] the answer appears to be <100 mg/dl (a 2-digit LDL!). Evidence from the 7-nation study,[16] Framingham study,[17,18] and Multiple Risk Factor Intervention Trial (MRFIT)[19–22] support the view that if the serum LDL cholesterol is <100 mg/dl (and the high-density lipoprotein [HDL] cholesterol level is >20 mg/dl*) atherosclerotic plaques large enough to produce clinical events are rare. (When the serum LDL cholesterol is about 100, the total cholesterol is usually about 150 mg/dl.) Pure vegetarians (assuming that they do not have familial hypercholesterolemia and do not eat too much saturated vegetable fats) usually have total cholesterol levels <150 mg/dl and LDL cholesterol levels <100 mg/dl. Most persons on our planet actually have serum LDL cholesterol levels <100 mg/dl, and few of them have atherosclerotic events. It is the adults in the developed world who have the higher levels. If it is advisable to decrease the serum LDL cholesterol level to <100 mg/dl after a heart attack, surely it must be useful to seek that level before a heart attack, and then the atherosclerotic event would be unlikely.

It is useful to know what cholesterol number is needed to prevent an atherosclerotic event. The recommendation to lower the LDL cholesterol to <160 mg/dl if the LDL is >190 mg/dl, and no other atherosclerotic risk factors or events are present, is simply inadequate. Most coronary events occur in persons with serum LDL cholesterol levels between 130 and 160 mg/dl. The LDL cholesterol goal of 130 mg/dl for the individual with ≥2 non-LDL risk factors (systemic hypertension, man ≥55 years, woman ≥45 years, cigarette smoking, diabetes mellitus, low [<35] serum HDL cholesterol) is too inadequate a goal to prevent atherosclerotic events.

The LDL cholesterol goal of <100 mg/dl for everybody, irrespective of whether they have other risk factors or have had an atherosclerotic event, would not only greatly simplify the guidelines, but if carried out, would dramatically improve our health. In other words, the goal would be the same for both primary and secondary prevention.

I am not oblivious to the fact that the LDL cholesterol goal of <100 mg/dl is simply unobtainable for most United States adults, but nevertheless, it is useful to know what number is necessary to prevent our most common fatal disease. Most Americans do not achieve the present generous goal recommendations for cholesterol with diet and/or drug therapy. Whether or not we are willing to alter our diet sufficiently and/or to spend the money necessary to obtain the lipid-lowering drugs, and then take them religiously to achieve this goal is up to us. If the lipid-lowering drugs were treated like coronary angioplasty or coronary bypass (i.e., the Federal Government pays the bill from age 65 on), the problem would be lessened to some extent. The cost of 1 coronary stent would buy enough statin drug for a patient for well over a year!

One could argue that it is unnecessary to eliminate atherosclerosis because we need to obliterate >75% of the cross-sectional area of an arterial lumen before organ ischemia can be a consequence. Thus, we can fill up most of the arterial lumen without functional consequence. On the other hand, it would appear that "plaque begets more plaque" and, just like the stock market, we cannot predict when we have reached the 75% cross-sectional area limit (or know when a stock has reached its peak).

One could also argue that if LDL cholesterol of <100 mg/dl was used as the goal that too many Americans would be frightened unnecessarily. An estimated 25% of American adults, 40 million persons, have serum total cholesterol levels >240 mg/dl, which means nearly all of them have high LDL cholesterol levels. A low percent of Americans >40 years

*The serum HDL cholesterol level is often <35 mg/dl when the serum total cholesterol is <150 mg/dl. Mautner et al[23] studied a patient with severe coronary artery disease who underwent coronary bypass despite a serum total cholesterol averaging 72 mg/dl and an HDL cholesterol averaging 1 mg/dl (40 different determinations). Selecting an HDL cholesterol level >20 mg/dl takes into account these kind of cases. The total/HDL cholesterol ratio is not as useful when the total cholesterol is <150 mg/dl as it is when it is >200 mg/dl.

of age have serum LDL cholesterol levels <100 mg/dl (and most of them are vegetarians or on a statin drug). Physicians who decrease their own serum LDL cholesterol levels to <100 mg/dl probably have a better chance of selling patients on their plan compared with physicians with higher LDL cholesterol levels.

As a rule, the most costly part of our meals is the flesh we consume. Meatless meals are inexpensive meals. If the money we use to purchase and eat the muscles of cows, pigs, chickens, turkeys, and fish were put into vegetables, fruits, and lipid-lowering drugs, our health would skyrocket. I am not naive enough to believe that Americans will suddenly become vegetarians, but there is simply no reason why flesh is necessary for each of our 21 weekly meals. If we could decrease flesh consumption to 7 meals a week that would be a splendid start, and the cows, pigs, chickens, turkeys and fish would leap for joy. There is still a holocaust going on—just ask the cows (100,000/day killed in the USA) or pigs (250,000/day) or chickens (15,000,000/day). The healthier are our nonhuman animals, the healthier are the human ones. We kill them, and, then, they kill us! When we are kind to them, they are kind to us.

The goal, I say, for everyone, is to have LDL cholesterol <100!

William C. Roberts

William Clifford Roberts, MD
Baylor University Medical Center
Dallas, Texas 75246

1. Expert Panel on Detection, Evaluation, and Treatment of High Blood Cholesterol in Adults. Summary of the second report of the National Cholesterol Education Program (NCEP) expert panel on detection, evaluation, and treatment of high blood cholesterol in adults (adult treatment panel II). *JAMA* 1993;269: 3015–3023.

2. Expert Panel on Detection, Evaluation and Treatment of High Blood Cholesterol in Adults. National Cholesterol Education Program: second report of the expert panel on detection, evaluation, and treatment of high blood cholesterol (adult treatment Panel II). *Circulation* 1994;89:1329–1445.

3. Pyörälä K, de Backer G, Graham I, Poole-Wilson P, Wood D, on behalf of the Task Force. Prevention of coronary disease in clinical practice. Recommendations of the Task Force of the European Society of Cardiology, European Atherosclerosis Society and European Society of Hypertension. *Eur Heart J* 1994;15:1300–1331.

4. Garber AM, Browner WS. American College of Physicians Guidelines for using serum cholesterol, high-density lipoprotein cholesterol, and triglyceride levels as screening tests for preventing coronary heart disease in adults. *Ann Intern Med* 1996;124:515–517.

5. Fuster V, Pearson TA. 27th Bethesda Conference: matching the intensity of risk factor management with the hazard for coronary disease events. *J Am Coll Cardiol* 1996;27:957–1047.

6. Singh RB, Mori H, Chen J, Mendis S, Moshiri M, Zhu S, Kim SH, Sy RG, Faruqui AM. Recommendations for the prevention of coronary heart disease in Asians: a scientific statement of the International College of Nutrition. *J Cardiovasc Risk* 1996;3:489–494.

7. Grundy SM, Balady GJ, Criqui MH, Fletcher G, Greenland P, Hiratzka LR, Houston-Miller N, Kris-Etherton P, Krumholz HM, LaRosa J, Ockene IS, Pearson TA, Reed J, Smith SC Jr, Washington R. When to start cholesterol-lowering therapy in patients with coronary heart disease: a statement for healthcare professionals from the American Heart Association Task Force on Risk Reduction. *Circulation* 1997;95:1683–1685.

8. Grundy SM, Balady GJ, Criqui MH, Fletcher G, Greenland P, Hiratzka LR, Houston-Miller N, Kris-Etherton P, Krumholz HM, LaRosa J, Ockene IS, Pearson TA, Reed J, Smith SC Jr. Washington R. Guide to primary prevention of cardiovascular diseases. *Circulation* 1997;95:2329–2331.

9. Cleeman JI, Grundy SM. National cholesterol education program recommendations for cholesterol testing in young adults: a science-based approach. *Circulation* 1997;95:1646–1650.

10. Cullen P, Assmann G. Treatment goals for low-density lipoprotein cholesterol in the secondary prevention of coronary heart disease: absolute levels or extent of lowering? *Am J Cardiol* 1997;80:1287–1294.

11. Cullen P, Funke H, Schulte H, Assmann G. Lipoproteins and cardiovascular risk—from genetics CHD prevention. *J Atherosclerthromb* 1997;4:51–58.

12. Recommendations of the Second Joint Task Force of the European and other Societies on Coronary Prevention. Prevention of coronary heart disease in clinical practice. *Eur Heart J* 1998;19:1434–1503.

13. Pyörälä K, Wood D. Prevention of coronary heart disease in clinical practice. European recommendations revised and reinforced. *Eur Heart J* 1998;19:1413–1415.

14. Law MR, Thompson SG. By how much and how quickly does reduction in serum cholesterol concentration lower risk of ischemic heart disease? *Br Med J* 1994;308:367–373.

15. Grundy SM. Statin trials and goals of cholesterol-lowering therapy. *Circulation* 1998;97:1436–1439.

16. Keys A. Seven Countries. A Multivariate Analysis of Death and Coronary Heart Disease. Cambridge, Massachusetts: Harvard University Press 1980:381.

17. Kannel WB, Castelli WP, Gordon T, McNamara PM. Serum cholesterol, lipoproteins, and the risk of coronary heart disease: the Framingham Study. *Ann Intern Med* 1971;74:1–12.

18. Anderson KM, Castelli WP, Levy D. Cholesterol and mortality: 30 years of follow-up from the Framingham Study. *JAMA* 1987;257:2176–2180.

19. Multiple Risk Factor Intervention Trial Research Group. Multiple risk factor trial: risk factor changes and mortality results. *JAMA* 1982;248:1465–1477.

20. Stamler J, Wentworth D, Neaton JD, for the MRFIT Research Group. Is relationship between serum cholesterol and risk of premature death from coronary heart disease continuous and graded? Findings in 356,222 primary screenees of the Multiple Risk Factor Intervention Trial (MRFIT). *JAMA* 1986;256:2823–2828.

21. Multiple Risk Factor Intervention Trial Research Group. Mortality after 16 years for participants randomized to the Multiple Risk Factor Intervention Trial. *Circulation* 1996;94:946–951.

22. Gotto AM. The Multiple Risk Factor Intervention Trial (MRFIT). A return to a landmark trial. *JAMA* 1997;277:595–597.

23. Mautner GC, Sanchez JA, Rader DJ, Mautner GC, Ferrans VJ, Fredrickson DS, Brewer HB Jr, Roberts WC. The heart in Tangier disease. Severe coronary atherosclerosis with near absence of high-density lipoprotein cholesterol. *Am J Clin Path* 1992;98:191–198.

An Address to the Dallas, Texas, Rotary Club on 19 May 1999

One half of us in this room will die from cardiovascular disease! Cardiovascular disease will cost us this year 100 billion dollars or approximately $625 for every adult over 20 years of age in this country. And we are all paying these bills whether we have heart disease or not because 46 million Americans under age 65 have no medical insurance and that number is increasing by 1.5 million each year. Atherosclerotic coronary artery disease—our most common cardiovascular disease—kills early. The average age of death from this condition in men is 60, and in women, 69. That means, of course, that half of the men with fatal coronary artery disease never reach their 60th birthday, the age of many of our best CEOs. And *atherosclerosis*, the medical word for "hardening of the arteries," is not a hereditary disease. As we have learned from Brown and Goldstein of this city, atherosclerosis is of genetic origin in at most 1 of 200 persons and maybe in no more than 1 of 500! The rest of us determine whether we get it or not when we pull our chair up to the table 21 times a week. And neither is atherosclerosis a degenerative disease, as I was taught in medical school.

If cardiovascular disease is neither the consequence of our genetic makeup (with some exceptions) nor the consequence of our arteries simply wearing out, what is it due to and can we prevent it or arrest it?

Before attempting to answer these 2 questions, perhaps it would be useful to review briefly what has been accomplished in cardiovascular disease this century. The recording of blood pressure did not begin until the first decade of this century. Its usefulness was first recognized in the operating room and it did not become a part of the routine physical examination until about 1920. The frequent measuring of blood cholesterol did not begin until the 1950s. Although angina pectoris—transient chest pain with exertion—had been recognized in the late 1700s, it was not until this century that angina was clearly recognized to be the consequence of severe narrowing of the coronary arteries. Heart attack—or "acute myocardial infarction," as it is known medically—was believed to be always fatal until 1912 when it was first diagnosed during life. It was not until the late 1920s, however, before acute myocardial infarction was commonly diagnosed clinically.

My father, the first cardiologist in the South, had a heart attack in 1937. Treatment consisted of complete bed rest in the hospital for 1 month, then bed rest at home for another 2 months, and gradual progression in physical activities for the next 9 months. That was standard. Four years earlier he had been president of the American Heart Association so he knew the proper therapy for heart attack.

Then, just 2 years later—1939—a pathology study demonstrated that an acute myocardial infarction healed in 2 months. Those 10 months at home for my father therefore were a waste. When his second and fatal attack occurred in 1941, the only therapy available was morphine, digitalis, and nitroglycerin. The hospital offered no more benefits than home, and that is where he chose to die.

When President Kennedy was killed in 1963, there were no coronary care units, no coronary angiography, no coronary bypass, no cardiac transplantation, no echocardiography, no nuclear cardiographic studies, no reported studies demonstrating the usefulness of lowering blood cholesterol, no β-blocker or calcium blocker drugs or cholesterol lowering drugs or ACE inhibitors or thrombolytic drugs. Furthermore, no multicenter, placebo-controlled, double-blind clinical trials had been performed in heart disease. In other words, present-day cardiology has come about only in the last 35 years.

But can we afford present-day cardiology? The procedures take place in hospitals, by far the most expensive hotels in the world. All procedures are attempts to repair the wrecks. But can we prevent the wrecks from occurring in the first place? I say "yes," but that "yes" is contingent on each of us doing our part. We cannot leave our cardiovascular health entirely to our physicians or to our hospitals. They are primarily in the repair business, not in the prevention business.

Now to the cause of atherosclerosis. Evidence connecting elevated blood cholesterol and atherosclerosis is solid. The link began in 1908 when some Russian physiologists fed egg yolks, essentially pure cholesterol, to rabbits and produced atherosclerotic plaques similar to those occurring in humans. Atherosclerosis it turns out is a disease affecting only herbivores. You can feed a dog or cat all the cholesterol and saturated fat you wish and you cannot produce an atherosclerotic plaque. Of course, when human beings eat large quantities of cholesterol and saturated fat, atherosclerotic plaques are produced in abundance. The next link came from the biochemists who found cholesterol within the atherosclerotic plaques. Then it was learned that the higher the blood cholesterol level, the greater the chance of having symptomatic atherosclerosis, the greater the chance of dying from it, and the greater the quantity of atherosclerotic plaque at autopsy. In the past 10 years it has been learned unequivocally that lowering our blood cholesterol level, either before or after a heart attack, lowers significantly the chance of having a first or a repeat heart attack.

Cardiovascular preventive treatment through the years has focused primarily on *decreasing the risk* of developing atherosclerotic coronary artery disease rather than on *preventing or arresting* it. In 1970, the world's cholesterol guru stated that he did not worry about the total cholesterol level in a person over 50 unless it was >300 mg/dl and yet, only 1% of our population has levels this high and nearly 50% of us die from cardiovascular disease. By 1980, the "worry level" was down to 240; by 1990, it was down to 200, and the "worry number" in my view will continue to fall. The average total cholesterol in persons aged 20 to 75 in the USA is now 212 mg/dl, and, nevertheless, nearly half of us die from cardiovascular disease.

What cholesterol number is needed such that no atherosclerotic plaques form in our arteries? Pediatricians do not talk in terms of decreasing the risk of measles, mumps, or whooping cough. They talk in terms of total prevention. We need to do the same with atherosclerosis. Evidence is strong that the total cholesterol number must be <150 mg/dl and the LDL cholesterol (the bad one), <100 for plaques not to form. Vegetarians have these numbers! When we are born our blood total cholesterol is about 75 and our LDL cholesterol is about 50. By 2 weeks of life, both of these numbers have doubled and they usually remain at these doubled levels until we are 18 when both begin to rise.

What can each of us do to either prevent or arrest the atherosclerotic process in us? To bring our total cholesterol number to <150 we must considerably reduce the quantity of cholesterol, saturated fat, and calories we consume each week. Cholesterol comes entirely from animals and their products, about 45% from eggs and about 45% from cows, including their muscles, milk, butter, and cheese. Most of us now consume only about 300 mg of cholesterol daily, the equivalency of 3 toothpicks.

Our biggest problem is not the quantity of cholesterol we consume but the quantity of fat we consume. Although the percent of calories from fat has decreased in recent years, because we are eating far more calories than in the past, the quantity of fat consumed continues to rise. About a third of the fat we consume comes from cows. A deck of cards weighs approximately 75 g. That should be our daily limit, and we all would be healthier if we could limit it to 50 g daily (<2 ounces).

And we need to decrease the quantity of calories consumed each week. This reduction, of course, is not easy for any of us, but you gentlemen and ladies are the leaders of this city and you must set the example. No nation in the history of the planet has witnessed the degree of overweightness occurring in the USA. At least 60% of our adults are overweight and half of them are frankly obese, meaning >20% over ideal body weight.

I'll give you my plan: I weigh each morning upon arising. My maximal weight number is 170 pounds (I am 6 feet tall), and if I am over 170 I am particularly careful that day. For breakfast I generally have a banana with grapefruit juice. For lunch I generally have 3 vegetables. For dinner I generally have what I wish. With rare exception, I limit flesh to fish. I avoid eating between meals and at bedtime and I make desserts special occasions. I plan for holiday feasts or other special occasions by limiting calories before and after such events.

Why is control of body weight so important? The more we weigh, the sooner we die! Excess weight raises our blood cholesterol, our blood pressure, our blood sugar, and it leads to many diseases, such as diabetes. The easiest way to control weight is to eat vegetables and fruits. Long-term pure vegetarians are lean and they rarely have atherosclerosis. Furthermore, they have a very low frequency of high blood pressure, diabetes, certain cancers (including breast, bowel, and prostate gland), appendicitis, diverticulosis, gallstones, kidney stones, osteoarthritis, and osteoporosis. Vegetarianism is inexpensive medicine. Exercise producing fitness clearly makes us healthier but exercise without reducing caloric intake sheds few pounds. We have to walk or run 35 miles to loose 1 pound!

I doubt if many of us will leave this hall today and suddenly become pure vegetarians. But there is no reason why we need flesh 21 times a week. If we could reduce that to 5 or 7 times a week the health of this nation would skyrocket. And our cows would be much happier. Their holocaust continues. We have 100 million cows in the USA, and every day we kill 100,000 of them. We bring them into fenced lots their last 5 to 6 months of life, and feed them 20 to 25 pounds of grain and soybean every day. Why? To make them fat so that they taste better. And then, we kill them, and then, they kill us! We also kill 300,000 hogs and about 15,000,000 chickens each day in the USA. McDonalds now has 25,000 outlets; a new one opens every 3 days somewhere in the world. And we wonder why we have so much atherosclerosis.

A word on the cholesterol-lowering drugs. They are called statin drugs. You know them as *Mevacor*, *Pravacol*, *Zocor*, *Lescol*, *Lipitor*, and *Baycol*. These are miracle drugs. They are to atherosclerosis what penicillin was to infectious disease! They can lower our LDL cholesterol by as much as 60%. And they are some of the safest drugs we have. We need not fear these drugs. They have the capacity to decrease heart attacks by >50%, and as a bonus, they also decrease the frequency of strokes by about 30%.

A short word on blood pressure. Stroke is mainly

the consequence of elevated blood pressure. Heart disease, in contrast, is mainly the consequence of elevated blood cholesterol. Our blood pressure should be <135/85 mm Hg. If the pressure is elevated we need to take an antihypertensive medicine every day.

In summary, we all need to know our blood cholesterol number and if it is elevated we need to get it down. It is the best personal insurance we can buy. We also need to know our blood pressure number and if it is elevated we need to get it down. A stroke is worse than a heart attack and it can be prevented. And losing weight lowers both blood cholesterol and blood pressure! We need to be as familiar with our cardiovascular numbers as with our investments. We can never enjoy the latter if we are not here.

William Clifford Roberts, MD
Baylor University Medical Center
Dallas, Texas 75246

High Salt Intake, Its Origins, Its Economic Impact, and Its Effect on Blood Pressure

A number of years ago, when dining, I would cover the food on my plate with a heavy dose of salt before taking a single bite. After a while, I noted my blood pressure was a bit elevated and I abruptly stopped adding salt at the table. Within a month I found that I did not miss the added salt one iota. Unfortunately, salt added at the table accounts for only about 15% of the salt most Americans consume. Why is it that salt, so beneficial as a preservative and added to food for thousands of years, should only in recent years be discovered to be so harmful? MacGregor and de Wardener[1] in 1998 published a splendid book entitled *Salt, Diet & Health: Neptune's Poisoned Chalice: the Origins of High Blood Pressure*. The information that follows is taken entirely from their work, which describes how humans became addicted to salt, how it played an important economic and historical role, and how it became recognized as being so deleterious to our health.

SALT ADDICTION

Salt, of course, means sodium chloride, which is 40% sodium and 60% chloride. For 5,000,000 years our ancestors ate a diet to which no salt was added! Humans, like other mammals, relied on the small amounts of salt naturally present in food to provide enough to regulate the amount of fluid in our bodies. Powerful mechanisms for conserving salt within our bodies were developed. The addition of salt to food began 5,000 to 10,000 years ago, and then the problem of getting rid of the excess was produced. Our consumption of salt today is 10 to 20 times greater than 5,000 to 10,000 years ago. Because it had been geared to conserve salt, the human body found it difficult to dispose of this relatively sudden, in evolutionary terms, increase in salt intake. The result was a general rise in blood pressure. Those who had the greatest difficulty in getting rid of the excess salt had the greatest rise. Systemic hypertension is the major cause of stroke, of aortic dissection, a major contributor to aortic aneurysm, and an accelerator of atherosclerosis.

Humans are genetically programmed to eat about 1 gram (g) of salt daily, not the 10 we now average daily in the USA. The rise in salt intake was due to several factors but mainly to salt's ability to preserve food. The rise was then reinforced by an acquired addiction for salt which is now maintained, in large part (80%), by the consumption of processed foods. Until 8 to 4 million years ago, fruit was the main food of mammals. Later, when the human and ape lines diverged, the human line, our ancestors, began to eat a modest amount of meat until 1.8 to 1.6 million years ago when *Homo erectus* began to consume more meat as evidenced by the large accumulations of animal remains in archaeological sites. These hunter-gatherers lived in areas where there were large numbers of grazing animals. Their diets eventually consisted of 50% meat and 50% plants. If the wild animals our ancestors hunted had the same contents of minerals as in present-day cows and sheep, the intake of salt in paleolithic times was <1 g/day. Because the hunter-gatherers also consumed large quantities of vegetables and fruits, the potassium content of their diet was approximately 16 times greater than their salt intake. Potassium, in contrast to salt, lowers blood pressure. Our potassium intake now is considerably less and lower than that of salt.

The consumption of salt began to rise when the combined effects of overhunting, climate changes, and population growth led to the introduction of agriculture. During the first few 1,000 years after the advent of agriculture, the intake of meat declined and the proportion of vegetable food in the diet increased by up to 90%. These early farmers probably consumed about the same amount of salt as did their hunter-gathering ancestors (<1 g/day). Plants contain very little salt, so herbivores, in contrast to carnivores, may suffer from salt deficiency and will travel miles to salt licks. But, the amount of salt consumed by herbivores from salt licks is modest and there is no evidence that their total salt intake exceeded that of carnivores, the salt needs of which are satisfied by the salt contained in meat and blood. (Carnivores do not search for salt but they visit salt licks in hopes of making a meal of salt-seeking herbivores.)

The increased intake of salt by humans initially was the discovery that meat and other foods could be preserved by placing them into concentrated salt solutions. Nomads hunted and ate the meat within a few hours of the kill. When the wide herds migrated, the nomads moved with them. In contrast, the farmers were tied to their fields, making it difficult for them to acquire fresh meat. The need arose to preserve food during the winter, an essential element for survival. Preservation was achieved by soaking meat in brine. Salt permeates food and makes bacterial life impossible. Salt preservation was used in Egypt by at least 2,000 BC. Additionally, highly salted food suppresses the salt taste buds in the mouth so that natural foods become insipid and unappetizing. The result was that salt would then be added to unsalted food to bring it up to the same concentration as that of the preserved food.

The addiction for salt also must have been exacerbated by its increasing availability. The change from a nomadic to an agricultural way of life gave rise to settled communities, between which trade began to flourish. Salt became a precious article of commerce. About 1,000 years ago, salt intake in the Western world had risen to about 5 g/day. It continued to rise until the 19th century when, in Europe, it was about 18 g/day. In the 16th century in Sweden, daily salt intake rose to 100 g/day due to the high consumption of salted fish. The worldwide reduction to an average of 10 g/day during the 20th century is probably the result of the introduction of refrigeration.

Throughout the world there are still many isolated populations which continue to eat a low salt diet, 0.05 to 2 g/day. They are more fit and have little to no cardiovascular disease compared with populations consuming an average of 10 g of salt per day. Numidian nomads and certain Bedouins, who feed on fish and roasted meat, never eat salt with food. Eskimos who have not been in contact with Western civilization have a strong dislike for salt and avoid foods in which saltiness is detected.

Addiction to salt has been introduced subsequently to many of these isolated tribes and also, inadvertently, to a colony of chimpanzees, the species phylogenetically closest to humans. In the wild, chimpanzees eat a vegetable and fruit diet (low salt, high potassium). For many years a colony of chimpanzees in San Antonio, Texas, in addition to fruit and vegetables, ate 1 to 2 kg of biscuits per day and they provided 6 to 12 g of salt per day, the same high intake as in humans. (These biscuits also provided a potassium intake of 6 to 11 g/day.) The high content of salt given the chimpanzees was based on the prevailing assumption that because the average intake of salt in humans is around 10 g/day, that this should be normal for chimpanzees, our nearest relatives who are near our weight. The chimpanzees then were given biscuits identical to the original ones except that they contained a low salt content (0.5 g/day). They refused the low salt biscuits and rapidly lost weight. Thus, these chimpanzees had become so addicted to the taste of high salt biscuits that they found the taste of low salt biscuits so repellent that they preferred to do without!

In 1853, Lehmann, a physiologist, asserted that humans had no need to add salt to natural food. He had noted that most animals in freedom or captivity did well on natural food without the addition of salt. He admitted that some herbivores (e.g., cow and deer) ate salt eagerly when they were offered it or when they came across it in salt licks, but he believed that there was no proof that they needed it. At the time, Lehmann was a voice crying in the wilderness, but today most veterinarians have similar views.

Addiction to a high salt intake in modern humans is induced early in life. Newborn infants are either indifferent to or avoid moderate to high concentrations of salt, but by 2 or 3 years of age children commonly prefer salty foods over the same foods without salt. It appears that the ability to taste salt develops in infants after 4 months of life. It is uncertain whether this preference for salt develops because of maturation in the infant's ability to detect salt, which they then find pleasurable, or whether, as is more probable, the normal high salt content of food given to children conditions them to its taste. Some investigators have reported that a preference for a salty food in infants can be induced by only 1 exposure to the salted food. It is hardly surprising, therefore, that as these children get older, their addiction for salty foods, fanned by commerce, worsens. Urinary salt excretion (virtually all salt consumed is excreted in the urine) was reported in 4- to 6-year-old children in 1986 in the UK. The mean 24-hour salt excretion was 4 g; their mean body weight was 21 kg. Although difficult to compare salt excretion in young children with that of adults, when compared for an equivalent muscle mass, salt excretion was 3.5 times greater in the children than the average excretion in adults, an indication of an enormous salt intake in the children.

SALT AS A REVERED SUBSTANCE

The usefulness of salt for purifying and preserving food raised it to a revered substance. In some cultures, salt was used to ward off the evil eye, and this belief stemmed from the belief that the devil was actually afraid of salt. Throughout history, salt has been seen as an emblem of hospitality. The Romans considered salt to be a sacred article of food, and it was a matter of religious principle with them to see that no other dish was placed upon the table before the salt was in position. For centuries, the wealthy placed silver saltcellars in the middle of the table, and they served as a symbol of friendship and hospitality. The saltcellar was a sign that the guest had been invited in love. That it was the last article to be removed was to remind guests that while meals may come to an end, friendship is perpetual. The emblematic saltcellar increasingly became a decorative art of beauty. The rank of guests at a banquet in England was indicated by their place at the table with reference to the saltcellar. Salt also constituted the essence of things, particularly of life itself. Christ told his disciples, "Ye are the salt of the earth," i.e., the best of the human race. And again, referring to them he asked, "If the salt has lost its savour wherewith shall it be salted?"

Salt rapidly moved from the magical to the medicinal. Salt was used extensively throughout history in the belief that it prevented and cured certain diseases. It was thought that the corruption of a corpse in the grave was due in part to worms and that salt delayed this corruption. Salt, therefore, was used to treat the living suffering from worms.

Salt also was considered a symbol of procreation and reproduction. The sea, with its wealth of fish, was believed, because of its saltiness, to be a fructifying creative element. Feeding a dog salt was believed to increase the number of puppies. Ships carrying salt were believed to cause the mice in the holes to multiply far more than on ships carrying non-salt cargoes. Eating salt was believed to cause mice to become impregnated. Salt also was connected with barrenness, presumably because of the empty isolation of salty deserts and other places where an excess of salt prevents all growth, and it was used by women to prevent barrenness. The dread of impotence on the marriage night (an embarrassment known at one time as the "ligature") could be allayed if one or both partners carried some salt in their pockets or on their clothes or the wife had salt in her shoe. Salt was considered to have an exciting influence on the nervous system, arousing passion and desire.

The veneration of salt by humans is perhaps best illustrated by the association of salt with most forms of religion. The earlier gods were worshiped as the givers of the fruits of the earth, and this included "bread and salt." Salt was an essential constituent of sacrificial offerings in ancient Egypt, Greece, Rome, and Judaism. In the Roman Catholic Church, salt was introduced as a purifying substance for baptisms in about the 4th century, and it has played a prominent part in certain rituals since.

SALT'S POLITICAL AND ECONOMIC IMPACT

The presence of salt often determined the site of settlements and their prosperity. Where salt was plentiful societies tended to be free, independent, and democratic, but where it was scarce ". . . he who controlled the salt controlled the people." The ample supply of salt along the shores of the Mediterranean and the North Sea was associated with free societies. In Rome, salt was often given to the people by the government. In contrast to the liberal societies associated with the relatively ample supply of salt, in the ancient river valley civilizations of the Nile, in Babylon, Mexico, Peru, and some part of China, the scarcity of salt led to its being monopolized by the rulers and priests. They kept the salt in heavily guarded stores and were thus able to manipulate their unfortunate salt-addicted populations, who were entirely dependent on them to satisfy their craving and their absolute need for salt to preserve meat and fish. The need for salt for preservation and the desire for its taste has always been so great that for nearly 4,000 years governments found it profitable to control its availability. The immense wealth and prosperity of several empires, including the Chinese and Venetian, were entirely based on salt. The industrial importance of salt remains embedded in the names of certain towns that were big producers of salt: Salins in France, Salzburg in Austria, Salzkotten in Prussia, Saltdean in England, Saltcoats in Scotland, and Saltville in Virginia, and towns the names of which begin with *Hal* (the Greek for salt), Halle, Hallstadt, and Hallein.

There are 2 infamous centers of industrial salt production, mentioned in the Old Testament, Sodom and Gomorrah, which lay at the southern end of the Dead Sea. The citizens of Sodom and Gomorrah indulged in certain sexual habits which were disapproved of in Heaven. God therefore decided to destroy them. One man named Lot, however, together with his wife and 2 daughters, were led to safety by an angel. They were instructed not to look back at the town they were leaving. Unfortunately, Lot's wife could not resist 1 backward glance, and she was immediately turned into a pillar of salt. This biblical incident has been depicted in many medieval stained-glass windows, engravings, and paintings.

Salt was often a cause of conflict and at other times influenced the course of a war. In earlier times there were vicious local wars for the possession of salt springs and surface deposits of salt, particularly in Central Europe. The dominance of England in salt export during the 19th century not only had a profound effect on India but also on the American Civil War. In 1861, there was no refrigeration and canning had not been invented. Salt was needed for the preservation of meat, poultry, and fish, and for the preparation of leather. The hides used to make the harnesses for the thousands of mules pulling supply wagons were kept in brine until they were tanned. The South needed about 300 million pounds of salt per year for a population of 9 million, half of whom were in the Army. By 1860, people in the USA were consuming more salt than any other country, an average of 50 pounds (23 kilograms) per person per year. All meat and fish were either smoked or packed in brine. The monthly allowance for a Confederate soldier in 1864 was 1.5 pounds (680 g) of salt, which, if it were all consumed, would give a minimum of 23 g of salt per day, 4 times the current recommendation of 6 g/day. The South's sources of salt were well below these needs. Its principal salt-producing areas were in Wilmington, North Carolina, which was lost early in the war, and in Saltville, West Virginia. Most of the South's salt requirements before the war had come by sea from England. When the war started, the North blockaded the southern ports and the South's supply of salt suddenly stopped. The lack of salt severely interrupted the preservation of meat, and its absence in food lowered the morale of the population and that of the soldiers. Some individuals cornered the available salt, which raised its price. The border dividing the Union from the Confederacy stretched for hundreds of miles and made trade between the 2 relatively easy.

Blockade running was common along the coast. A profitable run for the North was to transport contraband goods, including salt, to Cuba where they were picked up by Southern blockade-running ships. A host of illicit traders prospered on both sides. Rhett Butler in *Gone with the Wind* is a prototype of the affluent, glamorous salt-blockade runner. A successful run was an event of major local importance and was reported in the local journals. General Sherman, who purposely made war against civilians because they supplied the armies he was fighting, was the first to urge the federal authorities to decree that salt be contraband. He asserted that salt was as much a contraband of war as gunpowder. The South, to overcome its grave shortage, used desperate measures. They attempted to obtain salt by boiling seawater at various sites along the West Coast of Florida where there were forests near the beaches to supply the necessary fuel. However, these sites were regularly destroyed by the North's Navy, and, as usual, they were back in production within a few days, but the price paid by the South to keep up the production of salt was crippling. The North considered that the destruction of salt stores and the harassment of its production were equal to the winning of battles and were worth the cost of the military operations involved. It has been claimed that the lack of salt, by diverting much of the South's men and money from the first objective of war—to defeat the enemies' Army—was an important contribution to the South's defeat.

SALT AND BLOOD PRESSURE

The earliest comment relating dietary salt to blood pressure was by the Chinese in 1700 BC: ". . . if large amounts of salt are taken, the pulse will stiffen or harden." It was not until nearly 3,500 years later, when Richard Bright of Guy's Hospital in London suggested in 1836 that the blood pressure of patients with severe renal disease might be elevated. Later, another physician at Guy's Hospital noted that high blood pressure also could occur in individuals whose kidneys looked normal. Today, the latter are said to have *essential* or *primary* hypertension, i.e., of unknown cause, by far the commonest form of high blood pressure, accounting for 95% of all cases in humans and affecting 10% to 15% of the world's population of 6.2 billion people. Essential hypertension is characterized by a gradual increase in blood pressure with age so that by age 60, 50% of the population in the Western World have levels >140/90 mm Hg. In the remaining 5% of the hypertensive population, the rise in blood pressure is due to some form of renal or endocrine disease and the high pressure is then known as *secondary* hypertension. In secondary hypertension the importance of dietary salt in causing blood pressure to rise is well established. The importance of dietary salt in essential hypertension has been more difficult to discern.

The connection between salt and high blood pressure was first demonstrated in France in 1904 by Ambard and Beaujard. These investigators studied for 3 weeks 6 patients with high blood pressure from essential hypertension. They varied the intake of salt by means of 3 diets: one contained little salt but 2 liters of milk per day; the second also contained little salt but, in addition to milk, contained much protein, meat, and many eggs; the third diet consisted of the same amounts of milk as the first plus 2 liters of salty broth containing 10.5 g of salt. Salt balance was measured by estimating the amount of salt in the urine each day. They found that when the diet contained little salt, more salt was excreted in the urine than was eaten so that the patient was in negative sodium balance. The blood pressure fell even though the intake of protein was considerable. (Protein excess at the time was considered the cause of systemic hypertension.) When the diet was high in salt, less salt was excreted in the urine so that the patient was in positive sodium balance, i.e., retaining salt, and the blood pressure rose even when the protein intake was low. Ambard and Beaujard concluded that they had demonstrated a close relation between salt balance and blood pressure.

During the following 20 years, salt deprivation was used to lower blood pressure, mainly in patients with renal disease, but with poor results. Allen and Scherril, in 1922, described the effect of a low salt diet in 180 patients with severe essential hypertension. They were all given a normal protein intake. The blood pressure returned to normal in 19%. In 42%, the fall in blood pressure and the relief of symptoms were sufficient to be regarded as therapeutically successful. Complete failure occurred in 30%. These authors concluded that essential hypertension was a "salt nephritis." Houghton, also in 1922, discussed all the effects of salt reduction in several forms of hypertension and proposed that a rise in blood pressure is "a tertiary condition of which the immediate cause is a larger salt intake than the damaged kidneys can excrete." This is a modern view.

Despite the work of Ambard and Beaujard, Allen and Scherril, Houghton, and a few others, the connection between salt intake and hypertension continued to be denied. The position was finally clarified by Kempner in 1948. He treated hypertensive patients with a diet containing <0.5 g of salt, 20 g of protein, and little fat. It consisted of rice and fruit. Kempner was most interested in the relatively low protein content of his diet and he was reluctant to admit that it might be the low salt of the diet that lowered blood pressure. He attributed such an assertion to others who used his diet. It is ironic that Kempner is now remembered as the person who demonstrated beyond any shadow of doubt that high blood pressure can often be lowered by a low salt diet. Kempner's diet was so low in salt that the 24-hour urinary excretion of salt at the end of 2 months usually fell to <0.25 g. Kempner published the effect of his diet on 500 patients with essential hypertension. The article illustrated by blood pressure charts showing relentless falls in blood pressure, chest radiographs showing pronounced reductions in heart sizes, electrocardiograms showing gross abnormalities reverting to normal, and photographs of damaged retinae that dramatically improved. There is no doubt that Kempner's rice diet achieved remarkable and sustained results. He made no mention, however, of how difficult it was to get patients to follow his rice diet or of the complications associated with such severe and rapidly induced reductions in salt intake. One reason he was so successful using his diet, when others failed, was that he collected all the urine excreted each day from each patient so that by the time he saw them in the ward he knew how much salt they had excreted and therefore how much salt they had eaten. Kempner's reaction when they had erred was such that the patients were unlikely to err again. His use of salt restriction at the time was the only therapeutic maneuver available to lower blood pressure. When oral diuretics were introduced in the mid-1950s, the increased urinary excretion of salt was considered a satisfactory alternative to a low salt diet and a much more convenient way of dealing with the habitual high consumption of salt.

Because diuretics have adverse consequences, moderate dietary salt restriction (to 3 to 6 g/day) to control blood pressure in essential hypertension has been advocated. Numerous trials have shown that such reductions decrease blood pressure greatest in the elderly and in those with the highest pressures.

A link between salt and blood pressure also can be demonstrated by measuring the small changes in blood pressure that are rapidly induced by an abrupt change in salt intake or salt output, for example, an intravenous infusion of saline or the administration of a diuretic. Individuals in whom these interventions cause the least change in blood pressure are termed *salt resistant*, and individuals in whom larger changes are produced are referred to as *salt sensitive* and are considered by some to be more likely to develop hypertension later in life. There is little evidence, however, that the immediate response of blood pressure to such sudden drastic changes in salt status indicates how the blood pressure of an individual responds to a lifetime's exposure to a high salt diet.

The effect of a reduction in dietary salt intake on systemic arterial pressure has been measured in normal newborn babies, school children, and adults. Nonhuman animal studies also have shown that young animals are much more sensitive to the level of dietary salt intake than adults, and that even a transient rise in intake early in life may increase their response to a high intake later in life. In a large study of 750 children, a reduction in salt intake from 9 to 7 g/day induced a significant fall in blood pressure after 6 months. In a similar study involving 32 adults (average age 40 years), reduction in salt from 9 to 4 g/day caused a significant fall in blood pressure at 12 weeks and the fall in pressure was correlated with the fall in salt excretion. In normal circumstances, salt excretion is almost the same as salt intake. In a study of adults 60 to 78 years old, a reduction in salt intake from 10 to 5 g/day for 4 weeks reduced systolic pressure by 8 mm Hg and diastolic pressure by 4 mm Hg, similar to reductions achieved by blood pressure–lowering drugs. The extent of the fall in blood pressure was the same whether the subject started with a high or a normal blood pressure.

Severe increases in salt intake for a few days have little effect on normal blood pressure. In young adults, 28 g of salt per day was required to cause a rise in blood pressure. In subjects aged ≥50 years, however, only 20 g/day for a few days was necessary to cause a rise in blood pressure. It appears, therefore, that the effect of a sudden rise in dietary salt intake on normal blood pressure during a person's life varies and is most pronounced in the very young and after age 50.

A well-documented connection between systemic hypertension and dietary salt intake has been demonstrated in normal dogs, rabbits, rats, baboons, and chimpanzees. The work on rats and chimpanzees is the most relevant to essential hypertension. A study performed in 1951 found that the substitution of a 1% salt solution for drinking water produced hypertension in the chicken, rat, and rabbit. Whatever experimental method was used to induce secondary hypertension (e.g., by partially obstructing a renal artery), it was facilitated by increasing the salt intake and prevented by salt restriction.

Experiments in chimpanzees strongly reinforced the proposal that essential hypertension is due to the prevailing high intake of salt. Chimpanzees normally consume a diet low in salt, but when their salt intake increases to that of present-day humans they, like humans, develop hypertension. Again like humans, a number of chimpanzees do not develop high blood pressure on the high salt diet. The rise in pressure was gradual and it was still rising 18 months after they started eating the high salt diet. Upon returning to a diet that contained <0.5 g of salt per day, blood pressure fell to its original level.

There have been nearly 40 accounts of certain primitive populations in which blood pressure did not rise with age—in other words, they did not have essential hypertension. Their dietary intake of salt was <3 g/day, in a few it was <1 g/day, and in 1 it was about 0.5 g/day. Studies of populations with a high prevalence of hypertension (some Japanese and Portuguese communities) have shown high intakes of salt. In 1 study, salt intake averaged 26 g/day. In between are the bulk of westernized societies that consume 7 to 12 g/day (average 10). The connection between salt intake and hypertension in these intermediate populations is evident but more difficult to discern mainly because of the narrow range of salt intake.

The Yanomamo Indians are probably the most primitive native tribe in the world. They live in about 100,000 square miles along the border between Venezuela and Brazil. There are approximately 18,000 individuals scattered through the Amazon rain forest in about 200 villages with 40 to 200 persons in each. They have been described as seminomadic "slash and burn" agriculturists living on a diet of locally produced crop and game supported by wild fruits and insects. Their staple foods are cooked bananas and manioc. In most villages there is little access to salt, refined sugar, alcohol, or dairy products. In one group of 206 persons aged 20 to 50 years, which comprised all the adults from 3 villages, the mean 24-hour urinary excretion of salt was 0.5 g/day, with a potassium excretion of 3 g/day. The mean weight of the men (50 kg) was about the same as that of chimpanzees. Their blood pressure was much lower than that found in western populations and there was no rise in blood pressure with increasing age. Their blood pressure, just like that of the Western world, is approximately 90/60 mm Hg at birth and that is their blood pressure their entire lives. The Yanomamos probably represent the ultimate human example of the importance of salt on blood pressure.

Although numerous studies have confirmed that there is a significant relation between salt intake (measured as 24-hour salt excretion) and blood pressure, 1 obstacle has bothered a great many researchers and continues to do so. It is that within a single community there is no relation between blood pressure and the salt intake of its individuals. There are many reasons for this apparent lack of correlation between blood pressure and the intake of salt within individuals of a single community. Blood pressure varies from day to day in an individual. The day-to-day fluctuations in salt ingested and excreted by each person in any one 24-hour period varies enormously (3 to 18 g/day). Such variations depend on the type of food eaten the previous day and its salt content. To obtain an accurate estimate of an individual's average salt excretion, it is necessary to measure the salt excretion on >5 occasions, which is not practical when studying large numbers of people. Such large methodologic difficulties mask the detection of differences between subjects.

The relation of blood pressure to salt intake was studied extensively by Dahl. Over a number of years, he and his associates measured the blood pressure and the 24-hour urinary excretion of salt in Alaskan Eskimos, Marshall Islanders in the Pacific, and employees at the Brookhaven Laboratory in the USA where Dahl worked. Correlation between the average daily salt intake and the prevalence of hypertension in these different centers was excellent. The Eskimos, whose salt intake was about 4 g/day, had no hypertension. The Japanese had the highest salt intake and the highest prevalence of hypertension, and the other 3 were in between. Although the relation between salt intake and blood pressure was not evident within the individuals in most populations, salt intake controlled blood pressure. He studied Brookhaven's employee use of salt at the table. He classified the subjects into 3 groups: (1) those who did not add and had never added salt to food; (2) those who added salt to food only if, after first tasting it, found it insufficiently salty for their palate; and (3) those who added salt to food without first tasting it. Although the mean blood pressures of the 3 groups were similar, fewer persons had high blood pressure among the group with low salt intake (group 1).

SALT AND HYPERTENSION IN AFRICAN-AMERICANS

African-Americans have the highest prevalence of high blood pressure in the world. The prevalence of high blood pressure is nearly twice as high among African-Americans than in Caucasian Americans (38% vs 20%) and 2 to 4 times higher than in West Africans. The degree of hypertension appears to collate with the darkness of skin color. The blood pressure of African-Americans also is more sensitive to increases in salt intake than that of American whites, and they retain an intravenous load of salt far longer than whites. Conversely, it is easier to lower the blood pressure of African-Americans with a diuretic. Thus, African-Americans have an enhanced ability to retain salt or they have a diminished ability to get rid of a high salt intake.

A hypothesis to explain the high prevalence of hypertension in African-Americans proposes that the process of enslavement decimated those who were least able to conserve salt so that the survivors were individuals who were best able to conserve salt. For 300 years, between 1500 and 1800, over 12,000,000 black people were transported against their will from the West Coast of Africa to the Western Hemisphere. Most went to South America, but 6% of the total, estimated to be about 430,000, ended up in North America. Many came from vary low salt areas in West Africa, such as the sub-Sahara Savanna. Those who already had the best ability to conserve salt would have had a better chance of surviving the voyage, but this would also have made them and their descendants more likely to develop a higher blood pressure subsequently when exposed to a high salt intake.

The slaves were conquered by African neighbors to the north and east. After capture they were force-marched 100 to 200 miles to the coast by African slave handlers. There they were confined to crowded huts known as barracoons to wait several weeks or months for the ships to take them away. The death rate from the point of capture to the coast was about 10%, and another 10% died in the barracoons. Conditions on board ship were terrible and, on average, 15% died during the 2-month crossing. Another 5% died while waiting in the USA to be sold, and a further 10% died in the first 2 years when they were being "seasoned" to their new environment. Thus, on average, only 60% of those captured survived >2 years. The causes of death were most often due to an illness associated with loss of salt and water. There was the heat and excessive sweating during the forced marches to the coast and the incarceration in the unventilated barracoons and ships' holds. During the sea voyage, vomiting due to seasickness was common. Diarrhea was always rife and it was the predominant cause of death. This hypothesis suggests that the possession of kidneys with ability to hold on to salt would have increased the chances of surviving. It is this selective survival among the descendants of the surviving slaves of genes responsible for an increased ability to hold on to salt that is now responsible for the exceptionally high prevalence of hypertension in African-Americans.

MECHANISM FOR SALT'S EFFECT ON BLOOD PRESSURE

The lack of an obvious mechanism whereby salt intake controls blood pressure has been 1 factor that has delayed acceptance of the relation between the 2. In essential hypertension in humans, in secondary hypertension in humans associated with overt renal disease, and in hereditary hypertension in rats, the kidney has difficulty excreting salt, and this sets in motion a train of events that causes the blood pressure to rise. The observations upon which this evidence is based can be divided into those which show that the rise in blood pressure is due to an abnormal kidney and those which demonstrate that the kidney has a diminished ability to excrete salt. When blood pressure rises, it causes widespread changes, particularly in the kidney, which it sometimes even destroys. Therefore, the evidence that is pertinent to the search for the initial cause of the rise in pressure has to be distinguished from the changes produced by high blood pressure itself. This distinction is most easily made by studying the human or nonhuman animals who are going to develop hypertension but before the actual development of hypertension.

Confirmation that the initiating trigger that causes blood pressure to rise in hypertensive strains of rats and in essential hypertension is in the kidney has been obtained by kidney cross transplant experiments. The animal experiments consist of cross-transplanting 1 kidney from 1 animal (the donor) to another (the recipient) in which the kidneys have been removed. The kidney may come from either a prehypertensive strain rat or from a normotensive control animal. When a kidney from a prehypertensive hypertensive strain rat is transplanted into a control normotensive rat, the blood pressure rises. When a kidney from a control rat is transplanted into a prehypertensive hypertensive strain rat, the blood pressure does not rise. If a kidney from a normotensive rat is placed into a hypertensive strain when it has already developed high blood pressure, the blood pressure comes down. These experiments demonstrate that blood pressure follows the kidney.

Similar results have been obtained in humans with essential hypertension. In 6 black patients with terminal renal failure due to prolonged essential hypertension, the blood pressure fell to normal and remained normal for many years after receiving a kidney from a young normotensive donor. In another investigation, the blood pressure of the parents of the donors of kidneys and the recipients were measured. The patients who received a kidney from a donor from a family with high blood pressure needed significantly more blood pressure–lowering therapy than those who received a kidney from a family with normal blood pressure.

There is some evidence that normotensive children of parents with essential hypertension have difficulty excreting salt. Compared with control subjects, intravenous administration of a salt solution at a certain rate to normotensive first-degree relatives of patients with essential hypertension leads to a rise in blood pressure and reduced salt excretion. An increase in salt intake to 16 g/day for 7 days causes an increase in blood pressure in normotensive offspring of hypertensive patients, but does not raise the blood pressure of normotensive offspring of normotensive parents. These observations suggest that although the kidney in essential hypertension looks normal, it has an inherited impaired ability to excrete salt. It is now evident that the difficulty in excreting sodium by normal-looking kidneys of young patients with essential hypertension and of prehypertensive hypertensive strain rats is due to the presence of many intrinsic renal functional abnormalities. There are disturbances of kidney blood flow and of several locally produced kidney hormones and other substances that control salt excretion. Thus, the rise in pressure in essential hypertension depends on the magnitude of the excess salt intake, the type of severity and combination of intrinsic renal abnormalities that impair the kidney's ability to excrete salt, and the number of years the individual has had this conflict. The exact mechanism whereby the kidney's difficulty to excrete salt raises the blood pressure is not known.

COMMERCIAL REASONS FOR HIGH SALT FOODS

The above evidence indicates a strong connection between salt intake and blood pressure. Why then is so much salt continually added to foods? The first is taste. Tomato juice without salt is virtually intolerable for example. The food industry is more than happy to agree in public that taste is the major reason why they add salt to food. The other 2 reasons, however, are entirely commercial and for most foods are the real reason the food industry wants the intake of salt to remain high. The salt content of food is an important determinant of the amount of water the food contains, and it increases the weight of food at very little cost. If the salt content of sausages is increased from 0.5% to 2.5%, which is the usual concentration of salt in sausages, the water content is increased by approximately 20%. Far less salt could be added if other flavors were substituted, but because this would reduce the weight of the sausage, consumers would expect the price to fall. They would resist paying the same amount for a lighter sausage.

The second commercial reason is that salt increases thirst. In most temperate climates the body needs about a liter of fluid a day. If the consumption of salt is increased, the salt concentration of the body will tend to rise, which stimulates thirst and therefore the amount one drinks. There is a direct relation between salt intake and fluid intake. It is not surprising that in pubs there are often free supplies of salted peanuts and potato chips, and that many of the soft drink manufacturers, some of whom also make alcoholic drinks, own companies that specialize in the manufacture of highly salted snacks. If salt intake were to be reduced, those companies would lose hundreds of millions of dollars in sales of soft drinks!

The salt extractors and the salt manufacturers in the USA finance a public relations body known as the Salt Institute, which provides a one-sided story supporting the high salt content of processed food. The Institute propagates the view that there is a considerable debate within the medical and scientific community as to whether any relation exists between hypertension and sodium intake in the general population and that a decrease in sodium intake may result in a rise or a decrease in blood pressure for some and an increase in blood pressure in others and no significant fall in blood pressure for most. This view is very reminiscent of that taken by the tobacco industry for many decades regarding the danger or the lack thereof of cigarettes. The Salt Institute, which seemed to know about the Intersalt study (the worldwide investigation on the relation of salt excretion to blood pressure) in advance of its publication, turned the study on its head and interpreted it in a way exactly opposite to that of the authors, that salt intake had no relation to blood pressure. The Institute's attempts to discredit the Intersalt study have continued unrelentingly.

The Salt Institute, a large snack company, and the Dairy Council in the USA have been very much involved in putting forward another concept, that what really raises blood pressure is not a high salt intake but a low calcium intake and that eating more calcium (e.g., milk has a high content of calcium) would solve the blood pressure problem. Giving calcium to patients with high blood pressure, however, has not lowered it and indeed there is little or no relation between calcium intake and blood pressure in different populations. The Salt Institute then argued that a very high calcium intake lowered blood pressure in individuals who were already on a high salt intake. This has not proven to be the case. A high salt intake is an important aggravating factor in bone demineralization, and reducing salt intake is likely to have a greater beneficial effect on bone density than increasing calcium intake. The food industry's next rather rash maneuver was to assert that a moderate reduction in salt intake may be dangerous. Close analyses of the study cited in support failed to back up this claim.

DECREASING SALT INTAKE

Since there is little doubt that increased salt intake increases blood pressure, what steps can we take to decrease the intake of salt? There are at least 3:

1. *Do not add salt at the table.* It is not impolite not to pass the salt shaker! Sauces that are also added to food or added at the table, such as tomato ketchup, are also usually high in salt. Adding salt at the table is essentially a habit. This was clearly demonstrated in a study in an Australian canteen where the hole in the saltcellar was reduced. As a result, the habitual unthinking number of shakes delivered only half the quantity of salt. No one noticed any difference.
2. *Stop adding salt when cooking.* This is more difficult because it requires the agreement of the person who does the cooking in the household. At first the food will taste bland. Two to 4 weeks later, however, as the sensitivity of the salt taste receptors in the mouth become more sensitive to the taste of salt in the usual concentrations, it is more pleasant. (It is the same as giving up sugar in tea or coffee—initially it is difficult, but later the taste of sugar in tea or coffee is unpleasant.) Salt is often added inadvertently; all stock cubes, gravy browning, soy sauce, and ready-prepared mustard all contain large amounts of salt and should be avoided.
3. *Avoid manufactured foods or processed foods that have had salt added.* This is by far the most difficult step because many processed foods are not labeled with their salt content and if they are labeled, the labels tend to be confusing. Instead of being labeled as the amount of salt or equivalent of salt, they are labeled as sodium and in most countries as grams of sodium per 100 g of food. Buying as much fresh food as possible or foods that are not processed with salt or if processed have <0.1 g of sodium per 100 g of food is useful, but few processed foods achieve such low concentrations.

The labeling system in the USA is cumbersome. The packet is labeled with the percent of the daily dietary intake that eating 1 portion of that food contributes to the recommended dietary intake (6 g of salt per day). An average packet of salted crisps contains 2 g of salt, which would account for 33% of the recommended daily salt intake. The idea behind this food-labeling system is that one can then add up all of these percentages and work out whether one's salt intake for the day is above or below the recommended intake.

Foods with a low salt content are fresh and frozen vegetables. Vegetables in tin cans generally have salt added. Fresh meat is low in salt. All uncooked pasta, rice, olive oil, rapeseed oil, unsalted nuts, fruit juices, tea, coffee, and most alcoholic drinks are low in salt. In contrast, foods that have a high salt content include: meat products (e.g., bacon, ham, cured meat, canned meat, sausages, paté), smoked fish and fish in tin cans, instant noodles and soups, tinned or packet soups, stock cubes, gravy brownings, yeast extracts, meat extracts, vegetable juices, soy sauce, and salted fish.

Most fast foods contain large amounts of salt as well as saturated fat. A hamburger with french fries generally contain approximately 5 g of salt.

CONCLUSION

Salt and blood pressure go together. The more salt we take in, the higher our blood pressure. Systemic hypertension is the major cause of stroke, of aortic dissection, a major contributor to aortic aneurysm, and an accelerator of atherosclerosis. We all must decrease our salt intake! As Freis stated in 1976: ". . . the evidence is very good . . . that reduction of salt in the diet to below 2 g/day would result in the prevention of essential hypertension and its disappearance as a major public health problem."[2] Sacks and colleagues[3] 25 years later appear to support this earlier recommendation.

Thank you Drs. MacGregor and de Wardener for producing such a splendid book.

William Clifford Roberts, MD
Editor in Chief
Baylor Heart & Vascular Hospital
Baylor University Medical Center
Dallas, Texas

1. MacGregor GA, de Wardener HE. Salt, Diet & Health: Neptune's Poisoned Chalice: The Origins of High Blood Pressure. Cambridge, UK: Cambridge University Press, 1998:233.

2. Freis ED. Salt, volume and the prevention of hypertension. *Circulation* 1976;53:589–595.

3. Sacks FM, Svetkey LP, Vollmer WM, Appel LJ, Bray GA, Harsha D, Obarzanek E, Conlin PR, Miller ER III, Simons-Morton DG, Karanja N, Lin P-H. Effects on blood pressure of reduced dietary sodium and the dietary approaches to stop hypertension (DASH) diet. *N Engl J Med* 2001;344:3–10.

The Heart at Necropsy in Massive Obesity (>300 pounds or >136 kilograms)

A 52-year-old African-American man, who weighed 580 pounds (264 kg) and was 72 inches tall (body mass index = 79 kg/m^2!), was hospitalized because of increasing dyspnea. He had been known to have systemic hypertension, sleep apnea, and diabetes mellitus. He never had symptoms or objective evidence of myocardial ischemia. The serum total cholesterol was 142, low-density lipoprotein cholesterol 40, high-density lipoprotein cholesterol 17, and triglycerides 242 mg/dl. An echocardiogram disclosed the left ventricular ejection fraction to be 62%. Twelve days after admission he was found dead in bed. Autopsy disclosed massive pulmonary embolism without pulmonary infarction. The heart weighed 780 g, but did not float in water. The epicardium and the 4 cardiac valves were normal. The walls of the ventricles were devoid of foci of necrosis and fibrosis. The major epicardial coronary arteries were all large and devoid of atherosclerotic plaques. Likewise, the aorta contained few atherosclerotic plaques.

There are relatively few necropsy data on the status of the heart at necropsy in massively obese subjects. Amad et al,[1] in 1965, described findings at necropsy in 6 patients aged 35 to 65 years (mean 47), who weighed from 308 to 495 pounds (140 to 225 kg): the hearts in the 3 women weighed 400, 500, and 620 g and the hearts in the 3 men, 450, 900, and 1,100 g. The weights had been taken from autopsy reports. These authors excluded patients "who had clinical signs or pathologic evidence of coronary atherosclerosis or who had systemic arterial pressures ≥150/90 mm Hg." The number of patients excluded was not described. By gross examination, none of their patients had fatty infiltration into myocardium or grossly visible foci of myocardial necrosis or fibrosis.

Warnes and Roberts,[2] in 1984, described 12 patients at necropsy aged 25 to 59 years (mean 37; 5 women and 7 men) who weighed from 312 to >500 pounds (mean 381). Five patients had died suddenly, 2 of chronic congestive heart failure, 1 of acute myocardial infarction, 1 of aortic dissection, 1 of an intracerebral bleed, 1 of drug overdose, and 1 shortly after ileal bypass. Only 2 of the 12 patients had 1 or more epicardial coronary arteries narrowed >75% in cross-sectional area by atherosclerotic plaque and those 2 were the only 2 with left ventricular foci of either necrosis or fibrosis. Of the 2 patients with narrowing 76% to 100% in cross-sectional area by plaque, each patient had both the right and left anterior descending coronary arteries narrowed to this degree. Of the 48 major epicardial coronary arteries in the 12 patients (4/patient), 4 were narrowed at some point 76% to 100% in cross-sectional area by atherosclerotic plaque. A total of 664 five-mm segments were examined from 11 hearts (mean 60/patient). Only 2 patients had any 5-mm segments narrowed 76% to 100% in cross-sectional area. Of the 664 five-mm coronary segments, 431 (65%) were narrowed 0% to 25% in cross-sectional area; 143 (21%), 26% to 50%; 73 (11%), 51% to 75%; and 17 (3%) were narrowed 76% to 100%. The hearts in the 12 patients were all heavier than normal (380 to 990 g [mean 616]). The subepicardial adipose tissue by visual inspection appeared to be increased in 9 of the 12 patients, but in no patient did the heart float in water.

The average age of death in the 12 patients described by Warnes and Roberts was only 37 and only 1 patient was >50 years of age. That fact may be a major reason for the mild amount of coronary atherosclerosis found in these patients. The 2 with symptomatic fatal coronary disease were aged 42 and 59 years. In none of the 12 patients reported by Warnes and Roberts or in the 6 patients reported by Amad et al were serum cholesterol values available.

No other reports on the heart at necropsy in massively obese persons have appeared since 1984. It appears that the massively obese person usually dies from a noncoronary cause before significant coronary atherosclerosis has had time to develop.

William C. Roberts

William Clifford Roberts, MD
Editor in Chief
Baylor Heart & Vascular Institute
Baylor University Medical Center
Dallas, Texas

1. Amad KH, Brennan JC, Alexander JK. The cardiac pathology of chronic exogenous obesity. *Circulation* 1965;32:740–745.

2. Warnes CA, Roberts WC. The heart in massive (more than 300 pounds or 136 kilograms) obesity: Analysis of 12 patients studied at necropsy. *Am J Cardiol* 1984;54:1087–1091.

Getting More People on Statins

Statins have been available in the United States since 1987, and yet 15 years later most patients who have had atherosclerotic events and/or diabetes mellitus, or who are at high risk for atherosclerotic events are not on statin therapy despite its proven benefit in decreasing first and repeat atherosclerotic events. The following are my recommendations for increasing the numbers of patients on statin therapy.

1. *Shift the emphasis from secondary prevention and diabetes mellitus to primary prevention.* Do not wait to start statin therapy until after an atherosclerotic event has occurred or diabetes mellitus has appeared. By the time either has appeared ≥1 major epicardial coronary arteries have been narrowed >75% in cross-sectional area by atherosclerotic plaque.[1,2] Guidelines for lipid-lowering therapy, formulated by the Adult Treatment Panel of the National Cholesterol Education Committee in 1988, and revised in 1993 and in 2001, are based on *decreasing the risk* of developing first and repeated atherosclerotic events.[3] Because it is rarely genetic in origin (the familial variety is present in only about 1 in 500 people[4]), atherosclerosis in my view needs to be approached not primarily from the standpoint of decreasing risk but from the standpoint of actually preventing and/or arresting plaque formation. Pediatricians do not talk in terms of decreasing the risk of measles, mumps, pertussis, and polio. They focus on total prevention of these conditions. The same approach can be applied to atherosclerosis.

But what serum cholesterol numbers are necessary to prevent atherosclerotic plaques from forming? The evidence is substantial that if over decades serum total cholesterol is <150 mg/dl, the low-density lipoprotein (LDL) cholesterol <100 mg/dl, and the high-density lipoprotein (HDL) cholesterol >20 mg/dl, the chances of forming atherosclerotic plaques are slim. (I realize that many readers will be shocked by the mention of an HDL cholesterol of only >20 mg/dl. But this number is only used when the total cholesterol is <150 mg/dl and the LDL cholesterol is <100 mg/dl.[5] If the total cholesterol is 200 mg/dl and the HDL cholesterol is only 21 mg/dl, an atherosclerotic event is likely.) Because about 45% of adults in the Western World die from cardiovascular disease, these numbers need to be the goals of *all adults*, not just adults with atherosclerotic events and/or diabetes mellitus, and now lipid-lowering agents, which can achieve these goals in most patients, are available. Thus, lower the bar for those eligible for statin therapy!

But how can these therapies be afforded the argument goes? These numbers can be achieved by following a vegetarian-fruit diet, which is the least expensive route. If that route is unsatisfactory simply decreasing the quantity of flesh (muscle) consumed by one half would free up enough money to purchase the lipid-lowering agent(s). We seem to afford arterial angioplasty and stents, bypass, endarterectomy and resection, and expensive diagnostic tests, and pacemakers and defibrillators without excessive thought, and yet there is no evidence that either arterial angioplasty or bypass prolongs life. In contrast, lipid-lowering therapy prolongs life by decreasing atherosclerotic events including stroke.[6–11] Thus, I say serum LDL cholesterol should be <100 mg/dl, total cholesterol <150 mg/dl, and HDL cholesterol >20 mg/dl for everybody. By doing this, the guidelines would be immediately simplified, and there would be no separation of so-called primary and secondary prevention or distinction between diabetics and nondiabetics.

The average LDL cholesterol in persons in coronary care units with acute coronary syndromes is about 145 mg/dl, and yet according to the most recent guidelines an LDL cholesterol of 159 mg/dl in a patient with only 1 or no other risk factor is considered "borderline" and not worthy of lipid-lowering drug therapy. This recommendation makes little sense to me. The Heart Protection Study[11] demonstrated a significant reduction in first and repeat atherosclerotic events by simvastatin therapy in patients with pretreatment serum LDL cholesterol levels ≤115 mg/dl. In contrast to lipid-lowering agents, aspirin is recognized to decrease atherosclerotic events irrespective of the platelet count or the "stickiness" of platelets. Likewise, the prophylactic value of lowering an elevated systemic arterial pressure is well recognized irrespective of the magnitude of blood pressure elevation.

2. *Eliminate the need for titration of statin drugs.* This is done by starting the patient initially on the proper dose, i.e., the one that lowers the LDL cholesterol to <100 mg/dl. A major reason patients do not achieve this LDL cholesterol goal is that the statin dose is too low and the dose is never raised. If the initial LDL cholesterol level is 185 mg/dl, for example, a drop of slightly >45% will be necessary to achieve an LDL cholesterol of <100 mg/dl. As shown in Table 1 that would require 40 mg of atorvastatin or 80 mg of simvastatin.

In contrast to statins, niacin therapy needs to be titrated, starting with a low dose (such as 500 mg) and gradually increasing to 1,500 mg if necessary. Likewise, fibrates might best be titrated—at least when added to a statin drug.

TABLE 1 Comparative Efficacy of the Five Currently Available Statin Drugs

Statin Drug (mg)					Serum Cholesterol	
Atorvastatin (Lipitor)	Simvastatin (Zocor)	Lovastatin (Mevacor)	Provastatin (Pravachol)	Fluvastatin (Lescol)	Total	LDL
5	10	20	20	20	22%↓	27%↓
10	20	40	40	80	27%↓	34%↓
20	40	80	80		32%↓	41%↓
40	80				37%↓	48%↓
80					42%↓	55%↓

Modified from Roberts WC. The rule of 5 and the rule of 7 in lipid-lowering by statin drugs. *Am J Cardiol* 1997;80:106–107.

3. *Eliminate the requirement for liver function tests.* The concern of hepatic dysfunction by physicians and patients frightens patients, and yet acute liver failure produced by a statin drug is incredibly rare (1/1 million patient-treatment years), a rate approximately equal to the rate of idiopathic acute liver failure.[12] The evidence that liver failure is ever the result of statin therapy is at best tenuous! Minor elevations in hepatic enzymes, i.e., serum alanine aminotransferase enzyme (ALT), occur in 2.6 % and 5.0% of patients on lovastatin 20 and 80 mg/day, respectively.[12] These elevations are reversible with continuing therapy, are dose related, and are probably related to the cholesterol lowering per se![12] (Elevation of the serum aminotransferase [AST] levels can occur with either muscle or liver injury and is thus less specific than elevation of the ALT level.[13]) In all of the 5-year, double-blind, placebo-controlled statin trials,[6–11] no patient was permitted in the trial if his/her baseline ALT or AST was >3 times the upper limit of normal. When these trials were initiated, it was not appreciated that hepatitis C was common (estimated 3 million patients in the United States) or that fatty liver, a cause of ALT elevation, was present in probably 50% of patients with diabetes mellitus, and there are an estimated 17 million diabetics in the USA. Alcoholism can also alter hepatic enzymes and there are probably 10 to 12 million habitual alcoholics in the United States. In other words, there are several causes for elevation of serum ALT. The danger for a patient with an elevated serum LDL cholesterol is arterial not hepatic! Additionally, there is no evidence that statins further elevate ALT when the level of this enzyme is raised by another condition.[12]

The requirement to do liver function tests in patients on statins needs to be removed from the package insert! If this were done, the money now applied to tests for hepatic dysfunction could be applied to purchasing the drug, and a malpractice worry would be removed from the concern of physicians, and worry about potential liver damage could be removed from the concern of both patients and physicians. There is no logic in requiring liver function tests periodically for patients on statins but not for patients on fibrates or niacin. Television ads that call attention to the potential danger of statins to the liver frightens patients unnecessarily and many patients appear to worry more about their liver than they do their arteries. This worry may be one reason why about 50% of patients on statins discontinue them in 1 year.

The only major concern of statin therapy is *myopathy* and that occurs in about 1 in 10,000 person-years, a multifold risk less than the consequences of accumulating atherosclerotic plaques in arteries.[12] In contrast, the risk of myopathy for patients on a fibrate is nearly 7/10,000 person-years.[12] For the general population, which is not on either a statin or a fibrate, the risk is 0.2/10,000 patient-years.[12] Elevation (<3 times the upper limit of normal) of the serum creatine phosphokinase (CPK) occurs in as many as 30% of dyslipidemic patients not taking lipid-lowering agents.[13] The risk of myopathy is less than that of a major bleed in patients taking aspirin or a nonsteroidal anti-inflammatory drug.

In summary, atherosclerosis needs to be viewed as a potentially preventable disease. Atherosclerosis needs to be discussed in terms of plaque prevention, not in terms of decreasing risk. This means that LDL cholesterol in all adults needs to be <100 mg/dl with HDL cholesterol as high as possible but at least >20 mg/dl when the total cholesterol is <150 mg/dl. If patients are started on the dose of statin that lowers the LDL cholesterol to <100 mg/dl *from the beginning*, this action will usually eliminate the need for statin titration. Baseline and periodic liver function tests also need to be eliminated because the evidence that statin therapy alters them is tenuous and the fright produced in patients from worry about their liver may play a role in their discontinuing statin therapy. Monitoring for hepatotoxicity is ineffectual in preventing serious liver disease and it may increase the risk of atherosclerotic events because of needless discontinuation of cholesterol-lowering therapy for false-positive results in patients who are benefiting from statin treatment. And finally, statin drugs not only decrease the frequency of coronary events but also stroke (by 30%).

William C. Roberts

William Clifford Roberts, MD
Editor in Chief
Baylor Heart & Vascular Institute
Baylor University Medical Center
Dallas, Texas

1. Roberts WC. Qualitative and quantitative comparison of amounts of narrowing by atherosclerotic plaques in the major epicardial coronary arteries at necropsy in sudden coronary death, transmural acute myocardial infarction, transmural healed myocardial infarction and unstable angina pectoris. *Am J Cardiol* 1989;64:324–328.

2. Waller BF, Palumbo PJ, Lie JT, Roberts WC. Status of the coronary arteries at necropsy in diabetes mellitus with onset after age 30 years. Analysis of 229 diabetic patients with and without clinical evidence of coronary heart disease and comparison to 183 control subjects. *Am J Med* 1980;69:498–506.

3. Expert Panel on Detection, Evaluation, and Treatment of High Blood Cholesterol in Adults. Executive summary of the third report of the National Cholesterol Education Program (NCEP) expert panel on detection, evaluation, and treatment of high blood cholesterol in adults (Adult Treatment Panel III). *JAMA* 2001;285: 2486–2497.

4. Brown MS, Goldstein JL. How LDL receptors influence cholesterol and atherosclerosis. *Sci Am* 1984;251:58–66.

5. Mautner SL, Sanchez JA, Rader DJ, Mautner GC, Ferrans VJ, Fredrickson DS, Brewer HB Jr, Roberts WC. The heart in Tangier disease. Severe coronary atherosclerosis with near absence of high-density lipoprotein cholesterol. *Am J Clin Pathol* 1992;191–198.

6. Scandinavian Simvastatin Survival Study Group. Randomised trial of cholesterol lowering in 4444 patients with coronary heart disease: the Scandinavian Simvastatin Survival Study (4S). *Lancet* 1994;344:1383–1389.

7. Shepherd J, Cobbe SM, Ford I, Isles CG, Lorimer AR, Macfarlane PW, McKillop JH, Packard CJ, for the West of Scotland Coronary Prevention Study Group. Prevention of coronary heart disease with pravastatin in men with hypercholesterolemia. *N Engl J Med* 1995;333:1301–1307.

8. Sacks FM, Pfeffer MA, Moye LA, Rouleau J, Rutherford JD, Cole T, Brown L, Warnica JW, Arnold JM, Wun CC, Davis BR, Braunwald E. The effect of pravastatin on coronary events after myocardial infarction in patients with average cholesterol levels. Cholesterol and Recurrent Events Trial investigators. *N Engl J Med* 1996;335:1001–1009.

9. The Long-Term Intervention with Pravastatin in Ischaemic Disease (LIPID) Study Group. Prevention of cardiovascular events and death with pravastatin in patients with coronary heart disease and a broad range of initial cholesterol levels. *N Engl J Med* 1998;339:1349–1357.

10. Downs JR, Clearfield M, Weis S, Whitney E, Shapiro DR, Beere PA, Langendorfer A, Stein EA, Kruger W, Gotto AM Jr, for the AFCAPS/TexCAPS Research Group. Primary prevention of acute coronary events with lovastatin in men and women with average cholesterol levels. Results of AFCAPS/TexCAPS. *JAMA* 1998;279:1616–1622.

11. Heart Protection Study Collaborative Group. MRC/BHF Heart Protection Study of cholesterol lowering with simvastatin in 20536 high-risk individuals: a randomized placebo-controlled trial. *Lancet* 2002;360:7–22.

12. Tolman KG. The liver and lovastatin. *Am J Cardiol* 2002;89:1374–1380.

13. Dujovne CA. Side effects of statins: hepatitis versus "transaminitis"—myositis versus "CPKitis." *Am J Cardiol* 2002;89:1411–1413.

Miscellany

ANOTHER WIN FOR STATINS

The Anglo-Scandinavian Cardiac Outcomes Trial—Lipid-Lowering Arm (ASCOT-LLA) involved nearly 20,000 hypertensive patients aged 40 to 79 years with at least 3 other cardiovascular risk factors.[1,2] The patients were randomized to 1 of 2 antihypertensive regimens, 1 arm treated with a calcium antagonist (amlodipine) plus an angiotensin-converting enzyme (ACE) inhibitor (perindopril) and the other arm treated with a β blocker (atenolol) plus a diuretic (doxazosin). Half of the patients in each hypertensive arm—about 5,000 patients per arm—were treated with atorvastatin 10 mg daily, and the other half received placebo. The criteria for inclusion in the study were an untreated systolic blood pressure ≥160 mm Hg or a diastolic pressure ≥100 mm Hg or both, or a treated systolic blood pressure ≥140 mm Hg or diastolic ≥90 mm Hg or both. Total cholesterol concentrations had to be ≤250 mg/dl (≤6.5 mmol/L), and patients could not be taking a statin or fibrate upon enrollment. All patients also had to have at least 3 of these 11 risk factors: left ventricular hypertrophy, other electrocardiographic abnormalities, type 2 diabetes mellitus, peripheral arterial disease, previous stroke or transient ischemic attack, male sex, age ≥55 years, microalbuminuria or proteinuria, smoker, ratio of plasma total cholesterol to high-density lipoprotein cholesterol ≥6, or family history of premature coronary heart disease.

The study stopped after 3.3 years for the 5,000 subjects in each arm of the study who were receiving atorvastatin because by that time 100 primary events had occurred in the atorvastatin group compared with 154 events in the placebo group (36% less). This benefit emerged in the first year of follow-up. In each of the 2 atorvastatin arms, the relative risk reduction in fatal and nonfatal stroke was 27% (89 atorvastatin vs 121 placebo), total cardiovascular events were reduced by 21% (389 atorvastatin vs 486 placebo), and total coronary events were reduced by 29% (178 atorvastatin vs 247 placebo). There were 185 deaths in the atorvastatin group and 212 in the placebo group (13% less). Atorvastatin lowered the mean serum total cholesterol from 212 to 162 mg/dl (26% decrease) and the low-density lipoprotein cholesterol from 131 to 90 mg/dl (31% decrease).

This study is important for atorvastatin because the only previous long-term study of atorvastatin included a small number of patients (about 300). The ASCOT-LLA study shows that atorvastatin has long-term outcome benefits similar to those provided by simvastatin, pravastatin, and lovastatin.

USEFULNESS OF STATINS FOR PREVENTING CARDIOVASCULAR EVENTS IN PERSONS WITH MILD CHRONIC RENAL INSUFFICIENCY

Tonelli and colleagues[3] for the Cholesterol and Recurrent Events (CARE) Trial Investigators found 1,711 participants who had chronic renal insufficiency with a creatine clearance ≤75 ml/min. These patients were a subgroup of the 4,159 patients in the trial that compared pravastatin (40 mg daily) with placebo in patients with previous myocardial infarction and total plasma cholesterol levels <240 mg/dl. After a mean follow-up of 59 months, the incidence of death from coronary artery disease or nonfatal acute myocardial infarction was lower in participants receiving pravastatin than those receiving placebo. Likewise, pravastatin was associated with a lower frequency of other coronary events and coronary revascularization, but not with total mortality or stroke. These data indicate that pravastatin is effective and safe for secondary prevention of cardiovascular events in persons with mild chronic renal insufficiency.

OBESITY'S EFFECT ON LIFESPAN

We all know the dangers of obesity, and we also know the difficulties of maintaining ideal body weight. Fontaine and colleagues[4] from Baltimore, Maryland, and Birmingham, Alabama, attempted to quantify the effect of obesity in terms of the expected number of years of life lost (YLL), defined as the difference between the number of years a subject would be expected to live if he or she were not obese and the number of years expected to live if the he or she were obese. The investigators used 4 large databases to derive YLL estimates for adults aged 18 to 85 years. Body mass index (BMI), divided into various categories, was used. BMI of 24 kg/m^2 was used as the reference category. The investigators found the optimal BMI (associated with the least YLL or greatest longevity) to be 23 to 25 kg/m^2 for whites and 23 to 30 kg/m^2 for blacks. For any degree of being overweight, younger adults generally had greater YLL than did older adults. The maximum YLL for white men and white women—aged 20 to 30 years with a severe level of obesity (BMI >45)—was 13 and 8 years, respectively. For men, this represented a 22% decrease in expected remaining lifespan. Blacks at younger ages with severe levels of obesity had a maximum YLL of 20 years for men and 5 years for women. Thus, obesity decreases life expectancy considerably, especially among younger adults.

OBSTRUCTIVE SLEEP APNEA AND HEART FAILURE

Sleep apnea occurs almost entirely in overweight persons, and heart failure is more common in overweight persons than in those at ideal body weight. Thus, the combination of obstructive sleep apnea and heart failure is not uncommon. Kaneko and colleagues[5] from Toronto studied 24 patients with obstructive sleep apnea and heart failure. Each patient underwent polysomnography, and the following morning their blood pressure and heart rate were measured by digital photoplethysmography and their left ventricular dimensions and ejection fractions were assessed by echocardiogram. The subjects were then randomly assigned to receive medical therapy alone (12 patients) or with the addition of continuous positive airway pressure (12 patients) for 1 month. In the control group who received only medical therapy, there were no significant changes in the severity of obstructive sleep apnea, daytime blood pressure, heart rate, left ventricular end-systolic dimension, or left ventricular ejection fraction during the study. In contrast, continuous positive airway pressure markedly reduced obstructive sleep apnea, daytime systolic blood pressure (126 to 116 mm Hg), heart rate (68 to 64 beats/min), and left ventricular end-systolic dimension (54 to 52 mm) and improved left ventricular ejection fraction (25% to 34%). Thus, continuous positive airway pressure is useful in patients with heart failure combined with obstructive sleep apnea.

SLEEP-DISORDERED BREATHING AMONG PROFESSIONAL FOOTBALL PLAYERS

Sleep-disordered breathing means apnea and hypopnea during sleep, and it affects about 4% of the general population. George and colleagues[6] from 3 different cities did overnight polysomnographic studies in 52 National Football League players. Offensive and defensive linemen accounted for 85% of the sleep-disordered breathing cases. Linemen also had the largest neck circumference (19 ± 1 in) and highest BMI (37 ± 3 kg/m^2). Both systolic blood pressure (129 ± 11 vs 122 ± 9 mm Hg) and diastolic blood pressure (84 ± 9 vs 77 ± 8 mm Hg) were significantly higher in linemen than in other players. The investigators estimated that the prevalence of sleep-disordered breathing among all professional football players was 14% and 34% within the high-risk group, mainly the linemen. This estimated prevalence is much higher than that found in men of similar age. The presence of sleep-disordered breathing is a known risk factor for the development of systemic hypertension, and treatment of sleep-disordered breathing will presumably reduce the risk of cardiovascular disease. The offensive linemen in the National Football League now average well over 300 lb, and the defensive linemen are not far behind. Professional football is not healthy for the heart or the joints.

C-REACTIVE PROTEIN (CRP)

An expert panel convened by the American Heart Association and the Centers for Disease Control and Prevention has issued recommendations about when to do the high-sensitivity CRP (hs-CRP) test, which costs between $15 and $20.[7] Their recommendations were: (1) widespread use of hs-CRP testing to screen the entire adult population to assess cardiovascular risk is inappropriate; (2) physicians should first assess traditional cardiovascular disease risk factors and calculate an absolute Framingham score before considering hs-CRP testing; (3) testing hs-CRP should be considered for patients at intermediate risk (10% to 20% risk of developing coronary heart disease in the next 10 years) as determined by the Framingham risk score; (4) two hs-CRP tests, averaged, fasting or nonfasting, optimally taken 2 weeks apart, provide a more stable estimate of hs-CRP than a single test; (5) a serum hs-CRP level of <1 mg/L is considered low risk, 1.0 to 3.0 is considered average risk, and >3.0 mg/L is considered high risk; and (6) a search should be made for an obvious source of infection or inflammation in patients with hs-CRP levels >10 mg/L; hs-CRP should then be measured again in 2 weeks.

FOOD PORTION SIZES

Although many believe that food portion sizes are increasing, no data have documented actual increases. Neilsen and Popkin[8] from Chapel Hill, North Carolina, compared food portion sizes consumed in the United States from 1977 to 1978 with those consumed by individuals in 1996. Consumption by over 63,000 persons aged ≥2 years were sampled. Portion sizes varied by food source, with the largest portions consumed at fast food establishments and the smallest at other restaurants. Between 1977 and 1996, food portion sizes increased inside and outside the home. The energy intake and portion size of salty snacks increased by 93 kcal (28 to 45 g), soft drinks by 49 kcal (387 to 588 ml), hamburgers by 97 kcal (162 to 198 g), French fries by 68 kcal (88 to 102 g), and Mexican food by 133 kcal (179 to 227 g). Thus, portion sizes and energy intake for specific food types have increased markedly during these 20 years, with the greatest increases being for food consumed at fast food establishments and in the home.

FAT CITY

For the third year in a row, *Men's Fitness* magazine has awarded Houston the dubious title of the fattest city in the United States among a list 25 cities.[9] The other 4 in the top 5 were Chicago, Detroit, Philadelphia, and St. Louis. Dallas ranked number 9.

CONTINUING DECREASE IN DEATH RATES FROM CORONARY HEART DISEASE

Fewer people are dying from coronary heart disease in most developed countries. Between 1988 and 1998, the death rate from heart disease in the United States decreased approximately 30%; in the United Kingdom 38%; in Denmark 49%; in Norway 45%; and in Australia 45%.[10] The improved outcomes are attributed to quicker diagnoses and treatment of recent-onset chest pain, more prompt use of thrombolytic agents and coronary angioplasty, and greater use of preventive drugs.

CHANGING INCIDENCE OF OUT-OF-HOSPITAL CARDIAC ARREST

Because the overall mortality from coronary heart disease in the United States has been decreasing, it follows that the incidence of out-of-hospital cardiac arrest must also be decreasing. A study from Finland described a marked decrease in out-of-hospital cardiac arrest in a 5-year period (1994 to 1999), and another study in Sweden showed a decrease during a 17-year period. Cobb and colleagues[11] compared out-of-hospital cardiac arrest cases during 21 years (1979 to 2000) in Seattle, Washington. The annual incidence of cardiac arrest with ventricular fibrillation as the first identified rhythm decreased by about 56% and was most evident in men. When all treated arrests (including asystole) with presumed cardiac etiology were considered, the incidence decreased by 43% in men but negligibly in women. Thus, in Seattle and hopefully in other parts of the country, there has been a major decline in the incidence of out-of-hospital ventricular fibrillation and in all cases of cardiac arrest presumably due to heart disease.

TREATING SYSTEMIC HYPERTENSION WITH DIURETICS, ACE INHIBITORS, AND CALCIUM ANTAGONISTS

In late 2002, the Antihypertensive and Lipid-Lowering Treatment To Prevent Heart Attack Trial (ALLHAT) involved >42,000 patients from the United States and Canada and compared the diuretic chlorthalidone with an ACE inhibitor (lisinopril) and a calcium antagonist (amlodipine).[12] (The α-adrenergic receptor inhibitor arm was stopped early because of adverse events.) ALLHAT concluded that chlorthalidone was more effective for blood pressure control and for outcomes than was lisinopril or amlodipine.

In early 2003, the Second Australian National Blood Pressure Study (ANBP2) trial was reported.[13] It involved just over 6,000 patients who were followed by 1,594 family practitioners in Australia for a median of 4.1 years. The ANBP2 trial indicated that enalapril, the ACE used, had an outcome advantage over hydrochlorothiazide, the diuretic used. Thus, the conclusions of these 2 trials are diametrically opposed to one another.[14] The ALLHAT trial used chlorthalidone, the ANBP2 trial, hydrochlorothiazide. No head-to-head trials have compared the efficacy of and outcomes with these 2 diuretics. ALLHAT used lisinopril, whereas ANBP2 used enalapril as the ACE inhibitor. Likewise, no head-to-head comparisons have been done on the long-term efficacy of and outcomes with these 2 ACE inhibitors. In both trials, other antihypertensive medicines were frequently used to achieve blood pressure goals, and the use of these additional agents compound the complexities of comparisons between these trials. In the ALLHAT trial, the diuretic-based regimen was more efficacious in blood pressure lowering and in the percentage of patients in whom the blood pressure goal was achieved compared with the lisinopril and amlodipine arms. In the ANBP2 trial, there were similar reductions in blood pressure in the chlorothiazide and lisinopril arms. In the ALLHAT trial, the primary outcome of death from coronary causes or nonfatal myocardial infarction was similar in the 3 treatment arms, but when the primary and secondary cardiovascular events were combined, the outcomes favored chlorthalidone. The primary outcome in the ANBP2 trial was the total number of fatal and nonfatal cardiovascular events, and here enalapril performed better than chlorothiazide. So take your choice. I take an ACE, an aldosterone receptor blocker, and hydrochlorothiazide (12.5 mg), and my pressure is 115/75 mm Hg.

ALCOHOL, STROKE, AND ACUTE MYOCARDIAL INFARCTION

Stroke is the third leading cause of death and a major cause of disability in the United States. Approximately 30% of stroke survivors are permanently disabled and 20% require institutionalized care. Stroke also, of course, is a huge financial burden for patients, their families, and the health care system. The direct and indirect cost of stroke in the United States in 2002 was estimated to be $50 billion. Over the past 20 years, many observational epidemiologic studies have examined the role of alcohol as both a risk factor and a potential protective factor for stroke.

Studies investigating the association between moderate consumption of alcohol and stroke have reported conflicting results. Reynolds and colleagues[15] from New Orleans, Louisiana, performed a meta-analysis of 35 observational studies (cohort or case control) to examine the relative risk of stroke at various levels of alcohol consumption. Compared with abstainers, those who consumed >60 g of alcohol per day had an increased relative risk of total stroke (64% increase), ischemic stroke (69% increase), and hemorrhagic stroke (18% increase), whereas consumption of <12 g/day was associated with a reduced relative risk of total stroke (17% decrease) and ischemic stroke (20% decrease). Consumption of 12 to 24 g/day was associated with a reduced relative risk of ischemic stroke (28% decrease). These results indicate that heavy alcohol consumption increases the relative risk of stroke, whereas light or moderate alcohol consumption may protect against total and ischemic stroke.

Although moderate consumption of alcohol confers a decreased risk of acute myocardial infarction, the role that the type of beverage consumed, the pattern of drinking, and whether the alcohol is consumed with meals or not is unclear. Mukamal and colleagues[16] from Boston, Massachusetts, studied the association of alcohol consumption and acute myocardial infarction in 38,077 male health professionals who were free of cardiovascular disease and cancer at baseline. During the 12-year follow-up (1986 to 1998) there were 1,418 cases (4%) of acute myocardial infarction. Compared with men who consumed alcohol less than once per week, men who consumed alcohol 3 to 4 or 5 to 7 days per week had decreased risks of acute myocardial infarction (32% decrease and 37% decrease, respectively). The risk was similar in men who consumed <10 g of alcohol per drinking day and those who consumed ≥30 g per drinking day. No single type of beverage conferred additional benefit nor did consumption with meals.

Thus, in men, consumption of alcohol at least 3 to 4 days a week was inversely associated with the risk of myocardial infarction. Neither the type of beverage nor the portion consumed with meals substantially altered this association. Men who increased their alcohol consumption by 12.5 g daily during a 40-year period had a further decreased risk of acute myocardial infarction. (A 5-oz [150 ml] glass of wine contains about 20 g of alcohol, a 12-oz [355 ml] container of beer contains approximately 14 g of alcohol, and a 50-ml glass of spirits contains 20 g of alcohol.)

NEPHRON NUMBER AND SYSTEMIC HYPERTENSION

Brenner and colleagues[17–19] proposed nearly 20 years ago that a low number of nephrons increases the risk of systemic hypertension and progressive renal disease. This hypothesis was based on observations that rat strains with a high complement of nephrons were less susceptible to progressive renal disease. Conversely, in both nonhuman animals and in humans, a decrease in the number of nephrons is associated with systemic hypertension and increased risk of progressive renal disease. Keller and colleagues[20] from Germany designed a study to test the hypothesis that a reduced number of nephrons contributes to essential hypertension in the general population. Using a 3-dimensional stereologic method, they compared the number and volume of glomeruli in 10 white patients aged 35 to 59 years with essential hypertension or left ventricular hypertrophy or both and renal arteriolar lesions with the number and volume in 10 normotensive subjects matched for sex, age, height, and weight. All 20 subjects had died in accidents. Patients with hypertension had significantly fewer glomeruli per kidney than matched normotensive controls (median 702,379 vs 1,429,200). Patients with hypertension also had a greater glomerular volume than did the controls (median 6.50×10^{-3} mm^3) but very few obsolescent glomeruli. These data support the hypothesis that the number of nephrons is reduced in white patients with essential hypertension.

Finding obsolescent glomeruli in hypertensive kidneys implies ongoing nephron loss, meaning that persons with hypertension most likely had not lost glomeruli over time but rather had a smaller number at birth. What determines nephron number? All studies to date according to Ingelfinger[21] show that there is a variation among phenotypically normal persons, with some having more nephrons than others. "Perinatal programming," the term coined to describe the observation that events during gestation can have far-reaching effects into adulthood, was first proposed by Barker and colleagues in 1989 when they observed an inverse relation between birth weight and cardiovascular disease in a cohort of middle-aged British men. Clinical and experimental data amassed since that observation suggest that alterations in intrauterine nutrition, especially protein calorie restriction, may "program" the fetus for later susceptibility to systemic hypertension, cardiovascular disease, and stroke. Studies in experimental models show directly that relatively minor insults, such as protein restriction, can result in fewer nephrons. The concepts of perinatal programming and hyperfiltration fit well together: persons who undergo intrauterine stress, even fairly subtle, may not develop a full complement of nephrons. Over time, the compensatory efforts of the kidney go awry, leading to increased filtration by each nephron, then subtle dysfunction and scarring and, ultimately, hypertension. Ingelfinger suggested that improved nutrition for pregnant women may prevent decreased nephron endowment, which, in turn, may decrease the frequency of systemic hypertension in susceptible offspring during their adult lives.

William C. Roberts

William Clifford Roberts, MD
Editor in Chief
Baylor Heart & Vascular Institute
Baylor University Medical Center
Dallas, Texas

1. Sever PS, Dahlöf B, Poulter NR, Wedel H, Beevers G, Caulfield M, Collins R, Kjeldsen SE, Kristinsson A, McInnes GT, et al, for the ASCOT Investigators. Prevention of coronary and stroke events with atorvastatin in hypertensive patients who have average or lower-than- average cholesterol concentrations in the Anglo-Scandinavian Cardiac Outcomes Trial—Lipid Lowering Arm (ASCOT-LLA): a multicentre randomized controlled trial. *Lancet* 2003;361:1149–1158.

2. Sever PS, Dahlöf B, Poulter NR, Wedel H, Beevers G, Caulfield M, Collins R, Kjeldsen SE, Kristinsson A, McInnes GT, et al, for the ASCOT Investigators. Rationale, design, methods and baseline demography of participants of the Anglo-Scandinavian Cardiac Outcomes Trial. *J Hypertension* 2001;19:1139–1147.

3. Tonelli M, Moyé L, Sacks FM, Kiberd B, Curhan G, for the Cholesterol and Recurrent Events (CARE) Trial Investigators. Pravastatin for secondary prevention of cardiovascular events in persons with mild chronic renal insufficiency. *Ann Intern Med* 2003;138:98–104.

4. Fontaine KR, Redden DT, Wang C, Westfall AO, Allison DB. Years of life lost due to obesity. *JAMA* 2003;289:187–193.

5. Kaneko Y, Floras JS, Usui K, Plante J, Tkacova R, Kubo T, Ando S, Bradley TD. Cardiovascular effects of continuous positive airway pressure in patients with heart failure and obstructive sleep apnea. *N Engl J Med* 2003;348:1233–1241.
6. George CFP, Kab V, Levy AM. Increased prevalence of sleep-disordered breathing among professional football players. *N Engl J Med* 2003;348:367–368.
7. Pearson TA, Mensah GA, Alexander RW, Anderson JL, Cannon RO III, Criqui M, Fadl YY, Fortmann SP, Hong Y, Myers GL, et al. Markers of inflammation and cardiovascular disease. Application to clinical and public health practice. A statement for healthcare professionals from the Centers for Disease Control and Prevention and the American Heart Association. *Circulation* 2003;107:499–511.
8. Nielsen SJ, Popkin BM. Patterns and trends in food portion sizes, 1977–1998. *JAMA* 2003;289:450–453.
9. Lozano JA. Houston gains its 3rd 'fat city' title. *The Dallas Morning News* January 3, 2003.
10. Kmietowicz Z. UK lags behind many European countries in reducing deaths from heart disease. *BMJ* 2003;326:242.
11. Cobb LA, Fahrenbruch CE, Olsufka M, Copass MK. Changing incidence of out-of-hospital ventricular fibrillation, 1980–2000. *JAMA* 2002;288:3008–3013.
12. The ALLHAT Officers and Coordinators for the ALLHAT Collaborative Research Group. Major outcomes in high-risk hypertensive patients randomized to angiotensin-converting enzyme inhibitor or calcium channel blocker vs diuretic. The Antihypertensive and Lipid-Lowering Treatment to Prevent Heart Attack Trial (ALLHAT). *JAMA* 2002;288:2981–2997.
13. Wing LMH, Reid CM, Ryan P, Beilin LJ, Brown MA, Jennings GLR, Johnston CI, McNeil JJ, Macdonald GJ, Marley JE, Morgan TO, West MJ, for the Second Australian National Blood Pressure Study Group. A comparison of outcomes with angiotensin-converting-enzyme inhibitors and diuretics for hypertension in the elderly. *N Engl J Med* 2003;348:583–592.
14. Frohlich ED. Treating hypertension—What are we to believe? *N Engl J Med* 2003;348:639–641.
15. Reynolds K, Lewis LB, Nolen JDL, Kinney GL, Sathya B, He J. Alcohol consumption and risk of stroke. A meta-analysis. *JAMA* 2003;289:579–588.
16. Mukamal KJ, Conigrave KM, Mittleman MA, Camargo CA Jr, Stampfer MJ, Willett WC, Rimm EB. Roles of drinking pattern and type of alcohol consumed in coronary heart disease in men. *N Engl J Med* 2003;348:109–118.
17. Hakim RM, Goldszer RC, Brenner BM. Hypertension and proteinuria: long-term sequelae of uninephrectomy in humans. *Kidney Int* 1984;25:930–936.
18. Brenner BM, Garcia DL, Anderson S. Glomeruli and blood pressure: less of one, more of the other? *Am J Hypertens* 1988;1:335–347.
19. Brenner BM, Chertow GM. Congenital oligonephropathy and the etiology of adult hypertension and progressive renal injury. *Am J Kidney Dis* 1994;23:171–175.
20. Keller G, Zimmer G, Mall G, Ritz E, Amann K. Nephron number in patients with primary hypertension. *N Engl J Med* 2003;348:101–108.
21. Ingelfinger JR. Is microanatomy destiny? *N Engl J Med* 2003;348:99–100.

The Metabolic Syndrome

At my weekly conference with the cardiology fellows recently, I asked them how many times they had diagnosed "the metabolic syndrome" in the past year and written the diagnosis in the patient's record. It was apparent from their answers that none had. One of the better parts of the Third Report of the National Cholesterol Education Program Expert Panel on Detection, Evaluation, and Treatment of High Blood Cholesterol in Adults (Adult Treatment Panel III) was placing proper emphasis on this syndrome.[1] The Panel's definition of the metabolic syndrome included 3 of the following 5 factors: (1) *abdominal obesity*: waist circumference in men >102 cm (>40 inches) and in women >88 cm (>35 inches); (2) *serum triglycerides* >150 mg/dl (>3.82 mmol/L); (3) *high-density lipoprotein (HDL) cholesterol* <40 mg/dl (<1.03 mmol/L) in men and <50 mg/dl (<1.30 mmol/L) in women; (4) *systemic arterial blood pressure* ≥130/≥85 mm Hg; and (5) *fasting blood glucose* ≥110 mg/dl. The Panel noted that waist circumference was correlated better with abdominal obesity than body mass index.

Before the metabolic syndrome can be treated properly, it needs to be diagnosed. Overweightness is so common now in the US that it is overlooked. Waist measurement, much less body mass index, infrequently appears on office or hospital patient records. Serum triglyceride levels of 151 to 200 mg/dl (1.7 to 2.3 mmol/L) are considered normal by many physicians and most laboratories report triglycerides between 151 and 200 mg/dl as normal. Serum HDL cholesterol levels >35 mg/dl, systemic blood pressures <140/90 mm Hg, and fasting blood glucose ≤125 mg/dl are considered normal by most physicians. Thus, diagnosis of the metabolic syndrome does not require a great deal of abnormality among these 5 factors. As a consequence, >50 million Americans have the metabolic syndrome.[2] Additionally, >80% of adults with the metabolic syndrome have a high percentage of their low-density lipoprotein particles small and dense rather than large and buoyant, and the smaller particles are the more atherogenic ones.

The best treatment of the metabolic syndrome is weight loss, but, of course, this therapy is the hardest to administer and the least successful. Weight loss—even as little as 5% to 10% of body weight—decreases serum triglycerides, glucose, and blood pressure, raises HDL cholesterol, and improves the quality of life.[3,4] Lowering fat intake and/or adding orlistat therapy (which decreases fat absorption about 30%) lowers triglycerides, as do statins, fibrates, niacin, and ezetimibe.[5,6] Niacin also enlarges low-density lipoprotein particle size.

For better control of present and future atherosclerotic cardiovascular disease, the metabolic syndrome needs to be diagnosed and treated more often.

William C. Roberts

William Clifford Roberts, MD
Editor in Chief
Baylor Heart & Vascular Institute
Baylor University Medical Center
Dallas, Texas

1. Expert Panel on Detection, Evaluation, and Treatment of High Blood Cholesterol in Adults. Executive summary of the Third Report of the National Cholesterol Education Program (NCEP) Expert Panel on Detection, Evaluation, and Treatment of High Blood Cholesterol in Adults (Adult Treatment Panel III). *JAMA* 2001;285:2486–2497.
2. Park Y-W, Zhu S, Palaniappan L, Heshka S, Carnethon MR, Heymsfield SB. The metabolic syndrome. Prevalence and associated risk factor findings in the US population from the Third National Health and Nutrition Examination Survey, 1988–1994. *Arch Intern Med* 2003;163:427–436.
3. Heymsfield SB, Segal KR, Hauptman J, Lucas CP, Boldrin MN, Rissanen A, Wilding JPH, Sjöström L. Effects of weight loss with orlistat on glucose tolerance and progression to type 2 diabetes in obese adults. *Arch Intern Med* 2000;160: 1321–1326.
4. Rössner S, Sjöström L, Noack R, Meinders AE, Noseda Gon behalf of the , European Orlistat Obesity Study Group. Weight loss, weight maintenance, and improved cardiovascular risk factors after 2 years treatment with Orlistat for obesity. *Obes Res* 2000;8:49–61.
5. Elam MB, Hunninghake DB, Davis KB, Garg R, Johnson C, Egan D, Kostis JB, Sheps DS, Brinton EAfor the , ADMIT Investigators. Effect of niacin on lipid and lipoprotein levels and glycemic control in patients with diabetes and peripheral arterial disease. The ADMIT Study: a randomized trial. *JAMA* 2000;284: 1263–1270.
6. Gagné C, Gaudet D, Bruckert Efor the , Ezetimibe Study Group. Efficacy and safety of ezetimibe coadministered with atorvastatin or simvastatin in patients with homozygous familial hypercholesterolemia. *Circulation* 2002;105:2469–2475.

Two More Drugs for Dyslipidemia

During the last 16 years, 7 statin drugs have been introduced into the USA for treatment of dyslipidemia. Of the 7, one (cerivastatin, Baycol®) was withdrawn 4 years after its introduction because of a large number of cases of fatal and nonfatal rhabdomyolysis. Of the 4 statins (lovastatin, pravastatin, simvastatin, and fluvastatin) introduced in the USA before 1997, all have proven to be safe and efficacious. Atorvastatin, the world's best selling drug, was introduced in 1997, the same year that cerivastatin appeared in the USA market, and it too has proved to be very efficacious and safe,[1] and to have results of long-term outcome studies similar to those observed with lovastatin, pravastatin, and simvastatin.[2,3] Since 1997, only 1 new statin has been introduced into the USA and that was rosuvastatin (Crestor®) in 2003. This piece summarizes some features of this newest statin and also discusses briefly some characteristics of ezetimibe (Zetia®), the other drug for dyslipidemia also introduced into the USA in 2003.

Rosuvastatin calcium, compared to the other 5 presently available statin drugs possesses the following features[4]: (1) it is the most efficacious statin for lowering serum total cholesterol; (2) it is the most efficacious statin for lowering serum low-density lipoprotein (LDL) cholesterol; (3) it is most efficacious statin for lowering serum non–high-density lipoprotein (HDL) cholesterol; (4) it is the most efficacious statin, along with atorvastatin, for lowering serum triglycerides; (5) it has safety features in its 5 to 40 mg dose range similar to those of the other 5 presently available statins; and (6) it has few interactions with other drugs, and those it does have are similar to those found with most of the other presently available statins.

The efficacy of the 5 to 40 mg doses of rosuvastatin compared with that of the other 5 statins are summarized in Table 1. Rosuvastatin at the 5 mg dose lowers LDL cholesterol an average of about 42%; at 10 mg, 48%; at 20 mg, 55%; and at 40 mg, 63%.[4] Rosuvastatin increases HDL cholesterol more than any of the other statins and that increase is dose-related. Simvastatin also increases HDL cholesterol as the dose of simvastatin increases.[5] The increase with simvastatin is greatest in patients with low baseline HDL cholesterol levels. Atorvastatin, in contrast, has decreasing effects on HDL cholesterol as the dose of atorvastatin increases.[5]

Now to the potential downsides of rosuvastatin. First, there are no long-term outcome studies with this new statin. Significant long-term studies on atorvastatin, however, were not available until 6 years after its introduction,[3] but, nevertheless, this excellent agent skyrocketed to the number 1 position in sales within months after its initial launch. In contrast to the situation with the other 6 statins, however, long-term studies were underway with rosuvastatin before it was approved by the Federal Drug Administration (FDA); thus, the results of these studies will be available in another 3 or so years. Second, long-term safety of rosuvastatin has not yet been determined. Rosuvastatin, however, had been used in >10,000 subjects before its approval in the USA, a number far in excess of patients studied in other statin trials before the statin was approved. Because the FDA had been burned by the particularly toxic effects of cerivastatin, which subsequently was withdrawn from the marketplace, rosuvastatin received a particularly careful scrutiny by the FDA before giving its approval.

One side effect noted before approval with rosuvastatin therapy was proteinuria/microscopic hematuria in a small percent (<1%) of patients taking this drug. This complication, however, was noted to occur primarily in the patients receiving the 80 mg dose, and, as a consequence, that dose of rosuvastatin was not approved by the FDA. At doses of 5 to 40 mg, the frequency of proteinuria in patients on rosuvastatin appears to be similar to that of the other statins, and the possible appearance of proteinuria is also mentioned in the package inserts of some of the other statins. Studies have shown in certain non-human animals (opossum) that the proteinuria is the result of lack of adequate reabsorption of both high and low molecular weight proteins in the proximal renal tubules. The proteinuria is not due to excessive filtration at the glomerular level. Furthermore, the proteinuria/microscopic hematuria is transient and does not lead to renal dysfunction, i.e., elevation of the serum creatinine level. There is some evidence that rosuvastatin is nephroprotective as demonstrated by the decrease in the serum creatine level in many patients after institution of rosuvastatin therapy. This finding also has been observed with atorvastatin, simvastatin, and pravastatin. Additionally, patients with proteinuria at baseline have been observed to have less proteinuria after initiation of rosuvastatin therapy. The appearance of proteinuria with all statins at most doses (compared with no proteinuria at baseline) is <1% and usually no more than 0.6%, the latter percent being that seen also in the placebo groups.

It is unlikely that rosuvastatin possesses the particularly toxic characteristics possessed by cerivastatin. First, rosuvastatin is relatively hydrophilic, just as is pravastatin, a characteristic possibly favoring safety.

TABLE 1 Comparative Efficacy of the 6 Currently Available Statin Drugs

Statin Drug (mg)						Serum Cholesterol	
Rosuvastatin (Crestor®)	Atorvastatin (Lipitor®)	Simvastatin (Zocor®)	Lovastatin (Mevacor®)	Pravastatin (Pravachol®)	Fluvastatin (Lescol®)	Total	LDL
—	—	10	20	20	40	22%↓	27%↓
—	10	20	40	40	80	27%↓	34%↓
5	20	40	80	80	—	32%↓	41%↓
10	40	80	—	—	—	37%↓	48%↓
20	80	—	—	—	—	42%↓	55%↓
40	—	—	—	—	—	47%↓	63%↓

All the other statins are relatively lipophilic, and cerivastatin was the most lipophilic of all statins. The amount of statin available in the bloodstream (bioavailability) was by far the greatest with cerivastatin of any of the statins, namely 60%, whereas the bioavailability of rosuvastatin is 20% and all the other proven safe statins are also 20% to <5% (simvastatin). The frequency of hepatic serum transaminase elevations and the frequency of myopathy/rhabdomyolysis in patients on rosuvastatin (5 to 40 mg doses) have been low and comparable to that of the other 5 presently available statin drugs.[6,7]

Ezetimibe (Zetia®), a cholesterol absorption blocker acting in the small intestine, was also introduced in 2003. It is available only in the 10 mg dose and as monotherapy lowers serum total cholesterol about 13%; LDL cholesterol, about 18%; triglycerides, about 8%, with little effect on HDL cholesterol.[8–13] When combined with any statin drug, the effect of ezetimibe on these lipoproteins is amplified, such that the LDL cholesterol reduction jumps to 25%, the triglycerides decrease to 14%, and the HDL cholesterol increases to an average of 3%. Because 10 mg of atorvastatin or 20 mg of simvastatin lowers LDL cholesterol an average of 34%, the combination of either of these statins at these doses with 10 mg of ezetimibe lowers LDL cholesterol an average of 58% with an HDL cholesterol increase being an average of 9%. (The lowering of the serum triglyceride level is baseline dependent, such that levels <100 mg/dl at baseline usually are unaffected, whereas levels >200 mg/dl at baseline might be lowered by the combination by as much as 30% or so.) Because only about 20% of the ezetimibe in the small intestine is absorbed into the systemic circulation, specifically the enterohepatic circulation, the drug has no major side effects. Additionally, the side effects of the statin drugs at the lower doses are essentially the same as placebo. Thus, the combination of ezetimibe plus statin (at a relatively low dose) provides serum LDL cholesterol reductions of >50%, reductions available only with atorvastatin 80 mg (55%↓) and rosuvastatin 20 mg (55%↓) and 40 mg (63%↓). The mechanism of action of ezetimibe and the statins are entirely different, a factor favoring the combination rather than a high-dose statin. Most adults in the USA would benefit greatly from a 50%+ reduction in serum LDL cholesterol!

Because the lower the serum LDL cholesterol levels, the lower the occurrence of atherosclerotic events, I predict, in contrast to *The Lancet* editors (unsigned editorial)[14] that both rosuvastatin and ezetimibe will prove to be highly effective agents and, in the end, that combination lipid-lowering therapy—just like in the treatment of high blood pressure—will win out over monotherapy for patients with dyslipidemia. With any new drug, of course, it is wise to be cautious, particularly in view of the superb efficacious and safety records of the presently available lipid-lowering drugs. Therefore, at this time I would tend to limit, except in very unusual circumstances, the use of rosuvastatin to the 5, 10, and 20 mg doses and avoid the 40 mg dose. I see no downside from the 10 mg ezetimibe tablet.

William C. Roberts

William Clifford Roberts, MD*
Editor in Chief
Baylor Heart & Vascular Institute
Baylor University Medical Center
Dallas, Texas

1. Newman CB, Palmer G, Silbershatz H, Szarek M. Safety of *atorvastatin* derived from analysis of 44 completed trials in 9,416 patients. *Am J Cardiol* 2003;92:670–676.
2. Mikhailidis DP, Wierzbicki AS. The GREek Atorvastatin and Coronary-heart-disease Evaluation (GREACE Study). *Curr Med Res Opin* 2002;18:215–219.
3. Sever PS, Dahlöf B, Poulter NR, Wedel H, Beevers G, Caulfield M, Collins R, Kjeldsen SE, Kristinsson A, McInnes GT, Mehlsen J, Nieminen M, O'Brien E, Östergren J, for the ASCOT Investigators. Prevention of coronary and stroke events with atorvastatin in hypertensive patients who have average of lower-than-average cholesterol concentrations, in the Anglo-Scandinavian Cardiac Outcomes Trial–Lipid Lowering Arm (ASCOT-LLA): a multicentre randomized controlled trial. *Lancet* 2003;361:1149–1158.
4. Jones PH, Davidson MH, Stein EA, Bays HE, McKenney JM, Miller E, Cain VA, Blasetto JW, for the STELLAR Study Group. Comparison of efficacy and safety of *rosuvastatin* versus *atorvastatin*, *simvastatin*, and *pravastatin* across doses (STELLAR Trial). *Am J Cardiol* 2003;93:152–160.
5. Kastelein JJP, Isaacsohn JL, Ose L, Hunninghake DB, Frohlich J, Davidson MH, Habib R, Dujovne CA, Crouse JR III, Liu M, Melino MR, O'Grady L,

*WCR has no stocks in any pharmaceutical or medical device company. He is on the speakers' lists of several pharmaceutical companies, including Merck, Merck/Schering Plough, Pfizer, and Schering Plough. WCR has received grants from Bristol-Myers Squibb, Merck, and Pfizer (Parke-Davis). He also is on the advisory board of Johnson-Johnson/Merck, which is attempting to get lovastatin approved for over-the-counter use.

Mercuri M, Mitchel YB, and Simvastatin Atorvastatin HDL Study Group. Comparison of effects of *simvastatin* versus *atorvastatin* on high-density lipoprotein cholesterol and apolipoprotein A-1 levels. *Am J Cardiol* 2000;86:221–223.
6. Gaist D, Garcia Rodríguez LA, Huerta C, Hallas J, Sinsrup SH. Lipid-lowering drugs and risk of myopathy: a population-based follow-up study. *Epidemiology* 2001;12:565–569.
7. Staffa JA, Chang J, Green L. Cervastatin and report of fatal rhabdomyolysis. *N Engl J Med* 2002;346:539–540.
8. Sudhop T, Lütjohann D, Kodal A, Igel M, Tribble DL, Shah S, Perevozskaya I, von Bergmann K. Inhibition of intestinal cholesterol absorption by ezetimibe in humans. *Circulation* 2002;106:1943–1948.
9. Gagńe C, Bays HE, Weiss SR, Mata P, Quinto K, Melino M, Cho M, Musliner TA, Gumbiner B, for the Ezetimibe Study Group. Efficacy and safety of *ezetimibe* added to ongoing statin therapy for treatment of patients with hypercholesterolemia. *Am J Cardiol* 2002;90:1084–1091.
10. Dujovne CA, Ettinger MP, McNeer JF, Lipka LJ, LeBeaut AP, Suresh R, Yang B, Veltri EP, for the Ezetimibe Study Group. Efficacy and safety of a potent new selective cholesterol absorption inhibitor, in *ezetimibe*, in patients with primary hypercholesterolemia. *Am J Cardiol* 2002;90:1092–1097.
11. Davidson M, McGarry T, Bettis R, Melani L, Lipka LJ, LeBeaut AP, Suresh R, Sun S, Veltri EP, on behalf of the Ezetimibe Study Group. Ezetimibe co-administered with simvastatin in patients with primary hypercholesterolemia. *J Am Coll Cardiol* 2002;40:2125–2134.
12. Knopp RH, Gitter H, Truitt T, Bays H, Manion CV, Lipka LJ, LeBeaut AP, Suresh R, Yang B, Veltri EP, for the Ezetimibe Study Group. Effects of ezetimibe, a new cholesterol absorption inhibitor, on plasma lipids in patients with primary hypercholesterolemia. *Eur Heart J* 2003;24:729–741.
13. Ballantyne CM, Houri J, Notarbartolo A, Melani L, Lipka LJ, Suresh R, Sun S, LeBeaut AP, Sager PT, Veltri EP, for the Ezetimibe Study Group. Effect of ezetimibe coadministered with atorvastatin in 628 patients with primary hypercholesterolemia: a prospective, randomized double-blind trial. *Circulation* 2003; 107:2409–2415.
14. The Lancet. The statin wars: why AstraZeneca must retreat. *Lancet* 2003; 362:1341.

The Amish, Body Weight, and Exercise

When discussing the need to lose weight, a common remark is "I need to do more exercise." For most of us, little weight is lost by exercise unless we do a lot of it. Pushing away from the table is usually the best type of exercise for most of us to lose weight. But there are exceptions. In general, we need to walk 35 miles to lose 1 pound, and if we trod those type distances daily, calorie consumption can be essentially whatever we want it to be. A good example are the Amish.

Bassett and colleagues[1] studied 98 Old Order Amish adults aged 18 to 75 years including 53 men and 45 women, all of whom lived in an Amish community in Southeastern Ontario, Canada. Most were farmers. The 98 participants represented 42% of the 455 people in the Amish community. A pedometer was given to each of the 98 and they recorded the number of steps per day and their physical activities for 1 week. The average numbers of steps per day during that week was 18,425 for the men and 14,196 for the women. The men reported 10 hours per week of vigorous physical activity, 43 hours of moderate physical activity, and 12 hours per week of walking. Women reported 3.4 hours per week of vigorous physical activity, 39 hours of moderate physical activity, and nearly 6 hours per week of walking. A total of 25% of the men and 27% of the women were overweight (body mass index $\geq$25 kg/m^2) but none of the men and only 9% of the women were obese (body mass index $\geq$30 kg/m^2). Thus, only 4% of these Amish adults were obese compared with about 30% of the US adult population.

I wear a step counter pedometer also every day and I average about 7,500 steps daily. Most of that is simply walking around the large Baylor University Medical Center. I try not to eat between meals or at bedtime and eat desserts sparingly. I also try to avoid the white starches. In contrast, these Amish men and women, who average 18,000 or 14,000 steps daily, eat meat, potatoes, gravy, cakes, pies, and eggs. But they are moving on their feet all day. Each 2,000 steps averages 1 mile. The men are walking about 9 miles on average each day and the women, about 7 miles each day. Each mile uses about 100 calories. The men by their walking alone use up 900 calories daily and the women, 700 calories daily. Vigorous and moderately vigorous physical activity eats up even more calories. The Amish appear to be more modern than we give them credit for. All of us need to acquire some Amish habits.

A piece in *Obesity Research* evaluated state-by-state expenditures related to weight problems.[2] States spend an average of about 5% of their health care dollars for medical costs on obesity-related disease. California is number 1, spending nearly $8 billion annually or 5.5% of its total medical spending. Texas is third, spending $4.3 billion on obesity-related problems or 6.1% of its total medical spending. Obesity costs the US about $40 billion a year or about $175 per person in health care related expenditures. Maybe the best way for the US to decrease its health care costs is for each 1 of us to lose $\geq$10 pounds. Ideal body weight is the most healthful thing for any of us. The most attractive dress and the most handsome suit is ideal body weight! By losing weight, our blood cholesterol, our blood pressure, and our blood sugar drop. Thus, we decrease our chance of getting atherosclerotic diseases, high blood pressure and all its consequences (particularly stroke and aortic dissection), and diabetes mellitus with all of its consequences. Those of us in the health care arena need to set the example. When doctors quit smoking, the lay public noticed. Setting ideal body weight examples for patients might be the best medicine of all.

William C. Roberts

William Clifford Roberts, MD
Editor in Chief
Baylor Heart & Vascular Institute
Baylor University Medical Center
Dallas, Texas

1. Bassett DR Jr, Schneider PL, Huntington GE. Physical activity in an Old Order Amish Community. *Med Sci Sports Exercise* 2004;36:79–85.
2. Costs of obesity. *Advocacy Weekly*, January 26, 2004.

Over-the-Counter Statin Drug

The statin drugs are the most effective drugs ever created for preventing and arresting atherosclerosis, the biggest killer of adults in the Western World. Indeed, it can be said that the statin drugs are to atherosclerosis what penicillin was to infectious disease. The first statin, namely, lovastatin (Mevacor), was introduced in the USA in 1987, and subsequently, 6 others (pravastatin, simvastatin, fluvastatin, atorvastatin, cerivastatin [withdrawn 4 years later], and rosuvastatin) have appeared. Several 2-, 3-, and 5-year studies have shown that these drugs are enormously effective in preventing first and repeat atherosclerotic events. Despite the proven effectiveness of these drugs, they are underutilized in patients with proven atherosclerotic events, in patients with diabetes mellitus, and in subjects with particular risks of developing these events. A group particularly neglected for this therapy are subjects whose serum low-density lipoprotein (LDL) cholesterol is from 130 to 170 mg/dl and who are free of an atherosclerotic event and of diabetes mellitus. An estimated 18 million Americans are at this risk level and are eligible for lipid-lowering therapy. Unfortunately, only about 4 million of them are currently on lipid-lowering therapy.

Three randomized controlled mega trials now unequivocally demonstrate reduction in risk of atherosclerotic events in primary prevention: the West of Scotland Coronary Atherosclerosis Prevention Study (WOSCOPS), the Air Force/Texas Coronary Atherosclerosis Prevention Study (AFCAPS/Tex CAPS), and the Anglo-Scandinavian Cardiac Outcomes Trial (ASCOT); these trials also show that these drugs are quite safe (rhabdomyolysis in 1/10,000 users).

In an attempt to fill this treatment gap in patients at low to moderate risk, 2 pharmaceutical companies (Johnson & Johnson/Merck and Bristol Myers Squibb [BMS]) have approached the Federal Drug Administration (FDA) regarding the possibility of making available a statin drug for over-the-counter (OTC) use. In 1998, the Mevacor OTC Board of Advisors of Johnson & Johnson/Merck was formed.* This advisory board has met biannually since 1998. The first switch application was submitted to the FDA in 1999 for lovastatin 10 mg and (by BMS) for pravastatin 10 mg. The FDA's Advisory Committee in July 2000 recommended further study of consumer behavior and more proof of benefit in the target population.

As a consequence of the compelling AFCAPS/Tex CAPS data, which included 6,605 intermediate risk patients (10-year risk for coronary heart disease of ≤20% and ≥2 atherosclerotic risk factors) treated with 20 to 40 mg/day of lovastatin and resulted in a 37% relative risk reduction for a first major coronary event, the Mevacor OTC group, with input from the FDA, recommended increasing the OTC lovastatin dose to 20 mg daily for low to moderate risk populations based on the National Cholesterol Education Committee's Adult Treatment Panel III guidelines. Additionally, Mevacor Self-Management System was developed to educate and guide appropriate consumer behavior.

The result was the CUSTOM trial, which is described in detail in this issue. The CUSTOM trial in essence demonstrates that most consumers appropriately chose whether or not to use Mevacor OTC, that most users achieved beneficial lipid lowering with lovastatin 20 mg (comparable to that seen in randomized controlled clinical trials), that most consumers appropriately managed their treatment over time, that the Mevacor OTC Self-Management System generated large numbers of consumer interactions with health care professionals (as directed by the label), that heart-healthy lifestyle behaviors (diet and exercise) were maintained or improved, and that consumers can safely manage their use of Mevacor OTC over time.

While the CUSTOM study was being reviewed for publication, simvastatin (Zocor) 10 mg became available to the public in the United Kingdom without a prescription. The UK government hopes making it easier for individuals to acquire a low-cost statin (<$1.00 per day) will increase the drug's use and reduce cardiovascular mortality and morbidity in that nation. The UK is the first nation to approve over-the-counter statin availability. If lovastatin is approved for OTC use in the USA, it will be the first drug approved in this manner for *long-term* use, not for an acute condition. I hope the FDA in 2005 will look favorably for OTC statin therapy also in the USA.

William C. Roberts

William Clifford Roberts, MD*
Editor in Chief
Baylor Heart & Vascular Institute
Baylor University Medical Center
Dallas, Texas

*WCR serves on the Mevacor OTC Board of Advisors of Johnson & Johnson/Merck and has done so since 1998. He also has served in an advisory capacity to Pfizer for selected studies. He has received grants in the past from Parke-Davis (Pfizer) and Bristol-Myers-Squibb. He is on the teaching faculties of several pharmaceutical companies, including Merck, Merck/Schering Plough, Schering Plough, Pfizer, and AstraZeneca. He does not own stock in any pharmaceutical or medical device company.

Managing Patients With High Blood Pressure Before the Introduction of Antihypertensive Drugs

The seventh report of the Joint National Committee on Prevention, Detection, Evaluation, and Treatment of High Blood Pressure listed 66 antihypertensive drugs with 27 combinations (24 with a diuretic) for treating patients with systemic hypertension.[1] The first effective drugs for lowering an elevated blood pressure came in the 1950s—thiazide diuretics, rauwolfia alkaloids, ganglion blockers, and sympathetic antagonists. So how were patients with elevated blood pressures managed before that time? My father, Stewart R. Roberts (1878 to 1941),[2] authored an article on hypertension in 1936 and devoted 1 page to its management.[3] Under the subheading "Treatment of Essential Hypertension," he wrote the following:

> "...There is no drug that once and for all will break the grip of the vasomotor center on its subservient nerves and reduce a high pressure to a normal pressure. There is no method of living and no diet that will do this. The best we can do is to attempt to control the blood pressure with an attitude of mind, a poise, an external and internal calmness, reasonable food, sedative drugs and perhaps vasodilators from time to time. The treatment of essential hypertension is no simple matter. An inflamed appendix can be cut out and removed and the patient and the surgeon are through with it forever, but an essential hypertension is a functional evil of vascular mechanics that the victim has to live with and his physician has to do the best he can with. The following are guiding points:
>
> 1. Peace, poise and contentment of mind. Go slow and go easy each day. Avoid the drive toward a far-off triumph as riches, power, position and scholarship. Have a great faith. Be more content with life. And make less effort for the things of life. Do the day's work and after that one has only to live until bedtime.
>
> 2. Stabilize the emotions. Keep them under control. Every emotion, however good, is to be retained within the high inclosure of peace. This is a high art. The emotions of happiness as well as the emotions of evil are to remain within reasonable bounds. Hypertension itself certainly stimulates the emotions, nervousness, anger, resentment, elation and sometimes consternation. "Let sleeping dogs lie." Close the back door. Be done with the past. Let your emotions sit on the front porch and look to the rising sun.
>
> 3. Put chains on the instinct. Leave fear and preservation to the gods. Be neither on the defensive nor on the offensive. One is a long time dead. And one is still alive. Be on good terms with the instinct of hunger. Do not worry about what you shall eat nor what you shall drink. The details are relatively unimportant. The quantity and the mass are very important. Slowly bring your weight to normal, if one is fat. Be reasonable at the table, not over active. Push your chair back after you have eaten to live. Seek pleasure elsewhere than at the table. Let the third instinct of sex be within reasonable bounds. Nature may aid you here anyway. Be more thinking and considerate of yourself and less instinctive.
>
> 4. Care for your body, not for your desires. The pressure falls during sleep and rest and before a good fire on a winter night. Go to bed sooner and go elsewhere less. A 20 minute warm tub bath at bedtime and a long night's sleep are hard to improve upon. A nap after lunch of 30 minutes to an hour, and train yourself to it, may cause a drop of 5 to 30 mm. from the morning tension. Walking is your best exercise, avoiding shortness of breath. Hurry and worry will undo all else. Horseback riding is not bad; lifting is.
>
> Something that sooths—an automobile ride, a book is another, a game is another. Open bowels daily, and drink water and eat fruits freely. If you can draw in some of your efforts, do so. Go home sooner and leave your work where you work. Tobacco is a vasoconstrictor and is to be avoided.
>
> 5. There are four drugs that appear useful. The most useful treatment is rarely mentioned. This is the example, the teaching, the strength, the influence and the psychotherapy of an understanding physician. He may not be able to reduce the patient's blood pressure to any great degree, but he can reduce the patient to that life of poise that will enable him to withstand his pressure. Sometimes this is more important than reducing the pressure, particularly if it is all that can be done. (a) A sedative is valuable. Phenobarbital in half-grain doses at bedtime or after meals or after lunch and supper, or in larger individuals a grain at bedtime is a psychic sedative, slightly sleep producing, of several hours' influence and is invaluable. (b) Chloral hydrate in doses of 5 to 10 grains at bedtime or twice daily is useful for variable periods. It lacks the cumulative influence of the bromides and in these doses has no depressing influence upon the heart. (c) Of vasodilators there are two that are often of aid: erythrol tetranitrate in one-half grain doses (30 mg.) or nitroglycerin in 1/200 grain doses (0.3 mg.) are safe, can be taken for long periods and do permit some vasodilation. One of these may be given after breakfast and after supper, or once daily at bedtime. The nitroglycerin in this small dose is best given after meals. It does not cause headaches and it does take the edge off the tension of the circulation. Bleeding at intervals aids some extreme cases. Finally, when the symptoms of an insidious heart strain begin, the activities and the efforts of the patient should be restricted to a smaller circle. As these increase the circle of activity decreases, until finally the third stage with heart failure demands a treatment for angina or for cardiac asthma or for congestive

heart failure or for nephritis or for cerebral hemorrhage as indicated in the individual case."

William Clifford Roberts, MD
Editor in Chief
Baylor Heart and Vascular Institute
Baylor University Medical Center
Dallas, Texas

1. Joint National Committee. The seventh report of the Joint National Committee on Prevention, Detection, Evaluation, and Treatment of High Blood Pressure (JNC-7 Express). *JAMA* 2003;289:2560–2571.
2. Roberts CS. Life and Writings of Stewart R. Roberts, MD. Georgia's First Heart Specialist. 1993:138.
3. Roberts SR. Hypertension. *J Med Assoc Georgia* 1936;25:413–417.

Systemic Hypertension: Some Observations

An article from this pen 30 years ago provided some evidence that systemic hypertension was a greater risk factor for development of other cardiovascular diseases than previously indicated.[1] That evidence was primarily increased cardiac mass (>350 g in adult women; >400 g in adult men) in a very high percentage of patients with non-traumatic sudden death; angina pectoris; acute myocardial infarction and certain of its complications (rupture, left ventricular aneurysm, mitral regurgitation); fusiform, saccular and dissecting aneurysm of the aorta; cerbrovascular accidents; renal failure; and many cases of aortic valve stenosis and mitral anular calcium. These earlier observations have been reinforced subsequently.

It is estimated in the USA that there are about 65 million adults with systemic hypertension, 15 million who have survived ≥1 coronary events, 17 million with diabetes mellitus, 5 million with heart failure, 5 million with strokes, and 8 million with atrial fibrillation. Thus, more adults in the USA have elevated (>140/90 mm Hg) systemic blood pressure (BP) than all the patients with coronary heart disease, diabetes mellitus, heart failure, strokes, and atrial fibrillation combined. Yet, other than hyperlipidemia (low-density lipoprotein cholesterol >100 mg/dl), elevated systemic arterial BP is our most common cardiovascular condition, proper treatment of which prevents or certainly sharply decreases strokes, aortic dissections, both systolic and diastolic heart failure, and chronic renal failure.

In the late 1970s, of every 100 US adults with high BP, only 50 knew that they had it, only 30 of the 50 received ≥1 antihypertensive drugs, and only 15 of the 30 being treated had their BP "controlled" (<140/90 mm Hg).[2] Today, awareness, treatment, and control are not much better: of every 100 with elevated BP, 70 are aware that they have it, 50 are receiving therapy, and 30 are controlled, a 50% increase in the "control" group in the last 30 years, but still 70% are receiving inadequate antihypertensive therapy or none at all.[2–4]

Complications of elevated BP begin to arise when the BP passes 115/75 mm Hg.[2] For every 20 mm Hg increase in the peak systolic pressure or 10 mm Hg increase in the end-diastolic pressure, the complication rate (stroke, heart failure, renal failure, aortic dissection) doubles. Thus, at 135/85 mm Hg, the risk is 2 times that at 115/75 mm Hg and yet that level is considered "normal." At 155/95 mm Hg, the risk increases 4 times and at 175/105 mm Hg, the risk is 8 times that at the 115/75 mm Hg level. It is much less expensive to treat high BP than to treat a stroke, or heart or renal failure, or aortic dissection.

In the Western World, the systolic BP tends to rise with age such that by age 60, 50% of Americans have a systolic pressure >140 mm Hg, and by age 100, 90% have an elevated systolic pressure.[5,6] In other words, one's age minus 10% generally indicates the percent of older individuals in the USA with systolic hypertension. The diastolic BP works in the opposite way. Most persons <50 years of age with hypertension have the diastolic form, i.e., diastolic BP >90 mm Hg. From age 50 to 60 years the diastolic BP tends to level off, and after age 60 it tends to gradually decline. Because in older individuals the systolic BP tends to increase progressively with age and the diastolic BP tends to decrease progressively with age, the pulse pressure, the difference between the peak systolic and the end diastolic systemic BP, tends to rise progressively with age.

Although many studies have shown the systolic BP to be more predictive of untoward events (stoke, heart failure, renal failure, aortic dissection) than the diastolic BP, most studies examining the effects of "controlling" BP by ≥1 antihypertensive agents have focused on the diastolic rather than the systolic BP. (The Federal Drug Administration until the last decade or so also insisted on using the diastolic BP as the marker of a drug's effectiveness, despite the finding in the Framingham study >30 years ago showing the systolic pressure to be more predictive of untoward events than was the diastolic BP.) Indeed, after the systolic BP, the pulse pressure is more predictive of untoward events and the diastolic BP, the least predictive.[2]

Although a blood pressure of 140/90 mm Hg has been used as the cut off between normal and elevated BP, the BP level, just like the low-density-lipoprotein cholesterol level, is a continium, the higher the level, the greater the risk. The systemic BP at birth is about 90/60 mm Hg, a level often characterized in adults in the USA as "shock", but in societies where no salt is eaten, or at least the salt level is so low that it cannot be measured, the BP does not rise with age and remains at about 90/60 mm Hg throughout life. Thus, a systolic BP of 140 mm Hg is 36% higher than what our systolic BP probably should be. Fittingly, the Joint National Committee (JNC) on prevention, detection, evaluation and treatment of high BP (JNC 7) defined "normal" BP as that <120/<80 mm Hg.

Many things we do in living our lives effect our BP.[7] Weighing too much, smoking cigarettes, eating high-fat and high sodium calories, drinking alcohol and caffeine, stress, and taking non-steroidal anti-inflammatory medications all raise our BP. In contrast, bed rest, sleep, losing weight, relaxation, exercise, vegetarian-fruit (fiber) diet, garlic, omega-3 polyunsaturated fatty acids, potassium, magnesium, vitamin C, marital harmony, and owning a pet all lower our BP.

Although systolic hypertension is more common than diastolic hypertension, the latter is far more easily controlled by antihypertensive drugs than is the systolic pressure. Isolated systolic hypertension (>160/<90 mm Hg) (stage 2 hypertension[2]) is particularly resistant to control and, with few exceptions, requires ≥2 antihypertensive drugs.

The JNC 7 report[2] published May 21, 2003—a splendid document—lists 66 individual oral antihypertensive agents and 27 combination oral antihypertensive agents containing 2 drugs in 1 pill. Of the 27 combinations, 24 contain a diuretic as 1 of the 2 drugs and the other 3 include a calcium antagonist with either an angiotensin-converting enzyme inhibitor or an angiotensin receptor blocker. The latter 3 combinations can lower the systolic BP about 30 mm Hg and the diastolic BP about 15 mm Hg. Few patients with hypertension can have the elevated BP "controlled" (<140/90 mm Hg) with a single antihypertensive drug; most require ≥2 drugs. The type(s) of drug(s) chosen is not nearly as important as administering ≥1 drug and convincing patients that the best anti-stroke, anti-heart failure insurance is taking the antihypertensive drug(s) every day. And 70% of the hypertensive patients in the USA are not being "controlled." We all can do better.

William Clifford Roberts, MD
Editor in Chief
Baylor Heart and Vascular Institute
Baylor University Medical Center
Dallas, Texas

1. Roberts WC. The hypertensive diseases. Evidence that systemic hypertension is a greater risk factor to the development of other cardiovascular diseases than previously suspected. *Am J Med* 1975;59:523–532.
2. Chobanian AV, Bakris GL, Black HR, Cushman WC, Green LA, Izzo JL, Jones DW, Materson BJ, Oparil S, Wright JT Jr., Roccella EJ, and the National High Blood Pressure Education Program Coordinating Committee. The seventh report of the Joint National Committee on Prevention, Detection, Evaluation, and Treatment of High Blood Pressure. *JAMA* 2003;289:2560–2572.
3. Burt VL, Whelton P, Roccella EJ, Brown C, Jeffrey A, Higgins M, Horan MJ, Labarthe D. Prevalence of hypertension in the US adult population: results from the third National Health and Nutrition Examination Survey, 1988–1991. *Hypertension* 1995;25:305–313.
4. Lloyd-Jones DM, Evans JC, Larson MG, O'Donnell CJ, Roccella EJ, Levy D. Differential control of systolic and diastolic blood pressure. Factors associated with lack of blood pressure control in the community. *Hypertension* 2000;36:594–599.
5. Franklin SS, Gustin W IV, Wong ND, Larson MG, Weber MA, Kannel WB, Levy D. Hemodynamic patterns of age-related changes in blood pressure: the Framington Heart Study. *Circulation* 1997;96:308–315.
6. Sagie A, Lason MG, Levy D. The natural history of borderline isolated systolic hypertension. *N Engl J Med* 1993;329:1912–1917.
7. Kaplan KM. Kaplan's Clinical Hypertension. 8th Ed. Philadelphia: Lippincott Williams & Wilkins, 2002:550.

Atherosclerosis: Its Cause and Its Prevention

I recently spoke at a university hospital and began the presentation by asking the audience to name the atherosclerotic risk factors. Various members of the audience spoke up, and the following was the order in which the risk factors were announced. I wrote them on the flip chart (easel) I used for the presentation: (1) family history, (2) diabetes mellitus, (3) cigarette smoking, (4) high blood pressure, (5) inactivity, (6) overweight, (7) aging, (8) malism, and (9) increased serum cholesterol. I then asked if atherosclerosis was a multifactorial disease or a unifactorial one. The answer universally was multifactorial. I then went down the list of 9 risk factors asking the same question of each, "Does this factor have to be present for atherosclerosis to occur?" The answer for each was "No" except for the last one, namely, hypercholesterolemia. But if that is the case, why was abnormal cholesterol not mentioned as #1 rather than #9? I have experienced the same scenario on many occasions. I believe a strong case can be made for there being a single absolute atherosclerotic risk factor and that atherosclerosis does not occur when that factor is missing.[1] Of course, all of these factors are determined by how they are defined; therefore, the definitions of each are crucial.

Although present in many patients, a family history of cardiovascular disease, however, that is defined, is certainly not necessary. When in medical school, I was taught that atherosclerosis was a degenerative disease, the consequence of living on planet Earth. Certainly that is not the case. Although more common in older people, young adults are not immune to atherosclerotic events. And men do not have a monopoly on plaques. Cardiovascular disease is the most common cause of death in women residing in the Western World. Juvenile diabetes mellitus (type 1) is a genetic problem: type 2 diabetes is a consequence of excessive weight, and cholesterol numbers are virtually never normal (to be defined later) in that situation. Cigarette smoking and/or elevated blood pressures are frequent in some societies where atherosclerotic events are rare. Exercise is quickly nullified by stopping at a fast-food outlet (meaning quick plaques) on the way home from the run. Although most patients with atherosclerotic events are overweight, an increased waist measurement is not a requirement for plaques to form.

Evidence That Cholesterol Causes Atherosclerosis

If *dyslipidemia* is the cause of atherosclerosis what evidence might be presented to the jury that indeed cholesterol is the villain? In my view, there are 4 facts supporting the proposition that cholesterol is the cause of atherosclerosis.[2]

(1) Atherosclerosis is easily produced in non-human herbivores (e.g., rabbits, monkeys) by feeding them a high cholesterol (e.g., egg yokes) or high saturated fat (e.g., animal fat) diet. These studies initially were done by some Russian physiologists beginning nearly 100 years ago.[3,4] And atherosclerosis was not produced in a minority of rabbits fed these diets. No, it was produced in 100% of the animals! Indeed, atherosclerosis is one of the easiest diseases to produce experimentally, but the experimental animal must be an herbivore. It is not possible to produce atherosclerosis in a carnivore, with one exception, and that is in carnivores who have hypothyroidism due to thyroidectomy. The only condition I can think of which is easier to produce experimentally than atherosclerosis is an endocrine deficiency. If the thyroid gland is removed, the consequence is hypothyroidism unless the thyroid hormone is replaced.

In contrast to feeding cholesterol and/or saturated fat, it is not possible to produce atherosclerotic plaques in herbivores by raising the blood pressure chronically or by blowing cigarette smoke in their faces for their entire lifetimes, or by somehow raising their blood glucose levels without simultaneously feeding an atherogenic diet. Few audiences I speak to remember the absolute ease with which atherosclerosis can be produced experimentally.

Although presently it is commonly stated that "atherosclerosis is an inflammatory disease," I am unconvinced that inflammation or infection actually play a role in the production of atherosclerotic plaques.[5–8] Inflammatory cells are infrequent in plaques of coronary arteries studied at necropsy or in endarterectomy specimens. When present, the few mononuclear cells, even giant cells, appear to be a reaction to the deposits of lipid (pultaceous debris) present in the plaque. "Inflammation" appears to be a surrogate for elevation of serum C-reactive protein or various cytokines (interleukins-1 and-6, tumor necrosis factor, etc.), not for inflammatory cells in plaques. Thus, it is a definition situation, and the morphologic definition of inflammation is not applicable.

(2) Cholesterol is present in the plaques. Several studies in the 1930s nicely demonstrated that experimentally produced plaques in herbivores were similar to plaques in humans.[9,10]

(3) Populations with relatively high serum cholesterol levels compared to populations with relatively low serum cholesterol levels have a much higher frequency of atherosclerotic events, a much higher frequency of dying from these events, and a much greater quantity ("burden") of

plaque in their arteries. This factor was nicely supplied by the 7-Countries study[11] *and the Framingham study among others.*[12,13]

(4) Lowering serum total cholesterol and low-density lipoprotein (LDL) cholesterol levels decrease first and repeat atherosclerotic events.[14–31] *Additionally, plaque size may decrease.*[32–34]

In my view, the connection between cholesterol elevation and atherosclerotic plaques is clear and well established.[2] Atherosclerosis is a cholesterol problem! If one has elevated cholesterol and also has an elevated blood pressure, or smokes cigarettes, or has an elevated blood sugar, these additional factors serve to amplify the cholesterol damage but they by themselves do not produce arterial plaques! Societies with a high frequency of systemic hypertension or a high frequency of cigarette smoking but low serum cholesterol levels rarely get atherosclerosis.

Differences Between Herbivores and Carnivores

Because humans get atherosclerosis, and atherosclerosis is a disease only of herbivores, humans also must be herbivores.[35] Most humans, of course, eat flesh, but that act does not make us carnivores. Carnivores and herbivores have different characteristics. (1) The *teeth* of carnivores are sharp; those of herbivores, flat (humans have some sharp teeth but most are flat for grinding the fruits, vegetables, and grains we are built to eat). (2) The *intestinal tract* of carnivores is short (about 3 times body length); that of herbivores, long (about 12 times body length). (Since I am 6 feet tall my intestinal tract should be about 60 feet long. As a consequence if I eat bovine muscle [steak], it could take 5 days to course through those 20 yards.) (3) *Body cooling* for carnivores is done by panting because they have no ability to sweat; although herbivores also can pant, they cool their bodies mainly by sweating. (4) *Drinking fluids* is by lapping them for the carnivore; it is by sipping them for the herbivore. (5) *Vitamin C* is made by the carnivore's own body; herbivores obtain their ascorbic acid only from their diet. Thus, although most human beings think we are carnivores or at least conduct their lives as if we were, basically humans are herbivores. If we could decrease our flesh intake to as few as 5 to 7 meals a week our health would improve substantially.

Conditions Uncommon in Human Non-Flesh Eaters

Some extremely common conditions in the Western World are relatively uncommon in purely or predominately vegetarian-fruit eating societies.[36–39] These include: (1) *severe atherosclerosis* and its devastating consequences (heart attacks, brain attacks, etc.)[40,41]; (2) *systemic hypertension*: in societies who eat not enough salt for it to be measurable, the systemic arterial blood pressure is usually about 90/60 mm Hg, a level near what it is at birth, but a level in the Western World often associated with shock[42–48]; (3) *stroke*[49]; (4) *obesity*[50]; (5) *diabetes mellitus*[51–53]; (6) *some common cancers* (colon, breast, prostate gland)[54–69]; (7) *constipation, cholecystitis, gallstones, appendicitis, diverticulosis, hemorrhoids, inguinal hernia, varicose veins*[70,71]; (8) *renal stones*[72]; (9) *osteoporosis* and *osteoarthritis*[73–76]; (10) *salmonellosis* and *trichinosis*; and (11) *cataracts and macular degeneration.*[77,78]

Cholesterol Numbers Needed to Prevent and Arrest Atherosclerotic Plaques

The guidelines for cholesterol modifying therapy published in 1988, 1993, and 2001, and modified subsequently, brought some rationale into the arena of who should and who should not be treated with "life-style changes" and/or lipid-lowering drugs or both.[79–83] These guidelines, however, were based exclusively on the concept of "decreasing risk" of events, not decreasing the formation of plaques. Because atherosclerosis is rarely genetic in origin (1 in 500),[84] and because the pharmaceutical industry has provided us with truly miracle drugs for lowering serum LDL cholesterol levels, it is time to switch gears from the concept of decreasing risk of atherosclerotic events to actual prevention of atherosclerotic plaques.[85] To make this change the guideline-recommended numbers must be lowered substantially.

According to the published guidelines, initiation of lipid-modifying drug therapy should be based on the serum LDL cholesterol level and the presence or absence of other atherosclerotic risk factors.[79–82] Lipid-lowering drug therapy is recommended in persons with only 1 or no non-LDL cholesterol risk factors if the LDL cholesterol is >190 mg/dl with a goal of <160 mg/dl. But, the most common LDL cholesterol number in people with heart attacks is about 140 mg/dl so this recommendation is not "preventive." If >1 non-LDL-cholesterol risk factor is present then the LDL cholesterol drug-treatment number is >160 mg/dl with the goal of <130 mg/dl. If a patient has a coronary event, however (or is at high risk of an atherosclerotic event, such as having diabetes mellitus or a previous non-coronary atherosclerotic event), the LDL cholesterol goal is <100 mg/dl (with an "option" of <70 mg/dl).[83] If it is useful for the LDL cholesterol to be <100 mg/dl *after* a heart attack, surely it must be useful for the LDL cholesterol to be <100 mg/dl *before* a heart attack! Therefore, in my view, the goal for all populations—not just those with heart or brain attacks or diabetes mellitus or non-coronary atherosclerotic events—needs to be LDL cholesterol <100 mg/dl and ideally <70 mg/dl. If such a goal was created, the great scourge of the Western World would be essentially eliminated, "primary" and "secondary" prevention would be the same, and >100 million Americans—rather than the present 13 million—would need to be on a statin drug with or without ezetimibe or be pure vegetation-fruit eaters.

Thus, although not clearly established at this time, to prevent atherosclerotic plaques, the serum LDL cholesterol needs to be <70 mg/dl, the serum total cholesterol certainly <150 mg/dl, and the high-density lipoprotein (HDL) cholesterol >20 mg/dl. The latter—surely a surprise to most readers—is in patients with a serum total cholesterol level of about 130 mg/dl, and a LDL cholesterol level about 60 mg/dl. Exactly what HDL cholesterol level is required to prevent plaques is unclear at this time, but clearly if the LDL cholesterol is very low (e.g., 50 mg/dl) then a low HDL cholesterol—as long as it is >20 mg/dl—appears not to be dangerous. Ideal may be equal serum HDL and LDL cholesterol levels or a HDL cho-

Table 1
Statins and their equivalent efficacious doses, their effects on total (TC) and low-density lipoprotein (LDL) cholesterol, and effect on LDL cholesterol by ezetimibe alone and in combination with a statin

Statin (mg)									
Rosuvastatin Crestor®	Atorvastatin Lipitor®	Simvastatin Zocor®	Lovastatin Mevacor®	Pravastatin Pravacol®	Fluvastatin Lescol®	↓ TC‡	↓ LDL‡	↓ LDL by Ezetimibe 10 mg	Total LDL ↓ by Statin + Ezetimibe 10 mg‡
1.25*	5	10	20	20	40	22%	27%	18%	45%
2.5†	10	20	40	40	80	27%	34%	18%	52%
5	20	40	80	80	—	32%	41%	14%	55%
10	40	80	—	—	—	37%	48%	12%	60%
20	80	—	—	—	—	42%	55%	10%	65%
40	—	—	—	—	—	47%	60%	10%	70%

* Not available.
† The 2.5-mg tablet is available in Japan but not in other countries.
‡ These reductions are ±3%.

lesterol greater than LDL cholesterol. In summary, the recommended guideline numbers—particularly those for primary prevention—are those for decreasing the risk of atherosclerosis events, not for preventing formation of atherosclerotic plaques.

The Rule of 5 and the Rule of 7 in Lipid-Lowering Therapy and the Goal for All

The statin drugs, in my view, are the best cardiovascular drugs ever created, in that they have the greatest potential to prevent atherosclerotic plaques and their complications, and they also have the greatest potential to arrest plaque formation, and therefore, to prevent additional atherosclerotic events. The statin drugs are to atherosclerosis what penicillin was to infectious diseases.[86] Despite their being truly miracle drugs, they are terribly underutilized and underdosed.

The average serum LDL cholesterol level in American adults is about 130 mg/dl. Therefore, if we want to prevent plaque formation in the USA, most of us will need a 50% LDL cholesterol reduction! As shown in Table 1, that goal can be achieved by 3 doses of statin monotherapy (rosuvastatin 20 and 40 mg daily or atorvastatin 80 mg daily) or by adding ezetimibe 10 mg to all statin doses except the lowest level of recommended statin doses.[87] Because titration is often neglected, starting the dose from the beginning that achieves the preventive goal (LDL cholesterol <70 mg/dl) appears reasonable. Most American adults have life insurance, which, in actuality, is death insurance. The insured pays for the policy, dies, and then someone else gets the money. The statin drugs–with or without ezetimibe–represent true life insurance. The taker of the drug lives longer and is able to provide for his/her family longer. They are safe.[88–105] (Myopathy occurs 1 in 10,000 persons.) The risk of taking the drug is far less than the atherosclerotic consequences that might occur from not taking the drug! Of course, a vegetarian-fruit diet is the least expensive and safest means of achieving the plaque-preventing LDL goal, but few in the Western World are willing to live on the herbivore diet[106,107] If we did so, however, we would prevent the daily killing in the USA of 100,000 cows, of 300,000 pigs, and of 15 to 20 million chickens!

Conclusion

Thanks to the pharmaceutical industry, we now have the armamentarium to change our cardiovascular health. We will not do so by waiting to treat our serum LDL cholesterol levels until an atherosclerotic event occurs or by using guidelines such as LDL cholesterol >190 or >160 mg/dl before lipid-lowering drug therapy is initiated. The blowing up of balloons or the placing of stents in our arteries or the performing of bypass operations (with all of their damaging incisions [e.g., median sternotomy]) can be prevented or their need enormously reduced if the statin drugs ± ezetimibe are utilized in proper doses to produce serum LDL cholesterol levels low enough where atherosclerotic plaques do not form. Life insurance policies are often purchased by individuals in their 20s. Statin drugs ± ezetimibe can be started at the same time because they—along with antihypertensive drugs—represent true life insurance. And to smoke cigarettes or to eat excess calories or not to put on a seatbelt in an automobile or airplane or to ride a motorcycle or not to control our cholesterol numbers is simply not to use our brain as it was intended to be used!

William Clifford Roberts, MD
Baylor Heart & Vascular Institute
Baylor University Medical Center
Dallas, Texas

1. Roberts WC. Atherosclerotic risk factors—are there ten or is there only one? *Am J Cardiol* 1989;64:552–554.
2. Roberts WC. Factors linking cholesterol to atherosclerotic plaques. *Am J Cardiol* 1988;62:495–499.
3. Anitschkow N, Chalatow S. On experimental cholesterin steatosis and its significance in the origin of some pathological processes. *Centralbl f allg Path u path Anat* 1913;24:1–9.
4. Anitschkow N. Experimental atherosclerosis in animals. In Arteriosclerosis: A Survey of the Problem. E.V. Cowdry, editor. Macmillan, New York. 1933:271–322.
5. Ridker PM, Cushman M, Stampfer MJ, Tracy, RP, Hennekens CH. Inflammation, aspirin, and the risk of cardiovascular disease in apparently healthy men. *N Engl J Med* 1997;336:973–979.
6. Ridker PM, Rifai N, Pfeffer MA, Sacks FM, Moye LA, Goldman S, Flaker GC, Braunwald E, for the Cholesterol and Recurrent Events (CARE) Investigators. Inflammation, pravastatin, and the risk of coronary events after myocardial infarction in patients with average cholesterol levels. *Circulation* 1998;98:839–844.

7. Ross R. Atherosclerosis: an inflammatory disease. *N Engl J Med* 1999;340:115–126.
8. Ridker PM, Rifai N, Rose L, Buring JE, Cook NR. Comparison of C-reactive protein and low-density lipoprotein cholesterol levels in the prediction of first cardiovascular events. *N Engl J Med* 2002;347: 1557–1565.
9. Leary T. Experimental atherosclerosis in the rabbit compared with human (coronary) atherosclerosis. *Arch Path* 1934;17:453–492.
10. Leary T. Atherosclerosis, the important form of atherosclerosis, a metabolic disease. Eleventh Ludrig Hektoen Lecture of the Frank Billings Foundation of the Institute of Medicine of Chicago. *JAMA* 1935;105:475–481.
11. Keys A. SEVEN COUNTRIES. A Multivariate Analysis of Death and Coronary Heart Disease. Cambridge, Massachusetts: Harvard University Press 1980:381.
12. Kannel WB, Castelli WP, Gordon T, McNamara PM. Serum cholesterol, lipoprotein, and the risk of coronary heart disease: the Framingham study. *Ann Intern Med* 1971:74:1–12.
13. Castelli WP. Epidemiology of coronary heart disease: The Framingham Study. *Am J Med* 1984;76(2A):4–12.
14. Miettinen M, Turpeinen O, Karvonen MJ, Elosuo R, Paavilainen E. Effects of cholesterol-lowering diet on mortality from coronary heart-disease and other causes: a twelve-year clinical trial in men and women. *Lancet* 1972;2:835–838.
15. Turpeinen O. Effect of cholesterol-lowering diet on mortality from coronary heart disease and other causes. *Circulation* 1979;59:1–7.
16. Multiple Risk Factor Intervention Trial Research Group. Multiple risk factor intervention trial: risk factor changes and mortality results. *JAMA* 1982;248:1465–1477.
17. From the Lipid Metabolism-Atherogenesis Branch, National Heart, Lung, and Blood Institute, Bethesda, MD. The Lipid Research Clinics Coronary Primary Prevention Trial Results. 1. Reduction in incidence of coronary heart disease. *JAMA* 1984;251:351–364.
18. The Lipid Research Clinics Coronary Primary Prevention Trial Results. 1. The relationship of reduction in incidence of coronary heart disease to cholesterol lowering. *JAMA* 1984;251:365–374.
19. Frantz ID Jr, Dawson EA, Ashman PL, Gatewood LC, Bartsch GE, Kuba K, Brewer ER. Test of effect of lipid lowering by diet on cardiovascular risk: the Minnesota Coronary Survey. *Arteriosclerosis* 1989;9:129–135.
20. Scandinavian Simvastatin Survival Study Group. Ramdomised trial of cholesterol lowering in 4444 patients with coronary heart disease; the Scandinavian Simvastatin Survival Study (4S). *Lancet* 1994;334: 1383–1389.
21. Shepherd J, Cobbe SM, Ford I, Isles CG, Lorimer AR, MacFarlane PW, McKillop JH, Packard CJ, for the West of Scotland Coronary Prevention Study Group. Prevention of coronary heart disease with pravastatin in men with hypercholesterolemia. *N Engl J Med* 1995; 333:1301–1307.
22. Sacks FM, Pfeffer MA, Moye LA, Rouleau JL, Rutherford JD, Cole TG, Brown L, Warnica JW, Arnold JMO, Wun CC, David BR, Braunwald E, for the Cholesterol and Recurrent Events Trial Investigators. The effect of pravastatin on coronary events after myocardial infarction in patients with average cholesterol levels. *N Engl J Med* 1996;335:1001–1009.
23. The Long-Term Intervention with Pravastatin in Ischaemic Disease (LIPID) Study Group. Prevention of cardiovascular events and death with pravastatin in patients with coronary heart disease and a broad range of initial cholesterol levels. *N Engl J Med* 1998;339:1349–1357.
24. Downs JR, Clearfield M, Weis S, Whitney E, Sharpiro DR, Beere PA, Langendorfer A, Stein EA, Kruyer W, Gotto AM Jr, for the AF-CAPD/TexCAPS Research Group. Primary prevention of acute coronary events with lovastatin in men and women with average cholesterol levels: results of AFCAPS/TexCAPS. *JAMA* 1998;279:1615–1622.
25. LaRosa JC, He J, Vupputuri S. Effect of statins on risk of coronary disease: a meta-analysis or randomized controlled trials. *JAMA* 1999; 282:2340–2346.
26. Gotto AM Jr, Whitney E, Stein EA, Shapiro DR, Clearfield M, Weis S, Jou JY, Langendorfer A, Beere PA, Watson DJ, Downs Jr, De Cani JS. Relation between baseline and on-treatment parameters and first acute major coronary events in the Air Force/Texas Coronary Atherosclerosis Prevention Study (AFCAPS/TexCAPS). *Circulation* 2000;101:477–484.
27. Heart Protection Study Collaborative Group. MRC/BHF Heart Protection Study of cholesterol-lowering with simvastatin in 20,536 high-risk individuals: a randomized placebo-controlled trial. *Lancet* 2002;360:7–22.
28. Heart Protection Study Collaborative Group. MRC/BHF Heart Protection Study of cholesterol-lowering with simvastatin in 5963 people with diabetes: a randomized placebo-controlled trial. *Lancet* 2003; 361:2005–2016.
29. Sever PS, Dahlof B, Poulter NR, Wedel H, Beevers G, Caulfield M, Collins R, Kjeldsen SE, Kristinsson A, McInnes GT, Mehlsen J, Nieminen M, O'Brien E, Ostergren J, ASCOT Investigators. Prevention of coronary and stroke events with atorvastatin in hypertensive patients who have average or lower-than-average cholesterol concentrations, in the Anglo-Scandinavian Cardiac Outcomes Trial-Lipid Lowering Arm (ASCOT-LLA): a multicentre randomized controlled trial. *Lancet* 2003;361:1149–1158.
30. Collin R, Armitage J, Parish S, Sleight P, Peto R, for the Heart Protection Study Collaborative Group. Effects of cholesterol-lowering with simvastatin on stroke and other major vascular events in 20,536 people with cerebrovascular disease or other high-risk conditions. *Lancet* 2004;363:757–767.
31. Cannon CP, Braunwald E, McCabe CH, Rader DJ, Rouleau JL, Belder R, Joyal SV, Hill KA, Pfeffer MA, Skene AM. Pravastatin or Atorvastatin Evaluation and Infection Therapy—Thrombolysis in Myocardial Infarction 22 Investigators. Intensive versus moderate lipid lowering with statins after acute coronary syndromes. *N Engl J Med* 2004;350:1495–1504.
32. Nissen SE, Tuzcu EM, Schoenhagen P, Brown BG, Ganz P, Vogel RA, Crowe T, Howard G, Cooper CJ, Brodie B, Grines CL, DeMaria AN, for the REVERSAL Investigators. Effect of intensive compared with moderate lipid-lowering therapy on progression of coronary atherosclerosis: a randomized controlled trial. *JAMA* 2004;291:1071–1080.
33. Nissen SE, Tuzcu EM, Schoenhagen P, Crowe T, Sasiela WJ, Tsai J, Orazem J, Magorien RD, O'Shaughnessy C, Ganz P, for the Reversal of Atherosclerosis with Aggressive Lipid Lowering (REVERSAL) Investigators. Statin therapy, LDL cholesterol, C-reactive protein, and coronary artery disease. *N Engl J Med* 2005;352:29–38.
34. Nissen SE, Nicholls SJ, Sipahi I, Libby P, Raichlen JS, Ballantyne CM, Davignon J, Erbel R, Fruchart JC, Tardif J, Schoenhagen P, Crowe T, Cain V, Wolski K, Goormastic M, Tuzcu EM, for the ASTEROID Investigators. Effect of very high-intensity statin therapy on regression of coronary atherosclerosis. The ASTEROID Trial. *JAMA* 2006;295;13:E1–E10.
35. Roberts WC. We think we are one, we act as if we are one, but we are not one. *Am J Cardiol* 1990;66:1402.
36. Steiner PE. Necropsies on Okinawans. Anatomic and pathologic observations. *Arch Pathol* 1946;42:359–380.
37. Eaton SB, Konner M, Shostak M. Stone Agers in the fast lane: chronic degenerative diseases in evolutionary perspective. *Am J Med* 1988;84:739–749.
38. McCullough ML, Feskanich D, Stampfer MJ, Rosner BA, Hu FB, Hunter DJ, Vriyam JN, Colditz GA, Willett WC. Adherence to the dietary guidelines for Americans and risk of major chronic disease in women. *Am J Clin Nutr* 2000;72:1214–1222.
39. McCullough ML, Feskanich D, Rimm EB, Giovannucci EL, Ascherio A, Variyam JN, Spiegelman D, Stampfer MJ, Willett WC. Adherence to the dietary guidelines for Americans and risk of major chronic disease in men. *Am J Clin Nutr* 2000;72:1223–1231.
40. Law MR, Morris JK. By how much does fruit and vegetable consumption reduce the risk of ischaemic heart disease? *Eur J Clin Nutr* 1998;52:549–556.
41. Hu FB, Stampfer MJ, Manson JE, Rimm EB, Colditz GA, Speizer FE, Hennekens CH, Willett WC. Dietary protein and risk of ischemic heart disease in women. *Am J Clin Nutr* 1999;70:221–227.
42. Obarzanek E, Velletri PA, Cutler JA. Dietary protein and blood pressure. *JAMA* 1961;275:1598–1603.
43. Oliver WJ, Cohen EL, Neel JV. Blood pressure, sodium intake and sodium related hormones in the Yanomamo Indians, a "no-salt" culture. *Circulation* 1975;52:146–151.
44. Meneely GR, Battarbee HD. High sodium-low potassium environment and hypertension. *Am J Cardiol* 1976;38:768–785.

45. Antonios TT, MacGregor GA. Deleterious effects of salt intake other than effects on blood pressure. *Clin Exp Pharmacol Physiol* 1995; 22:180–184.
46. Stamler J, Caggiula A, Grandits GA, Kjelsberg M, Cutler JA. Relationship to blood pressure of combinations of dietary macronutrients. Findings of the Multiple Risk Factor Intervention Trial (MRFIT). *Circulation* 1996;94:2417–2423.
47. MacGregor GA, deWardner HE. Salt, Diet and Health. Neptune's Poisoned Chalice: The Origins of High Blood Pressure. Cambridge, UK: Cambridge University Press 1998:233.
48. Washburn S, Burke GL, Morgan T, Anthony M. Effect of soy protein supplementation on serum lipoproteins, blood pressure, and menopausal symptoms in perimenopausal women. *Menopause* 1999;6:7–13.
49. Joshipura KJ, Ascherio A, Manson JE, Stampfer MJ, Rimm EB, Speizer FE, Hennekens CH, Spiegelman D, Willett WC. Fruit and vegetable intake in relation to risk of ischemic stroke. *JAMA* 1999; 282:1233–1239.
50. Must A, Apadano J, Coakley EH, Field AE, Golditz G, Dietz WH. The disease burden associated with overweight and obesity. *JAMA* 1999;282:1523–1529.
51. O-Dea K, Traianedes K, Ireland P, Niall M, Sadler J, Hopper J, DeLuise M. The effects of diet differing in fat, carbohydrate, and fiber on carbohydrate and lipid metabolism in type 2 diabetes. *J Am Diet Assoc* 1989;89:1076–1086.
52. Feskens EJ, Bowles CH, Krombout D. Inverse association between fish intake and risk of glucose intolerance in normoglycemic elderly men and women. *Diabetes Care* 1991;14:935–941.
53. Salmeron J, Manson JE, Stampfer MJ, Colditz GA, Wing AL, Willett WC. Dietary fiber, glycemic load, and risk of non-insulin-dependent diabetes mellitus in women. *JAMA* 1997;277:472–477.
54. Mills PK, Annegers JR, Phillips RL. Animal product consumption and subsequent fatal breast cancer risk among Seventh-day Adventists. *Am J Epidemiol* 1988;127:440–453.
55. Block G, Patterson B, Subar A. Fruit, vegetables, and cancer prevention: a review of the epidemiological evidence. *Nutr Cancer* 1992; 18:1–29.
56. Hunter DJ, Willett WC. Diet, body size, and breast cancer. *Epidemiol Rev* 1993;15:110–132.
57. Ames BN, Gold LS, Willett WC. The causes and prevention of cancer. *Proc Natl Acad Sci USA* 1995;92:5258–5265.
58. Willett WC, Hunter DJ. Prospective studies of diet and breast cancer. *Cancer* 1994;74(3 suppl):1085–1089.
59. Martin-Moreno JM, Willett WC, Gorgojo L, Banegas JR, Rodriguez-Artalejo F, Fernandez-Rodrigues JC, Maisonneuve P, Boyle P. Dietary fat, olive oil intake and breast cancer risk. *Int J Cancer* 1994; 58:774–780.
60. Yuan JM, Wang QS, Ross RK, Henderson BE, Yu MC. Diet and breast cancer in Shanghai and Tianjin, China. *Br J Cancer* 1995;71: 1353–1358.
61. Jacobs DR Jr, Marquart L, Slavin J, Kushi LH. Whole grain intake and cancer: an expanded review and meta-analysis. *Nutr Cancer* 1998;30:85–96.
62. Giovannucci E, Rimm EB, Wolk A, Ascherio A, Stampfer MJ, Colditz GA, Willett WC. Calcium and fructose intake in relation to risk of prostate cancer. *Cancer Res* 1998;58:442–447.
63. Norrish AE, Skaeff CM, Arribas GL, Sharpe SJ, Jackson RT. Prostate cancer risk and consumption of fish oils: a dietary biomarker-based case-control study. *Br J Cancer* 1999;81:1238–1242.
64. Holmes MD, Stampfer MJ, Colditz, GA, Rosner B, Hunter DH, Willett WC. Dietary factors and the survival of women with breast carcinoma. *Cancer* 1999;86:826–835.
65. Holmes MD, Hunter DJ, Colditz GA, Stampfer MJ, Hankinson SE, Speizer FE, Rosner B, Willett WC. Association of dietary intake of fat and fatty acids with risk of breast cancer. *JAMA* 1999;281:914–920.
66. Zhang S, Hunter DJ, Hankinson SE, Giovannucci EL, Rosner BA, Golditz GA, Speizer FE, Willett WC. A prospective study of folate intake and the risk of breast cancer. *JAMA* 1999;281:1632–1637.
67. Franceschi S, Favero A. The role of energy and fat in cancers of the breast and colon-rectum in a southern European population. *Ann Oncol* 1999;10(suppl 6):61–63.
68. Fuchs CS, Giovannucci EL, Colditz GA, Hunter DJ, Stampfer MJ, Rosner B, Speizer FE, Willett WC. Dietary fiber and the risk of colorectal cancer and adenoma in women. *N Engl J Med* 1999;340:169–176.
69. Michels KB, Giovannuci E, Joshipura KJ, Rosner BA, Stampfer MJ, Fuchs CS, Colditz GA, Speizer FE, Willett WC. Prospective study of fruit and vegetable consumption and incidence of colon and rectal cancers. *J Natl Cancer Insti* 2000;92:1740–1752.
70. Sweeney M. Constipation: diagnosis and treatment. *Home Care Provid* 1997;2:250–255.
71. Aldoori WH, Giovannucci EL, Rockett HR, Sampson L, Rimm EB, Willett WC. A prospective study of dietary fiber types and symptomatic diverticular disease in men. *J Nutr* 1998;128:714–719.
72. Curhan GC, Willett WC, Rimm EB, Spiegelman D, Stampfer MJ. Prospective study of beverage use and the risk of kidney stones. *Am J Epidemiol* 1996;143:240–247.
73. Cummings SR, Nevitt MC, Browner WS, Stone K, Fox KM, Ensrud KE, Cauley J, Black D, Vogt TM. Risk factors for hip fracture in white women. Study of Osteoporotic Fractures Research Group. *N Engl J Med* 1995;332:767–773.
74. Feskanich D, Willett WC, Stampfer MJ, Colditz GA. Protein consumption and bone fractures in women. *Am J Epidemiol* 1996;143: 472–479.
75. Munger RG, Cerhan JR, Chiu BC. Prospective study of dietary protein intake and risk of hip fracture in postmenopausal women. *Am J Clin Nutr* 1999;69:147–152.
76. Tucker KI, Hannan MT, Chen H, Cupples LA, Wilson PW, Kiel DP. Potassium, magnesium, and fruit and vegetable intakes are associated with greater bone mineral density in elderly men and women. *Am J Clin Nutr* 1999;69:727–736.
77. Sommerburg O, Keunen JE, Bird AC, van Kuijk FJ. Fruits and vegetables that are sources for lutein and zeaxanthin: the macular pigment in human eyes. *Br J Ophthalmol* 1998;82:907–910.
78. Jacques PF. The potential preventive effects of vitamins for cataract and age-related macular degeneration. *Int J Vitam Nutr Res* 1999;69: 198–205.
79. National Cholesterol Education Program. Report of the NCEP Expert Panel on Detection, Evaluation, and Treatment of High Blood Cholesterol in Adults. *Arch Intern Med* 1988;148:36–39.
80. Expert Panel on Detection, Evaluation, and Treatment of High Blood Cholesterol in Adults. Summary of the second report of the National Cholesterol Education Program (NCEP) Expert Panel on Detection, Evaluation, and Treatment of High Blood cholesterol in Adults (Adult Treatment Panel II). *JAMA* 1993;269:3015–3023.
81. Sempos CT, Cleeman JL, Carroll MD, Johnson CL, Bachorik PS, Gordon DJ, Burt VL, Briefel RR, Brown CD, Lippel K, Rifkind BM. Prevalence of high blood cholesterol among US adults. An update based on guidelines from the second report of the National Cholesterol Education Program Adult Treatment Panel. *JAMA* 1993;269: 3009–3014.
82. Executive Summary of the Third report of the National Cholesterol Education Program (NCEP) Expert Panel on Detection, Evaluation, and Treatment of High Blood Cholesterol in Adults (Adult Treatment Panel III). *JAMA* 2001;285:2486–2497.
83. Grundy SM, Cleeman JL, Merz CN, Brewer HB Jr, Clark LT, Hunninhake DB, Pasternak RC, Smith SC Jr, Stone NJ, for the Coordinating Committee of the National Cholesterol Education Program. Implications of recent clinical trials for the National Cholesterol Education Program Adult Treatment panel III guidelines. *Circulation* 2004;110:227–239.
84. Brown MS, Goldstein JL. How LDL receptor influence cholesterol and atherosclerosis. *Sci Amer* 1984;251(5)58–66.
85. Roberts WC. Shifting from decreasing risk to actually preventing and arresting atherosclerosis. *Am J Cardiol* 1999;83:816–817.
86. Roberts WC. The underused miracle drugs. The statin drugs are to atherosclerosis what penicillin was to infectious disease. *Am J Cardiol* 1996;78:377–378.
87. Roberts WC. The rule of 5 and the rule of 7 in lipid-lowering by statin drugs. *Am J Cardiol* 1997;80:106–107.
88. Davidson MH, Stein EA, Hunninghake DB, Ose L, Dujovne CA, Insull W Jr, Bertolami M, Weiss SR, Kastelein JJ, Scott RS, Campodonico S, Escobar ID, Schrott HG, Bays H, Stepanavage ME, Wu M, Tate AC, Melino MR, Kush D, Mercuri M, Mitchel YB. Lipid-altering efficacy and safety of simvastatin 80 mg/day: worldwide long-term experience in patients with hypercholesterolemia. *Nutr Metab Cardiovasc Dis* 2000;10:253–262.

89. Grundy SM. Can statins cause chronic low-grade myopathy (editorial)? *Am Intern Med* 2002;137:617–618.
90. Ballantyne CM, Corsini A, Davidson MH, Holdaas H, Jacobson TA, Leitersdorf E, Marz W, Reckless JP, Stein EA. Risk for myopathy with statin therapy in high-risk patients. *Arch Intern Med* 2003;163: 553–564.
91. Jones PH, Davidson MH, Stein EA, Bays HE, McKenney JM, Miller E, Cain VA, Blasetto JW. Comparison of the efficacy and safety of rosuvastatin versus atorvastatin, simvastatin and pravastatin across doses (STELLAR Trial). *Am J Cardiol* 2003;92:152–160.
92. Thompson PD, Clarkson P, Karas RH. Statin-associated myopathy. *JAMA* 2003;289:1681–1690.
93. Sheperd J, Hunninghake DB, Stein EA, Kastelein JJP, Harris S, Pears J, Hutchinson HG. Safety of Rosuvastatin. *Am J Cardiol* 2004;94: 882–888.
94. Ballantyne CM, Blazing MA, King TR, Brady WE, Palmisano J. Efficacy and safety of ezetimibe co-administered with simvastatin compared with atorvastatin in adults with hypercholesterolemia. *Am J Cardiol* 2004;93:1487–1494.
95. Grundy SM. The issue of statin safety: where do we stand? *Circulation* 2005;111:3016–3019.
96. Alsheikh-Ali AA, Ambrose MS, Kuvin JT, Karas RH. The safety of rosuvastatin as used in common clinical practice: a postmarketing analysis. *Circulation* 2005;111:3051–3057.
97. Waters DD. Safety of high-dose atorvastatin therapy. *Am J Cardiol* 2005;96(suppl):69F–75F.
98. Davidson MH, Clark JA, Glass LM, Kanumalla A. Statin safety: an appraisal from the adverse event reporting system. *Am J Cardiol* 2006;97(suppl):32C–43C.
99. Thompson PD, Clarkson PM, Rosenson RS. An assessment of statin safety by muscle experts. *Am J Cardiol* 2006;97(suppl):69C–76C.
100. Cohen DE, Anania FA, Chalasani N. An assessment of statin safety by hepatologists. *Am J Cardiol* 2006;97(suppl):77C–81C.
101. Kasiske BL, Wanner C, O'Neill WC. An assessment of statin safety by nephrologists. *Am J Cardiol* 2006;97(suppl):82C–85C.
102. McKenney JM, Davidson MH, Jacobson TA, Guyton JR. Final conclusions and recommendations of the National Lipid Association Statin Safety Assessment Task Force. *Am J Cardiol* 2006;97(suppl): 89C–94C.
103. Ferdinand KC, Clark LT, Watson KE, Neal RC, Brown CD, Kong BW, Barnes BO, Cox WR, Zieve FJ. Isaacsohn J, Ycas J, Sager PT, Gold A, for the ARIES Study Group. Comparison of efficiacy and safety of rosuvastatin versus atorvastatin in African-American patients in a six-week trial. *Am J Cardiol* 2006;97:229–235.
104. Jones PH, Davidson MH, Reporting rate of rhabdomyolysis with fenofibrate + statin versus gemfibrozil + any statin. *Am J Cardiol* 2005;95:120–122.
105. Ornish D. Can life-style changes reverse coronary atherosclerosis? *Hosp Pract* 1991;26:(5):123–126, 129–132.
106. Leaf A. Dietary prevention of coronary heart disease: The Lyon Diet Heart Study. *Circulation* 1999;99:733–735.
107. Denke MA. Diet, lifestyle, and nonstatin trials: review of time to benefit. *Am J Cardiol* 2005;96(suppl):3F–10F.

Evaluating Lipid-Lowering Trials in the Twenty-First Century

It's these large, multicenter, double-blind, often placebo-controlled clinical trials that have the greatest impact on how medicine now is practiced. With lipid-lowering drugs, the trials are of 2 basic types: (1) the outcome trials, listed in Table 1,[1–11] and (2) the imaging trials, listed in Table 2.[12–17]

To evaluate such a trial appropriately, it is important to know the number of subjects and/or patients in the trial; their age and gender distributions; whether or not there was preexisting cardiovascular disease, diabetes mellitus, renal disease, valvular heart disease, or none of these; the length of the study; whether the study was or was not stopped early; whether the study drug was compared with placebo, with another drug, or simply with a lower dose of the same drug; the doses of the drug or drugs studied; the end points of the trial; the percentages of events (in outcome trials) in the study and control groups; the absolute and relative differences in the percentages of events between groups at the end of the study period; and the baseline and final serum lipid values in the study patients and the controls.

The outcome trials usually involve several thousand patients, who are followed usually for 2 to 5 years, and have primary end points that usually include various combinations of cardiovascular death, all-cause death, nonfatal acute myocardial infarction, stroke, hospitalization for unstable angina pectoris, and revascularization (percutaneous coronary intervention, coronary artery bypass grafting, and/or peripheral arterial procedures). These trials are usually very expensive and usually sponsored by single pharmaceutical companys. At least 11 major outcome trials have been published during the present decade (Table 1).

In contrast to the outcome trials, the imaging trials (Table 2) involve far fewer patients (usually <1,000), followed for a far shorter time period, and as a consequence, they are far less expensive. Those reported have focused on the coronary artery (intravascular ultrasonic imaging) or on the carotid artery (intima-media thickness [IMT]) and the change in plaque volume (on intravascular ultrasound) or in IMT in millimeters from baseline to the end of the trial.

The initial results of the major lipid-lowering trials are usually published in the major general medical journals. Each of the 17 trials briefly summarized in Tables 1 and 2 were published in the *New England Journal of Medicine* (7 trials), *JAMA* (6 trials), or *The Lancet* (4 trials). Because these journals are provided to the press shortly before publication, the results of major trials appear in the news media across the country, and the first appearance of the results of the trials for many physicians is in the media. Most media reports of trials focus on the single trial whose results have just appeared and do not give the necessary perspective of the new trials results compared with similar previous trial publications. And it is crucial not to draw absolute conclusions from single trials!

Three trials in recent times have received particular, and in my view unwarranted, attention. One was the Ezetimibe and Simvastatin in Hypercholesterolemia Enhances Atherosclerosis Regression (ENHANCE) trial, an imaging (carotid IMT) trial comparing simvastatin 80 mg plus ezetimibe 10 mg with simvastatin 80 mg in 720 patients followed for a mean of 2 years after the baseline IMT study.[16] All patients had baseline low-density lipoprotein (LDL) cholesterol levels >300 mg/dl. (Most physicians do not have a single patient in their practices with a baseline LDL cholesterol level that high!) The LDL cholesterol level in the combination-therapy group decreased from 319 to 141 mg/dl (a 56% decrease), and that in the simvastatin-only group decreased from 318 to 193 mg/dl (a 39% decrease). There was no significant difference in mean carotid IMT or in events between the 2 treatment groups.

The ENHANCE trial was presented at the Annual Scientific Sessions of the American College of Cardiology, with virtually no debate after presentation. Its publication prompted a committee of the American College of Cardiology to recommend using ezetimibe only as a lipid-lowering agent of last resort, preferring higher dose statins, niacin, fibrates, and bile acid resins before prescribing ezetimibe. This recommendation, in my view, loses sight of the lipid-lowering goal, which is maximal benefit with minimal risk. There is no evidence to date that ezetimibe (for which approximately 80% is not absorbed from the gut) is hazardous. At the lower doses of statins, ezetimibe provides an average 18% further reduction in serum LDL cholesterol, and thus it is a "statin-sparing" drug. And the side effects of statins are dose related: the higher the dose, the greater the potential for side effects. In contrast to the average 18% additional reduction with ezetimibe 10 mg, colestipol can also provide an 18% reduction in LDL, but it requires a dose of 30,000 mg to achieve the same percentage reduction, and cholestyramine at 24,000 mg/day will also give an 18% average LDL reduction. When a 10-mg tablet will give the same LDL reduction as multiple pills amounting to 30,000 or 24,000 mg, it is obvious which drug is preferable. Thank you, "expert committee," but I will stay with ezetimibe, with its good efficiency and safety and lack of side effects.

Numerous editorials followed in various medical journals.[18–25] Many physicians switched many patients away from Vytorin (Merck/Schering-Plough Pharmaceuticals, Whitehouse Station, New Jersey), the combination of ezetimibe and simvastatin in 1 pill, and almost certainly, the number and percentage of patients lowering their LDL cholesterol to

Table 1
Cardiovascular outcome studies with lipid-lowering agents in the first decade of the 21st century

								Events			Mean LDL-C (mg/dl)			
											Patients		Controls	
Study	Year of Publication	Journal of Publication	No. of Subjects	Subjects	Age (yrs)	Length of Study (yrs)	Comparison Agents (mg)	Patients	Control	Relative Risk Reduction	Baseline	End	Baseline	End
MIRACL[1]	2001	*JAMA*	3,086	ACS	Mean 65	0.31	A 80 vs P	14.80%	17.40%	↓16%	124	72	124	135
HPS[2]	2002	*Lancet*	20,526	CAD, PVD, stroke, DM	40–80	5	S 40 vs P	7.60%	9.10%	↓17%	131	90	131	129
ASCOT-LLA[3]	2003	*Lancet*	10,305	SH	40–79	Median 3.3*	A10 vs P	1.90%	3.00%	↓31%	133	90	133	126
PROVE-IT[4]	2004	*NEJM*	4,162	ACS	Mean 58	Mean 2	A 80 vs pravastatin 40	19.7%	22.3%	↓14%	106	62	106	95
CARDS[5]	2004	*Lancet*	3,838	DM	40–75	Median 3.9*	A 10 vs P	9.4%	13.4%	↓37%	117	81	117	120
A to Z[6]	2004	*JAMA*	4,497	ACS	Mean 61	0.5–2	S 40 to S 80 vs P to S 20	14.4%	16.7%	↓11%†	112	66	111	81
TNT[7]	2005	*NEJM*	10,001	CAD, PVD, stroke, DM	Mean 61	Median 4.9	A 80 vs A 10	8.7%	10.9%	↓22%	97	77	98	97
IDEAL[8]	2005	*JAMA*	8,888	MI	<80	Median 4.8	A 80 vs S 20	9.3%*	10.4%*	↓11%†	122	81	121	104
SPARCL[9]	2006	*NEJM*	4,731	Stroke, TIA	Mean 63	Median 4.9	A 80 vs P	11.2%	13.1%	↓16%	133	43	134	129
SEAS[10]	2008	*NEJM*	1,873	AS	Mean 67	Median 4.3	S 40 + E 10 vs P	35.3%	38.2%	↓9%†	140	75	139	134
JUPITER[11]	2008	*NEJM*	17,802	Healthy	Median 66	Median 1.9*	R 20 vs P	0.016%	0.028%	↓47%	108	55	108	109

A = atorvastatin; ACS = acute coronary syndrome; AS = aortic stenosis; CAD = coronary artery disease; DM = diabetes mellitus; LDL = low-density lipoprotein cholesterol; MI = myocardial infarction; P = placebo; PVD = peripheral vascular disease; R = rosuvastatin; S = simvsatatin; SH = systemic hypertension; TIA = transient ischemia attack.

* Stopped early - Study planned for 5 years.

† Not significant.

Table 2
Imaging studies in the first decade of the 21st century using statin drugs

									Plaque Change			LDL-C (mg/dl)			
												Patients		Controls	
Study	Year of Publication	Journal of Publication	Type Study	Artery Studied	No. of Subjects	Mean Age (yrs)	Length of Study (yrs)	Comparison Agents (mg)	Patients	Control	Type of Patients	Baseline	End	Baseline	End
ASAP[12]	2001	*Lancet*	IMT	Carotid	325	30–70	2	A 80 vs S 40	↓0.031% (mm^3)	↑0.036% (mm^3)	FH	309	150	322	187
REVERSAL[13]	2005	*NEJM*	IVUS	Coronary	502	56	1.5	A 80 vs pravastatin 40	↓0.2% (mm^3)	↑5.1% (mm^3)	CAD*	150	79	150	110
ASTEROID[14]	2006	*JAMA*	IVUS	Coronary	349	58	2	R 40 vs P	↓0.98% (mm^3)	—	CAD*	130	61	—	—
METEOR[15]	2007	*JAMA*	IMT	Carotid	984	37	2	R 40 vs P	↓0.0014% (mm)	↑0.0131% (mm)	Healthy	155	78	154	152
ENHANCE[16]	2008	*NEJM*	IMT	Carotid	720	48	2	S 80 + E 10 vs S 80	↓0.0111% (mm)	↑0.0058% (mm)	FH	319	141	318	193
SANDS[17]	2008	*JAMA*	IMT	Carotid	499	56	3	Aggressive vs standard	↓0.012% (mm)	↑0.038% (mm)	DM	104	72	104	104

A = atorvastatin; CAD = coronary artery disease; DM = diabetes mellitus; FH = familial hypercholesterolemia; IMT = intimal medial thickness; IVUS = intravascular ultrasonic imaging; LDL = low-density lipoprotein cholesterol; P = placebo; R = rosuvastatin; S = simvastatin.

* By angiogram.

<100 or <70 mg/dl decreased. Maximum benefit was eliminated by a perceived lack of benefit!

Now, why was the ENHANCE trial a negative one? There has been considerable public discussion of this point. I believe the difference between the 2 arms—simvastatin 80 mg plus ezetimibe 10 mg versus simvastatin 80 mg—was not great enough in the 2 years of the study to show IMT regression or lack of progression when the IMTs of the carotid arteries at baseline were essentially normal. Two preceding carotid IMT trials, each also 2 years in duration, had shown significant difference in the primary end points. In Antioxidant Supplementation in Atherosclerosis Prevention (ASAP),[12] the same patients were studied, but the potency difference between the study drug (atorvastatin 80 mg) and the control drug (simvastatin 40 mg) was 4 times, and in Measuring Effects on Intima-Media Thickness: An Evaluation of Rosuvastatin (METEOR),[15] rosuvastatin 40 mg (its maximal dose) was compared with placebo! In the ENHANCE trial, the potency difference between the study group (simvastatin 80 mg plus ezetimibe 10 mg) and the control group (simvastatin 80 mg) was inadequate. If the dose of simvastatin in the control group had been 20 or 40 mg, the study may have shown positive results, and there would not have been such commotion in the medical and media communities.

On January 8, 2009, the United States Food and Drug Administration's safety review committee reported that it had completed its review of the ENHANCE trial comparing Vytorin with Zocor (simvastatin; Merck & Company, Whitehouse Station, New Jersey) and concluded that it supported the continued use of Vytorin.[26] Pending the results of the Improved Reduction of Outcomes: Vytorin Efficacy International Trial (IMPROVE-IT), involving 18,000 patients and expected to be completed in 2012, the agency advised that "based on currently available data, patients should not stop taking Vytorin or other cholesterol lowering drugs."

A more recent trial, Simvastatin and Ezetimibe in Aortic Stenosis (SEAS), showed a slight increase in cancer (105 vs 70 cases) during the median 4.3 years of the trial, and that of course led to a safety scare.[10] This outcome trial involved patients with valvular aortic stenosis: 333 received simvastatin 40 mg plus ezetimibe 10 mg versus placebo. The trial failed to show slowed progression of aortic stenosis in the treatment group and also showed no reduction in events due to aortic stenosis (although it did show a decrease in myocardial ischemic events). The mean age of patients in this trial was 67 years. Aortic stenosis in this age group is associated with heavy calcific deposits, and it seems unlikely that lipid lowering at this stage would be beneficial. In contrast, lipid-lowering therapy in a 20-year-old patient with a bicuspid aortic valve might prove useful in preventing or delaying the development of aortic stenosis. The cancer scare caused by the results of this trial was of course attributed to ezetimibe, because none of the simvastatin monotherapy trials had shown an increase in cancer. As a consequence, Richard Peto (probably the world's premier statistician) and colleagues[25] compared the incidence of cancer in the SEAS trial of 1,873 patients followed for a mean of 4.1 years with cancer data from 2 large ongoing trials: the Study of Heart and Renal Protection (SHARP), involving 9,264 patients with a mean follow-up so far of 2.7 years, and the IMPROVE-IT trial, currently involving 11,353 patients with a mean follow-up so far of 1 year. In SHARP and IMPROVE-IT combined, there was no overall excess of cancer (313 cases in the treatment group vs 326 cases in the control group) and no particular excess of cancer at any particular site. Peto et al[25] concluded that "the available results from these 3 trials do not provide credible evidence of any adverse effect of ezetimibe on rates of cancer."

The third of the lipid-lowering trials that has received enormous medical and media editorial attention is Justification for the Use of Statins in Primary Prevention: An Intervention Trial Evaluating Rosuvastatin (JUPITER), an outcome trial involving 17,802 apparently healthy men and women (mean age 66 years with serum LDL cholesterol levels <130 mg/dl [mean 108] and high-sensitivity C-reactive protein levels ≥2 mg/dl [median 4.2]).[11] The treatment group received rosuvastatin 20 mg/day (vs placebo). The trial was stopped after 1.9 years (maximum 5). In the treatment group, LDL cholesterol levels were reduced by 50% (to 55 mg/dl) and C-reactive protein levels by 37% (to 1.8 mg/dl). The combined primary end point of myocardial infarction, stroke, arterial revascularization, hospitalization for unstable angina pectoris, or death from cardiovascular causes was reduced by 41%, including a 48% reduction in stroke and a 20% reduction in death from any cause. These are spectacular results and indicate that lowering LDL cholesterol into the range of 50 to 59 mg/dl leads to major reductions quickly in major cardiovascular events and fewer needs for hospitalization or cardiovascular procedures.

How was JUPITER (published in the *New England Journal of Medicine* on November 20, 2008) received by the media? In an unsigned editorial[27] in the *New York Times* on November 17, 2008, titled "Who Should Take a Statin?" the *Times* concluded that "before rushing ahead [giving several million more people statins] it will be crucial to establish who might really benefit. . . . the long-term safety of drastically lowering cholesterol levels [must be established] before committing patients who have no clinical signs of disease to decades of drug treatment." Statins have been available in the United States now for 22 years, and this miracle drug, which actually can and does prevent heart and brain attacks, still is greatly underprescribed and underdosed in millions of people who need it. Statins are the best life insurance against atherosclerotic events ever created, but they are not useful if they are not taken. Only pure vegetarians for practical purposes do not need statins. Most of the rest of us do!

The November 17, 2008, edition of the *New York Times* also included a piece titled "A Call for Caution in the Rush to Statins" by Tara Parker-Pope.[28] She suggested that "statins (like Crestor, from AstraZeneca, and Lipitor, from Pfizer) are far from magic pills. While they clearly save lives in people with a previous heart attack or other serious heart problems, for an otherwise healthy person the potential benefit remains small." Where is she coming from? She went on, "And because of the way the Jupiter results were reported, many healthy people are likely to get an exaggerated view of statins' benefits. While the investigators reported an impressive-sounding [her word] 50 percent reduction in the risk of serious heart problems among the statin users, in reality everyone in the study had a low risk to begin with." But those who took the drug got a much lower risk!

And *USA Today* on February 2, 2009, had its say in a piece titled "That Bad Cholesterol Just Got Worse" by Steve Sternberg.[29] The same critical theme followed. Why keep shooting down a miracle? We all—if we continue our present habits—can choose angioplasty and stents or bypass or lower our LDL drastically. I prefer the latter.

William Clifford Roberts, MD
Baylor Heart and Vascular Institute
Baylor University Medical Center
Dallas, Texas 75246

1. Schwartz GG, Olsson AG, Ezekowitz MD, Ganz P, Oliver MF, Waters D, Zeiher A, Chaitman BR, Leslie S, Stern T. Effects of atorvastatin on early recurrent ischemic events in acute coronary syndromes. The MIRACL Study: a randomized control trial. *JAMA* 2001;285(13):1711–1718.
2. Heart Protection Study Collaborative Group. MRC/BHF Heart Protection Stdy of cholesterol-lowering with simvastatin in 5963 people with diabetes: a randomized placebo-controlled trial. *Lancet* 2003;361:2005–2016.
3. Sever PS, Dahlöf B, Poulter NR, Wedel H, Beevers G, Caulfield M, Collins R, Kjeldsen SE, Kristinsson A, McInnes GT, Mehisen J, Neiminen M, O'Brien E, Östergren J. Prevention of coronary and stroke events with atorvastatin in hypertensive patients who have average or lower-than-average cholesterol concentrations, in the Anglo-Scandinavian Cardiac Outcomes Trial - Lipid Lowering Arm (ASCOT-LLA): a multicentre radomised controlled trial. *Lancet* 2003;361:1149–1158.
4. Cannon CP, Branwald E, MCCabe CH, Rader DJ, Rouleau JL, Belder R, Joyal SV, Hill KA, Pfeffer MA, Skene AM, for the Pravastatin or Atorvastatin Evaluation and Infection Therapy Thrombolysis in Myocardial Infarction 22 Investigators. *N Engl J Med* 2004;350:1495–1504.
5. Colhoun HM, Betteridge DJ, Durrington PN, Hitman GA, Neil HAW, Livingstone SJ, Thomason MJ, Mackness MI, Charleton-Menys V, Fuller JH, on behalf of the CARDS Investigators. Primary prevetion of cardiovascular disease with atorvastatin in type 2 diabetes in the Collaborative Atorvastatin Diabetes Study (CARDS): multicentre randomized placebo-controlled trial. *Lancet* 2004;364:685–696.
6. de Lemos JA, Blazing MA, Wiviott SD, Lewis EF, Fox KAA, White HD, Rouleau JL, Pedersen TR, Gardner LH, Mukherjee R, Ramsey KE, Palmisano J, Bilheimer DW, Pfeffer MA, Califf RM, Braunwald E, for the A to Z Investigators. Early intensive vs a delayed conservative simvastatin strategy in patients with acute coronary syndromes. Phase Z of the A to Z Trial. *JAMA* 2004;292:1307–1316.
7. LaRosa JC, Grundy SM, Waters DD, Shear C, Barter P, Fruchart JC, Gotto AM, Greten H, Kastelein JJP, Shepherd J, Wenger N, for the Treating to New Targets (TNT) Investigators. Intensive lipid lowering with atorvastatin in patients with stable coronary disease. *N Engl J Med* 2005;352:1425–1435.
8. Pedersen TR, Faergeman O, Kastelein JJP, Olsson AG, Tikkanen MJ, Holme I, Larsen L, Bendiksen FS, Lindahl C, Szarek M, Tsai J, for the Incremental Decrease in End Points Through Aggressive Lipid Lowering (IDEAL) Study Group. *JAMA* 2005;294:2437–2445.
9. Amareco P, Bogosslavsky J, Callahan A III, Goldstein LB, Hennerici M, Rudolph AE, Sillesen H, Simunovic L, Szarek M, Welch KMA, Zivin JA. High-dose atorvastatin after stroke or transient ischemic attack. The Stroke Prevention by Aggressive Reduction in Cholesterol Levels (SPARCL) Investigators. *N Engl J Med* 2006;355:549–559.
10. Rossebø AB, Pedersen TR, Boman K, Brudi P, Chambers JB, Egstrup K, Gerdts E, Gohlke-Bärwolf C, Holme I, Kesäniemi YA, Malbecq W, Nienaber CA, Ray S, Skjrpe T, Wachtell K, Willenheimer R, for the SEAS Investigators. Intensive lipid lowering with simvastatin and ezetimibe in aortic stenosis. *N Engl J Med* 2008;359:1343-1356.
11. Ridker PM, Danielson E, Fonseca FAH, Genest J, Gotto AM Jr, Kastelein JJP, Koenig W, Libby P, Lorenzatti AJ, MacFadyen JG, Nordestgaard BG, Shepherd J, Willerson JT, Glynn RJ, for the JUPITER Study Group. Rosuvastatin to prevent vascular events in men and women with elevated C-reactive protein. *N Engl J Med* 2008;359:2195–2207.
12. Smilde TJ, van Wissen S, Wollershein H, Kastelein JJP, Stalenhoef AFH. Effect of aggressive versus conventional lipid lowering on atherosclerosis progression in familial hypercholesterolaeia (ASAP): a prospective, randomized, double-blind trial. *Lancet* 2001;357:577–581.
13. Nissen SE, Tuzcu EM, Schoenhagen P, Crowe T, Sasiela WJ, Tsai J, Orazem J, Magorien RD, O'Shaughnessy C, Ganz P, for the Reversal of Atherosclerosis with Aggressive Lipid Lowering REVERSAL Investigators. Statin therapy, LDL cholesterol, C-reactive protein, and coronary artery disease. *N Engl J Med* 2005;352:29–38.
14. Nissen SE, Nicholls SJ, Sipahi I, Libby P, Raichlen JS, BAllantyne CM, Davignon J, Erbel R, Fruchart JC, Tardif JC, Schoenhagen P, Crowe T, Cain V, Wolski K, Goormastic M, Tuzcu EM, for the ASTEROID Investigators. Effect of very high-intensity statin therapy on regression of coronary atherosclerosis. *JAMA* 2006;295:1556–1565.
15. Crouse JR III, Raichlen JS, Riley WA, Evans GW, Palmer MK, O'Leary DH, Grobbee DE, Bots ML, for the METEOR Trial. Effect of Rosuvastatin on progression of carotid intima-media thickness in low-risk individuals with subclinical atherosclerosis. *JAMA* 2007; 297:1344–1353.
16. Kastelein JJP, Akdim F, Stroes ESG, Zwinderman AH, Bots ML, Stalenhoef AFH, Visseren FLJ, Sijbrands EJG, Trip MD, Stein EA, Gaudet D, Duivenvorden R, Veltri EP, Marais AD, de Groot E, for the ENHANCE Investigators. Simvastatin with or without ezetimibe in familial hypercholesterolemia. *N Engl J Med* 2008;358:1431–1443.
17. Howard BV, Roman MJ, Devereux RB, Fleg JL, Galloway JM, Henderson JA, Howard WJ, Lee ET, Mete M, Poolaw B, Ratner RE, Russell M, Silverman A, Sylianou M, Umans JG, Wang W, Weir MR, Weissman NJ, Wilson C, Yeh F, Zhu J. Effect of lower targets for blood pressure and LDL cholesterol on atherosclerosis in diabetes. The SANDS randomized trial. *JAMA* 2008;299(14):1678–1689.
18. Musunuru K, Blumenthal RS. Another perspective on ENHANCE: What was not discussed and communicated. Cardiology (published by The American College of Cardiology) April 2008:14–17.
19. Adams SL. ENHANCE panel advises cardiologists to use statins, scale back ezetimibe use. CardiologyToday.com May 2008; pg 10.
20. Mitka M. Cholesterol drug controversy continues. *JAMA* 2008; 299(19):2266.
21. Davidson MH. Interpreting the ENHANCE Trial. Is ezetimibe/simvastatin no better than simvastatin along? Lessons learned and clinical implications. *Cleve Clin J Med* 2008;75(7):479–482, 486–488, 490–491.
22. Steinberg D. Simvastatin with or without ezetimibe in familial hypercholesterolemia. *N Engl J Med* 2008;359(5):529–533.
23. Editorial. Intensive lipid intervention in the Post-ENHANCE Era. *Mayo Clin Proc* 2008;83(8):867–869.
24. Toth PP, Maki KC. A commentary on the implications of the ENHANCE (Ezetimibe and Simvastatin in hypercholesterolemia enhances atherosclerosis regression) trial: Should ezetimibe move to the "back of the line" as a therapy for dyslipidemia? *J Clin Lipidol* 2008;2(5):313–317.
25. Peto R, Emberson J, Landray M, Baigent C, Collins R, Clare R, Calif R. Analyses of cancer data from three ezetimibe trials. *N Engl J Med* 2008;359:1357–1366.
26. U.S. Food and Drug Administration. Follow-up to the January 25, 2008 early communication about an ongoing data review for ezetimibe/simvastatin marketed as Vytorin), ezetimibe (marketed as Zetia), and Simvastatin (marketed as Zocor). http://www.fda.gov/cder/drug/early_comm/ezetimibe_simvastatin.html.
27. Editorial. Who Should Take a Statin? New York Times, November 17, 2008.
28. Parker-Pope T. A Call for Caution in the Rush to Statins. New York Times, November 17, 2008.
29. Sternberg S. That bad cholesterol just got worse. USA Today. February 2, 2009.

It's the Cholesterol, Stupid!

During the 1992 presidential campaign in the United States, the Clinton campaign slogan was "It's the economy, stupid" and that phrase apparently was helpful in getting Mr. Clinton elected president. Several recent publications have been highly critical of some lipid-lowering trials using statin drugs and have debased the cholesterol "hypothesis" on atherosclerosis.[1–3]

What is the evidence that "elevated cholesterol" causes atherosclerosis? There are 4 supporting arguments in my view.[4–7] (1) Atherosclerotic plaques are easily produced experimentally in herbivores (e.g., rabbits, monkeys) simply by feeding these animals cholesterol (e.g., egg yolks) or saturated fats. Indeed, atherosclerosis is probably the second easiest disease to produce experimentally. (The first is an endocrine deficiency—simply excise an endocrine gland.) (2) Cholesterol is present in atherosclerotic plaques in experimentally produced atherosclerosis and in plaques in human beings. (3) Societies and subjects with high serum cholesterol levels (total and low-density lipoprotein [LDL] cholesterol) compared to populations and subjects with low levels have a high frequency of atherosclerotic events, a high frequency of dying from these events, and a large quantity (burden) of plaque in their arteries. (The best study in my view supporting this thesis is the Seven-Country study.[8–10]) (4) Lowering total and LDL cholesterol levels decrease the frequency of atherosclerotic events, the chances of dying from these events, and the quantity of plaques in the arteries. No one has produced atherosclerosis experimentally by increasing arterial blood pressure or glucose levels or by blowing smoke in the faces of rabbits their entire lifetime or by stressing these animals. The only way to produce atherosclerosis experimentally is by feeding high-cholesterol and/or high–saturated fat diets to herbivores. (Atherosclerosis is not a disease of carnivores and it is not possible to produce atherosclerosis in carnivores [dogs, cats, tigers, lions, etc.] unless the thyroid gland is removed or made dysfunctional before a high-cholesterol or high–saturated fat diet is administered.[11])

Why has the proved causal relation between abnormal serum LDL cholesterol and atherosclerosis been so difficult to accept by so many extremely intelligent physicians? One factor, in my view, is that this cholesterol–atherosclerosis causal relation has been diluted by the concept of multiple atherosclerotic risk factors and the idea that atherosclerosis is a multifactorial disease. The Framingham study, which has taught us all so much, introduced the concept of "risk factors" and fostered the view that the larger the number of risk factors present, the greater the chance of atherosclerotic events.[12] As a consequence, increased cholesterol became just 1 of several risk factors and was perceived as essentially having no more influence than increased systolic blood pressure, diabetes mellitus ("glucose intolerance"), cigarette smoking, abdominal obesity or lack of regular physical activity, family history, or left ventricular hypertrophy except in younger patients.[13] The view that atherosclerosis is a multifactorial disease has muddled the waters in my view. This is not to say that cigarette smoking, increased blood pressure, diabetes mellitus or obesity, and inactivity are not harmful—of course they are—but if serum LDL cholesterol is <60 mg/dl or serum total cholesterol is <150 mg/dl, there is no evidence (with extremely rare exceptions[14]) in my view that these other risk factors cause atherosclerosis.

A second factor is the introduction and propagation of the thesis that atherosclerosis is an inflammatory disease.[15] Yes, a few mononuclear cells are regularly seen in experimentally produced atherosclerotic plaques but not commonly in plaques of patients with fatal coronary disease or in plaques excised by endarterectomy.[16,17] Yes, some blood inflammatory markers are commonly increased in patients with atherosclerotic events. However, many patients have atherosclerotic events when high-sensitivity C-reactive protein (hs-CRP) is normal (<1 mg/dl) and patients with the highest levels of hs-CRP (e.g., those with rheumatoid arthritis or systemic lupus erythematosus) have only a slightly higher frequency of atherosclerotic events than do others of similar age and gender with normal or near normal hs-CRP levels. The same principle, however, does not apply to cholesterol. Patients with the highest serum levels of total and LDL cholesterol, namely those patients with homozygous familial hypercholesterolemia, have an incredibly high frequency of atherosclerotic events and they have these events at very young ages—teenage years.[18] In addition, patients with the next highest serum LDL cholesterol levels, namely those with heterozygous familial hypercholesterolemia, have atherosclerotic events often in their 30s and 40s.

A third factor preventing acceptance of the causal relation between abnormal serum LDL cholesterol and atherosclerosis has been the observation that of adults with nonfamilial hypercholesterolemia but similar levels of serum LDL cholesterol, some develop atherosclerotic events and others do not. It is in this group particularly in my view that the other risk factors and high-density lipoprotein cholesterol levels come into play. Of 2 patients of similar age and gender and similar serum LDL cholesterol levels, say 130 mg/dl, the patient whose systolic systemic blood pressure is 170 mm Hg versus the other patient with a systolic pressure of 115 mm Hg is at much greater risk of an atherosclerotic event. Cigarette smoking may work in similar fashion. Nevertheless, if serum LDL cholesterol is <60 mg/dl, maybe <50 mg/dl, irrespective of degree of blood pressure increase or number of cigarettes smoked daily, atherosclerotic plaques do not develop.

Another factor may be the use of multiple atherosclerotic risk factors in guidelines for who to treat and who not to treat with lipid-lowering drugs. Although guidelines do focus on serum LDL cholesterol level, the number of other risk factors present play a prominent role in this therapeutic decision.[19] If no other nonlipid risk factors are present or only if 1 non-LDL cholesterol risk factor is present and there have been no previous atherosclerotic events and diabetes mellitus is not present, the magical drug treatment number is an LDL cholesterol ≥190 mg/dl. Refraining from drug intervention until this very high LDL cholesterol level is reached plays down or even nullifies the importance of cholesterol in preventing events. (It is important to realize that the lipid-lowering drug guidelines [1988, 1993, 2001, and 2004] have to do only with decreasing atherosclerotic events. They do not concern themselves with preventing atherosclerotic plaques in the first place. Of course, if atherosclerotic plaques are prevented, atherosclerotic events do not occur!)

Such high guideline drug treatment levels keep, in my view, many patients deserving of lipid-lowering drug therapy from receiving these magical agents.[20] The danger of high cholesterol levels to longevity were recognized by life insurance companies in the 1930s but not by physicians. The normal range of serum total cholesterol in laboratory reports for decades was listed as 150 to 300 mg/dl. In 1972, 1 of the world's most prominent lipidologists reported that his total cholesterol "worry level" for patients was a value >300 mg/dl. If the expert uses such high levels, what importance can be placed on cholesterol by the nonexpert community? Incidentally, for the first several decades of the Framingham study, increased cholesterol was defined as a serum total cholesterol level >250 mg/dl. At this level, it is easy to understand how this risk factor did not separate itself from the others.

It is time to move on from a goal "to decrease risk" to a goal "to prevent plaques."[21] To do so requires much lower levels of LDL cholesterol than advocated by guideline publications. My goal for all subjects worldwide is a serum LDL cholesterol ≤100 mg/dl and ideally <60 mg/dl. The beauty of the Justification for Use of Statins in Prevention: an Intervention Trial Evaluating Rosuvastatin (JUPITER) is that it dramatically demonstrates what incredible decreases in events can be produced in a short period (<2 years) by decreasing LDL cholesterol by 50% even when starting from a level considered by many to be normal (<130 mg). The mean level (108 mg/dl) might be considered "good" or even "great" by many physicians but its lowering to 55 mg/dl (by rosuvastatin 20 mg/dl) decreased all events by >40%, indeed nearly 50%, including a decrease in stroke by 48%! This trial beautifully shows that we can drastically decrease or even prevent atherosclerotic events and expensive procedures by taking a single pill every day and do it safely. Most Americans will not reach JUPITER treatment levels (LDL cholesterol 55 mg/dl) by diet alone. Statin drugs have been ingested by humans for nearly 30 years and their safety and thus benefit/risk ratio may be the best of any proved-useful medication. Toxicity resides mainly in atherosclerosis, not in the drug.

I consider it unfortunate that there continues to be so much criticism of statin drugs, which I consider to be the best cardiovascular drugs ever created.* These drugs can prevent first and subsequent atherosclerotic events, they can lower cardiovascular and all-cause mortality rates, they have the capacity to decrease the quantity of atherosclerotic plaques already present, and by decreasing the frequency of myocardial infarcts they decrease the frequency of heart failure and malignant ventricular arrhythmias. Their ability to decrease serum levels of CRP may have benefits not yet fully appreciated. The discoverer of the first statin drug (Akira Endo, PhD) is deserving of the Nobel Prize for medicine!

The lower the LDL cholesterol, the better, and this principle has been established repeatedly despite voices of the anticholesterol, antistatin fallacy mongers! *It's the cholesterol, stupid*!

William Clifford Roberts, MD
Baylor Heart and Vascular Institute
Baylor University Medical Center
Dallas, Texas

1. Green LA. Cholesterol-lowering therapy for primary prevention: still much we don't know. *Arch Intern Med* 2010;170:1007–1008.
2. Ray KK, Seshasai SR, Erqou S, Sever P, Jukema JW, Ford I, Sattar N. Statins and all-cause mortality in high-risk primary prevention: a meta-analysis of 11 randomized controlled trials involving 65,229 participants. *Arch Intern Med* 2010;170:1024–1031.
3. de Lorgeril M, Salen P, Abramson J, Dodin S, Hamazaki T, Kostucki W, Okuyama H, Pavy B, Rabaeus M. Cholesterol lowering, cardiovascular diseases, and the rosuvastatin–JUPITER controversy: a critical reappraisal. *Arch Intern Med* 2010;170:1032–1036.
4. Roberts WC. Atherosclerotic risk factors: are there ten or is there only one? *Am J Cardiol* 1989;64:552–554.
5. Roberts WC. Atherosclerosis: its cause and its prevention. *Am J Cardiol* 2006;98:1550–1555.
6. Steinberg D. The Cholesterol Wars. The Skeptics vs. the Preponderance of Evidence. Amsterdam: Elsevier, 2007:227.
7. Truswell AS. Cholesterol and Beyond. The Research on Diet and Coronary Heart Disease 1900–2000. Sydney: Springer, 2010:227.
8. Keys A. Seven Countries. A Multivariate Analysis of Death and Coronary Heart Disease. Cambridge, MA: Harvard University Press, 1980:381.

* I have no investments in pharmaceutical or device companies, I receive no grants from them, and I am on no advisory boards of industry. I do, however, give talks periodically sponsored by pharmaceutical companies.

9. Verschurer WM, Jacobs DR, Bloemberg BP, Kromhout D, Menotti A, Aravanis C, Blackburn H, Buzina R, Dontas AS, Fidanza F. Serum total cholesterol and long-term coronary heart disease in different cultures. Twenty-five-year follow-up of the seven countries study. *JAMA* 1995;274:131–136.
10. Kromhout D, Menotti A, Blackburn H, eds. The Seven Countries Study. A Scientific Adventure in Cardiovascular Disease Epidemiology. Bilthoven, The Netherlands: Marjan Nijssen-Kramer, 1993:219.
11. Anitschkow NN. A history of experimentation on arterial atherosis in animals. In: Blumenthal HT, ed. Cowdry's Arteriosclerosis. A Survey of the Problem Springfield, IL: Charles C Thomas, 1967:21–44.
12. Kannel WB, Dawber TR, Kagan A, Revotskie N, Stokes J III. Factors of risk in the development of coronary heart disease—six year follow-up experience. The Framingham Study. *Ann Intern Med* 1961;55: 33–50.
13. Kannel WB, Castelli WP, Gordon T. Cholesterol in the prediction of atherosclerotic disease: new perspectives based on the Framingham Study. *Ann Intern Med* 1979;90:85–89.
14. Mautner SL, Sanchez JA, Rader DJ, Mautner GC, Ferrans VJ, Fredrickson DS, Brewer HB Jr, Roberts WC. The heart in Tangier disease: severe coronary atherosclerosis with near absence of high-density lipoprotein cholesterol. *Am J Clin Pathol* 1992;98:191–198.
15. Libby P, Ridker PM, Maseri A. Inflammation and atherosclerosis. *Circulation* 2002;105:1135–1143.
16. Roberts WC. Qualitative and quantitative comparison of amounts of narrowing by atherosclerotic plaques in the major epicardial coronary arteries at necropsy in sudden coronary death, transmural acute myocardial infarction, transmural healed myocardial infarction and unstable angina pectoris. *Am J Cardiol* 1989;64:324–328.
17. Roberts WC, Turnage TA II, Whiddon LL. Quantitative comparison of amounts of cross-sectional area narrowing in coronary endarterectomy specimens in patients having coronary artery bypass grafting to amounts of narrowing in the same artery in patients with fatal coronary artery disease studied at necropsy. *Am J Cardiol* 2007;99:588–592.
18. Sprecher DL, Schaefer EJ, Kent KM, Gregg RE, Zech LA, Hoeg JM, McManus B, Roberts WC, Brewer HB, Jr. Cardiovascular features of homozygous familial hypercholesterolemia: analysis of 16 patients. *Am J Cardiol* 1984;54:20–30.
19. Grundy SM, Cleeman JL, Merz CN, Brewer HB Jr, Clark LT, Hunninhake DB, Pasternak RC, Smith SC Jr, Stone NJ, for the Coordinating Committee of the National Cholesterol Education Program. Implications of recent clinical trials for the National Cholesterol Education Program Adult Treatment Panel III guidelines. *Circulation* 2004;110:227–239.
20. Roberts WC. The underused miracle drugs: the statin drugs are to atherosclerosis what penicillin was to infectious disease. *Am J Cardiol* 1996;78:377–378.
21. Roberts WC. Shifting from decreasing risk to actually preventing and arresting atherosclerosis. *Am J Cardiol* 1999;83:816–817.

Determining the Quantity of Alcohol Consumed

Questioning patients about their consumption of alcohol (ethanol) is an important part of history taking. To determine the specific quantity, it is essential to understand how much alcohol is in a bottle of spirits or a bottle of wine or a bottle of beer, and the container sizes in which they are consumed. I am reminded of the executive who asked his assistant to come into his office: "Aren't you proud of me?" he asked. "I am down to 1 cup of coffee a day." An enormous cup—probably holding 3,000 ml—was sitting on his desk.

Spirits: The small containers of spirits provided by commercial airline carriers to individual passengers contain 50 ml. Because the 50 ml generally contains 40% alcohol (80 proof), there is 20 ml (2/3 oz) of alcohol in each small bottle. The usual 750-ml bottle of spirits purchased in a store contains 40% alcohol or 300 ml of alcohol, an amount equal to 15 of the 50-ml bottles of spirits.

Wine: The small bottles of wine provided by commercial airline carriers to individual passengers contain 187 ml, and because they consist usually of about 13.5% alcohol, those containers provide 25 ml of alcohol. The usual bottle of wine purchased in a store contains 750 ml, the same quantity as the usual bottle of spirits, but the alcohol content is usually about 13.5%. Thus, the quantity of alcohol in a 750-ml bottle of wine is approximately 100 ml, such that consuming an entire bottle of wine (750 ml) provides essentially the same quantity of alcohol as does consuming 5 50-ml bottles of spirits. Four of the 187-ml bottles of wine are equivalent to the 750-ml sized bottle.

Beer: The alcoholic content of beer varies, but most commonly in the United States, it is about 5% by volume. Thus, a 12 fl oz (355-ml) bottle or can contains 18 ml of ethanol, such that the alcohol content of 5 beers roughly equals drinking a full 750-ml bottle of wine or a third of a 750-ml bottle of spirits.

Alcohol equivalence: In general, drinking 12 oz of beer equals drinking 5 oz of wine or 1.5 oz of spirits. Or, 285 ml of beer = 120 ml of wine = 30 ml (a single jigger) of spirits. It is easier to keep track of beers drunk than wine or spirits, particularly in homes or at parties. Wine glasses are often refilled before they are emptied, and wine glasses vary considerably in size (4, 5, 8, 12, 16, and 20 oz). Glasses are generally more filled with red wine than with white wine. Becoming savvy to glass size obviously is important. Some hosts and party providers measure spirits before glasses are filled, others do not. Thus, knowing glass sizes and watching the servers is helpful in estimating quantities of alcohol consumed.

Calories in alcohol: They amount to 7 calories per milliliter or gram of alcohol. Thus, a 50-ml bottle of spirits with 40% by volume alcohol (80 proof; 20 ml of alcohol) provides 140 cal, and most spirit pourers provide at least this amount per cocktail. An ounce of 80-proof (40% alcohol) whiskey, gin, vodka, rum, tequila, or brandy contains 65 cal. Liqueurs (Drambuie, Cointreau, Kahlua) contain about 125 cal/oz. A 5-oz glass of red or dry white wine, sherry, or champagne contains about 100 cal. A regular 12-oz (355-ml) bottle or can of beer contains 150 cal, and "light" beer 110 cal. And beer and wine also provide calories in the nonalcohol portions of those drinks. Thus, although a little alcohol may be useful for our coronary arteries, lots of alcohol is bad for our brains, livers, and bellies.

William Clifford Roberts, MD
Baylor Heart and Vascular Institute
Baylor University Medical Center
Dallas, Texas

Two Observations Suggesting That We Die in Ventricular Systole

Does it take more energy for the cardiac ventricles to contract or to relax? And if it takes more energy for the ventricles to relax than to contract, would it be reasonable to believe that we die in ventricular systole rather than in ventricular diastole?

Two observations suggest that we die in ventricular systole. One, as illustrated in the accompanying Figures 1 to 5, if the minute size of the left ventricular cavity represents ventricular diastole, what size could possibly represent ventricular systole? Two, the thickness of the left ventricular free wall at necropsy corresponds to the thickness measured during life by echocardiogram during ventricular systole, not during ventricular diastole.[1]

If the left ventricle is dilated during life, it will also be dilated after death, and therefore in these circumstances, it is not possible to know at necropsy that death occurred during ventricular systole. When the left ventricular cavity is of normal size during life, however, the left ventricular cavity is small or minute after life.

William Clifford Roberts, MD
Baylor Heart and Vascular Institute
Baylor University Medical Center
Dallas, Texas 75246
E-mail: wc.roberts@baylorhealth.edu.

1. Maron BJ, Henry WL, Roberts WC, Epstein SE. Comparison of echocardiographic and necropsy measurements of ventricular wall thicknesses in patients with and without disproportionate septal thickening. *Circulation* 1977;55:341–346.

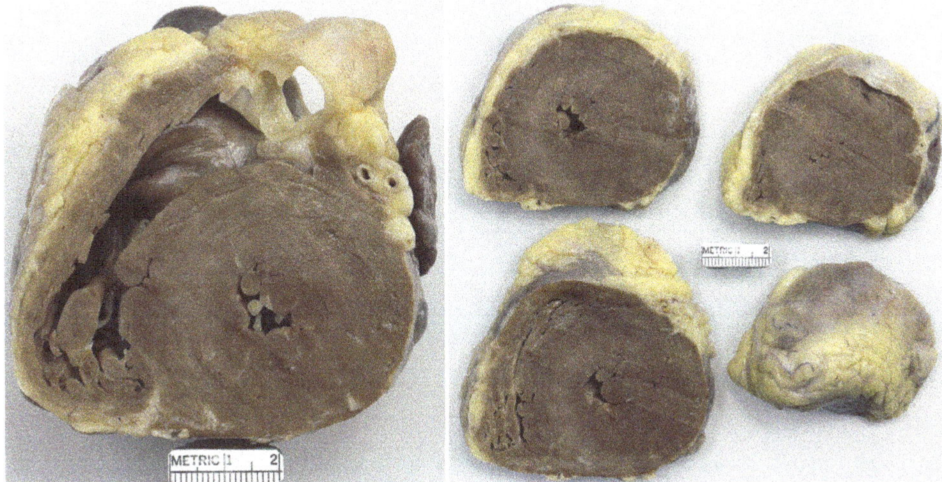

Figure 1. Cross sections of the cardiac ventricles cut parallel to the posterior atrioventricular sulcus in a 76-year-old hypertensive woman who died suddenly after hospitalization for what turned out to be acute aortic dissection. There was a through-and-through tear in the ascending aorta leading to hemopericardium. The heart weighed 310 g. The left ventricular cavity is minute.

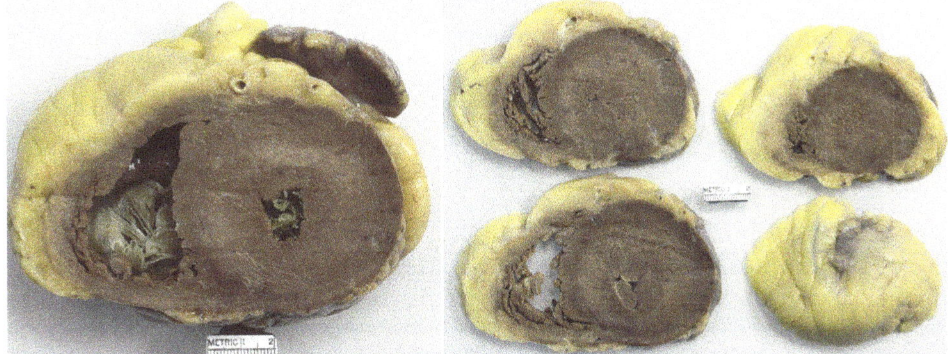

Figure 2. Cross section of the cardiac ventricles in a 69-year-old obese, hypertensive woman who died of an ischemic bowel after a recent stroke. The heart weighed 515 g, and she weighed 250 lb. The sections of cardiac ventricles show a minute left ventricular cavity. The heart floated in water due to the excessive subepicardial adipose tissue (body mass index 39 kg/m^2).

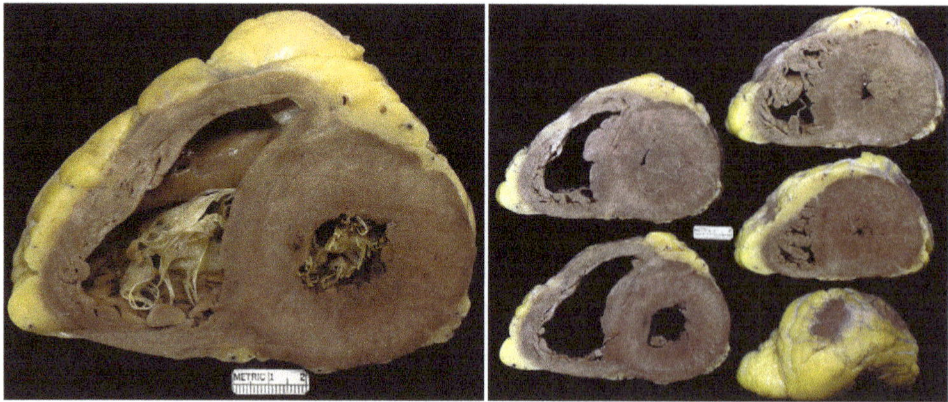

Figure 3. Cross sections of the cardiac ventricles in a 75-year-old man who died suddenly in a hospital restroom after admission for a non–ST-segment elevation acute myocardial infarction. The left ventricular cavity is very small at the base and minute elsewhere. The heart weighed 560 g.

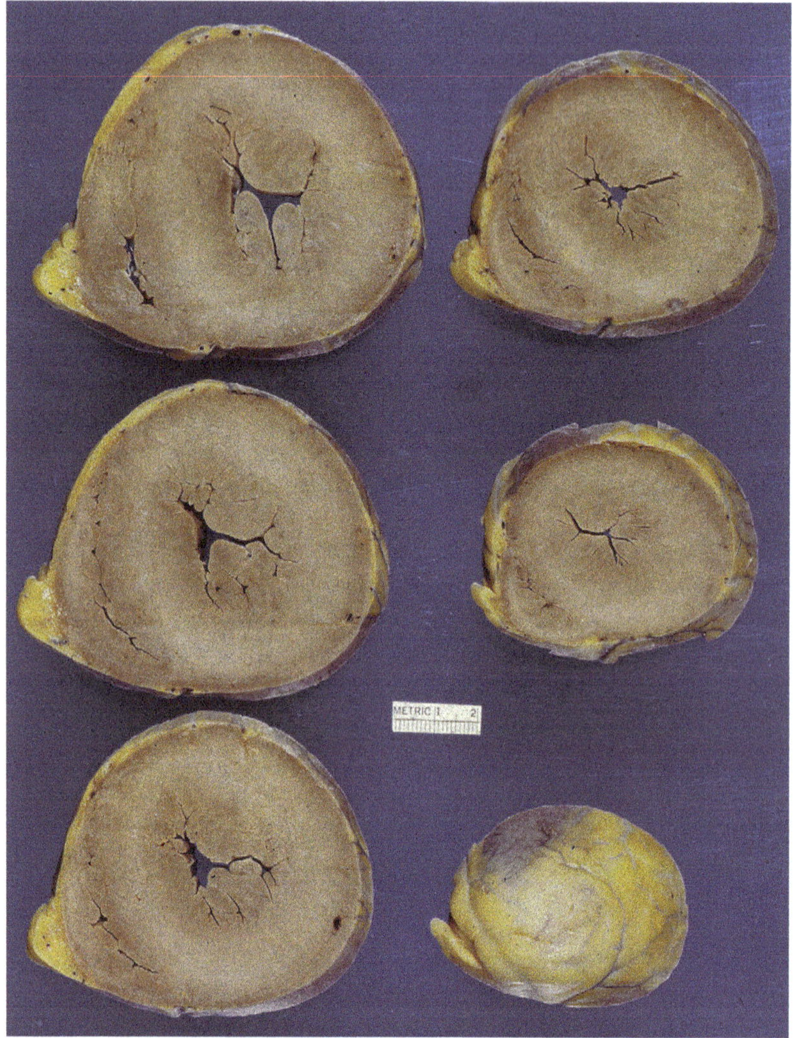

Figure 4. Cross sections of the cardiac ventricles in a 70-year-old man who had had several dizzy spells in the previous 3 months. The lumen of the right carotid artery was found to have a diameter reduction narrowing of 75%, and a carotid endarterectomy was performed. Three hours later, he had fatal cardiac arrest. Necropsy showed the aortic valve to be extremely stenotic. Both ventricular cavities were minute. The heart weighed 495 g.

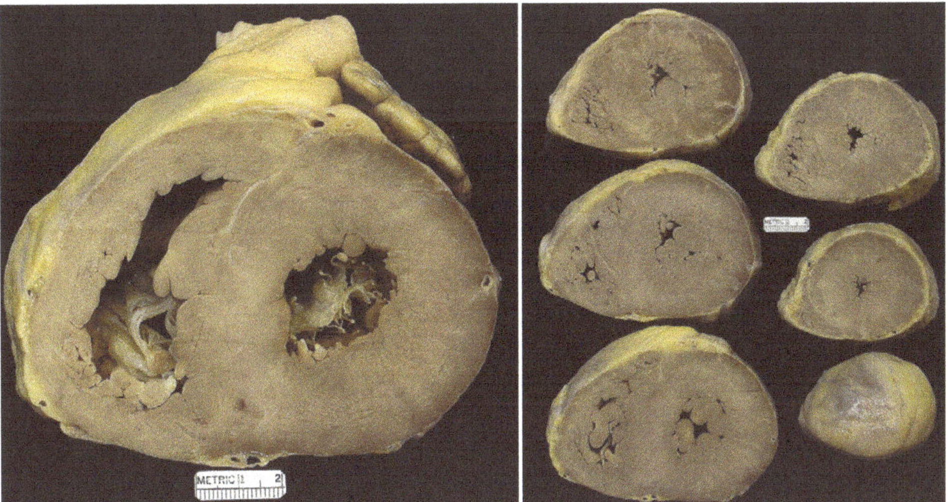

Figure 5. Cross sections of the cardiac ventricles in a 55-year-old man who died of systemic AL amyloidosis with diffuse involvement of the heart. The heart weighed 625 g. The left ventricular cavity is minute except in the most basal portion *(upper photo)*.

Cardiovascular Disease

Mitral Commissurotomy—Still a Good Operation

Recently, I examined an operatively excised, severely stenotic mitral valve that was free of calcific deposits (by radiography of the excised valve) and of associated mitral regurgitation (by left ventricular angiography). The patient had no evidence of dysfunction of either the tricuspid or aortic valves. I asked the surgeon who had performed the mitral valve replacement (MVR) why that procedure was performed rather than mitral valve commissurotomy (MVC). I was surprised to hear that he "rarely did MVC anymore" and that he had "more confidence in MVR than in MVC." He had used a mechanical prosthesis for the MVR, which necessitated anticoagulant therapy for the rest of this 36-year-old woman's life. When I mentioned that chronic anticoagulant therapy would not have been necessary had MVC been performed, he responded that "MVR was still worth the difference." I disagree, and so does Bonchek[1] in the editorial in this issue.

In 1978, Lachman and I[2] radiographed 164 operatively excised stenotic mitral valves and quantitated the amount of calcific deposits in them. Of the 164 valves, 14 had absent and 43 minimal calcific deposits on x-ray examination of the excised valve. Of the 57 patients with absent or minimal calcific deposits, 37 had moderate to severe mitral regurgitation, and therefore, each clearly warranted MVR. The remaining 20 had absent or minimal calcific deposits and absent or minimal mitral regurgitation as determined by left ventricular angiography; nevertheless, MVR had been performed. We analyzed retrospectively those 20 patients to examine if MVR was preferable to MVC.[3]

To answer this question unequivocally, the stenotic mitral valves in patients who had only commissurotomy would have to be studied morphologically and radiographically in the same manner as those that were excised and replaced. Obviously, the nonexcised valve cannot be examined in the same manner as the excised valve. Nevertheless, the ideal valve for MVC in the past has been considered to be the stenotic one that is free of calcific deposits, free of significant mitral regurgitation, and mobile. The excised mitral valves in the 20 patients whom we[3] analyzed were free of calcific deposits by preoperative examination (or nearly so by radiography of the excised valve, a far more sensitive technique than x-ray or fluoroscopy through the chest wall), and none had significant regurgitation by left ventricular angiography. The degree of mobility was infrequently described in the operative note. All 20 patients analyzed would probably have been acceptable candidates for MVC in the pre-valve replacement era. Why, then, might valve replacement be performed with its prosthetic- or bioprosthetic-related complications rather than MVC in this circumstance?

Of the 20 patients studied by Lachman and me,[3] several reasons appeared to account for MVR rather than MVC: (1) *Another cardiac valve was also replaced* (13 patients). Therefore, if the patient is required to have anticoagulant therapy for a prosthesis in the tricuspid or aortic valve position, MVR may be the more reasonable procedure and will avoid the risk of significant regurgitation or incomplete relief of the stenosis by MVC. (2) *Cardiopulmonary bypass was used* (all 20 patients). This procedure obviously allows visual inspection of the valve, something not possible when MVC is done as a "closed" procedure. I suspect that the visually inspected stenotic mitral valve is more frightening to the observer than is the palpated stenotic valve. Thus, visual inspection alone, particularly when valve replacement is a reasonable and uncriticized option, may push the surgeon toward replacement rather than simple commissurotomy in some patients. (3) *Some surgeons had relatively little experience with MVC* (17 patients). Of the 20 patients we analyzed, 17 were operated on by surgeons <40 years old when the operation was done. As pointed out by Bonchek,[1] younger surgeons have had much less experience with MVC than with MVR. (4) *Dissatisfaction with attempted MVC* (3 patients). (5) *Previous MVC had been performed* (11 patients). Although there is disagreement on this point, a mitral valve that has had a commissurotomy and later becomes severely stenotic can nevertheless have another MVC as long as calcific deposits are absent and regurgitation is absent or minimal. (6) *Incorrect identification of mitral calcific deposits* (2 patients). A calcific deposit was described in the mitral leaflets at operation, but x-ray of the excised valve showed that it was devoid of calcium.

Each of these 6 factors contributed in ≥1 of the 20 patients analyzed to the final operative decision of MVC rather than MVR. Even though MVC has been performed for >30 years, the mere alternative of MVR appears to have somewhat altered the definition of the mitral valve previously considered ideal for MVC. We need to return to the earlier definition of the ideal mitral valve suitable for MVC.

References

1. **Bonchek LI.** Current status of mitral commissurotomy: indications, techniques and results. Am J Cardiol 1983;52:411–414.
2. **Lachman AS, Roberts WC.** Calcific deposits in stenotic mitral valves. Extent and relationship to age, sex, degree of stenosis, cardiac rhythm, previous commissurotomy and left atrial body thrombus from study of 164 operatively-excised valves. Circulation 1978;57:808–815.
3. **Roberts WC, Lachman AS.** Mitral valve *commissurotomy* versus *replacement*. Considerations based on examination of operatively excised stenotic mitral valves. Am Heart J 1979;98:56–62.

William C. Roberts

William C. Roberts, MD
Editor-in-Chief

The "Blessing" Of Angina Pectoris

The use of the word "blessing" when speaking of angina pectoris needs considerable explanation because the patient who has angina clearly does not consider him-self/herself "blessed." But when applied on a *relative* rather than on an *absolute* basis, there is justification for the use of this word. Over 95% of patients with atherosclerotic coronary heart disease (CAD) present clinically in 1 of 3 ways: acute myocardial infarction (AMI), cardiac arrest (sudden coronary death) or angina pectoris.

Although the amount of left ventricular myocardium lost is variable, AMI indicates permanent, irreplaceable loss of ventricular myocardium. The amount of myocardium lost is generally much less in the patients with so-called uncomplicated AMI compared to those in whom the acute event is complicated by cardiogenic shock or in whom chronic intractable congestive heart failure, with or without aneurysmal formation, is a late consequence. Irrespective of the size of the AMI, however, the patient whose initial manifestation of atherosclerotic CAD is AMI begins a symptomatic course with a partially but permanently damaged left ventricle, and therapy thereafter—either medical or surgical or both—is usually not as beneficial as in the patient with symptomatic CAD without permanent left ventricular damage.

The patient whose initial manifestation of atherosclerotic CAD is fatal cardiac arrest has no opportunity to receive long-term medical or surgical therapy irrespective of the presence or absence of underlying previous (clinically silent) myocardial damage. About 50% of successfully resuscitated survivors of cardiac arrest are left with no apparent permanent left ventricular damage.

Thus, relative to the initial clinical appearance of atherosclerotic CAD as manifested by AMI or fatal cardiac arrest, the patient whose initial clinical manifestation of CAD is angina pectoris (or nonfatal cardiac arrest) is "blessed." Angina, of course, in about 90% of the patients, indicates the presence of severe narrowing of ≥ 1 major epicardial coronary artery and is the result of *transient*, not permanent, myocardial ischemia. The left ventricular myocardium at the time of the initial appearance of angina is usually normal, or if a scar (indicative of a previously silent AMI which healed) is present, it is usually small and infrequently results in left ventricular dysfunction.[1] Thus, the patient with initial angina can undergo the definitive diagnostic study—selective coronary angiography—before the occurrence of permanent significant left ventricular damage. Of all patients with symptomatic CAD, those who deserve the most "aggressive" diagnostic and therapeutic approaches, unless contraindicated by extremely advanced age, presence of another more life-threatening condition or simply no desire on the part of the patient, are the patients whose only manifestation of atherosclerotic CAD is *unequivocal* angina pectoris. If I develop angina pectoris as the first manifestation of CAD, I want a coronary angiogram. Only 1 test during life can determine the presence or absence of significant coronary narrowing unequivocally and that is injection of contrast material into the coronary arteries. Angiography demonstrates the presence of normal (a 10% occurrence) or abnormal (a 90% occurrence) coronary arteries and if abnormal, the degree of, and the distribution of, the narrowings. In my view, most patients with significant (>50% diameter reduction) narrowing of ≥ 1 vital coronary arteries should be treated definitively at this juncture (before significant left ventricular damage has occurred from subsequent AMI or subsequent cardiac arrest). The most definitive therapy, of course, is dilatation of or bypass of the coronary narrowings.

In summary, *the initial appearance of angina pectoris is the time to do coronary angiography and if significant and appropriately located coronary narrowing is present, unless other factors preclude its performance, the time to dilate or to bypass the narrowing.* This aggressive approach initially almost certainly will delay for a reasonable period in most patients the occurrence of sudden coronary death (the most frequent cause of death in patients with angina) and permanent myocardial damage from AMI.

1. **Roberts WC.** The coronary arteries and left ventricle in clinically isolated angina pectoris. Circulation 1976;54:388–390.

William C. Roberts

William C. Roberts, MD
Editor-in-Chief

The 2 Most Common Congenital Heart Diseases

In virtually every article or book I have read on the frequency of the various congenital anomalies of the heart and great vessels, ventricular septal defect has been listed as the most frequent anomaly. But ventricular septal defect is not nearly as frequent as *mitral valve prolapse* (MVP) or *bicuspid aortic valve* (BAV). MVP occurs clinically in at least 5% of persons older than 20 years of age[1] and the congenitally BAV occurs in at least 1%, possibly as high as 1.5%, of persons older than 20 years.[2] Although fusion of 1 of 3 commissures may occur in a normally formed 3-cuspid aortic valve and this fusion yields an acquired BAV, the congenitally BAV is generally readily discernible from the acquired 1 and there is no disagreement on the congenital nature of this 2-cuspid aortic valve, which may or may not have a raphe in 1 of its 2 cusps.[2] MVP, in contrast, has not generally been thought of as a congenital anomaly because a systolic click and/or a late systolic precordial murmur is rarely if ever present from birth. On occasion, however, necropsy in infants has revealed the presence of MVP even though signs of mitral valve dysfunction may not have been detected clinically.[3]

I like to put both MVP and BAV in the category of "congenital anomalies present at birth but usually clinically silent until adulthood."[4] Although both conditions predispose to infective endocarditis, infection is not the major complication of either. The most common complication of MVP is mitral regurgitation, but usually it is mild and its usual mechanism is "overshooting" of 1 mitral leaflet during ventricular systole. Severe mitral regurgitation is an infrequent consequence, and when it occurs its mechanism is usually mitral anular dilatation[5]; less frequently, rupture of chordae tendineae, usually spontaneous, i.e., not secondary to infective endocarditis.[5] We recently found MVP to be the most frequent cause of *isolated* (normal aortic valve function) *pure* (no element of mitral stenosis) mitral regurgitation severe enough to warrant mitral valve replacement in patients older than 20 years.[5]

Although some patients with BAV develop pure aortic regurgitation, some secondary to infective endocarditis and some not.[6] the most common complication of BAV is not pure regurgitation but stenosis.[2] Indeed, the BAV is the underlying aortic valve structure in about 60% of patients aged 16 to 65 years with aortic stenosis severe enough to warrant aortic valve replacement or severe enough to be fatal.[2]

Thus, although the frequency of rheumatic heart disease is diminishing in the Western world, the frequency of MVP and BAV likely will not diminish because each of them represents congenitally defective or malformed tissue. Not only are MVP and BAV the most frequent congenital heart conditions, but after hypertensive and coronary heart diseases, MVP and BAV may be the most common cardiac conditions observed in adults 65 years of age and younger in the Western world. Thus, adult cardiologists do indeed see many patients with "congenital heart disease," patients who usually do not manifest cardiac dysfunction during childhood, and therefore their "congenital heart disease" is usually not detected by pediatric cardiologists. The presence or absence of MVP and BAV should be determined in all our patients, and, if either is present, prophylactic antibiotics against infective endocarditis appears warranted in each condition.

William C. Roberts

William C. Roberts, MD
Editor-in-Chief

References

1. **Procacci PM, Savran SV, Schreiter SL, Bryson AL.** Prevalence of clinical mitral-valve prolapse in 1169 young women. N Engl J Med 1976;294: 1086–1088.
2. **Roberts WC.** The congenitally bicuspid aortic valve. A study of 85 autopsy cases. Am J Cardiol 1970;26:72–83.
3. **Roberts WC, Honig HS.** The spectrum of cardiovascular disease in the Marfan syndrome: a clinico-morphologic study of 18 necropsy patients and comparison to 151 previously reported necropsy patients. Am Heart J 1982; 104:115–135.
4. **Roberts WC.** Congenital cardiovascular abnormalities usually "silent" until adulthood: morphologic features of the floppy mitral valve, valvular aortic stenosis, hypertrophic cardiomyopathy, sinus of Valsalva aneurysm, and the Marfan syndrome. In: Roberts WC, ed. Congenital Heart Disease in Adults. Philadelphia: F. A. Davis Co, 1979:407–453. (Cardiovascular Clinics 1979;10[1]:1–574.
5. **Waller BF, Morrow AG, Maron BJ, Del Negro AA, Kent KM, McGrath FJ, Wallace RB, McIntosh CL, Roberts WC.** Etiology of clinically isolated, severe, chronic pure mitral regurgitaiton: analysis of 97 patients over 30 years of age having mitral valve replacement. Am Heart J 1982;104:276–288.
6. **Roberts WC, Morrow AG, McIntosh CL, Jones M, Epstein SE.** Congenitally biscuspid aortic valve causing severe, pure aortic regurgitation without superimposed infective endocarditis. Analysis of 13 patients requiring aortic valve replacement. Am J Cardiol 1981;47:206–209.

When I Have an Acute Myocardial Infarction Take Me to the Hospital That Has a Cardiac Catheterization Laboratory and Open Cardiac Surgical Facilities

When a sick person is taken to a hospital in an ambulance, the driver is required in most cities to transport this passenger to the nearest hospital irrespective of the diagnostic and therapeutic facilities present in that hospital. If available somewhere in the local community, when and if I develop an acute myocardial infarction (AMI), I want to be transported by ambulance *to the nearest hospital that has a cardiac catheterization laboratory and open cardiac surgical facilities*. If coronary flow is to be predictably reinstituted, appropriate therapy must be started within 6 hours after onset of the pain of AMI. If the passenger having an AMI is initially taken to a hospital where these facilities are unavailable, later transfer to a hospital equipped for invasive cardiologic procedures causes an additional delay that may prevent early reestablishment of coronary flow.

Another reason for wanting the patient with an AMI to be located in a hospital containing a cardiac catheterization laboratory is for definitive diagnostic procedures if certain complications arise. Additionally, cardiac angiographic and hemodynamic studies just before discharge from the hospital are important and useful in many patients with AMI, and some of these patients deserve coronary dilatation or bypass procedures during hospitalization for AMI.

I realize that it is impossible for all patients having an AMI in the USA to be treated in a hospital having a cardiac catheterization laboratory and open-cardiac surgical facilities; use of either or both during AMI has not been proved at this time to increase long-term survival after AMI. No data are available comparing mortality rates of patients with AMI treated in hospitals that have catheterization laboratories and cardiac operative facilities with those that do not. Nevertheless, in my view, in large metropolitan areas, patients with AMI ideally should be brought to hospitals with invasive cardiologic and cardiac surgical facilities. Without these invasive facilities, patients with AMI simply do not have access to today's presently available maximal care. With the introduction of coronary thrombolytic and dilating procedures, the traditionally diagnostic cardiac catheterization laboratory also is becoming a therapeutic laboratory, and committees determining certificates of need for various hospitals must recognize this fact.

Thus, for me, when and if I have an AMI, please, ambulance driver, *take me to the hospital that has a cardiac catheterization laboratory and a cardiac surgical unit even if that hospital is not the closest one.*

William C. Roberts

William C. Roberts, MD
Editor-in-Chief

The Worst Heart Disease

Although the public may lump all diseases of the heart under the term "heart disease," obviously there are many varieties of cardiac disease, and most allow long-term survival. The average age of death among patients with coronary disease, for example, is 60 years, or 15 years below average life expectancy. Among patients with congenital heart disease, survival may be quite limited. The congenital malformation associated with the shortest life span, and, indeed, of all cardiac diseases the one allowing shortest survival, is *aortic valve atresia.*[1,2] This condition also is the most common cause of death from cardiovascular disease in the first week of life, and it is extremely rare for any infant with this malformation to live longer than 1 month. Most, of course, never leave the hospital after birth. This anomaly, illustrated in Figures 1 and 2, consists of total absence of the aortic valve and, with rare exception, the left ventricle is extremely small and often only slit-like. The mitral valve may or may not be atretic. Blood flows from pulmonary veins into left atrium and then across to the right side of the heart, usually through a valvular-incompetent patent foramen ovale. From the right atrium, blood flows into right ventricle and out into pulmonary trunk and into the systemic circuit through a patent ductus arteriosus. Thus, all blood exiting from the heart exits via the pulmonary trunk. In this circumstance the only purpose of the ascending aorta, which is severely hypoplastic, is to supply the coronary arteries. Because flow to the lungs is excessive, these infants usually die from pulmonary edema.

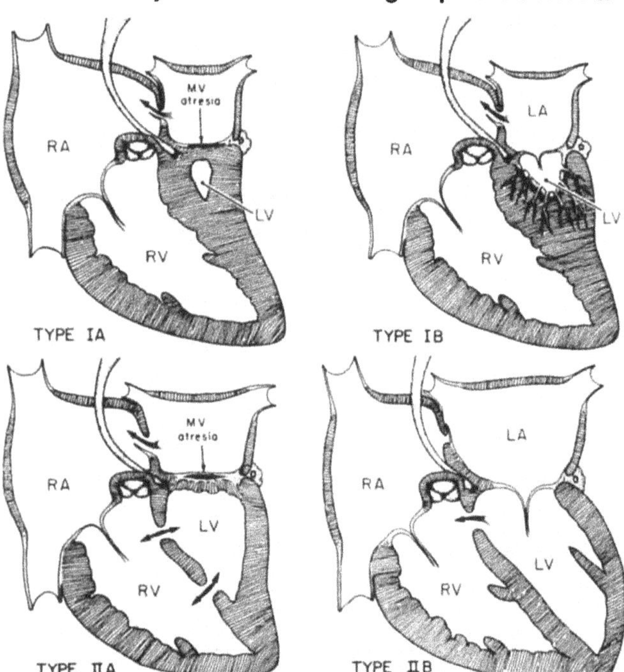

FIGURE 1. The 2 basic types and subtypes of aortic valve atresia. I have studied 85 patients with aortic-valve atresia at necropsy; 81 (95%) had either type IA or IB, and 4 had type IIA or IIB. LA = left atrium; LV = left ventricle; M.V. = mitral valve; RA = right atrium; RV = right ventricle. Reproduced, with permission of the authors and publisher, from Am J Cardiol 1976;37:753–756.

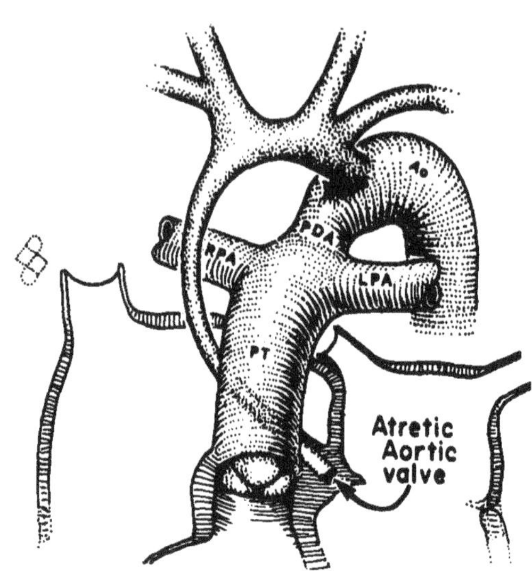

FIGURE 2. The great arteries in aortic valve atresia. The ascending aorta is extremely small and the pulmonary trunk (PT) is quite large. All blood enters the systemic arteries through the patent ductus arteriosus (PDA). Ao = descending thoracic aorta; LPA and RPA = left and right main pulmonary arteries, respectively. Reproduced, with permission of the authors and publisher, from Am J Cardiol 1976;37:753–756.

Aortic valve atresia may be difficult to diagnose clinically. It should be suspected in any newborn, however, having cardiorespiratory difficulties. As with any condition affecting the aortic valve, 75% are males. A precordial murmur may be absent. Although usually present and occasionally severe, cyanosis also may be absent and the arterial oxygen saturation may be almost normal. Echocardiography is helpful in diagnosis. Operative therapy, thus far, has been unsuccessful. Cardiac transplantation is probably the only potentially useful operative procedure.

In summary, of all cardiac conditions, aortic valve atresia is the worst, i.e., it allows the shortest survival.

William C. Roberts

William C. Roberts, MD
Editor-in-Chief

1. **Roberts WC, Perry LW, Chandra RS, Myers GE, Shapiro SR, Scott LP.** Aortic valve atresia: a new classification based on necropsy study of 73 cases. Am J Cardiol 1976;37:753–756.
2. **Perry LW, Scott LP III, Shapiro SR, Chandra RS, Roberts WC.** Atresia of the aortic valve with ventricular septal defect. A clinicopathologic study of four newborns. Chest 1977;72:757–761.

I Still Prefer *Ventricular Premature Complex*

A frequent finding on electrocardiograms are 1 or more abnormal QRS-T complexes in the same lead. The abnormal complexes have greater heights, greater widths, less straight sides, and broader peaks than their normal counterparts; they are not preceded by a P wave, and the direction of the T wave is usually opposite that of the QRS. Additionally, the abnormal QRS-T complex usually occurs earlier than would the normal complex and the interval between the preceding normal QRS complex is the same when more than 1 abnormal but similar QRS complex is recorded in the same electrocardiogram.

Despite the frequent occurrence of these bizarre QRS-T complexes, there appears to be little agreement as to the best name to call them.[1] As pointed out by Schamroth,[2] the first term used to describe them was *extrasystole*, a word coined by Engelmann in 1896 and continued by such authorities as Pan, MacKenzie, Rihl, Wenckeback and Lewis. Other terms followed, some consisting of 2 words such as *ectopic beat* or *contraction* and *premature beat* or *contraction*. Most terms, however, consisted of 3 words, 2 of which were *ventricular* and *premature*, with most authorities placing the word premature before ventricular. The choice of the third word in this triumvirate has varied and has included *beat*, *contraction*, *complex*, *deflection*, *impulse*, *activation*, *discharge* and *depolarization*.

Schamroth[2] argued for the term *ventricular extrasystole* on the basis of 4 factors: (1) Historic precedent. (2) Use of the word *beat* or *contraction* is improper. (3) "Ventricular premature contractions" have at least 6 causes, only 1 of which is a ventricular extrasystole. (An ectopic and premature ventricular electrical impulse with fixed coupling of the preceding event. He used the term "ectopic ventricular beats" for ventricular ectopic activity not fulfilling this definition.) (4) *Economy of language.* "Ventricular extrasystole" consists of only 2 words, whereas "premature ventricular contraction," 3 words. But Schamroth and many others before him have pointed out that the word *extrasystole* is incorrect because the abnormal QRS complex is only rarely a true extra or additional systole; it merely comes early and replaces the normal systole. Schamroth argues, however, that "The prefix *extra* in the context of extrasystole does not mean addition, but rather outside the normal, as in extracurricular or extraordinary." Julian[3] counters this argument: "But surely if these words mean 'outside the curriculum' or 'outside the ordinary', extrasystole must mean 'outside systole'? (?diastole)." Nikolic[4] also argues that Schamroth's definition of "extrasystole" to always involve "fixed coupling to a mechanical 'preceding beat' in the belief that 'complete ventricular activation resulting in a beat is necessary to precipitate or force the ensuing extrasystole' . . . is not always true, since extrasystoles are observed during electromechanical dissociation . . . [and] since electrical re-entry does not necessarily require any mechanical events. The fixity of coupling, itself, need not be confined to extrasystoles, since it may occur with the even less euphonious parasystoles."

Both Schamroth[2] and Julian[3] oppose use of the word "contraction" as in "premature atrial or ventricular contraction" because it describes the mechanical consequences only, which do not always occur. In the editorial elsewhere in this issue, Brugada and Wellens[5] provide elegant reasons why the term beat or contraction is not proper to describe "ventricular premature electrical stimuli resulting in a QRS complex in the surface electrocardiogram." These authors recommend *ventricular premature depolarization* as the most reasonable descriptive term. But depolarization is an electrophysiologic phenomenon; it is a process of neutralizing polarity and the process cannot be seen; the abnormal QRS complex, however, is visible. (It is similar to the use of the word *calcification*, which is the process of calcifying. The consequence of calcification is calcific deposits, which are visible, but the process itself is not visible.)

Despite these objections as delineated by Brugada and Wellens, Julian,[3] nevertheless, favors the use of the word "beat" as one of the descriptive terms:

> Beat is commonly used to describe both the electrical phenomenon and its mechanical consequences and has the advantage of simplicity and brevity. It has been objected that 'beat' implies mechanical activity, but like 'rhythm' itself, it is used as a mechanical analogy without necessarily having such an implication. The term 'beat' is generally understood and extensively used by distinguished authorities of many different nationalities . . . The word 'beat' can then be qualified by the use of further descriptive words such as 'ventricular' to define its source,

'early' to define its timing, or 'escape' to define its mechanism or in combination, as in 'late ventricular escape beat.'

Brugada and Wellens' arguments against the use of the word "beat," however, are convincingly reasonable to me. Most important, a beat is not seen on an electrocardiogram. Thus, I shall stay with the term ventricular premature *complex*. The normal QRS on the surface electrocardiogram, as pointed out by Brugada and Wellens, is called a complex. Why not call the abnormal QRS a complex also? A complex is visible. Clearly, a beat, contraction, depolarization or systole are not visible on the surface electrocardiogram. Julian[3] argues against the word "complex" because it ". . . can only be applied to the electrographic appearance and not to the fundamental phenomenon or to its other consequences." This argument, in my view, is why "complex" is the proper term, not why it is not. Nikolic[4] also argues for use of the word "complex": "It is short, euphonious and flexible enough to figure in conducted and non-conducted, atrial and ventricular, premature or late complexes." Julian,[6] however, further argues against use of the term complex: "Complex is commonly used as an adjective by American arrhythmologists to imply complicated and potentially sinister, and as a noun to indicate a complex whole. Thus, we may refer to an episode of multiform ventricular ectopic beats as a complex of complex complexes!"

It is preferable, in my view, to place the word "ventricular" before the word "premature" so that "ventricular premature complex" can flow parallel with ventricular tachycardia and ventricular fibrillation or any type of ventricular ectopic activity. Its proper abbreviation therefore is VPC, not PVC. And another minor deficiency of the term "ventricular extrasystole" is that its abbreviation, VE, may get confused with "ventricular ectopy," which, as pointed out by Spodick,[7] is one of our worst cardiologic terms because it means "misplaced ventricle" and has nothing to do with arrhythmia.

William C. Roberts

William C. Roberts, MD
Editor in Chief

References

1. Tenth Bethesda Conference on Optimal Electrocardiography of the American College of Cardiology. Task Force I. Standardization of terminology and interpretation. Am J Cardiol 1978;41:130–145.
2. **Schamroth L.** Premature ventricular contraction or ventricular extrasystole. Am J Cardiol 1083;51:1783–1784.
3. **Julian DG.** A complex matter. Eur Heart J 1984;5:513–514.
4. **Nikolic G.** A complex matter. Eur Heart J 1984;5:864.
5. **Brugada P, Wellens HJJ.** To beat or not to beat. Arguments for use of the term *ventricular premature depolarization.* Am J Cardiol 1985;55:1113–1114.
6. **Julian DG.** Editor's reply. Eur Heart J 1984;5:864.
7. **Spodick DH.** Cardiolocution. The cardiologist's assault on English. Am J Cardiol 1981;48:973–974.

The Silver Anniversary of Cardiac Valve Replacement

The year was 1960. Forty-three-year-old John Fitzgerald Kennedy was elected president of the USA; 16-year-old Bobby Fischer successfully defended his US chess championship; *To Kill a Mockingbird* by Harper Lee and *The Rise and Fall of the Third Reich* by William Shirer were published; birth control pills were made available to the public; Polaris missiles were successfully fired from a submerged atomic submarine; the International System of Units (SI), based on the metric system, was adopted as the worldwide standard at a General Conference on Weights and Measures; Theodore Maiman, physicist, developed the first LASER (*L*ight *A*mplification by *S*timulated *E*mission of *R*adiation), and successful, i.e., prolonged survival, cardiac valve replacement occurred. When the annals of cardiology are written, 1960 will be remembered as the time that cardiac valve replacement became a predictably successful reality. Since 1960, over 1 million dysfunctioning native cardiac valves have been replaced with a mechanical prosthesis or a bioprosthesis (tissue valve). If lasers prove successful for coronary artery disease, 1960 will acquire additional importance for cardiology.

Dwight Harken was the first to use a mechanical prosthesis successfully in the natural anatomic cardiac valve position. Charles Hufnagel in October 1952 had used a caged-ball prosthesis in the descending thoracic aorta for severe aortic regurgitation but the insertion in this position of course only partially decreased the amount of regurgitant flow during ventricular diastole.[1] It was obvious that the prosthesis had to be inserted proximal to the coronary arterial ostia to completely relieve the regurgitant flow and to have any effect in patients with aortic valve stenosis. The lucite ball used initially by Hufnagel was eventually changed by him to a hollow nylon core covered by silicone rubber so that it would be less noisy and also so that it would be isobaric with blood. Hufnagel gave Harken several of his hollow-nylon-silicone-rubber-covered poppets and Harken used them in his stainless steel double-caged prosthesis. Later, he used solid silicone rubber poppets. The outer cage prevented the poppet from touching the wall of aorta in its excursion. Harken's first aortic valve replacement using the caged-ball prosthesis with an Ivalon® aorta-widening gusset extending cephalad from the prosthetic attachment ring was unsuccessful.[2] His second patient, a 32-year-old woman who had had a previous transaortic valvuloplasty, underwent successful aortic valve replacement on March 10, 1960. Harken was nearly 50 years old at the time. The patient later developed significant peribasilar prosthetic regurgitation and the prosthesis was replaced in 1963. This patient is still alive in 1985. Harken had 2 survivors among his first 7 patients having aortic valve replacement with his caged-ball prosthesis.[3] The second successful operation was performed on June 7, 1960. This patient developed prosthetic endocarditis 23 years later, the prosthesis was replaced, and this patient is still alive in 1985. Thus, the initial prosthesis was in place for 23 years, the longest any prosthetic valve had been in place, and the poppet at reoperation "looked good." Neither of Harken's first 2 successful human aortic-valve-replacement patients ever received anticoagulants and neither apparently has had embolic complications.

The first successful mitral valve replacement was performed by Albert Starr in September 1960.[4] Although successful aortic valve replacement had never been accomplished in nonhuman animals before Harken's success in patients, Starr had successfully used a caged-ball prosthesis in dogs for mitral valve replacement before his attempt in humans. Indeed, he had canine survivors of mitral valve replacement with caged-ball prostheses for many months before he attempted, at the encouragement of his cardiologist colleague, Herbert Griswald, mitral valve

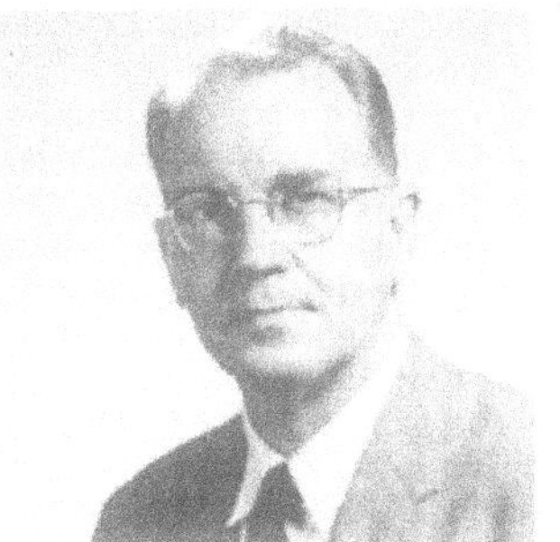
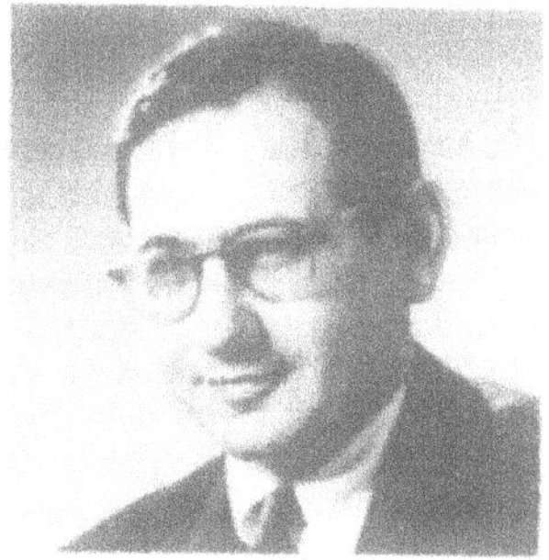

Dwight Harken (**left**) and Albert Starr (**right**) about the time of their first successful cardiac valve replacement.

replacement in a human patient. His first mitral valve replacement with a fully engineered caged-ball prosthesis was in a 33-year-old woman who had an air embolus at operation and she died 10 hours later. The second patient in whom 34-year-old Albert Starr performed mitral valve replacement was a 52-year-old truck dispatcher, who also received a caged-ball prosthesis, and he lived for 15 years thereafter. After Starr presented his results of mitral valve replacement in March 1961 before the American Surgical Association, Michael E. DeBakey[5] commented as follows: "I must say that this paper persuades me to reevaluate my attitude toward ball valves. I have been somewhat prejudiced against them because of my very early experience with their use in changing the directional flow in blood pumps. Our most recent experience with the use of such ball valves, as in the Hufnagel valve in aortic insufficiency, also tended to make me somewhat prejudiced . . . Nonetheless, it seems to me that this is very impressive work on the part of Drs. Starr and Edwards . . ."

Shortly after that surgical meeting, Starr visited Boston and observed Harken insert his double caged-ball prosthesis into the aortic valve position in a patient. At the time Starr became convinced that his fully engineered, single unit, caged-ball prosthesis, which he had used in the mitral position, also could be adapted to the aortic valve position. Thus, he and his engineering associate, Lowell M. Edwards,* also developed a factory-complete, caged-ball prosthesis for use in the aortic valve position and Starr later successfully used it for aortic valve replacement.

During the past 25 years Starr has continued to use the caged-ball prosthesis (Starr-Edwards) as his first choice among mechanical prosthetic valves. Harken, in contrast, later considered the caged-ball type to be far less desirable than some tilting disc prostheses.

Although other varieties of caged-ball prostheses (Magovern, Smeloff-Cutter, Braunwald-Cutter and DeBakey) followed the Harken and Starr-Edwards models, all but the Starr-Edwards type were discontinued. The Starr-Edwards caged-ball prosthesis underwent several changes before returning to an early model. The early processing procedures for the silicone rubber poppets proved to be poor and as a consequence many of the silastic poppets inserted before 1967 swelled by adsorbing lipids and some impacted in the cage; or they shrank or cracked and some dislodged from the cage. Although there have been some surface abrasion injuries, some to an extent that has allowed expulsion of the poppet from the cage, degeneration (variance) of the silicone rubber poppet of the fatty infiltration type has not been reported since the processing of the silicone was finally standardized in 1966. The use of cloth on the metallic struts as a means to decrease prosthetic thrombus in the Starr-Edwards model proved not to be an improvement. The hollow, metallic poppet, introduced almost simultaneously with the cloth covering of the metallic struts, caused disruption of the cloth on both base and stents, and this poppet and the cloth covering on the stents and the metallic studs on the metallic base have all been discontinued. Thus, a full circle has occurred with the caged ball. The only one presently manufactured in the USA is the model introduced in late 1965 and it consists of a silicone rubber poppet and non–cloth-covered stents and base (M 6120 in the mitral valve position and A 1260 in the aortic valve position).

Other prosthetic cardiac valves followed the caged ball. The first was a nontilting caged disc (1965), which was utilized by most surgeons only in the atrioventricular valve positions.[7,8] This prosthesis proved to be highly thrombogenic and obstructive and its use has virtually disappeared. The next development was the tilting disc and the Björk-Shiley prosthesis proved to be highly effective.[9–11] And, in the late 1970s, another tilting disc appeared, this one with a bileaflet configuration, the St. Jude Medical Prosthesis; it is the least obstructive and the least damaging to blood elements of any of the prosthetic valves.[12]

Tissue values, of course, also have been used as replacements for dysfunctioning native aortic valves. Aortic valve homografts were first used for aortic valve replacement in the early 1960s.[13–15] The initial results were gratifying: The valve lesions were usually ameliorated and anticoagulant therapy was not required. The problem proved to be accelerated wear with development of aortic regurgitation.[16–19] Other tissue valves followed, namely fascia lata, dura mater, parietal pericardium (human and bovine) and porcine aortic valve. The fascia lata and dura mater valves rapidly proved to be poor valve substitutes because they became stiff and relatively immobile. The porcine xenograft and bovine parietal pericardial valves preserved in glutaraldehyde and attached to a semiflexible stent proved to be effective.[20] (The porcine bioprosthesis failed quickly when preserved in formalin.[21])

I have examined at necropsy well over 1,000 hearts containing 1 or more prosthetic or bioprosthetic cardiac valves.[22–47] From my vantage point some views on cardiac valve replacement have been acquired and some of them are discussed in the remainder of this piece.

* Mr. Edwards at the time was a retired electrical engineer. During World War II he had designed a special airplane fuel pump that greatly contributed to the war effort. This pump handled mixtures of fuel in liquid and vapor phases. After retirement, as head of his own development company, he desired to continue to apply his knowledge by any contribution he might make to medicine. In 1958, he began working with Dr. Starr. Mr. Edwards, using his own laboratory facilities, was able to fabricate rapidly many prototype mitral valves for Dr. Starr to insert in experimental animals. Together, Edwards and Starr progressed through Teflon,® Lucite,® and silicone leaflet and ball-valve designs, and finally settled on a Teflon-rimmed stainless steel cage enclosing a silicone rubber ball.[6]

1. *Perform cardiac valve replacment only when absolutely necessary.* When I was a student in Emory medical school, the chief of surgery, J. D. Martin, often stated: "Never remove someone's stomach unless it is absolutely necessary." Certainly the same can be said of a cardiac valve. Except possibly in patients with severe, usually pure, aortic regurgitation, cardiac valve replacement should be reserved for patients with clear-cut evidence of significant cardiac dysfunction (functional class III or IV, New York Heart Association classification). Cardiac valvular operations that preserve the native valve, in my view, should be performed more often. Mitral valvuloplasty (commissurotomy) now is too often displaced in favor of mitral valve replacement,[48,49] and mitral and tricuspid valve reparative operations for pure regurgitation probably are too often displaced by valve replacement. Tricuspid valve replacement for pure tricuspid regurgitation secondary to mitral valve disease usually can be avoided. The tricuspid valve position simply is not ideal for either a mechanical prosthesis as a bioprosthesis.

2. *If anticoagulants are going to be administered chronically postoperatively* (because of "chronic atrial fibrillation or a huge left atrial cavity"), *a mechanical prosthesis, not a bioprosthesis, should be used for valve replacement.* The only advantage of a bioprosthesis is that use of this type of substitute cardiac valve does not require the use of anticoagulants. If anticoagulants are going to be used chronically postoperatively, use of a bioprosthesis cannot be justified.

3. *In patients having double- or triple-valve replacement, either mechanical prostheses or bioprostheses, not both, should be used in all native valve positions.* Utilizing a mechanical prosthesis in one valve position and a bioprosthesis in another is illogical because anticoagulants will be required because of the mechanical prosthesis. All bioprostheses will wear out if the patients survive long enough, and presently available mechanical valves are far more resistant to wear. Thus, because anticoagulants will have to be given if one of the native valves is replaced by a prosthesis, all valves replaced should be replaced by a mechanical prosthesis, or bioprostheses should be used for all native valves replaced.

4. *Bioprostheses should never be used in patients younger than age 20 years and, if possible, not in patients younger than age 30 years.*[37] Because not all patients can take anticoagulants, bioprosthetic (tissue) cardiac valves must be available, but except in older persons or in women wanting pregnancy or in vigorous outdoor persons in whom chronic anticoagulation might have excessively dangerous consequences, bioprostheses should be second-line rather than first-line cardiac valve substitutes. Persons having third or fourth valve replacements need mechanical prostheses, not bioprostheses, because each operation is more dangerous than the preceding one, and bioprostheses wear out.

5. *It is better to err on the side of using smaller-sized prostheses rather than larger-sized prostheses.* After deciding which type of prosthesis or bioprosthesis to utilize in a particular patient, the next most important decision is which size of prosthesis or bioprosthesis to use.[34] Although the sizing is generally not done until cardiotomy or aortotomy has been performed, the size of a substitute valve chosen should take into consideration the lean weight of the patient and the type of hemodynamic valvular lesion present and, in my view, roughly decided on before the patient and the surgeon enter the operating room. Volume lesions, of course, if chronic, dilate the ventricular cavity and usually the ascending aorta, and consequently larger-sized prostheses can usually be used. Pressure lesions, in contrast, mitral stenosis or aortic stenosis, or both, may not be associated with left ventricular dilatation and, consequently, a smaller-sized prosthesis or bioprosthesis will be required for the mitral position. Although the aortic root is usually dilated in chronic, isolated aortic stenosis and/or isolated regurgitation, when combined with chronic mitral valve stenosis or regurgitation, the aortic root is usually not dilated irrespective of whether the aortic valve is stenotic or purely regurgitant. Thus, in patients with combined mitral and aortic valve stenosis, or combined mitral and aortic regurgitation or mixed lesions, a smaller-sized prosthesis or bioprosthesis usually is preferred in the aortic valve position.

6. *Refrain from doing mitral valve replacement in the presence of massive mitral anular calcium.*

7. *Use interrupted sutures only for insertion of either prosthetic or bioprosthetic cardiac valves.* A single break of a continuous suture, despite 4 or 8 interrupted sutures, can produce massive regurgitation.

8. *Operative preciseness is far more important during insertion of tilting disc prostheses than during insertion of caged-ball prostheses.* A single suture may cause irreversible interference to closure of an occluder of a disc valve but may have no effect with a caged-ball prosthesis.[38] Careful orientation is far more important with tilting-disc prostheses than with caged-ball ones. The margin of error, in other words, is less with tilting-disc prostheses compared to caged-ball prostheses or bioprostheses.

9. *Predictably successful cardiac valve replacement can be achieved most often by surgeons who frequently perform cardiac valve replacement.* Although over 50% of prosthetic and bioprosthetic cardiac valves are supplied to surgeons who order relatively few substitute valves, predictably successful cardiac valve replacement cannot be obtained by an operator who only occasionally performs cardiac valve replacement. Predictable success requires a good prosthesis or bioprosthesis, a properly-sized

prosthesis or bioprosthesis, an absence of significant, associated, unpalliated valvular or coronary heart disease, or both, a good surgeon and good postoperative care.

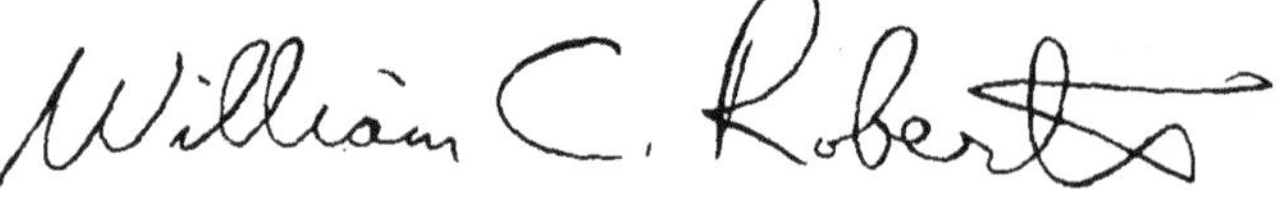

William C. Roberts, MD
Editor in Chief

References

1. **Hufnagel CA, Harvey WP.** The surgical correction of aortic regurgitation. Preliminary report. Bull Georgetown Univ Med Ctr 1953;6:60–61.
2. **Harken DE, Soroff HS, Taylor WJ, Lefemine AA, Gupta SK, Lunzer S.** Partial and complete prostheses in aortic insufficiency. J Thorac Cardiovasc Surg 1960;6:744–762.
3. **Harken DE, Taylor WJ, LeFemine AA, Lunzer S, Low HBC, Cohen ML, Jacobey JA.** Aortic valve replacement with a caged ball valve. Am J Cardiol 1962;9:292–299.
4. **Starr A, Edwards ML.** Mitral replacement. Clinical experience with a ball-valve prosthesis. Ann Surg 1961;154:726–740.
5. **DeBakey ME.** Discussion of Albert Starr's presentation. In Ref. 4:740.
6. **Blalock A.** Cardiovascular surgery, past and present. J Thorac Cardiovasc Surg 1966;51:153–167.
7. **Hufnagel CA, Conrad PW.** Comparative study of some prosthetic valves for aortic and mitral replacement. Surgery 1965;57:205–210.
8. **Kay EB, Suzuki A, Demaney M, Zimmerman HA.** Comparison of ball and disc valves for mitral valve replacement. Am J Cardiol 1966;18:504–514.
9. **Wada J.** Knotless suture method and Wada hingeless valve. Jpn J Thorac Surg 1967;15:88–94.
10. **Kaster RL, Lillehei CW.** A new cageless free-floating pivoting disc prosthetic heart valve: design, development and evaluation, Stockholm, 1967, Digest of the 7th International Conference on Medical and Biological Engineering: 387.
11. **Bjork VO.** A new tilting disc valve prosthesis. Scand J Thorac Cardiovasc Surg 1969;3:1–10.
12. **Nicoloff DM, Emery RW, Arom KV, Northrup WF III, Jorgensen CR, Wang Y, Lindsay WG.** Clinical and hemodynamic results with the St. Jude Medical cardiac valve prosthesis. A three-year experience. J Thorac Cardiovasc Surg 1981;82:674–683.
13. **Ross DN.** Homograft replacement of the aortic valve. Lancet 1962;2: 487.
14. **Duran CG, Gunning AJ.** A method for placing a total homologous aortic valve in the subcoronary position. Lancet 1962;2:488–489.
15. **Barratt-Boyes BG.** Homograft aortic valve replacement in aortic incompetence and stenosis. Thorax 1964;19:131–150.
16. **Ross D.** Biologic valves. Their performance and prospects. Circulation 1972;45:1259–1272.
17. **Angell WW, Shumway NE, Kosek JC.** A five-year study of viable aortic valve homografts. J Thorac Cardiovasc Surg 1972;64:329–339.
18. **Wallace RB, Londe SP, Titus JL.** Aortic valve replacement with preserved aortic valve hemografts. J Thorac Cardiovasc Surg 1974;67:44–52.
19. **Wallace RB.** Tissue valves. Am J Cardiol 1975;35:866–871.
20. **Reis RL, Hancock WD, Yarbrough JW, Glancy DL, Morrow AG.** The flexible stent. A new concept in the fabrication of tissue heart valve prostheses. J Thorac Cardiovasc Surg 1971;62:683–695.
21. **Yarbrough JW, Roberts WC, Reis RL.** Structural alterations in tissue cardiac valves implanted in patients and in calves. J Thorac Cardiovasc Surg 1973;65:364–375.
22. **Roberts WC, Morrow AG.** Mechanisms of acute left atrial thrombosis after mitral valve replacement. Pathologic findings indicating obstruction to left atrial emptying. Am J Cardiol 1966;1:497–503.
23. **Roberts WC, Morrow AG,** Late postoperative pathologic findings after cardiac valve replacement. Circulation 1967;36:I-48–I-62.
24. **Roberts WC, Morrow AG.** Causes of early postoperative death following cardiac valve replacement. Clinico-pathologic correlations in 64 patients studied at necropsy. J Thorac Cardiovasc Surg 1967;54:422–437.
25. **Roberts WC, Morrow AG.** Anatomic studies of hearts containing caged-ball prosthetic valves. Johns Hopkins Med J 1967;121:271–295.
26. **Roberts WC, Morrow AG.** Compression of anomalous left circumflex coronary arteries by prosthetic valve fixation rings. J Thorac Cardiovasc Surg 1969;57:834–838.
27. **Shepard RL, Glacy DL, Stinson EB, Roberts WC.** Hemodynamic confirmation of obstruction to left ventricular inflow by a caged-ball prosthetic mitral valve. Case report. J Thorac Cardiovasc Surg 1973;65:252–254.
28. **Roberts WC, Bulkley BH, Morrow AG.** Pathologic anatomy of cardiac valve replacement: a study of 224 necropsy patients. Prog Cardiovasc Dis 1973;15:539–587.
29. **Roberts WC.** Operative treatment of hypertrophic obstructive cardiomyopathy. The case against mitral valve replacement. Am J Cardiol 1973; 32:377–381.
30. **Seningen RP, Bulkley BH, Roberts WC.** Prosthetic aortic stenosis. A method to prevent its occurrence by measurement of aortic size from preoperative aortogram. Circulation 1974;49:921–924.
31. **Fishbein MC, Roberts WC, Golden A, Hufnagel CA.** Cardiac pathology after aortic valve replacement using Hufnagel trileaflet prostheses: a study of 20 necropsy patients. Am Heart J 1975;89:443–448.
32. **Roberts WC, Fishbein MC, Golden A.** Cardiac pathology after valve replacement by disc prosthesis. A study of 61 necropsy patients. Am J Cardiol 1975;35:740–760.
33. **Roberts WC, Hammer WJ.** Cardiac pathology after valve replacement with a tilting disc prosthesis (Bjork-Shiley type). A study of 46 necropsy patients and 49 Bjork-Shiley prostheses. Am J Cardiol 1976;37:1024–1032.
34. **Roberts WC.** Choosing a substitute cardiac valve: type, size, surgeon. Am J Cardiol 1976; 38:633–644.
35. **Spray TL, Roberts WC.** Structural changes in porcine xenografts used as substitute cardiac valves. Gross and histologic observations in 51 glutaraldehyde-preserved Hancock valves in 41 patients. Am J Cardiol 1977; 40:319–330.
36. **Ferrans VJ, Spray TL, Billingham ME, Roberts WC.** Structural changes in glutaraldehyde-treated porcine heterografts used as substitute cardiac valves. Transmission and scanning electron microscopic observations in 12 patients. Am J Cardiol 1978;41:1159–1184.
37. **Geha AS, Laks H, Stansel HC Jr, Cornhill JF, Kilman JW, Buckley MJ, Roberts WC.** Late failure of porcine valve heterografts in children. J Thorac Cardiovasc Surg 1979;78:351–364.
38. **Waller BF, Jones M, Roberts WC.** Postoperative aortic regurgitation from incomplete seating of tilting-disc occluders due to overhandling knots or long sutures. Chest 1980;78:565–568.
39. **Roberts WC.** Complications of cardiac valve replacement: characteristic abnormalities of prostheses pertaining to any or specific site. Am Heart J 1982;103:113–122.
40. **Roberts WC, Isner JM, Virmani R.** Left ventricular incision midway between the mitral anulus and the stumps of the papillary muscles during mitral valve excision with or without rupture or aneurysmal formation: analysis of 10 necropsy patients. Am Heart J 1982;104:1278–1287.
41. **Warnes CA, Scott ML, Silver GM, Smith CW, Ferrans VJ, Roberts WC.** Comparison of late degenerative changes in porcine bioprostheses in the mitral and aortic valve position in the same patient. Am J Cardiol 1983; 51:965–968.
42. **Silver MA, Oranburg PR, Roberts WC.** Severe mitral regurgitation immediately after mitral valve replacement with a parietal pericardial bovine bioprosthesis. Am J Cardiol 1983;52:218–219.
43. **Warnes CA, McIntosh CL, Roberts WC.** Wear of the metallic studs on the composite seat of the 2320 Starr-Edwards aortic valve and its clinical consequences. Am J Cardiol 1983;52:1062–1065.
44. **Cohen SR, Silver MA, McIntosh CL, Roberts WC.** Comparison of late (62 to 140 months) degenerative changes in simultaneously implanted and explanted porcine (Hancock) bioprostheses in the tricuspid and mitral valve positions in six patients. Am J Cardiol 1984;53:1599–1602.
45. **Ross EM, Roberts WC.** A precaution when using the St. Jude Medical prosthesis in the aortic valve position. Am J Cardiol 1984;54:231–233.
46. **Silver MA, Cohen SR, McIntosh CL, Cannon RO III, Roberts WC.** Late (5 to 132 months) clinical and hemodynamic results after either tricuspid valve replacement or anuloplasty for Ebstein's anomaly of the tricuspid valve. Am J Cardiol 1984;54:627–632.
47. **Lester WM, Roberts WC.** Fatal bioprosthetic regurgitation immediately after mitral and tricuspid valve replacements with Ionescu-Shiley bioprostheses. Am J Cardiol 1985;55:590–592.
48. **Roberts WC, Lachman AS.** Mitral valve *commissurotomy* versus *replacement*. Considerations based on examination of operatively excised stenotic mitral valves. Am Heart J 1979;98:56–62.
49. **Roberts WC.** Mitral commissurotomy—still a good operation. Am J Cardiol 1983;52:A9–A10.

Mitral Valve Prolapse and Systemic Hypertension

In the USA there are approximately 160 million persons over 20 years of age (total population = 238 million). Of the 160 million, an estimated 8 million (5%) have auscultatory evidence of mitral valve prolapse (MVP) and 60 million (37%) have systemic hypertension (SH) (arterial pressure ≥140/90 mm Hg). Accordingly, of the 8 million with MVP, nearly 3 million (0.37 × 8) have SH, and of the 60 million with SH, 3 million (0.05 × 60) have MVP. The number of persons, therefore, with both MVP and SH in the USA is substantial.

Except in the person with left ventricular outflow obstruction, the systemic peak systolic arterial pressure is identical to the left ventricular peak systolic pressure, which of course is the pressure that closes the mitral valve orifice during ventricular systole. The normal mitral valve withstands elevation of the left ventricular peak systolic pressure without development of mitral regurgitation unless mitral anular calcific deposition is heavy, a process which is more frequent in hypertensive than in normotensive persons.[1] But how well does the defective, i.e., prolapsed or floppy, mitral valve tolerate chronic elevation of the left ventricular peak systolic pressure? My answer is "poorly," and the reason is because the associated SH (specifically, the elevated left ventricular systolic pressure) greatly increases the frequency of spontaneous rupture of mitral chordae tendineae, an occurrence virtually limited to patients with preexisting MVP. Jeresaty and associates[2] found underlying MVP in 23 (92%) of 25 patients with spontaneous rupture of mitral chordae tendineae and Hickey and associates[3] found underlying MVP in 29 (94%) of 31 patients with spontaneous rupture of mitral chordae tendineae. In an earlier study,[4] my colleagues and I examined 60 operatively excised purely regurgitant prolapsed mitral valves: 13 had ruptured chordae tendineae and of these, 11 (85%) had had SH before valve replacement; of the remaining 47 valves, none had ruptured chordae tendineae and only 11 (23%) of them had had SH preoperatively.

The normal mitral leaflets, as with the leaflets of all 4 cardiac valves, consist of 2 components: the fibrosa and the spongiosa. The fibrosa consists of collagen fibrils and the spongiosa, of an acid mucopolysaccharide material. In MVP the collagen fibrils of both the leaflets and chordae tendineae are defective[5] and probably, at least initially, decreased in number, and the spongiosa material, the "weaker" of the 2 components, is present in excessive amounts. It is reasonable to believe that the weaker the mitral leaflet and chordal structures, the greater the effect on them of the left ventricular systolic pressure, and the greater the mitral closing pressure the greater its effect on the defective mitral leaflet and chordal structures.

In summary, the normal mitral valve tolerates elevated left ventricular systolic pressures (mitral closing pressures) well, i.e., without creating mitral regurgitation and without rupturing mitral chordae tendineae. The prolapsed mitral valve, in contrast, contains defective collagen fibrils and excess spongiosa and it appears to withstand elevated left ventricular systolic pressures poorly as manifested by a high frequency of spontaneous rupture of chordae tendineae (and probably also by an increased degree of leaflet prolapse). Thus, proper treatment of SH may prevent or delay the appearance of severe mitral regurgitation that occurs in some patients with MVP.

William C. Roberts

William C. Roberts, MD
Editor in Chief

1. **Roberts WC.** Morphologic features of the normal and abnormal mitral valve. Am J Cardiol 1983;51:1005–1028.
2. **Jeresaty RM, Edwards JE, Chawla SK.** Mitral valve prolapse and ruptured chordae tendineae. Am J Cardiol 1985;55:138–142.
3. **Hickey AJ, Wilcken DEL, Wright JS, Warren BA.** Primary (spontaneous) chordal rupture: relation to myxomatous valve disease and mitral valve prolapse. JACC 1985;5:1341–1346.
4. **Waller BF, Morrow AG, Maron BJ, Del Negro AA, Kent KM, McGrath FJ, Wallace RB, McIntosh CL, Roberts WC.** Etiology of clinically isolated, severe, chronic, pure mitral regurgitation: an analysis of 97 patients over 30 years of age having mitral valve replacement. Am Heart J 1982;104:276–288.
5. **Renteria VG, Ferrans VJ, Jones M, Roberts WC.** Intracellular collagen fibrils in prolapsed ("floppy") human atrioventricular valves. Lab Invest 1976; 35:439–443.

Effects of Antihypertensive Therapy on Blood Lipid Levels

In the 1970s "massive" educational and therapeutic programs were carried out in the USA to determine how many of its citizens had systemic hypertension and to treat effectively those who did. These programs have been highly successful. The major direct consequence of systemic hypertension, namely stroke, is clearly decreasing in frequency; dissection of the aorta, another direct consequence of systemic hypertension, may be decreasing in frequency; and the frequency of fatal coronary artery disease is decreasing, but how much of its decrease is attributable to better control of systemic hypertension is uncertain.

In the 1980s, the emphasis has switched from blood pressure lowering to blood lipid lowering. The results of the Lipid Research Clinics Coronary Primary Prevention Trial (LRC-CPPT) were published in January 1984 and they established conclusively that the lowering of the plasma total cholesterol level, at least when initially considerably elevated (>265 mg/dl), was associated with a decrease in heart attack frequency.[1] Armed with this information, the National Heart, Lung, and Blood Institute has instituted a "massive" educational program involving both medical-care providers and patients to identify all citizens in the USA with hypercholesterolemia and to treat effectively those above certain levels (roughly total plasma cholesterol >220 mg/dl for persons <30 years of age and >240 mg/dl for persons >40 years of age). The results of this campaign on the blood cholesterol levels will not be known for several years, but any population-wide lowering of the blood cholesterol levels surely will have important beneficial effects on the frequency of symptomatic coronary artery disease.

The most important finding from the LRC-CPPT was that every 1% decrease in the plasma total cholesterol level was associated with a 2% decrease in the frequency of fatal coronary artery disease and/or nonfatal acute myocardial infarction (Figure). This monumental study (3,086 men enrolled, 193,000 clinic visits, 1,055,000 clinic data forms, 341,000 blood tests, 72,000 electrocardiograms, and >$150 million cost)—the most important cardiologic study of this decade in my view—also showed that the appearance of angina pectoris or congestive heart failure or resuscitated cardiac arrest or a positive exercise stress test, and the need for coronary artery bypass grafting was significantly less in the group randomized to lipid-lowering therapy (cholestyramine) compared to the group randomized to placebo.

A corollary to this finding would be that every 1% increase in plasma total cholesterol level would be associated with a 2% increase in heart attack frequency (Figure). Although this "corollary" is unproven, it is established that the risk of heart attack is proportional to the serum (or plasma) total cholesterol level—the higher the level, the greater the risk.[2]

Thus, for patients receiving therapy for any condition for many years, it is important that the blood lipid levels (at least the total cholesterol and the low-density lipoprotein [LDL] cholesterol) do not increase. The largest group of patients most likely to receive medical therapy over many years, of course, is that with systemic hypertension and most patients

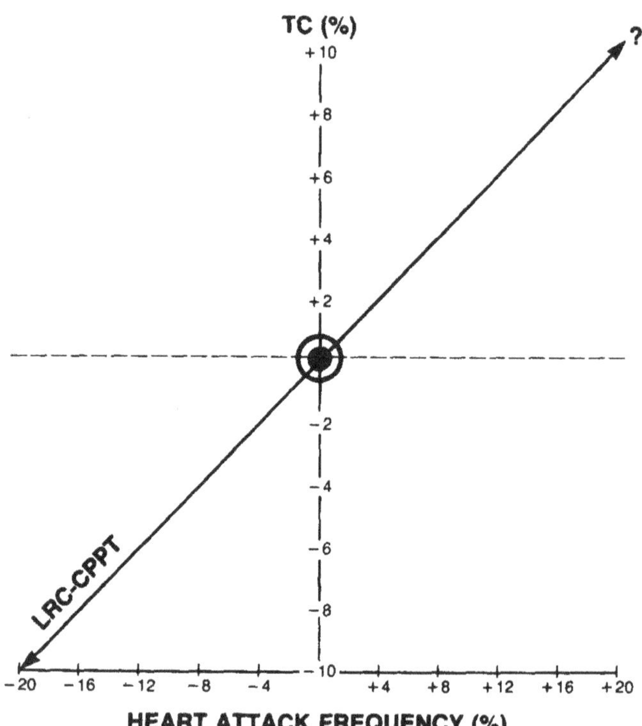

FIGURE. Effect of increasing or decreasing plasma total cholesterol (TC) level on heart attack frequency. LRC-CPPT = Lipid Research Clinics Coronary Primary Prevention Trial.

with systemic hypertension are asymptomatic. Of the 160 million USA citizens >20 years of age, it is estimated that 60 million (37%) have a systemic arterial blood pressure >140/90 mm Hg. It is also known that persons with untreated systemic hypertension have higher total and LDL-cholesterol and lower HDL-cholesterol than normotensive subjects of similar age and sex.[3]

Several studies have examined the effects of various antihypertensive medicines on blood lipid levels. Most studies have showed that *diuretics* during the first 12 months of therapy raise the blood total and LDL-cholesterol levels and lower the HDL-cholesterol levels.[4–17] These levels, however, appear to return to baseline or below by 12 months and do not increase to 4 years thereafter.[16] *Beta blockers* without intrinsic sympathomimetic activity (ISA) raise the blood triglyceride level, lower the HDL-cholesterol level, raise the total to HDL-cholesterol ratio, and have little or no effect on the total or LDL-cholesterol levels; β blockers with ISA, however, do not raise the blood triglyceride or lower the HDL-cholesterol levels and they do not change or they slightly lower the total and LDL-cholesterol levels.[18–21] The short-term elevations of blood lipid levels by diuretics appear to be reversed by administering an ISA β blocker simultaneously.[22] *Calcium-channel blockers* and *converting enzyme inhibitors* do not adversely effect blood lipid levels short-term; long-term data are not yet available.[23]

Most studies on the effects of antihypertensive drugs on the blood lipid levels are short term (≤12 months), most did not have 3 different determinations of the blood lipid levels before initiation of antihypertensive therapy—a requirement to be reasonably (75%) certain of the baseline level[24]—, some were not randomized prospective studies, and most were complicated by more than 1 drug being given simultaneously. Thus, more information is required to be certain of long-term effects of various antihypertensive medicines on blood lipid levels. It would be ideal to have a drug that not only decreased elevated blood pressure levels but simultaneously lowered blood lipid levels. But lacking this ideal antihypertensive agent at present, it is important that blood pressure lowering not be accompanied by blood lipid raising.

William C. Roberts

William C. Roberts, MD
Editor-in-Chief

References

1. Lipid Research Clinics Program. The Lipid Research Clinics Coronary Primary Prevention Trial Results. I. Reduction in incidence of coronary heart disease. II. The relationship of reduction in incidence of coronary heart disease to cholesterol lowering. JAMA 1984;251:351–374.
2. Grundy SM. Can dietary change prevent coronary heart disease? Prog Cardiol 1981;10:13–21.
3. MacMahon SW, Macdonald GJ, Blacket RB. Plasma lipoprotein levels in treated and untreated hypertensive men and women. The National Heart Foundation of Australia Risk Factor Prevalence Study. Arteriosclerosis 1985;5:391–396.
4. Schoenfeld MR, Goldberger E. Hypercholesterolemia induced by thiazides: a pilot study. Curr Ther Res 1964;6:180–184.
5. Ames RP, Hill P. Elevation of serum lipid levels during diuretic therapy of hypertension. Am J Med 1976;61:748–757.
6. Kannel WB, Gordon T, McGee D. Diuretics and serum cholesterol. Lancet 1977;1:1362–1363.
7. Helgeland A, Hjermann I, Holme I, Leren P. Serum triglycerides and serum uric acid in untreated and thiazide-treated patients with mild hypertension. The Oslo study. Am J Med 1978;64:34–38.
8. Goldman AI, Steel BW, Schnaper HW, Fritz A, Frohlich ED, Perry MH. Serum lipoprotein levels during chlorthalidone therapy: a Veterans Administration–National Heart, Lung, and Blood Institute cooperative study on antihypertensive therapy: mild hypertension. JAMA 1980;244:1691–1695.
9. Grimm RH, Leon AS, Hunninghake DB, Lenz K, Hannan P, Blackburn H. Effects of thiazide diuretics on plasma lipids and lipoproteins in mildly hypertensive patients: a double-blind controlled trial. Ann Intern Med 1981;94:7–11.
10. Amery A, Birkenhager W, Bulpitt C, Clement D, Deruyttere M, de Schaepdryver A, Dollery C, Fagard R, Furette F, Forte J. Influence of antihypertensive therapy on serum cholesterol in elderly hypertensive patients. Acta Cardiol 1982;37:235–244.
11. Veterans Administration Cooperative Study Group on Antihypertensive Agents. Comparison of propranolol and hydrochlorothiazide for initial treatment of hypertension. I. Results of short-term titration with emphasis on racial differences in response. II. Results of long-term treatment. JAMA 1982;248:2004–2011.
12. Williams WR, Borhani NO, Schnaper HW, Schneider KA, Slotkoff L. On behalf of the Hypertension Detection and Follow-Up Program (HDFP) Cooperative Group. The relationship between diuretics and serum cholesterol in HDFP participants (abstr). JACC 1983;1:623.
13. Lasser NL, Grandits G, Caggiula AW, Cutler JA, Grimm RH Jr, Kuller LH, Sherwin RW, Stamler J. Effects of antihypertensive therapy on plasma lipids and lipoproteins in the Multiple Risk Factor Intervention Trial. Am J Med 1984;76:suppl 2A:52–66.
14. Ames RP. Coronary heart disease and the treatment of hypertension: impact of diuretics on serum lipids and glucose. J Cardiovasc Pharmcol 1984;6:S466–S473.
15. Weinberger MH. Antihypertensive therapy and lipids. Evidence, mechanisms, and implications. Arch Intern Med 1985;145:1102–1105.
16. Burris JF, Freis ED. Thiazides do not cause long-term increases in serum lipid concentrations. Arch Intern Med 1985;145:2264–2266.
17. Wallace RB, Hunninghake DB, Chambless LE, Heiss G, Wahl P, Barrett-Connor E. A screening survey of dyslipoproteinemias associated with prescription drug use. The Lipid Research Clinics Program Prevalence Study. Circulation 1986;73:suppl I:I-70–I-79.
18. van Brummelen P. The relevance of intrinsic sympathomimetic activity for β-blocker-induced changes in plasma lipids. J Cardiovasc Pharm 1983;5:S51–S55.
19. Leren P. Effect of alpha- and beta-blocker therapy on blood lipids: European experience. Am J Med 1984;76:67–71.
20. Giuntoli F, Scalabrino A, Galeone F, Birindelli A, Natali A, Panigada G, Saba P. Antihypertensive and metabolic effects of a long-term treatment with acebutolol. Curr Ther Res 1984;36:188–194.
21. Lehtonen A. Effect of beta blockers on blood lipid profile. Am Heart J 1985;109:1192–1196.
22. Schiffl H, Weidmann P, Mordasini R, Riesen W, Bachmann C. Reversal of diuretic-induced increases in serum low-density-lipoprotein cholesterol by the betablocker pindolol. Metabolism 1982;31:411–415.
23. Pool PE, Seagren SC, Salel AF, Skalland ML. Effects of diltiazem on serum lipids, exercise performance and blood pressure: randomized, double-blind, placebo-controlled evaluation for systemic hypertension. Am J Cardiol 1985;56:86H–91H.
24. Blackburn H. Coronary risk factors. How to evaluate and manage them. Eur J Cardiol 1975;2/3:249–283.

Sudden Cardiac Death: Definitions and Causes

The phrase "sudden death" has been used by lay and medical persons for nearly 450 years. It has many definitions. "Sudden death" might be a game played to break a tie or the extra minutes of play added to a tied game, the winning team being the first team to score. In medicine "sudden death" generally denotes death which is *nonviolent* or nontraumatic, which is *unexpected*, which is *witnessed* and which is *instantaneous* or occurs within a few minutes of an abrupt change in previous clinical state. In heart disease the word "cardiac" is usually placed between the words "sudden" and "death," and the phrase "sudden cardiac death" usually is applied to persons who die suddenly from atherosclerotic coronary artery disease.[1] Necropsy studies of persons dying suddenly from cardiac disease, however, disclose many causes of "sudden cardiac death," and, therefore, greater specificity is required in terms to prevent confusion (Figure). Of persons dying suddenly from cardiovascular disease, the cause may be *cardiac* or *noncardiac*. The cardiac causes may be subdivided into *coronary* and *noncoronary*. Of the coronary causes, atherosclerosis is, of course, by far the most common, and the term *atherosclerotic sudden coronary death* may be applied to them.[2–18] In young persons particularly, several *nonatherosclerotic* coronary conditions, mainly coronary anomalies, cause sudden death.[19–28] Of the cardiac but noncoronary causes of sudden death, the most common are cardiomyopathy, particularly hypertrophic cardiomyopathy,[29–39] and valvular heart disease, most commonly the conditions causing left ventricular outflow obstruction,[40–50] sometimes associated with prosthetic or bioprosthetic heart valves.[51] Also, there are noncardiac but vascular causes of sudden death.[52–55] Some cardiac arrhythmic causes of sudden death not necessarily associated with morphologic abnormalities, e.g., prolonged QT interval syndrome, do not appear in the accompanying figure.[19,56–59]

Some examples of the many causes of sudden cardiac death:

(1) A 13-year-old athletic boy, the son of a former professional football player, collapsed while jogging and died. He had always been asymptomatic. His brother, a year older, had died a year earlier also while jogging. M.M.'s electrocardiogram 6 months earlier was considered "abnormal" but his left ventricular pressure was normal and there was no obstruction to left ventricular outflow.

(2) A 17-year-old girl, who ran 40 miles weekly, suddenly collapsed and died just after crossing the finish line of a 3-mile race. She had been "healthy" all of her life.

(3) A 19-year-old male midshipman was always asymptomatic until he suddenly collapsed and died while sitting on a bench immediately after running around the track several times. On admission examination a year earlier, electrocardiogram had shown ventricular premature complexes and left-axis deviation. The heart was of normal size by chest roentgenogram. The blood pressure was 135/80 mm Hg.

(4) A 28-year-old woman, well all her life, suddenly collapsed and died while running for a bus.

(5) A 28-year-old man died suddenly while pushing a brick-loaded wheelbarrow. He had been well until 2 days earlier when he complained of "pain in his neck," but this did not prevent him from performing his usual construction job activities.

(6) A 33-year-old woman, a domestic, collapsed while at work and died immediately. She had been healthy all her life.

(7) A 44-year-old woman, a secretary, collapsed while walking in her office and died. She had been asymptomatic all her life but on routine examination several years earlier was found to have precordial murmurs (each grade 2/6) consistent with "aortic stenosis and regurgitation." Chest radiograph had shown mild cardiomegaly and electrocardiogram had shown left ventricular hypertrophy.

(8) A 44-year-old male taxicab driver was well until about 1 hour before death when he became enraged because his taxicab was bombarded by snowballs thrown by 3 youths. One snowball entered an open window and hit him in the face, knocking off his glasses. He immediately radioed the police, who arrived several minutes later and apprehended the youths. The police described the taxicab driver as "livid with rage" over the incident and advised him to leave the scene. Thirty minutes later he radioed his dispatcher that he was having breathing difficulties. He arrived at the dispatcher's office a few minutes later, collapsed, and died.

(9) A 60-year-old male school teacher had been well all his life except for recognized systemic hypertension until a

few minutes before death, when he became enraged when trying to prevent 2 students in the school gymnasium from fighting. He finally broke up the fight and, while walking away from the event minutes later, collapsed and died.

(10) An 81-year-old woman, who had had a pacemaker inserted for complete heart block 23 months earlier, collapsed and died while climbing a flight of stairs in her home. During the preceding 2 days, she had noted excessive fatigue, nausea and vomiting.

The cause of death in each of the above 10 patients was different and had not a necropsy been performed, the cause of death could not have been accurately predicted. Patient 1 had *hypertrophic cardiomyopathy*. Patient 2 had *congenital hypoplasia of both right and left circumflex coronary arteries with inadequate perfusion of the posterior wall of the left ventricle.*[19] Patient 3 had *origin of the left main coronary artery from the right sinus of Valsalva with coursing of the left main between the pulmonary trunk and ascending aorta.*[23] Patient 4 had *isolated coronary arterial dissection* involving the left anterior descending and left circumflex coronary arteries.[28] Patient 5 had extensive *cardiac sarcoidosis.*[35] Patient 6 had a *ruptured sinus of Valsalva aneurysm* (into the pericardial sac rather than into the right side of the heart).[60] Patient 7 had *congenital origin of the left main coronary artery from the pulmonary trunk.*[24] Patient 8 had *atherosclerotic coronary artery disease* with severe narrowing of each of the 3 major coronary arteries. Patient 9 had a large heart (550 g [normal ≤400 g]) from *systemic hypertension* but no significant coronary arterial narrowing or other recognized cause of sudden death.[61] Patient 10 had severe *coronary arterial atherosclerosis* with *acute myocardial infarction* complicated by *rupture of the left ventricular free wall* and hemopericardium. Tests of the pacemaker after death disclosed that it had functioned normally.

In any study discussing sudden death from cardiovascular disease, the word *sudden* needs defining. The World Health Organization has used a 24-hour definition of sudden, meaning, of course, death occurring within 24 hours of an abrupt change in previous clinical status.[62] When this definition of sudden is used, many cases of acute myocardial infarction are intermixed with cases of sudden atherosclerotic coronary death unassociated with myocardial necrosis. Because it takes over 6 hours for histologic evidence of myocardial necrosis to be apparent and because most persons who die suddenly do so within an hour of change in previous clinical status, the 6-hour definition for "sudden" when applied to "atherosclerotic sudden coronary death" more clearly separates the infarct cases from the noninfarct ones.[2,4,16,17]

Although the term sudden implies *unexpected*, in only a quarter of victims of atherosclerotic coronary artery disease is sudden death the initial manifestation of coronary artery disease, and therefore, truly unexpected. Sudden death in patients with angina pectoris or healed myocardial infarction is really not so unexpected. Likewise, in persons with hypertrophic cardiomyopathy and certain forms of valvular heart disease, death suddenly is always a shock but, in actuality, not so unexpected.

Although sudden death is usually reserved for *nonviolent* or nontraumatic deaths, various mentally or even physically traumatic events can precipitate sudden death.[63,64]

The term "sudden death" is often used for persons in hospitals who are found dead, most often in their beds. I try to reserve the term "sudden death" for persons who have fatal or nonfatal cardiac arrest *outside* the hospital or at least

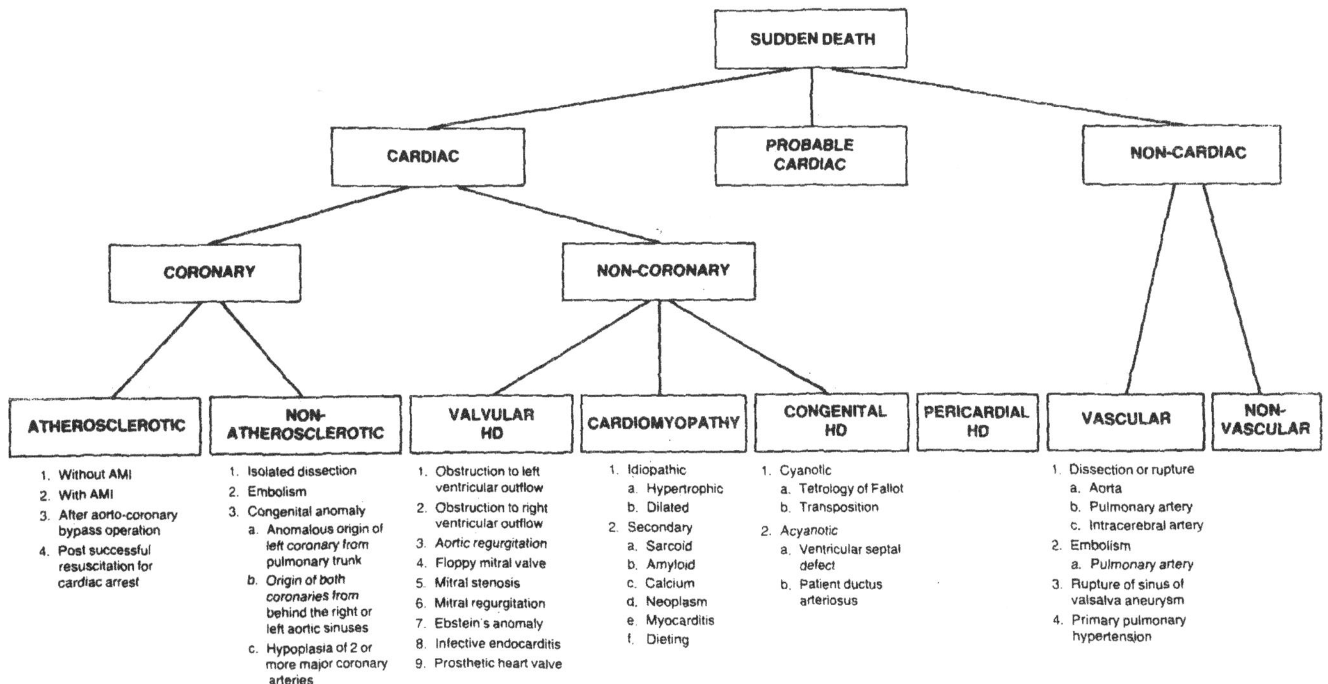

whose symptoms of cardiovascular dysfunction appear initially while outside a hospital. Some of these victims, of course, are rushed to hospitals, where fatal cardiac arrest occurs shortly after arrival.

I have examined many manuscripts that have used the phrase "sudden death" as a *cause* of death: "Patient so and so died of sudden death or patient so and so had sudden death but lived"! Obviously, the term "sudden death" should be used only as a *mode* of death or otherwise lawyers and editors will have a field day.

The use of the term "sudden death" in persons who are successfully resuscitated is not recommended. The use of the term *nonfatal cardiac arrest* (to contrast with *fatal cardiac arrest*) is preferable in this circumstance.

In summary, sudden cardiac death has many causes. Atherosclerotic coronary artery disease, obviously, is by far the most common cause of "sudden cardiac death," but the latter term is not synonmous with atherosclerotic coronary artery disease. "Sudden coronary death" is not ideal either because not all sudden coronary deaths are the result of atherosclerotic narrowing, but "sudden coronary death" is more precise than "sudden cardiac death." Sudden death is not always so *sudden*, or so *unexpected*, or *witnessed* and indeed it may be caused by or precipitated by mental or physical violence. Thus, greater precision is needed when discussing "sudden cardiac death."

William C. Roberts

William C. Roberts, MD
Editor in Chief

References

1. Eisenberg MS, Bergner L, Hallstrom AP, Cummins RO. *Sudden cardiac death. Sci Am 1986(May);254:37–43.*
2. Roberts WC, Buja LM. *The frequency and significance of coronary arterial thrombi and other observations in fatal acute myocardial infarction. A study of 107 necropsy patients. Am J Med 1972;52:425–443.*
3. Bulkley BH, Roberts WC. *Atherosclerotic narrowing of the left main coronary artery. A necropsy analysis of 152 patients with fatal coronary heart disease and varying degrees of left main narrowing. Circulation 1976;53: 823–828.*
4. Roberts WC, Jones AA. *Quantitation of coronary arterial narrowing at necropsy in sudden coronary death. Analysis of 31 patients and comparison with 25 control subjects. Am J Cardiol 1979;44:39–45.*
5. Waller BF, Roberts WC. *Sudden death while running in conditioned runners aged 40 years or over. Am J Cardiol 1980;45:1292–1300.*
6. Brosius FC Jr, Blackbourne BD, Roberts WC. *Death in the disco. Chest 1980;78:321–323.*
7. Walker BF, Csere RS, Baker WP, Roberts WC. *Running to death. Chest 1981;79:346–349.*
8. Brosius FC III, Waller BF, Roberts WC. *Radiation heart disease. Analysis of 16 young (aged 33 to 50 years) necropsy patients who received over 3,500 rads to the heart. Am J Med 1981;70:519–530.*
9. Cabin HS, Roberts WC. *Fatal cardiac arrest during cardiac catheterization for angina pectoris: analysis of 10 necropsy patients. Am J Cardiol 1981;48:1–8.*
10. Roberts WC, Maron BJ. *Sudden death while playing professional football. Am Heart J 1981;102:1061–1063.*
11. McManus BM, Waller BF, Graboys TB, Mitchell JH, Siegel RJ, Miller HS Jr, Froelicher VF, Roberts WC. *Exercise and sudden death. Part I. Current Prob Cardiol 1981;6(9):1–89.*
12. McManus BM, Waller BF, Graboys TB, Mitchell JH, Siegel RJ, Miller HS Jr, Froelicher VF, Roberts WC. *Exercise and sudden death. Part II. Current Prob Cardiol 1982;6(10):1–57.*
13. Roberts WC, Curry RC Jr, Isner JM, Waller BF, McManus BM, Mariani-Constantini R, Ross AM. *Sudden death in Prinzmetal's angina with coronary spasm documented by angiography. Analysis of three necropsy patients. Am J Cardiol 1982;50:203–210.*
14. Warnes CA, Kishel JC, Roberts WC. *Fatal cardiac arrest during cardiac catheterization for angina pectoris. A marker of quadruple vessel disease. Chest 1983;84:631–632.*
15. Sprecher DL, Schaefer EJ, Kent KM, Gregg RE, Zech LA, Hoeg JM, McManus B, Roberts WC, Brewer HB Jr. *Cardiovascular features of homozygous familial hypercholesterolemia: analysis of 16 patients. Am J Cardiol 1984;54:20–30.*
16. Warnes CA, Roberts WC. *Sudden coronary death: relation of amount and distribution of coronary narrowing at necropsy to previous symptoms of myocardial ischemia, left ventricular scarring and heart weight. Am J Cardiol 1984;54:65–73.*
17. Warnes CA, Roberts WC. *Comparison at necropsy by age group of amount and distribution of narrowing by atherosclerotic plaque in 2995 five-mm long segments of 240 major coronary arteries in 60 men aged 31 to 70 years with sudden coronary death. Am Heart J 1984;108:431–435.*
18. Warnes CA, Roberts WC. *Sudden coronary death: comparison of patients with to those without coronary thrombus at necropsy. Am J Cardiol 1984; 54:1206–1211.*
19. Maron BJ, Roberts WC, McAllister HA, Rosing DR, Epstein SE. *Sudden death in young athletes. Circulation 1980;62:218–229.*
20. Maron BJ, Epstein SE, Roberts WC. *Causes of sudden death in competitive athletes. JACC 1986;7:204–214.*
21. Roberts WC, Siegel RJ, Zipes DP. *Origin of the right coronary artery from the left sinus of Valsalva and its functional consequences: analysis of 10 necropsy patients. Am J Cardiol 1982;49:863–868.*
22. Roberts WC, Robinowitz M. *Anomalous origin of the left anterior descending coronary artery from the pulmonary trunk with origin of the right and left circumflex coronary arteries from the aorta. Am J Cardiol 1984;54:1381–1383.*
23. Barth CW III, Roberts WC. *Left main coronary artery originating from the right sinus of Valsalva and coursing between the aorta and pulmonary trunk. JACC 1986;7:366–373.*
24. Roberts WC. *Major anomalies of coronary arterial origin seen in adulthood. Am Heart J 1986;111:in press.*
25. Roberts WC, Silver MA, Sapala JC. *Intussusception of a coronary artery associated with sudden death in a college football player. Am J Cardiol 1986;57:179–180.*
26. Roberts WC. *Coronary embolism: a review of causes, consequences, and diagnostic considerations. Cardiovasc Med 1978;3:699–710.*
27. Waller BF, Dixon DS, Kim RW, Roberts WC. *Embolus to the left main coronary artery. Am J Cardiol 1982;50:658–660.*
28. Bulkley BH, Roberts WC. *Dissecting aneurysm (hematoma) limited to coronary artery. A clinicopathologic study of six patients. Am J Med 1973;55:747–756.*
29. Roberts WC, Ferrans VJ. *Pathologic anatomy of the cardiomyopathies. Idiopathic dilated and hypertrophic types, infiltrative types and endomyocardial disease with and without eosinophilia. Hum Pathol 1975;6:287–342.*
30. Maron BJ, Roberts WC, Edwards JE, McAllister HA, Foley DD, and Epstein SE. *Sudden death in patients with hypertrophic cardiomyopathy: characterization of 26 patients without functional limitation. Am J Cardiol 1978;41:803–810.*
31. Maron BJ, Lipson LC, Roberts WC, Savage DD, Epstein SE. *"Malignant" hypertrophic cardiomyopathy: identification of a subgroup of families with unusually frequent premature death. Am J Cardiol 1978;41:1133–1140.*
32. Maron BJ, Tajik AJ, Ruttenberg HD, Graham TP, Atwood GF, Victoria BE, Lie JT, Roberts WC. *Hypertrophic cardiomyopathy in infants: clinical features and natural history. Circulation 1982;65:7–17.*
33. Maron BJ, Roberts WC, Epstein SE. *Sudden death in hypertrophic cardiomyopathy: a profile of 78 patients. Circulation 1982;65:1388–1394.*
34. Maron BJ, Epstein SE, Roberts WC. *Hypertrophic cardiomyopathy: a common cause of sudden death in the young competitive athlete. Eur Heart J 1983;4:suppl F:135–144.*
35. Roberts WC, McAllister HA Jr, Ferrans VJ. *Sarcoidosis of the heart. A clinicopathologic study of 35 necropsy patients (group I) and review of 78 previously described necropsy patients (group II). Am J Med 1977;63:86–108.*
36. Virmani R, Bures JC, Roberts WC. *Cardiac sarcoidosis: a major cause of sudden death in young individuals. Chest 1980;77:423–428.*
37. Saffitz JE, Sazama K, Roberts WC. *Amyloidosis limited to small arteries causing angina pectoris and sudden death. Am J Cardiol 1983;51:1234–1235.*
38. Roberts WC, Waller BF. *Cardiac amyloidosis causing cardiac dysfunction: analysis of 54 necropsy patients. Am J Cardiol 1983;52:137–146.*
39. Saffitz JE, Ferrans VJ, Rodriquez ER, Lewis FR, Roberts WC. *Histiocytoid cardiomyopathy: a cause of sudden death in apparently healthy infants. Am J Cardiol 1983;52:215–217.*
40. Morrow AG, Fort L III, Roberts WC, Braunwald E. *Discrete subaortic stenosis complicated by aortic valvular regurgitation. Clinical, hemodynamic, and pathologic studies and the results of operative treatment. Circulation 1965;31:163–171.*
41. Roberts WC, Morrow AG. *Aortico-left ventricular tunnel. A cause of massive aortic regurgitation and of intracardiac aneurysm. Am J Med*

1965;39:662-667.

42. Roberts WC. *The structure of the aortic valve in clinically-isolated aortic* stenosis. *An autopsy study of 162 patients over 15 years of age.* Circulation *1970;42:91-97.*

43. Roberts WC. The congenitally bicuspid aortic valve. A study of 85 autopsy *cases. Am J Cardiol 1970;26:72-83.*

44. Roberts WC. Anatomically isolated aortic valvular disease. The case *against its being of rheumatic etiology. Am J Med 1970;49:151-159.*

45. Roberts WC, Perloff JK, Constantino T. Severe *valvular aortic stenosis in patients over 65 years of age. A clinicopathologic* study. *Am J Cardiol* 1971;27:497-506.

46. Falcone MW, Roberts WC, Morrow AG, Perloff JK. *Congenital aortic stenosis resulting from unicommissural valve. Clinical and anatomic features in twenty-one adult patients. Circulation 1971;44:272-280.*

47. Roberts WC, Dangel JC, Bulkley BH. *Non-rheumatic valvular cardiac disease. A clinicopathologic survey of 27 different conditions causing valvular dysfunction.* Cardiovasc Clin 1973;5:333-446.

48. Maron BJ, Redwood DR, Roberts WC, Henry WL, Morrow AG, Epstein SE. *Tunnel subaortic stenosis. Left ventricular outflow tract obstruction produced by fibromuscular tubular narrowing. Circulation* 1976;54:404-416.

49. Roberts WC. *Morphologic features of the normal and abnormal mitral valve.* Am J Cardiol 1983;51:1005-1028.

50. Roberts WC. *The 2 most common congenital heart diseases.* Am J Cardiol 1984;53:1198.

51. Roberts WC. *The silver anniversary of cardiac valve replacement.* Am J Cardiol 1985;56:503-506.

52. Roberts WC. *The aorta: its acquired diseases and their consequences as viewed from a morphologic perspective.* In: Lindsay J Jr, Hurst JW, eds. The Aorta. *New York: Grune & Stratton, 1979:51-117.*

53. Roberts WC. *Aortic dissection: anatomy, consequences, and causes.* Am Heart *J 1981;101:195-214.*

54. Waller BF, Reis RL, McIntosh CL, Epstein SE, Roberts WC. The Marfan *cardiovascular disease without the Marfan syndrome.* Chest 1980;77:533-540.

55. Roberts WC, Honig HS. *The spectrum of cardiovascular disease in the Marfan syndrome: a clinico-morphologic study of 18 necropsy patients and comparison to 151 previously reported necropsy patients.* Am Heart J 1982;104:115-135.

56. Isner JM, Sours HE, Paris AL, Ferrans VJ, Roberts WC. *Sudden, unexpected death in avid dieters using the liquid-protein-modified-fast diet. Observations in 17 patients and the role of the prolonged QT interval. Circulation* 1979;60:1401-1412.

57. Siegel RJ, Cabeen WR Jr, Roberts WC. *Prolonged QT interval-ventricular tachycardia syndrome from massive rapid weight loss utilizing the liquid-protein-modified-fast diet: sudden death with sinus node ganglionitis and neuritis.* Am Heart J 1981;102:121-123.

58. Isner JM, Roberts WC, Heymsfield SB, Yager J. *Anorexia nervosa and sudden death.* Ann Intern Med 1985;102:49-52.

59. McManus BM, Fleury TA, Roberts WC. *Fatal catecholamine crisis in pheochromocytoma: curable cause of cardiac arrest.* Am Heart J 1981; 102:930-932.

60. Roberts WC. *Congenital cardiovascular abnormalities usually "silent" until adulthood: morphologic features of the floppy mitral valve, valvular aortic stenosis, hypertrophic cardiomyopathy, sinus of Valsalva aneurysm, and the Marfan syndrome.* In: Roberts WC, ed. Congenital Heart Disease in Adults. *Philadelphia: FA Davis, 1979:407-453* (Cardiovasc Clin 10;[1]:-574).

61. Roberts WC. The hypertensive diseases. *Evidence that systemic hypertension is greater risk factor to the development of other cardiovascular diseases than previously suspected.* Am J Med 1975;59:523-532.

62. *Classification of atherosclerotic lesions. Report of a study group.* WHO Techn Rep Ser 1958 (No. 143).

63. Engel GL. *Sudden and rapid death during psychological stress. Forklore or folk wisdom?* Ann Intern Med 1971;74:771-782.

64. Engel GL. *Psychologic stress, vasodepressor (vasovagal) syncope, and sudden death.* Ann Intern Med 1978;89:403-412.

A Simple Histologic Classification of Pulmonary Arterial Hypertension

For many years students of congenital heart disease were unable to explain the differences in survival patterns in patients with similar-sized isolated communications between systemic and pulmonary circulations. In 1927 Moschcowitz[1] suggested that the explanation may be the presence of pulmonary hypertension in some patients with shunts and its absence in others. In 1935, Brenner[2] described histologic features of the normal pulmonary arteries and veins. In 1936, Parker and Weiss[3] at the Boston City Hospital described changes in the parenchyma and vessels of lungs in patients with mitral stenosis. In the late 1940s, Edwards,[4] who also trained at the Boston City Hospital in the late 1930s, began describing anatomic changes in the pulmonary vasculature in patients with congenital heart disease, and he too attributed the changes to the effects of pulmonary hypertension. In 1958, Heath and Edwards[5] proposed an anatomic classification of hypertensive pulmonary changes (Fig. 1). Their classification was based primarily on observations of necropsy patients with large ventricular septal defect or patent ductus arteriosus having *pulmonary hypertension from birth*, but a few patients had primary pulmonary hypertension.

Although the Heath and Edwards classification brought organization to a complex subject, reevaluation nearly 30 years later indicates that their classification has certain deficiencies. Considerable overlap exists between their grades 2 and 3 and grades 4 and 5. *Alveolar hemosiderosis* (grade 5) does not concern a pulmonary artery and it may occur in patients without pulmonary arterial hypertension. In my view, a classification of pulmonary arterial changes should not include changes in alveolar spaces (hemosiderosis). Their grade 6 category implies that grades 1 through 5 are prerequisites, when, in actuality, necrotizing vasculitis may occur in the absence of grades 1 to 5 and it may occur in the absence of pulmonary hypertension. A classification of hypertensive changes in the pulmonary arteries should be applicable, of course, to all patients with pulmonary hypertension irrespective of its cause and irrespective of whether the hypertension is congenital or acquired in origin.

The classification of pulmonary arterial changes recommended herein consists of only 3 grades, and is based on histologic alterations irrespective of the etiology of or the time of appearance of the pulmonary arterial hypertension. The major changes in the pulmonary arteries include: (1) *medial thickening* (MT), (2) *intimal thickening* (IT), and (3) *plexiform lesion* (PL) (Fig. 2). Grade I includes MT only; grade II, MT plus IT; and grade III, MT plus IT plus PL (Fig. 3). Neither arteritis (vasculitis) nor hemosiderosis are included in the grading system.

Medial thickening: This indicates an increase in the thickness of the media of a pulmonary artery or of a pulmonary arteriole, or both. Whether this occurs entirely from hypertrophy of smooth muscle cells or from both hypertrophy and hyperplasia is unclear. Thus, the reason for the phrase *medial thickening* rather than *medial hypertrophy*.

Intimal thickening: There are 2 types of intimal thickening: the cellular variety, in which the proliferated intima consists primarily of smooth-muscle cells with collagen in between, and the acellular variety, which consists mostly of dense fibrous (collagen) tissue with minimal or no smooth muscle cells.

Plexiform lesion: This is an aneurysmal or glomus-like structure that emerges at more-or-less right angles to a muscular pulmonary artery. Just after origin of the right-angle branch it suddenly bulges into a plexus of channels, the walls of which consist primarily of fibrous tissue covered by endo-

Basis of Grades of Hypertensive Pulmonary Vascular Disease Found in Association with Large Ventricular Septal Defects and Functionally Related Diseases

	Grade of hypertensive pulmonary vascular disease					
	1	2	3	4	5	6
Type of intimal reaction	←None→					
		←	←	Cellular	→	→
			←	Fibrous and fibroelastic	→	→
				←	Plexiform lesion	→
State of media of arteries and arterioles	←	←	Hypertrophied	→	→	→
			←	Some generalized dilatation	→	→
				←	Local "dilatation lesions"*	→
					← Pulmonary hemosiderosis†	→
						←Necrotizing arteritis→

*Vein-like branches of hypertrophied muscular pulmonary arteries, angiomatoid lesion, and cavernous lesion

†Associated with distended, thin-walled, arterial vessels throughout the lung

FIGURE 1. Classification of hypertensive pulmonary vascular changes by Heath and Edwards in 1958.[5] Reproduced with permission of the publisher.

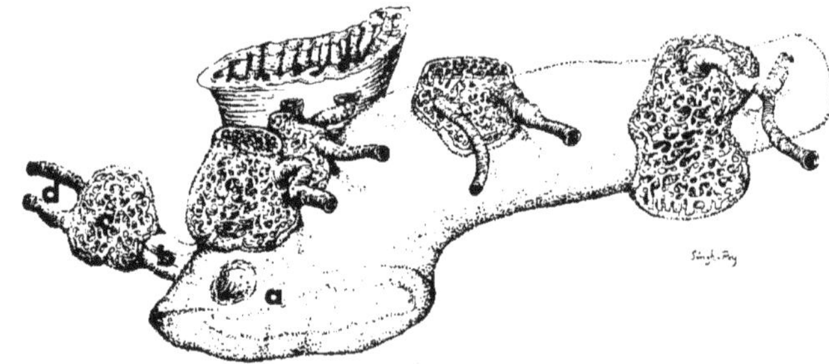

FIGURE 2. Drawing from Moschcowitz et al[10] of plexiform lesions arising from a muscular pulmonary artery. Reproduced with permission of the publisher.

CHANGE (S)	GRADE	MORPHOLOGY
Normal or Thin-Walled	0	
Medial Thickening (MT)	I	
MT + Intimal Thickening (IT)	II	
MT + IT + Plexiform Lesion	III	

FIGURE 3. Types of grading of the morphologic pulmonary artery changes from Virmani and Roberts.[12] Reproduced with permission of the publisher.

thelial cells. The PL gives rise to thin-walled channels, probably dilated arterioles, which rapidly branch into alveolar septal capillaries. These thin-walled channels when considerably dilated have been called *dilatation lesions.*

Proposed causes: *Medial thickening* is a response of the arterial wall to increased pressure and therefore occurs only in patients with pulmonary arterial hypertension. Medial thickening is never simply a normal consequence of aging. *Intimal thickening* is not necessarily the consequence of pulmonary arterial hypertension, but it is accelerated by elevation of pulmonary arterial pressure. Cellular and acellular IT is frequently observed in older persons, most of whom have normal pulmonary arterial pressures.[6] The occurrence of IT combined with MT, however, is indicative of pulmonary hypertension. *Plexiform lesions* occur only in patients with severe pulmonary hypertension, but most patients with severe pulmonary hypertension do not have them. Plexiform lesions occur in patients with large intravascular shunts or primary pulmonary hypertension or pulmonary embolic or thrombotic disease, but they do not occur in patients in whom the severe pulmonary hypertension is secondary to left-sided cardiac disease (e.g., mitral stenosis). Plexiform lesions do not occur if the cause of the pulmonary hypertension is located distal to the pulmonary capillary level or, stated differently, if the pulmonary arterial hypertension is the consequence of pulmonary venous hypertension. For a PL to occur, the cause of the hypertension must originate at the capillary or recapillary level.[7]

The exact cause of PLs is unknown. Serial sections of lung at sites of a PL generally show extreme narrowing or almost total obstruction of the lumen of the muscular pulmonary artery distal to the origin of the small muscular pulmonary artery or arteriole which is the site of the PL. Kanjuh and colleagues[8] suggested that the PL was a consequence of a *jet lesion* caused by blood rapidly changing its course because of the distal obstruction of the relatively large muscular pulmonary artery distal to the site of the PL. Thus, the PL might act as a dissipator of the extremely high pulmonary arterial pressure. Others have suggested that the PL represents a site of *anastomoses of pulmonary arteries and veins*[9] or it is a *congenital malformation.*[10] PL, however, has never been observed in the lungs at birth; the earliest it has been observed is at 2 months of age.[11] The PL may represent an aneurysm formed at sites of *congenitally underdeveloped or weak media* (analogous to the formation of an intracerebral berry aneurysm in systemic hypertension), the aneurysm later being filled by thrombus, which organizes into multiple minute vascular channels.[12,13] Wagenvoort and Wagenvoort[14] proposed that the PL represents a site of healed necrotizing arteritis. The inflammation weakens the arterial wall, which focally expands, fibrin and platelets are deposited in the aneurysm, and organization of the thrombus produces multiluminal channels lined by endothelial cells.

Whatever its cause, the PL represents irreversible pulmonary hypertension, whereas MT alone or MT plus IT indicates that the pulmonary hypertension is reversible.

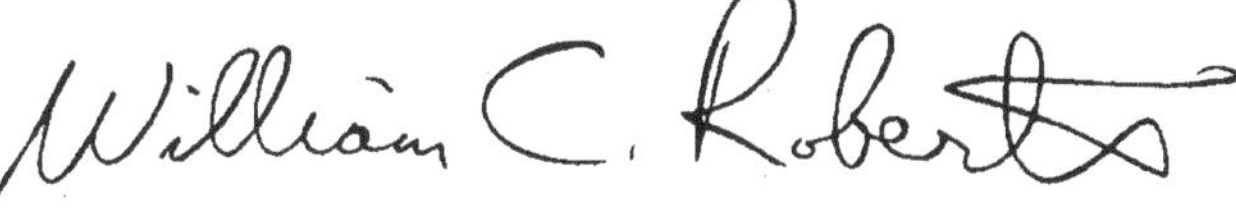

William C. Roberts, MD
Editor in Chief

References

1. Moschcowitz E. Hypertension of the pulmonary circulation; its causes, dynamics and relation to other circulatory states. Am J Med Sci 1927;174:388–406.
2. Brenner O. Pathology of the vessels of the pulmonary circulation. Arch Intern Med 1935;56:211–237, 457–497, 724–752, 976–1014, 1189–1241.
3. Parker F, Weiss S. The nature and significance of the structural changes in the lungs in mitral stenosis. Am J Pathol 1936;12:573–598.
4. Edwards JE. Functional pathology of the pulmonary vascular tree in congenital cardiac disease. Circulation 1957;15:164–196.
5. Heath D, Edwards JE. The pathology of hypertensive pulmonary vascular disease. A description of six grades of structural changes in the pulmonary arteries with special reference to congenital cardiac septal defects. Circulation 1958;18:533–547.
6. Wagenvoort CA, Wagenvoort N. Age changes in muscular pulmonary arteries and arterioles. Arch Pathol 1965;79:524–528.
7. Roberts WC, Fredrickson DS. Gaucher's disease of the lung causing severe pulmonary hypertension with associated acute recurrent pericarditis. Circulation 1967;35:783–789.
8. Kanjuh VI, Sellers RD, Edwards JE. Pulmonary vascular plexiform lesion. Arch Pathol 1964;78:513–522.
9. Hufner RF, McNicol CA. The pathologic physiology of microscopic pulmonary vascular shunts. AMA Arch Pathol 1958;65:554–560.
10. Moschcowitz E, Rubin E, Strauss L. Hypertension of the pulmonary circulation due to congenital glomoid obstruction of the pulmonary arteries. Am J Pathol 1961;39:75–93.
11. Hruban Z, Humphreys EM. Congenital anomalies associated with pulmonary hypertension in an infant. Arch Pathol 1960;70:766–779.
12. Virmani R, Roberts WC. Pulmonary arteries in congenital heart disease: a structure-function analysis. In: Roberts WC, ed. Adult Congenital Heart Disease. Philadelphia: FA Davis, 1987:77–131.
13. Naeye RL, Vennart GP. Structure and significance of pulmonary plexiform structures. Am J Pathol 1960;36:593–621.
14. Wagenvoort CA, Wagenvoort N. Pathology of Pulmonary Hypertension. New York: Wiley & Sons, 1977.

The Senile Cardiac Calcification Syndrome

Calcific deposits in the heart are common in older individuals residing in areas where symptomatic atherosclerosis is common. The most common location of the calcific deposits is the *epicardial coronary arteries*. Calcific deposits in coronary arteries are located in intimal plaques, not in media, and therefore, their presence indicates the presence of atherosclerosis. In younger individuals, calcific deposits in epicardial coronary arteries not only indicate the presence of atherosclerotic plaques, but they nearly always indicate the presence of significant luminal narrowing of the arteries containing the calcified plaques. In persons >65 years of age, however, calcific deposits in epicardial coronary arteries do not necessarily indicate the existence of severe luminal narrowing.[1]

A second common site of cardiac calcific deposits is the *mitral anular area*. "Mitral anular calcium" (MAC) is really a misnomer because if calcific deposits were limited to the anulus they would not be visible grossly. The calcific deposits in actuality are located between the undersurface of the posterior mitral leaflet and the mural endocardium of left ventricular wall in apposition to posterior mitral leaflet.[2,3] These calcific deposits usually are located only behind the posterior mitral leaflet and because this leaflet has a C-shaped circumferential attachment to the anulus, the "anular" calcium, if extensive, has a C-shaped configuration. Rarely, the calcium also extends across anterior mitral leaflet to form an "O."[4] When these calcific deposits are small, no hemodynamic consequence results. If the calcific deposits are large, mild to moderate regurgitation may occur and, on rare occasion, actual "mitral" stenosis.[5] In older individuals with mitral "anular" calcium, the anular circumference is virtually never dilated, whereas in younger individuals, particularly those with mitral valve prolapse, the anulus may be dilated.[6–8] Mitral valve replacement in the setting of heavy mitral anular calcium can be hazardous.

The third common site of calcium in the heart in elderly individuals is the *aortic valve cusps*.[9] These calcific deposits are located nearly entirely on the aortic aspects of the cusps, and whether or not the valve is stenotic is determined by the quantity of calcium deposited. Large quantities of calcium impart an immobility to the cusps, which can prevent their opening adequately during ventricular systole. Calcific aortic valve disease in the elderly usually is not associated with commissural fusion and, therefore, the cusps coapt properly with each other during ventricular diastole and aortic regurgitation usually is absent or minimal.[9]

The fourth common location of calcific deposits in the elderly heart is the *left ventricular papillary muscles*, limited to their apical portions.[10] The papillary muscles are the last portions of the heart to be perfused with arterial blood, and, therefore, if any portion of the heart is likely to be short-changed of oxygenated blood, they are it, particularly the posteromedial papillary muscle, which has a single arterial supply, in contrast to the double coronary arterial supply of the anterolateral papillary muscle. Calcific deposits in the apices of the papillary muscles appear to have no functional consequence.

Calcific deposits in the coronary arteries are a manifestation of atherosclerosis, and thus the factors that predispose to noncalcific atherosclerosis also predispose to calcific atherosclerosis. the major predisposing factor, of course, is an elevated (>150 mg/dl) blood total cholesterol level. Because only 5% of Americans over 40 years of age have a total cholesterol level <150 mg/dl, 95% of the population >40 years of age are candidates for atherosclerosis extensive enough to produce luminal narrowing of 1 or more major coronary arteries.

It is my understanding that mitral anular calcium and aortic valve calcium are rare in elderly individuals residing in areas of the world where total blood cholesterol levels are <150 mg/dl. Because calcific deposits in the mitral anular area and in the aortic valve cusps are observed only in populations that develop significant coronary atherosclerosis, it is reasonable to suspect that the cause of the mitral anular calcium and the aortic valve cuspal calcium in the elderly is similar, namely, that the mitral anular and aortic cuspal calcium in the elderly is a form of atherosclerosis. Further support for this view is the frequent occurrence of calcific deposits in the coronary artery, mitral anular area and aortic valve in the same person (Fig. 1). In a study from my laboratory of necropsy persons age >65 years, 100% of those with mitral anular or aortic valve cuspal calcium also had calcific deposits in one or more coronary arteries.[3] Furthermore, of 100 persons >65 years of age with mitral anular calcium, 75 also had aortic cuspal calcium.[3]

The factors that predispose to atherosclerosis in the coronary arteries also predispose to calcific deposits in the mitral anular region and in the aortic valve cusps. Patients with extreme hypercholesterolemia (total cholesterol >500 mg/dl—type II homozygous hyperlipoproteinemia) develop severe coronary atherosclerosis by age 15 years and also calcific aortic valve stenosis in the teens.[11] Mitral anular calcium also occurs in these individuals in the teens.[11] Patients with systemic hypertension have a higher frequency of mitral anular and aortic valve calcific deposits than normotensive persons of similar age and sex.[3,12] Any condition causing hypercalcemia may lead to calcific deposits in the epicardial coronary arteries, mitral anular area, and aortic valve cusps.[13] Patients with diabetes mellitus have more coronary atherosclerosis and, specifically, more calcific deposits in these arteries than do nondiabetic persons of similar age and sex.[14–16] Diabetes mellitus patients also have more mitral anular and aortic cuspal calcific deposits than do nondiabetic persons of similar age and sex.[3]

Another factor suggesting that coronary atherosclerosis, mitral anular calcium and aortic valve calcium in the elderly have a similar etiology is a similar surface appearance of all 3 structures before the calcific deposits form. Specifically, during the teens, 20s and 30s, focal yellow deposits are observed on the endothelium of the epicardial coronary arteries, on the ventricular surfaces of the posterior mitral leaflet, and on the aortic aspects of each of the aortic valve cusps. These yellow deposits, of course, are foam cells. These collections of foam cells represent early or "young" atherosclerotic lesions. Experimentally induced systemic arterial atherosclerosis also is associated with deposition of fatty plaques on the aortic surfaces of the aortic valve cusps and on the ventricular surface of the posterior mitral leaflet.[17] As the fatty plaques get larger, their nutritional needs appear not be be fulfilled, and they degenerate into calcific deposits.

In persons under 65 years of age symptomatic coronary artery disease and clinical evidence of aortic valve stenosis is considerably more frequent in men than in women.[18–22] After age 65, however, the frequency of symptomatic coronary artery disease is nearly similar in men and women, and, likewise, after age 65 years, the frequency of aortic valve stenosis is similar in men and women.[9] After age 65, the frequency of mitral anular calcium is also similar in men and women, but of those persons with "massive" quantities of calcium in the mitral anular area, far more are women than men.[3]

Diagnosis of aortic valve stenosis in the elderly is more difficult than is this diagnosis in younger person.[2] The reason is not entirely certain, but the different configuration of the stenotic aortic valve in elderly compared to that in younger individuals almost certainly is a factor. In the elderly, the aortic valve is usually (90%) 3-cuspid, the calcific deposits are limited to the aortic aspects of the cusps, the commissures are not fused, and aortic regurgitation is usually absent.[9] In the younger individuals, the stenotic aortic valve commonly is congenitally bicuspid and associated regurgitation as the rule rather than the exception.[21] Another factor is that most (75%) of the elderly individuals also have mitral anular calcium, which can also produce a precordial systolic murmur, and few younger persons with aortic valve stenosis have mitral anular calcium.[3] Third, the systemic systolic pressure is usually normal (<140 mm Hg) in younger individuals with aortic valve stenosis, but it often is >140 mm Hg in the older patients.[9] An older individual may have aortic valve stenosis despite the presence of systemic hypertension! And finally, the cardiac output generally is lower and the distance from precordium to heart is greater in older compared to young individuals and these 2 factors may decrease the intensity of the systolic precordial murmur.

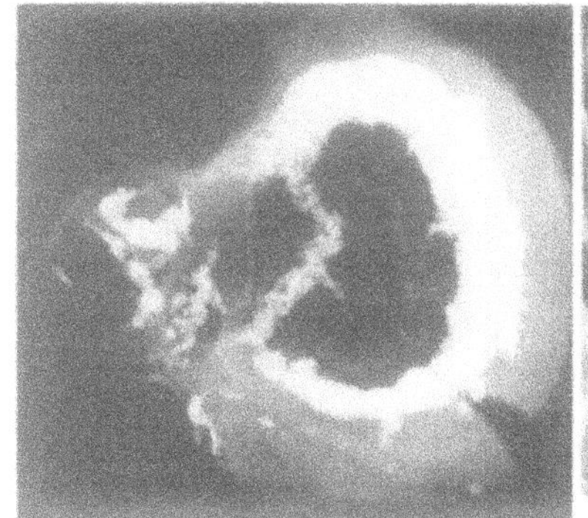
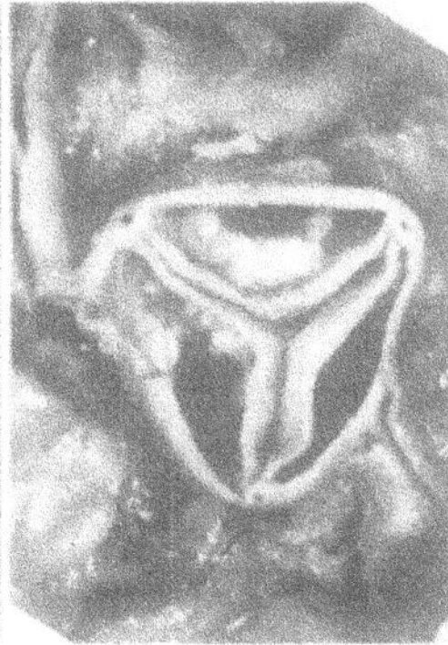

FIGURE 1. Radiograph of heart (*left*) and aortic valve (*right*) in an 82-year-old woman (NNMC #A70-200) who died of caecal volvulus. She never had symptoms of cardiac dysfunction, yet she has massive calcific deposits in the mitral "anular" region, across the anterior mitral leaflet, in the aortic valve cusps, and in the epicardial coronary arteries. The calcium in the aortic valve is located entirely on the aortic aspects of the cusps. None of the 3 commissures are fused, and therefore there was no aortic regurgitation. Reproduced with permission from Roberts and Perloff.[2]

Thus, cardiac calcium is not good. It may narrow the coronary arteries, mitral valve orifice and aortic valve orifice and it may prevent either or both of these valvular orifices from closing completely. It is reasonable to believe that both mitral anular and aortic cuspal calcific deposits in the elderly have the same etiology as the coronary atherosclerotic plaques because the 3 are commonly present in the same heart and the predisposing factors of all 3 are the same.

William C. Roberts, MD
Editor in Chief

References

1. Waller BF, Roberts WC. *Cardiovascular disease in the very elderly. Analysis of 40 necropsy patients aged 90 years or older.* Am J Cardiol 1983;51:403–421.
2. Roberts WC, Perloff JK. *Mitral valvular disease. A clinicopathologic survey of the conditions causing the mitral valve to function abnormally.* Ann Intern Med 1972;77:939–975.
3. Roberts WC. *Morphologic features of the normal and abnormal mitral valve.* Am J Cardiol 1983;51:1005–1028.
4. Roberts WC, Waller BF. *Mitral valve "annular" calcium forming a complete circle or "O" configuration: clinical and necropsy observations.* Am Heart J 1981;101:619–621.
5. Hammer WJ, Roberts WC, De Leon AC Jr. *"Mitral stenosis" secondary to combined "massive" mitral anular calcific deposits and small, hypertrophied left ventricles.* Am J Med 1978;64:371–376.
6. Roberts WC, Dangel JC, Bulkley BH. *Non-rheumatic valvular cardiac disease: a clinicopathologic survey of 27 different conditions causing valvular dysfunction.* Cardiovasc Clin 1973;5:333–446.
7. Roberts WC, Honing HS. *The spectrum of cardiovascular disease in the Marfan syndrome: a clinico-morphologic study of 18 necropsy patients and comparison to 151 previously reported necropsy patients.* Am Heart J 1982;104:115–135.
8. Waller BF, Morrow AG, Maron BJ, Del Negro AA, Kent KM, McGrath FJ, Wallace RB, McIntosh CL, Roberts WC. *Etiology of clinically isolated, severe, chronic, pure mitral regurgitation: analysis of 97 patients over 30 years of age having mitral valve replacement.* Am Heart J 1982;104:276–288.
9. Roberts WC, Perloff JK, Costantino T. *Severe valvular aortic stenosis in patients over 65 years of age. A clinicopathologic study.* Am J Cardiol 1971;27:497–506.
10. Roberts WC, Cohen LS. *Left ventricular papillary muscles. Description of the normal and a survey of conditions causing them to be abnormal.* Circulation 1972;46:138–154.
11. Sprecher DL, Schaefer EJ, Kent KM, Gregg RE, Zech LA, Hoeg JM, McManus B, Roberts WC, Brewer HB Jr. *Cardiovascular features of homozygous familial hypercholesterolemia: analysis of 16 patients.* Am J Cardiol 1984;54:20–30.
12. Roberts WC. *The hypertensive diseases. Evidence that systemic hypertension is a greater risk factor to the development of other cardiovascular diseases than previously suspected.* Am J Med 1975;59:523–532.
13. Roberts WC, Waller BF. *Effect of chronic hypercalcemia on the heart. An analysis of 18 necropsy patients.* Am J Med 1981;71:371–384.
14. Curry RC Jr, Roberts WC. *Status of the coronary arteries in the nephrotic syndrome. Analysis of 20 necropsy patients aged 15 to 35 years to determine if coronary atherosclerosis is accelerated.* Am J Med 1977;63:183–192.
15. Crall FV Jr, Roberts WC. *The extramural and intramural coronary arteries in juvenile diabetes mellitus. Analysis of nine necropsy patients aged 19 to 38 years with onset of diabetes before age 15 years.* Am J Med 1978;64:221–230.
16. Waller BF, Palumbo PJ, Lie JT, Roberts WC. *Status of the coronary arteries at necropsy in diabetes mellitus with onset after age 30 years. Analysis of 229 diabetic patients with and without clinical evidence of coronary heart disease and comparison to 183 control subjects.* Am J Med 1980;69:498–506.
17. Thubrikar MJ, Deck JD, Aouad J, Chen JM. *Intramural stress as a causative factor in atherosclerotic lesions of the aortic valve.* Atherosclerosis 1985; 55:299–311.
18. Roberts WC, Buja LM. *The frequency and significance of coronary arterial thrombi and other observations in fatal acute myocardial infarction. A study of 107 necropsy patients.* Am J Med 1972;52:425–443.
19. Roberts WC. *Anatomically isolated aortic valve disease. The case against its being of rheumatic etiology.* Am J Med 1970;49:151–159.
20. Roberts WC. *The structure of the aortic valve in clinically isolated aortic stenosis. An autopsy study of 162 patients over 15 years of age.* Circulation 1970;42:91–97.
21. Roberts WC. *The congenitally bicuspid aortic valve. A study of 85 autopsy cases.* Am J Cardiol 1970;26:72–83.
22. Falcone MW, Roberts WC, Morrow AG, Perloff JK. *Congenital aortic stenosis resulting from unicommissural valve. Clinical and anatomic features in twenty-one adult patients.* Circulation 1971;44:272–280.

Good-Bye to Thoracotomy for Cardiac Valvulotomy

The introduction of cardiac catheterization in the early 1940s revolutionized diagnostic cardiology.[1] Successful closed pulmonic and mitral valvulotomy in the late 1940s opened the heart to the surgeon.[2–4] The introduction of cardiopulmonary bypass in the mid 1950s revolutionized treatment of intracardiac congenital anomalies.[5] The creation of a good substitute cardiac valve in 1960 revolutionized the treatment of valvular regurgitation, aortic valve stenosis and mitral stenosis associated with either heavy calcific deposits and/or regurgitation.[6,7] In the mid-1960s, the catheter balloon was introduced as a means of opening the atrial septum to allow better mixing of blood in infants with complete transposition of the great arteries and similar anomalies.[8] The introduction of selective coronary angiography in the early 1960s made possible the introduction of aortocoronary bypass in the late 1960s and it revolutionized the treatment of coronary heart disease.[9,10] This coronary revolution continued with the introduction of percutaneous transluminal coronary angioplasty in the late 1970s in which an inflated elongated balloon was used to dilate narrowed coronary arteries. Now, in the mid-1980s, the balloon catheter is revolutionizing the therapy of stenotic cardiac valve disease.

Although started exclusively as a diagnostic laboratory, the catheter balloon has added a major therapeutic dimension to the catheterization laboratory. The balloon which Rashkind and Miller[8] used for atrial septostomy was egg-shaped when inflated. In retrospect, the balloon atrial septostomy was more of a landmark in cardiology than originally believed. A printer's error in a legend to a figure in the article by Rashkind and Miller in 1966 changed "magnified" to "magnificent" (". . .a magnificent view of the catheter tip with the balloon. . .") and today this word appropriately describes the first and subsequent therapeutic benefits of the intracardiac catheter balloon.

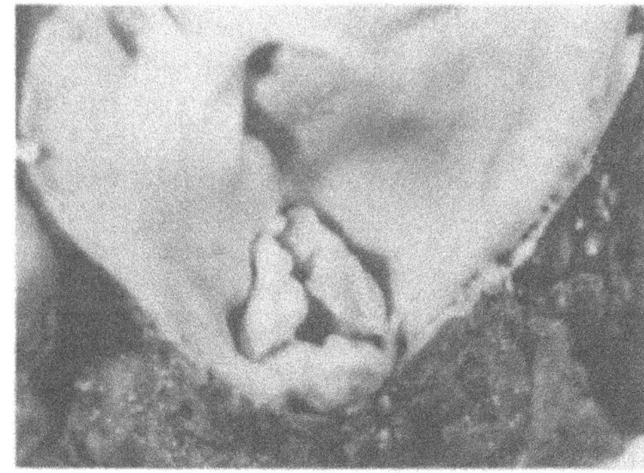

FIGURE 1. Congenital valvular pulmonic stenosis in a 43-year-old woman who died shortly after valvulotomy via thoracotomy. Reproduced with permission from Roberts WC, Dangel JC, Bulkley BH. *Nonrheumatic valvular cardiac disease: a clinicopathologic survey of 27 different conditions causing valvular dysfunction. Cardiovasc Clin 1973;5:333–446.*

The latest use of the catheter balloon, of course, is to dilate stenotic cardiac valves. Just like the initial use of the balloon catheter was by a pediatric cardiologist for congenital heart disease, successful balloon catheter valvulotomy also was first achieved by a pediatric cardiologist for congenital heart disease, specifically pulmonic valve stenosis by Kan and associates[11] in 1982 (Fig. 1). Numerous subsequent reports[12–43] followed and it is now clear, with one possible exception, that catheter balloon valvulotomy is the *procedure of choice* for patients with pulmonic valve stenosis.[44] The exception may be the patients in whom the obstruction results from a dysplastic pulmonic valve. The peak systolic gradient reduction using balloons 20 to 40% larger than the diameter of the root of the pulmonary trunk is roughly equivalent to that of surgery (about a 75% reduction).[44]

The stenotic *aortic* valve in *infants and children* was subjected to the balloon catheter initially by Lababidi,[45] and subsequently this procedure has been performed successfully in infants and children in other centers.[46–51] In general, the peak systolic pressure gradient is reduced about 50%. It is likely, however, that the percent gradient reduction will increase as better balloon catheters and probably larger ones are developed. It is only a matter of time before the U.S. Food and Drug Administration will approve balloon aortic valvuloplasty for infants and children as it already has approved balloon pulmonic valvuloplasty.

In 1986, Cribier and associates[52] extended percutaneous transluminal valvuloplasty to aortic valve stenosis *in adults*, and subsequently this procedure has been performed in adults in several other medical centers[53–55] (Fig. 2 to 6). Most adults reported have been over 65 years of age and the peak systolic gradient reduction has been about 50% (Fig. 2 and 3).

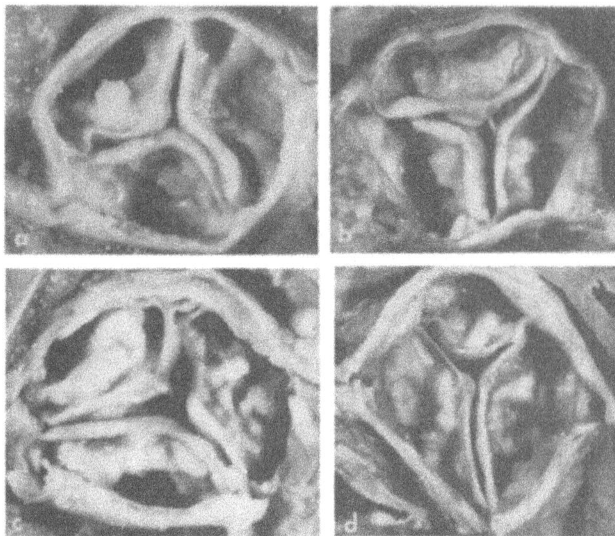

FIGURE 2. Three-cuspid stenotic aortic valves from 4 elderly patients. *a*, an 83-year-old woman; *b*, an 81-year-old woman; *c*, an 85-year-old woman; *d*, an 80-year-old man. Except for slight fusion of 1 commissure in *c*, none of the commissures are fused. Despite the calcific deposits on the aortic aspects of the cusps, these valves have been amenable to balloon valvuloplasty. Reproduced with permission from Roberts et al.[73]

FIGURE 3. Stenotic 3-cuspid aortic valves with fusion of 1 or 2 of the 3 commissures in 4 older patients. *a*, a 66-year-old man; *b*, a 70-year-old woman. *c*, a 76-year-old woman. *d*, an 82-year-old man. The commissural fusion, a relatively uncommon finding in stenotic aortic valves in patients older than 65 years of age, may limit the effectiveness of balloon valvuloplasty. Reproduced with permission from Roberts et al.[73]

The stenotic *mitral* valve was first subjected to percutaneous transluminal balloon valvuloplasty by Inoue and associates[56] in 1984, and subsequently this procedure has been performed in several centers[57–68] (Fig. 7 and 8). This procedure requires crossing the atrial septum by the balloon catheter. Even in the presence of calcific deposits in the mitral leaflets, the mean diastolic pressure gradient between left atrium and left ventricle can be expected to fall by 50% and by much more in the noncalcified valves.

Thus, balloon valvuloplasty in infants, children and adults in pulmonic, aortic and mitral positions is effective. It relieves or decreases symptoms of cardiac dysfunction, it decreases gradients across stenotic valves, and it increases valve areas. And the safety of the procedure is remarkable. Symptoms or signs compatible with dislodgment of calcific fragments or other material from the valve have been rare, significant regurgitation has been rare, and thoracotomy and cardiotomy or aortotomy has been avoided. The mechanism of the balloon dilatation appears to be identical to that produced by operative finger "fracture" or metallic instrument dilatation. The potential of restenosis after balloon valvuloplasty is as yet unknown, but I suspect that it will be similar to that from valvuloplasty after thoracotomy, namely, to be expected if the patient survives a sufficient period. Whereas thoracotomy can be performed a limited number of times in a lifetime, balloon valvuloplasty, just like coronary angioplasty, can be performed on several occasions.

When valvuloplasty (commissurotomy) via thoracotomy was introduced in 1948, this procedure proved to be extremely effective in mitral valves which were severely stenotic, devoid of calcific deposits, and free of associated significant mitral regurgitation. After mitral valve replacement became common in the 1960s, and along with a reduction in the frequency of mitral stenosis because of a decreasing frequency of rheumatic heart disease, mitral valvuloplasty became an infrequent operation. I have examined a number of operatively excised mitral valves in the past 15 years that preoperatively were purely stenotic or nearly so, that contained no calcific deposits by fluoroscopy, that were

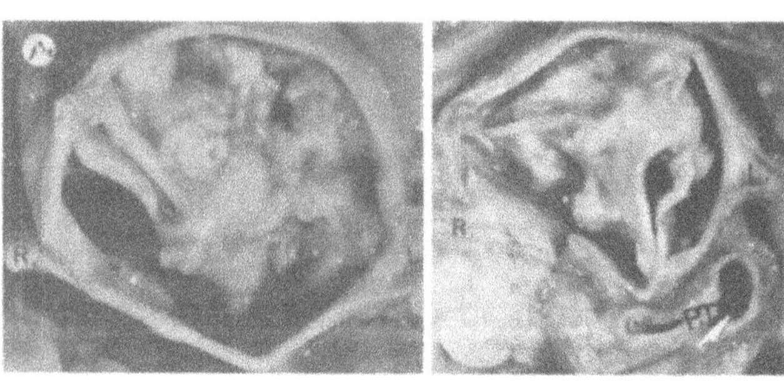

FIGURE 4. Congenitally unicuspid stenotic aortic valves. *Left*, in a 48-year-old man and *right*, in a 62-year-old man. It is unlikely that these congenitally unicuspid stenotic valves can have much gradient reduction by balloon valvuloplasty. L = left coronary arteries; PT = pulmonary trunk; R = right coronary arteries. Reproduced with permission from Falcone MW, Roberts WC, Morrow AG, Perloff JK. *Congenital aortic stenosis resulting from a unicommissural valve. Clinical and anatomic features in twenty-one adult patients. Circulation 1971;41:272–280.*

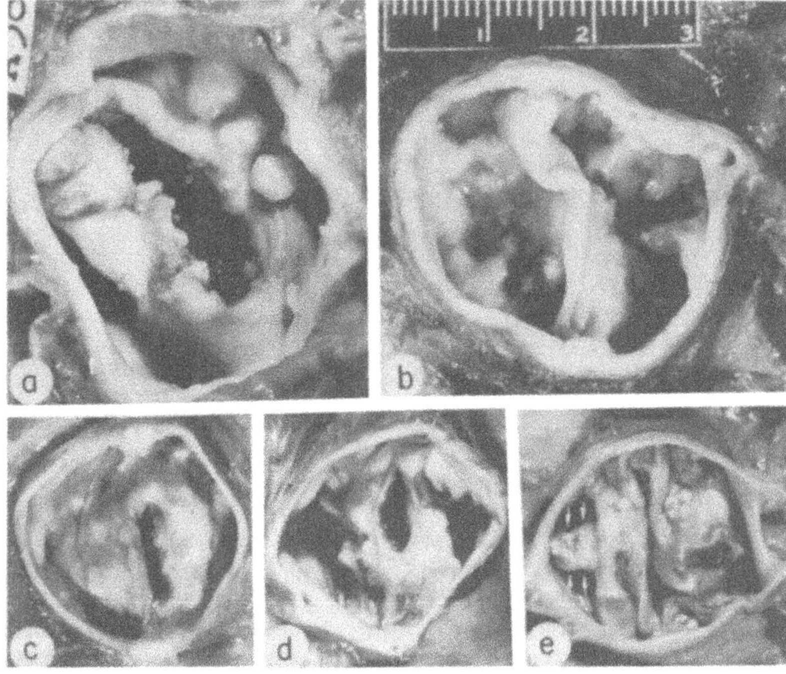

FIGURE 5. Congenitally bicuspid severely stenotic aortic valves in 5 patients. *a*, a 35-year-old man. *b*, a 54-year-old man. The peak systolic pressure gradient across this valve was 70 mm Hg. *c*, a 35-year-old man. The peak systolic pressure gradient was 92 mm Hg. *d*, a 54-year-old man. *e*, a 79-year-old woman. All 5 valves are heavily calcified and severely stenotic. I doubt if balloon valvuloplasty could satisfactorily dilate these valves. Reproduced with permission from Roberts WC.[71]

free or nearly so of associated mitral regurgitation by left ventricular angiography, and, nevertheless, the valve was excised[69] (Fig. 7). Balloon valvuloplasty may prevent operative valvuloplasty in the future and reserve operation for the patient who requires valve replacement because of stenosis associated with heavy calcific deposits or with significant associated regurgitation, or for the patient with pure valvular regurgitation (no element of stenosis).

It will be splendid to allow the young woman with mitral stenosis to have a balloon valvuloplasty during the child-bearing years and a valve replacement after age 40. Likewise, to prevent an open aortic valvulotomy in the first 20 years of life may allow a single aortic operation, valve replacement, in mid- or later adulthood for the person with symptomatic aortic stenosis early in life.

Balloon mitral or aortic valvuloplasty, of course, will not be a curative procedure. The value stenosis will eventually return just like it does after valvuloplasty via thoracotomy. But valve replacement is not a curative procedure either. All mechanical valves require anticoagulants forever thereafter, and all tissue valves eventually wear out and a subsequent operation is necessary if the patient survives a sufficient period. Anticoagulants are not required after percutaneous transluminal balloon valvuloplasty. Hospitalization may be reduced by this latter procedure to a couple of days. The pain and problems of thoracotomy are prevented.

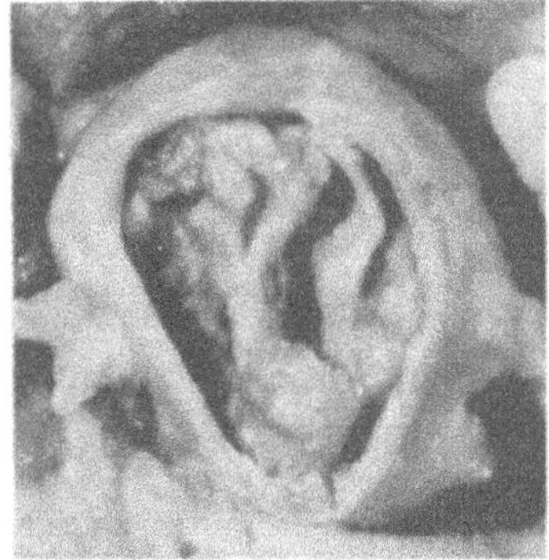

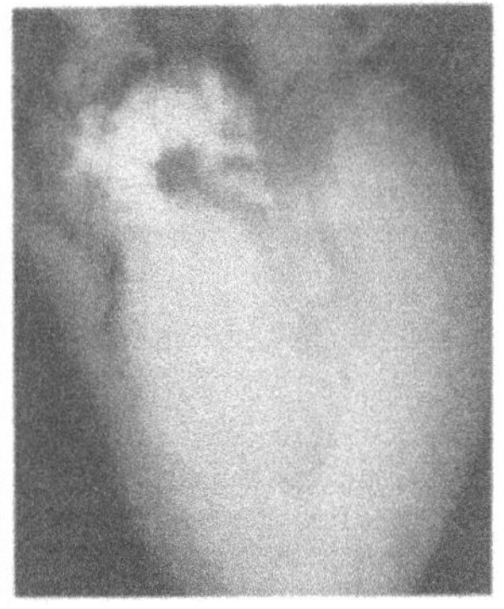

FIGURE 6. A congenitally malformed, probably bicuspid, severely stenotic aortic valve (*left*) in a 54-year-old man with radiograph of the heart specimen (*right*). Masses of rock, such as shown here, surely will not be amenable to balloon valvuloplasty. The peak systolic pressure gradient between left ventricle and aorta was 84 mm Hg. Reproduced with permission from Roberts WC. *Renal hemosiderosis (blue kidney) in patients with valvular heart disease. Am J Pathol 1966;48:409–419.*

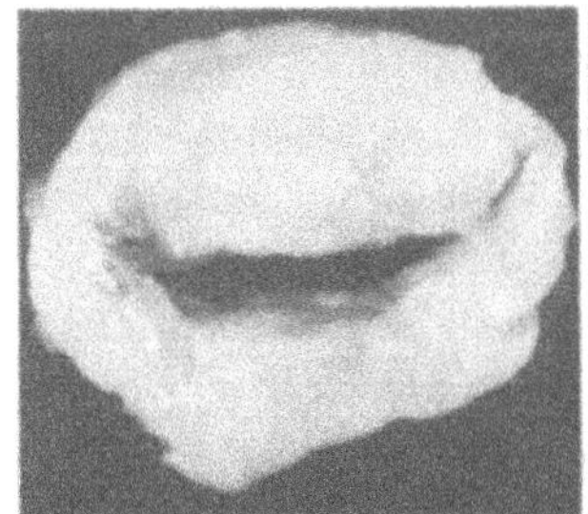

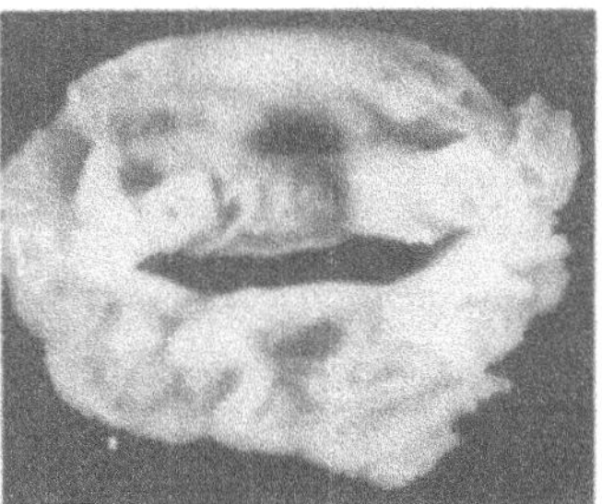

FIGURE 7. Operatively excised stenotic mitral valve in a 60-year-old woman. *Left*, atrial aspect; *right*, ventricular aspect. Radiograph of the operatively excised valve disclosed that it was devoid of calcific deposits and left ventricular angiography preoperatively disclosed mild mitral regurgitation. The mean diastolic pressure gradient between pulmonary artery wedge position and left ventricle was 14 mm Hg. This type valve would appear to be ideal for catheter balloon valvuloplasty.

Some stenotic cardiac valves almost surely will not respond favorably to balloon valvuloplasty (Fig. 3 to 6, 8). The most common structure underlying the stenotic aortic valve in the presence of an anatomically normal mitral valve is the bicuspid condition in the age group 16 to 65 years[70–72] (Fig. 5 and 6). These valves often become extensively calcified by age 40 to 50 years. I suspect that valve replacement will prove to be the initial procedure of choice in them. In contrast, 90% of persons with aortic valve stenosis over 65 years of age have a 3-cuspid aortic valve, usually without commissural fusion, and most of them appear to respond favorably to balloon valvuloplasty[73] (Fig. 2). About 10% of persons over 65 years of age with aortic stenosis, however, have a bicuspid aortic valve, and I suspect that these individuals will not have an effective gradient reduction by balloon dilatation.

In recent years I have witnessed aortic valve replacement in patients with peak systolic pressure gradients across the aortic valve of <50 mm Hg, and without significant associated aortic regurgitation. The reason aortic valve replacement was done was because coronary artery bypass grafting was warranted and in this circumstance ignoring the aortic valve disease seemed inadvisable. The availability of the balloon catheter may prevent both valve replacement and coronary bypass for some patients with combined valvular and coronary disease.

Balloon valvuloplasty for mitral stenosis in third world countries will be exceedingly useful. In this group, both calcific deposits in the mitral leaflets and associated severe mitral regurgitation is uncommon. Mitral stenosis in the Western world is decreasing in frequency except in the older age group. The older group of patients—usually women—also may be good candidates for the catheter balloon rather than the knife and finger.

In conclusion, the balloon catheter has converted the catheterization laboratory from purely a diagnostic to a diagnostic plus a therapeutic laboratory. Balloon valvuloplasty is now the procedure of choice for patients with pulmonic valve stenosis. It also, I suspect, will prove to be the procedure of choice for aortic valve stenosis causing symptoms of cardiac dysfunction in the first 2 decades of life. It is highly likely that balloon valvuloplasty will prove to be the procedure of choice for mitral stenosis unassociated with heavy calcific deposits or significant mitral regurgitation. In the older age group, despite calcific deposits, balloon valvuloplasty may prove to be the initial procedure of choice for both stenotic mitral and aortic valves. The heavily calcified congenitally unicuspid and bicuspid aortic valve almost certainly will not be the ideal valve for balloon valvuloplasty, and I suspect that valve replacement will remain the procedure of choice for persons with this underlying valve structure. It will only be a matter of time before combined mitral and aortic stenosis in the same patient will be subjected to the balloon catheter and I predict that the balloon will prove effective in many of them. The technology for balloon valvuloplasty is changing rapidly and better results than those currently reported may be expected in the future.

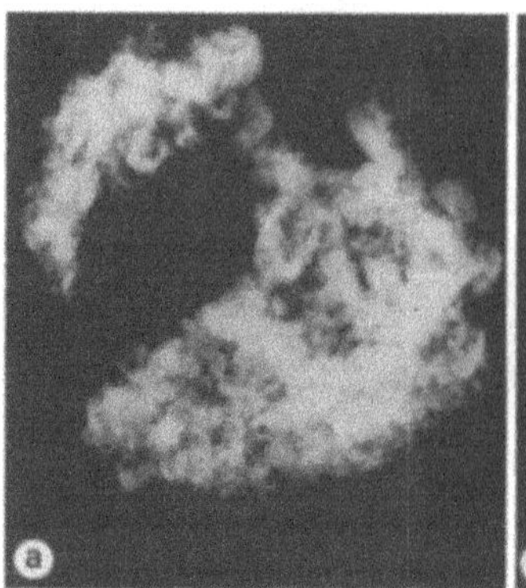

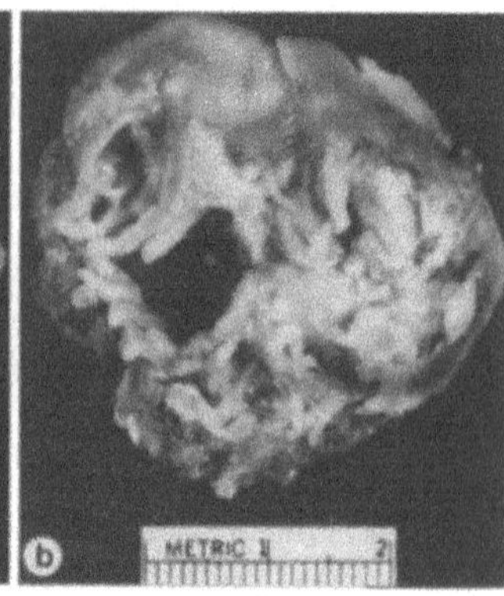

FIGURE 8. Operatively excised severely stenotic and heavily calcified mitral valve in a 26-year-old man. The mean diastolic pressure gradient between pulmonary artery wedge position and left ventricle was 15 mm Hg. This degree of calcium would appear to severely limit the effectiveness of catheter balloon valvuloplasty. Reproduced with permission from Lachman AS, Roberts WC. *Calcific deposits in stenotic mitral valves. Extent and relation to age, sex, degree of stenosis, cardiac rhythm, previous commissurotomy and left atrial body thrombus from study of 164 operatively-excised valves. Circulation 1978;57:808–815.*

William C. Roberts, MD
Editor in Chief

1. Cournand A, Ranges HA. *Catheterization of the right auricle in man. Proc Soc Exp Biol Med 1941;46:462–464.*
2. Brock RC. *Pulmonary valvulotomy for the relief of congenital pulmonary stenosis. Report of three cases. Br Med J 1948;1:1121–1126.*
3. Harken DW, Ellis LB, Ware PF, Norman LR. *The surgical treatment of mitral stenosis. I. Valvuloplasty. N Engl J Med 1948;239:801–809.*
4. Bailey CP. *The surgical treatment of mitral stenosis (mitral commissurotomy). Dis Chest 1949;15:377–384.*
5. Gibbon JH Jr. *Application of a mechanical heart and lung apparatus to cardiac surgery. Minn Med 1954;37:171–185.*
6. Harken DE, Soroff HS, Taylor WJ, Lefemine AA, Gupta SK, Lunzer S. *Partial and complete prosthesis in aortic insufficiency. J Thorac Cardiovasc Surg 1960;40:744–752.*
7. Starr A, Edwards ML. *Mitral replacement: clinical experience with a ball valve prosthesis. Ann Surg 1961;154:726–740.*
8. Rashkind WJ, Miller WW. *Creation of an atrial septal defect without thoracotomy. A palliative approach to complete transposition of the great arteries. JAMA 1966;196:991–992.*
9. Sones FM Jr, Shirey EK. *Cine coronary arteriography. Mod Concepts Cardiovasc Dis 1962;31:735–738.*
10. Favaloro RG. *Saphenous vein graft in the surgical treatment of coronary artery disease: operative technique. J Thorac Cardiovasc Surg 1969;58:178–185.*
11. Kan JS, White RI Jr, Mitchell SE, Gardner TJ. *Percutaneous balloon valvuloplasty: a new method for treating congenital pulmonary valve stenosis. N Engl J Med 1982;307:540–542.*
12. Pepine CJ, Gessner IH, Feldman RL. *Percutaneous balloon valvuloplasty for pulmonic valve stenosis in the adult. Am J Cardiol 1982;50:1442–1445.*
13. Fontes VF, Sousa JE, Pimentel-Filho WA, Buchler JR, da Silva MV, Bembom MC. *Pulmonary balloon valvuloplasty. Report of a case. Arq Bras Cardiol 1983;41:49–52.*
14. Lababidi Z, Wu JR. *Percutaneous balloon pulmonary valvuloplasty. Am J Cardiol 1983;52:560–562.*

15. Tynan M, Jones O, Joseph MC, Deverall PB, Yates AK. *Relief of pulmonary valve stenosis in first week of life by percutaneous balloon valvuloplasty. Lancet 1984;1:273.*

16. Kan JS, White RI Jr, Mitchell SE, Anderson JH, Gardner TJ. *Percutaneous transluminal balloon valvuloplasty for pulmonary valve stenosis. Circulation 1984;69:554-560.*

17. Rocchini AP, Kveselis DA, Crowley D, Dick M, Rosenthal A. *Percutaneous balloon valvuloplasty for treatment of congenital pulmonary valvular stenosis in children. JACC 1984;3:1005-1012.*

18. Fontes VF, Sousa JE, Esteves CA, Silva MV, Bembom MC, Silva MA, Cano M, Pontes SC JR. *Pulmonary valvuloplasty with the balloon catheter. An alternative in the treatment of pulmonary valve stenosis. Arq Bras Cardiol 1984;42:249-253.*

19. Abkin KH, Gotman LN. *Roentgenoendovascular valvuloplasty of isolated pulmonary stenosis by balloon dilatation. Khirurgiia (Mosk) 1984;6:91-93.*

20. Shuck JW, McCormick DJ, Cohen IS, Oetgen WJ, Brinker JA. *Percutaneous balloon valvuloplasty of the pulmonary valve: role of right to left shunting through a patent foramen ovale. JACC 1984;4:132-135.*

21. Bussmann WD, Sievert H, Reifart N. *Percutaneous bursting of the pulmonary valve. Deutsch Med Wochenschr 1984;109:1106-1108.*

22. Walls JT, Lababidi Z, Curtis JJ, Silver D. *Assessment of percutaneous balloon pulmonary and aortic valvuloplasty. J Thorac Cardiovasc Surg 1984;88:352-356.*

23. de Ubago JL, Figueroa A, Colman T, Lamelas R, Gallo JI, Diaz del Rio A, Duran CM. *Percutaneous pulmonary valvuloplasty using a balloon catheter. Rev Esp Cardiol 1984;37:354-358.*

24. Corbelli JC, Sterba R, Moodie DS. *Percutaneous balloon valvuloplasty for congenital pulmonary valve stenosis. Cleve Clin Q 1984;51:541-544.*

25. Ben-Shachar G, Cohen MH, Sivakoff MC, Portman MA, Riemenschneider TA, Van-Heeckeren DW. *Development of infundibular obstruction after percutaneous pulmonary balloon valvuloplasty. JACC 1985;5:754-756.*

26. Hess J, Mooyaart EL, Karliczek GF, Bergstra A, Landsman ML, Kuipers JR. *Percutaneous transluminal balloon valvuloplasty as a new treatment method in pulmonary valve stenosis. Ned Tijdschr Geneeskd 1985;129:403-406.*

27. Latson LA, Cheatham JP, Gumbiner CH, Hofschire PJ, Kugler JD, Fleming W. *Percutaneous balloon valvuloplasty for congenital pulmonary valve stenosis. Nebr Med J 1985;70:76-79.*

28. Benson LN, Smallhorn JS, Freedom RM, Trusler GA, Rowe RD. *Pulmonary valve morphology after balloon dilatation of pulmonary valve stenosis. Cathet Cardiovasc Diagn 1985;11:161-166.*

29. Tynan M, Baker EJ, Rohmer J, Jones OD, Reidy JF, Joseph MC, Ottenkamp J. *Percutaneous balloon pulmonary valvuloplasty. Br Heart J 1985;53:520-524.*

30. Rey C, Marache P, Matina D, Mouly A. *Percutaneous transluminal valvuloplasty in pulmonary stenosis. Apropos of 24 cases. Arch Mal Coeur 1985;78:703-710.*

31. Khalilullah M, Bahl VK, Choudhary A, Yadav BS, Babu MR, Natarajan D, Kaul UA, Arora R. *Pulmonary balloon valvuloplasty for the nonsurgical management of valvular pulmonary stenosis. Indian Heart J 1985;37:150-153.*

32. Kveselis DA, Rocchini AP, Snider AR, Rosenthal A, Crowley DC, Dick M II. *Results of balloon valvuloplasty in the treatment of congenital valvar pulmonary stenosis in children. Am J Cardiol 1985;56:527-532.*

33. Miller GA. *Balloon valvuloplasty and angioplasty in congenital heart disease. Br Heart J 1985;54:285-289.*

34. Sullivan ID, Robinson PJ, Macartney FJ, Taylor JF, Rees PG, Bull C, Deanfield JE. *Percutaneous balloon valvuloplasty for pulmonary valve stenosis in infants and children. Br Heart J 1985;54:435-441.*

35. Macaya C, Perez de la Cruz JM, Prieto J, Melgares R, Cutillas N, Santalla A, Bermudez R, Azpitarte J. *Percutaneous transluminal valvuloplasty with the balloon catheter in congenital stenosis of the pulmonary valve. Res Esp Cardiol 1985;38:408-414.*

36. Bussmann WD, Sievert H, Reifart N, Kober G, Satter P, Kaltenbach M. *Percutaneous pulmonary valvuloplasty. Z Kardiol 1985;74:718-721.*

37. McCredie RM, Swinburn MJ, Lee CL, Warner G. *Balloon dilatation pulmonary valvuloplasty in pulmonary stenosis. Aust NZ J Med 1986;16:20-23.*

38. Berland J, Cribler A, Champoud O, Barbe P, Letac B. *Balloon catheter dilation of severe pulmonary restenosis 11 years after surgical valvulotomy. Arch Mal Coeur 1986;79:385-389.*

39. Sutton TM, Carlson R, Bayron H, Griese GG. *Balloon pulmonary valvuloplasty for treatment of congenital pulmonary stenosis. Wis Med J 1986;85:30-32.*

40. Vitek B, Suchanek M. *Balloon dilatation (valvuloplasty) of valvular stenosis of the pulmonary artery. Cesk Pediatr 1986;41:268-270.*

41. Yeager SB, Neal WA, Balian AA, Gustafson RA. *Percutaneous balloon pulmonary valvuloplasty. W Va Med J 1986;82:169-171.*

42. Ali-Khan MA, Yousef SA, Mullins CE. *Percutaneous transluminal balloon pulmonary valvuloplasty for the relief of pulmonary valve stenosis with special reference to double-balloon technique. Am Heart J 1986;112:158-166.*

43. Radtke W, Keane JF, Fellows KE, Lang P, Lock JE. *Percutaneous balloon valvotomy of congenital pulmonary stenosis using oversized balloons. JACC 1986;8:909-915.*

44. Locke JE, Keane JF, Fellows KE. *The use of catheter intervention procedures for congenital heart disease. JACC 1986;6:1420-1423.*

45. Lababidi Z. *Aortic balloon valvuloplasty. Am Heart J 1983;106:751-752.*

46. Labadibi Z, Wu JR, Walls JT. *Percutaneous balloon aortic valvuloplasty: results in 23 patients. Am J Cardiol 1984;53:194-197.*

47. Rupprath G, Neuhaus KL. *Percutaneous balloon valvuloplasty for aortic valve stenosis in infancy. Am J Cardiol 1985;55:1655-1656.*

48. Sanchez GR, Mehta AV, Ewing LL, Brickley SE, Anderson TM, Black IF. *Successful percutaneous balloon valvuloplasty of the aortic valve in an infant. Pediatr Cardiol 1985;6:103-106.*

49. Walls JT, Lababidi Z, Curtis JJ, Silver D. *Assessment of percutaneous balloon pulmonary and aortic valvuloplasty. J Thorac Cardiovasc Surg 1984;88:353-356.*

50. Macaya C, Santalla A, Perez de la Cruz JM, Prieto J, Melgares R, Cutillas N, Castillo C, Azpitarte J. *Percutaneous transluminal valvuloplasty with the balloon catheter in congenital stenosis of the aortic valve. Rev Exp Cardiol 1985;38:396-399.*

51. Choy M, Beekman RH, Rocchini AP, Crowley DC, Snider AR, Dick M II, Rosenthal A. *Percutaneous balloon valvuloplasty for aortic stenosis in infants and children. Am J Cardiol 1987;59:in press.*

52. Cribier A, Savin T, Saoudi N, Rocha P, Berland J, Letac B. *Percutaneous transluminal valvuloplasty of acquired aortic stenosis in elderly patients: an alternative to valve replacement? Lancet 1986;1:63-67.*

53. Sievert H, Kaltenbach M, Bussman WD, Kober G. *Percutaneous valvuloplasty of the aortic valve in adults. Deutsch Med Wochenschr 1986;111:504-506.*

54. McKay RG, Safian RD, Lock JE, Mandell VS, Thurer RL, Schnitt SJ, Grossman W. *Balloon dilatation of calcific aortic stenosis in elderly patients: postmortem, intraoperative, and percutaneous valvuloplasty studies. Circulation 1986;74:119-125.*

55. Isner JM, Salem DN, Desnoyers MR, Hougen TJ, Makkey WC, Pandian NG, Eichhorn EJ, Konstam MA, Levine HJ. *Treatment of calcific aortic stenosis by balloon valvuloplasty. Am J Cardiol 1987;59:in press.*

56. Inoue K, Owaki T, Nakamura T, Kitamura F, Miyamoto N. *Clinical application of transvenous mitral commissurotomy by a new balloon catheter. J Thorac Cardiovasc Surg 1984;87:394-402.*

57. Reifart N, Nowak B, Baykut D, Sarai K, Satter P, Kaltenbach M, Bussmann WD. *In vitro study of transvenous commissurotomy in severe mitral valve stenosis using the balloon catheter. Z Kardiol 1985;74:234-237.*

58. Reifart N, Nowak B, Baykut D, Bussman WD, Kaltenbach M. *Experimental mitral valvuloplasty of fibrotic and calcified valves with balloon catheters. JACC 1985;5:448.*

59. Lock JE, Khalilullah M, Shrivastava S, Bahl V, Keane JF. *Percutaneous catheter commissurotomy in rheumatic mitral stenosis. N Engl J Med 1985;313:1515-1518.*

60. Babic UU, Pejcic P, Djurisic Z, Vucinic M, Grujici SM. *Percutaneous transarterial balloon valvuloplasty for mitral valve stenosis. Am J Cardiol 1986;57:1101-1104.*

61. Al Zaibag M, Al Kasab S, Ribeiro PA, Al Fagih M. *Percutaneous double-balloon mitral valvotomy for rheumatic mitral valve stenosis. Lancet 1986; 1:757-761.*

62. McKay RG, Lock JE, Keane JF, Safian RD, Aroesty JM, Grossman W. *Percutaneous mitral valvuloplasty in an adult patient with calcific rheumatic mitral stenosis. JACC 1986;7:1410-1415.*

63. Palacios IF, Lock JE, Keane JF, Block PC. *Percutaneous transvenous balloon valvotomy in a patient with sever calcific mitral stenosis. JACC 1986;7:1416-1419.*

64. Kveselis DA, Rocchini AP, Beekman R, Snider AR, Crowley DN, Dick M, Rosenthal A. *Balloon angioplasty for congenital and rheumatic mitral stenosis. Am J Cardiol 1986;57:348-350.*

65. de Ubaga JLM, Colman T, Figueroa A, de Prada JAV, Bardaji JL, Martin-Duran R, Gomez-Duran CM. *Percutaneous balloon valvulotomy in calcific and fibrotic rheumatic mitral stenosis. Am J Cardiol 1987;59:in press.*

66. Block PC, Palacious IF, Jacobs ML, Fallon JT. *Mechanism of percutaneous mitral valvotomy. Am J Cardiol 1987;59:in press.*

67. Kaplan JD, Isner JM, Karas RH, Halaburka KR, Konstam MA, Hougen TJ, Cleveland RJ, Salem DN. *In vitro analysis of mechanisms of balloon valvuloplasty of stenotic mitral valves. Am J Cardiol 1987;59:in press.*

68. Pandian NG, Isner JM, Hougen TJ, Desnoyers MR, McInerney K, Salem DN. *Percutaneous balloon valvuloplasty of mitral stenosis aided by cardiac ultrasound. Am J Cardiol 1987;59:in press.*

69. Roberts WC, Lachman AS. *Mitral valve commissurotomy versus replacement. Considerations based on examination of operatively excised stenotic mitral valves. Am Heart J 1979;98:56-62.*

70. Roberts WC. *The structure of the aortic valve in clinically-isolated aortic stenosis. An autopsy study of 162 patients over 15 years of age. Circulation 1970;42:91-97.*

71. Roberts WC. *The congenitally bicuspid aortic valve. A study of 85 autopsy cases. Am J Cardiol 1970;26:72-83.*

72. Roberts WC. *Anatomically isolated aortic valvular disease. The case against its being of rheumatic etiology. Am J Med 1970;49:151-159.*

73. Roberts WC, Perloff JK, Costantino T. *Severe valvular aortic stenosis in patients over 65 years of age. A clinicopathologic study. Am J Cardiol 1971;27:497-506.*

Examining Operatively Excised Cardiac Valves

Recently, I received a letter from a cardiovascular surgeon (Henry E. Martinez, MD, Amarillo, Texas) describing how operatively excised cardiac valves are handled by the pathologist at his hospital and inquiring whether or not I agreed with the method of handling. His letter stated "...we have rules in our hospital that require that all cardiac valves excised be sent to the pathologists for processing. There they are fixed and slide preparations are made. The pathologist then looks at the slides, sends a detailed report and accompanying bill to the patient. It has been my opinion for a long time that these reports are of no

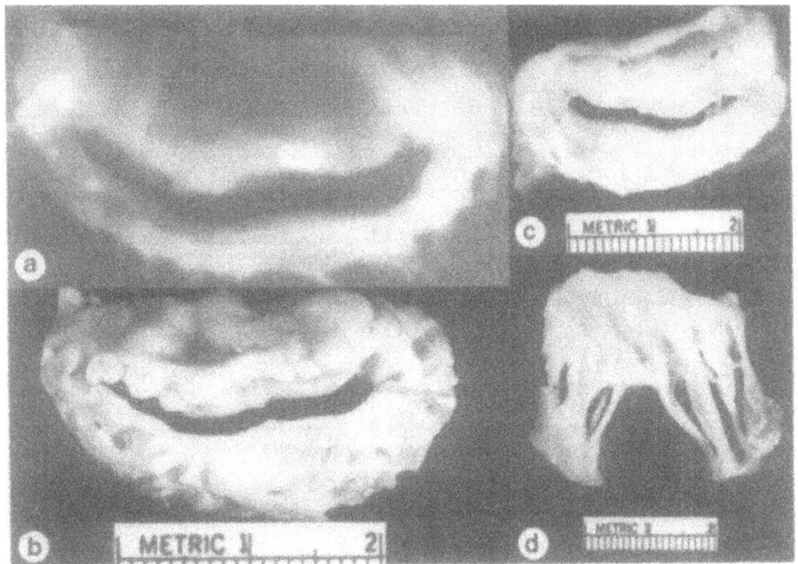

FIGURE 1. Operatively excised severely stenotic mitral valve in a 63-year-old woman (S67-815) who several years earlier had undergone mitral commissurotomy. *a*, radiograph showing 2 minute-sized calcific deposits. *b*, view of ventricular aspect after excision of chordae tendineae and papillary muscles. *c*, view of atrial aspect. *d*, view of anterior mitral leaflet and its attached chordae tendineae. This would have been a good valve for repeat commissurotomy either by finger, instrument or balloon. There was no mitral regurgitation.

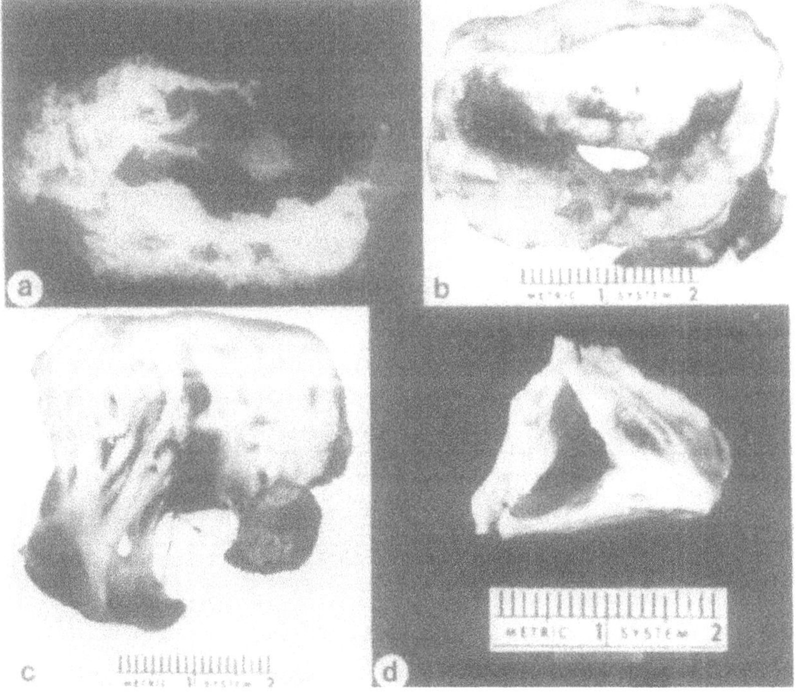

FIGURE 2. Operatively excised severely stenotic mitral valve (*a*, *b* and *c*) and stenotic and regurgitant aortic valve (*d*) in a 30-year-old woman (S74-5035). *a*, radiograph of mitral valve showing heavy calcific deposit. *b*, mitral valve from left atrial aspect. *c*, mitral valve showing ventricular aspect of the anterior mitral leaflet and its attached chordae tendineae and papillary muscle. *d*, aortic aspect of a 3-cuspid aortic valve with fusion of 1 of the 3 commissures. A suture was placed at the sites of the nonfused commissures so that the photograph could show how the valve appeared when intact.

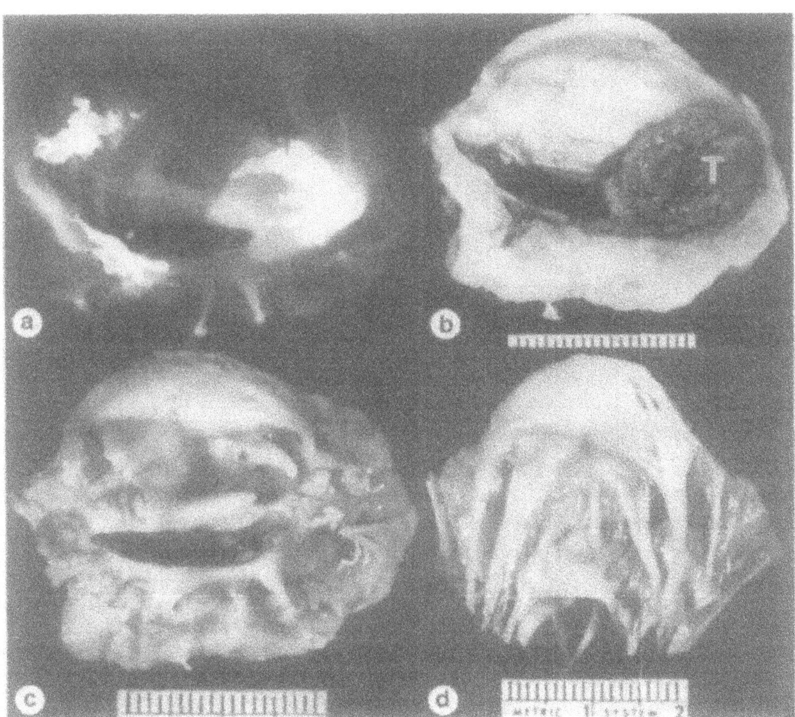

FIGURE 3. Operatively excised severely stenotic mitral valve in a 72-year-old woman (S76-76). *a*, radiograph showing 3 calcific deposits. *b*, view from atrial aspect showing a thrombus (T) at the anterolateral commissure. *c*, view from ventricular aspect. *d*, view of ventricular aspect of anterior mitral leaflet. Neither papillary muscle had been excised. Balloon valvulotomy would be undesirable in the presence of thrombus adjacent to the valve orifice, but fortunately, thrombus at this location is rare.

value. . .in the patient's subsequent course or in educating the medical personnel associated with the patient."

I agree completely with Dr. Martinez and discussed this subject in an article in 1966.[1] In my laboratory, the only operatively excised cardiac valves that are divided into smaller pieces for histologic examination are those with obvious vegetations or those suspected of containing vegetative material, and these type valves are relatively infrequently seen. The final anatomic diagnosis of all other operatively excised cardiac valves is based entirely on gross inspection, and no histologic sections are prepared.

In my view, the surgeon should make every attempt to excise the cardiac valve intact. During the past 25 years, I have examined hundreds of cardiac valves excised by a number of different surgeons. Usually, it is possible to identify the operating surgeon by examining the operatively excised valve. Some surgeons virtually routinely excise the valve intact; others virtually never excise the valve intact. It is likely that the chance of dislodgment of fragments of the valve is less when the valve is removed intact than when it is removed in multiple pieces. In the 1960s most operatively excised mitral valves received in my laboratory contained portions of both papillary muscles. Today, papillary muscles are less often excised, and therefore, accuracy in detecting ruptured chordae tendineae is less than in the early period of valve replacement. Also today, portions of the posterior mitral leaflet are often not excised when valve replacement is performed for pure mitral regurgitation.

The most important procedure to be performed on the operatively excised valve is a good photograph of it (Fig. 1 to 5). Ideally, the photograph should be a part of the official report describing gross anatomic features of the excised valve. In my laboratory, all stenotic and most purely regurgitant operatively excised valves are x-rayed, and these radiographs provide precise records of the presence and the amount of calcific depos-

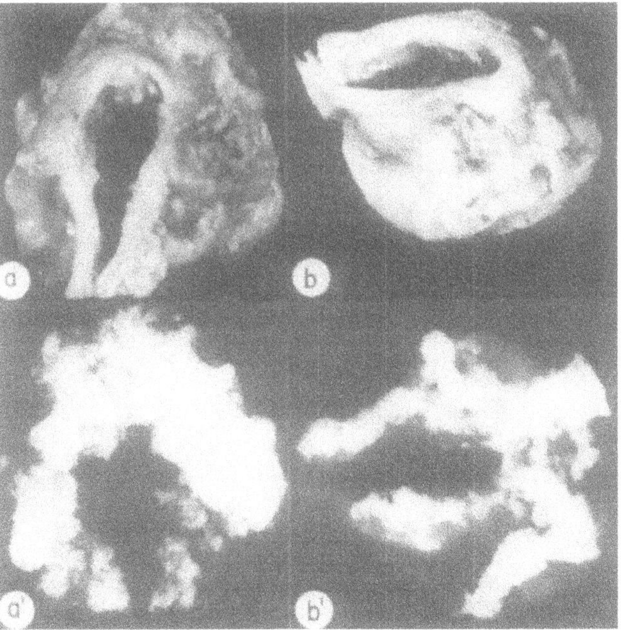

FIGURE 4. Operatively excised, heavily calcified, stenotic, congenitally unicommissural and unicuspid aortic valves from each of 2 patients. *a* and *a'*, view of valve from aortic aspect and radiography of it in a 53-year-old man (S69-2699). *b* and *b'*, view of valve and radiograph of it from a 41-year-old man (S70-3087). Histologic sections of these valves would, of course, not have shown that the underlying malformation was a congenital one and that the valve consisted of a single cusp rather than the usual 3 cusps. (Reproduced with permission from Falcone MW, Roberts WC, Morrow AG, and Perloff JK. Congenital aortic stenosis resulting from a unicommissural valve. Clinical and anatomic features in twenty-one adult patients. Circulation 1971;44:272–280).

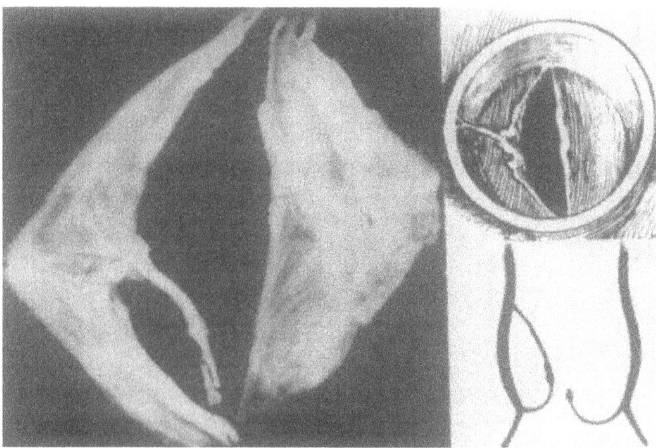

FIGURE 5. Operatively excised, purely regurgitant, congenitally bicuspid aortic valve in a 26-year-old man (A66-6). One of the cusps was attached to the wall of aorta cephalad to the sinotubular junction as shown in the drawing. (The photograph of the noncalcified valve is reproduced with permission from reference 6.)

its. Finally, all operatively excised valves are retained. This retention and storage of all valves allows studies of the causes of the various types of valvular dysfunction during different periods and other clinicomorphologic studies.[2–19]

In summary, the operatively excised cardic valve should not be processed as a "routine surgical specimen." The most precise morphologic diagnosis results from careful gross inspection of the valve and not from histologic examination of sections of it. Photographs of the valve provide the most effective record of the pathologic findings, and permit correlations between the anatomic abnormalities and clinical, hemodynamic and operative findings.

William C. Roberts

William C. Roberts, MD
Editor in Chief

1. Roberts WC, Morrow AG. *Cardiac valves and the surgical pathologist. Arch Pathol 1966;82:309–313.*

2. Roberts WC, Buchbinder NA. *Healed left-sided infective endocarditis: a clinicopathologic study of 59 patients. Am J Cardiol 1977;40:876–888.*

3. Lachman AS, Roberts WC. *Calcific deposits in stenotic mitral valves. Extent and relation to age, sex, degree of stenosis, cardiac rhythm, previous commissurotomy and left atrial body thrombus from study of 164 operatively-excised valves. Circulation 1978;57:808–815.*

4. Covarrubias EA, Sheikh MU, Isner J, Gomes M, Hufnagel CA, Roberts WC. *Calcific pulmonic stenosis in adulthood. Treatment by valve replacement (porcine xenograft) with postoperative hemodynamic evaluation. Chest 1979;75:399–402.*

5. Roberts WC, Lachman AS. *Mitral valve commissurotomy versus replacement. Considerations based on examination of operatively excised stenotic mitral valves. Am Heart J 1979;98:56–62.*

6. Roberts WC, Morrow AG, McIntosh CL, Jones M, Epstein SE. *Congenitally bicuspid aortic valve causing severe, pure aortic regurgitation without superimposed infective endocarditis. Analysis of 13 patients requiring aortic valve replacement. Am J Cardiol 1981;47:206–209.*

7. Waller BJ, Morrow AG, Maron BJ, Del Negro AA, Kent DM, McGrath FJ, Wallace RB, McIntosh CL, Roberts WC. *Etiology of clinically isolated, severe, chronic, pure mitral regurgitation: analysis of 97 patients over 30 years of age having mitral valve replacement. Am Heart J 1982;104:276–288.*

8. Waller BF, Kishel JC, Roberts WC. *Severe aortic regurgitation from systemic hypertension. Chest 1982;82:365–368.*

9. Waller BF, McManus BM, Roberts WC. *Mitral valve stenosis produced by or worsened by active bacterial endocarditis. Chest 1982;82:498–500.*

10. Byram MT, Roberts WC. *Frequency and extent of calcific deposits in purely regurgitant mitral valves: analysis of 108 operatively excised valves. Am J Cardiol 1983;52:1059–1061.*

11. Waller BF, Maron BJ, Del Negro AA, Gottdiener JS, Roberts WC. *Frequency and significance of M-mode echocardiographic evidence of mitral prolapse in clinically isolated pure mitral regurgitation: analysis of 65 patients having mitral valve replacement. Am J Cardiol 1984;53:139–147.*

12. Day PJ, Roberts WC. *Relation of level of total serum cholesterol to amount of calcific deposits in operatively excised stenotic mitral valves: analysis of 155 cases. Am J Cardiol 1984;53:157–159.*

13. Subramanian R, Olson LJ, Edwards WD. *Surgical pathology of pure aortic stenosis: a study of 374 cases. Mayo Clin Proc 1984;59:683–690.*

14. Olson LJ, Subramanian R, Edwards WD. *Surgical pathology of pure aortic insufficiency: a study of 225 cases. Mayo Clin Proc 1984;59:835–841.*

15. Jeresaty RM, Edwards JE, Chawla SK. *Mitral valve prolapse and ruptured chordae tendineae. Am J Cardiol 1985;55:138–142.*

16. Subramanian R, Olson LJ, Edwards WD. *Surgical pathology of combined aortic stenosis and insufficiency: a study of 213 cases. Mayo Clin Proc 1985;60:247–254.*

17. Hanson TP, Edwards BS, Edwards JE. *Pathology of surgically excised mitral valves: one hundred consecutive cases. Arch Pathol Lab Med 1985; 109:823–828.*

18. Peterson MD, Roach RM, Edwards JE. *Types of aortic stenosis in surgically removed valves. Arch Pathol Lab Med 1985;109:829–832.*

19. Roberts WC, McIntosh CL, Wallace RB. *Mechanisms of severe mitral regurgitation in mitral valve prolapse determined from analysis of operatively excised valves. Am Heart J 1987;113:1316–1323.*

The Logic of Using Either Two Mechanical Valves or Two Bioprosthetic Valves for Replacement of Both Mitral and Aortic Valves

N.G., a 53-year-old woman, at age 26 had mitral commissurotomy for mitral stenosis and at age 41 the stenotic mitral valve was replaced with a bioprosthesis (Hancock) and the regurgitant aortic valve, with a Bjork-Shiley prosthesis. At age 52, the bioprosthesis in the mitral position had degenerated (severely regurgitant) and it was now replaced with a St. Jude medical prosthesis. Multiple complications occurred postoperatively and she died in February 1988, 40 days after the third cardiac operation. Had the mitral valve been replaced 11 years earlier with a prosthetic rather than a bioprosthetic valve, it is unlikely that a third operation would have been required. After the second operation, she received daily warfarin therapy because of the prosthetic valve in the aortic valve position.

This case is not an infrequent occurrence. Among 54 patients having simultaneous replacement of both mitral and aortic valves and studied later at necropsy by Roberts and Sullivan,[1] 38 (70%) had mechanical prostheses in both valve positions, 4 (8%) had bioprostheses in both valve positions and 12 (22%) had 1 mechanical prosthesis and 1 bioprosthesis. To utilize a bioprosthesis in 1 left-sided valve position and a mechanical prosthesis in the other left-sided valve position is illogical because the advantages of each type of substitute valve are lost by the presence of the other type of substitute valve. The advantage, of course, of a mechanical prosthesis is that it should not wear out; its disadvantage is that all patients having one need long-term anticoagulant (warfarin) therapy. In contrast, the advantage of the bioprosthesis is that patients having one do not need long-term anticoagulant therapy; the disadvantage of the bioposthesis is that it wears out if the patient lives long enough, usually 5 to 15 years, and then another operation is required. Thus, the placing of 1 bioprosthetic valve and 1 mechanical valve in the same patient translates into the loss for the patient of each of the advantages of the mechanical and bioprosthetic valves, and at the same time, the gain for the patient of the disadvantages of each of the 2 types of substitute cardiac valves. Either both left-sided valve substitutes should be mechanical prostheses or both should be bioprostheses!

William C. Roberts

William C. Roberts, MD
Editor in Chief

1. Roberts WC, Sullivan MF. *Clinical and necropsy observations early after simultaneous replacement of the mitral and aortic valves. Am J Cardiol 1986;58:1067–1084.*

Reprinted from the April 1, issue of **The American Journal of Cardiology,** A Yorke Medical Journal,
Published by Cahners Publishing Company. a Division of Reed Publishing USA, 249 West 17th Street, New York, N.Y., 10011.

Defining Idiopathic Dilated Cardiomyopathy: A Courtroom Discussion

Doctor, how do you define the condition idiopathic dilated cardiomyopathy (IDC)?

I define IDC as heart muscle disease unassociated with coronary, valvular, hypertensive, pericardial, congenital or pulmonary heart disease or with an infiltrative myocardial disease.

Doctor, you have defined IDC by what it is not. Before we discuss what it is, let's delve into each of these "unassociated conditions" to make certain we agree on what "unassociated" means. You say unassociated with coronary artery disease? Does this mean "absent" coronary disease?

Because coronary arterial atherosclerosis is so prevalent in adults living in the Western world it is not realistic to believe that coronary artery disease is actually "absent". It is better to say "insignificantly narrowed" epicardial coronary arteries.

Then neither the word "unassociated" nor "absent" is appropriate in characterizing the status of the epicardial coronary arteries in patients with IDC. What degree of luminal narrowing do you consider "significant"?

Because flow through an artery is not compromised until >75% of the lumen's cross-sectional area is obliterated, it is reasonable to consider >75% cross-sectional area narrowing as "significant" and lesser degrees of narrowing as "insignificant".

At present the only means of determining coronary arterial narrowing during life is by angiography, and the unit of angiographic narrowing is diameter reduction, not cross-sectional area reduction. Thus, what is a 75% cross-sectional area narrowing equivalent to in terms of diameter narrowing?

In general, a 75% cross-sectional area narrowing is equivalent to a 50% diameter narrowing. This equivalency assumes that the coronary artery is relatively straight (and obviously the right and left circumflex coronary arteries are not straight) and that the lumen is central or nearly so (and the lumen is central in only about 30% of significantly narrowed epicardial coronary arteries). Nevertheless, some demarcation definition is needed and the 50% diameter reduction is reasonable.

Therefore, doctor, if 1 or more epicardial coronary arteries is narrowed at some point >50% in diameter at angiography, then the diagnosis of IDC cannot be made. Is that correct?

Yes. But, because coronary arterial disease is so common in our society a few patients with "IDC" will have associated coronary artery disease. Nevertheless, it is improper to diagnose IDC in the presence of "significant" coronary arterial narrowing.

Doctor, now let's move to another "unassociated condition", namely valvular heart disease. I understand that most patients with IDC have precordial murmurs and other evidences of mitral and/or tricuspid valve regurgitation sometime during their courses? Thus, is not atrioventricular valve regurgitation valvular heart disease? What do you mean then by "unassociated with valvular heart disease"?

Yes, it is true that most patients with IDC develop atrioventricular valve regurgitation but this regurgitation is functional or nonorganic; i.e., it is caused by the dilation of the cardiac ventricles, not by primary disease of the valvular leaflets and/or chordae tendineae.

Then "unassociated valvular heart disease" means lack of intrinsic disease of the valvular leaflets and/or chordae, even though the degree of valvular regurgitation may be equal to or even greater than in patients with primary valvular disease. Is that correct?

Yes. But quantitating the degree of tricuspid or mitral valve regurgitation is difficult. Furthermore, valvular repair or replacement is contraindicated in patients with IDC although at times the degree of regurgitation might be considerable.

If atrioventricular valve regurgitation in patients with IDC is not due to primary valve disease, then what is the mechanism of the regurgitation?

The mechanism of the tricuspid valve regurgitation is different from that of the mitral regurgitation. The tricuspid valve regurgitation results from dilatation of the tricuspid valve anulus. Normally the tricuspid valve anulus is ≤11 cm in circumference; in patients with IDC the circumference may increase to as much as 16 cm, depending on the original size of the heart. Whenever the right ventricular cavity dilates the tricuspid valve anulus dilates, and the amount of anular circumference dilatation is roughly proportional to the amount of right ventricular cavity dilatation.

The mitral regurgitation in IDC, in contrast, is never the result of mitral anular dilatation.[1,2] Normally, the mitral anulus is about 9 cm in circumference, and in IDC, the anular circumference rarely increases to more than about 11 cm. The maximal transverse dilatation of the left ventricle takes place in the midportion of the cavity or about half way between the mitral valve anulus and the left ventricular apex. The midcavity dilatation causes the papillary muscles to move outwardly from the cavity's center and this outward movement pulls the chordae tendineae toward the ventricle's mural endocardium which in turn pulls the margins of the posterior and anterior mitral leaflets away from one another with resulting regurgitation. An additional factor is the elongation of the left ventricular cavity from the mitral anulus to apex, a distance equivalent to that distance from the base of the right aortic valve cusp to left ventricular apex. As this longitudinal distance increases the stumps of both left ventricular papillary muscles move away from the mitral anulus or toward the left ventricular apex. This movement, in turn, pulls the chordae tendineae and their attached leaflets closer to the left ventricular mural endocardium, further increasing the regurgitant area of the mitral orifice during ventricular systole.

Doctor, how is secondary atrioventricular valvular regurgitation as occurs in patients with IDC distinguished clinically from primary valvular regurgitation as occurs, for example, in patients with mitral valve prolapse?

Sometimes this distinction is not easy clinically, especially if the murmur of mitral regurgitation is present when the patient with IDC is first seen. In general, the intensity of the precordial murmur of primary mitral regurgitation is louder than that of secondary mitral regurgitation. The echocardiogram is helpful in this distinction. In IDC, the left ventricular wall contracts poorly whereas in primary mitral regurgitation, left ventricular contraction usually is good. In chronic primary mitral regurgitation, the left atrial cavity is usually larger than in secondary mitral regurgitation associated with IDC. If there is associated aortic valve regurgitation, diagnosis of IDC is inappropriate, and mitral regurgitation when present in this circumstance is more liable to be primary rather than secondary. Any dysfunction of a semilunar cardiac valve is incompatible with IDC. Neither the ascending aorta nor the pulmonary trunk dilate in IDC whereas one or both may dilate in patients with primary valve disease. In the Western world mitral valve prolapse is now the most common cause of primary, pure (no associated valve stenosis) mitral regurgitation and when the regurgitation is severe the mitral anulus is usually considerably dilated.[3–5] Thus, in contrast to earlier teachings, the only condition associated with severe mitral anular dilatation is mitral valve prolapse and IDC is rarely if ever associated with a functionally significant increase in mitral anular circumference.

Doctor, now let's move to another "unassociated condition", namely systemic hypertension. You stated earlier that systemic hypertension was absent in patients with IDC and yet some patients with IDC have histories of systemic hypertension or actually elevated systemic arterial pressures early in their courses or during periods of particularly severe congestive heart failure. How do you explain these apparent discrepancies?

Yes, all of your statements about systemic hypertension in IDC are true. Most patients with systemic hypertension who develop severe chronic congestive heart failure, however, have underlying atherosclerotic coronary artery disease and usually one or more healed myocardial infarcts, which may or may not have been clinically apparent. As the cardiac output in these patients with "ischemic cardiomyopathy" progressively falls the systemic arterial pressure also progressively falls because systemic hypertension requires both an increased peripheral vascular resistance and a normal or increased cardiac output. Although nearly 10% of patients with IDC may also have grossly visible left ventricular scars, the scars are small, in contrast to the patients with ischemic cardiomyopathy, and focal wall motion abnormalities are uncommon in IDC whereas they are common in ischemic cardiomyopathy. In contrast to ischemic cardiomyopathy, the epicardial coronary arteries are not significantly narrowed in IDC and clinical events characteristic of acute myocardial infarction are nearly nonexistent in IDC, whereas, of course, they are common in patients with ischemic cardiomyopathy.[7,8] As the congestive heart failure worsens in both IDC and in ischemic cardiomyopathy the systemic arterial pressure falls so that during the last 3 months of life the systemic arterial pressure in both conditions is typically about 90/60 mm Hg. The distinction between IDC and ischemic cardiomyopathy, therefore, is not on the basis of previous or present levels of systemic arterial pressure but on the basis of the presence or absence of coronary arterial narrowing and a history of an event characteristic of acute myocardial infarction that healed.

Doctor, are there any circumstances where the systemic arterial pressure progressively increases along with a progressive increase in congestive heart failure?

Yes. The most common is chronic renal disease. Typically, as the renal disease worsens the systemic arterial pressure progressively rises and, finally, features of congestive heart failure appear and progress. Some of these latter features may be consequences of retained body fluids as renal output diminishes. Hemodialysis is changing this picture a bit. Nevertheless, the heart in chronic renal failure is one of increased mass and increased ventricular cavity size, features characteristic of IDC. Diagnosis of IDC, however, is inappropriate in the presence of chronic renal disease either clinically or at necropsy.

Doctor, now let's move to another "unassociated cardiac condition", namely pericardial heart disease. Are pericardial effusions common in patients with IDC?

Yes. Pericardial effusions are common in patients with chronic congestive heart failure from any cause, just as effusions into pleural spaces and into abdominal cavity are common in patients with heart failure. The effusions are serous and those into the pericardial cavity rarely are more than 200 ml, and they are never associated with tamponade. Normally, the pericardial sac contains up to 50 ml of serous fluid ("the oil of the heart" to decrease friction between the visceral and parietal pericardia) and an increase of 3 or 4 times over several months is of no functional consequence.

Thus, doctor, it is not correct to say "absent" pericardial disease. Some abnormality is present, namely serous effusions, but the abnormality is of no functional consequence. Are there any other pericardial abnormalities in patients with IDC?

No. Fibrin deposits on the pericardial surfaces and pericardial friction rubs are absent in patients with IDC. Likewise, neither the parietal nor the visceral pericardia are thickened in IDC. Nevertheless, particularly before the advent of echocardiography, patients with IDC sometimes were misdiagnosed as having "constrictive pericarditis" (better termed "constrictive pericardial disease") and thoracotomy was performed. Hemodynamically, constrictive pericardial disease can mimic IDC. Thoracotomy and pericardiectomy are the treatments for the former, but thoracotomy obviously is contraindicated in IDC. Thus, clinically significant pericardial heart disease is absent in IDC, but pericardial heart disease often is a diagnostic consideration in these patients.

Doctor, now let's move to another "unassociated condition", namely congenital heart disease. Does the absence of congenital heart disease indicate that IDC cannot be present at birth? Is IDC ever of congenital origin?

Yes. In a rare patient IDC manifests itself early in life and when this occurs it is possible that IDC was present from birth and is therefore congenital in origin in this circumstance. Furthermore, IDC occurs occasionally in more than 1 family member and in this circumstance it is "familial" and therefore possibly congenital. In contrast to IDC, which is rarely congenital or familial, hypertrophic cardiomyopathy is usually familial and occasionally manifests itself from the time of birth. Therefore, although hypertrophic cardiomyopathy is usually classified under myocardial diseases of uncertain origin, it is also congenital heart disease and indeed one of the more common varieties of congenital heart disease. Although the cardiac abnormality usually is present from the time of birth, it usually does not manifest itself until adulthood.

Doctor, now let's move to another "unassociated condition", namely pulmonary parenchymal or vascular disease. How much lung disease do you allow to be present and still diagnose IDC?

Sometimes a lot and sometimes very little. Many men, and in some studies most men,[6] with IDC are habitual alcoholics and the frequency of heavy cigarette smoking is much higher in chronic alcoholics than in nonalcoholics. Accordingly, the frequency of parenchymal pulmonary disease is fairly frequent in older adults with IDC. In general, parenchymal pulmonary disease may increase pulmonary arterial pressure and lead to cor pulmonale. Although cor pulmonale typically causes dilation of only the right side of the heart, an occasional patient with cor pulmonale also has a dilated left ventricular cavity and this circumstance can lead to confusion with IDC. The patient with severe parenchymal lung disease should be excluded from consideration of having IDC.

Pulmonary emboli with and without pulmonary infarcts are common in patients with IDC and this complication of IDC obviously should not exclude diagnosis of the underlying condition. Thrombi in the right ventricular cavity and in the right atrial appendage are common in IDC and are the likely sources of the pulmonary emboli. Elevation of the pulmonary arterial pressure may also occur in IDC as a consequence of the elevated pulmonary venous pressures from elevated left ventricular filling pressures.

Doctor, now let's move to another "unassociated condition", namely infiltrative heart disease. Obviously, the presence of amyloid fibrils, sarcoid granulomas or iron in the heart excludes the diagnosis of IDC. Which of the infiltrative diseases is most commonly confused with IDC?

Cardiac *sarcoidosis*.[9] This infiltrative cardiomyopathy may cause severe dilatation of both ventricular cavities, ventricular arrhythmias and conduction disturbances in the absence of palpable lymph nodes or radiographically visible pulmonary lesions, and, therefore, it can readily mimic IDC. It is important not to misdiagnose cardiac sarcoidosis as IDC because the sarcoid granuloma usually are responsive to corticosteroid therapy, whereas, short of cardiac transplantation, there is no specific therapy for IDC. Biopsy of a lymph node more likely will lead to diagnosis of sarcoidosis than will endomyocardial biopsy. Cardiac *hemosiderosis*,[10] even though it too may produce severe ventricular cavity dilatation, is rarely confused with IDC because of a history of repeated blood transfusions unassociated with bleeding diastasis or evidence of hemochromatosis (hepatic cirrhosis, diabetes mellitus, etc.) Cardiac *amyloidosis* is rarely confused with IDC because the cardiac ventricular cavities are not dilated in this condition (unless another cardiac disease is also present like atherosclerotic coronary artery disease) and these patients are generally much older than the IDC patients. Amyloid heart disease is far more likely to be confused with hypertrophic cardiomyopathy than with IDC.

Doctor, does the presence of inflammatory infiltrates in the interstitium of the ventricular walls exclude the diagnosis of IDC?

No. For years many investigators believed that myocarditis (interstitial inflammatory cells associated with necrotic myocardial fibers) was a precursor of IDC. With some exceptions, endomyocardial biopsy in patients with IDC has failed to disclose the presence of interstitial inflammatory cells in patients with IDC. In 1 necropsy study of 152 patients with IDC, only 5 had interstitial myocardial inflammatory cell infiltrates and in them the infiltrates were small, mononuclear and located in areas where fibrous tissue was increased.

Doctor, does the presence of certain systemic diseases or diseases that affect primarily noncardiac organs or tissues prevent the diagnosis of IDC?

Yes and no. The presence of *diabetes mellitus* does not. It is generally believed that patients with diabetes have an increased frequency of clinically significant atherosclerosis compared to nondiabetics of similar age and sex. Of 152 recently reported necropsy patients with IDC,[6] 8 had associated diabetes mellitus, and none, of course, had significant narrowing of a major epicardial coronary artery and none had abnormalities of the intramural coronary arteries.

Three neurologic conditions—namely, Duchenne's type of muscular dystrophy, Friedreich's ataxia and myotonia congenita—occasionally are associated with dilatation of both cardiac ventricles, depressed ventricular function, arrhythmias and conduction disturbances, and abnormalities of some intramural coronary arteries. The dilated cardiomyopathy observed in these 3 neurologic conditions is probably related to the neurologic disease, and, therefore, the use of the word "idiopathic" to precede the phrase "dilated cardiomyopathy" in them is inappropriate.

Some patients with chronic anemia, for example, congenital hemolytic anemia or sickle-cell anemia, develop dilated ventricular cavities, precordial murmurs consistent with tricuspid and/or mitral regurgitation, and depressed ventricular function. Despite a similar morphologic appearance of the heart, diagnosis of IDC in the setting of chronic severe anemia is inappropriate.

Doctor, let's move the discussion from what IDC is not to what it is. What has to be present before IDC is present?

Both ventricular cavities must be dilated, the cardiac mass must be increased and the cardiac output must be decreased. Also, the dilatation of both ventricles is roughly to the same degree. The circumstance where 1 cardiac ventricle is enormously dilated and the other one is only slightly dilated is not IDC. A condition that causes dilatation of only 1 cardiac ventricle is not IDC. Both atrial cavities also are dilated. It is likely that the atrial dilatation simply follows the ventricular dilatation.

The weight of the heart at necropsy in IDC is always increased. Although total cardiac mass is increased, the thickness of the left and right ventricular walls may not be greater than normal. Indeed, in IDC usually the maximal thickness of the right ventricular free wall is ≤5 mm and that of the left ventricular free wall is ≤15 mm. The maximal thickness of the left ventricular free wall and ventricular septum in IDC is similar.

Some athletes have hearts with dilated ventricular cavities and increased mass but in them the cardiac output is normal or even supernormal. In IDC, cardiac output is depressed. The ventricles dilate in IDC as systolic function worsens, which in turn causes increased end-systolic volume, and this leads to further ventricular dilatation.

Doctor, could you summarize your definiton of IDC?

IDC is a heart muscle disease of uncertain origin characterized by dilatation of both ventricular cavities, by increased cardiac mass and by depressed cardiac output. IDC is unassociated with significant narrowing of 1 or more epicardial coronary arteries; with primary valvular heart disease; with systemic hypertension; with functionally significant pericardial heart disease; with congenital defects or anomalies of cardiac septa or great arteries or veins; or with myocardial infiltrative diseases, such as sarcoid, amyloid and iron. IDC should not be considered in the presence of severe parenchymal pulmonary disease or in the presence of conditions that affect primarily noncardiac organs or tissues such as chronic anemia and the neurogenic heart diseases.

Doctor, is the "definition of a disease" the same as "criteria for diagnosis of a disease"?

No. A definition of a disease is a description of what the disease is and is independent of the means by which the disease is diagnosed. A definition may change as more information is gained about the disease. Criteria for diagnosis of a disease, in contrast, are dependent on the symptoms and physical signs produced by a disease and on the findings produced by laboratory tests and various "instruments of precision" that are helpful in diagnosing the disease. The laboratory tests and "instruments of precision" change periodically and when they do the criteria for diagnosis of a disease also may change.

Thank you doctor.

William C. Roberts

William C. Roberts, MD
Editor in Chief

1. Roberts WC, Cohen LS. Left ventricular papillary muscles. Description of the normal and a survey of conditions causing them to be abnormal. *Circulation 1972;46:138–154.*

2. Roberts WC, Perloff JK. Mitral valvular disease. A clinicopathologic survey of the conditions causing the mitral valve to function abnormally. *Ann Intern Med 1972;77:939–975.*

3. Waller BJ, Morrow AG, Maron BJ, Del Negro AA, Kent KM, McGrath FJ, Wallace RB, McIntosh CL, Roberts WC. Etiology of clinically isolated, severe, chronic, pure mitral regurgitaton: analysis of 97 patients over 30 years of age having mitral valve replacement. *Am Heart J 1982;104:276–288.*

4. Roberts WC, McIntosh CL, Wallace RB. Mechanisms of severe mitral regurgitation in mitral valve prolapse determined from analysis of operatively excised valves. *Am Heart J 1987;113:1316–1323.*

5. Roberts WC, Honig HS. The spectrum of cardiovascular disease in the Marfan syndrome: a clinico-morphologic study of 18 necropsy patients and comparison to 151 previously reported necropsy patients. *Am Heart J 1982;104:115–135.*

6. Roberts WC, Siegel RJ, McManus BM. Idiopathic dilated cardiomyopathy: analysis of 152 necropsy patients. *Am J Cardiol 1987;60:1340–1355.*

7. Ross EM, Roberts WC. Severe atherosclerotic coronary artery disease, healed myocardial infarction and chronic congestive heart failure: analysis of 81 patients studied at necropsy. *Am J Cardiol 1986;57:44–50.*

8. Ross EM, Roberts WC. Severe atherosclerotic coronary arterial narrowing and chronic congestive heart failure without myocardial infarction: analysis of 18 patients studied at necropsy. *Am J Cardiol 1986;57:51–56.*

9. Roberts WC, McAllister HA Jr, Ferrans VJ. Sarcoidosis of the heart. A clinicopathologic study of 35 necropsy patients (group I) and review of 78 previously described necropsy patients (group II). *Am J Med 1977;63:86–108.*

10. Buja LM, Roberts WC. Iron in the heart. Etiology and clinical significance. *Am J Med 1971;51:209–221.*

11. Roberts WC, Waller BF. Cardiac amyloidosis causing cardiac dysfunction: analysis of 54 necropsy patients. *Am J Cardiol 1983;52:137–146.*

The Echocardiographic Diseases

A 72-year-old obese, hypertensive and diabetic woman was hospitalized for increasing dyspnea. The electrocardiogram disclosed no abnormalities. By chest radiograph the lung fields were "clear" and the cardiac silhouette was of normal size. The M-mode echocardiogram disclosed no abnormalities, but the 2-dimensional echocardiogram showed a small mass in the right atrium. The transesophageal echocardiogram disclosed that the mass was attached by a fairly wide stalk to the fossa ovale region of the atrial septum, that it occupied <20% of the area of the right atrium, that it did not extend caudally to the level of the tricuspid valve anulus, and that it contained calcific deposits. The 2.0 cm, 20 g right atrial mass was operatively excised, and histologic examination disclosed it to be a myxoma.

Did the presence of a mass in the right atrium warrant its excision? The mass did not come close to the tricuspid valve anulus, much less protrude through the tricuspid valve orifice. The mass was firmly attached by a relatively broad base to the atrial septum. The right atrial cavity was larger than normal and therefore the mass could not possibly obstruct flow through this cavity and it was several centimeters from the orifices of the vena cava. The presence of calcific deposits in the mass indicated that the mass had been in the right atrium for a long time. There were no indications that portions of the mass had been dislodged and embolized to a pulmonary artery. The pulmonary arterial and right-sided cardiac pressures were normal. The increasing dyspnea in the patient could not justifiably be attributed to the right atrial mass.

Through the years I have seen several small *left* atrial myxomas at necropsy, so small that they could not possibly have caused cardiac dysfunction. They had not been diagnosed during life because an echocardiogram had not been performed. They were incidental necropsy findings and they had nothing to do with the patients' deaths.

The echocardiogram has almost revolutionized cardiac diagnosis. The transesophageal technique is so sensitive and its pictures so vivid that it is almost like "feeling" the heart itself. Some diseases are diagnosed now more often by echocardiogram than by any other means. These diseases include *mitral valve proplapse*, *hypertrophic cardiomyopathy*, extensive *cardiac amyloidosis*, *intracavitary masses* including thrombi, and benign and malignant neoplasms including atrial myxomas, cardiac *valvular vegetations and calcific deposits*, *mitral anular calcium* and probably *mitral stenosis*, *bicuspid aortic valves*, *dysfunctioning prosthetic* and *bioprosthetic valves*, *aneurysms of the ascending or descending thoracic aorta*, and some *pericardial disorders*. The echocardiogram is far better than the electrocardiogram in determining the presence or absence of cardiac hypertrophy. It is wonderful for determining the sizes of the cardiac cavities and whether or not the ventricular walls are contracting well. It is excellent in locating localized ventricular wall protrusions (aneurysms). For congenital heart disease, the echocardiogram—not cardiac catheterization—is now often the definitive diagnostic procedure. The echocardiogram does not compete as yet with the angiogram in determining the presence or absence of coronary artery disease, but that too may eventually change. In a way the echocardiogram is a "live autopsy" in that it provides both anatomic and functional information on the heart. The Doppler technique provides splendid information on blood flow through the heart, whether the valves are stenotic or incompetent or both, and the degree of that valvular dysfunction.

But is the echocardiogram diagnosing too much "disease"? Is it a too sensitive diagnostic instrument? If a mass is diagnosed, irrespective of its size or whether it is causing dysfunction, does the diagnosis itself mandate the excision of the mass, as in the 72-year-old woman described earlier? I remember a report several years ago where a nodule was detected on the mitral valve by echocardiogram. The nodule was operatively excised and it was a benign fibrous nodule (elastofibroendothelioma), and it had caused no dysfunction. Intracardiac thrombi have been operatively excised on other occasions.

I salute the echocardiogram and the splendid diagnostic and prognostic information that it provides. I worry sometimes that this apparatus has become so good that it leads at times to operative interventions that may not be warranted.

William C. Roberts, MD
Editor in Chief

Living with a Congenitally Bicuspid Aortic Valve

A healthy, weight-lifting, athletic, 32-year-old former fellow of mine while spending time recently in an echocardiography laboratory had an esophageal echocardiogram "to see what it was like". To his surprise, the echocardiogram disclosed that he had a bicuspid aortic valve, which was noncalcified and competent. He called to relay this news and we discussed how he might prevent complications from developing on the congenitally malformed valve. I recommended the following:

Avoid infection. Prophylactic antibiotics obviously are required during dental and other operative procedures. Sir William Osler was the one who pointed out in 1885 the extreme propensity of the bicuspid aortic valve to be the site of infective endocarditis.[1–3] Certainly one with a bicuspid aortic valve should not use illicit drugs intravenously. Opiate addicts with bicuspid aortic valves do not live long.[4,5]

Discontinue lifting weights. This type of exercise puts undue stress, i.e., pressure, although for short periods, on the aortic valve.

Maintain a normal systemic blood pressure. Although the bicuspid aortic valve probably is not affected adversely by the left ventricular systolic pressure irrespective of its level, the level of the valve's closing pressure, i.e., the aortic diastolic pressure, probably plays a prominent role in determining whether the bicuspid valve becomes stenotic, or purely regurgitant (without superimposed infective endocarditis) or functions normally throughout life.

Keep the heart rate relatively slow. It is reasonable to believe that if the aortic valve closes only 55 times a minute rather than 75 times a minute (a 27% heart rate reduction) that the wear and tear received by the aortic valve from the aorta's closing pressure would be reduced. The best way to produce a relatively slow heart rate is by various aerobic exercises. Although the heart rate increases during the exercise, the total 24-hour heart beats probably would be reduced substantially. Beta-blocker therapy could be useful to achieve this objective.

Keep the serum total cholesterol level relatively low. The major reason a bicuspid aortic valve becomes stenotic is because large calcific deposits develop on the aortic aspects of the cusps and the large deposits impart an immobility to the cusps which prevent their opening adequately during ventricular systole.[1–3] Thus, prevention of calcific deposits is essential for prevention of stenosis. In older persons in the Western world it is common to develop calcific deposits on the aortic aspects of the aortic valve cusps, on the ventricular aspects of the posterior mitral leaflet (mitral "anular" calcium), and in atherosclerotic plaques in the coronary arteries (as well as in plaques in other arteries).[6] The development of calcific deposits on the aortic valve, mitral anulus and coronary arteries with age occurs only in those populations with serum total cholesterol levels >150 mg/dl and usually in those persons with levels >200 mg/dl. Thus, maintaining a low serum total cholesterol level prevents calcific deposits on a normally formed aortic valve, and therefore it is reasonable to believe that maintaining a low level would have similar effect on a bicuspid aortic valve. Calcific deposits are never present on the aortic valve at birth; they are always acquired. Calcific deposits are less common on stenotic mitral valves (rheumatic origin) in persons residing in the undeveloped nations of the world (where the serum total cholesterol levels often are <150 mg/dl) than in persons in the Western World where these levels are usually >150 mg/dl. Thus, maintaining a relatively low serum total cholesterol level might deter calcific deposition on a bicuspid aortic valve, and if no calcium, no stenosis. Preventing calcific deposits, however, would not prevent the development of pure aortic regurgitation or infective endocarditis.[7,8]

Try to forget that the aortic valve is bicuspid. As long as the bicuspid valve functions normally there is nothing to worry about, and no one can predict which bicuspid aortic valve will function normally for a full lifetime and which one will become stenotic, purely regurgitant (without superimposed infective endocarditis) or infected. In other words, the natural history of a congenitally bicuspid aortic valve is unknown. It appears that about 1% of live births have a congenitally bicuspid valve. If that be the case about 50 million (of 5 billion) persons on planet earth have a congenitally bicuspid aortic valve, and about 2.5 million persons in the USA have a bicuspid aortic valve. What percentage of them in a lifetime will develop stenosis, pure regurgitation, infection, or no complications is unknown. Thus, life must continue and the focus must be on things other than the bicuspid aortic valve. Even with the worst scenario, aortic valve replacement is usually highly successful.

The echocardiogram will continue to detect abnormalities in the heart that at the time cause no trouble. As a consequence, this instrument at times will produce worry and concern in both patient and physician. It also can provide superb information on the natural history of many cardiac abnormalities.

William C. Roberts

William Clifford Roberts, MD
Editor in Chief

1. Roberts WC. The congenitally bicuspid aortic valve. A study of 85 autopsy cases. *Am J Cardiol 1970;26:72–83.*
2. Roberts WC. Anatomically isolated aortic valvular disease. The case against its being of rheumatic etiology. *Am J Med 1970;49:151–159.*
3. Roberts WC. The structure of the aortic valve in clinically-isolated aortic stenosis. An autopsy study of 162 patients over 15 years of age. *Circulation 1970;42:91–97.*
4. Dressler FA, Roberts WC. Infective endocarditis in opiate addicts: analysis of 80 cases studied at necropsy. *Am J Cardiol 1989;63:1240–1257.*
5. Dressler FA, Roberts WC. Modes of death and types of cardiac diseases in opiate addicts: analysis of 168 necropsy cases. *Am J Cardiol 1989;64:909–920.*
6. Roberts WC. The senile cardiac calcification syndrome. *Am J Cardiol 1986;58:572–574.*
7. Roberts WC, Morrow AG, McIntosh CL, Jones M, Epstein SE. Congenitally bicuspid aortic valve causing severe, pure aortic regurgitation without superimposed infective endocarditis. Analysis of 13 patients requiring aortic valve replacement. *Am J Cardiol 1981;47:206–209.*
8. Arnett EW, Roberts WC. Pathology of active infective endocarditis: a necropsy analysis of 192 patients. *Thorac Cardiovasc Surg 1982;30:327–335.*

Coronary "Lesion," Coronary "Disease," "Single-Vessel Disease," "Two-Vessel Disease": Word and Phrase Misnomers Providing False Impressions of the Extent of Coronary Atherosclerosis in Symptomatic Myocardial Ischemia

Coronary arterial angiography in patients with symptomatic myocardial ischemia generally discloses a significant narrowing in 1 or more of the 4 major (right, left main, left anterior descending and left circumflex) epicardial coronary arteries. The degree of narrowing is determined by measuring the transverse dimension of the opacified narrowed lumen and comparing this dimension to an adjacent lumen which is considered to be angiographically normal or nearly so. Thus, if the luminal diameter of the narrowing is 1 mm and the diameter of the adjacent lumen is 3 mm, the diameter reduction is considered to be about 70%. This degree of narrowing frequently is described as a "70% lesion" and the artery containing the "lesion" is spoken of as being "diseased." If only 1 of the 4 major coronary arteries contains a "significant lesion" (most commonly considered to be a narrowing >50% in diameter), then the patient is described as having "1-vessel or single vessel disease." If >1 major epicardial coronary artery contains a "lesion" >50% in diameter, the patient is considered to have "multivessel disease." If 2 arteries contain a "significant lesion" then the patient is spoken of as having "2-vessel disease"; if 3 arteries contain a "significant lesion," then the phrase "3-vessel disease" is applied. If 4 arteries contain "significant lesions," the phrase "4-vessel disease" has rarely been applied. Most commonly in this circumstance the patient is spoken of as having "left main disease," meaning that the lumen of the left main coronary artery is narrowed >50% or >70% in diameter. Whenever, however, the lumen of the left main coronary artery is narrowed >50% or >70% in diameter, the lumens of the other 3 major coronary arteries also are narrowed to a similar extent, and, therefore, the phrase "4-vessel disease" is usually applicable in this circumstance.[1]

I have problems with the use of the words "lesion" and "disease" in the above described circumstances, and also problems with the phrases "1-vessel disease," "2-vessel disease," and "3-vessel disease." The reason for concern is that the word "lesion" implies the presence of abnormality at one site and the absence of abnormality at another site. Numerous necropsy studies in patients >30 years of age with fatal coronary artery disease, irrespective of the type of fatal coronary event, have disclosed that the atherosclerotic process, in essentially all patients, is diffuse and extensive.[2] Furthermore, intravascular ultrasonic imaging in patients with symptomatic myocardial ischemia also has shown that the coronary atherosclerotic process is diffuse and extensive. Thus, the diffuse nature of coronary atherosclerosis as observed at necropsy in patients with fatal coronary artery disease also has been confirmed to be present during life. It no longer can be surmised, therefore, that the diffuse nature of coronary atherosclerosis is limited to patients with fatal coronary artery disease. Furthermore, the same diffuse process of coronary atherosclerosis is observed at necropsy in patients with previous symptomatic myocardial ischemia but who died from a non-cardiac cause.[3]

Thus, the word "lesion" to describe an angiographic narrowing is not incorrect, but its implication, that "lesions" are not present elsewhere in that artery or in another artery, is incorrect. I prefer the use of the word "narrowing" to describe angiographic luminal reductions because lesions are present in all segments of the epicardial artery. Some "lesions" result in luminal narrowings ≤25% in diameter; others result in narrowings 26 to 50% in diameter; others 51 to 75%, and still others produce narrowings of 76 to 100%. The continual use of the word "lesion" instead of the words "significant narrowing" leads many to believe that coronary atherosclerosis in persons with symptomatic myocardial ischemia is a focal process, and this belief is incorrect.

The word "disease" is not correct when applied to a "significant narrowing." "Disease" is a word to be applied to the general condition which, in this case of course, is "atherosclerosis." The word "disease" is incorrectly applied when describing the most severely narrowed site in the artery. Thus, neither the word "lesion" nor "disease" is correct because the condition is not limited to a single location in any one artery.

The phrases "single-vessel disease" (1-vessel disease), "double-vessel disease" (2-vessel disease), "triple-vessel disease" (3-vessel disease) are not ideal because they

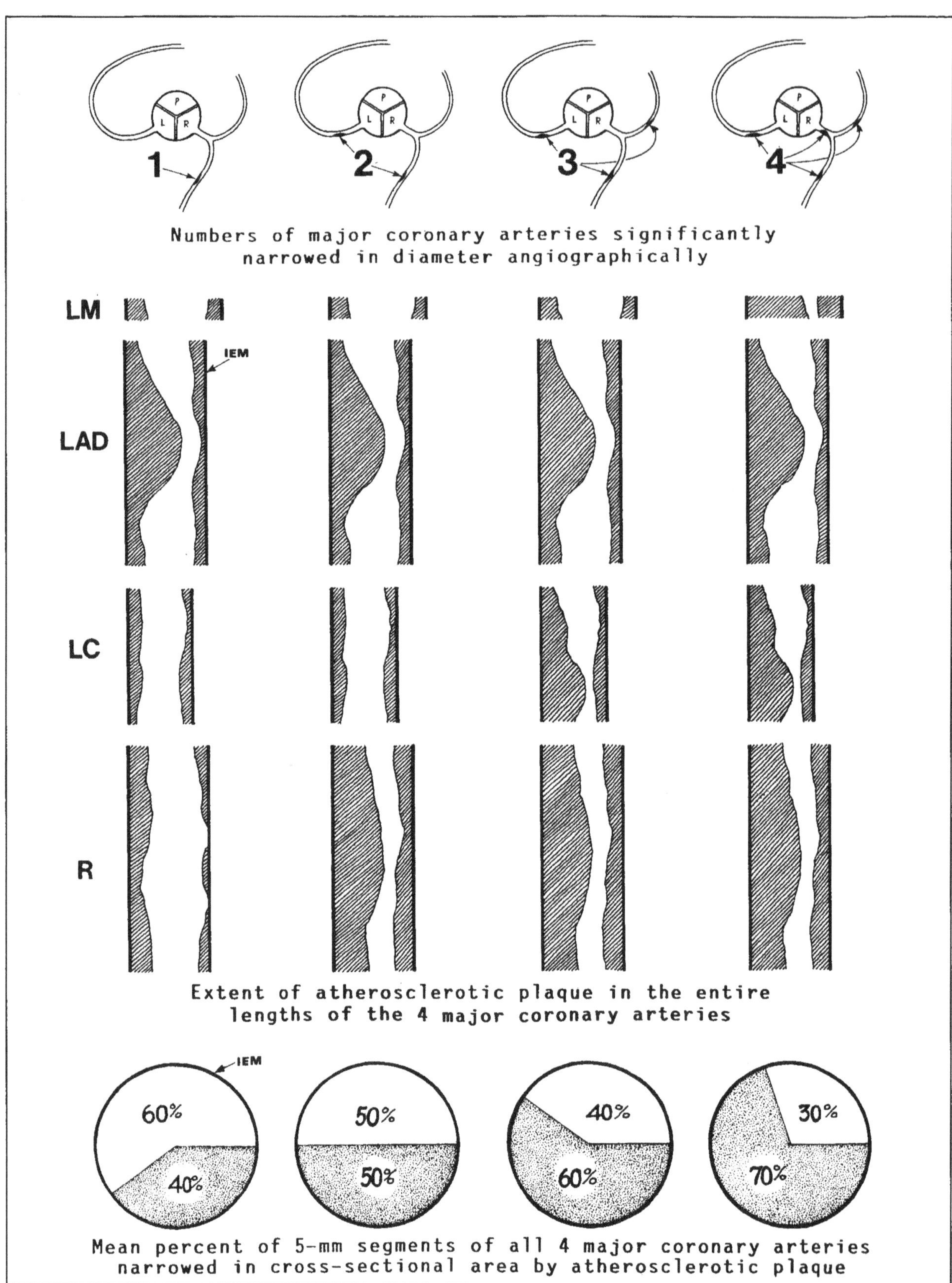

FIGURE 1. Diagram showing numbers of coronary arteries significantly narrowed by angiogram (*top*), the amounts of plaque in the entire lengths of the 4 major (left main [LM], left anterior descending [LAD], left circumflex [LC], and right [R]) epicardial coronary arteries (*middle*), and a cross-sectional area view (*bottom*) of the average amount of plaque in each 5-mm segment of the entire lengths of the 4 major coronary arteries according to the numbers of major arteries significantly narrowed by angiogram.

imply that the atherosclerotic process involves some and spares other coronary arteries. In persons over 30 years of age with symptomatic myocardial ischemia, a "significant narrowing" by angiography occasionally is limited to a single major coronary artery, but the other major coronary arteries are not "free of disease"; they simply have atherosclerotic plaques which reduce the luminal diameter <50% (or whatever definition is selected for "significant narrowing"). The significant narrowing or narrowings represent only the sites of the largest atherosclerotic plaques; the other sites also contain plaques, but they are smaller ones, and consequently produce less luminal narrowing. Whenever any plaque in a coronary artery is large enough to cause "significant narrowing" at any site, it is best to assume that all portions of the epicardial coronary arteries also contain plaque. Thus, if 1 major epicardial coronary artery is significantly narrowed (the narrowing may be shorter in length than 1 cm) and the lengths of the right (10 cm), left anterior descending (10 cm), left circumflex (6 cm), and left main (1 cm) coronary arteries are placed together, all 27 cm contain atherosclerotic plaques of varying sizes (Figure 1). The sites of "significant narrowing" merely represent the largest mountains in the 27-cm chain. Even in the patient with "significant narrowing" of a single major coronary artery, the amount of plaque present in all 4 major coronary arteries as a proportion of the total potential lumen (that enclosed by the internal elastic membrane) of all 4 arteries probably represents about 40% (Figure 1). In the patient with significant narrowing by angiogram of 2 major coronary arteries, the other major arteries always contain plaque in each of their 5-mm long segments. In this circumstance, the amount of plaque present in all 4 major arteries, as a proportion of the total potential lumen, probably represents at least 50%. In the patient with significant narrowing by angiogram of 3 major arteries (right, left anterior descending, left circumflex), the amount of plaque present in all 4 major arteries, as a proportion of the total potential lumen, probably represents at least 60%. In the patient with significant narrowing by angiogram of all 4 major coronary arteries, the amount of plaque present in all 4 arteries, as a proportion of the total potential lumen, probably represents at least 70%. Thus, the more arteries containing a "significant narrowing" at any site in the artery, the greater the amount of total plaque in that artery and in the "insignificantly narrowed" arteries.

Not only are virtually all 5-mm long segments of the 4 major epicardial coronary arteries sites of atherosclerotic plaque in patients with symptomatic or fatal myocardial ischemia, but a certain threshold of total luminal narrowing appears to be required to produce fatal or non-fatal myocardial ischemia. By study of each 5-mm long segment of each of the 4 major epicardial coronary arteries in various subsets of coronary patients, the lumens in about a third of the entire lengths of the 4 arteries are narrowed >75% in cross-sectional area by plaque and another third are narrowed 51–75% in cross-sectional area by plaque.[2] Although some patients with fatal coronary events have considerably less quantities of plaque in the coronary arteries, others have considerably more quantities of plaque, to such an extent at times that <20% of the potential lumen of the 4 major coronary arteries is not obliterated by plaque.

Thus, coronary atherosclerosis in patients with fatal or symptomatic myocardial ischemia is ***a diffuse and extensive process***. Knowledge that the plaque deposits are extensive and diffuse might cause some to question the rationale of coronary bypass or coronary angioplasty. These procedures, however, have proved their value irrespective of the extent of the atherosclerotic process. Nevertheless, the extensive nature of the process suggests that only a fine line separates adequate myocardial oxygenation from inadequate myocardial oxygenation and that small structural alterations can produce large functional differences. Because such large amounts of coronary plaque are required before evidence of myocardial ischemia results, it is possible that relatively small changes in our dietary habits could have relatively large effects on the sizes of plaques in our coronary arteries.

William C. Roberts

William Clifford Roberts, MD
Editor in Chief

1. Bulkley BH, Roberts WC. Atherosclerotic narrowing of the left main coronary artery. A necropsy analysis of 152 patients with fatal coronary heart disease and varying degrees of left main narrowing. *Circulation 1976;53:823–828.*
2. Roberts WC. Qualitative and quantitative comparison of amounts of narrowing by atherosclerotic plaques in the major epicardial coronary arteries at necropsy in sudden coronary death, transmural acute myocardial infarction, transmural healed myocardial infarction and unstable angina pectoris. *Am J Cardiol 1989;64:324–328.*
3. Virmani R, Roberts WC. Non-fatal healed transmural myocardial infarction and fatal non-cardiac disease. Qualification and quantification of coronary arterial narrowing and of left ventricular scarring in 18 necropsy patients. *Br Heart J 1981;45:434–441.*

The Best Anti-Heart Failure Agent Will Be a Lipid-Lowering Agent

In December 1990 this column contained a piece entitled "The Best Antiarrhythmic Agent Will Be a Lipid-Lowering Agent."[1] Its point was that although there were many causes of malignant or potentially malignant ventricular arrhythmias, atherosclerotic coronary artery disease was by far the most common (>75%). And the frequency of symptomatic and fatal myocardial ischemia increases as the amount of plaque in our coronary arteries increases. And the amount of plaque increases as our total and low-density lipoprotein levels in the serum increase and as the high-density lipoprotein cholesterol level decreases. If the percentage of calories from fat diminished in our diets from approximately 40% to about 10%, our serum total cholesterol levels and the frequency of symptomatic and fatal myocardial ischemia would drop to rates where malignant ventricular arrhythmias would not be problems. Because reducing our percentage of calories from fat by 75% is unrealistic for most of us, the lipid lowering drugs are needed.

In conjunction with low fat–low cholesterol diets, lipid-lowering agents slow, retard, and reverse the atherosclerotic process, and, therefore, delay, retard, and prevent the formation of atherosclerotic plaques by lowering our total and low-density lipoprotein serum levels and by raising our high-density lipoprotein levels. The lower the total and low-density lipoprotein serum levels, the less the atherosclerotic plaque and the less the chance of developing malignant and potentially malignant arrhythmias.

The same argument can be made with respect to congestive heart failure. Since atherosclerotic coronary artery disease is its most common cause in the Western world, it too could be prevented or delayed by earlier therapy directed at lowering the low-density lipoprotein cholesterol and raising the high-density cholesterol levels. When congestive heart failure occurs in vegetarian societies its etiology nearly always is a condition other than atherosclerosis. In the Western world I suspect that more congestive heart failure will be prevented by lipid-lowering medicines earlier than will be helped by the more conventional anticongestive heart failure medicines later.

In summary, lipid-lowering agents should also be viewed as anti-heart failure agents, and I predict that they will prove to be the best anti-heart failure agents.

William C. Roberts

William Clifford Roberts, MD
Editor in Chief

1. Roberts WC. The best antiarrhythmic agent will be a lipid-lowering agent. *Am J Cardiol* 1990;66:1402.

A Unique Heart Disease Associated With a Unique Cancer: Carcinoid Heart Disease

LOCATION OF THE CARCINOID PRIMARY TUMOR

Carcinoid tumors are never primary in the heart and they infrequently metastasize to the heart. Nevertheless, patients with *ileal* carcinoid, the location of the primary tumor in nearly all patients who develop the carcinoid syndrome (flushing and diarrhea), when hepatic metastases are present, often develop distinctive lesions in the heart, always located in the right side of the heart, and occasionally also on the left side of the heart[1-3] (Figure 1). Patients with carcinoid tumor primary in the *ovary* associated with carcinoid heart disease are extremely rare, but in this circumstance typical carcinoid cardiac lesions may develop unassociated with hepatic carcinoid metastases, because the venous drainage from the ovaries is into the inferior vena cava.[4,5] When the primary carcinoid tumor arises in a pulmonary *bronchus*, the carcinoid lesions may be limited to the left-sided cardiac valves. In this circumstance, the liver may be devoid of carcinoid metastases. If hepatic carcinoid metastases are present and if carcinoid heart disease occurs, the distinctive fibrous lesions always involve the right side of the heart with or without involvement of one or both left-sided valves.

MORPHOLOGIC CHARACTERISTICS OF THE CARCINOID CARDIAC LESIONS

The distinctive carcinoid cardiac lesions consist of deposits of fibrous tissue *devoid of elastic fibers* on the ventricular aspect of the tricuspid valve leaflets and on the arterial aspect of the pulmonic valve cusps.[1-3,6] Occasionally, deposits also are seen on the ventricular aspects of the mitral leaflets and, very rarely and usually to a small extent, on the aortic aspects of the aortic valve cusps. Most patients with carcinoid heart disease have the distinctive fibrous lesions limited to the right side of the heart. Much less often, patients with right-sided lesions also have similar lesions on the left side of the heart, but in this circumstance the left-sided lesions are always smaller and of no functional significance. In the setting of bronchial carcinoid, the mitral valve lesions, however, may be so extensive that mitral stenosis has been a consequence, and right-sided carcinoid lesions may be absent.

COMPARISON OF CARCINOID SYNDROME PATIENTS WITH AND WITHOUT CARCINOID HEART DISEASE

Ross and Roberts[3] studied at necropsy 36 patients with the carcinoid syndrome, 21 (57%) of whom did and 15 (43%) of whom did not have carcinoid heart disease. The 2 groups were similar in mean age (54 vs 55 years), duration of clinical illness (4.7 vs 6.3 years), body weight (50 vs 52 kg), systemic blood pressure (117/77 vs 128/77 mm Hg), blood hematocrit (37% vs 36%), total serum protein (6.0 g/dl), and serum albumin (2.2 vs 2.6 g/dl). The 2 groups were significantly different in the frequency of the presence of precordial murmurs consistent with tricuspid regurgitation and/or pulmonic stenosis (95% vs 13%), cardiomegaly by chest radiography (38% vs 0), low voltage on electrocardiogram (47% vs 0), and location of the primary site of the carcinoid tumor. Total 12-lead electrocardiographic QRS voltage[3] was similar in each group (105 vs 132 mm) (10 mm = 1 mV). Of the patients with carcinoid heart disease, 43% died of cardiac causes; in contrast, none of those without carcinoid heart disease died of cardiac causes. Of the 21 subjects with carcinoid heart disease, 7 had left-sided cardiac involvement, but in none was it of functional significance. Thus, although carcinoid heart disease frequently is the cause of death in patients with the carcinoid syndrome, the development of carcinoid heart disease appears to be unrelated to the duration of symptoms of the carcinoid syndrome.

Clinical diagnosis of carcinoid heart disease can usually be established by noninvasive means. *Auscultation*, of course, is the first clue. In 20 (95%) of the 21 subjects studied by Ross and Roberts[3] with carcinoid heart disease and in 5 (33%) of the 15 subjects without carcinoid heart disease, 1 or more precordial murmurs were recorded. Of the 20 subjects with precordial murmurs and carcinoid heart disease, 8 had both systolic and diastolic murmurs and 12 had only systolic murmurs; of the 5 subjects with precordial murmurs but without carcinoid heart disease, the murmurs in all were systolic only. Thus, nearly all patients with carcinoid heart disease have precordial murmurs, and when the murmur has a diastolic component, diagnosis of carcinoid heart disease usually can be made with confidence.

The *systemic arterial blood pressure* is not helpful in either diagnosing carcinoid syndrome or distinguishing those with from those without carcinoid heart disease. Only 3 of the 36 subjects studied by Ross and Roberts[3] had indirect systolic systemic ar-

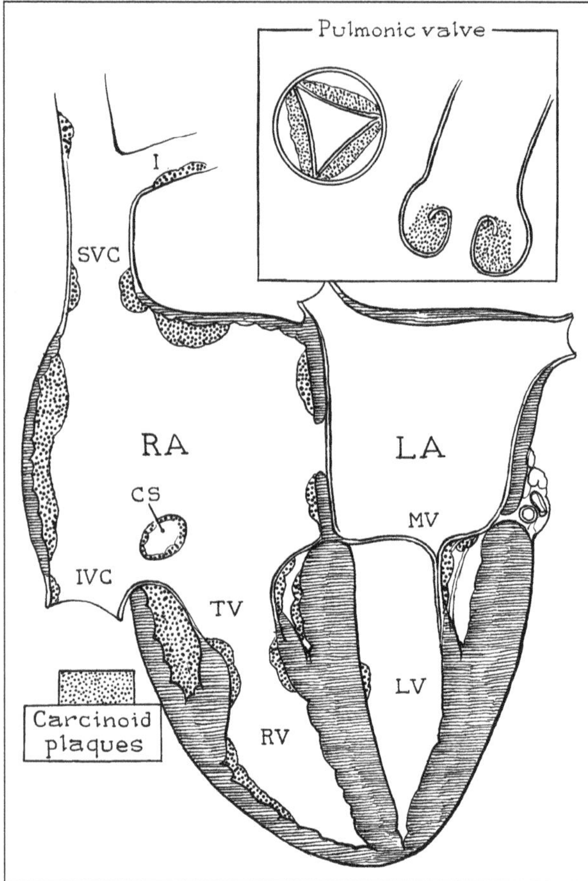

FIGURE 1. Diagram showing location of carcinoid fibrous plaques in *carcinoid heart disease.* CS = coronary sinus ostium; I = innominate vein; IVC = inferior vena cava; LA = left atrium; LV = left ventricle; MV = mitral valve; RA = right atrium; RV = right ventricle; SVC = superior vena cava; TV = tricuspid valve. Reproduced with permission from Ross EM and Roberts WC.[3]

terial pressures >140 mm Hg and/or diastolic arterial pressures >90 mm Hg: 1 of the 21 with and 2 of the 15 without carcinoid heart disease. The average peak systolic pressure was 117 mm Hg in the 21 subjects with and 128 mm Hg in the 15 subjects without carcinoid heart disease; the average diastolic pressure in both groups was 77 mm Hg.

Chest radiography is helpful in diagnosing carcinoid heart disease. The cardiothoracic ratio was >0.50 in 8 (38%) of the 21 subjects with carcinoid heart disease and in none of 15 subjects without carcinoid heart disease. Thus, the cardiothoracic ratio is not a very sensitive test for carcinoid heart disease, but it is specific.

The *resting electrocardiogram* is somewhat useful in distinguishing the subjects with from those without carcinoid heart disease. The sum of the QRS voltage in leads I, II, and III was ≤15 mm in 9 of the 21 subjects studied by Ross and Roberts[3] with and in none of the 15 subjects without carcinoid heart disease. The sum of the total 12-lead QRS voltage ranged from 58 to 227 mm (10 mm = 1 mV) in 34 subjects, and the mean values were not significantly different between the 2 groups (105 vs 132 mm) (normal >175 mm).[7] Evidence of right ventricular hypertrophy was rare. The R wave was greater than the S wave in either leads V_1 or V_2 in only 4 of the 19 subjects with and in none of the 15 subjects without carcinoid heart disease. Despite right atrial dilatation in the subjects with carcinoid heart disease, all 19 with and all 15 without carcinoid heart disease had sinus rhythm. The R-R interval was normal (≤0.20 seconds) in 18 of 19 subjects with and in 14 of 15 subjects without carcinoid heart disease. The width of the QRS complex was normal (≤0.12 second) in all subjects, irrespective of whether or not they had carcinoid heart disease. Thus, other than the higher frequency of low voltage in the subjects with carcinoid heart disease, the electrocardiogram was not helpful in distinguishing subjects with from those without carcinoid heart disease.

MORPHOLOGIC FEATURES OF CARCINOID HEART DISEASE

All of the 21 patients with carcinoid heart disease studied by Ross and Roberts[3] had involvement of both tricuspid and pulmonic valves by carcinoid plaques, and 19 of them also had carcinoid plaques on the mural endocardium of the right atrium and usually also on the mural endocardium of the right ventricle. The number of subjects with right-sided valvular dysfunction as a consequence of the carcinoid plaques on the valvular leaflets is less certain because of the relative difficulty in diagnosing by auscultation mild degrees of tricuspid and pulmonic valve dysfunction. In 2 of the 21 subjects with right-sided carcinoid heart disease, the degree of morphologic involvement of both valves was minimal and valvular function clearly was not affected. Of the remaining 19 subjects, 18 had precordial systolic and/or diastolic murmurs of grade 2/6 or greater intensity.

Although the composition and location of the carcinoid plaques on both right-sided cardiac valves are similar, the functional consequences of the carcinoid plaques are different. The deposits occur nearly entirely on the downstream side of the valvular leaflets, i.e., on the ventricular aspects of the septal and posterior tricuspid leaflets and on the pulmonary arterial side of the pulmonic valve cusps. On the anterior tricuspid valve leaflet, the deposits can be on both sides. The consequences of the "downstream" deposition is an adherence of the leaflet to the underlying mural endocardium (tricuspid septal and posterior leaflets) or to the underlying pulmonary arterial endothelium (pulmonic valve) via the carcinoid plaques. The fibrous tissue of the carcinoid plaque acts as a constricting substance such that the "ring" of both right-sided cardiac valves is made smaller than normal and at the same time leaflet mobility is diminished. The consequence is tricuspid regurgitation with or without some degree of stenosis. Nearly all patients with pure tricuspid regurgitation (no element of stenosis) have dilated valve rings, but patients with some degree of stenosis in addition to regurgitation do not have dilated annuli. Patients with carcinoid heart disease follow this principle.

Thus, patients with carcinoid heart disease have much more tricuspid regurgitation than stenosis, but usually there is some degree of stenosis, albeit small.

In contrast to the tricuspid valve, the dominant functional pulmonic valve lesion is stenosis, although all patients with stenosis have some degree of pulmonic regurgitation. The reason for the difference—compared with the tricuspid valve—is that the orifice of the normal pulmonic valve is much smaller initially than the orifice of the tricuspid valve. Thus, the constriction by deposition of carcinoid plaques within the pulmonic sinuses causes constriction of the pulmonic root with the production of pulmonic stenosis. Because the distal portions of the pulmonic cusps are inverted toward the sinuses and the mobility of the cusps is lost, some degree of regurgitation is inevitable in these patients who have any degree of pulmonic stenosis.

Although combined lesions of both mitral and aortic valves are fairly common as a consequence of either rheumatic heart disease or infective endocarditis, or both, combined lesions of both tricuspid and pulmonic valves are rare, and carcinoid is the only condition in which uniformly both—not just 1—right-sided valves are involved. The 2 dominant functional consequences of right-sided carcinoid heart disease are pulmonic stenosis and tricuspid regurgitation. These 2 lesions in the same patient are particularly unfavorable because the pulmonic stenosis increases the degree of tricuspid regurgitation. A commonly employed method of producing chronic congestive heart failure in experimental animals is by banding the pulmonary trunk to create pulmonic stenosis, and excising or destroying 1 or more tricuspid valve cusps to make the valve purely regurgitant. Thus, right-sided carcinoid heart disease in essence creates this experimental model. If a patient with carcinoid heart disease had only dysfunction of the pulmonic or the tricuspid valve, probably the functional consequence would be insignificant. It is the combination of both right-sided valvular lesions—namely pulmonic stenosis and tricuspid regurgitation—that has the potential of being devastating.

ECHOCARDIOGRAPHIC FEATURES OF CARCINOID HEART DISEASE

Echocardiography, particularly cross-sectional, is helpful in diagnosing carcinoid heart disease. Callahan and associates[8] described retrospectively echocardiographic features in 20 patients with the carcinoid syndrome. By physical examination, 15 patients had a diagnosis of carcinoid heart disease and the other 5 did not. Both M-mode and cross-sectional echocardiographic examinations in the latter 5 patients disclosed no abnormal findings. Of the 15 patients with auscultatory evidence of carcinoid heart disease, 5 had normal M-mode and cross-sectional echocardiographic findings. The other 10, all of whom had tricuspid regurgitation by physical examination, had dilated right ventricular cavities, abnormal motion of the ventricular septum, and of the 9 in whom the tricuspid valve leaflets were visualized by cross-sectional echocardiography, strikingly abnormal tricuspid leaflets (thickened and retracted with fixed orifice). The pulmonic valve cusps were not visualized in any patient by M-mode echocardiography, but in the 4 in whom they were visualized by cross-sectional echocardiography, the pulmonic valve cusps were abnormal in each.

Howard and associates[9] prospectively examined by cross-sectional echocardiography 14 patients with the carcinoid syndrome, and 8 had definite abnormalities of 1 or both right-sided cardiac valves. Clinically, 7 had auscultatory evidence of tricuspid regurgitation including 1 with a diastolic rumble, and 5 of them had diffusely thickened and retracted tricuspid valve leaflets; the other 9 patients had normal tricuspid valves by echocardiography. Four patients by auscultation had evidence of pulmonic stenosis with or without pulmonic regurgitation. The pulmonic valve cusps were visualized by echocardiogram in 7 patients: 2 had retracted pulmonic cusps with decreased systolic motion (1 of whom had pulmonic stenosis by auscultation) and 5 had normal cusps (none of whom had auscultatory evidence of pulmonic stenosis).

Transesophageal echocardiography has proved to be more useful than transthoracic echocardiography for diagnosis of carcinoid heart disease. Lundin and associates[10] detected by the transesophageal approach tricuspid regurgitation in 22 (71%) of 31 patients with ileal carcinoid versus 18 (57%) by the transthoracic investigation. The transesophageal images allowed measurement of the thicknesses of the atrioventricular valve leaflets, and also the inner layer of the right atrial walls. The mean thicknesses of the anterior tricuspid leaflets were significantly greater than that of the anterior mitral leaflets, a difference not seen in controls. The patients with functional signs of severe carcinoid heart disease had significantly thicker mean right atrial inner layers than did those with less or no signs of right-sided cardiac disease.

Doppler echocardiography also has proved useful for diagnosis of carcinoid heart disease. Pellikka and colleagues[11] studied by echocardiogram 132 patients with the carcinoid syndrome and found that 74 (56%) had echocardiographic, including Doppler, features of carcinoid heart disease: 72 patients (97%) had shortened and thickened tricuspid valve leaflets; all 74 (100%) had Doppler evidence of tricuspid regurgitation (moderate or severe in 62 [90%]). Severe tricuspid regurgitation was characterized by a dagger-shaped Doppler spectral profile with an early peak pressure and rapid decline. The pressure half time was prolonged, a finding consistent with associated tricuspid valve stenosis. The pulmonic valve cusps were thickened, retracted, and immobile in 36 patients (59%) and the valve was so small that it could not be visualized in an additional 29 patients (39%). Of the 47 patients who had Doppler examination of the pulmonic valve, regurgitation was found in 38 (81%) and stenosis was present in 25

(53%). Left-sided valvular involvement was present in 5 patients (7%), 4 of whom had a patent foramen ovale or carcinoid metastases in the lung. Myocardial carcinoid tumor metastases were found in 3 (4%) of the 74 patients. Small pericardial effusions were present in 10 patients (14%). The patients with and without echocardiographic evidence of carcinoid heart disease did not differ with regard to sex, age, location of the primary tumor, duration of symptoms, or signs of the carcinoid syndrome (dermal flushing, diarrhea). Dyspnea was more frequent in those with than in those without carcinoid heart disease (54% vs 27%). Precordial murmurs were more frequent in those with than in those without carcinoid heart disease (92% vs 43%). Three-year survival of patients with compared to those without echocardiographic evidence of carcinoid heart disease was reduced (31% vs 68%).

MAGNETIC RESONANCE IMAGING AND COMPUTED TOMOGRAPHY IN CARCINOID HEART DISEASE

Magnetic resonance imaging and *computed tomography* also may be helpful in diagnosing carcinoid heart disease.[12] Although the findings usually simply corroborate those seen by echocardiography, supplemental information occasionally is supplied.

SERUM AND URINE TESTS IN CARCINOID HEART DISEASE

Measurement of circulating *serotonin* (5-hydroxytryptamine) or its principal metabolite, *5-hydroxyindole acetic acid* (5-HIAA), of course, is helpful in diagnosing the carcinoid syndrome, but it may not be helpful in differentiating the patients with and without carcinoid heart disease.[13] Roberts and Sjoerdsma[1] in their early (1964) study of 17 necropsy patients with the carcinoid syndrome, 9 with and 8 without carcinoid heart disease, found no significant difference in the urinary levels of 5-HIAA in those patients with and in those without carcinoid heart disease. More recently (1989), Himelman and Schiller[14] found higher peak levels of urinary 5-HIAA in their 17 patients with echocardiographic evidence of carcinoid heart disease and more severe hepatic dysfunction than in their 13 patients without carcinoid heart disease (331 ± 231 mg vs 58 ± 78 mg). Lundin and associates[15] studied 68 patients with proven mid-gut carcinoid tumors, 50 of whom had the carcinoid syndrome. Of the 68 patients, 61 (89%) had elevated urinary 5-HIAA levels. The 18 patients with advanced right-sided valve disease had significantly higher mean 5-HIAA urinary levels than did the patients without right-sided lesions or functionally insignficant ones (800 vs 210 μmol/day). Pellikka and associates[11] also observed higher levels of urinary 5-HIAA in their 74 patients with echocardiographic evidence of carcinoid heart disease than in their 58 patients without evidence of heart disease but with the carcinoid syndrome (270 vs 131 mg/day). The study by Robiolio et al,[16] utilizing the Duke Carcinoid Database of 604 patients with carcinoid tumors, found both plasma serotonin (1,130 vs 426 pmol/ml) and urinary 5-HIAA (219 vs 55 mg/day) strikingly higher in the 19 patients with proven carcinoid heart disease than in the 585 patients with carcinoid tumors (only some of whom had the carcinoid syndrome [flushing and diarrhea] but no carcinoid heart disease). Flushing and diarrhea was almost 3 times more common in patients with carcinoid heart disease than in those without the characteristic cardiac disease.

Other circulating substances have been found to be elevated in patients with carcinoid heart disease. Lundin and associates[15] found, for example, significantly higher plasma levels of *tachykinins neuropeptide K* and *substance P* in their patients with ileal carcinoid tumors with the most severe right-sided heart disease. Lundin and colleagues[17] found significantly higher plasma *atrial natriuretic peptide levels* in their patients with ileal carcinoid tumors with the most severe right-sided heart disease.

HEMODYNAMIC AND ANGIOGRAPHIC OBSERVATIONS IN CARCINOID HEART DISEASE

There are surprisingly few reported hemodynamic and angiographic observations in patients with carcinoid heart disease. Biörck and colleagues[18] in 1952 described a boy with "unusual cyanosis . . . with pulmonary stenosis and tricuspid insufficiency" who died shortly after injection of contrast material into the right ventricular cavity. Schwaber and Lukas[19] in 1962 described "hyperkinemia" associated with considerable cardiac failure in a patient with the carcinoid syndrome without associated carcinoid heart disease. Of the 17 necropsy patients with carcinoid heart disease described by Roberts and Sjoerdsma[1] in 1964, none had had cardiac catheterization performed, and of the 36 patients with carcinoid syndrome reported in 1986 by Ross and Roberts,[3] only 3 had had cardiac catheterization and 2 of them had been reported earlier by Roberts and colleagues.[2] In each of their 2 patients the right atrial pressures were quite high; the a-wave was 24 and the v-wave 34 mm Hg in 1 patient and 18 and 23 mm Hg, respectively, in the other patient. The latter patient had a right ventricular pressure of 45/13 mm Hg and a pulmonary arterial pressure of 20/8 mm Hg with a normal cardiac index (3.2 L/min/m^2). Each of the 2 patients had extensive right atrial carcinoid deposits. The authors suggested that the right atrial plaques make this chamber relatively inelastic and consequently not able to distend or to contract normally. This reduction in right atrial elasticity or distensibility significantly alters the hemodynamic findings in the right atrial pulse. Thus, in each of the 2 patients there was a greater elevation in right atrial pressures than would have been expected from the sizes of the tricuspid valve orifices observed at necropsy. These authors speculated that even mild tricuspid valve carcinoid disease might produce significant elevation of right atrial pressures because of associated right atrial carcinoid plaques, whereas an equal degree of rheumatic tricuspid disease might not cause right atrial hypertension.

More hemodynamic information was reported when valve replacement or valvuloplasty became a more common form of therapy in carcinoid heart disease. The degree of both tricuspid valve stenosis and pulmonic valve stenosis in patients with carcinoid heart disease appears to be rather small. The mean diastolic gradient between right atrium and right ventricle is usually $<$10 mm Hg, and the peak systolic pressure gradient between right ventricle and pulmonary trunk is nearly always $<$50 mm Hg, the latter, of course, being far less than that in the usual patient with congenital pulmonic valve stenosis. Because carcinoid involvement of both the tricuspid and pulmonic valves causes the cusps to retract toward their margins of attachment, the valvular orifices become fixed in an open position, which necessitates some degree of regurgitation of each valve. Because the tricuspid valve ring is initially much larger than the pulmonic valve "ring," similar degrees of deposition of carcinoid plaques on each of these 2 valve leaflets results in very different hemodynamic consequences. Stenosis is the major hemodynamic lesion involving the pulmonic valve, and regurgitation is the major hemodynamic lesion involving the tricuspid valve. The combination of pulmonic stenosis and tricuspid regurgitation is a very unfavorable hemodynamic combination because the former worsens the latter.

OPERATIVE TREATMENT OF CARCINOID HEART DISEASE

Cardiac valve replacement and/or *valvuloplasty* has been performed in some patients with carcinoid heart disease since 1963.[20] Most reports have been single case studies and these were reviewed by Ross and Roberts[3] up to 1985. In 1990 Lundin and associates[21] replaced both tricuspid and pulmonic valves with tissue valves in 4 patients: 1 died 5 days postoperatively and the other 3 were free of evidence of cardiac dysfunction 10, 12, and 38 months postoperatively. These authors also summarized outcomes in 25 previously reported patients having cardiac valve replacement for carcinoid heart disease. Knott-Craig and colleagues[22] reported results of mechanical valve replacement of the tricuspid valve in 10 patients combined with pulmonic valvectomy in 9 and pulmonic valve replacement (homograft) in 1: 4 patients died early and the remaining 6 were alive at 4, 4, 4, 7, 24, and 46 months postoperatively. These authors also reviewed 28 previously reported patients who had had tricuspid valve replacement for carcinoid heart disease. There was no significant difference in survival of patients with a bioprosthesis versus a mechanical prosthesis in the tricuspid valve position. For the entire group of 38 patients having tricuspid valve replacement for carcinoid heart disease, the 4-year survival was 48 ± 13%.

Connolly and colleagues[23] reported 26 patients having cardiac valve replacement for carcinoid heart disease and compared results with those in 40 patients with the carcinoid syndrome not having a cardiac operation. Nine patients (35%) died in the early postoperative period: of the 17 survivors, 8 were alive at a mean follow-up of 28 months and each of the 8 were symptomatically improved. The only predictor of operative mortality was low voltage (sum of QRS in I, II, and III $\leq$15 mm) on the preoperative electrocardiogram. Predictors of late survival included a lower preoperative urinary 5-HIAA level. And finally, Robiolio and associates[24] using the Duke Carcinoid Database, described results of bioprosthetic replacement of the tricuspid valve in 8 patients (2 also had open pulmonic valvuloplasty): 5 died within 30 days of the operation; 2 of the 3 survivors lived $>$10 years. Review of their 8 patients and 39 previously published valve replacement cases for carcinoid heart disease disclosed a 30-day mortality of 56% for patients $>$60 years of age and zero for those $\leq$60 years of age. Thus, although valve replacement may afford prolonged palliation for carcinoid heart disease, it is associated with a significant mortality risk.

A potential danger in using a bioprosthesis or any type of tissue valve for valve replacement in a patient with carcinoid heart disease is involvement of the bioprosthetic cusps by the same characteristic carcinoid fibrotic process that affected the native valves. Schoen and colleagues[25] described at necropsy typical carcinoid plaques on the cusps of the bioprosthesis in the tricuspid valve position, although bioprosthetic function at this time appeared to have been normal. Ridker and associates[26] described a patient who had replacement of the tricuspid valve with a porcine bioprosthesis and pulmonic valvulotomy, and when studied 11 years later had a stenotic (10 mm Hg mean diastolic gradient) bioprosthesis in the tricuspid valve position. The bioprosthesis was excised at reoperation and its cusps were thickened by both calcific deposits and typical carcinoid fibrous plaques. Ohri and colleagues[27] described typical carcinoid plaques that had developed on the cusps of a cryopreserved allograft which had been used to replace a native pulmonic valve only 3 months earlier because of carcinoid involvement. The patient continued to have pulmonary hypertension postoperatively and soon after operation developed pulmonic regurgitation which progressively worsened.

Balloon valvulotomy also has been performed in patients with carcinoid heart disease, and the results are mixed. Grant et al[28] reported 2 patients and each had balloon dilatation of stenotic pulmonic valves resulting from carcinoid heart disease. One patient had symptomatic benefit for 2 months and the other had no improvement. Onate and associates[29] performed balloon valvuloplasty of both tricuspid and pulmonic valves in 2 patients: 1 was not improved and the second became asymptomatic. Hargreaves and colleagues[30] described successful balloon dilatation of the pulmonic valve resulting from carcinoid heart disease.

William C. Roberts

William Clifford Roberts, MD
Editor in Chief
Baylor University Medical Center
Dallas, Texas 75246

1. Roberts WC, Sjoerdsma A. The cardiac disease associated with carcinoid syndrome (carcinoid heart disease). *Am J Med* 1964;36:5–34.
2. Roberts WC, Mason DT, Wright LD Jr. The non-distensible right atrium of carcinoid disease of the heart, *Am J Clin Pathol* 1965;44:627–631.
3. Ross EM, Roberts WC. The carcinoid syndrome: comparison of 21 necropsy subjects with carcinoid heart disease to 15 necropsy subjects without carcinoid heart disease. *Am J Med* 1986;79:339–354.
4. Oei SG, Kloosterman MD, Verhoeven ATHM. Primary ovarian carcinoid tumor in combination with carcinoid heart disease: a case report, *Eur J Obstet Gyn Reprod Biol* 1989;31:185–188.
5. Wilkowske MA, Hartmann LC, Mullany CJ, Behrenbeck T, Kvols LK. Progressive carcinoid heart disease after resection of primary ovarian carcinoid. *Cancer* 1994;73:1889–1991.
6. Ferrans VJ, Roberts WC. The carcinoid endocardial plaque. An ultrastructural study. *Human Pathol* 1976;7:387–409.
7. Odom H II, Davis JL, Dinh H, Baker BJ, Roberts WC, Murphy ML. QRS voltage measurements in autopsied men free of cardiopulmonary disease: a basis for evaluating total QRS voltage as an index of left ventricular hypertrophy. *Am J Cardiol* 1986;58:801–804.
8. Callahan JA, Wroblewski EM, Reeder GS, Edwards WD, Seward JB, Tajik AJ. Echocardiographic features of carcinoid heart disease. *Am J Cardiol* 1982;50:762–768.
9. Howard RJ, Drobac M, Rider WD, Keane TJ, Finlayson J, Silver MD, Wigle ED, Rakowski H. Carcinoid heart disease: diagnosis by two-dimensional echocardiography. *Circulation* 1982;66:1059–1065.
10. Lundin L, Landelius J, Andren B, Oberg K. Transesophageal echocardiography improves the diagnostic value of cardiac ultrasound in patients with carcinoid heart disease. *Br Heart J* 1990;64:190–194.
11. Pellikka PA, Tajik AJ, Khandheria BK, Seward JB, Callahan JA, Pitot HC, Kvols LK. Carcinoid heart disease. Clinical and echocardiographic spectrum in 74 patients. *Circulation* 1993;87:1188–1196.
12. Mirowitz SA, Gutierrez FR. MR and CT diagnosis of carcinoid heart disease. *Chest* 1993;103:630–631.
13. Oates JA. The carcinoid syndrome. *N Engl J Med* 1986;315:702–704.
14. Himelman RB, Schiller NB. Clinical and echocardiographic comparison of patients with the carcinoid syndrome with and without carcinoid heart disease. *Am J Cardiol* 1989;63:347–352.
15. Lundin L, Norheim I, Landelius J, Öberg K, Theodorsson-Norheim E. Carcinoid heart disease: relationship of circulating vasoactive substances to ultrasound-detectable cardiac abnormalities, *Circulation* 1988;77:264–269.
16. Ribiolio PA, Rigolin VH, Wilson JS, Harrison JK, Sanders LL, Bashore TM, Feldman JM. Carcinoid heart disease. Correlation of high serotonin levels with valvular abnormalities detected by cardiac catheterization and echocardiography. *Circulation* 1995;92:790–795.
17. Lundin L, Öberg K, Landelius J, Hansson HE, Wilander E, Theordorsson E. Plasma atrial natriuretic peptide in carcinoid heart disease, *Am J Cardiol* 1989;63:969–972.
18. Biörck G, Axen O, Thorson A. Unusual cyanosis in a boy with congenital pulmonary stenosis and tricuspid insufficiency. Fatal outcome after angiocardiography. *Am Heart J* 1952;44:143–148.
19. Schwaber JR, Lukas DS. Hyperkinemia and cardiac failure in the carcinoid syndrome, *Am J Med* 1962;32:846–853.
20. Wright PW, Mulder DG. Carcinoid heart disease. Report of a case treated by open heart surgery. *Am J Cardiol* 1963;12:864–868.
21. Lundin L, Hansson H-E, Landelius J, Öberg K. Surgical treatment of carcinoid heart disease. *J Thorac Cardiovasc Surg* 1990;100:552–561.
22. Knott-Craig CJ, Schaff HV, Mullany CJ, Kvols LK, Moertel CG, Edwards WD, Danielson GK. Carcinoid disease of the heart. Surgical management of ten patients. *J Thorac Cardiovasc Surg* 1992;104:475–481.
23. Connolly HM, Nishimura RA, Smith HC, Pellikka PA, Mullany CJ, Kvols LK. Outcome of cardiac surgery for carcinoid heart disease. *J Am Coll Cardiol* 1995;25:410–416.
24. Robiolio PA, Rigolin VH, Harrison JK, Lowe JE, Moore JO, Bashore TM, Feldman JM. Predictors of outcome of tricuspid valve replacement in carcinoid heart disease. *Am J Cardiol* 1995;75:485–488.
25. Schoen FJ, Hausner RJ, Howell JF, Beazley HL, Titus JL. Porcine heterograft valve replacement in carcinoid heart disease. *J Thorac Cardiovasc Surg* 1981;81:100–105.
26. Ridker PM, Chertow GM, Karlson EW, Neish AS, Schoen FJ. Bioprosthetic tricuspid valve stenosis associated with extensive plaque deposition in carcinoid heart disease. *Am Heart J* 1991;121:1835–1838.
27. Ohri SK, Schofield JB, Hodgson H, Oakley CM, Keogh BE. Carcinoid heart disease: early failure of an allograft valve replacement. *Ann Thorac Surg* 1994;58:1161–1163.
28. Grant SCD, Scarffe JH, Levy RD, Brooks NH. Failure of balloon dilatation of the pulmonary valve in carcinoid pulmonary stenosis. *Br Heart J* 1992;67:450–453.
29. Onate A, Alcibar J, Inguanzo R, Pena N, Gochi R. Balloon dilatation of tricuspid and pulmonary valves in carcinoid heart disease. *Texas Heart Inst J* 1993;20:115–119.
30. Hargreaves AD, Pringle SD, Boon NA. Successful balloon dilatation of the pulmonary valve in carcinoid heart disease. *Intern J Cardiol* 1994;45:150–151.

Primary and Secondary Neoplasms of the Heart

In the last 40 years cardiac neoplasms have progressed from clinical curiosities described primarily in numerous case reports with diagnosis mainly at autopsy to fairly rapid antemortem diagnosis and frequent curative operative therapy. Diagnosis has been greatly facilitated by 2-dimensional echocardiography and, in select cases, the use of magnetic resonance imaging or computed tomography.

CLASSIFICATION

There is no perfect classification for cardiac neoplasms. Like any organ or tissue, neoplasms involving the heart may be primary or secondary. The primary ones may be benign or malignant and the secondary or metastatic ones are, by definition, malignant. The metastatic neoplasms are far more frequent than are the primary neoplasms by at least a 30 to 1 ratio.[1,2] The various frequencies of the primary benign and primary malignant tumors vary from report to report, approximately 0.1% to 0.3% in most autopsy series. A recent list of primary benign neoplasms gathered by investigators at the Armed Forces of Pathology is listed in Table I, and those primary malignant tumors encountered are listed in Table II.[3] The frequencies of the metastatic neoplasms also vary from report to report, but nearly all studies have listed carcinoma of the lung as the most commonly encountered metastatic tumor at autopsy followed by cancer of the breast, lymphoma, and leukemia (Table III). The order of frequency of metastases is different, however, if the frequency of each different type of tumor with metastasis to the heart is determined. For example, Table IV lists the frequencies of metastases to the heart in each of 100 cases of each of 20 separate tumors: melanoma has the highest frequency of metastases to the heart followed by malignant germ cell tumor, leukemia, lymphoma, cancer of the lung, and then the various sarcomas.[3]

LOCATION OF CARDIAC NEOPLASMS

Cardiac neoplasms may involve only the endocardium, only the myocardium, only the epicardium, or various combinations (Figure 1). By far the most common location of metastatic cardiac neoplasm is epicardium.[4] Neoplasms limited to parietal pericardium without extension into epicardium are not considered cardiac neoplasms. The epicardial tumor deposits may be multifocal or single, or they may be extensive and essentially diffuse or nearly so. Likewise, the intramyocardial masses may be focal or multifocal. The most common location for intramyocardial masses is left ventricular free wall and ventricular septum, portions of the heart, of course, with the greatest myocardial mass. The endocardial neoplasms are the intracavitary ones. They may involve a single cardiac cavity or >1. They may be limited to either the right or left side of the heart or they may involve both. It is the intracavitary tumors that produce obstruction to inflow into the heart or into a ventricular cavity or outflow from a ventricular cavity. The intracavitary neoplasms are the ones that may partially dislodge and produce either pulmonary or systemic emboli, or both. The intracavitary deposits are the ones with the potential of producing the triad of obstruction, embolization, and constitutional symptoms.

TABLE I Primary *Benign* Neoplasms of the Heart (1976–1993)*

Tumor†	Total	Surgical	Autopsy	Age ≤15 Years at Diagnosis
Myxoma	114	102	12	4
Rhabdomyoma	20	6	14	20
Fibroma	20	18	2	13
Hemangioma	17	10	7	2
Atrioventricular nodal	10	0	10	2
Granular-cell	4	0	4	0
Lipoma	2	2	0	0
Paraganglioma	2	2	0	0
Myocytic hamartoma	2	2	0	0
Histiocytoid cardiomyopathy	2	0	2	2
Inflammatory pseudotumor	2	2	0	1
Fibrous histiocytoma	1	0	1	0
Epitheloid hemangio-endothelioma	1	1	0	0
Bronchogenic cyst	1	1	0	0
Teratoma	1	0	1	1
Totals	199	146 (73%)	53 (27%)	45 (23%)

*Modified from: Burke A, Virmani R. Atlas of Tumor Pathology. Tumors of the Heart and Great Vessels. Washington, DC: Armed Forces Institute of Pathology 1996:231.

†Excludes papillary fibroelastoma and lipomatous hypertrophy of the atrial septum.

Tumor	Total	Surgical	Autopsy	Age ≤15 Years at Diagnosis
Sarcoma	137 (95%)	116	21	11 (8%)
Angio	33	22	11	1
Unclassified	33	30	3	3
Fibrous histiocytoma	16	16	0	1
Osteo	13	13	0	0
Leiomyo	12	11	1	1
Fibro	9	9	0	1
Myxo	8	8	0	1
Rhabdomyo	6	2	4	3
Synovial	4	4	0	0
Lipo	2	0	2	0
Schwannoma	1	1	0	0
Lymphoma	7 (5%)	1	6	0
Totals	144 (100%)	117 (81%)	27 (19%)	11 (8%)

TABLE II Primary *Malignant* Tumors of the Heart (1976–1993)*

*Modified from: Burke A, Virmani R. Atlas of Tumor Pathology. Tumors of the Heart and Great Vessels. Washington, DC: Armed Forces Institute of Pathology 1996:231.

TABLE III Metastatic Neoplasms in the Heart at Necropsy—Order of Frequency of Cancers Encountered*

Primary Tumor	Total Autopsies	Metastases to Heart
1. Lung	1,037	180 (17%)
2. Breast	685	70 (10%)
3. Lymphoma	392	67 (17%)
4. Leukemia	202	66 (33%)
5. Esophagus	294	37 (13%)
6. Uterus	451	36 (8%)
7. Melanoma	69	32 (46%)
8. Stomach	603	28 (5%)
9. Sarcoma	159	24 (15%)
10. Oral cavity & tongue	235	22 (9%)
11. Colon & rectum	440	22 (5%)
12. Kidney	114	12 (11%)
13. Thyroid gland	97	9 (9%)
14. Larynx	100	9 (9%)
15. Germ cell	21	8 (38%)
16. Urinary bladder	128	8 (6%)
17. Liver & biliary tract	325	7 (2%)
18. Prostate gland	171	6 (4%)
19. Pancreas	185	6 (3%)
20. Ovary	188	2 (1%)
21. Nose (interior)	32	1 (3%)
22. Pharynx	67	1 (1%)
23. Miscellaneous	245	0
	6,240	653 (10%)

*Modified from: Burke and Virmani (who combined studies of McAllister HA and Fenoglio JJ Jr). Tumors of the Cardiovascular System Atlas of Tumor Pathology. Washington, DC: Armed Forces Institute of Pathology 1978: 111–119; and Mukai K, Shinkai T, Tominaga K, Shomosato Y. The incidence of secondary tumors of the heart and pericardium: a 10-year study. *Jpn N Clin Oncol* 1988;18:195–201.

SPECIFIC BENIGN PRIMARY CARDIAC NEOPLASMS

Myxoma: Myxomas are by far the most common type of primary cardiac tumor and 75% of them are located in the left atrial cavity (Figure 2), about 23% in the right atrial cavity (Figure 3), and about 2% in a ventricular cavity.[4–16] On rare occasion, the tumor is present in more than 1 cavity.[17] Generally, the neoplasm when located in the left atrium produces symptoms when it reaches about 70 g in size. Those in the right atrium that produce symptoms are usually about twice as large and sometimes several-fold larger. The cell of origin of the myxoma is still unclear.[5] How fast atrial myxomas grow has never been clarified. An attempt to answer this question was provided by a

TABLE IV *Metastatic* Neoplasms in the Heart at Necropsy: Order of Frequency of Metastases of Each Different Primary Tumor

Primary Tumor	Number of Autopsies	Percentage With Metastases to Heart*
Melanoma	100	46%
Germ cell	100	38%
Leukemia	100	33%
Lymphoma	100	17%
Lung	100	17%
Sarcoma	100	15%
Esophagus	100	13%
Kidney	100	11%
Breast	100	10%
Mouth & tongue	100	9%
Thyroid gland	100	9%
Uterus	100	8%
Urinary bladder	100	6%
Stomach	100	5%
Colon & rectum	100	5%
Prostate gland	100	4%
Pancreas	100	3%
Nose (interior)	100	3%
Ovary	100	1%
Pharynx	100	1%
Miscellaneous	100	0

*These percentages were obtained by combining studies by McAllister and Fenoglio and by Mukai et al. (see Table III).

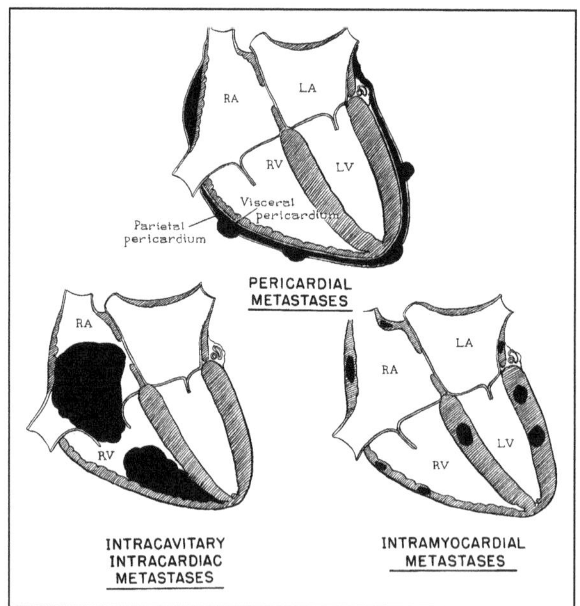

FIGURE 1. Diagram showing various locations of cardiac neoplasms involving the heart. LA = left atrium; LV = left ventricle; RA = right atrium; RV = right ventricle.

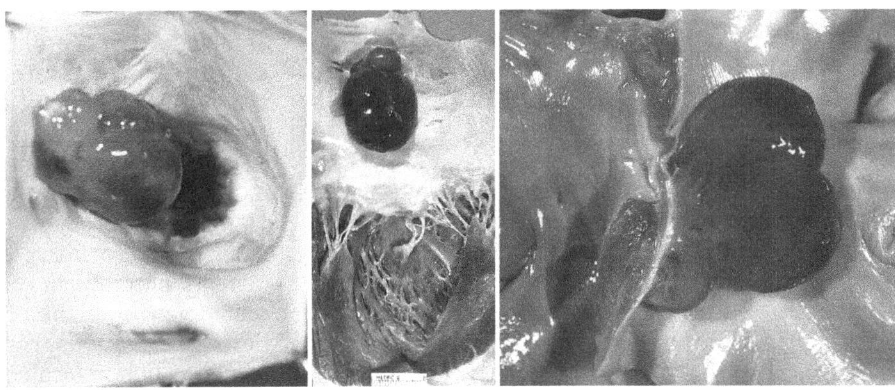

FIGURE 2. Clinically silent left atrial *myxoma* in a 60-year-old woman (A69-275) who died of metastatic carcinoid. The myxoma was not large enough to prolapse through the mitral orifice during ventricular diastole. *Left;* view from cephalad portion of the left atrium. *Center;* view of opened left atrium, mitral valve, and left ventricle. *Right;* longitudinal view showing attachment of the myxoma to the atrial septum by a relatively broad base. (Reproduced with permission from Ferrans VF and Roberts WC[5]).

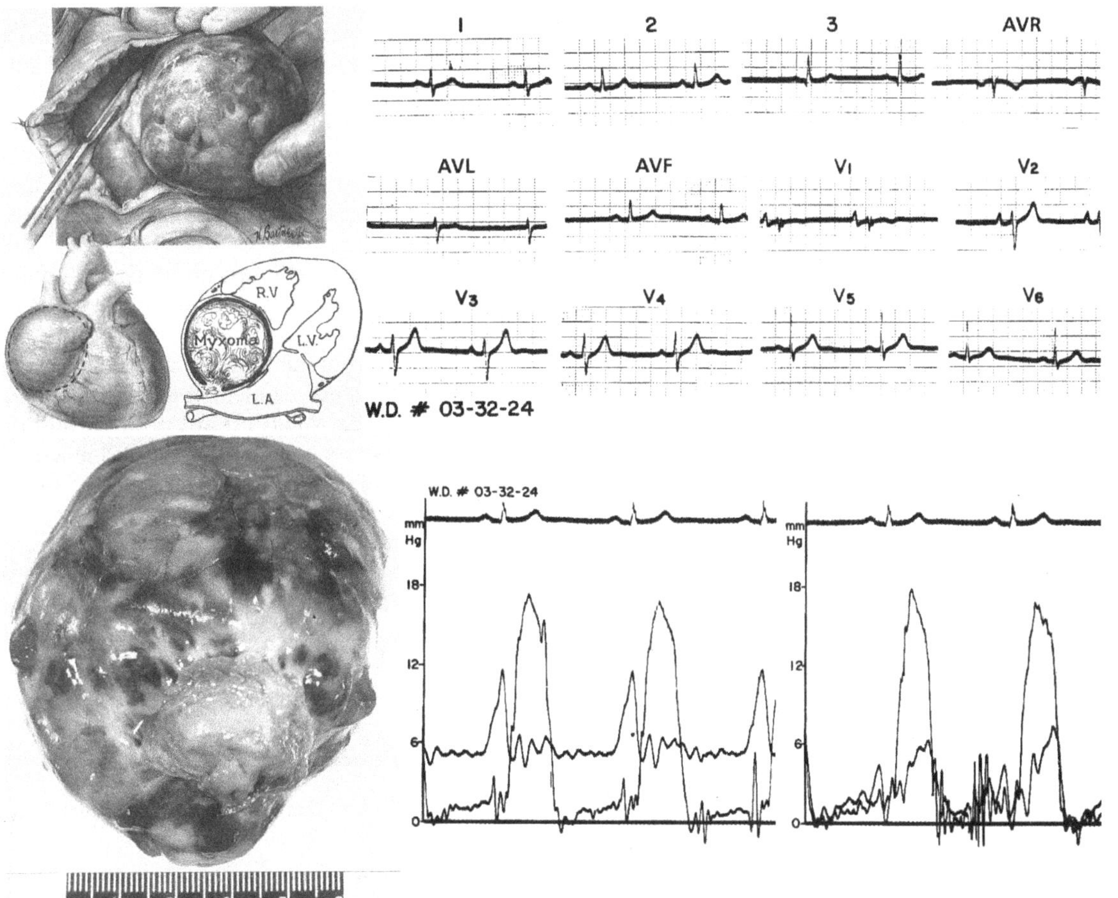

FIGURE 3. *Myxoma* excised from the right atrium from a 46-year-old man (S61-980) who had had evidence of cardiac dysfunction for 12 years. The tumor was attached to the atrial septum by a relatively small stalk (*lower left*). The myxoma weighed 142 g and its largest diameter was 8 cm. *Upper right;* electrocardiogram, Lower right; simultaneous right atrial and right ventricular pressure tracings before and after excision of the myxoma.

study that examined size of recurrent myxomas and divided that size in grams by the interval between the first operation and the second one.[18] It was estimated that recurrent left atrial myxomas grow on average of 0.15 cm/month or 1.8 cm/year, or an average of 1.2 g/month or 14 g/year. Whatever the exact growth rate may be, it appears that both recurrent and initial left atrial myxomas grow rather rapidly. Morphologic diagnosis of myxoma is readily made by gross inspection, and their appearance is clearly different from thrombi. The surface is smooth but irregular, shiney, and usually multicolored. Some contain calcific deposits, sometimes extensive ones, and those with calcific deposits appear to embolize very infrequently. The calcium may limit the growth potential of a myxoma. Attachment is nearly always to the atrial septum if the tumor is in the left atrium and the stalk is most commonly much smaller than the maximal diameter of the mass. On occasion, the site of attachment to the atrial septum is broad. The mean age of patients with sporadic myxoma is 56 years and 70% are women.

Familial cardiac myxomas constitute approxi-

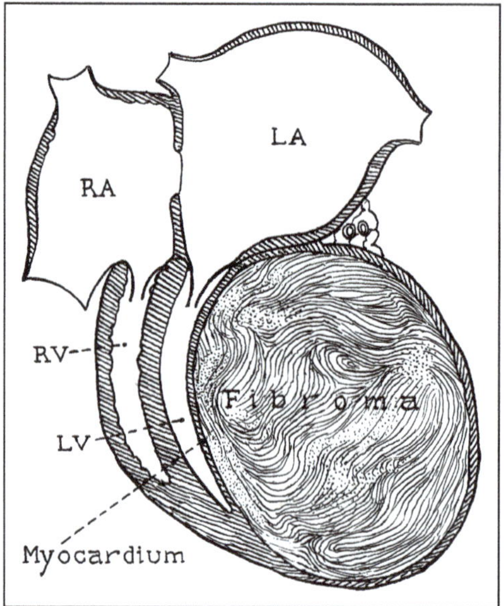

FIGURE 4. Diagram of an intramyocardial *fibroma* seen at necropsy in a 5-month-old boy (A-07-92) who was found dead in his crib. The neoplasm had been diagnosed by biopsy during the child's first few days of life. It was considered nonresectable.

mately 10% of all patients with myxomas and the transmission is an autosomal dominant one. The familial myxomas occur in younger patients (mean age 25) than the nonfamilial ones and they have less female gender predominance. The myxomas in the familial syndrome are much more liable (50% of the time) to be multiple and to have a ventricular cavity location (13% as compared with about 2% in the nonfamilial or sporadic patients with myxomas). These patients typically have exterior facial freckling; they have noncardiac myxomas (breast or skin) and also endocrine neoplasms. Both the NAME (nevi, atrial myxoma, neurofibromata, and ephelides) and the LAMB (lentigines, atrial myxoma, and balloon nevi) syndromes are associated with the familial variety of cardiac myxoma. Chromosomal abnormalities for atrial myxoma on chromosome 2 (Carney's) and chromosome 12 (Kiras-genes) have been described.

Myxomas probably present the most varied clinical picture of all primary cardiac neoplasms.[6,8,9] Several major syndromes have been observed including presentation with signs of emboli, obstruction to blood flow, and various constitutional syndromes. Fragments of tumor located in the right side of the heart may embolize to the lungs and those in the left side of the heart, of course, to various systemic organs. Diagnosis may be made on occasion by finding typical myxomatous endothelial-like cells which are elongated and spindle shaped with round or oval nuclei and prominent nucleoli in operatively removed emboli. Obstruction to blood flow may occur at the orifice of any valve, most commonly, of course, the mitral valve. Interference with flow through the mitral orifice may mimic signs of mitral stenosis, including signs of pulmonary congestion, diastolic apical rumble, opening snap, and accentuated first heart sounds. A murmur of mitral regurgitation may also be present as a result of chronic damage to the valve leaflets or to interference with proper closure of the valve by tumor. Differentiation between left atrial tumor and primary mitral stenosis is suggested by the influence of position on symptoms and on the intensity of the precordial murmurs and the opening snap.

The constitutional symptoms associated with atrial myxomas are protean and include fever, weight loss, Raynaud's phenomenon, digital clubbing, anemia, elevated erythrocyte sedimentation rate, elevated leuko-

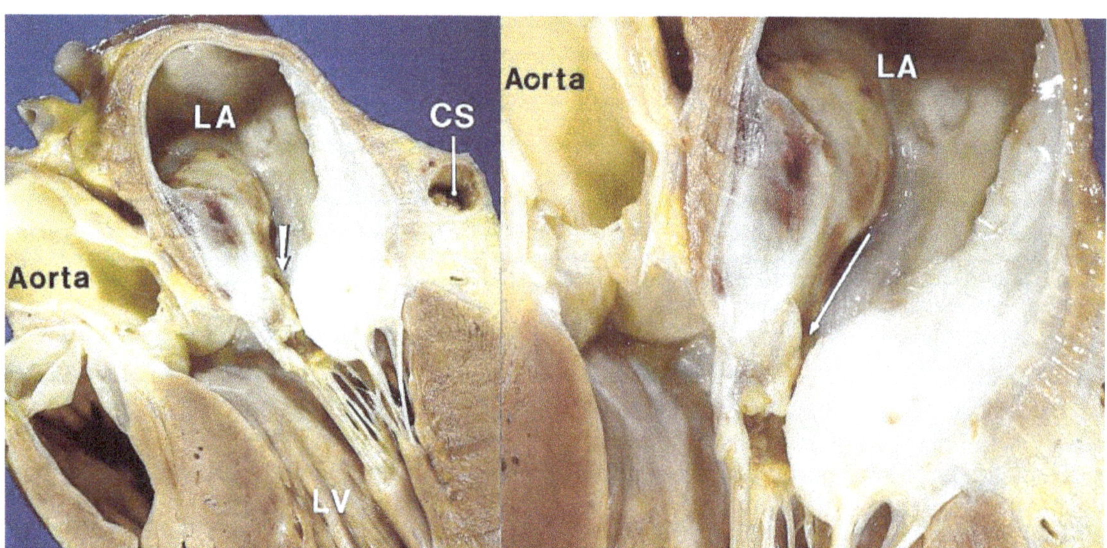

FIGURE 5. *Primary cardiac sarcoma,* undifferentiated type, causing mitral stenosis in a 46-year-old woman (A90-2) who had been well until 8 months before death. Cardiac catheterization disclosed a 20-mm Hg mean diastolic gradient between the pulmonary artery wedge position and left ventricle (LV). Right ventricular pressure was 105/18 mm Hg. The neoplasm is located in the walls of the left atrium (LA) and in both anterior and posterior mitral leaflets. The patient is described in detail elsewhere)[39] CS = coronary sinus. (Reproduced with permission from Domanski et al[39].)

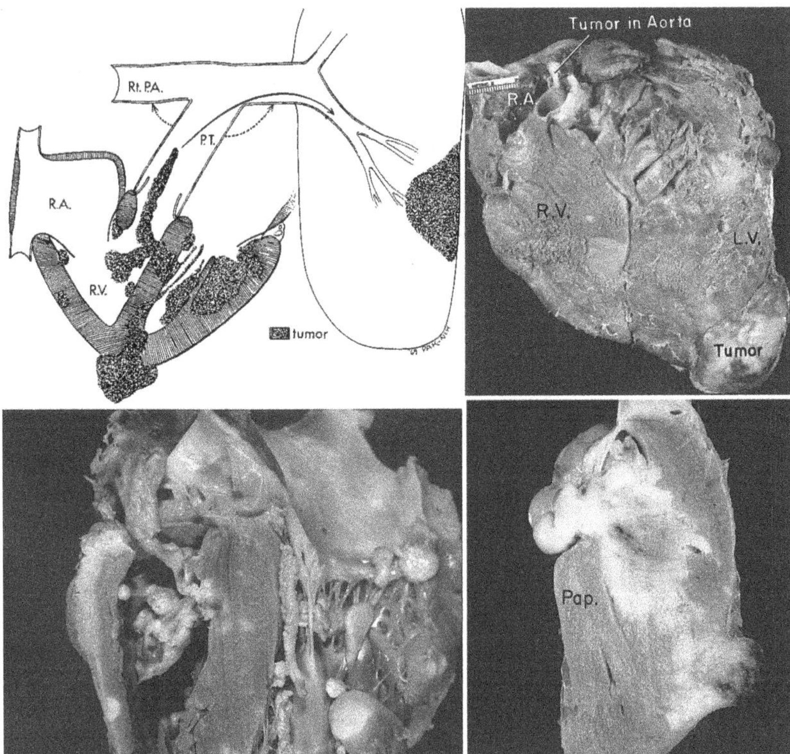

FIGURE 6. ***Primary cardiac sarcoma,*** **undifferentiated type, with neoplastic emboli to lungs and other organs in a 26-year-old man (A69-149) who had been well until 3 months before death.** ***Upper right;*** **exterior of heart containing blood, fibrin, and tumors.** ***Lower left;*** **opened right ventricle (R.V.), left ventricle (L.V.), left atrium, and aortic valve showing numerous tumor deposits.** ***Lower right;*** **section of left ventricular wall showing neoplasm extending through the entire wall and with extension beneath posterior mitral leaflet and through the epicardium. Pap. = papillary muscle; RA = right atrium; Rt. P.A. = right pulmonary artery.**

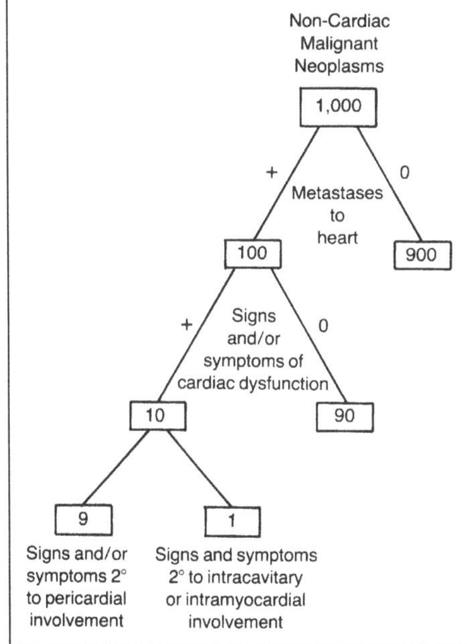

FIGURE 7. Diagram showing the relative frequency of cardiac metastases producing cardiac dysfunction.

cyte count, decreased platelet count, positive seroreactive protein, and abnormal serum proteins (usually increased gamma globulins). These constitutional symptoms may mimic infective endocarditis, collagen vascular disease, or occult malignancy.

Right atrial myxoma has occasionally migrated to the left atrial cavity via a patent foramen ovale with resultant systemic hypoxemia.[19,20]

The proper treatment of myxoma in any cavity of the heart is operative resection because there is no medicine known to shrink myxomas or to prevent their continued growth.[4,10] Some surgeons advise a biatrial approach for full visualization of both sides of the heart and then complete removal of a left or right atrial myxoma, excising the full thickness of the atrial septum if the neoplasm is attached to the region of the fossa ovalis. If a large portion of the atrial septum is removed, a cloth patch or parietal pericardium must be used to close the defect. Because fragmentation and embolization of the tumor is an ever present threat, vigorous palpation and other manipulations of the heart should be avoided until cardiopulmonary bypass is initiated. Most surgeons usually induce ventricular standstill with cardioplegia solution before manipulating the heartto reduce the possibility of fragmentation of portions of the tumor. Left atrial myxomas have been removed successfully during pregnancy. On occasion, an atrioventricular valve has been so traumatized by the tumor's prolapsing through it during ventricular diastole that valve excision and replacement is necessary. Fortunately, recurrences of atrial myxomas are rare, and if they do recur, it is usually within 4 years after the initial resection.

Rhabdomyoma: The most common cardiac neoplasm in infants and children is rhabdomyoma.[21] There is some question as to whether this particular tumor is a true neoplasm or actually resembles a hamartoma. These neoplasms are usually multiple, most often involve the ventricular myocardium, and project into the cavity or move freely as a pedunculated mass.[22–24] Associated *tuberous sclerosis* is present in about one third of the patients. The diagnosis is suggested by the presence of yellow-brown angiofibromas (''adenoma sebaceum'') on the face, sublingual fibromas around the fingernails, café au lait spots, and subcutaneous nodules. Presenting symptoms may be caused by obstruction to inflow into or outflow from the ventricles, arrhythmias, atrioventricular block, pericardial effusion, and even sudden death.[25] These neoplasms may mimic pulmonic valve stenosis and produce hypoxic spells, resembling those seen in tetralogy of Fallot. These neoplasms are usually readily diagnosed by echocardiography, angiog-

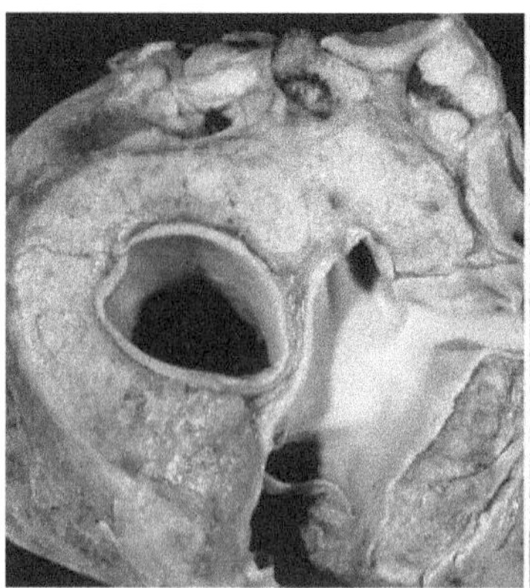

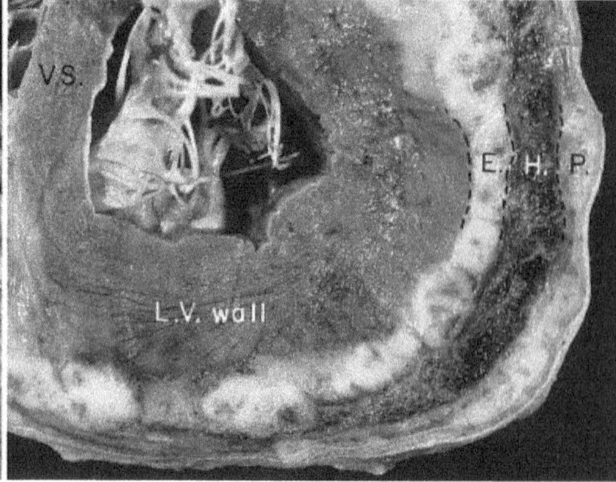

FIGURE 8. Metastatic *squamous-cell carcinoma of the lung* in a 61-year-old man (67A-531). Cardiac tamponade was the immediate cause of death. The entire heart and great vessels were encased in tumor. (Reproduced with permission from: Roberts WC, Spray TL. Pericardial heart disease. *Curr Prob Cardiol* 1977; (June);2(3):1–71.)

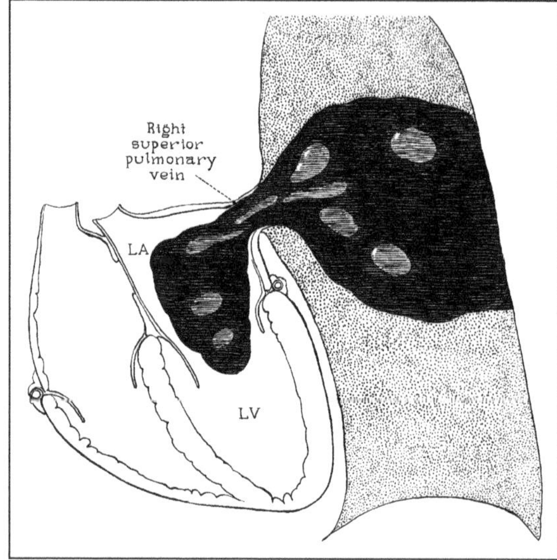

FIGURE 9. *Sarcoma,* undifferentiated type, in *lung* (primary uncertain) in a 29-year-old woman (A21-83) in whom echocardiogram disclosed tumor in the left atrium (LA) moving about "like a yo-yo." The left lung and its left atrial extension were operatively excised. LV = left ventricle.

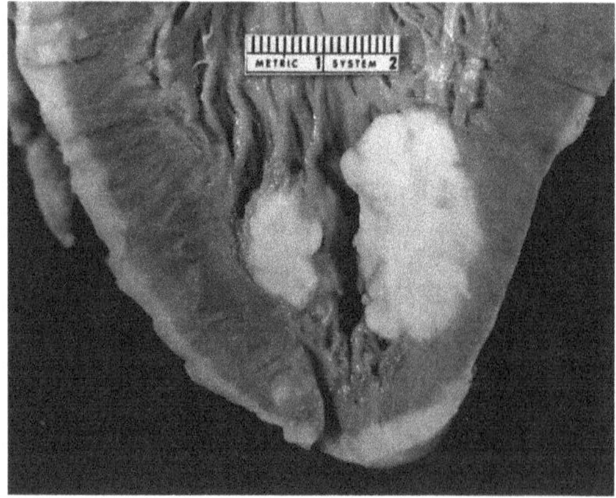

FIGURE 10. Opened left ventricle showing 2 asymptomatic apical neoplastic deposits from *adenocarcinoma in the lung* in a 59-year-old woman (A73-62). Another silent metastasis was in the right ventricular outflow tract but no metastasis was present in epicardium.

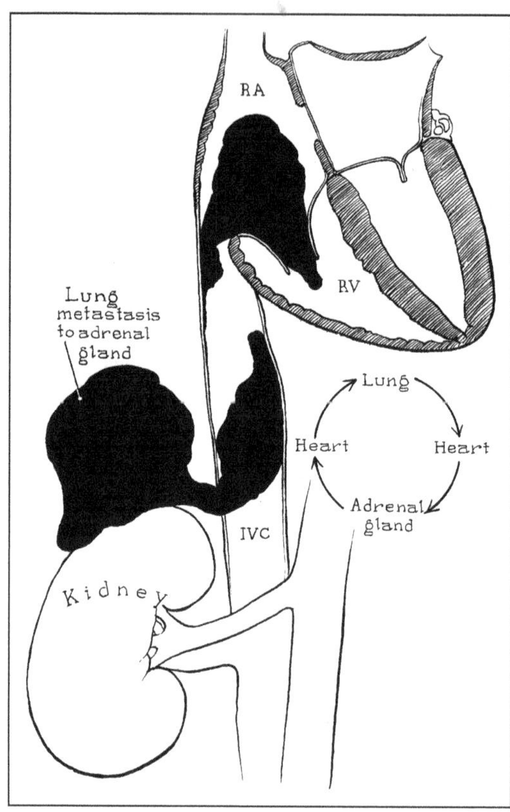

FIGURE 11. Diagram of metastatic *cancer of the lung* to the right adrenal gland with extension into the inferior vena cava (IVC) and then into the right atrium (RA) and right ventricle (RV) in a 57-year-old man (DCVAH #84A-121). Echocardiogram showed the right atrial mass which prolapsed through the tricuspid valve in atrial diastole.

raphy, or magnetic resonance imaging. Prenatal detection of intracardiac rhabdomyoma by intrauterine echocardiography has been reported with successful operative removal. The occurrence of more than 1 tumor does not prevent operative intervention. On rare occasion, these tumors have produced ventricular tachycardia in infants, and this arrhythmia has disappeared following successful operative removal.

Fibroma: Fibromas are usually intramural within a ventricular wall (Figure 4).[3,26] Most also occur in infants and children. Calcific deposits may be present within the neoplasm. Sudden death has occurred in about one third of the patients, presumably the result of a conduction defect or arrhythmia or obstruction to outflow from a ventricle. Left-axis deviation has been seen on electrocardiogram. Total or partial resection

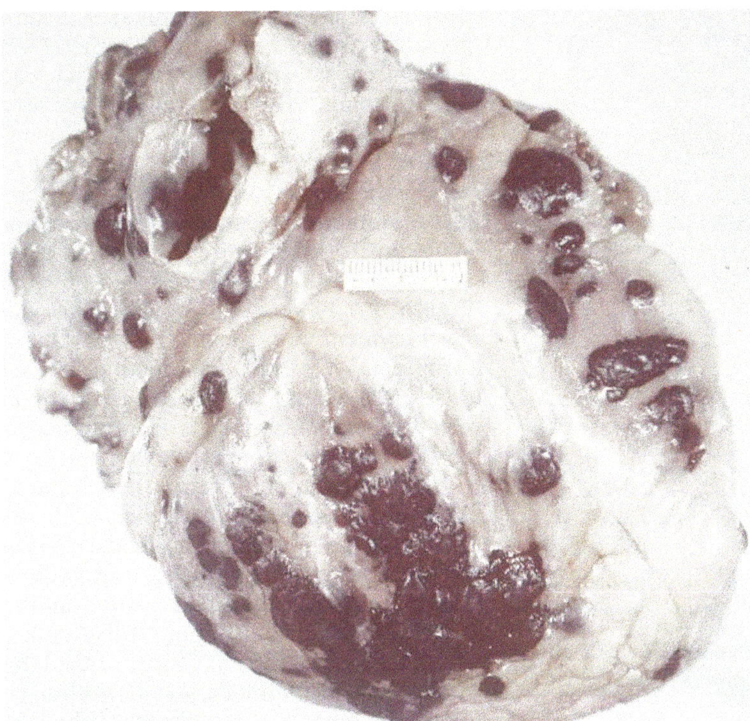

FIGURE 12. Exterior of posterior surface of the heart with clinically silent multiple metastases of *melanoma* in a 33-year-old man (A77-220).

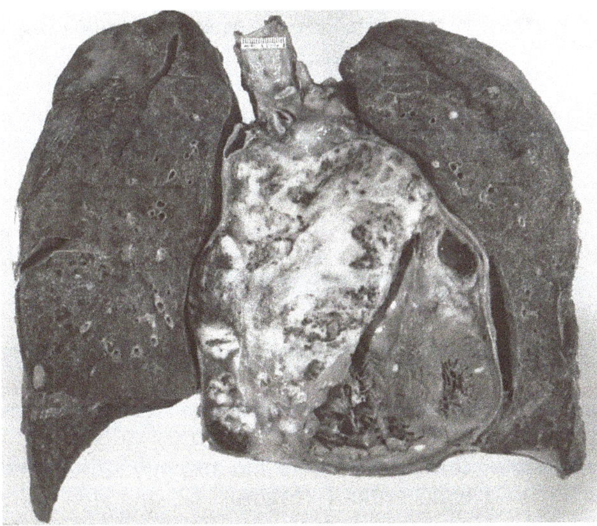

FIGURE 13. Metastatic *melanoma* to the heart in a 53-year-old man (A75-41). During life a pericardial friction rub was audible and the neck veins were quite distended. The parietal pericardium is everywhere adherent to epicardium. The superior vena cava, right atrium, right ventricle, and pulmonary trunk were severely compressed by the tumor. (Reproduced with permission from: Roberts WC, Spray TL. Pericardial heart disease. Curr Probl Cardiol 1977;(June);2(3)1–71.)

of the neoplasm may relieve obstruction with an excellent probability of long-term survival.

Lipoma: Lipomas involving the heart may be extremely small and represent incidental necropsy findings, or they may be massive.[27–30] The largest cardiac neoplasm ever reportedly apparently was an intrapericardial lipoma. They may be mistaken for pericardial cysts, they may cause pericardial effusion, or they may be asymptomatic and are suggested by a widened mediastinum on chest radiograph. Intramyocardial lipomas are encapsulated and usually small. Lipomas also have been located on cardiac valves and here they may simulate vegetations or myxomas.[29] Magnetic resonance imaging permits preoperative identification of these fatty tumors.

Hemangioma: These tumors are best diagnosed by coronary angiography which yields a characteristic "tumor blush." Spontaneous resolution without treatment has been reported. Total excision is usually not possible.

SPECIFIC MALIGNANT PRIMARY CARDIAC NEOPLASMS

Angiosarcoma: Nearly all primary malignant cardiac neoplasms are sarcomas, and the most frequent one is angiosarcoma.[31–35] It characteristically originates from the right atrium. The large quantity of vascular channels within these tumors and the subsequent large quantity of blood flowing through them may produce a continuous precordial murmur. About 25% of all angiosarcomas will, at least in part, be intracavitary, producing valvular obstruction, right-sided heart failure, and hemorrhagic pericardial tamponade. The course is rapid with widespread metastases and operative intervention is usually unsuccessful.

Rhabdomyosarcoma: Rhabdomyosarcoma is the second most frequent primary sarcoma of the heart, and, like angiosarcoma, it is most common in males.[36–38] In contrast, however, to angiosarcoma, no single cardiac chamber has a predilection for this neoplasm. Indeed, the neoplasm may be in all 4 cardiac chambers, or at least in more than 1, and obstruction may occur in 1 or more valve orifices. Again, prognosis is poor, survival is short, and operative intervention is usually futile.

Miscellaneous: Fibrosarcoma, liposarcoma, primary malignant lymphoma, and occasional sarcomas of other cell types constitute the remaining but infrequent primary malignant cardiac neoplasms (Figures 5 and 6). All of these neoplasms may obstruct valvular orifices or obliterate chambers and/or produce peripheral emboli.[39] Hypertrophic cardiomyopathy has been suggested by heavy tumorous infiltrations into the ventricular septum.[40]

METASTATIC NEOPLASMS TO THE HEART

Metastatic or secondary tumors of the heart with a primary in another body organ or tissue are far more frequent than are primary tumors of the heart.[41] The

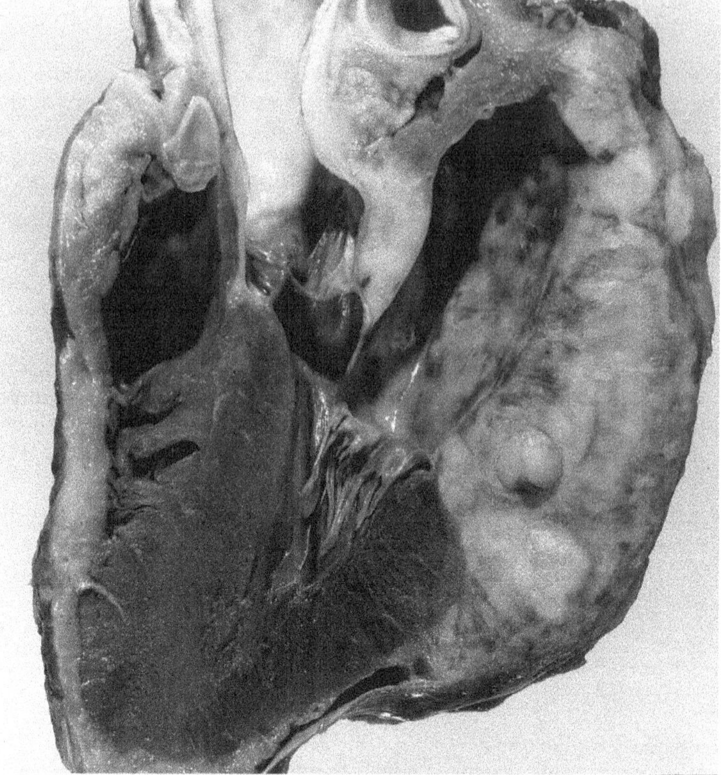

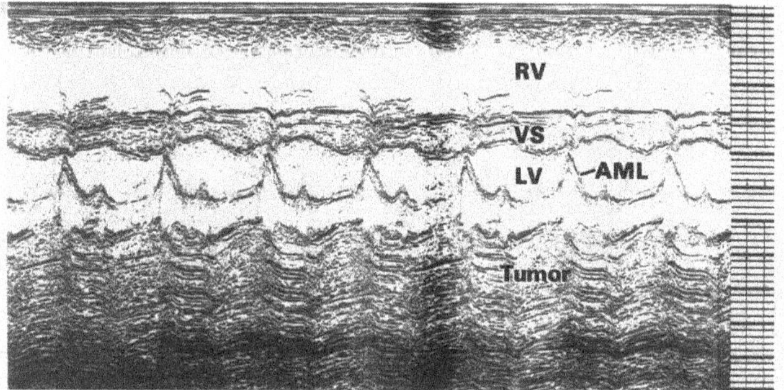

FIGURE 14. *Cardiac histiocytic lymphoma* in a 64-year-old woman (A77-172) who had had evidence of congestive heart failure for 7 months. The cause of the heart failure was not apparent until necropsy. The patient is described in detail elsewhere.[57] *Upper;* longitudinal view of heart showing posterior wall of left atrium to be massively thickened by the neoplasm. *Lower;* echocardiogram showing the tumor behind the more basal portion of left ventricle (LV). AML = anterior mitral leaflet; RV = right ventricle; VS = ventricular septum. (Reproduced with permission from Roberts et al.[57])

secondary tumors are far more commonly carcinomas than sarcomas simply because carcinomas are far more common than are sarcomas. Diagnosis can be suspected whenever cardiac manifestations occur in a patient diagnosed with a primary tumor in an organ or tissue other than the heart. The development of cardiac enlargement, tachycardia, arrhythmias, or heart failure in the presence of neoplasm elsewhere in the body is highly suggestive of cardiac metastases. Only rarely is metastatic tumor limited to the heart. Thus, the presence of metastatic tumor in the heart usually indicates widespread metastases in a number of body organs. On rare occasion, cardiac involvement may be the first or only expression of a noncardiac primary neoplasm. The most common sign is tamponade.[42] Direct invasion of the heart via the vena cava or pulmonary veins may lead to obstruction of an atrioventricular valve as well as to pulmonary or systemic emboli, or both.[43–45]

Only a minority of patients with metastases to the heart develop signs and/or symptoms of cardiac dysfunction as a result of the cardiac metastases. As shown in Figure 7, only about 10% of patients with cardiac metastases develop signs and/or symptoms of cardiac dysfunction, and of them 90% result from pericardial involvement and only about 10% from intracavitary or intramyocardial involvement.

Specific types of metastatic neoplasms to the heart: *Carcinoma of the lung* and *carcinoma of the breast* tend to invade parietal pericardium and then visceral pericardium leading to myocardial constriction and/or pericardial effusion (Figure 8). Another common presentation of cancer of the lung is to invade the pulmonary veins within the lung with spread of the cancer within the lumen of the pulmonary veins into the left atrium, which in turn can continue into the mitral orifice sometimes causing obstruction of that orifice (Figure 9).[46,47] Isolated or multiple left ventricular neoplastic deposits also are common (Figure 10). Metastatic cancer from the lung to the adrenal gland also may extend into the inferior vena cava and then into the right side of the heart (Figure 11), just as can primary adrenal gland or renal cancer.[48] Cancer of the lung or breast surrounding the main right or left pulmonary artery can lead to pulmonary arterial obstruction.[49]

Melanoma has the highest frequency of metastases to the heart per 100 cases of any neoplasm.[50,51] The metastases may be anywhere in the heart and usually melanotic metastases invade the walls of all 4 cardiac chambers and also epicardium and endocardium (Figures 12 and 13). The cancers in these patients are in so many body organs that the presence of the neoplasm in the heart is almost incidental.

Leukemia commonly invades the heart.[52] In the days before platelet transfusions, extensive hemorrhages into the myocardial walls and into endocardium and epicardium was commonly found in patients with fatal leukemia of various types. Histologically, leukemic infiltration between myocardial cells is quite common and sometimes gross deposits of leukemic cells are visible within the heart. A few patients with leukemia present with pericardial effusion, which is usually hemorrhagic. Large calcific deposits in the right side of the heart have been reported.[53]

Lymphoma also has a very high frequency of metastases to the heart.[54–59] Nearly 25% of patients with

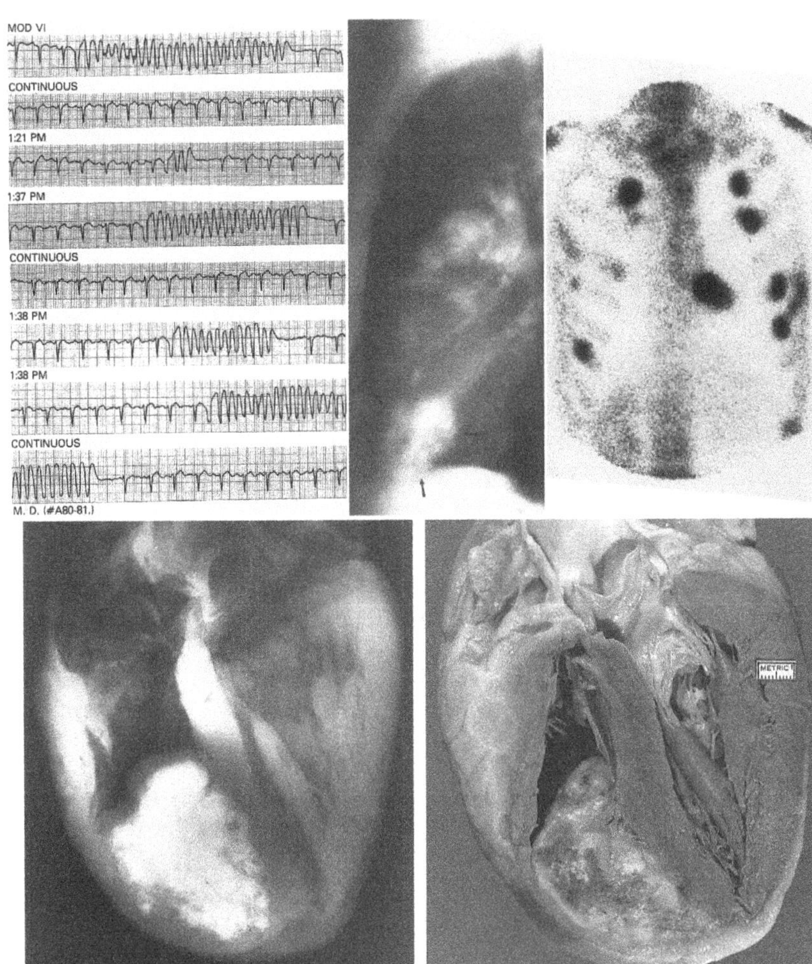

FIGURE 15. ***Osteogenic sarcoma*** **to the heart in a 39-year-old woman (A80-81) with a large calcified tumor in the right ventricle. This patient, who was ill for 20 months, had episodic ventricular tachycardia (*upper left*) during her last 20 months. *Upper middle;* lateral chest radiograph showing a calcified tumor (*arrows*) in the right ventricle (*lower left and lower right*). The computed tomogram (*upper right*) also shows the calcified right ventricular tumor as well as multiple metastases in the lungs and bones. The patient is described elsewhere.[60] (Reproduced with permission from Seibert et al.[60])**

lymphomas of various types have lymphoma involving epicardium, myocardium, or endocardium, or combinations (Figure 14). In contrast to leukemic involvement, the lymphomatous deposits are usually grossly discernible.

Some cancers, like *osteognic sarcoma,* may have calcium within them (Figure 15).[60,61]

NON-NEOPLASTIC CONDITIONS IN THE HEART OR PERICARDIUM FREQUENTLY MISTAKEN FOR CARDIAC NEOPLASM

Pericardial cyst: Pericardial or mesothelial cysts are the most frequent benign "tumors" of the pericardium. These cysts are generally asymptomatic and found on "routine" chest radiograph.[62] About a quarter of the patients, however, develop various symptoms including chest pain, dyspnea, cough, and tachycardia as a consequence of a pericardial cyst. The cysts are usually outside the pericardial cavity and, therefore, they really should not be considered "cardiac tumors."

Teratoma: Teratomas are actually extracardiac in at least 99% of the cases, but still within the pericardial cavity.[63–65] They arise and receive their blood supply from the ascending aorta or pulmonary trunk, presumably through the vasa vasorum. Most are found in infants and children and primarily in females. Recurrent serious pericardial effusion in children should suggest intrapericardial teratoma. Because these tumors may become quite large, they may cause compression of various cardiac chambers with subsequent symptoms therefrom.

Lipomatous hypertrophy of the atrial septum: Massive fatty infiltration of the atrial septum is an extremely common condition occurring almost exclusively in persons over 50 years of age, and usually over 65 years of age (Figure 16).[66] These lesions are essentially limited to obese people and they are always associated with enormous quantities of subepicardial adipose tissue, particularly enormous amounts of adipose tissue in the atrioventricular sulci. These hearts are almost always so fat that they float in water.[67] Normally the atrial septum is <1 cm in thickness. In patients with lipomatous hypertrophy of the atrial septum, the atrial septum cephalad to the fossa ovale may be as thick as 7 cm and the portion of atrial septum caudal to the fossa ovali may be as thick as 4 cm. Enormous infiltration of fat in the atrial septum may be associated with atrial arrhythmias. It is probably the only atrial arrhythmia that is treatable, possibly curable, by transient starvation. The importance of lipomatous hypertrophy of the atrial septum in the context of "cardiac tumors" is that these patients should not be operated on to remove fat from the atrial septum. The treatment is simply weight loss. These fatty deposits may be diagnosed by echocardiography or computed tomography or magnetic resonance imaging.[68,69] Fat in the subepicardial adipose tissue has been confused by echocardiogram with pericardial effusion.[70]

Papillary fibroelastomas: These small avascular growths with multiple papillary fronds are located mainly on cardiac valves. They are common in older individuals. These lesions will be discussed in a future from-the-editor column.

Thrombi: These masses when within an intracardiac cavity may be indistinguishable from neoplasm by

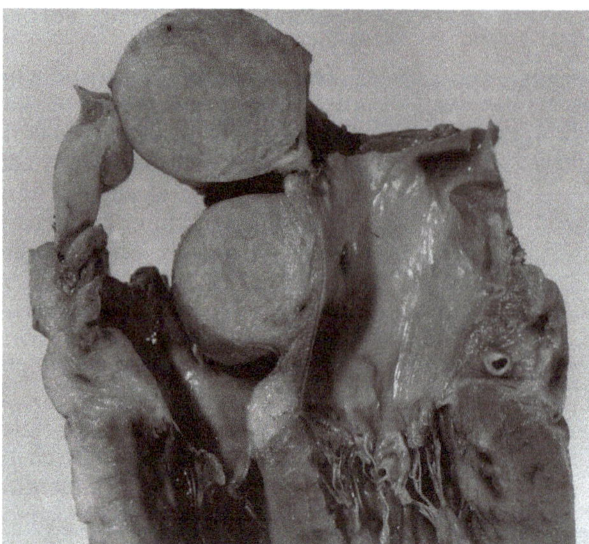

FIGURE 16. *Lipomatous hypertrophy of the atrial septum* in a 74-year-old woman (GT #77A-42) with huge fatty deposits in the atrial septum (except for the fossa ovale area). (Reproduced with permission from: Shirani J, Roberts WC.[66])

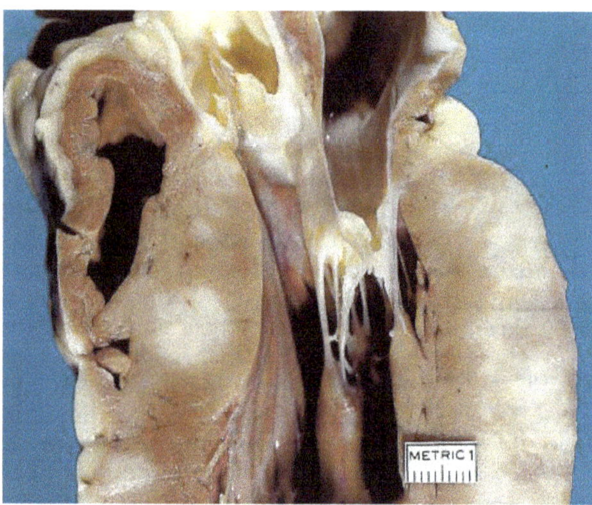

FIGURE 17. Longitudinal view of heart in a 27-year-old woman (DCMEO #83-10-670) with *cardiac sarcoidosis* simulating cardiac neoplasms.

echocardiogram or radiograph. Grossly, however, they are very different.

Sarcoid: When located in myocardium, sarcoid granuloma may grossly resemble neoplasm (Figure 17).[71–73]

CONSEQUENCES OF THERAPY FOR NEOPLASMS IN THE HEART OR MEDIASTINUM

Radiation heart disease: Radiation heart disease was first recognized after radiation therapy for Hodgkin's disease.[74–78] Some of the earlier patients with Hodgkin's disease received 8,000 rads, and that quantity of radiation caused consequences to pericardium, myocardium, and endocardium. The most common manifestation of radiation heart disease is pericardial effusion. The mechanism of the effusion is unclear. Fibrin deposits occur on both the visceral and parietal aspects of the pericardia. Because coronary arteries are located in subepicardial adipose tissue, they often receive the effects of radiation. Many patients have been reported to have coronary arterial narrowing at a very young age after radiation therapy, particularly patients with Hodgkin's disease. The intimal plaques resulting from radiation heart disease in actuality cannot be distinquished from plaques occurring from typical atherosclerosis. The distinguishing features of radiation heart disease involving the coronary arteries is extensive fibrous thickening of the adventitia, and also loss, focally or diffsely, of internal and external elastic membranes, particularly the latter. Narrowing of coronary ostia also are common in radiation heart disease. Radiation also can cause considerable scarring within the subepicardial adipose tissue. The second most common manifestation of radiation heart disease is mural endocardial thickening, most commonly of the right atrium and ventricle, but focally also in the left ventricle. The third most common manifestation of radiation heart disease is interstitial fibrosis and, depending on the portal of entry, it usually involves the anterior wall of the right ventricle more than any other portion of the heart.

Cardiac hemorrhages: Thrombocytopenia, particularly if persistent, often results in focal epicardial, myocardial, and mural endocardial hemorrhages. If the hemorrhages are located in conduction tissue, various degrees of heart block or arrhythmias may be the consequence.

Cardiac infection: The most common cardiac infections today in cancer patients are myocardial abscesses and mural endocardial and epicardial abscesses. These are particularly prevalent in patients with prolonged leukopenia.[79,80] Patients having unsuccessful bone-marrow transplantation are particularly prone to these infections, which usually are produced by fungi, not bacteria. Gas gangrene may involve the heart as well as most other body organs and tissues.[81]

Cardiac adiposity or the corticosteroid-treated heart: Patients with various types of cancers, particularly those with leukemia and lymphoma, and those developing cancer after transplantation of 1 or more body organs, usually receive corticosteroid therapy for prolonged periods. The consequence is excessive deposition of fat in the heart, mainly in the subepicardial areas.[82] These hearts may become so fatty that they float in water (buffalo hump of the heart), and this excessive subepicardial adipose tissue may simulate pericardial effusion.

Cardiac hemosiderosis: Normally the human body contains approximately 4 g of iron. If the deposits increase to about 25 g, iron deposits then are usually found within myocardial cells. Patients who receive 100 units of blood without associated bleeding diatheses can acquire approximately 25 g of iron within the body organs and tissues. In some patients with cancer, particularly leukemia, this situation may exist and the result is cardiac hemosiderosis.[83] These patients may be asymptomatic or they may develop features of dilated cardiomyopathy with heart failure. At times, ventricular arrhythmias may be a consequence. Myocardial restriction as a result of myocardial ironic deposits has occurred, but dilation is far more common.[84]

Anthracycline chemotherapy (doxorubicin and daunorubicin): Cardiac toxicity is a well-recognized complication of these agents and is frequently the dose-limiting factor in their administration.[85–87] Clinical toxicity is usually manifested by evidence of impaired left ventricular systolic function. Morphologic signs of toxicity may be present when clinical signs of toxicity are absent.

William Clifford Roberts, MD,
Editor in Chief
Baylor Cardiovascular Institute
Baylor University Medical Center
Dallas, Texas 75246

1. Lam KY, Dickens P, Chan ACL. Tumors of the heart. A 20-year experience with review of 12485 consecutive autopsies. *Arch Pathol Med* 1993;117:1027–1031.
2. Reynan K. Frequency of primary tumors of the heart. *Am J Cardiol* 1996;77: 107.
3. Burke A, Virmani R. Atlas of Tumor Pathology. Third Series Fascicle 16. Tumors of the Heart and Great Vessels. Washington, DC: Armed Forces Institute of Pathology 1996:231.
4. Bahnson HT, Spencer FC, Andrus EC. Diagnosis and treatment of intracavitary myxomas of the heart. *Ann Surg* 1957;145:915–926.
5. Ferrans VJ, Roberts WC. Structural features of cardiac myxomas. Histology, histochemistry, and electron microscopy. *Human Pathol* 1973;4:111–146.
6. Peters MN, Hall RJ, Cooley DA, Leachman RD, Garcia E. The clinical syndrome of atrial myxoma. *JAMA* 1974;230:695–701.
7. Morgan DL, Palazola J, Reed W, Bell HH, Kindred LH, Beauchamp GD. Left heart myxomas. *Am J Cardiol* 1977;40:611–614.
8. St. John Sutton MG, Mercier L-A, Giuliani ER, Lie JT. Atrial myxomas. A review of clinical experience in 40 patients. *Mayo Clin Proc* 1980;55:371–376.
9. Markel ML, Waller BF, Armstrong WF. Cardiac myxoma. A review. *Medicine* 1987;66:114–125.
10. Murphy MC, Sweeney MS, Putnam JB Jr, Walker WE, Frazier OH, Ott DA, Cooley DA. Surgical treatment of cardiac tumors: a 25-year experience. *Ann Thorac Surg* 1990;49:612–618.
11. Tazelaar HD, Locke TJ, McGregor CGA. Pathology of surgically excised primary cardiac tumors. *Mayo Clin Proc* 1992;67:957–965.
12. Burke AP, Virmani R. Cardiac myxomas: a clinicopathologic study. *Am J Clin Pathol* 1994;100:671–680.
13. Morrow AG, Kahler RL, Reis RL. Primary myxoma of the right ventricle. Clinical, hemodynamic and angiographic findings before and following operative treatment. *Am J Med* 1966;40:954–960.
14. Hickie JB, Gibson H, Windsor HM. "The wrecking ball": right atrial myxoma. *Med J Aust* 1970;2:82–86.
15. Hada Y, Wolfe C, Murray GF, Craig E. Right ventricular myxoma. Case report and review of phonocardiographic and auscultatory manifestations. *Am Heart J* 1980;100:871–877.
16. Massumi R. Bedside diagnosis of right heart myxomas through detection of palpable tumor shocks and audible plops. *Am Heart J* 1983;105:303–310.
17. Leonhardt ET, Kullenberg KP. Bilateral atrial myxomas with multiple arterial aneurysms—a syndrome mimicking polyarteritis nodosa. *Am J Med* 1977; 62:792–794.
18. Malekzadeh S, Roberts WC. Growth rate of left atrial myxoma. *Am J Cardiol* 1989;64:1075–1076.
19. Talley RC, Baldwin BJ, Symbas PN, Nutter DO. Right atrial myxoma. Unusual presentation with cyanosis and clubbing. *Am J Med* 1970;48:256–260.
20. Goldschlager A, Popper R, Goldschlager N, Gerbode F, Prozan G. Right atrial myxoma with right to left shunt and polycythemia presenting as congenital heart disease. *Am J Cardiol* 1972;30:82–86.
21. Chan HSL, Sonley MJ, Moës CAF, Daneman A, Smith CR, Martin DJ. Primary and secondary tumors of childhood involving the heart, pericardium, and great vessels. A report of 75 cases and review of the literature. *Cancer* 1985;56: 825–836.
22. Fenoglio JJ Jr, McAllister HA, Ferrans VJ. Cardiac rhabdomyoma: a clinicopathologic and electron microscopic study. *Am J Cardiol* 1976;38:241–251.
23. Smythe JF, Dyck JD, Smallhorn JF, Freedom RM. Natural history of cardiac rhabdomyoma in infancy and childhood. *Am J Cardiol* 1990;66:1247–1249.
24. Burke AP, Virmani R. Cardiac rhabdomyoma, a clinicopathologic study. *Mod Pathol* 1991;4:70–74.
25. Biancaniello TM, Meyer RA, Gaum WE, Kaplan S. Primary benign intramural ventricular tumors in children: pre- and post-operative electrocardiographic, echocardiographic, and angiocardiographic evaluation. *Am Heart J* 1982;103:852–857.
26. Williams DB, Danielson GK, McGoon DC, Feldt RH, Edwards WD. Cardiac fibroma. Long-term survival after excision. *J Thorac Cardiovasc Surg* 1982;84: 230–236.
27. Estevez JM, Thompson DS, Levinson JP. Lipoma of the heart. Review of the literature and report of 2 autopsied cases. *Arch Pathol* 1964;77:638–642.
28. Moulton AL, Jaretzki A III, Bowman FO Jr, Silverstien EF, Bregman D. Massive lipoma of the heart. *NY State J Med* 1976;76:1820–1825.
29. Dollar AL, Wallace RB, Kent KM, Burkhart MW, Roberts WC. Mitral valve replacement for mitral lipoma associated with severe obesity. *Am J Cardiol* 1989;64:1405–1407.
30. Shirani J, Roberts WC. Epicardial Lipoma. *Am Heart J* 1993;126:1030.
31. Bear PA, Moodie DS. Malignant primary cardiac tumors. The Cleveland Clinic Experience, 1956–1986. *Chest* 1987;92:860–862.
32. Putman JB Jr, Sweeney MS, Colon R, Lanza LA, Frazier OH, Cooley DA. Primary cardiac sarcomas. *Ann Thorac Surg* 1991;51:906–910.
33. Burke AP, Cowan D, Virmani R. Primary sarcomas of the heart. *Cancer* 1992;69:387–395.
34. Glancy DL, Morales JB, Roberts WC. Angiosarcoma of the heart. *Am J Cardiol* 1968;21:413–419.
35. Herrmann MA, Shankerman RA, Edwards WD, Shub C, Schaff HV. Primary cardiac angiosarcoma: a clinicopathologic study of six cases. *J Thorac Cardiovasc Surg* 1992;103:655–664.
36. Shrivastava S, Jacks JJ, White RS, Edwards JE. Diffuse rhabdomyomatosis of the heart. *Arch Pathol Lab Med* 1977;101:78–90.
37. Hajar R, Roberts WC, Folger GM Jr. Embryonal botryoid rhabdomyosarcoma of the mitral valve. *Am J Cardiol* 1986;57:376.
38. Hui KS, Green LK, Schmidt WA. Primary cardiac rhabdomyosarcoma: definition of a rare entity. *Am J Cardiovasc Pathol* 1988;2:19–29.
39. Domanski MJ, Delaney TF, Kleiner DE Jr, Goswitz M, Agatston A, Tucker E, Johnson M, Roberts WC. Primary sarcoma of the heart causing mitral stenosis. *Am J Cardiol* 1990;66:893–895.
40. Isner JM, Falcone MW, Virmani R, Roberts WC. Cardiac sarcoma causing "ASH" and simulating coronary heart disease. *Am J Med* 1979;66:1025–1030.
41. Abraham DP, Reddy V, Gattusa P. Neoplasms metastatic to the heart: review of 3314 consecutive autopsies. *Am J Cardiovasc Pathol* 1990;3:195–198.
42. Adenle AD, Edwards JE. Clinical and pathologic features of metastatic neoplasms of the pericardium. *Chest* 1982;81:166–169.
43. MacLowry JD, Roberts WC. Metastatic choriocarcinoma of the lung. Invasion of pulmonary veins with extension into the left atrium and mitral orifice. *Am J Cardiol* 1966;18:938–941.
44. Labib SB, Schick EC Jr, Isner JM. Obstruction of right ventricular outflow tract caused by intracavitary metastatic disease: analysis of 14 cases. *J Am Coll Cardiol* 1992;19:1664–1668.
45. Domanski MJ, Cunnion RE, Fernicola DJ, Roberts WC. Fatal cor pulmonale caused by extensive tumor emboli in the small pulmonary arteries without emboli in the major pulmonary arteries or metastases in the pulmonary parenchyma. *Am J Cardiol* 1993;72:233–234.
46. Onuigbo WI. Direct extension of cancer between pulmonary veins and the left atrium. *Chest* 1972;62:444–446.
47. Weg IL, Mehra S, Azueta V, Rosener F. Cardiac metastasis from adenocarcinoma of the lung. Echocardiographic-pathologic correlation. *Am J Med* 1986;80:108–112.
48. Kadir S, Coulam CM. Intracaval extension of renal cell carcinoma. *Cardiovasc Intervent Radiol* 1980;3:180–183.
49. Waller BF, Fletcher RD, Roberts WC. Carcinoma of the lung causing pulmonary arterial stenosis. *Chest* 1981;79:589–591.
50. Glancy DL, Roberts WC. The heart in malignant melanoma. A study of 70 autopsy cases. *Am J Cardiol* 1968;21:555–571.
51. Waller BV, Gottdiener JS, Virmani R, Roberts WC. The "charcoal heart". Melanoma to the cor. *Chest* 1980;77:671–676.
52. Roberts WC, Bodey GP, Wertlake PT. The heart in acute leukemia. A study of 420 autopsy cases. *Am J Cardiol* 1968;21:388–412.
53. Waller BF, Roberts WC. Systolic clicks caused by rocks in the right heart chambers. *Am Heart J* 1981;102:459–460.
54. Roberts WC, Glancy DL, DeVita VT Jr. Heart in malignant lymphoma

(Hodgkin's disease, lymphosarcoma, reticulum cell sarcoma and mycosis fungoides). A study of 196 autopsy cases. *Am J Cardiol* 1968;22:85–107.
55. Terry LN, Kligerman MM. Pericardial and myocardial involvement by lymphomas and leukemias. *Cancer* 1970;25:1003–1008.
56. McDonnell PJ, Mann RB, Bulkley BH. Involvement of the heart by malignant lymphoma: a clinicopathologic study. *Cancer* 1982;49:944–951.
57. Roberts CS, Gottdiener JS, Roberts WC. Clinically undetected cardiac lymphoma causing congestive heart failure. *Am Heart J* 1990;120:1239–1242.
58. Holladay AO, Siegel RJ, Schwartz EA. Cardiac malignant lymphoma in acquired immune deficiency syndrome. *Cancer* 1992;70:2203–2207.
59. Moore JA, DeRan BP, Minor R, Arthur J, Fraker TD. Transesophageal echocardiographic evaluation of intracardiac lymphoma. *Am Heart J* 1992;124: 514–516.
60. Seibert KA, Rettenmier CW, Waller BF, Battle WE, Levine AS, Roberts WC. Osteogenic sarcoma metastatic to the heart. *Am J Med* 1982;73:136–141.
61. Burke AP, Virmani R. Osteosarcomas of the heart. *Am J Surg Pathol* 1991;15:289–295.
62. Feigin DS, Fenoglio JJ, McAllister HA, Madewell JR. Pericardial cysts: a radiologic-pathologic correlation and review. *Radiology* 1977;125:15–20.
63. Reynolds JL, Donahue JK, Pearce CW. Intrapericardial teratoma: a cause of acute pericardial effusion in infancy. *Pediatrics* 1969;4:71–78.
64. DeGeeter B, Kretz JG, Nisand I, Eisenmann B, Kieny MT, Kieny R. Intra-pericardial teratoma in a newborn infant: Use of fetal echocardiography. *Ann Thorac Surg* 1983;35:664–666.
65. Brabham KR, Roberts WC. Cardiac-compressing intrapericardial teratoma at birth. *Am J Cardiol* 1989;63:386–387.
66. Shirani J, Roberts WC. Clinical, electrocardiographic and morphologic features of massive fatty deposits (''lipomatous hypertrophy'') in the atrial septum. *J Am Coll Cardiol* 1993;22:226–238.
67. Roberts WC, Roberts JD. The floating heart or the heart too fat to sink: analysis of 55 necropsy patients. *Am J Cardiol* 1983;52:1286–1289.
68. Applegate PM, Taijk AJ, Ehman RL, Julsrud PR, Miller FA Jr. Two-dimensional echocardiographic and magnetic resonance imaging observations in massive lipomatous hypertrophy of atrial septum. *Am J Cardiol* 1987;59:489–491.
69. Kindman LA, Wright A, Tye T, Seale W, Appleton C. Lipomatous hypertrophy of the interatrial septum: characterization of transesophageal and transthoracic echocardiography, magnetic resonance imaging, and computed tomography. *J Am Soc Echocardiogr* 1988;1:450–454.
70. Isner JM, Carter BL, Roberts WC, Bankoff MS. Subepicardial adipose tissue producing echocardiographic appearance of pericardial effusion. Documentation by computed tomography and necropsy. *Am J Cardiol* 1983;51:565–569.
71. Roberts WC, McAllister HA Jr, Ferrans VJ. Sarcoidosis of the heart. A clinicopathologic study of 35 necropsy patients (group I) and review of 78 previously described necropsy patients (group II). *Am J Med* 1977;63:86–108.
72. Virmani R, Bures JC, Roberts WC. Cardiac sarcoidosis: a major cause of sudden death in young individuals. *Chest* 1980;77:423–428.
73. Shirani J, Roberts WC. Subepicardial myocardial lesions. *Am Heart J* 1993; 125:1346–1352.
74. Morton DL, Kagar AR, Roberts WC, O'Brien KP, Holmes EC, Adkins PC. Pericardiectomy for radiation-induced pericarditis with effusion. *Ann Thorac Surg* 1969;8:195–208.
75. Serpik A, Lowenbraum S, Sheinbrot S, Brace K, Belcher V, Roberts WC. Possible radiation pericarditis in Hodgkin's disease. *Cancer Chemo Report* 1970; 54:199–208.
76. McReynolds RA, Gold GL, Roberts WC. Coronary heart disease after mediastinal irradiation for Hodgkin's disease. *Am J Med* 1976;60:39–45.
77. Brosius FC III, Waller BF, Roberts WC. Radiation heart disease. Analysis of 16 young (aged 15 to 33 years) necropsy patients who received over 3,500 rads to the heart. *Am J Med* 1981;70:519–530.
78. Harvey LAC, DeMaio SJ, Roberts WC. Radiation-induced cardiovascular disease including stenosis of coronary ostium, coronary and carotid arteries, and aortic valve. *Baylor University Med Ctr Proc* 1994;7:33–36.
79. Ihde DC, Roberts WC, Marr KC, Brereton HD, McGuire WP, Levine AS, Young RC. Cardiac candidiasis in cancer patients. *Cancer* 1978;41:2364–2371.
80. Ross EM, Macher AM, Roberts WC. *Aspergillus Fumigatus* thrombi causing total occlusion of both coronary arterial ostia, all four major epicardial coronary arteries and coronary sinus and associated with purulent pericarditis. *Am J Cardiol* 1985;56:499–500.
81. Roberts WC, Berard CW. Gas gangrene of the heart in clostridial septicemia. *Am Heart J* 1967;74:482–488.
82. Bulkley BH, Roberts WC. The heart in systemic lupus erythematous and the changes induced in it by corticosteriod therapy. A study of 36 necropsy patients. *Am J Med* 1975;58:243–264.
83. Buja LM, Roberts WC. Iron in the heart. Etiology and clinical significance. *Am J Med* 1971;51:209–221.
84. Cutler DJ, Isner JM, Bracey AW, Hufnagel CA, Conrad PW, Roberts WC, Kerwin DM, Weintraub AM. Hemochromatosis heart disease: an unemphasized cause of potentially reversible restrictive cardiomyopathy. *Am J Med* 1980;69: 923–928.
85. Buja LM, Ferrans VJ, Mayer RJ, Roberts WC, Henderson ES. Cardiac ultrastructural changes induced by daunorubicin therapy. *Cancer* 1973;32:771–788.
86. Buja LM, Ferrans VJ, Roberts WC. Drug-induced cardiomyopathies. *Adv Cardiol* 1974;13:330–348.
87. Isner JM, Ferrans VJ, Cohen SR, Witkind BG, Virmani R, Gottdiener JS, Beck JR, Roberts WC. Clinical and morphologic cardiac findings after anthracycline chemotherapy. Analysis of 64 patients studied at necropsy. *Am J Cardiol* 1983;51:1167–1174.

Papillary Fibroelastomas of the Heart

These are small avascular growths with multiple papillary fronds most commonly located on cardiac valves, mainly the aortic and mitral (Figure 1).[1–4] They are never present at birth, but are seen, at least on valves, primarily in older persons. They consist of fibrous tissue covered by an elastic membrane which in turn is covered by endocardium. Occasionally (about 15%), they also occur on left ventricular and/or ventricular septal mural endocardium,[15–14] particularly in patients with small or relatively small ventricular cavities, such as in patients with mitral stenosis (Figure 2)[9,12,13] or hypertrophic cardiomyopathy (Figures 3 and 4).[5,11] When located on the aortic valve, they usually are located on the ventricular aspects of the cusps in the more central portions but they also occur on the aortic aspects of these cusps usually near the margins.[15–20] When occurring on the mitral valve leaflets, they are usually on the atrial aspects near the margins.[21–28] In patients with mitral stenosis or hypertrophic cardiomyopathy, however, they involve the ventricular aspects of the anterior mitral leaflet and they sometimes are seen on chordae tendineae and mural endocardium, particularly over the papillary muscles. These lesions appear to result from contact of one valve leaflet with another or one mural endocardial surface with another.

A number of patients have been reported with papillary fibroelastomas and evidence of *stroke*[19–21,26,27,29–33] or loss of vision.[34] Whether the stroke was connected in any way with the cardiac fibroelastomas is debatable (in my view). Some patients have been in their 20s or 30s without other predisposing features or findings commonly associated with cerebral infarction, and the occurrence of stroke in the younger age group certainly is suggestive of a connection. In contrast to myxoma, where myxomatous material has been seen in systemic emboli, however, histologic findings of papillary fibroelastomas have not been observed in a cerebral artery in a patient with stroke and cardiac papillary fibroelastomas. Furthermore, the papillary fibroelastomas are firmly attached to valvular or mural endocardium and, therefore, dislodgement of a fibroelastoma would appear extremely unlikely. Thrombus, however, is occasionally superimposed on papillary fibroelastomas and it may be that the thrombus is the material that is dislodged and responsible for the stroke.

Additionally, *angina pectoris*,[33] *acute myocardial infarction*,[35–38] and *sudden death*[39] have been observed in patients with cardiac papillary fibroelastomas, mainly on the aortic valve. These papillary

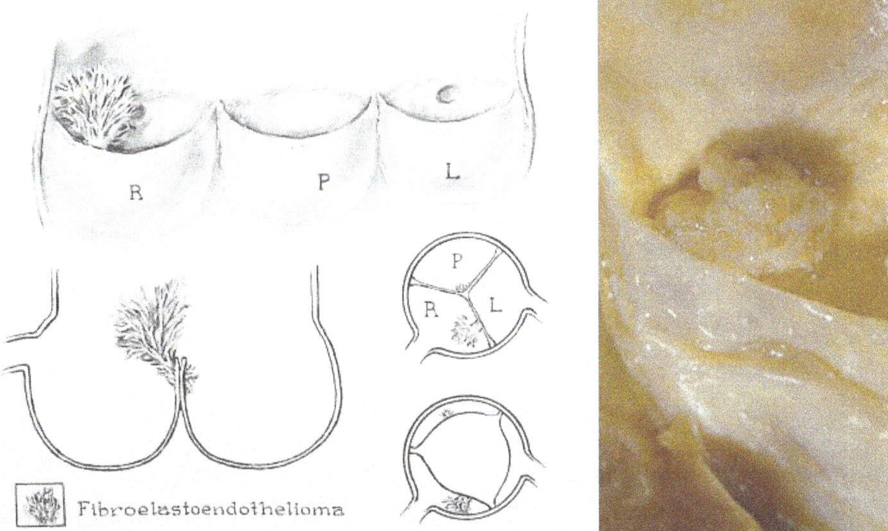

FIGURE 1. Fibroelastomas on the aortic valve in a 66-year-old man (FSH#85A-95) who had an *acute myocardial infarction* of the posterior left ventricular wall with subsequent fatal rupture of the posteromedial papillary muscle. The epicardial coronary arteries were severely narrowed by atherosclerotic plaque. *Left,* 1 fibroelastoma was located on the aortic aspect of the right (R) cusp, and during ventricular systole (*bottom right*), it was located close to the ostium of the right coronary artery. If the fibroelastoma had been located more centrally on the right cusp it theoretically could have contacted the ostium of the right coronary artery during ventricular systole. *Right,* photograph of the fibroelastoma on the right cusps. L = left cusp; P = posterior cusp.

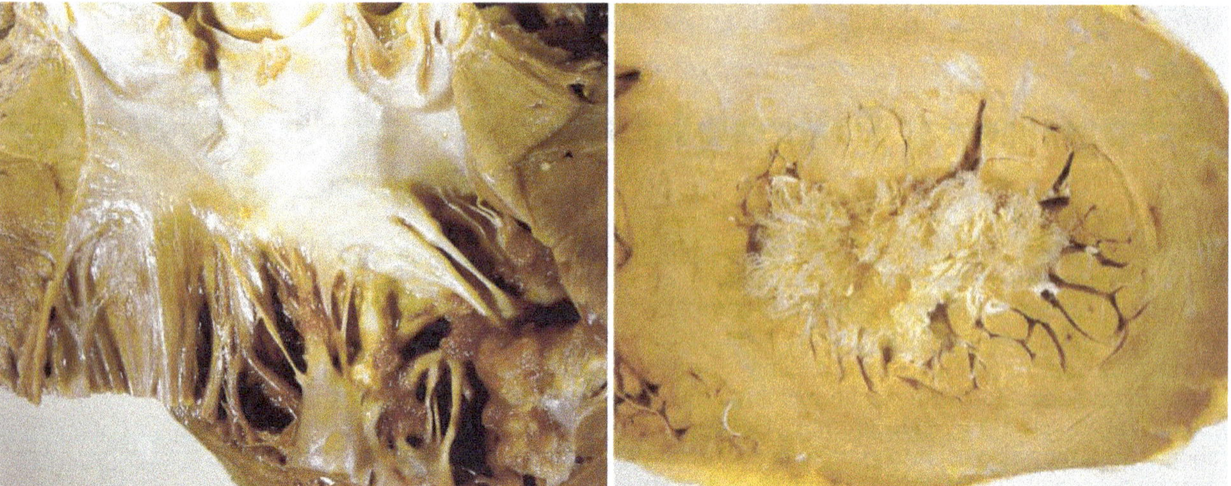

FIGURE 2. Multiple fibroelastomas in a 49-year-old woman (GT#83A-14) with *mitral stenosis. Left,* opened left ventricular outflow tract showing numerous elastofibromas attached to the ventricular aspect of the mitral leaflets and to their chordae tendineae and papillary muscles. One fibroelastoma is also located on the ventricular aspect of the posterior aortic valve cusp. *Right,* view of left ventricle showing papillary fibroelastomas filling the cavity.

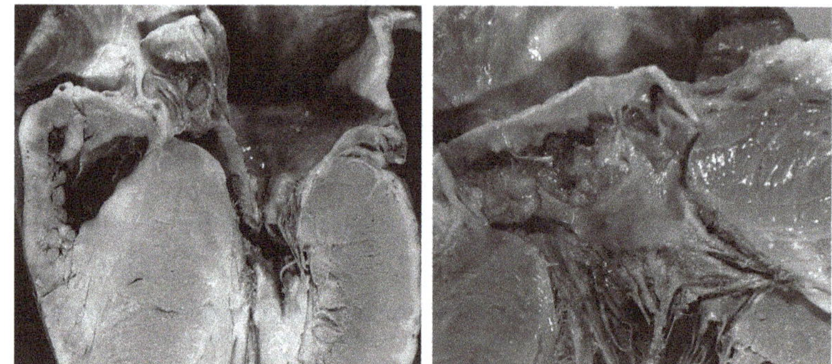

FIGURE 3. Multiple papillary fibroelastomas in a 36-year-old woman (A67-121) with *hypertrophic cardiomyopathy.* The left ventricular-aortic peak systolic pressure gradient was 75 mm Hg and the heart weighed 450 g. *Left,* longitudinal anterior to posterior cut exposing the left ventricular outflow tract, left atrium, and right ventricular outflow tracts. The fibroelastomas are located on the ventricular aspects of both anterior and posterior mitral leaflets and their chordae tendineae and papillary muscles and also on the aortic valve cusps. *Right,* opened aortic valve and left ventricular outflow tract demonstrating fibroelastomas on the ventricular aspects of all 3 aortic valve cusps, on the mural endocardium in apposition to anterior mitral leaflet, and also on the ventricular aspects of the anterior mitral leaflet.

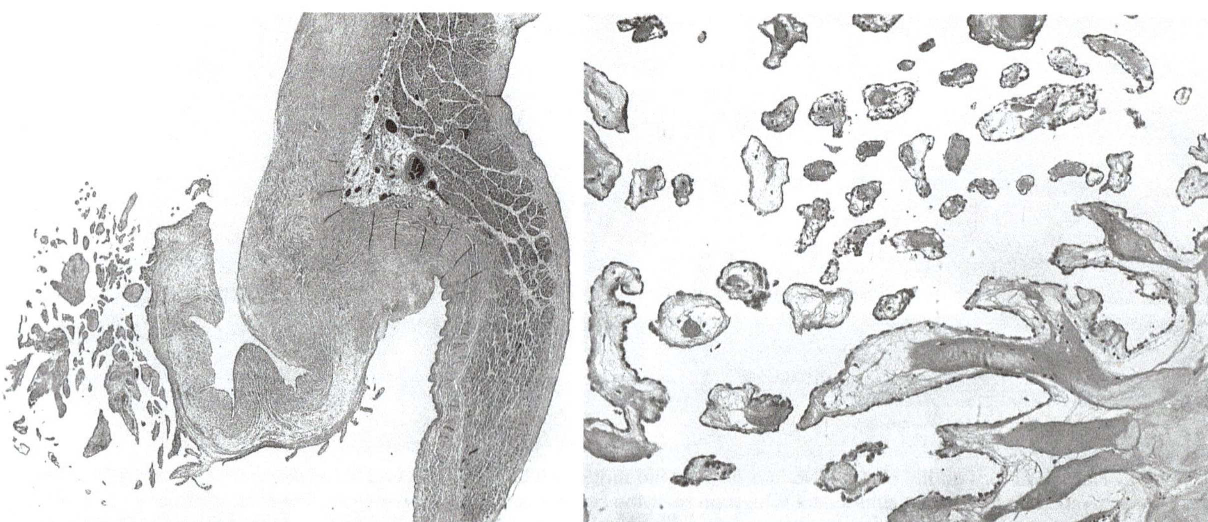

FIGURE 4. Photomicrographs of papillary fibroelastomas from the patient described in Figure 3. *Left,* view of aortic valve cusps with multiple fibroelastomas on the ventricular aspect of the cusps. *Right,* close-up view of the papillary fibroelastoma. Hematoxylin-eosin stains, left, ×15; right, ×84; reduced by 30%.

growths may also obstruct an aortic ostium of a coronary artery.[40,41]

On rare occasion, papillary fibroelastomas have been observed on the right side of the heart, mainly the tricuspid valve.[42–47]

Papillary fibroelastomas have been operatively excised from cardiac valves and/or mural endocardium in patients with evidence of stroke or other peripheral events and a few patients have had cardiac valve replacement.[9,11,13,14,19,20,22–24,29,30,34,37,41,45,47] When papillary fibroelastomas are detected by echocardiography in asymptomatic patients, operative excision rarely appears warranted. Whether operative excision or valve replacement is beneficial for papillary fibroelastomas in patients with cerebral or myocardial ischemic events is unsettled. I wonder if anticoagulation in these patients may be preferable to operative excision or valve replacement. There are no long-term follow-up studies available to answer these questions.

William C. Roberts

William Clifford Roberts, MD
Editor in Chief
Baylor Cardiovascular Institute
Baylor University Medical Center
Dallas, Texas 75246

1. Raeburn C. Papillary fibro-elastic hamartomas of the heart valves. *J Pathol Bacteriol* 1953;65:371–374.
2. Heath D, Best PV, Davis BT. Papilliferous tumors of the heart valves. *Br Heart J* 1961;23:20–24.
3. Nassar SGA, Parker JC Jr. Incidental papillary endocardial tumor. *Arch Pathol* 1971;92:370–376.
4. Fisbein MC, Ferrans VJ, Roberts WC. Endocardial papillary elastofibromas. Histologic, histochemical, and electron microscopical findings. *Arch Pathol* 1975;99:335–341.
5. Roberts WC. Valvular, subvalvular, and supravalvular aortic stenosis: morphologic features. *Cardiovasc Clin* 1973;5:97–126.
6. Heath D, Thompson IM. Papillary "tumors" of the left ventricle. *Br Heart J* 1965;29:950–954.
7. Burn CG, Bishop MB, Davies JNP. A stalked papillary tumor of the mural endocardium. *Am J Clin Pathol* 1969;51:344–346.
8. Flotte T, Pinar H, Feiner H. Papillary elastofibroma of the left ventricular septum. *Am J Surg Pathol* 1980;4:585–588.
9. Almagro UA, Perry LS, Choi H, Pintar K. Papillary fibroelastoma of the heart. Report of six cases. *Arch Pathol Lab Med* 1982;106:318–321.
10. Ong LS, Nanda NC, Barold SS. Two-dimensional echocardiographic detection and diagnostic features of left ventricular papillary fibroelastoma. *Am Heart J* 1982;103:917–918.
11. Topol EJ, Biern RO, Reitz BA. Cardiac papillary fibroelastoma and stroke. Echocardiographic diagnosis and guide to excision. *Am J Med* 1986;80:129–132.
12. Kalman JM, Lubicz S, Brennan JB, Vernon-Roberts E, Calafiore P. Multiple cardiac papillary fibroelastoma and rheumatic heart disease. *Aust N Z J Med* 1991;21:744–746.
13. Bedi HS, Sharma VK, Mishra M, Kasliwal RR, Trehan N. Papillary fibroelastoma of the mitral valve associated with rheumatic mitral stenosis. *Eur J Cardiothorac Surg* 1995;9:54–55.
14. Allen KB, Goldin M, Mitra R. Transaortic video-assisted excision of a left ventricular papillary fibroelastoma. *J Thorac Cardiovas Surg* 1996;112:199–201.
15. Campbell M, Carling W. Sudden death due to a fibrinous polyp of the aortic valve. *Guy's Hosp Rep* 1934;84:41–42.
16. Butterworth JS, Poindexter CA. Papilloma of cusp of the aortic valve: report of a patient with sudden death. *Circulation* 1973;48:213–215.
17. Cha SD, Incarvito J, Fernandez J, Chang KS, Maranhao V, Gooch AS. Giant Lambl's excrescences of papillary muscle and aortic valve: echocardiographic, angiographic, and pathologic findings. *Clin Cardiol* 1981;4:51–54.
18. Gopal A, Li Mandri G, King DL, Marboe C, Homma S. Aortic valve papillary fibroelastoma. A diagnosis by transthoracic echocardiography *Chest* 1994;105: 1885–1887.
19. Ragni T, Grande AM, Cappuccio G, Arbustini E, Grasso M, Tramarin R, Vigano M. Embolizing fibroelastoma of the aortic valve. *Cardiovasc Surg* 1994; 2:639–641.
20. Shahian DM, Labib SB, Chang G. Cardiac papillary fibroelastoma. *Ann Thorac Surg* 1995;59:538–541.
21. Fowles RE, Miller DC, Ebgert BM, Fitzgerald JW, Popp RL. Systemic embolization from a mitral valve papillary endocardial fibroma detected by two-dimensional echocardiography *Am Heart J* 1981;102:128–130.
22. Groton ME, Soltanzadeh H. Mitral valve fibroelastoma. *Ann Thorac Surg* 1989;47:605–607.
23. Gallo R, Kumar N, Prabhakar G, Awada A, Maalouf Y, Duran CM. Papillary fibroelastoma of mitral valve chorda. *Ann Thorac Surg* 1993;55:1576–1577.
24. Shapiro OM, Willimason WA, Dugan JM. Papillary fibroelastoma of the mitral valve. *Cardiovasc Surg* 1993;1:599–601.
25. Mann J, Parker DJ. Papillary fibroelastoma of the mitral valve. a rare cause of transient neurological deficits. *Br Heart J* 1994;71:6.
26. Pinelli G, Carteaux JP, Mertes PM, Civit T, Trinh A, Villemot JP. Mitral valve tumor revealed by stroke. *J Heart Valve Dis* 1995;4:199–201.
27. Zamora RL, Adelberg DA, Berger AS, Huettner P, Kaplan HJ. Branch retinal artery occlusion caused by a mitral valve papillary fibroelastoma *Am J Opthalmol* 1995;119:325–329.
28. Colucci V, Alberti A, Bonacina E, Gordini V. Papillary fibroelastoma of the mitral valve. A rare cause of embolic events. *Tex Heart Inst J* 1995;22:327–331.
29. McFadden PM, Lacy JR. Intracardiac papillary fibroelastoma: an occult cause of embolic neurologic deficit. *Ann Thorac Surg* 1987;43:667–669.
30. Brown RD Jr, Khandheria BK, Edwards WD. Cardiac papillary fibroelastoma: a treatable cause of transient ischemic attack and ischemic stroke detected by transesophageal echocardiography. *Mayo Clinic Proc* 1995;70:863–868.
31. Ighoghossian N, Trouillas P, Perinetti M, Barthelet M, Ninet J, Loire R. Lambl's excrescence: an uncommon cause of cerebral embolism. *Rev Neurol* 1995;151:583–585.
32. Kasarskis EJ, O'Connor W, Earle G. Embolic stroke from cardiac papillary fibroelastomas. *Stroke* 1988;19:1171–1173.
33. Zull DN, Diamond M, Beringer D. Angina and sudden death resulting from papillary fibroelastoma of the aortic valve. *Ann Emerg Med* 1985;14:470–473.
34. Shirani J, Bradlow JA, Metbeyeva P, Losada M, Factor SM, Strom JA, Sisto D. Transient loss of vision as the presenting symptom of papillary fibroelastoma of aortic valve. *Cardiovasc Pathol* 1997,6:237–240.
35. Richard J, Castello R, Dressler FA, Willman VL, Nashed A, Lewis B, Labovitz AJ. Diagnosis of papillary fibroelastoma of the mitral valve complicated by non-Q wave infarction with apical thrombus. trans-esophageal and transthoracic echocardiography study. *Am Heart J* 1993;126:710–712.
36. Etienne Y, Jobic Y, Houel JF, Barra JA, Boschat J, Meunier M, Penther P. Papillary fibroelastoma of the arotic valve with myocardial infarction: echocardiographic diagnosis and surgical excision. *Am Heart J* 1994;127:443–445.
37. Eckstein FS, Chafers HJ, Grote J, Mugge A, Borst HG. Papillary fibroelastoma of the aortic valve presenting with myocardial infarction. *Ann Thorac Surg* 1995;60:206–208.
38. Grote J, Mugge A, Schfers JH, Daniel WG, Lichtlen PR. Multiplane transesophageal echocardiography detection of a papillary fibroelastoma of the aortic valve causing myocardial infarction. *Eur Heart J* 1995;16:426–429.
39. Harris LS, Adelson L. Fatal coronary embolism from a myxomatous polyp of the aortic valve: an unusual cause of sudden death. *Am J Clin Pathol* 1965;43:61–64.
40. Boone S, Higginson LA, Walley VM. Endothelial papillary fibroelastoma arising in and around the aortic sinus, filling the ostium of the right coronary artery. *Arch Pathol Lab Med* 1992;116:135–137.
41. Mazzucco A, Bortolotti U, Thiene G, Dan M, Stritoni P, Scutari M, Stellin G. Left ventricular fibroelastoma with coronary embolization. *Eur J Cardiothorac Surg* 1989;3:471–473.
42. Anderson KR, Fiddler FI, Lie JR. Congenital papillary tumor of the tricuspid valve: an unusual cause of right ventricular outflow obstruction in a neonate with trisomy E. *Mayo Clin Proc* 1977;52:665–669.
43. Frumin H, O'Donnell L, Kerin NZ, Levine F, Nathan LE, Klein SP. Two-dimensional echocardiographic detection and diagnostic features of tricuspid papillary fibroelastoma. *J Am Coll Cardiol* 1983;2:1016–1018.
44. Mohan JC, Goel PK, Gambhir DS, Khanna SK, Arora R. Calcified mobile papillary fibroelastoma of the tricuspid valve a case report. *Indian Heart J* 1987;39:237–239.
45. Wolfe JT III, Finck SJ, Safford RE, Perselin ST. Tricuspid valve papillary fibroelastoma: echocardiographic characterization. *Ann Thorac Surg* 1991;51: 116–118.
46. Neerukonda SK, Jantz RD, Vijay NK, Narrod JA, Schoonmaker FW. Pulmonary embolization of papillary fibroelastoma arising from the tricuspid valve. *Tex Heart Inst J* 1991;18:132–135.
47. Ganjoo AK, Johnson WD, Gordon RT, Jain DP, Lang GE, Shankar VS. Tricuspid papillary fibroelastoma causing syncopal episodes. *J Thorac Cardiovasc Surg* 1996;112:551–553.

Fewer Hearts Than Earlier Predicted

The United Nations recently published ''World Population Prospects: The 1996 Revision.'' This book was reviewed by Ben Wattenberg in *The New York Times Magazine* of November 23, 1997. There is mounting evidence from both rich and poor nations strongly suggesting that the population explosion is fizzling! Never before have birthrates fallen so far, so fast, so low, for so long around the world as has occurred in the last 40 years. From 1950 to 1955, the global ''total fertility rate,'' the average number of children born per woman per lifetime, was 5. That was well above the so-called replacement rate of 2.1 children, the level needed to keep a population from falling over time, absent immigration. This scary growth continued for about 15 years, until by 1975 to 1980, the fertility rate had fallen to 4 children per woman, and by 1990–1995, the rate had fallen to just below 3. Today the total fertility rate is estimated to be 2.8 and sinking.

But what about women in the less developed countries? Even there, the fuse is sputtering. The fertility rate in less developed countries in 1965 to 1970 was 6 children per woman. Now it is 3 and falling more quickly than ever before. In some nations the numbers are even more striking. Italy, a Catholic country, has a fertility rate of 1.2 children per woman, the world's lowest rate and the lowest national rate ever recorded (absent famines, plagues, wars, or economic catastrophes). European birth rates of the 1980s, already at record breaking lows, fell another 20% in the 1990s to about 1.4 children per woman. With these rates, by the year 2060, Europe will have lost 24% of its people. Japanese and Russian rates are also at about 1.4 children. India's fertility rate now is lower than that in the USA in the 1950s. The rate in Bangladesh has fallen from 6.2 to 3.4 in just 10 years! Mexico has moved 80% of the way toward replacement level.

All this sounds a bit strange since the last 50 years have had the greatest population growth in history and such growth has not quite ended. What's happening is that 2 powerful trends—population explosion and the baby bust—are now at war. Although they can coexist for a while, it appears that the baby bust will win out eventually. From 1750 to 1950, global population increased from 1.0 to 2.5 billion. From 1950 to 2000, it will increase to 6 billion. In the USA in 1790, women bore an average of 7.7 children. Since 1972, the fertility rate in the USA has averaged 1.9 (among the lowest rates are those experienced by Jewish women and by black women with college degrees).

The UN projects that the global population in 2050 will be 9.4 billion people, and that prediction is based on the assumption that all nations will move to a fertility rate of about 2.1 children per woman. Based on current data, however, these projections may be far too high. Some projections by the year 2050 show the global population to be 7.7 billion, and that is based on an assumption that the global fertility rate will drop to 1.6 children per woman. This number is already the current rate in the developed nations. The assumption is that as nations modernize they will behave as modern nations. Already 51 nations, with 44% of the world's population, are at or below replacement. UN demographers also project that by 2010 to 2015, there will be 88 such nations, with 67% of the population at or below replacement levels.

What is causing the birth dearth? One factor surely is urbanization, reflecting the shift from wanting more children to help on the farm to wanting fewer mouths to feed in the city. Other factors include more education for women, legal abortion, higher incomes, unemployment yielding lower incomes, greater acceptance of homosexuality, new aspirations for women, better contraception (including ''morning after pills'' endorsed by new Food and Drug Administration guidelines), later marriages, difficulty conceiving at older ages, more divorce, and vastly lower infant mortality rates. When parents know their children will survive, fertility rates plummet.

When people have fewer babies and live longer, the median age of society climbs. In 1990, about 6% of the world's population was over age 65. By 2050, that figure will be about 18%. By having relatively fewer children, people today are eroding the population base that should pay for their pensions in their old age. In 1955, there were 9 American workers to support each Social Security recipient. Today, there are 3. By 2030, the number is expected to be 2.

For the environment, the prospect of fewer people than expected is good news. More people cause more pollution, more people use more resources, and more affluent people do more of both.

Consider geopolitics. In 1950, roughly 32% of the world's population lived in ''the West''—the modern nations of Europe, North America, and Japan. Today 20% do, and in 2050 it will be more like 12%. The West has been the driving force, of course, of modern civilization by inexorably pushing toward democratic values. Will that continue when its share of the total population is only 11%?

And the economic effects could be harsh. Businesses tend to do better when their population customer bases grow. For a while there will be plenty of extra customers coming on steam no matter what projection is used (two billion more even under the low scenario). In the past 50 years in America, the population has doubled. That escalator of consumer demand won't continue. American population in the next half century will probably grow much more slowly, perhaps by <30%, with most of the increase in the next 20 years. Europe may become an ever smaller picture postcard continent.

And what about psychological effects? There will be more and more people without brothers or sisters, uncles, aunts or cousins, children or grandchildren—lonelier people. Clergymen say that the saddest funerals are those in which the deceased has no offspring. There will be more and more people living alone.

William C. Roberts

William C. Roberts, MD
Editor in Chief
Baylor Cardiovascular Institute
Baylor University Medical Center
Dallas, Texas 75246

Fifty Years of Hypertrophic Cardiomyopathy†

In 1869, Liouville[1] and Hallopeau[2] each reported a patient who probably had hypertrophic cardiomyopathy (HC). The 2 investigators noted striking hypertrophy of the ventricular septum, and each considered the left ventricular outflow tract to be obstructed by the hypertrophied septal muscle; Hallopeau noted thickening of the anterior mitral leaflet in his 69-year-old patient.

In 1907, Schmincke[3] described severe hypertrophy of the ventricular septum in the hearts of 2 women aged 50 and 56 years. In addition to the septal thickening, the left ventricular free wall in each patient was severely hypertrophied. Schmincke considered the ventricular septal hypertrophy to be primary and of congenital origin, leading to obstruction to left ventricular ejection and to secondary hypertrophy of the left ventricular free wall.

After Schmincke's[3] report in 1907, a period of nearly 50 years elapsed before another probable report of this disease appeared. In 1952, Davies[4] described a family in which many members had heart disease and histories of sudden death and systolic precordial murmurs. At necropsy, the heart of 1 patient showed "diffuse sub-aortic stenosis" associated with left ventricular hypertrophy. Davies described an area of fibrosis of 4 cm^2 in the left ventricular outflow tract opposite the anterior mitral leaflet, a lesion highly suggestive of HC.

In 1957, Brock[5] operated on a 63-year-old woman thought to have a valvular aortic stenosis and systematic hypertension. At operation, however, the aortic valve was normal, and no obstruction to left ventricular outflow was encountered by dilating instruments, despite direct pressure tracings showing subvalvular obstruction. The patient died shortly after the operation, and necropsy showed a hypertrophied, nondilated left ventricular cavity and no subaortic fibrous stricture.

Although the cases reported by Liouville,[1] Hallopeau,[2] Schmincke,[3] Davies,[4] and Brock[5] were probable examples of HC, the comparative thicknesses of the ventricular septum and left ventricular free wall were not described by any of them. The first unequivocal description of HC was by Teare[6] in London, reported in the *British Heart Journal* in January 1958. Although Brock's clinical report was published in *Guy's Hospital Reports* in the final quarterly issue of 1957, Teare's report had been received by the journal in January 1957, before Brock operated on his patient, and Brock's publication did not appear, until 1958 although the date on the issue was 1957. Thus, it is fair to credit Teare with the first detailed anatomic description and to credit Brock with the first description of the functional nature of this entity. Teare described gross and histologic cardiac findings in 9 patients aged 14 to 45 years (average 26; 2 female, 7 male), 8 of whom died suddenly. Although he did not give measurements of the thicknesses of the ventricular septum and left ventricular free wall, Teare clearly indicated and illustrated that the septum was thicker than the left ventricular free wall and, indeed, called the condition asymmetrical hypertrophy of the heart. He considered the localized septal hypertrophy to be a "benign tumor" or "hamartoma." Teare observed on histologic examination "bizarre arrangements of muscle bundles" and "considerable variation in size" of the myocardial fibers in the ventricular septum. He also noted a similar disordered arrangement of muscle bundles in the adjacent anterior free wall of the left ventricle. In 1 patient, the posterior left ventricular free wall "appeared thinner than normal," and histologic examination of it showed normal arrangement and uniform size of the myocardial fibers. Although 1 of his 9 patients underwent valvulotomy for suspected mitral stenosis (this was the only patient in his study who had not died suddenly), there were no descriptions of the mitral valve, no mention of mural endocardial thickening in the left ventricular outflow tract, and no comments regarding the sizes of the various cardiac

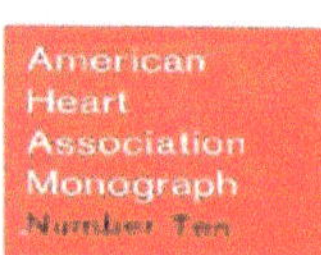

Idiopathic Hypertrophic Subaortic Stenosis

I. A Description of the Disease Based Upon an Analysis of 64 patients

Braunwald E, Lambrew CT, Rockoff SD, Ross J Jr, Morrow AG: pages 3-119

II. Operative Treatment and the Results of Pre- and Postoperative Hemodynamic Evaluations

Morrow AG, Lambrew CT, Braunwald E: pages 120-151

III. Intraoperative Studies of the Mechanism of Obstruction and Its Hemodynamic Consequences

Pierce GE, Morrow AG, Braunwald E: pages 152-213

Published by the AMERICAN HEART ASSOCIATION, INC

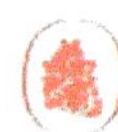

Figure 1. The 1964 monograph of 213 pages by Braunwald et al.[8–10]

Manuscript received November 6, 2008; revised manuscript received and accepted November 7, 2008.

†A modified version of this piece was presented on October 4, 2008, at a scientific symposium sponsored by the Eugene Braunwald Endowment for the Advancement of Cardiovascular Discovery and Care at the Brigham and Women's Hospital, Boston, Massachusetts.

Table 1
Cardiac findings in hypertrophic cardiomyopathy divided by presence or absence of cardiac operation

Characteristic	Cardiac Operation		
	0 (n = 153)	+ (n = 77)	Total (n = 230)
Dilated atria	98%	100%	99%
Increased heart weight	95%	96%	96%
Nondilated left ventricle	82%	75%	80%
Thickened anterior mitral leaflet	66%	94%	75%
Mural plaque, LV outflow tract	60%	93%	71%
VS larger than left ventricle	71%	63%	68%
Transmural scarring, VS and/or LV wall	42%	43%	42%
Disorganization, cardiac myocytes	95%	95%	95%
Intramural coronary disease	83%	83%	83%
Interstitial fibrosis, VS and LV wall	90%	90%	90%

LV = left ventricular; VS = ventricular septum.

Table 2
Gross cardiac findings by 3 age groups in 153 patients with hypertrophic cardiomyopathy without cardiac operations

Characteristic	Age Group (yrs)		
	≤10 (n = 15)	11–70 (n = 124)	>70 (n = 14)
Dilated atria	95%	100%	100%
Increased heart weight	80%	98%	86%
Nondilated left ventricle	73%	81%	93%
Thickened anterior mitral leaflet	27%	66%	100%
Mural plaque, LV outflow tract	27%	78%	100%
VS larger than left ventricle	73%	71%	79%
Transmural scarring, VS and/or LV wall	0%	45%	50%

LV = left ventricular; VS = ventricular septum.

Table 3
Complications of hypertrophic cardiomyopathy

Death: sudden and nonsudden
Atrial dilatation: atrial fibrillation
Mitral valve disease: mitral regurgitation
Fibrous thickening (anatomic systolic anterior motion)
Insertion, papillary muscle, into leaflet
Rupture of chordae tendineae
Prolapse
Annular calcification
Infective endocarditis
Papillary muscle calcification
Myocardial infarction: left ventricular dilation
Left ventricular apical diverticulum
Pulmonary hypertension
Aneurysm pulmonary arteries
Ossific nodules, lungs
Heart block and bundle branch block

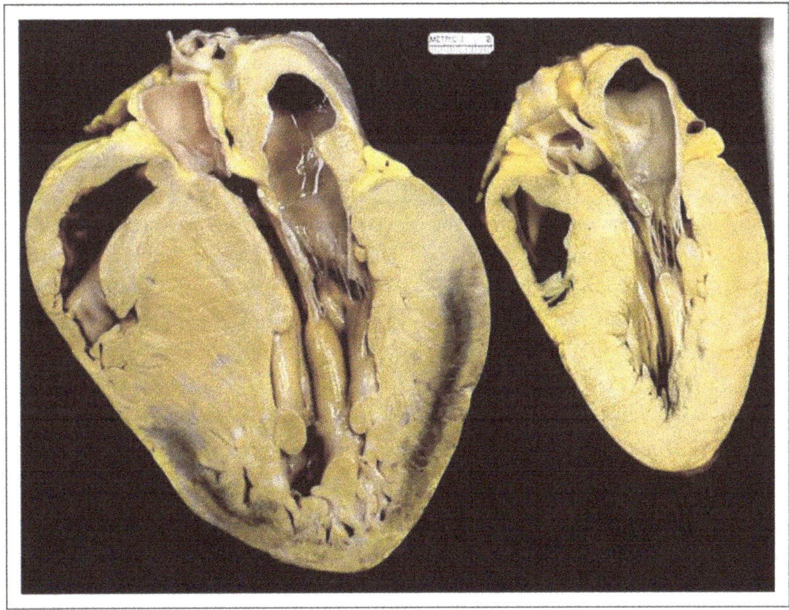

Figure 2. The hearts of 2 15-year-old male patients with HC, each of whom died suddenly. The heart on the *left* weighed 1,415 g, and the ventricular septum was much thicker than the left ventricular free wall. The heart on the right weighed 425 g, and the thicknesses of the ventricular septum and left ventricular free wall were similar.

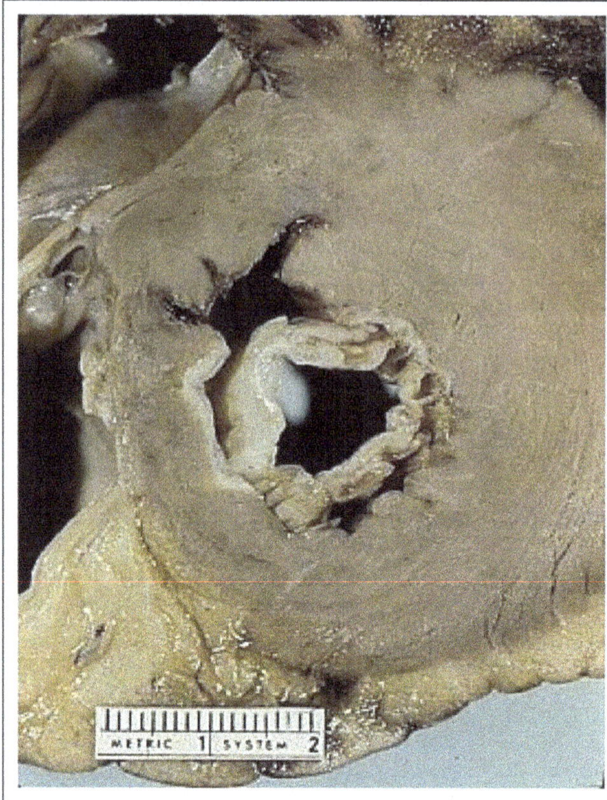

Figure 3. Heart of a patient who underwent partial ventricular septectomy and septotomy for HC. The septal mural endocardium and anterior mitral leaflet were thickened by fibrous tissue. The thickening represents the anatomic equivalent of systolic anterior motion of the anterior mitral leaflet.

chambers. Teare's report, however, established HC as a distinct entity.

Although these heretofore-mentioned reports, mainly necropsy ones, likely represent examples of the disease, HC was put on the clinical screen by Braunwald et al[7] in 1960, and by 1964, Braunwald et al[8–10] had reported extensive clinical and operative studies on 64 of these patients (Figure 1). This American Heart Association monograph included 213 pages of original work! No condition in the annals of medicine had been described so extensively in such a short period of time, and Dr. Braunwald deserves the credit. Indeed, as Dr. William Osler emphasized, "In science the credit goes to the man who convinces the world, not to the man to whom the idea first occurred."

Dr. Albert Schweitzer opined that "as we acquire more knowledge, things do not become more comprehensive, but more mysterious." Certainly this statement is applicable to HC as it has unfolded in the past 50 years.

Listed in Table 1 are morphologic features of 230 patients with HC studied at autopsy by the same investigator from 1959 to the present time.[11] The diversity of anatomic findings has altered the definition of this condition on several occasions. Essentially, none of the 10 morphologic features occurs in all patients. The ventricular septum is thicker than the left ventricular free wall in about two-thirds

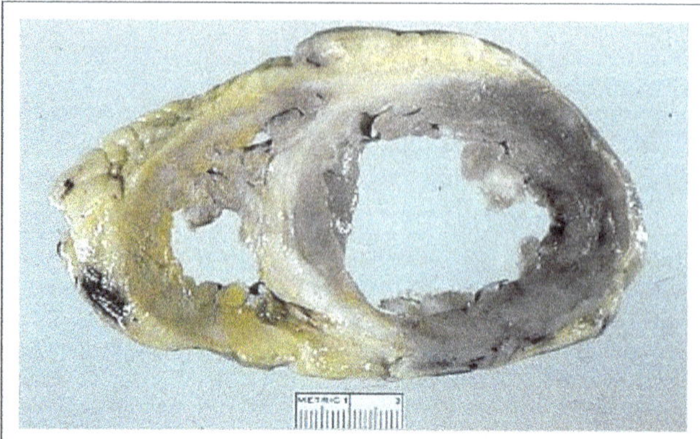

Figure 4. Transverse slice of the cardiac ventricles in a 46-year-old man with HC who developed extensive ventricular septal scarring and dilatation of both ventricular cavities. The resulting severe heart failure prompted cardiac transplantation. Reproduced with permission from *Am J Cardiol*.[22]

of patients, not 100%, as some originally thought. Cardiac mass is usually, but not always, increased.[12] This condition has produced the largest hearts known to humankind.[13]

Figure 2 shows the hearts of 2 15-year-old male patients with HC.[13,14] Both patients died suddenly. The heart on the left weighed 1,415 g, the heaviest I have ever seen. The ventricular septum was much thicker than the left ventricular free wall. The heart on the right weighed 425 g, or 30% of the heart on the left. The ventricular septum and left ventricular free wall were of similar thickness. Yet the 2 patients had the same condition, namely, HC.

The congenital condition, according to Dr. Barry Maron,[15] is present in 1 of 500 humans (the same prevalence, incidentally, as familial hyperlipidemia[16]). It can be manifested in newborns or not until the nonagenarian age group (Table 2).[15,17] It is of course a congenital heart disease, which usually is not manifested until adulthood.[18]

HC has many complications, and some are listed in Table 3. Sometimes a complication is the first clinical manifestation of the condition.

Figure 3 shows a heart in which the myectomy-myotomy procedure was performed. The operation was devised by Dr. Andrew G. Morrow,[9] who performed 299 of these operations and who himself had the disease. This operation is not for the occasional heart surgeon, which is 1 reason I predict that it will eventually vanish. Mitral valve replacement is not the proper operation, except in patients with very damaged mitral valves from infective endocarditis.[19,20]

Figure 4 shows the heart of a patient with HC who developed extensive ventricular septal scarring with ventricular cavity dilation, an occurrence, according to Dr. Maron, in 2% of these patients.[21] These patients are candidates for cardiac transplantation.[22]

In summary, HC was put on the diagnostic and therapeutic map by Dr. Braunwald and his colleagues[7–10] in the early 1960s. Much additional information, of course, has been learned subsequently. This condition produces the largest myofibers of any condition with or without the stimulus of ventricular outflow obstruction or elevation of ventricular peak systolic pressures. The ultimate therapy, in my view, will involve an agent that reduces myofiber size. Whether myofiber number is increased in HC remains unclear.

William Clifford Roberts, MD
Baylor Heart and Vascular Institute
Baylor University Medical Center
Dallas, Texas

1. Liouville H. Rétrécissement cardiaque sous aortique. *Gazette Med Paris* 1869;24:161–163.
2. Hallopeau M. Rétrécissement ventriculo-aortique. *Gazette Med Paris* 1869;24:683–684.
3. Schmincke A. Ueber linkseitigue muckulöse conusstenosen. *Disch Med Wochenschr* 1907;33:2082.
4. Davies LG. Familial heart disease. *Br Heart J* 1952;14:206–212.
5. Brock R. Functional obstruction of the left ventricle (acquired aortic subvalvular stenosis). *Guys Hosp Rep* 1957;106:221–238.
6. Teare D. Asymmetrical hypertrophy of the heart in young adults. *Br Heart J* 1958;20:1–18.
7. Braunwald E, Morrow AG, Cornell WP, Aygen MM, Hilbish TF. Idiopathic hypertrophic subaortic stenosis. Clinical, hemodynamic and angiographic manifestations. *Am J Med* 1960;29:924–925.
8. Braunwald E, Lambrew CT, Rockoff SD, Ross J Jr, Morrow AG. I. A description of the disease based upon an analysis of 64 patients. *Am Heart Assoc Monogr* 1964;10:IV3–IV119.
9. Morrow AG, Lambrew CT, Braunwald E. Operative treatment and the results of pre- and postoperative hemodynamic evaluations. *Am Heart Assoc Monogr* 1964;10:IV120–IV151.
10. Pierce GE, Morrow AG, Braunwald E. Intraoperative studies of the mechanism of obstruction and its hemodynamic consequences. *Am Heart Assoc Monogr* 1964;10:IV152–IV213.
11. Roberts CS, Roberts WC. Morphologic features (of hypertrophic cardiomyopathy). In: Zipes DP, Rowlands DJ, eds. Progress in Cardiology. Philadelphia, Pennsylvania: Lea & Febiger, 1989:3–32.
12. Olivotto I, Maron MS, Autore C, Lesser JR, Rega L, Casolo G, DeSantis M, Quarta G, Nistri S, Cecchi F, Salton CJ, Udelson JE, Manning WJ, Maron BJ. Assessment and significance of left ventricular mass by cardiovascular magnetic resonance in hypertrophic cardiomyopathy. *J Am Coll Cardiol* 2008; 52:559–566.
13. Roberts CS, Roberts WC. Hypertrophic cardiomyopathy as a cause of massive cardiomyopathy (>1000 g). *Am J Cardiol* 1989;64:1209–1210.
14. Maron BJ, Maron MS, Lesser JR, Hauser RG, Haas TS, Harrigan CJ, Appelbaum E, Main ML, Roberts WC. Sudden cardiac arrest in hypertrophic cardiomyopathy in the absence of conventional criteria for high risk status. *Am J Cardiol* 2008;101:544–547.
15. Maron BJ. Hypertrophic cardiomyopathy. A systemic review. *JAMA* 2002;287:1308–1320.
16. Brown MS, Goldstein JL. How LDL receptors influence cholesterol and atherosclerosis. *Sci Am* 1984;251:58–66.
17. Maron BJ, Tajik AJ, Ruttenberg HD, Graham TP, Atwood GF, Vitorica BE, Lie JT, Roberts WC. Hypertrophic cardiomyopathy in infants. Clinical features and natural history. *Circulation* 1982;65: 7–17.
18. Roberts WC. Congenital cardiovascular abnormalities usually silent until adulthood. In: Roberts WC, ed. Adult Congenital Heart Disease. Philadelphia, Pennsylvania: F.A. Davis, 1987:717–727.
19. Roberts WC. Operative treatment of hypertrophic obstructive cardiomyopathy. The case against mitral valve replacement. *Am J Cardiol* 1973;32:377–381.
20. Roberts WC, Kishel JC, McIntosh CL, Cannon RO III, Maron BJ. Severe mitral or aortic valve regurgitation, or both, requiring valve replacement for infective endocarditis complicating hypertrophic cardiomyopathy. *J Am Coll Cardiol* 1992;19:365–371.
21. Hecht GM, Klues HG, Roberts WC, Maron BJ. Coexistence of sudden cardiac death and end-stage heart failure in familial hypertrophic cardiomyopathy. *J Am Coll Cardiol* 1993;22:489–497.
22. Shirani J, Maron BJ, Canon RO III, Sheyda S, Roberts WC. Clinicopathologic features of hypertrophic cardiomyopathy managed by cardiac transplantation. *Am J Cardiol* 1993;72:434–440.

Forty-Five Years in the Cardiovascular Arena

In 1963, I was a cardiology fellow under Drs. Eugene Braunwald and Andrew G. Morrow in the National Heart Institute of the National Institutes of Health in Bethesda, Maryland. That was the year President John F. Kennedy was killed in Dallas, Texas. When he arrived at Parkland Hospital, there was no electrocardiograph in the emergency room.[1] What has occurred in cardiovascular medicine since that fatal November day in 1963 is astounding! No specialty in medicine has had such a transformation.

In 1963, a patient with an acute myocardial infarction (AMI) was treated about the same as when my father had his first heart attack in 1938, 25 years earlier. It was bed rest on the ward or in a private room, and that went on for a month. In 1963, there were no coronary care units, no echocardiograms, no intravascular ultrasonic imaging, no myocardial perfusion imaging (nuclear cardiology), no computed tomography, and no magnetic resonance imaging. Coronary angiography was being done in only 3 or 4 hospitals in all of the United States. And of course, there was no coronary angioplasty or coronary stenting or coronary bypass. Cardiac valve replacement had started only 3 years earlier, and repair techniques for atrioventricular valve regurgitation were yet to be developed. The aorta in its various segments was just beginning to be resected (by DeBakey and Cooley). Carotid endarterectomy was infrequent. Percutaneous techniques to open intracardiac obstructions or close intracardiac defects were unavailable. The Swan-Ganz catheter had not yet appeared. Pacemakers were available, but they weighed 8 times what they weigh today and lasted about a fifth as long. Implantable cardioverter defibrillators were unavailable, and indeed, external cardiac defibrillation had just begun (in 1960). Electrophysiologic techniques to determine sites of ventricular arrhythmias and catheter and operative ablation procedures were 20 years away. Heart transplantation was 5 years away.

And drugs for cardiovascular conditions were just beginning. The first antihypertensive drug had arrived just 10 years earlier. A β blocker had just arrived on the scene. There were no calcium channel blockers, angiotensin-converting enzyme inhibitors or angiotensin receptor blockers, or thienopyridines or glycoprotein IIb/IIIa inhibitors or direct thrombin inhibitors. Aspirin had not yet been recognized as a cardiac disease–preventive medication. Statins and ezetimibe were not yet discovered, and niacin had not yet been recognized as a lipid-altering agent. Digoxin, quinidine, and procaine amide were the mainstays of antiarrhythmic therapy. Lidocaine had just arrived.

Thrombolytic therapy for AMI was reported initially in 1976 by Chazov in a Russian medical journal, and the concept was lost until 5 years later, when Peter Rentrop injected streptokinase directly into the "infarct-related" coronary arteries in patients with AMIs.[2] He took patients with AMIs directly to the cardiac catheterization laboratory, and in some patients, he injected streptokinase directly into the totally occluded coronary arteries, while in some others, he injected nitroglycerin. In the streptokinase group, the arteries in most patients opened up quickly, but they did not do so in the patients in whom nitroglycerin had been injected. At repeat catheterization 7 days later, however, the infarct-related coronary arteries in the 2 groups were patent. Thus, in this initial study, Rentrop and colleagues demonstrated in patients with AMI that the infarct-related coronary artery was totally occluded at the onset of the infarction, that streptokinase dissolved the thrombus superimposed on the atherosclerotic plaque rather quickly, and that spontaneous lysis of the thrombus did occur, but its occurrence was too late to limit the size of the acute myocardial infarct.

It was not long, of course, before other thrombolytic agents were demonstrated to be better than streptokinase and also that the administration of the fibrinolytic agent by the intravenous route was as beneficial as by the intracoronary route. It was shown early that whatever the thrombolytic agent administered, the shorter the period from door to needle or from emergency medical service to needle, the better the outcome and that ideally, the time should be <30 minutes. Of course, some patients have contraindications to fibrinolysis (severe hypertension; possible aortic dissection; recent trauma, surgery, or bleeding; bleeding or clotting disorder; another life-threatening condition, etc.) and therefore their only hope of salvaging myocardium is primary percutaneous coronary intervention (PCI).

Although coronary angioplasty had been introduced in 1978, it took some time and major persistence by several investigators to convince the cardiovascular community that primary PCI provided better hospital and 1-year outcomes than intravenous thrombolysis, as long as the medical contact–to–balloon or door-to-balloon time was <90 minutes, and ideally, of course, the shorter the better. The invasive strategy is now the preferred therapy, assuming that skilled personnel and equipment are available and that medical contact–to–balloon or door-to-balloon time is <90 minutes.

Why has primary PCI proved to be better than thrombolysis? Some morphologic studies in the 1980s showed that the quantity of underlying plaque at the site of thrombi in patients with AMIs varies from about 30% to 95% of the cross-sectional area (averaging 80%) and therefore that the area occupied by thrombi ranges from 70% to only 5%

(averaging 20%).[3] Thus, thrombolytic therapy on average when successful opens up the artery only 20% in cross-sectional area, whereas PCI, ideally including initial evacuation of the thrombus, cracks the underlying plaque and therefore provides a much greater opening than thrombolysis alone.[4] Indeed, PCI opens the artery to a greater degree than it was before the AMI!

When I interned at Boston City Hospital in 1958, the hospital mortality in patients with AMI was about 35%. Today, without reperfusion, either by thrombolytic therapy or PCI, that mortality is about 25%. With successful thrombolysis alone, it is about 7%, and with PCI alone, it is about 5%, and even less when the thrombus is initially evacuated.

These results are of course remarkable. Patients with ventricular fibrillation before hospitalization and cardiogenic shock on admission continue to have very high hospital mortality rates. as do patients with right ventricular infarctions, ventricular rupture, and important mitral regurgitation. Better secondary prevention will continue to reduce the frequency of another atherosclerotic event, and better primary prevention would prevent many AMIs from ever occurring.

William Clifford Roberts, MD
Baylor Heart and Vascular Institute
Baylor University Medical Center
Dallas, Texas 75246

1. Jones RC. Assassination of a president. *Proc (Bayl Univ Med Cent)* 1999;12:97–99.
2. Rentrop P, Blanke H, Karsch KR, Kaiser H, Kostering H, Leitz K. Selective intracoronary thrombolysis in acute myocardial infarction and unstable angina pectoris. *Circulation* 1981;63:307–317.
3. Brosius FC III, Roberts WC. Significance of coronary arterial thrombus in transmural acute myocardial infarction. A study of 54 necropsy patients. *Circulation* 1981;63:810–816.
4. Potkin BN, Roberts WC. Effects of percutaneous transluminal coronary angioplasty on atherosclerotic plaques and relation of plaque composition and arterial size to outcome. *Am J Cardiol* 1988;62:41–50.

So You Want to See Your Heart

Recently, I was walking in the corridors of Baylor University Medical Center and suddenly was stopped and asked by a very kind man, "I understand, Dr. Roberts, that you have my heart?" He was Mr. Melvin A. Jones, who had undergone heart transplantation (number 437) at Baylor University Medical Center in 2003. I told him, "Of course I have your heart. We keep these specimens for various studies." We arranged for Mr. Jones to come to the weekly cardiac pathology conference, and accordingly he saw his heart (Figures 1 and 2). Mr. Jones is asymptomatic and is living a very active life. He indicated that he has had 5 new grandchildren since his heart transplantation!

William Clifford Roberts, MD
Baylor Heart and Vascular Institute, at Baylor University Medical Center, Dallas, Texas.

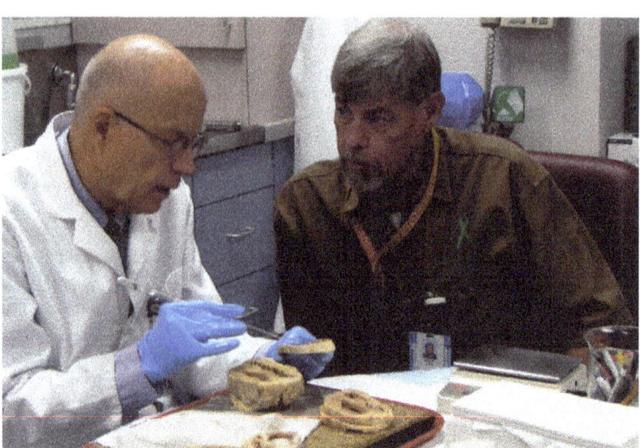

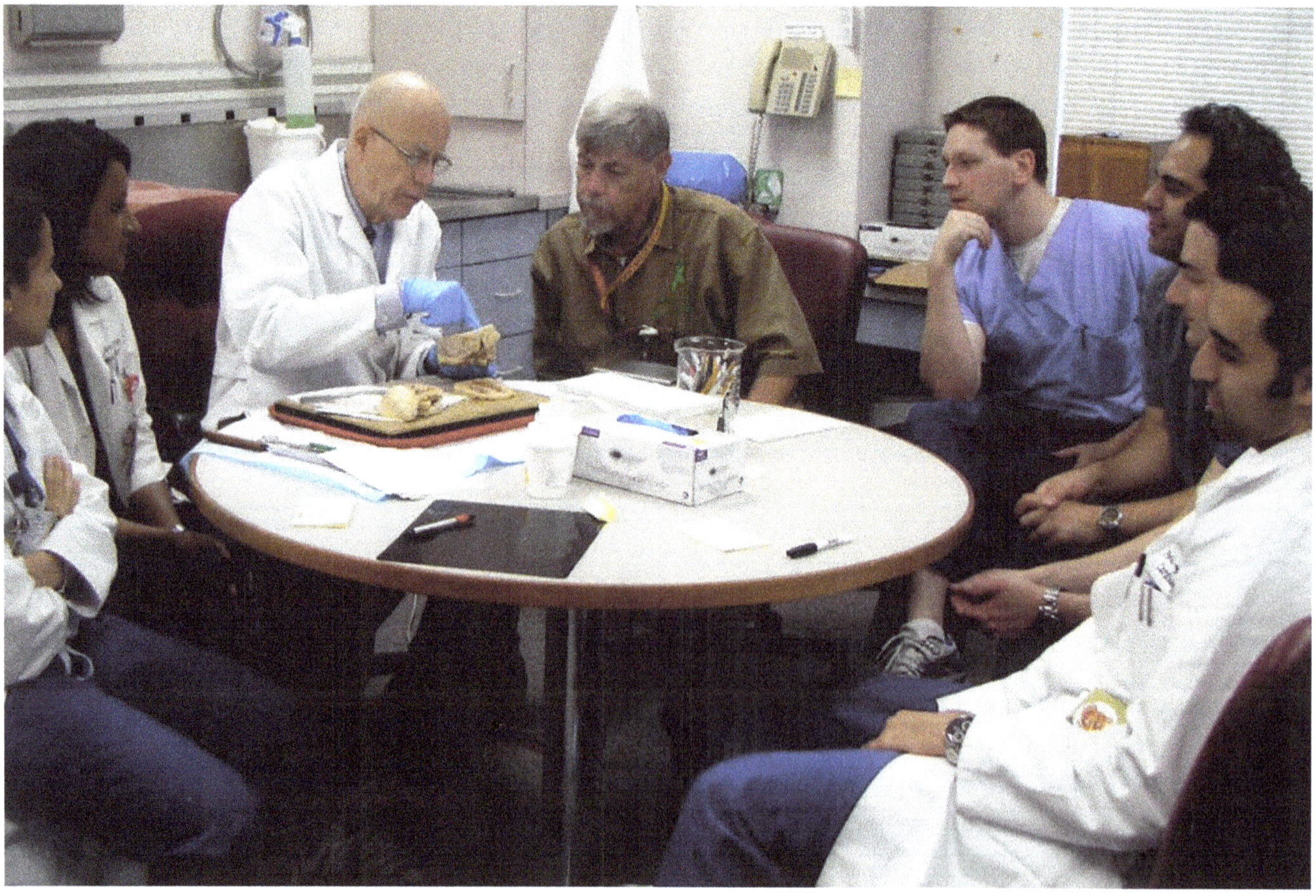

Figure 1. View of Mr. Jones looking at his own heart with Dr. Roberts. (Photograph by Jamie Ko.)

Figure 2. View of Baylor University Medical Center cardiology fellows also looking at the interaction. (Photograph by Jamie Ko.)

Prophylactic Replacement of a Dilated Ascending Aorta at the Time of Aortic Valve Replacement of a Dysfunctioning Congenitally Unicuspid or Bicuspid Aortic Valve

Recently, I examined a beautifully excised severely stenotic congenitally bicuspid aortic valve in a 64-year-old man who, at the same operation, had undergone excision of the ascending aorta, which, by preoperative imaging studies, had a maximal diameter of 4.3 cm. Histologically, the wall of the aorta was normal. Although the aortic valve replacement (AVR) was clearly appropriate, was excision of the ascending aorta justified on a prophylactic basis? I would argue that the latter should be reconsidered.

Before the 1990s, relatively few patients with stenotic or purely regurgitant congenitally malformed aortic valves also underwent concomitant resection of the dilated ascending aorta. During the 1990s, some prominent and persuasive cardiac surgeons began advocating prophylactic concomitant ascending aortic resection in these circumstances, mainly for 3 reasons. First, to prevent postoperative dilation of the ascending aorta in a previously normal sized aorta or to prevent additional dilation in an already dilated aorta; second, to prevent aortic dissection, which is recognized to occur more commonly in patients with congenitally unicuspid and bicuspid aortic valves than in patients with tricuspid aortic valves[1,2]; and, finally, to prevent rupture of the ascending aorta late postoperatively. The latter reason was because it is recognized that the media of the ascending aorta in patients with congenitally bicuspid aortic valves can be depleted of certain elements (elastic fibers, smooth muscle cells, collagen) and can be repleted with certain other elements (mucopolysaccharide material) compared to the aorta's structure in adults with tricuspid aortic valves[3] (except in those patients with the Marfan syndrome and the forme fruste variety of it,[4] cardiovascular syphilis,[5–7] and ankylosing spondylitis,[8] and giant-cell aortitis[9]).

But how often do these potential aortic complications (additional dilation, dissection, rupture) occur in patients who have had AVR because of a dysfunctioning congenitally malformed aortic valve (either unicuspid or bicuspid) without concomitant resection of the dilated ascending aorta? The answer is infrequently. The best data (largest number of patients and longest follow-up) supporting that view comes from an analysis of 1,286 patients (1,180 [92%] with aortic stenosis [AS], 85 [7%] with aortic regurgitation [AR], and 20 [1%] aortic valve dysfunction type not stated) who had undergone AVR at the Mayo Clinic from 1960 to 1995 because of a dysfunctioning bicuspid aortic valve, without concomitant resection of the ascending aorta, irrespective of its size.[10] The mean age at operation was 58 years (72% men). The follow-up period was 0 to 38 years (median 12). During that postoperative period (excluding the 36 who died early [2.8%] and the 26 lost to follow-up [2.6%]), documented aortic dissection occurred in 13 (1%) and additional aortic dilation (ascending aorta diameter reached ≥5.0 cm or >1.0 from that at the time of AVR) occurred in 127 (9.9%). Additionally, 11 (0.08%) of the 1,227 patients not dying early or lost to follow-up later underwent resection of the ascending aorta; in 9 of the 11, however, it was at the time of replacement of a malfunctioning mechanical prosthesis or a bioprosthesis in the aortic valve position.

Although 151 events affecting the ascending aorta occurred during the long follow-up period, 127 (84%) consisted of dilation of the aorta, something that can occur after any aortotomy, irrespective of the structure of the aortic valve, and dilation of the ascending aorta after an aortotomy in and of itself infrequently produces clinical consequences. Indeed, the 15-year all-cause survival was greater in the patients with "enlarged" aortas than in those with normal-size aortas at the time of AVR (56% vs 50%). Although the ascending aorta was later excised in 11 patients, that aortic resection probably would not have been done in 9 if excision of a dysfunctioning prosthesis or bioprosthesis had not been required. Additionally, aortotomy, performed with isolated AVR, causes proliferation of fibrous tissue around the aorta, making the aorta thicker than normal, and the resulting thicker wall almost surely is more difficult to rupture than an aortic wall of normal or less than normal thickness. Furthermore, any type of interruption of the wall of ascending aorta (be it for insertion of a saphenous vein conduit or arterial cannula or incision for AVR or for resection of an aortic tear in aortic dissection) increases the risk of late dissection or rupture, be it in patients with unicuspid, bicuspid or tricuspid aortic valves.[11]

Similar long-term follow-up after isolated AVR in patients with dysfunctioning tricuspid aortic valves without concomitant resection of ascending aorta was recently presented by Gaudino et al.[12] They described 93 consecutive patients (mean age 67 years; 74% men) undergoing isolated AVR for AS at their institution (Catholic University Rome) from January 1990 to December 2000. Preoperatively, the maximal diameter of the ascending aorta ranged from 5.0 to 5.9 cm (mean 5.6). The diagnosis of tricuspid aortic valve was confirmed in each patient at operation by visual inspection. The ascending aorta was neither replaced nor plicated. The 92 patients surviving the operation were followed up for a mean of 14.7 ± 4.8 years. During that period, 16 patients died (17%). In no case was death attributed to an aortic event. Indeed, no patient during the long follow-up experienced an acute ascending aortic rupture, dissection, or pseudoaneurysm formation. Also, during the follow-up, no patient required reoperation for thoracic aortic complications. Additionally, the diameter of the ascending aorta during the 10 years after AVR changed insignificantly (56 ± 2 mm preoperatively vs 57 ± 11 mm at the end of follow-up). The mean expansion rate of the ascending aorta was 0.3 ± 0.2 mm/year. Patients with connective tissue disorders such as the Marfan syndrome were excluded from their study. The report by Gaudino et al[12] included the largest number of patients with dilated ascending aortas and stenotic 3-cuspid aortic valves undergoing AVR alone and followed up for ≥10 years. The frequency of late ascending aortic complications is lacking in patients who have had combined AVR for dysfunctioning unicuspid, bicuspid, or tricuspid aortic valves and resection of the dilated ascending aortas with similarly long (10 to 15 years) follow-up.

Adding ascending aortic resection to AVR usually significantly increases the operative mortality. Data from the Society of Thoracic Surgeons database indicate that ascending aortic resection increases the operative risk by a factor of 2.78 compared to AVR alone.[13] I agree with McKeller et al[10] from the Mayo Clinic who stated: "The widespread adoption of an aggressive attitude toward [aortic] root replacement, therefore, may create more problems than it solves."

Another recent report also provides some evidence that prophylactic resection of the ascending aorta is probably performed too frequently (unnecessarily) in patients undergoing AVR for dysfunctioning congenitally malformed aortic valves.[14] The evidence is provided by a histologic study of operatively excised dilated (>4.5-cm) aortas in patients undergoing AVR for dysfunctioning unicuspid or bicuspid aortic valves. My colleagues and I examined histologically the operatively excised ascending aortas in 58 patients undergoing AVR for AS involving a congenitally unicuspid or bicuspid aortic valve and in 38 patients undergoing AVR for pure AR involving a bicuspid aortic valve.[14] All 96 patients by preoperative imaging studies had ascending aortas with diameters >4.5 cm. We found that dividing the patients into those with AS and those with pure AR, something that had not been done previously, was helpful in predicting whether the structure of the ascending aorta was likely to be normal, in which case its resection probably was not indicated, or abnormal, in which case its resection probably was indicated. In the 58 patients with AS, the structure of the aortic media was normal or nearly normal (consistent with aging) in all 14 patients with unicuspid aortic valves and in 39 (87%) of the 44 patients with bicuspid valves. In contrast, of the 38 patients with purely regurgitant congenitally bicuspid aortic valves (none had unicuspid valves), the aortic media was normal in 20 (53%) and abnormal in 18 (47%). These findings suggest that among patients with preoperative imaging studies showing the ascending aorta to have a diameter >4.5 cm, it is unlikely the ascending aorta requires resection if the congenitally malformed aortic valve is stenotic. However, aortic resection will be necessary in about 1/2 of the patients with purely regurgitant congenitally bicuspid valves. Unfortunately, among the patients with pure AR, no preoperative features were found to distinguish those with normal from those with abnormal aortic media histologically (judged exclusively by the degree, if any, of the loss of medial elastic fibers).

In summary, it is likely that too many dilated ascending aortas are being excised prophylactically in patients with aortic valve dysfunction involving a congenitally unicuspid or bicuspid aortic valve. The rates of late postoperative occurrence of aortic dissection and/or rupture are extremely low, and additional dilation of the ascending aorta after AVR infrequently produces deleterious clinical events. The histologic structure of the dilated ascending aorta is usually normal in patients with stenotic congenitally unicuspid or bicuspid aortic valves. In contrast, the aortic histologic structure is often (about 50%) abnormal in patients with dilated ascending aortas and purely regurgitant congenitally bicuspid aortic valves.

William Clifford Roberts, MD
Baylor Heart and Vascular Institute
Baylor University Medical Center
Dallas, Texas

1. Roberts CS, Roberts WC. Dissection of the aorta associated with congenital malformation of the aortic valve. *J Am Coll Cardiol* 1991;17:712–716.
2. Roberts CS, Roberts WC. Morphologic aspects of aortic dissection. In: Ernst CB, Stanley JC, eds. *Current Therapy in Vascular Surgery*. Philadelphia: B.C. Decker; 1991:245–151.
3. Fazel SS, Mallidi HR, Lee RS, Sheehan MP, Liang D, Fleishman D, Herfkens R, Mitchell RS, Miller DC. The aortopathy of bicuspid aortic valve disease has distinctive patterns and usually involves the transverse aortic arch. *J Thorac Cardovasc Surg* 2008;135:901–907.
4. Roberts WC, Honig HS. The spectrum of cardiovascular disease in the Marfan syndrome: a clinico-morphologic study of 18 necropsy patients and comparison to 151 previously reported necropsy patients. *Am Heart J* 1982;104:115–135.
5. Roberts WC, Ko JM, Vowels TJ. Natural history of syphilitic aortitis. *Am J Cardiol* 2009;104:1578–1587.
6. Roberts WC, Bose R, Ko JM, Henry AC, Hamman BL. Identifying cardiovascular syphilis at operation. *Am J Cardiol* 2009;104:1588–1594.
7. Roberts WC, Lensing FD, Kourlis H Jr, Ko JM, Newberry JW, Smerud MJ, Burton EC, Hebeler RF Jr. Full blown cardiovascular syphilis with aneurysm of the innominate artery. *Am J Cardiol* 2009;104:1595–1600.
8. Bulkley BH, Roberts WC. Ankylosing spondylitis and aortic regurgitation. Description of the characteristic cardiovascular lesion from study of eight necropsy patients. *Circulation* 1973;48:1014–1027.
9. Roberts WC, MacGregor RR, DeBlanc HJ Jr, Beiser GD, Wolff SM. The prepulseless phase of pulseless disease, or pulseless disease with pulses: a newly recognized cause of cardiac disease, monoclonal gammopathy and "fever of unknown origin." *Am J Med* 1969;46:313–324.
10. McKeller SH, Michelena HI, Li Z, Schaff HV, Sundt TM III. Long-term risk of aortic events following aortic valve replacement in patients with bicuspid aortic valves. *Am J Cardiol* 2010;106:1626–1633.
11. Muna WF, Spray TL, Morrow AG, Roberts WC. Aortic dissection after aortic valve replacement in patients with valvular aortic stenosis. *J Thorac Cardiovasc Surg* 1977;74:65–69.
12. Gaudino M, Anselmi A, Morelli M, Pragliola C, Tsiopoulos V, Glieca F, Possati G. Aortic expansion rate in patients with dilated post-stenotic ascending aorta submitted only to aortic valve replacement: long-term follow-up. *J Am Coll Cardiol* 2011;58:581–584.
13. Rankin JS, Hammill BG, Ferguson TB Jr, Glower DD, O'Brien SM, DeLong ER, Peterson ED, Edwards FH. Determinants of operative mortality in valvular heart surgery. *J Thorac Cardiovasc Surg* 2006;131:547–557.
14. Roberts WC, Vowel TJ, Ko JM, Filardo G, Hebeler RF Jr, Henry AC, Matter GJ, Hamman BL. Comparison of the structure of the aortic valve and ascending aorta in adults having aortic valve replacement for aortic stenosis versus for pure aortic regurgitation and resection of the ascending aorta for aneurysm. *Circulation* 2011;123:896–903.

International Cardiology

China and Chinese Cardiology

Lihui Wang is a 56-year-old Chinese physician (Fig. 1). She arises each morning at 6 in her 3-room apartment, shared until recently with her engineer husband and medical student son, exercises for 15 to 30 minutes, and leaves about 7:30 AM on her bicycle for the 10-minute ride to the Hospital of Beijing Medical University where she is Professor and Chairman of the Department of Medicine, Director of Cardiology, and President of the hospital. Despite her small stature (157 cm tall, 50 kg) and gentle composure, Professor Wang is clearly the dominant force in the 1,073-bed hospital which she directs. She performs rounds daily in the 6-bed cardiac care unit where about 100 patients with acute myocardial infarction are cared for each year. Her day at the hospital usually ends by 7:30 PM, but her briefcase accompanies her home on her bicycle. After a quick dinner, she is at her desk again by 9 to complete administrative tasks and she retires at midnight. This schedule is repeated 6 days a week. On Sunday she rests. Her salary is 230 Yuan a month (equivalent to 62 U.S. dollars) (3.71 Yuan = $1 U.S.), but the salary is adequate because rent of her apartment is only 5 Yuan; utilities, 5 Yuan; food, 40 Yuan; and about 20 Yuan is saved each month. Her son's tuition is paid by the state. Her salary is determined primarily by the number of years since graduation from medical school and to a small extent by her professional rank. She receives no additional income for being Chairman of the Department of Internal Medicine or Director of Cardiology or President of the Hospital. She will be eligible to retire at her present salary by age 62, but she has the option to work several years longer. She has 5 weeks of vacation and 7 national holidays each year. Professor Wang has had her hard times. During the Cultural Revolution's leveling process (1966 to 1976) in China, she was demoted to "cleaning woman" status and imprisoned in the hospital for 3 years.

I met Professor Wang and other Chinese cardiologists during a 6-day visit to Beijing and Shanghai, People's Republic of China, in May 1987 as one of a 5-man cardiologic teaching delegation (Fig. 2). I was "taken" by the warmth, openness, generosity, humility, honesty, kindness and strength of the Chinese people. During the meetings and hospital visits, the members of our delegation often were asked for suggestions as to how Chinese cardiology could be improved. But we can learn much from these Chinese. Alcoholism in their population is practically non-existent; opium, cocaine and marijuana use is absent; sexual promiscuity and divorce are rare; AIDS is non-existent; neurosis is rare; crime is virtually absent; although food is rationed and its prices controlled, starvation is a thing of the past; slums are gone or disappearing; health is generally good (life expectancy at birth is 66 years for men and 69 years for women), and expectations for improvements in life, liberty and happiness are high. The magnitude of their problems facing China, however, is mind-boggling:

1) *Population size.* There are over 1.1 billion people and 50% of them are under 21 years of age. Despite the governmental policy of only 1 child per couple initiated 8 years ago and apparently adhered to by 65% of the couples, China's population continues to increase: by 1,400 people every hour, by 34,000 every 24 hours, and by 15 million every year. Presently, there are 18 births and 7 deaths per 1,000 population.

2) *Food supply.* At the moment, it is adequate but it will not be so for long if the population continues to increase. Despite the large land area of China—slightly larger than that of the USA—only 12% of the land is arable, about a third less than in the USA, but the population of China is 4 times that of the USA. China consists mainly of mountains and deserts with 90% of the population inhabiting just over 15% of the total area. One-half of the land area of China contains only 4% of the population.

3) *Limited opportunities.* Despite enormous progress in education during the past 40 years (80% of the population was illiterate in 1949, whereas 80% are literate now), only 3% of Chinese youth enter college, whereas 40% do so in the USA. About 94% of China's children receive grammar (primary) school education but less than 50% of them finish high (middle) school. Nearly 5 million high school graduates apply for university and college, but only 275,000 (6%) gain a place. Only 8,500 positions are available for postgraduate training and 600,000 graduates apply for these positions (1 of every 14 gains a place). Thus, most Chinese are "peasants" (farmers) (80%) or (in urban areas) "workers." Their initial job is usually their lifelong and final job. The life of the peasants has been

Professor Lihui Wang.

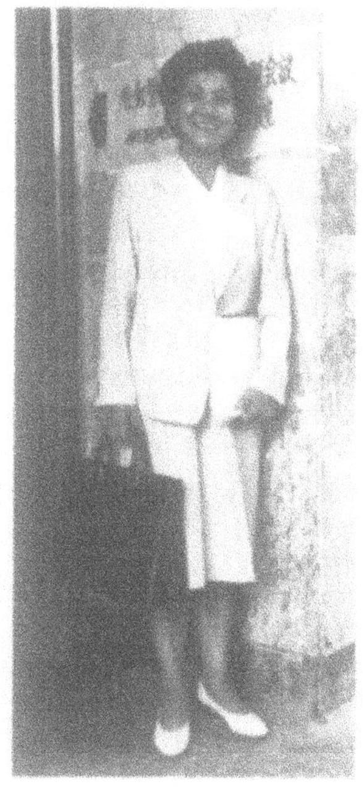

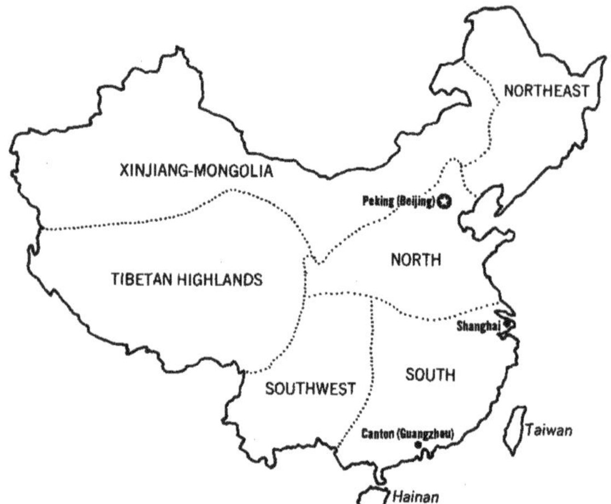

People's Republic of China.

improved enormously in recent years by the introduction of the incentive system and many such farmers have become comparatively wealthy. The city worker has little to no incentive program. Their salary from the state is small (about 65 Yuan [$18 US] a month) and it is not based on the quality or quantity of their work. There is change underway, however, to generate an incentive program for the workers.

4) *Spartan living conditions.* Apartments and houses in the cities are small, poorly furnished and "conveniences" are often shared with more than 1 family. There are more building cranes presently in Beijing, however, than in any city in the world and, therefore, living conditions are improving rapidly. Transportation in the major cities is primarily by bicycle and bus. Every family has at least 1 bike. If the private automobile becomes commonplace in China, the streets of large cities (15 have populations >1 million) will be clogged. Only 1,800 private cars are present in Beijing, a city of 8 million, and I never saw a gasoline service station while in either Beijing or Shanghai. Taxis are common, however, in both cities and virtually all large companies and hospitals have automobiles with drivers for their staff to use.

And now *Chinese cardiology.* Cardiovascular disease accounts for about 23% of the deaths in China and stroke (systemic hypertension) for about 20%.[1–5] Of the cardiovascular diseases, coronary artery disease is the most frequent.[1,6,7] Angina pectoris is far more common than is acute myocardial infarction. Although acute rheumatic fever is now infrequent, rheumatic heart disease is common. Congenital heart disease appears to affect their population as frequently as any other population.[8] Dr. Guan Han Zhou, a cardiovascular surgeon in Beijing, told me that only 200 coronary artery bypass grafting operations are performed in China each year and that most cardiovascular operations are for rheumatic or congenital heart diseases. In Shanghai, Dr. Hong-Shing Zhu told me that cardiovascular operations are infrequent in persons over 50 years of age. Aortic valve stenosis and mitral anular calcium are rare in their elderly, and both of these diseases in my view are secondary to atherosclerosis.[9] Likewise, fusiform abdominal aneurysm, a consequence of both atherosclerosis and systemic hypertension, is rare.[10]

Although coronary atherosclerosis is increasing in frequency in China—the price of progress—its frequency is much less at the moment than in the Western World. Nevertheless, small percentages mean large numbers of people when the population base is so large. It will be a long time before the frequency of coronary artery disease in China approaches that in the Western World. Obesity in China is rare. Over twice as much fish is consumed yearly as beef (5.2 vs 2.5 million metric tons). A large amount (17 million metric tons yearly) of pork, however, is eaten in China and the Chinese eat the fat as well as the muscle. The diet, however, is usually low in meat and consists primarily of rice, wheat, sweet potatoes and beans. Exercise is a necessity in China, not a luxury. Most person in cities use a bicycle to get to work. Most Chinese even in cities work outside. The day begins for most Chinese with some calisthenics, and virtually all adults under age 60 have jobs outside the home.

There are about 1.3 million physicians in China, and one-half of them are women. All are connected to a hospital where both in- and outpatients are seen. Private practice is virtually nonexistent. The numbers of cardiologists and cardiovascular surgeons are inadequate. Cardiac catheterization laboratories and cardiovascular surgical facilities are limited and the waiting time for these procedures is over 3 months. The diagnosis-related groups (DRGs) have not arrived in China. The usual hospital stay for an acute myocardial infarction is 28 days, and for a cardiovascular operation, 60 days. Patients apparently prefer the hospitals to their homes. Salaries for physicians usually begin at about 75 Yuan ($20 US) a month. A renowned 80-year-old university cardiologist in Shanghai told me that his salary was 350 Yuan ($75 US) a month, and that he was supplied with an automobile and a driver. In contrast, taxi cab drivers in Beijing and Shanghai commonly make 400 to 500 Yuan ($108 to $135 US) a month. Many farmers and shop-owners also are better paid than physicians. Cardiovascular surgeons and cardiologists have identical salaries.

The Western World has much to teach China and China has much to teach the Western World. It is wonderful that we can now communicate openly and freely with one another.

William C. Roberts

William C. Roberts, MD
Editor in Chief

1. Chen HZ, Lin YS, Dai RH, He WX, Yuan JG, Li JH, Wu SM, Yang YJ. *Changes in etiologic types of heart disease in Shanghai during the past 32 years. An analysis of 15,696 patients. Chin Med J 1985;98:151–156.*
2. Avolio AP, Deng FQ, Li WQ, Luo YF, Huang ZD, Xing LF, O'Rourke MF. *Effects of aging on arterial distensibility in populations with high and low prevalence of hypertension: comparison between urban and rural communities in China. Circulation 1985;71:202–210.*
3. Li SC, Schoenberg BS, Wang CC, Cheng XM, Bolis CL, Wang KJ. *Cerebrovascular disease in the People's Republic of China: epidemiologic and clinical features. Neurology 1985;35:1708–1713.*
4. Zhao GS, Yuan XY, Gong BQ, Wang SZ, Cheng ZH. *Nutrition, metabolism and hypertension. A comparative survey between dietary variables and blood pressure among three nationalities in China. J Clin Hypertens 1986;2:124–131.*
5. Huang YY. *Prevalence and unawareness of hypertension in the petrochemical industrial population in China. Prev Med 1986;15:643–651.*
6. No authors. *A pathological survey of atherosclerotic lesions of coronary artery and aorta in China. A coordination group in China. Pathol Res Pract 1985;180:457–462.*
7. Chen ZJ. *Sudden cardiac death in the People's Republic of China. Cor Vasa 1986;28:90–95.*
8. Lien WP, Chen JJ, Chen JH, Lin JL, Hsieh YY, Wu TL, Chu SH, Hung CR. *Frequency of various congenital heart diseases in Chinese adults: analysis of 926 consecutive patients over 13 years of age. Am J Cardiol 1986;57:840–844.*
9. Roberts WC. *The senile cardiac calcification syndrome. Am J Cardiol 1986;58:572–574.*
10. Roberts WC. *The hypertensive diseases. Evidence that systemic hypertension is a greater risk factor to the development of other cardiovascular diseases than previously suspected. Am J Med 1975;59:523–532.*

Japan and Japanese Medicine

Yazo Hirota is a 43-year-old cardiologist who directs the cardiac catheterization laboratory of the Third Division, Department of Internal Medicine, Osaka Medical College, Osaka, Japan. He is a native and resident of Kyoto. Six days a week he leaves his home shortly after 7 AM, taxis to the Kyoto train station, and boards the punctual 33-minute express to Osaka. He arrives at the hospital before 8 AM. Until 4 PM he either performs cardiac catheterizations or cares for patients or teaches, and from then until 8 or 9 PM he works in his research laboratory. After the evening train and taxi ride, he arrives home about 9 or 10 PM, showers and then soaks in a warm bath, visits briefly with his wife and 3 children (aged 8, 13 and 15 years), eats dinner and retires. This cycle continues for 6 days a week. Sunday is with the family.

Dr. Hirota is on the staff of a prominent university hospital connected with one of the national medical schools in Japan. As such, he receives a salary. The salaries of the university medical professors are similar in amount to those of nonmedical professors such as those in the English and History departments. Those physicians who have just completed their specialty training receive about 160,000 yen per month ($1,145) ($1 US = 140 yen), and a full professor, a rank rarely obtained before age 50, about 400,000 yen per month ($2,860.00). I met Dr. Hirota during a 3-day visit to Kyoto for a meeting in June 1987. We talked during a faculty dinner that included delicious filet mignon. It is a privilege to be served steak in Japan—I guess especially at a cardiology dinner. There are relatively few steer in Japan but those there are pampered; they are encouraged to drink large quantities of beer and many receive regular massages, both of which they believe increase the beef's succulence and tenderness.

Japan is an amazing country. Its geographic area is about the size of the state of California or the country of Finland, which has 4.5 million inhabitants, but Japan has 120 million, half the number in the USA. Japan consists of 4 large islands and about 3,000 smaller ones. About 71% of the land is mountainous and largely uninhabitable; the other 29% is relatively flat and contains all of the people, their living and working spaces and their farmlands. Thus, the place is crowded. Livable land is enormously expensive. The average home costs the equivalent of 7 years' salary of the owner. In contrast, in the USA the average home costs the equivalent of 3 years' salary. Furthermore, the average Japanese home is much smaller than the average American one. The average farm in Japan consists of 2.5 acres, and 40% of the arable land is used for cultivation of rice. Despite the relatively small space available, 72% of all agricultural foodstuffs and 90% of the fruit the Japanese consume is produced on Japanese land; and they catch more fish than any country. Of all countries to have a passion for golf it should not be Japan. Initiation fees at top private golf clubs are over $100,000 and a single round of golf for a visitor costs $250. This small lush green land has more active volcanoes than anywhere on earth, a serious quake every few years and about 1,000 tremors annually (all tall buildings are earthquake-constructed), about 6 typhoons a year, and frequent *tsuanmis*, huge sea waves, to 100 feet high, which slam ashore with devastating force.

The economic post–World War II miracle of Japan is well known. This despite the fact that virtually all major Japanese cities were burned out in World War II by 90,000 tons of bombs, mostly incendiaries dropped from B-29s. Two cities were obliterated by atom bombs. The road back was swift. General Douglas MacArthur, the Supreme Commander, initiated agricultural reform by transferring large portions of land held by long-entrenched landlords to the farmers and he broke up the great industrial complexes. A new Constitution offered a new type of government and the USA canceled most payments of war reparations. The Korean War in the early 1950s provided a boost to their new highly efficient factories, and for many years Japan reinvested huge proportions of their gross national product to further modernize old industries and bankroll new ones. And now the Japanese produce most of the world's videocassette recorders, transistor radios, tape machines, stereo sets, silicon memory chips and industrial robots. Despite having to import nearly all of its oil, natural gas and iron ore and 80% of its coal, Japan is the world's second largest steelmaker. (The USSR is first.)

So what kind of people are these Japanese? They all work enormously hard, and they have an enormous loyalty to the group of which they are a part (family, employer and his compa-

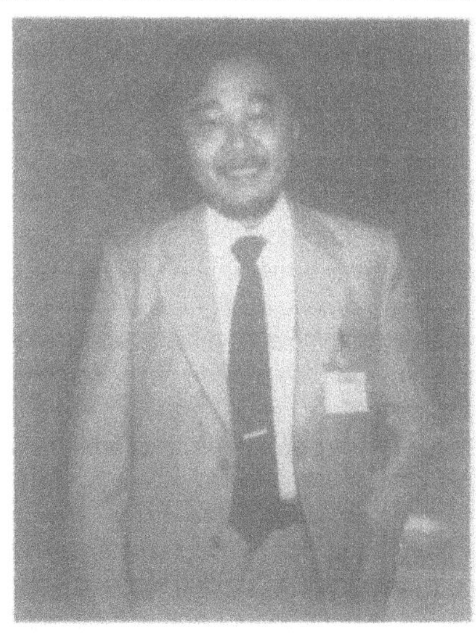

Yazo Hirota

ny, fellow employees, schoolmates, etc.). They demand excellence of effort from themselves, and they are kind, honest, polite and nondemanding of others. A recent survey showed that most (nearly 90%) are contented with their lives. Their society has been described as a *classless meritocracy.* The status, power and wealth a person attains is determined not by inheritance or family background but by success in a series of competitive examinations. Children take examinations to qualify for the best grammar schools, then for the best high schools and then for the universities. Student selections by the schools and universities are easy. Each school has a limited number of openings each year and counts down from the top of the best ranking to admit that number. Selections have nothing to do with teacher's recommendations, students' extracurricular activities, leadership qualities or personality. Thus, pressure to succeed in the examinations is immense. But for a modern Japanese, the rank and reputation of the university attended settles the course of future life. The blue-chip companies and top government ministries hire future managers almost exclusively from Tokyo University and a few others. Admission to one of these institutions puts one on "the fast escalator to the top." Mothers spend enormous amounts of time with their children to help them prepare for examinations because a mother's status and sense of achievement depend in large measure on her children's academic success. Despite the strain, students who have made it to a good high school or university have mastered a formidable body of knowledge. Japanese mathematics education, according to United Nations surveys, is the best in the world. International science tests have ranked Japanese students first in ability to understand and apply what they know. The Japanese high school students also delve more deeply into the history, geography and culture of foreign countries than most students in other countries. All Japanese elementary school students learn how to read music, to play a simple musical instrument, and to draw with a level of skill that in other countries would be considered evidence of innate artistic ability. Japanese schools also reinforce the pervasive belief that the group and the nation are more important than the individual. Discipline, filial piety, loyalty, honesty and respect are stressed. School children are responsible for keeping their schools clean. There are no other janitors.

How the Japanese have been able to excel at home and abroad so well has many reasons[1]: (1) *They buy rights to foreign technology when necessary.* They purchased from Western Electric the rights to the transistor for only $25,000! (2) *They spend heavily on research and development.* Most Japanese firms spend 6% of revenues, whereas the figure is 1% in the USA. As a result, the number of patents issued yearly to Japanese nationals by their government outstrips the number granted by the US Patent Office to American persons and firms, and Japan outpaces patents issued in the UK and France by a ratio of 7 to 1. (3) *They demand quality in their products.* Japanese customers insist on nothing but the best, and more than 85% of all goods made in Japan are earmarked for home consumption. Quality control is nearly a national passion. Fierce competition between Japanese companies demands a high level of inventiveness, rigid cost controls and excellent products. There are 11 auto companies in Japan, more than in any other country, and 8 more than in the USA. Each company survives by constantly striving to upgrade its products and to improve its production rates. A Japanese factory worker turns out considerably more goods per hour than his American or European counterpart. (4) *They have factories with the most efficient equipment.* They invented robots and they use more than in any other country, nearly 100,000. The robots are fast, clean, undemanding, precise, less expensive than human labor, tireless, and they never get bored. (5) *They save their money*—nearly 20% of their earnings—*and these huge annual savings serve as loans for capital investment.* (6) *They manage their companies on long-term bases.* Companies plan 5, 10, even 20 years ahead, and they do not have to report to shareholders every 3 months as in the USA. The Japanese are more interested in growth and market share than profits. (7) *They have a pro-business government rather than the opposite.* The Japanese civil service employs only the best of the university graduates and as a consequence it represents a national elite. (8) *They have cooperative unions that seek harmony, not disharmony.* Each company, not each industry, has its own union. What is good for the company is usually good for the union. (9) *They have company managers (white collar workers) and government bureaucrats who work efficiently and extremely long hours.* Both managers and workers are dedicated, uncomplaining and attentive to detail. Workers have a virtual guarantee of lifetime employment. This fact inspires an almost tribal sense of loyalty. Promotion is by seniority only (age plus length of service), so there is never embarrassment from reporting to younger persons. Women comprise 5% of managers and 40% of factory workers. The chief motivation in Japanese workers is the pervasive desire for group approval. Laziness is a cause for being ostracized from the group and being excluded from the group is the greatest humiliation that any Japanese can imagine. (10) *They make decisions in a careful, thought-out manner with much consultation and consensus of viewpoint.*

And now back to Japanese medicine. Obviously it is difficult to be accepted as a student in one of the 6-year national or *perfecture* (province or state) *medical schools; each perfecture* has at least 1 medical school. Nearly all medical school professors are graduates of 1 of the 10 or so most promiment medical schools. About one-third of the 75 or so medical schools are private and most of the students at the private schools are sons or daughters of physicians. These private schools are extremely expensive, >$60,000 per year, and the educational quality is inferior to that of the public or national schools.[2] Clinical training of all medical students in Japan is primarily by lecture and books. Dr. Jules Constant of Buffalo, New York, who has travelled to Japan yearly for 17 years to teach cardiovascular-examining skills to new house officers at several Japanese hospitals, told me that little ward experience is received by medical students, and they are not allowed to touch, i.e., examine patients. Their physical examination skills are not learned until after graduation!

The internship is virtually limited to a speciality area, internal medicine, surgery, etc. The house officers work hard, and they are paid overtime for work after 5 PM. The overtime is on an honor system. At the end of each month each house officer simply tells the hospital administrator the number of hours he/she worked overtime that month and that's it.

The Japanese physicians in private practice work longer hours as a rule than do the university physicians, and many may not arrive home until midnight, 6 days a week, and leave home in the early AM. But in contrast to the low salaries of the university physicians, the private physicians' incomes are 10 to 20 times larger. Physicians in Japan receive substantial tax benefits, more favorable than any other occupation in Japan, presumably because the Japanese revere authority and physicians there are considered to hold a privileged position. They also are at the top of a list of tax cheaters that the Japanese government publishes. The Japanese physician does not have to worry about malpractice or intraprofessional disciplinary measures (peer review), but strong ethical behavior is expected. Collection of the medical bill is not a problem. All employed (>97% of eligible citizens) are insured by either private (60 million persons) or governmental (45 million persons) programs. The cost of medical care in Japan in 1986 was $120 billion. For the private employed patient, 90% of medical costs now are paid by the insurance fund. For dependents of such an individual, 80% of the bill is paid by the insurance fund. The governmental insurance covers 70% of medical costs. All medical bills for persons aged 70 and over are covered by insurance. Private practitioners and medical corporations bill the insurance groups directly. The more drugs dispensed by the physician, the higher the bill. Laboratory tests and radiographic examinations also increase the bill, but not in proportion to the number of prescriptions written or minor procedures performed. It probably is reasonable to spend 10% of medical costs on drugs. In Japan the costs of drugs apparently frequently reaches 40% of the medical costs. In general, however, the fees that are controlled by the government are much lower than in the USA, despite the fact that most other "purchases" are much more expensive than in the USA.

Views differ on whether or not there are sufficient numbers of physicians in Japan. They number about 170,000 and they use 1.3 million hospital beds. The average stay in a hospital in Japan in 1985 was 39 days. Patients with acute myocardial infarction stay at least 30 days, and those having coronary artery bypass grafting, about 40 days. Insurance covers the stay, whether long or short. Housing in Japan is so crowded that it is difficult to care for the sick at home, and patients prefer to stay in the hospital to decrease the family burden. As everywhere in Japan, the hospitals are clean, comfortable, and the food is good. The consequence is that nearly all Japanese hospitals have full occupancy and fully paid-for beds. The full occupancy, however, produces a waiting list of about 30 days for cardiac catheterization and cardiac surgery in many hospitals. Profits are improved for hospitals by not running laboratories on a 24-hour basis. The equipment is modern and medicine is very technologically oriented. Life expectancy at birth in Japan is the highest in the world: 73 years for males and 80 years for females. There are 13 births per 1,000 population and 6 deaths per 1,000. Fifteen percent of the Japanese population is over age 60 and just over 20% is under age 15.

Cardiovascular diseases in Japan are similar to those in the Western world but their frequencies are a bit different. Systemic hypertension, as in the USA, is their most frequent cardiovascular disease and coronary artery disease is next.[3–7] Despite its increase in the past 20 years, however, the frequency of coronary artery disease remains much less than in the USA. The serum total cholesterol level has risen roughly in proportion to the increased frequency of coronary artery disease, and the high-density lipoprotein level has dropped,[8–14] but obesity is uncommon in Japan, red meat is too expensive, and "living on the floor" as they do in their homes keeps them in relatively good physical condition. Consequently, it will be a long time, in my view, before their frequency of coronary artery disease in Japan reaches that in the USA. Moreover, systemic hypertension is now better controlled than in the past and cigarette smoking is on the decline.

William C. Roberts

William C. Roberts, MD
Editor in Chief

1. Editors of Time-Life Books. *Japan. Alexandria, VA: Time-Life Books, 1985:160.*
2. Gillespie CA, Gillespie HE, Carr JE. *Contrasts between Japanese and American medical education and clinical practice. Milit Med 1984;149:393–396.*
3. Robertson TL, Kato H, Rhoads GG, Kagan A, Marmot M, Syme SL, Gordon T, Worth RM, Belsky JL, Dock DS, Miyanishi M, Kawamoto S. *Epidemiologic studies of coronary heart disease and stroke in Japanese men living in Japan, Hawaii and California. Incidence of myocardial infarction and death from coronary heart disease. Am J Cardiol 1977;39:239–243.*
4. Robertson TL, Kato H, Gordon T, Kagan A, Rhoads GG, Land CE, Worth RM, Belsky JL, Dock DS, Miyanishi M, Kawamoto S. *Epidemiologic studies of coronary heart disease and stroke in Japanese men living in Japan, Hawaii and California. Coronary heart disease risk factors in Japan and Hawaii. Am J Cardiol 1977;39:244–249.*
5. Reed DM, Feinleib M. *Changing patterns of cardiovascular disease in the Pacific basin: report of an international workshop. J Community Health 1983;8:182–205.*
6. Prentice RL, Shimizu Y, Lin CH, Peterson AV, Kato H, Mason MW, Szatrowski TP. *Serial blood pressure measurements and cardiovascular disease in a Japanese cohort. Am J Epidemiol 1982;116:1–28.*
7. Sugiura M, Matsushita S, Ueda K. *A clinicopathological study on valvular diseases in 3,000 consecutive autopsies of the aged. Jpn Circ J 1982;46:337–345.*
8. Sekimoto H, Goto Y, Goto Y, Naito C, Yasugi T, Okido M, Kuzuya F, Takeda R, Yamamoto A, Fukuzaki H, Kajiyama G, Kokubu T, Uzawa H, Mimura G, Shimada O. *Changes in serum total cholesterol and triglyceride levels in normal subjects in Japan in the past twenty years. Research committee on familial hyperlipidemia. Jpn Circ J 1983;47:1351–1358.*
9. Okuni M, Hayashi K, Kiryu S, Yamauchi K. *Risk factors of arteriosclerosis in Japanese children. Jpn Circ J 1980;44:69–75.*
10. Blackburn H. *Diet and atherosclerosis: epidemiologic evidence and public health implications. Prev Med 1983;12:2–10.*
11. Keys A, Menotti A, Aravanis C, Blackburn H, Djordevic BS, Buzina R, Dontas AS, Fidanza F, Karvonen MJ, Kimura N, Mohacek I, Nedeljkovic S, Puddu V, Punsar S, Taylor HL, Conti S, Dromhout D, Toshima H. *The seven countries study: 2,289 deaths in 15 years. Pre Med 1984;13:141–154.*
12. Yano Y, Irie N, Homma Y, Tsushima M, Takeuchi I, Nakaya N, Goto Y. *High density lipoprotein cholesterol levels in the Japanese. Atherosclerosis 1980;36:173–181.*
13. Ueshima H, Lida M, Shimamoto T, Konishi M, Tanigaki M, Nakanishi N, Takayama Y, Ozawa H, Kojima S, Komachi Y. *High-density lipoprotein cholesterol levels in Japan. JAMA 1982;247:1985–1987.*
14. Chiba K, Koizumi A, Kumai M, Watanabe T, Ikeda M. *Nationwide survey of high-density lipoprotein cholesterol among farmers in Japan. Prev Med 1983;12:508–522.*

The Kingdom of Saudi Arabia, Oil, Money and Cardiology

Muayed A. Al Zaibag (Figure) is a bright and vigorous 36-year-old Saudi physician who directs the Adult Cardiology Division of the Cardiac Department of the Armed Forces Hospital in Riyadh, Saudi Arabia. He arrives at the hospital in his Mercedes-Benz each day about 7 A.M. and leaves for home about 12 hours later. Dr. Zaibag recently directed an International Cardiology Symposium in Riyadh and invited me to attend. At the meeting results of balloon valvuloplasty of the tricuspid, pulmonic, mitral and aortic valves at the Armed Forces Hospital were presented by Zaibag and his colleagues and invitees from other countries discussed thrombolysis, coronary angioplasty and catheter procedures for closing intercirculatory shunts. Dr. Zaibag and his associates probably have done more catheter balloon valvuloplasties than any group in the world. His catheterization laboratories are the best money can buy. About 200 balloon valvuloplasty catheters of all sizes, each costing about $150, are available in his laboratory. Indeed, the most advanced diagnostic and therapeutic equipment is present throughout his hospital, and the latest technologic equipment appears to be present in most hospitals in Saudi Arabia.

The Cardiac Department at the Armed Forces Hospital includes 4 divisions: Adult Cardiology headed by Dr. Zaibag; Pediatric Cardiology headed by Dr. M.A. Ali Khan, an expatriate; Cardiac Surgery headed by 39-year-old Saudi Dr. Mohamed R. Al Fagih, who also is Chairman of the Cardiac Department; and Cardiac Anesthesiology. Dr. Al Fagih's surgical results appear to be outstanding.[1] In 1986, he and his colleagues performed 874 cardiac operations including repair of various congenital anomalies of the heart and great vessels in 365 patients (mortality 6%); valve repair or replacement in 243 (mortality 2%); coronary artery bypass grafting with or without repair of complications of acute myocardial infarction in 109 (mortality 6%) and miscellaneous procedures in 157. One operation was a cardiac transplant. The operating room suites also are the best money can buy.

Saudi Arabia is the twelfth largest country in the world, and occupies four-fifths of the Arabian peninsula. The land area is somewhere between 830,000 and 870,000 square miles, about one-third the size of the U.S.A., but larger than Western Europe, i.e., the combined surface areas of Portugal, Spain, France, United Kingdom, Ireland and Belgium.[2–6] Saudi Arabia is bordered by the Red Sea on the west, primarily the Persian Gulf on the east, Jordan, Iraq and Kuwait on the north, and Yemen, South Yemen and Omar on the south. It was created essentially from nothing in this century by one man. Although only 2% of the land is arable, Saudi Arabia is now the most valuable piece of real estate on earth.[3]

Abdul Aziz (Ibn Saud), who was born about 1880 (2 years after my father's birth), began putting the Kingdom together in 1902 when he captured the Riyadh area. Thirty years later most of the Arabian peninsula was his and he named the country The Kingdom of Saudi Arabia. Until his death at age 77 in 1953, Abdul Aziz personally controlled virtually every aspect of life in his country. But life was simple then. The entire Kingdom had a population of less than 1 million and most of the people were wandering Bedoins. The city of Riyadh, a medieval walled city surrounded by greenery and then stark desert, was made the capitol. Its population was less than 30,000. Every 3 or 4 weeks the mail was delivered from the coast by truck and was dumped in a pile at a corner of the main mosque.[3]

Abdul Aziz had 42 legitimate sons. The present King is the fourth Abdul Aziz son on the throne, and the royal family, all of whom are related to Abdul Aziz, now numbers more than 4,000.[3]

The Saudi government, headed by the King who usually also is Prime Minister, has 21 ministries and their heads form the Council of Ministers, which is the King's cabinet.[5,6] There is no constitution, no parliament, no political parties, no elections, no political prisoners and no income tax. Also, there are no cinemas, no theaters and no alcohol. Half the population, namely women, who live behind the veil, have few rights: a woman cannot be in the sole company of a man to whom she is not related or married; her dress is strictly regulated; she cannot drive an automobile; and she has restrictions on her ability to work and to socialize.[3,7] The Islamic religious code is the law of the land and all citizens are Moslems. Their religion allows men to have as many as 4 wives. The present population is estimated to be about 11 million, but probably as many as 4 million are expatriates working for varying periods in Saudi Arabia.[2–6] The Saudi population is homogeneous in culture, ethnicity and language.[8–11] Despite its great wealth, Saudi Arabia has many characteristics of underdeveloped nations; it is largely rural (70%) and is undergoing rapid urbanization. The life expectancy is relatively short (54 years), the birth rate (44/1,000 population), the death rate (13/1,000 population) and the infant mortality rate (152/1,000 births) are all high, while the literacy rate (30% of adults) is low.[5,6,12]

Saudi Arabia is divided into 4 provinces (Hijaz, the western; Najd, the central; Asir, the southwestern; and Hasa, the eastern) and each has an appointed governor (Emir). Each city, however, receives its funds from the central government, which provides all utilities and necessary services. Oil provides nearly all of the government's revenues which in turn through contracts, salaries, loans, subsidies and gifts are the prime source of wealth in the economy. Most Saudi citizens work for the government (Civil Service) or Armed Forces (including the National Guard) and are well paid. The rest are in private business, of which they are the majority owner. Much of their development is dependent on work done by expatriates.

Oil was initially found in 1859 in Pennsylvania and for most of the next 100 years the U.S.A. was the major producer of oil in the world. The U.S.A. and the U.S.S.R. remain the largest oil producers, but their reserves are diminishing each year. Oil was found in Saudi Arabia in 1938 and although nearly 35 billion barrels (each barrel is 44 gallons) of Saudi oil have since been produced, each year more oil is found in Saudi Arabia than is retrieved.[3,4] In 1960, their oil reserves were 53 billion barrels and by 1986, they had swollen to 169 billion barrels, a quarter of the world's total known reserves and almost double the reserves of any other country. Saudi Arabia has at least 50 years of oil in the ground, and probably much more, and it will have vast reserves long after the U.S.A. and U.S.S.R. run out. By 1985, fifty-nine commercial oil fields had been discovered in Saudi Arabia, but over two-thirds of them have been capped for later use (stopcocks in the sand).[4] The average Saudi oil well produces 10,000 barrels a day and the oil flows from most of them without being pumped.[3] Thus, their oil is the cheapest to produce in the world. The average oil well outside Saudi Arabia produces less than 100 barrels a day and most require pumps to get the oil to the surface.[3] Saudi Arabia needs only about 10,000 workers, less than 1% of its national labor force, to retrieve its oil, and until recently oil has accounted for 90% of its government's revenues and 98% of its exports.

With oil, of course, came money. In 1946, crude oil production in Saudi Arabia was about 170,000 barrels a day and each barrel yielded the country 17¢. During the 1960s, each barrel of oil was just under $2.00; in 1970 it rose to $3.00 a barrel; in October 1973 it was just over $5.00 a barrel and 2 months later it rose to over $11.00, nearly 6 times the price of 4 years earlier. By 1974 Saudi Arabia was producing nearly 8.5 million barrels a day. Before October 1973, Saudi Arabia had an annual income of just under $9 billion a year. By April 1974 annual revenues were running at $34 billion. In January 1979, a barrel of Saudi oil was selling for $13 and by April 1979, when Saudi Arabia was producing over 9.5 million barrels a day, it had risen to $28 a barrel. Saudi oil production peaked in 1980 at 10.5 million barrels a day and the oil glut in the 1980s has caused her present production to be less than 4 million barrels a day and the price has fallen to $15 to $20 a barrel. In the early 1980s, Saudi Arabia earned in less than 1 week what it earned in a year before the 1973 oil embargo.[3] At their peak in 1981 the Saudi government was receiving approximately $300 million a day for its oil, equivalent to about $75 a day for every Saudi man, woman and child. Its currency reserves are probably the largest single block of cash floating in the world's money markets. Indeed, men raised in goatskin tents now dominate the world's money market. In a single generation, Saudi Arabia has been transformed from one of the poorest countries in the world to the richest of all. With the present drop in oil produced and the price received for oil, the 1988 Saudi budget of nearly $38 billion will require the borrowing of $8 billion.

The sharp increase in the price of oil in the early 1970s created a unique problem for Saudi Arabia. The problem was not how to raise money but how to spend it. At first, she deposited much of the huge cash inflow into Western banks only to see its value erode by inflation. Saudi Arabia, therefore, turned to development of its "infrastructure"—industry, creation and expansion of cities, refineries, ports, houses, schools, universities, hotels, hospitals, roads, railroads, airports, telephones and royal palaces. The new buildings were the best money could buy. Two industrial cities, Yanbu on the Red Sea and Jubail on the Persian Gulf, were raised from the empty desert to recognizable identities in less than a decade. Riyadh virtually overnight became a modern city with heavy traffic. Only 30 years earlier it is said to have had only one 4-wheel motorized vehicle. The first paved road came to Saudi Arabia in 1955. By 1985, there were 30,000 kilometers of highway and the Saudis were becoming better drivers. Traffic-related accidents decreased from 40/1,000 cars in 1972 to 11/1,000 cars in 1986; injuries per 1,000 cars dropped from 36 to 8 and deaths from 5 to 1. The Saudi Airline by 1986 numbered more than 90 aircraft, including 10 Boeing 747s, which carry nearly 15 million passengers a year. New airports were built in most major cities. The new Jeddah International Airport, opened in 1981, is half as large again as Kennedy, LaGuardia, Newark, O'Hare and Los Angeles airports put together; the Riyadh Airport opened in 1983 is even larger and the Dhahran Airport is larger still.[3] In terms of numbers of passengers, however, none of these airports is among the world's 50 busiest.[5] The first school for girls opened in 1956 and now about 700,000 Saudi girls attend primary and secondary schools and many now go on to tertiary schools. The first Saudi university was opened in 1957 and now there are 7 and tuition is free. By 1990, more than 100,000 students will be attending universities.[4] With less money and high costs of its military (over one-third of its budget) the days of massive spending on roads, utilities, industries, universities and agriculture in Saudi Arabia, at least for the moment, are clearly over.

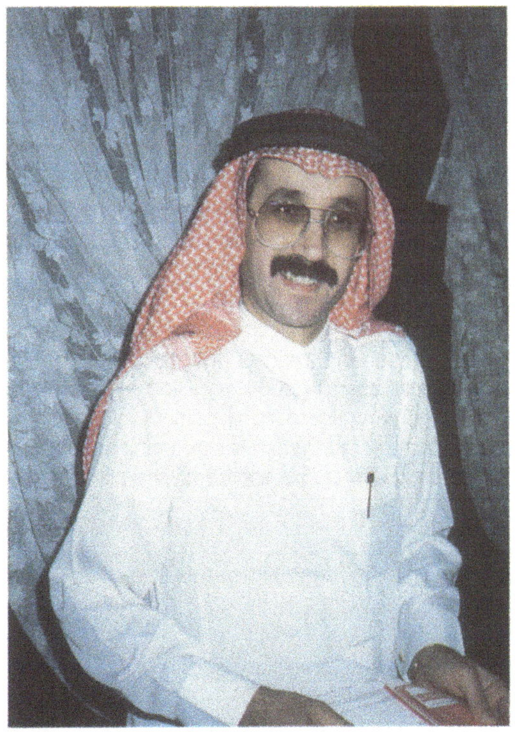

FIGURE. Dr. Muayed A. Al Zalbag.

Saudi Arabia has 4 medical schools, 1 in each province. The first class graduated in 1976; each graduates about 80 physicians a year and soon nearly 50% of the graduates will be women.[9–11] The medical school curriculum consists of 2 years in premedical courses, 2 years in medical (preclinical) courses and 2 years in clinical clerkships.The curriculum content resembles closely that found in the American and British medical education systems. In Saudi medical schools, all instruction, educational materials and examinations are in English. The female medical students are not permitted to intermingle with the male students; male instructors teach the female students in the preclinical years via television monitors while they teach the male students in person. Saudi Arabia currently is unable to provide training in medical and surgical specialities within its own borders for all its graduates. Consequently, many of its male graduates receive some training in other countries. (Saudi women physicians are prohibited from training in foreign lands unless accompanied by a male member of their family.) Medical students are paid with the understanding that they will practice medicine for 5 years in the public sector. After that some of them enter private practice and some actually leave medicine to become the legally and economically dominant "Saudi partner" in business ventures. There appears to be more financial reward in some of the nonmedical economic activities than in some medical practices. This gravition of some Saudi physicians into nonmedical businesses (automobile dealerships, apartment construction, video tape rentals, hotels) and into health-related businesses (establishment of private hospitals, clinics and pharmacies and importing of pharmaceuticals and medical equipment) is referred to as the "internal brain drain" in Saudi Arabia, and it will delay the time when Saudi patients are treated exclusively by Saudi physicians.[9] In 1981, there were about 5,300 physicians in Saudi Arabia but only about 10% were Saudis; the remainder were expatriate physicians mainly from Egypt, Pakistan and India. By 1990 it is estimated that the 4 Saudi medical schools will have graduated some 3,100 physicians.[11]

One of the greatest benefits flowing from Saudi Arabia's new wealth is the enormously improved health care that is free to all its citizens and to the nearly 1 million non-Saudi pilgrims who visit the Islamic holy places (Makkah and Medina) each year. By 1980, there were 87 well-equipped modern hospitals with almost 14,000 beds including a 1,000-bed hospital for tuberculosis and a 200-bed hospital for leprosy.[4] By 1986, the number of hospitals had increased to 157 with an estimated 29,000 beds, an average of 2.4 beds/1,000 population.[4] By 1990, the number of hospitals will be about 280 and the number of beds, about 55,000. Additionally, there are more than 1,450 primary health care centers. A comprehensive national medical record system is now being set up.[13] Virtually all nurses are expatriates but apparently there are plans to alter this situation.[7,14–17] (Likewise, all Saudi Airline stewardesses are expatriates.)

It is thought that many Saudi women hesitate to seek medical services to avoid what would be for them a very stressful encounter with a male physician.[8] Therefore, to facilitate access to medical care for a significant segment of the population and to preserve Islamic standards of sexual modesty, the Saudis are making some compromises in cultural tradition, women physicians being one of them.

Thus, in a single generation Saudi Arabia has become a world financial power and the leader of the Muslims who now number nearly 1 billion persons. It is good that the Royal family is sharing its wealth with its citizens.

William C. Roberts

William C. Roberts, MD
Editor in Chief

References

1. Mashat EM, Al-Fagih MR, Wareham EE. *Review of valvular cardiac surgery at the Riyadh Armed Forces Hospital. 1985;30:211–216.*
2. Azzi R. *Saudi Arabia: the Kingdom and its power. National Geographic 1980;158:286–333.*
3. Lacey R. *The Kingdom. Arabia & the House of Sa'ud. New York: Avon, 1981:631.*
4. Schofield D, Editor-in-Chief. *The Kingdom of Saudi Arabia, 7th edition. London: Stacey International, 1986:256.*
5. Hoffman MS, ed. *The World Almanac and Book of Facts 1987. New York: World Almanac, 1986:928.*
6. Johnson O, executive ed. *Information Please ALMANAC Atlas & Yearbook 1988, 41st edition. Boston: Houghton Mifflin, 1988:976.*
7. Milne M. *Practising overseas: there's more to it than the money. Can Med Assoc J 1986;135:1164–1171.*
8. Dubovsky SL. *Psychiatry in Saudi Arabia. Am J Psychiatry 1983;140:1455–1459.*
9. Searle CM, Gallagher EB. *Manpower issues in Saudi health development. Milbank Mem Fund Q Health Soc 1983;61:659–686.*
10. Gallagher EB, Searle CM. *Cultural forces in the formation of the Saudi medical role. Med Anthropol 1984;8:210–220.*
11. Gallagher EB, Searle CM. *Health services and the political culture of Saudi Arabia. Soc Sci Med 1985;21:251–262.*
12. Chattopadhyay K, Sengupta BS, Chattopadhyay C, Zaidi V. *Maternal mortality in Riyadh, Saudi Arabia. Br J Obst Gynecol 1983;90:809–814.*
13. Burney FA, Jamil ATM. *Computerized patient visit data analysis for the outpatient department of Jeddah General Hospital. J Med Systems 1984; 8:571–577.*
14. White J. *Advertisements for posts in Saudi Arabia. N Engl J Med 1983;309:991–992.*
15. Al-Matroudi M. *Employment in Saudi Arabia. N Engl J Med 1984; 311:263–264.*
16. Perkins MT. *Nursing inservice education in Saudi Arabia. J Cont Ed Nurs 1985;16:44–46.*
17. McFarlane C. *Working Abroad. Nursing Time 1987;83:26–28.*

Argentina and Argentine Cardiology

Jorge L. (Figure), a 44-year-old Assistant Professor of Medicine at the University of Buenos Aires, is in charge of the exercise laboratory of the hospital of the University of Buenos Aires (Hospital de Clínicas). Each morning with his 3 assistants he performs about 10 exercise stress tests and makes consultations to the 4 general medical services for the Division of Cardiology. After lunch he goes to his private office only a few blocks away and there he sees private patients until about 9 P.M. He then goes home except for 1 night a week when he lectures at a cardiac society meeting. Dinner with his wife and 2 daughters is usually about 10 P.M. and he retires to bed at midnight. On Saturdays and Sundays he usually makes hospital ward rounds to see his private patients. For his services at the University Hospital he receives $200 (US dollars) a month.

Jorge R. (Figure) is a 40-year-old cardiologist in the echocardiography laboratory at the same hospital. He also arises about 7 A.M. and arrives at the hospital about 8:30 A.M. He and the other 3 echocardiographic cardiologists perform about 15 echocardiograms each morning. (It is cost effective to the hospital for physicians to perform echocardiograms. There are no technicians.) He drives 30 minutes home to have lunch with his family, and, at 3 P.M., goes to his private office a block from home. There he sees patients until 7 or 8 P.M., and then home for dinner with his wife and 3 children at 9 P.M. For his work in the echocardiographic laboratory at the hospital he is paid $100 a month. In contrast to Jorge L., Jorge R. does not have a professional position in the medical school—although he teaches in the school—because he chose not to take the 4 years of courses on teaching required by the university for professional rank. Neither his pay nor his duties at the hospital, however, are affected by his not fulfilling the course work in techniques of teaching. The lack of professional rank prevents him from ever becoming chief of the cardiology division, but he says that position is of no interest to him.

I met Jorge L. and Jorge R. during a 2-day visit to Buenos Aires in May 1988. It was my fourth trip to Argentina and I will return as often as I am invited. Buenos Aires is one of the great cities on this planet, but it is a long way from the USA. Moscow is closer to New York City than is Buenos Aires, which is on the same latitude (35° South) as Capetown, South Africa, Sidney, Australia, and Auckland, New Zealand. Argentina has the potential to be one of the earth's great countries. Its land area is extensive, 1,000,000 square miles, one-third the size of the USA, and its soil is as fertile as any in the world.[1-3] Despite its being the eighth largest country in the world, Argentina's population is relatively small, only 33 million, 10 million of whom live in the Buenos Aires area and 2 million of whom live abroad.[4,5] The population is relatively homogenous; 97% are of European origin.[2] The average Argentine is said to be "an Italian who speaks Spanish and thinks British."[2] Over 90% of the population is Catholic. Growth rate is low, only 1% a year, and literacy rate is high, >90%.[4,5] Life expectancy for men is 67 years and for women, 73 years. The birth rate is 25/1,000, death rate 9/1,000 and infant mortality is 50/1,000 births.[4,5]

The northern portion of Argentina is heavily wooded and swampy (Gran Chaco); the central portion, where most of the people and cows live, is treeless and wheat or grass covered (6 feet thick topsoil) (pampas) and the southern portion is bleak, arid, cool (Patagonia) and contains millions of penguins and sheep.[3] Its western portion is mountainous and contains some of the best ski slopes and most spectacular scenery in the world. One snowy peak is nearly 23,000 feet high. The country produces enough oil for its own needs including enough for its 5 million motorized vehicles, and its agricultural output at one time was so great that Argentina was called "the breadbasket of the world."

Buenos Aires is a cosmopolitan city with 42 theaters, 200 movie houses, numerous museums and galleries and 150 parks. Its residents, called *Porteños* (of the port) are as educated, sophisticated and urbane as any on earth.[3] The classy *calle Florida*, a fashionable shopping street, competes well with those of Florence, Paris, London or New York. Few populations read more than do the Argentines. Philosophizing and flirting are said to be their 2 most popular activities, with soccer a close third.

Argentina won its independence from Spain in 1810. By 1880 it had killed nearly all Indians living in Argentina and the victorious military officers were rewarded by the government with huge parcels of land, commonly >100,000 acres. The country then began seeking immigrants from Europe and during the next decade about 1.5 million Spanish, Italians and some Germans and English settled in Argentina. The British built their railroads and later their telephone system, which facilitated rapid movement of their produce and cattle to port. By the early 20th century, Argentina was one of the 10 richest countries on earth.[1]

Today, Argentina—educated, sophisticated, homogenous and captivating—is broke. She is the third most

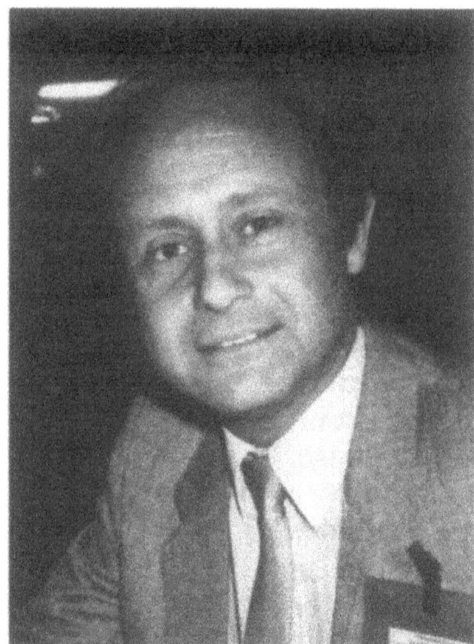

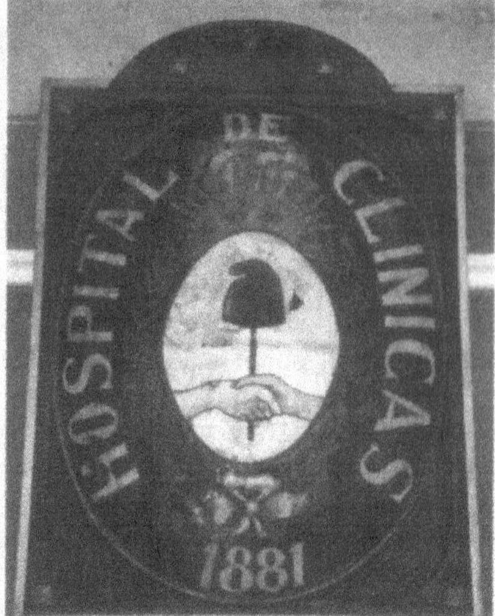

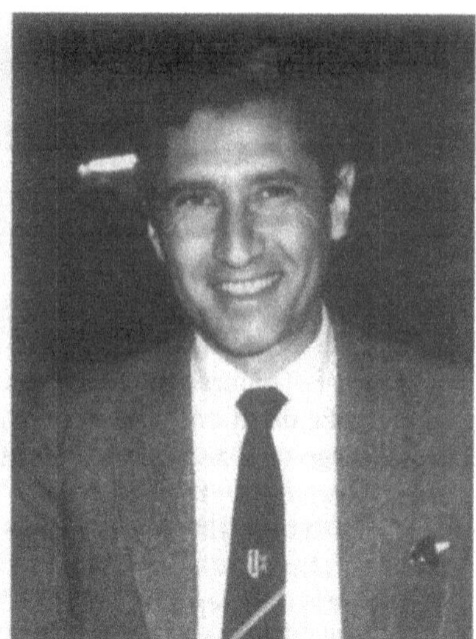

FIGURE. Jorge L. (*left*), Jorge R. (*right*) and the symbol of their hospital (*center*).

indebted nation in the world, owing $54 billion (US) dollars, and the interest on the debts takes 50% of her export income. What happened? Many blame the rule and residue of Juan Perón who came to power in 1946. He spent far more money than his government collected. Strong labor unions were established and output per worker fell. Perón was gone by 1955 but not his influence. His brief return in 1973 was as devastating as his earlier regime, and subsequent military regimes were just as corrupt and harsher. Democracy returned in 1983 but it will probably be many years before stable growth reappears. The annual inflation rate was nearly 700% in 1984 (about 2% a day) and down to 175% in 1987.

The unstable government and economy of Argentina during the past 50 years have had devastating effects on its medicine.[6] Argentina has 6 medical schools. The largest is the University of Buenos Aires, which has an open admission policy and free tuition and as a result its freshman class now contains about 5,000 students. (During Perón's last year in office [1974], the freshman medical school class at the University of Buenos Aires had 17,000 students, and 6 years later 2,500 graduated.) Now, by the beginning of the second year, the class size is down to 3,000; by the beginning of the fourth year (the first of the 3 clinical years), the class is down to 2,000, and after the sixth year, the number of graduates is about 1,500. Students are allowed to take the final examination for graduation up to 3 times. The other 5 medical schools have smaller graduating classes, each about 200 students, so that Argentina is producing each year about 2,500 new physicians. There are residency (no internships) slots in Argentina for only about 30% of its medical school graduates. Thus, 70% of the graduates go into practice directly from medical school, nearly always as salaried employees of 1 or several state or private health care institutions. The residency slots are awarded by scores on examinations and 1 interview and the training positions are usually in public hospitals.

One such hospital is that of the University of Buenos Aires, officially called Hospital de Clínicas José de San Martín. This hospital has a capacity for >1,000 beds but presently only 400 are used because of severe budgetary restrictions. With a few exceptions, equipment in the hospital is old. The exercise laboratory, which Jorge L. directs, has 2 treadmills. The echocardiographic laboratory, where Jorge R. works, has 2 machines doing both M-mode and cross-sectional echocardiography. The number of outpatients at this public hospital is large. In the hospital's cardiac catheterization laboratory about 15 procedures are done weekly and 2 to 3 open heart surgical procedures are performed weekly. The faculty at the University of Buenos Aires hospital is an A.M. one in that the faculty physicians are at the hospital from roughly 8 A.M. to 12 noon and then they go to their private offices after lunch. About half of the faculty have taken the necessary courses in teaching so that they have professional rank; the other half, who have equal teaching and service responsibilities, have not taken the courses in teaching and therefore they do not have professional rank. The faculty, professional rank or not, is paid $100 to $300 a month for work at the public hospital, after initially having worked for 5 or more years without pay. The large numbers of medical students prevent close supervision of students by the faculty. Ward rounds often consist of 1 faculty physician, 1 resident and 20 medical students. Lectures may be to as many as 1,500 students.

Cardiology training consists of 1 year of residency in internal medicine, 3 years of clinical training in cardiology, followed by 2 years of A.M. courses in cardiology at the University. When the clinical training is completed, however, there is no assurance of a faculty post and private practice in all cities in Argentina now is enormously competitive. Argentines who can afford private medicine are hospitalized in private hospitals that are far better equipped than are the public (teaching) hospitals. Most coronary bypass operations are performed at the private hospitals. The top 10 cardiovascular surgeons in Argentina may bill as much as $15,000 (US dollars) for a bypass operation for a private patient. Most patients, however, have some form of health insurance, and some of these policies pay as little as $700 for a bypass operation. About 5,000 coronary bypass operations and 90,000 percutaneous transluminal coronary angioplasty procedures were performed in Argentina in 1987. The bill to a private patient for coronary angioplasty is about $3,500. Most physicians in Argentina, however, are much poorer today than in the late 1960s;[6] the government pays only $3.00 for a private patient's visit to a private physician. Many physicians no longer recommend the medical profession to their children, and it will be many years before their outlook will change significantly either economically or academically.

Atherosclerotic coronary artery disease is the leading cause of death in Argentina, and, indeed, Argentine men have one of the highest coronary artery disease mortality rates (604/100,000) in the world.[7] The mortality rate for coronary artery disease in women (155/100,000) in Argentina is also one of the highest in the world.[7] The mean serum total cholesterol levels of Argentine middle-aged adults is high (241 ± 53 mg/dl in men and 235 ± 45 mg/dl in women).[8] Few people eat more beef than do the Argentines—an average of nearly 100 kg/capita/year. The calorie supply per capita in Argentina also is high (about 3,350), similar to that in the USA, West Germany, United Kingdom and Finland.[8] Systemic hypertension is frequent in Argentines, and only about 15% of its hypertensive patients are having their blood pressure controlled by antihypertensive agents.[8] Cigarette smoking is the rule among Argentine adults; the average number of cigarettes smoked is about 2,000/adult/year.[8] Forty percent of the adult Argentine population is overweight, and a similar percent of adults do not exercise.[8]

Argentine medicine has been enormously affected by the disruption in the Argentine government and economy. For medicine to return to its pre-1950 glory, the medical school faculty must be paid sufficiently so that private practice for half the day will be unnecessary; the number of its medical students must be enormously curtailed and stringent admission requirements must be established; modern diagnostic and therapeutic equipment is needed, and a drastic change in eating habits must occur for blood lipid and pressure levels to be drastically lowered. These changes unfortunately appear far away. The cheapest way for Argentina—as for any developed nation—to improve the health of its citizens is to decrease its intake of saturated fat, cholesterol and salt. For a nation raised on beef, butter, milk and cheese, the challenge is a great one.

William C. Roberts

William C. Roberts, MD
Editor in Chief

1. Scobie JR. *Argentina. A City and a Nation, second edition. New York: Oxford University Press, 1971:323.*
2. Nelson CB, editor. *Fodor's South America 1982. New York: Fodor's Modern Guides, Inc., 1982:630.*
3. La Argentina, un país maravilloso. *Buenos Aires: Manrique Zago, 1982:156.*
4. Johnson O, executive editor. *Information Please Almanac Atlas & Yearbook 1988, 41st edition. Boston: Houghton Mifflin, 1988:976.*
5. Hoffman MS, editor. *World Almanac and Book of Facts 1987. New York: World Almanac, 1987:928.*
6. Argentina: inflation vs medicine. *Medical World News 1976 (April 15):81–84.*
7. Hauger-Klevene, Balossi EC. *Coronary heart disease mortality and coronary risk factors in Argentina. Cardiology 1987;74:133–140.*
8. Neuman J, de Neuman MP, Valero E, Lindental D. *Epidemiology of coronary heart disease risk factors in a free-living population. Prev Med 1979;8:445–446.*

To Our Readers...

This issue inaugurates a redesign of the *Journal.* We hope you like it and we welcome your comments.

William C. Roberts

Brazil and Brazilian Cardiology

Dr. P. L. da Luz (Figure 1), a 48-year-old clinical cardiologist in Sao Paulo who spent 5 years in cardiology at Cedars-Sinai Hospital in Los Angeles earlier in his career, arises about 6:30 A.M. and arrives at the Joao Paulo II Heart Institute of the University of Sao Paulo's Hospital das Clinicas about 8:00 A.M. He is one of 200 physicians on the staff of the Heart Institute and he is one of few involved in research. He directs an active and productive research laboratory until about 2 P.M. Then he, like nearly all of his faculty colleagues, goes to his private office where he sees patients until about 8 or 9 P.M. Then home for dinner at about 9:30 with his lovely wife and 2 sons. Weekends are spent mainly relaxing and playing tennis. For his work at the Heart Institue Dr. da Luz is paid $1,000 (US dollars) a month.

I recently had a 3-day visit to Sao Paulo, my fourth trip to Brazil, where I participated in a cardiology meeting organized by Professor F. Pileggi (Figure 1), director of the Heart Institute, and Dr. da Luz. Sao Paulo is Brazil's big apple, the pride of Brazilians. Nothing of importance happens in Brazil that does not begin in Sao Paulo. Brazilia may be the country's capital, Rio de Janeiro may have the beauty, but politically, economically and culturally, Sao Paulo is the number 1 city in the country, the largest (14 million), the fastest growing and the wealthiest metropolis of all South America.[1] It is already 3 times the size of Paris, and by the year 2000 it is expected to have a population of 26 million.[1] Paulistanos, as natives of the city are called, work hard, play hard and demand the best in shopping, restaurants and entertainment. Sao Paulo is a cross between New York and Los Angeles. It sprawls over 590 square miles, is covered by a semipermanent blanket of smog and is connected by a giant freeway system. Concrete skyscrapers up to 42 stories high dominate the horizon, and traffic clogs the streets. Seventy percent of Sao Paulo inhabitants are descendents of immigrants, mainly from Portugal, Italy and Japan, and most arrived from 1885 to 1915.[1] Sao Paulo has 1.2 million Japanese, their largest community outside of Japan.[1] Another wave of Europeans arrived after World War II, while transplants from Brazil's interior and impoverished northeast arrive daily. The area is blessed with cheap electrical power, mainly hydroelectric, so industries thrive. Sao Paulo, 600 feet above sea level, has a direct "downhill" railway to the seaport town of Santos (only 30 miles away). Sao Paulo's elevation allows

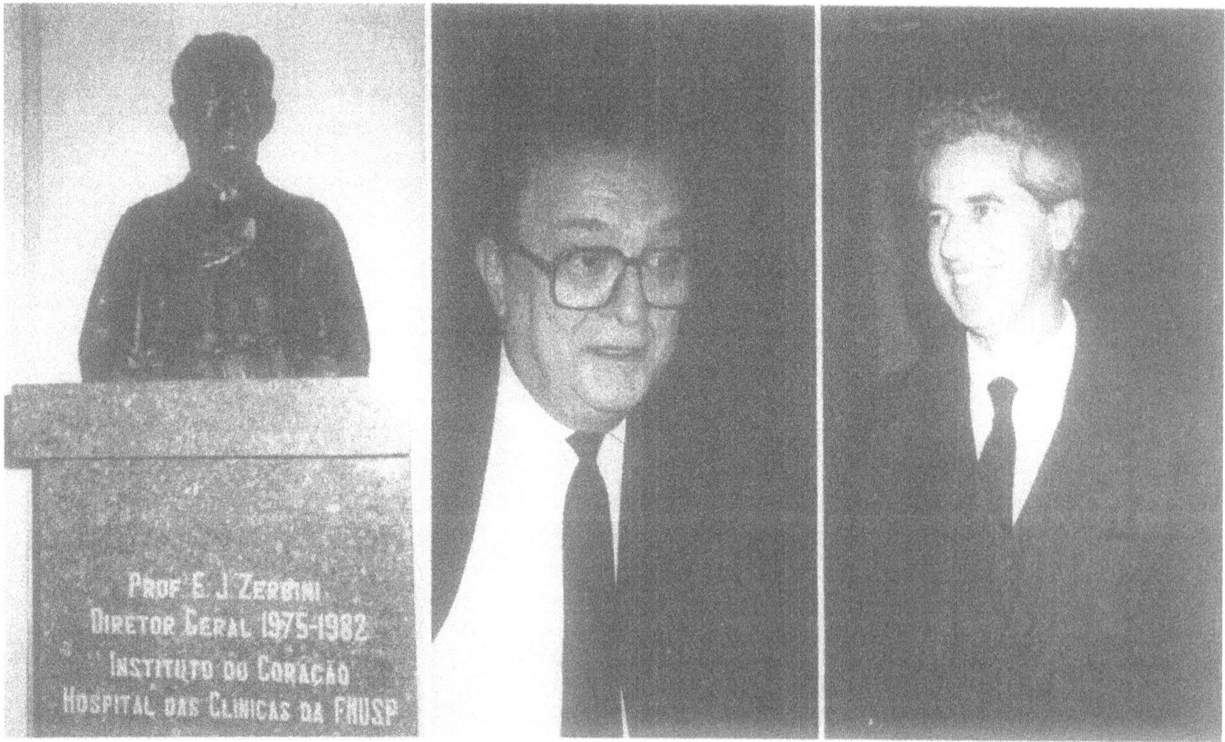

FIGURE 1. Statue of Professor E. J. Zerbini, the founder of the Joao Paulo II Heart Institute of the University of Sao Paulo's Hospital das Clinicas (*left*), Professor Fulvio Pileggi, the present director (*center*), and Dr. P. L. da Luz, a prominent member of the Institute's staff (*right*).

a drier climate than the rest of Brazil, and although 4 seasons occur in Sao Paulo, its plants and trees are green all year long.

The country of Brazil occupies nearly half the land area of the continent and produces 50% of the agricultural and industrial might of South America. Its land area is nearly 3,290,000 square miles, making it the fifth largest country in the world, with an area larger than that of the contiguous 48 states of the USA.[2,3] Despite its size, only 17% of the land is arable.[2,3] Its Atlantic coastline stretches 4,600 miles. The equator crosses near the northern border of Brazil, and the tropic of Capricorn, near the southern border. The *North* region (Figure 2) (42% of the country) is the heavily wooded Amazon basin, one of the least populated regions of the world and the source of half the oxygen on this planet.[4] The Amazon River is 4,000 miles long, 2,100 of which are located in Brazil.[5] The river, the largest in the world, is larger than the next 8 largest rivers in the world combined.[5] Its flow is 60 times greater than that of the Nile and 10 times greater than that of the Mississippi.[5] The Amazon is up to 2 miles wide and up to 200 feet deep.[5] Some of its feeder streams are larger than the Mississippi. In contrast to the wet Amazon region, which during rainy season floods the land for 50 miles on each side of the river, the *Northeast* region of Brazil is semiarid scrubland periodically parched by drought, and it is heavily settled and poor.[4,6] The *Southeast* region, which contains Rio de Janeiro, is mountainous and loaded with minerals, small (<15% of the land area) and crowded (33% of the population).[7] The *South*, where Sao Paulo is located, is the most highly developed part of Brazil. It has 10% of the land, 35% of the population and produces half of the nation's coffee, cotton, fruits and vegetables, and contains most of its industry.[1] The *Central West* region, where Brazilia is located, contains vast fields with short stubby trees, 22% of the land area and 5% of the population.[5,8]

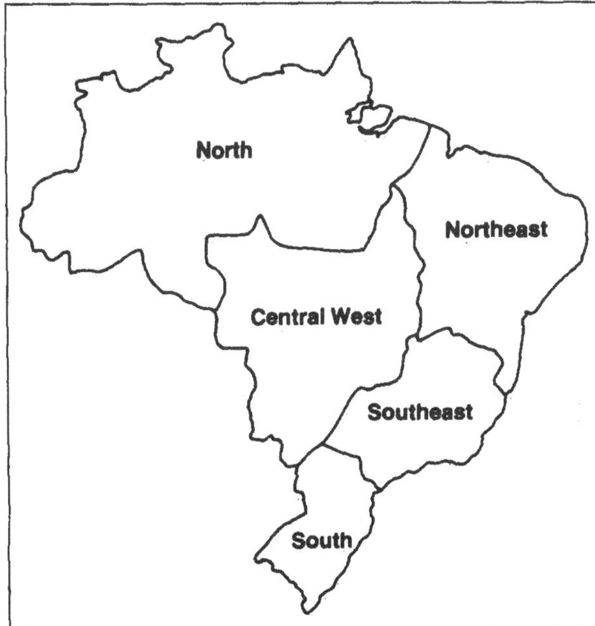

FIGURE 2. Map of the 5 major regions of Brazil.

Brazil has many similarities to the USA. Both are huge countries in both land and people. Brazil has a population of 140,000,000, the USA, 240,000,000. Both have heterogeneous populations, mainly from Europe and Africa. Brazil is 60% white, 26% mestizo and 11% black. The USA was discovered by the Spanish in 1492, and Brazil by the Portuguese in 1500. Both imported slaves from Africa. It took a civil war to abolish slavery in the USA in 1863, and it was done peacefully in Brazil in 1885. As in the USA, the European discoverers found many Indians, estimated to be 2 to 5 million, on the land that became Brazil.[9-11] The Indians in both countries died from white European's diseases and brutality so that today only about 190,000 to 230,000 Indians remain in Brazil. Initially, Brazil had its sugar cane in the northeast (today alcohol from the cane supplies 40% of the fuel for motorized vehicles in Brazil) and the USA had its tobacco in the southeast. Later, rubber in the Amazon became Brazil's gold, and now it is the industry and coffee in the south.

Today in Brazil a few have great wealth but most live in great poverty. Most Brazilians in the cities have an education that goes only to the eighth grade and most in the country's interior have <4 years of schooling.[1] The country is the developing world's largest debtor with about $110 billion owed to public and private foreign lenders.[12] The government is cash-strapped and only recently renegotiated a portion of its huge international debt so that it can again start paying its international bills and making domestic investments. It had stopped paying interest on its foreign debt about 19 months ago. Its inflation rate is sky high. In July 1988, the inflation rate was 24% in that month alone or nearly 1% a day, and it is likely that the inflation rate for all of 1988 will be over 300%. Its government spends too much money, and it is widely believed that its leaders place some of the public funds in their private accounts. The population growth rate is 2.5%, which means that there are about 3 million new Brazilians each year. About 40% of the population is <15 years of age.[3] There are not enough jobs for all the people and crime has become a problem. About 500,000 homeless children roam the streets of Sao Paulo and they live on their stolen wares, and in Rio the number is even greater. Rio de Janeiro is said to have more crime than any city in the world.

Despite these problems, Brazil is making giant strides. Already, its economy ranks eighth largest in the free world, and Brazilian exports sell well enough abroad that its trade balance is said to be positive.[1]

Medical care in the large cities of Brazil appears to be excellent. In some small interior towns medical care may be absent. In 1974, there were 63,000 physicians in Brazil.[1] Today, because of its 76 medical schools, about half of which are public (no tuition) and half of which are private, there are about 120,000 physicians, or about 8,000 new physicians each year. Now the large cities have too many physicians. For every place in the public (state) medical schools, there are about 40 applicants who take the written examination. Of them, 37 are eliminated and the remaining 3 take further examinations, and 1 of the 3 is chosen. The students enter the 6-year medical school immediately following completion of their 11 years of primary and secondary schools. The first 2 years of medical school are devoted to the basic sciences, the third and fourth years to clinical work and the last 2 years are a general medical "internship". Those graduates wishing to specialize do so after completion of the general medical internship.

There are 5,000 to 6,000 cardiologists in Brazil. After 1 year of a general medical residency, which begins after the 2-year internship, 2 years are spent in clinical cardiology. These 2 years do not involve time in cardiac catheterization, nuclear cardiology, echocardiography or electrophysiology, so to be a cardiologic subspecialist, 2 additional years in a subspecialty are required. In contrast to cardiologists in the USA, a hemodynamist in Brazil spends his/her entire time in the cardiac catheterization laboratory.

About 400 cardiac surgeons work in Brazil and they form about 50 "pump teams". Cardiac surgical training consists of 2 years of general surgery after the 2-year internship, followed by 5 years in thoracic and cardiac surgery. At the Heart Institute in Sao Paulo the staff surgeons operate until 3 or 4 P.M., and then go to private hospitals where additional cardiovascular operations are performed.

The enormously impressive Heart Institute of the University of Sao Paulo, where Dr. da Luz works, is a thoroughly modern facility, probably the largest center in the world devoted entirely to patients with heart disease. It was founded by Professor E. J. Zerbini in 1975 (Figure 1). It contains 260 beds and construction is underway to increase that number to >400. Its outpatient clinic is large and busy. Nearly everything in the institute is computerized. About 40 to 45 cardiac catheterizations are performed daily, including several coronary angioplasty procedures; about 100 echocardiograms, 100 radiographic studies, 25 nuclear cardiologic studies and 10 cardiac operations are also performed daily. Several cardiac transplants have been performed. About 60% of the patients have coronary artery disease,[13-15] 20% valvular heart disease,[16] 15% congenital heart disease and about 5% miscellaneous types.[17,18] Systemic hypertension also is common.[19-25] Chagas' disease now has been eradicated from Sao Paulo state, but patients in other areas of Brazil still acquire this condition and some of them make their way to the Heart Institute in Sao Paulo.[24,25] The institute has a large bioengineering section which makes and tests cardiac valves. The internationally prominent Dr. Adib Jatene directs this section and he is also head of the department of surgery. The anatomic pathology department of the Institute has 7 full-time pathologists and they perform >500 necropsies a year.

Coronary artery disease is the most common cardiac disease in the cities of Brazil. Steak, milk, butter and cheese are plentiful, but the rich, obviously, eat more of these fats than do the poor. Steaks were served at both the splendid dinners I attended in Sao Paulo with physicians of the Heart Institute and their elegantly dressed spouses. There are 12 McDonald's in Sao Paulo, and 1 of them is the largest McDonald's in the world. It appears that coronary artery disease will be a problem in Brazil for a long time to come.

Brazil is an exciting and vigorous country and I hope to return.

William C. Roberts

William C. Roberts, MD
Editor in Chief

1. Liounis A, editor. Fodor's Brazil 1988. *New York: Fodor's Travel Publications: 1988:214.*

2. Hoffman MS, editor. The World Almanac and Book of Facts 1987. *New York: World Almanac, 1986:928.*

3. Johnson O, editor. Information Please ALMANAC Atlas & Yearbook 1988, 41st edition. *Boston: Houghton Mifflin, 1987:976.*

4. de Sa Moreira C. Brazil. *Singapore: Tien Wah Press, 1978:151.*

5. McIntyre L. Amazon. The river sea. *National Geographic 1972;142:445–494.*

6. Wilson J, Gahan GW. Drought bedevils Brazil's Sertao. *National Geographic 1972;142:704–723.*

7. McDowell B, De Vore N III. Brazil's golden beachhead. *National Geographic 1978;153:246–276.*

8. McIntyre L. Treasure chest or Pandora's box? Brazil's wild frontier. *National Geographic 1977;152:684–719.*

9. von Puttkamer WJ. Brazil's Kreen-Akarores. Requiem for a tribe? *National Geographic 1975;147:254–268.*

10. von Puttkamer WJ. Brazil's Txukahameis. Good-bye to the Stone Age. *National Geographic 1975;147:270–282.*

11. Lea V, Branco MR. Brazil's Kayapo Indians. Beset by a golden curse. *National Geographic 1984;165:674–694.*

12. Blustein P. Brazil's high-stakes debt talks: throwing good money after bad? *Washington Post, May 24, 1988.*

13. de Lolio CA, de Souza JM, Laurenti R. Decline in cardiovascular disease mortality in the city of S. Paulo, Brazil, 1970 to 1983. *Rev Saude Publica 1986;20:454–464.*

14. Guzman SV, Lopez-Grillo L, Dorossiev DL, Feh'er J, Rosenthal J. Cardiac rehabilitation in different geographic areas. *Adv Cardiol 1986;33:142–151.*

15. Lessa I, Cortes E, Souza JA, Souza Filho J, Netto JP, Almida FA. Epidemiology of acute myocardial infarction in Salvador, Brazil. *Bull Pan Am Health Organ 1987;21:28–37.*

16. Zerbini EJ. Results of replacement of cardiac valves by homologous dura mater valves. *Chest 1975;67:706–710.*

17. Carvalho FR, Matos S, Victor EG, Saraiva L, Brindeiro Filho D, Maranhao E, Moraes CR. Phonomechanocardiographic findings in endomyocardial fibrosis. *Angiology 1984;35:63–70.*

18. Amorim DS. Current status of myocarditis and endomyocardial biopsy in Brazil. *Heart Vessels 1985;(suppl 1):79–82.*

19. Ribeiro MB, Ribeiro AB, Neto CS, Chaves CC, Kater CE, Iunes M, Saragoca MA, Zanella MT, Ancao MS, Marson O, Kohlmann O Jr, Franco RJ, Nunes SF, Ramos OL. Hypertension and economic activities in Sao Paulo, Brazil. *Hypertension 1981;3(6 pt 2):II-233–II-237.*

20. Barbosa CA, Morton NE, Wette R, Rao DC, Krieger H. Race, height, and blood pressure in Northeastern Brazil. *Soc Biol 1983;30:211–217.*

21. Ribeiro MB. Hypertension among female workers in Sao Paulo, Brazil. Predictors and joint effects. *Hypertension 1983;5(6 pt 3):V144–V148.*

22. Ramos O. Malignant hypertension: the Brazilian experience. *Kidney Int 1984;26:209–217.*

23. Ribeiro AB, Ribeiro MB. Epidemiological and demographic considerations. Hypertension in underdeveloped countries. *Drugs 1986;31(suppl 4):23–28.*

24. Lewinsohn R. Carlos Chagas (1879–1934): the discovery of Trypanosoma cruzi and of American trypanosomiasis (foot-notes to the history of Chagas's disease). *Trans R Soc Trop Med Hyg 1979;73:513–523.*

25. Maguire JH, Hoff R, Sherlock I, Guimaraes AC, Sleigh AC, Ramos NB, Mott KE, Weller TH. Cardiac morbidity and mortality due to Chagas' disease: prospective electrocardiographic study of a Brazilian community. *Circulation 1987;75:1140–1145.*

India and Indian Cardiology

S.T. (Figure 1), 47 years old, is chief, department of cardiology, Kilpauk Medical College, Madras, India. He arises Monday through Saturday at 5:30 A.M. and arrives at the University Hospital at about 8:30 A.M. There he teaches, administers the department, reads echocardiograms, advises trainees on patient management and occasionally performs cardiac catheterizations until about 4 P.M. when he goes to his office in his home. There he sees private patients until about 10 P.M. He then dines with his wife, son of 18 and daughter of 16. The type of patients seen at the university hospital and in his home are quite different. About 7 of every 10 patients at the university hospital have either rheumatic or congenital heart disease; about 7 of every 10 patients in his private office have coronary artery disease. For his work at the hospital, he is paid the equivalent of $300 (US dollars) a month. He lives fairly well because of the income from his private practice. (The local government now is considering rescinding the right of professors at his university the opportunity to do private practice.) Dr. S.T. retires each day about midnight. His only day "off" is Sunday, but on this day, he goes to private hospitals to see his private patients, usually numbering about 20.

J.N. (Figure 1), 35 years old, is one of 11 staff cardiologists at the All India Medical Institute in New Delhi. He arrives at the hospital 6 days a week at about 7:30 A.M. From 8 to 8:45 he and his colleagues review with Dr. H.D. Tandon, chairman of the cardiology department and chief of the cardiothoracic center, findings from the various cardiologic procedures performed the previous day. Twice weekly he works from 2 to 8 P.M. in the general cardiology clinic, once weekly in the acute rheumatic fever clinic and once weekly in the coronary artery disease clinic. One month a year he serves as the cardiology ward attendant, and 1 month a year he works exclusively in the cardiac catheterization laboratory. The remaining time is spent in investigative endeavors, most of which involve serial endomyocardial biopsies in patients with rheumatic fever, endomyocardial fibrosis and aortitis. During the 2 years that Dr. J.N. was waiting for a faculty position (assistant professor) in the cardiology department, he fulfilled requirements for a PhD degree. He is now on a salary that cannot be supplemented by private practice. For a nominal fee, he is provided living quarters on the hospital campus.

I met Dr. S.T. in Madras where he, with Dr. Natesa G. Pandian (Boston, Massachusetts), had organized a superb cardiologic meeting. I met Dr. J.N. in New Delhi where his chief, Dr. H.D. Tandon (Figure 1), had invited me to give a named lecture. Madras is India's fourth largest city, located on the Southeastern coast (Figure 2), with a population of about 4 million. Delhi, the capital located in the North, is more sophisticated, more beautiful and larger (7 million). The trip, my first to India, provided the opportunity to meet many Indians and to learn of their country and their medicine.

India's land area (>1,260,000 square miles) makes it the seventh largest country in the world.[1,2] In the North, the Himalayas separate India from China, and more mountains separate India from Burma on the East. Also on the East is Bangladesh, wedged between the 2 Indian states of Assam and West Bengal. In the Northwest, Pakistan and a small hook of Afghanistan border India and separate it from the USSR. Stretching southward, India crosses the Tropic of Cancer, then tapers off into a peninsula with the Arabian Sea to the West and the Bay of Bengal to the East. The Himalayan range is dramatically high (to 29,000 feet). The Indo-Gangetic plain beginning south of the Himalayas is a flat rich alluvial area watered by the Ganges and its tributaries. The Southern peninsula is a high plateau (Deccan) with coastal strips.

The population of India is about 800 million, making it the world's second most populated country.[1,2] The population was about 350 million when the British left in 1947. About 40% of the population is <15 years of age and only 3% are >65 years of age.[3] The average annual growth rate of the population is 2%, which means 16 million additional human beings each year.[3] The birth rate (number per 1,000 per year) is 33, death rate is 12 and growth rate is 21.[3] The average number of children born per woman is 5. The infant mortality per 1,000 live births is 95. The average life expectancy of both males and females is 53 years.[3]

The average per capita income is $270 (US dollars).[3] About 75% of the population live in rural areas and about 25% in urban areas.[1] The literacy rate of adults is 36%.[3] The number of university graduates and beyond is about 10 million.[3] The unemployment rate is high and many with jobs are underemployed. The Indians speak many languages. The official national language is Hindi, but English is the associate language and the single common language. In cities English is spoken or understood by most people; in rural areas English is rarely spoken or understood. There are 16 major regional languages plus 250 minor regional (district) languages. Private schools in the urban areas usually are taught in English, and public schools, usually in the regional language; those in rural areas, usually in the regional language.

Religion is a major force in India and plays an integral part in everyday life.[2] Its influence and symbolism are visible everywhere. On city pavements, religious paintings are created from chalk, colored powder and petals. Shrines, where people offer homage, are located in streets. Dashboards of taxicabs are decorated with pictures of gods. Homes often contain niches to hold sacred pictures or idols. Religious men dressed in saffron robes covering bodies smeared with ash are commonly seen: some are silent, some preach and some sing religious songs. Religion has been the greatest inspiration for its architecture. Numerous temples are encrushed with carvings of gods, animals, plants and religious motifs. Religious festivals and rites take place throughout the year. Roughly 83% of the people are Hindu, 12% Moslem, 3% Christian, 2% Sikh, and the Buddhist, Jains and Zoroastrians are each <1%.[2] Hinduism is one of the world's most powerful religious and social forces, ruling its adherents' entire lives from ceremonies performed at birth to food, clothing, employment, marriage and death. Islam came to India with the Moslem invaders. Their population of 77 million in India is about the same as that of Pakistan.

India has about 300,000 physicians practicing modern (allopathic) medicine (about 1 physician for each 3,000 people) and another 300,000 practicing the indigenous systems of medicine (homeopathy, Ayurveda, Uuani, Naturopathy and Siddha).[3] The country has 106 medical schools producing 13,000 graduates each year.[3] In most medical schools, 25% of the positions are reserved for women and 5% are reserved for foreign applicants (Indians residing in South Africa or Nepal, for example). The number of students in each medical school is variable. At Dr. J.N.'s All Indian Medical Institute only 35 students are in each class. At Dr. S.T.'s Kilpauk Medical College 150 students are in a class. The largest medical school has as many as 300 students per class, and most have about 125 students. Of the 106 medical schools, 4 are federal, 86 are state (23 states in India) and the remainder are private. In the state and federal schools, the tuition is only $20 (US dollars) a year. Food costs the student only $250 a year, and lodging only about $12 a year. The competition to get in medical school is fierce. For the 35 positions at the All India Medical Institute, the best medical school in India, there are about 15,000 applicants, and the other medical schools—all of which are larger—have up to 25,000 applicants. All applicants must have completed 10 years of primary and secondary school and 2 years of undergraduate work at a university. Medical school is 5 years. Internship is compulsory and is a rotating one. About 50% of those finishing the internship go directly into practice, most often on salary at a government- or industry-run clinic; a few go into private practice. The other 50% go from internship into specialty training.

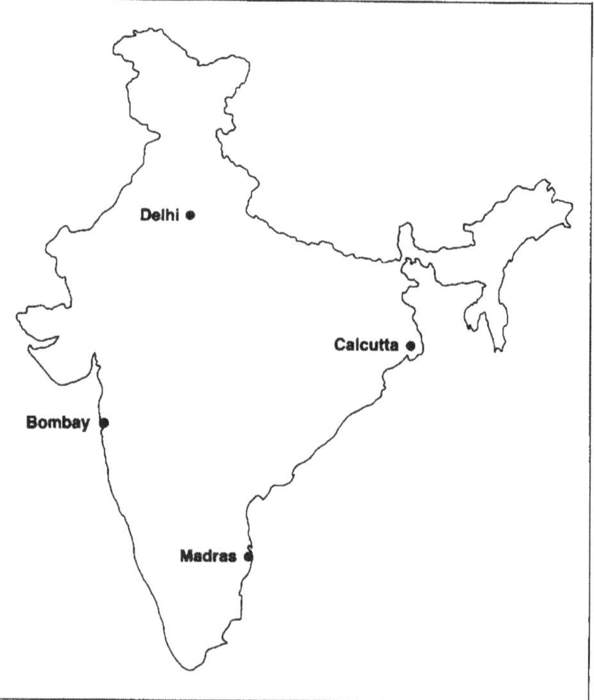

FIGURE 2. Map of India showing locations of the 4 largest cities.

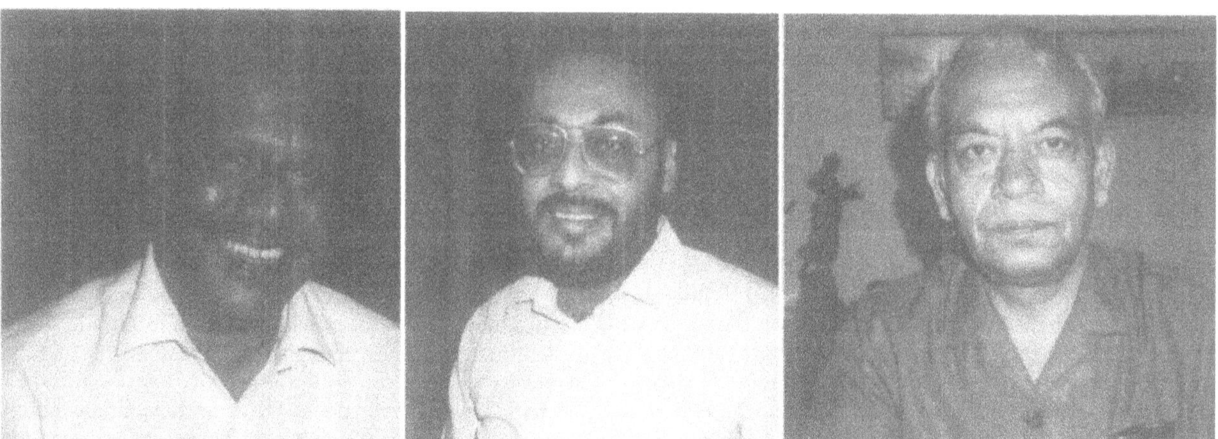

FIGURE 1. Photographs of Doctors S.T. (*left*), J.N. (*center*) and H.D. Tandon (*right*).

Trainees for specialty training are selected after written examinations and interviews. Both general internal medicine and general surgery require 3 years of training past internship. To become qualified in cardiology 3 years of cardiology fellowship are required, and to become qualified in cardiovascular surgery, 3 years of cardiovascular surgical training are necessary.

In the 12 cities in India with populations >1 million[3] there are too many physicians and it is difficult to begin a private practice. Many rural communities have no physicians despite the fact that there are about 40,000 unemployed physicians in India. Only about 25 fully qualified cardiologists and 25 fully qualified cardiovascular surgeons are produced each year in India. In all of India there are only about 200 board-certified cardiologists, although about 2,000 physicians call themselves cardiologists and limit their practices to cardiology. Only about 150 surgeons do cardiac operations in India, and of them only 115 are recognized by the Medical Council of India. Dr. Panangipalli Venugopal, chief of the cardiovascular surgical department at the All India Medical Institute, told me that there are 40 centers in India where cardiac operations are performed, but that only 15 of them meet optimal requirements (>200 open cardiac operations performed each year, etc.) delineated by The American College of Surgeons. Dr. Venugopal and his 6 associates have 4 operating rooms and they perform about 12 cardiac operations (8 open) each day. About a third are for coronary artery disease, a third for rheumatic heart disease and a third for congenital heart disease.

The cardiothoracic center of the All India Medical Institute is staffed by 11 full-time cardiologists and by 7 full-time cardiovascular surgeons. Each is on salary and each is supplied living quarters. Professor Tandon told me that several private cardiologists in New Delhi have a daily income equivalent to his monthly income. There are 90 cardiology beds and 90 cardiovascular surgery beds in the Cardiothoracic Center. Because the Institute, which has 2,000 total beds, is a federal hospital, patients come from the whole country. About 200 electrocardiograms, 25 echocardiograms, 50 chest radiographs, 6 exercise stress tests, 20 radionuclide studies, 7 cardiac catheterizations, 2 pacemaker insertions and 1 electrophysiologic study are performed each day.

Theoretically every Indian is entitled to receive free medical care. In the late 1970s, however, the most important hospitals began to levy direct charges to patients, usually in proportion to their means. At the All Indian Medical Institute all patients are charged for pharmaceuticals and for medical devices that are used by them and cannot be used by anyone else; for example, disposable oxygenators, artificial conduits, mechanical prosthetic valves and bioprostheses, balloon catheters for valvuloplasty, etc. Balloon catheters for percutaneous mitral valvulotomy in India cost 5,000 rupees; the entire cost for an operative closed mitral valvulotomy is 800 rupees, and, therefore, the latter procedure is performed far more commonly than the former. Most government employees have medical insurance that pays their medical bills. Employees in a few industries also have medical insurance, but most do not. The national railway company, the largest industry in India, has its own hospitals in big cities to provide free care for its employees; others can also be treated, but they have to pay. Most Indians in rural areas still rely on traditional medicine, which is cheap.

As in all developing countries, rheumatic fever and rheumatic heart disease are common in India.[4-12] It is estimated that >10 million of her children are afflicted. The frequency of congenital heart disease is probably similar to that in most other countries.[13-15] Systemic hypertension is not as common as in the Western world.[16-19] It is estimated that about 5% of its population >20 years of age have systemic arterial blood pressures >140/90 mm Hg. Although this percentage is much less than in the USA, 5% of 400 million still amounts to 20 million persons. Endomyocardial fibrosis, the condition initially described in Africa, is endemic in some areas in India.[20,21]

It is a bit surprising that coronary artery disease is as common as it is in India.[22-29] The meat of cows is rarely eaten in India, but there are over 180 million cows and their milk and butter are consumed freely. Cows are at peace in India in contrast to many in the USA. Gandhi said, "The greatness of a nation can be judged by the way its animals are treated" and the Indians do well with cows. It is not good, however, to be a chicken in India. During my 4 days in India, chicken was served at every meal, and it is by far the most common meat consumed in India. The chicken fat is eaten, not discarded. The goat is the second most common animal eaten in India. Coconut oil, which is 92% saturated fat, is the most common fatty acid consumed in India, presumably because it is relatively cheap. Many Hindus are vegetarians and obesity is uncommon.

India is a fast changing country. Many in the small rural villages are migrating to the large cities.[30-33] In big cities like Madras and New Delhi about 80% of the people live in houses or apartments with water and toilets. The rest live in huts or on streets, cook on open fires and have no electricity or water. In Bombay, and particularly in Calcutta, the situation is worse. By the year 2000, when India's population is expected to pass 1 billion, 3 cities—Bombay, Calcutta and New Delhi—are each projected to have at least 13 million, and more important, perhaps 95 cities are expected to top 1 million.[32,33] By 2000, about 30% or 300 million people will live in cities in India, and these figures mean massive traffic jams, crumbling, ill-maintained buildings and proliferating slums.[32,33] The situation in cities like Bombay and Calcutta is already so acute that progress is measured not in terms of new housing, but in the extent to which slums can be "regularized"—squatter's rights recognized and public water taps, community toilets and paved walkways with open sewers provided.[32,33] With rent control often limiting rents to 1948 levels, landlords often allow buildings to crumble, and then rebuild free of the rent restraints.

With these challenges to basic survival one has to question the need for cardiac surgery for a minute portion of the population.[34] Progress cannot come without population control, and this seems unlikely. India's problem also is a problem for the rest of us.

William C. Roberts

William C. Roberts, MD
Editor in Chief

1. Editors of Time-Life Books. India. *Alexandria, Virginia: Time-Life Books, 1987:160.*

2. Beresky AE, ed. Fodor's India Including Nepal. *New York: Fodor's Travel Publications, Inc., 1988:592.*

3. Pendse DR, editor, Statistical Outline of India 1988–89. *Bombay: Tata Services Limited, Department of Economics and Statistics, 1988:227.*

4. Nair DV, Kabir HA, Thankam S. Epidemiological survey of rheumatic heart disease in children at Alleppey. *Indian Heart J 1980;32:65–71.*

5. Koshi G, Benjamin V, Cherian G. Rheumatic fever and rheumatic heart disease in rural south Indian children. *Bull WHO 1981;59:599–603.*

6. Agarwal BL. Rheumatic heart disease unabated in developing countries. *Lancet 1981;2:910–911.*

7. Arora R, Subramanyam G, Khalilullah M, Gupta MP. Clinical profile of rheumatic fever and rheumatic heart disease: a study of 2,500 cases. *Indian Heart J 1981;33:264–269.*

8. Sanyal SK, Berry AM, Duggal S, Hooja V, Ghosh S. Sequelae of the initial attack of acute rheumatic fever in children from North India. A prospective 5-year follow-up study. *Circulation 1982;65:375–379.*

9. Padmavati S. The challenge of rheumatic fever and rheumatic heart disease in India. *Indian Heart J 1982;34:364–366.*

10. Mathur KS, Wahal PK. Epidemiology of rheumatic heart disease—a study of 29,922 school children. *Indian Heart J 1982;34:367–371.*

11. John S, Bashi VV, Jairaj PS, Muralidharan S, Ravikumar E, Sathyamoorthy I, Babuthaman C, Krishnaswamy S, Cherian G, Sukumar IP. Mitral valve replacement in the young patient with rheumatic heart disease. Early and late results in 118 subjects. *J Thorac Cardiovasc Surg 1983;86:209–216.*

12. Randhawa PS, Chopra P, Tandon HD. Pulmonary parenchymal changes in rheumatic mitral stenosis in India with special reference to the juvenile group. *Indian J Chest Dis Allied Sci 1983;25:273–279.*

13. Shrestha NK, Padmavati S. Congenital heart disease in Delhi school children. *Indian J Med Res 1980;72:403–407.*

14. Kinare SG, Sharma S. Congenital heart disease in first year of life (an autopsy study of 270 cases). *Indian J Pediatr 1981;48:745–754.*

15. Chadha SK, Thareja RN, Durairaj M, Alurkar VM, Rajan RS, Borcar JM, Palnitkar SD, Kelkar CK, Mitra TK, Khandekar SN, Prabhaharan SN, Kurian G. Surgery of congenital cardiac lesions in Armed Forces personnel. *Indian Heart J 1984;36:60–66.*

16. Wasir HS, Ramachandran P, Nath LM. Prevalence of hypertension in a closed urban community. *Indian Heart J 1984;36:250–253.*

17. Gupta SP, Siwac SB. Epidemiology of hypertension in a north Indian population based on rural-urban community surveys. *Jpn Heart J 1984;25:65–73.*

18. Wasir HS, Mohan JC. The challenge of mild hypertension. *Indian Heart J 1985;37:202–204.*

19. Sharma BK, Arora OP, Bansal BL, Sagar S, Khurana SK. Hypertension among the industrial workers and professional classes in Ludhiana, Punjab. *Indian Heart J 1985;37:380–385.*

20. Nair DV. Endomyocardial fibrosis in Kerala state. *Indian Heart J 1982; 34:412–417.*

21. Kartha CC, Sandhyamani S. An autopsy study of tropical endomyocardial fibrosis in Kerala. *Indian J Med Res 1985;82:439–446.*

22. Sharma SK, Shekhawat P, Madhok RK, Chadda VS, Goyal NK, Chadda S, Jain NC. Coronary prognostic index and early mortality of acute myocardial infarction. *Indian Heart J 1982;34:30–35.*

23. Kundu SC, Bhattacharjee TD, Banerjee D, Bose D, Ghosh S. Profile of myocardial infarction among the railroad workers in eastern India—a 6-year study. *Indian Heart J 1982;34:151–155.*

24. Kundu SC, Bhattacherjee TD, Majumdar S, Ghosh S, Banerjee D. Rehabilitation after myocardial infarction amongst the railroad workers in eastern India. *Indian Heart J 1983;35:98–102.*

25. Taskar SP, Iyyer IR, Nerurker SV, Sawant PN, Bhonsale DR, Kinare SG. Lipid profile in patients with myocardial infarction from the city of Bombay. *Indian Heart J 1983;35:169–171.*

26. Shanmugasundaram KR, Suresh S, Misra KP, Jayakrishnan TK. Plasma lipoprotein cholesterol in India in healthy persons and those with coronary heart disease. *Atherosclerosis 1983;46:129–135.*

27. Krishnaswami S, Richard J, Sathyamurthy I, Babu Uthaman C, Sukumar IP. Multivariate analysis of risk factors in coronary artery disease—predictive value in case detection in cardiovascular epidemiology. *Indian J Med Res 1984; 79:439–444.*

28. Kabi BC, Somani PN, Koteswara Rao GR. Serum triglyceride and lipoprotein cholesterol in male survivors of ischaemic heart disease in eastern Uttar Pradesh (North India). *Indian Heart J 1985;37:176–178.*

29. Agarwal OP. Prevention of atheromatous heart disease. *Angiology 1985; 36:485–492.*

30. White PT, Singh R. Why is it that Calcutta—the world's most maligned metropolis—is where so many people want to be? *National Geographic 1973 (April):534–563.*

31. Scofield J, Singh R. Bombay, the other India. *National Geographic 1981 (July):104–129.*

32. Weintraub RM. Burgeoning city slums change face of India. *The Washington Post 1988 (October 15):A1 and A22.*

33. Weintraub RM. "New Bombay" brings prosperity and problems to Indian villages. *The Washington Post, 1988 (October 16):A31 and A35.*

34. Meisner H. A cardiac surgeon in India. *Thorac Cardiovasc Surg 1980; 28:155–157.*

Bombay and a Congress on Coronary Artery Disease

7 February 1990 enroute Bombay, India, to Washington, DC: I am returning home after attending a World Congress on Coronary Heart Disease in Bombay, India. The President of the Congress was Dr. B.K. Goyal, President of the Heart Foundation of India, and the Secretary General was Dr. Lekha Pathak, Director of Cardiology at 1 of the 4 University of Bombay medical schools and the only female head of a university cardiology department in India. Dr. Denton A. Cooley from Houston, Texas, who has operated on several hundred Indians and is something of a hero in their country, was honored as the Patron of the Congress. The foreign invited guest speakers included 20 physicians from the USA, 5 from the United Kingdom, 2 from Canada, 2 from France, 2 from the USSR, and 1 each from the Netherlands, Denmark, Spain, Australia, and Jordan. The Congress was attended by about 1,200 physicians, nearly all from India. The meeting was held at the Taj Mahal Hotel, one of the finest hotels in the world, the older portion of which was opened in 1903.

Bombay is an island—originally 7 islands—separated by a winding creek from the subcontinent and located on India's western coast, the Arabian Sea. Landfill joined the 7 islands about 130 years ago. The island city occupies 169 square miles of land, one half of which represents landfill. Bombay is the commercial and financial capital of India, the richest city in Southern Asia, and one of the largest manufacturing centers in the East. It contains 15% of all factories in the country, 1 of every 10 manufacturing jobs, and its textile industry produces 40% of the country's cloth. Its 10 million people, making it larger than the entire country of Switzerland or Denmark or the Netherlands, represent about 1% of the country's population, but they pay about 40% of the country's taxes. The trend-setting Victorian City is also the Hollywood of India, which is the world's largest active cinema and video audience. Ten million Indians go to the movies every day and India produces about 800 films annually, twice as many as does the USA. As the gateway to India, Bombay handles 60% of India's international flights and 40% of its domestic airline traffic.

Because it is the most prosperous city in India, Bombay is inundated with persons seeking work from all over India, particularly from its own state, Maharashtra, and adjacent ones. It is estimated that about 1,000 Indians come to Bombay every day to settle permanently, and this migration has been going on for years. As a consequence, housing is totally inadequate and adequate housing is too expensive except for the well-to-do. In some areas of the city land costs $6,000/m^2$ and these soaring land values have led to the razing of hundreds of ornate, century old homes, created by the British in old Bombay. About 50% of the 10 million in Bombay live in heartrending slums and the poorest of the migrants find a place to live only on the sidewalks. These sidewalk sleepers, and there they urinate, defecate and fornicate, are estimated to number as high as 500,000. I nearly stumbled over a little boy, appearing to be about 7 years old, sleeping on the sidewalk less than 50 yards from the Taj Mahal Hotel, one of the most elegant in the world, where I was staying. The slum dwellers live primarily by begging or by distilling illicit liquor. The migrants into Bombay are more commonly men than women and the resulting male to female ratio in Bombay is 4 to 3. As a consequence, Bombay is said to have the largest red-light district in Asia. Because the migrants into Bombay during the past several decades have come from several states and various districts within them, at least 10 languages are spoken in Bombay, the main ones being Marathi, the language of the Maharashtra state, and Hindi. English is the main language of trade. Likewise, the religions of the Bombayites are varied. Hindu is the most common (nearly 85%) but Muslims, Sikhs (bearded and turbaned), Jains (an offshoot of the Hindu), Catholics (they frequently wear western dress), Koli (the fishermen), and Parsis (Jews) are all well represented. The Hindi are vegetarians, or at least they do not eat beef and they refuse to work in slaughter houses, and the Muslims shun pork. I was told by an Indian that I speak the Jain philosophy (the less animals we kill the healthier we are), and I was pleased by that comment.

Life in Bombay is difficult. There are too many people, too many motorized vehicles, too little breathable air, too much noise, too little space (for living or for playing), too much movement, too much talking. The streets of Bombay are simply bursting with chaos, commotion and color. It is overwhelming in a way. Yet things seem to work, as they work nowhere else in India. The trains and buses, for example, seem to run on time. About 4.5 million local Bombayites ride trains every day and 4 million ride buses every day. Over 6,000 trucks bring produce and other products into the city every day. Bombay is not only the major port for shipping and receiving products in and out of India, but it also serves as the major transfer point for commodities produced and consumed all over India. For example, steel produced in Calcutta to be used in Madras, both Eastern Indian cities, is first transported to the wharves or pauses in the wholesale warehouses of Bombay before going to Madras. The mushrooming population continues to encroach on the little remaining city land. Although the British created many parks, there now remains only 1 acre of open area—playing fields, parks, benches, traffic circles—for every 3,000 residents. London has 8 times as much. Thus, areas for sport are inadequate. On weekends and holidays, Chowputty Beach, Bombay's prime outdoor gathering place, is so crowded that space is available only for standing and the sand can hardly be seen. In an attempt to reduce traffic and train and bus crowding, working hours in many offices in Bombay are being staggered: some workers arrive at 8 A.M. and leave at 4 P.M.; others at 9 A.M. and leave at 5 P.M., others at 10 A.M. and leave at 6 A.M., etc.

About 150 certified cardiologists work in Bombay. The top ones work at 1 of the 4 university hospitals during the morning and early afternoon and then most go to their private offices for the later afternoon and early evening appointments. At the university, their salary is roughly equivalent to 300 US dollars a month. The top cardiologists can earn up to $7,000/month additionally in their private practices. At the government-owned and railway-owned hospitals, the physicians also earn about $300/month, but at the railway hospitals additional private practice is not permitted. The railway hospitals, however, provide their physicians with free housing on campus for their families and also free railway transportation anytime and anywhere in India. The working hours for these physicians also are regular, usually 9 A.M. to 5 P.M.

About 20 cardiac surgeons work in Bombay and cardiac operations are performed at 10 hospitals in Bombay: at each of the 4 university hospitals (all under the University of Bombay) and at 6 private hospitals. Surgeons at the university hospitals may or may not be able to have private practices at a private hospital, depending on their particular arrangement. Of the 20 surgeons, only about 10 have heavy operative loads. The most active cardiovascular surgeons earn about $20,000/month. The cost of a cardiac operation for a private patient in Bombay varies from $400 to $4,000, depending on the wealth of the patient. At the government and railroad hospitals, all care is "free" to the patient. Private insurance for nongovernment and nonrailway workers appears to be increasing. The total cost for a cardiac operation for a private patient in Bombay averages about $7,500, roughly 4 times less than in the USA. In Bombay, about 50% of the cardiac operations now are for coronary artery disease and the other 50% are equally split between congenital and valvular heart disease. The most common valve operation by far is mitral commissurotomy.

Coronary angioplasty is increasing in India. About 400 of these procedures were performed in 1989, half of them in Bombay.

With poverty everywhere and vegetarianism so prevalent, why is coronary artery disease so common in India and particularly in Bombay? There seems to be no question that coronary artery disease in Bombay is far more prevalent in the wealthy than in the poor and Bombay contains the largest number of wealthy people in India. Wealth attracts rich foods, which generally means those high in saturated fat and cholesterol. If only 1% of the population of Bombay is wealthy, this small percent still represents 100,000 people, but probably the upper 10% of persons in Bombay eat like the top 1%.

Vegetarianism in India, of course, is common because Hinduism is the largest religion in India. At each of the delicious cafeteria style lunches and dinners at the Congress in Bombay, large signs designated the vegetarian and the nonvegetarian dishes. Furthermore, the menus in the hotel restaurants clearly divided the vegetarian and nonvegetarian dishes. But the vegetation dishes served in Bombay are by no means fat free, for they are often cooked in animal fat and served with large amounts of cream and ghee (concentrated cream). Furthermore, coconut oil (92% saturated) and palm kernel oil (86% saturated) are commonly used on vegetables and other foods in India. Ice cream was served at each of the meals during the Congress and I noticed that many of those eating the vegetarian dishes were later filling their plates with ice cream and cake. Although McDonald's and Burger King have not been permitted to invade India, Bombay has its own Americanized versions in Pizza King and Big Bite. There both meat-containing and meatless hamburgers are available and both varieties contain a good bit of fat. Beef actually is the cheapest meat available in India: it costs $1.50/kg (in Japan a kilogram costs $70). It appears that "vegetarianism" is a bit contaminated in India.

India simply cannot afford coronary artery disease, the therapy of which is too expensive for a developing country. Much more important, however, is their mushrooming population. Their country may not be able to feed more than 1 billion people and that number is predicted by the year 2000. What happens to the kind, dignified, gracious, generous, warm and industrious people of Bombay may be a bellwether for predicting what will happen to the people in other megacities including Calcutta, Mexico City, Jakarta, Cairo, Addis Ababa, Sao Paulo, and even London, Los Angeles and New York. Elected politicians, however, do not win votes by telling couples how many children to have. Thus, India, the largest democracy in the world, I am afraid, will be unable to control its population. It is much easier to treat coronary artery disease than excessive reproduction, but the latter disease is a much more important one to control for India.

William C. Roberts

William Clifford Roberts, MD
Editor in Chief

Singapore and Singaporean Cardiology

Dr. P. J. (Figure 1) is a 39-year-old Chinese invasive cardiologist at the National University Hospital in Singapore and an Associate Professor of Medicine. He arises each day in his well-to-do flat at 7 A.M., leaves for the hospital at 7:30, and arrives at the hospital at 8:00 A.M. He usually spends the mornings in the catheterization laboratory, and in the afternoon he sees patients, teaches students and house officers, and leaves for home at 7:00 P.M., arriving about 7:30 P.M. Dinner has been prepared by his 34-year-old wife, the mother of 1 son and pregnant with another. After dinner there is more work until he retires at midnight. This routine continues Monday through Friday. Saturday, work in the hospital is from 8 A.M. to 1 P.M., and on Sundays he returns only to visit his private patients. For his work at the University Hospital he is paid the equivalent of $6,000 monthly, plus he is able to retain 80% of the professional fees for the private patients he sees. If he saw no private patients he would receive $1,500 monthly from the hospital. Because he sees private patients, his income from this activity is about $6,000 monthly, so that his total monthly income is about $12,000. In addition, he receives 42 days' vacation leave each year, 1 week of which is called compassionate leave (for illness in his family), and 2 weeks' leave each year for medical meetings. Also, he serves in the armed forces about 2 weeks a year because of his being in the reserves. Moreover, he receives 9 months every 5 years for sabbatical leave, during which time he is paid his full salary plus additional expense money of about $2,000 monthly. Twenty percent of his income is retained by the hospital, which adds another 20% each month. This money serves as his retirement, which is mandatory at age 60 and optional at age 55. The built-up retirement is paid at the time of retirement as a lump sum; it is not taxable; indeed, it is a tax deduction. He may also use all or portions of this money as a down payment for a home. As an interventional cardiologist his pay is higher than most other members of the department of medicine.

Dr. D. R. N. (Figure 1), a 45-year-old Chinese cardiologist, is in private practice. He was the first in Singapore to do coronary angioplasty and that was in 1984. Since then, about 2,000 angioplasty procedures have been done by the 12 invasive cardiologists in Singapore. As a private cardiologist he charges about $2,500 for coronary angioplasty, limited by all cardiologists thus far in Singapore to only 1 or 2 coronary arteries per patient. In his office he has all the modern cardiologic equipment, plus he dispenses—as do nearly all private physicians in Singapore (also in Malaysia, Hong Kong, and Japan)—drugs he prescribes to his patients. If he pays the pharmaceutical company $150 for a 100-tablet bottle of simvastatin, for example, he sells the filled bottle to a patient for $200. This custom is considered standard procedure in Singapore and Dr. D. R. N. receives about a third of his income from this activity. Despite his 7 office employees and his high-rent-district office, his overhead amounts to only 25% of his income. About 50% of his patients pay him during the time of the visit; the others later. Because malpractice law suits are nearly nonexistent in Singapore, malpractice insurance may not even be necessary. He does not have the perks of his university counterpart, Dr. P. J., but his income is considerably greater and he can work past the age of 60 if he wishes. His wife is a plastic surgeon and they have 3 children. Their home is one of the finest in Singapore.

I met Doctors P. J. and D. R. N. in Singapore in March 1991 while participating in the Third Asian Pa-

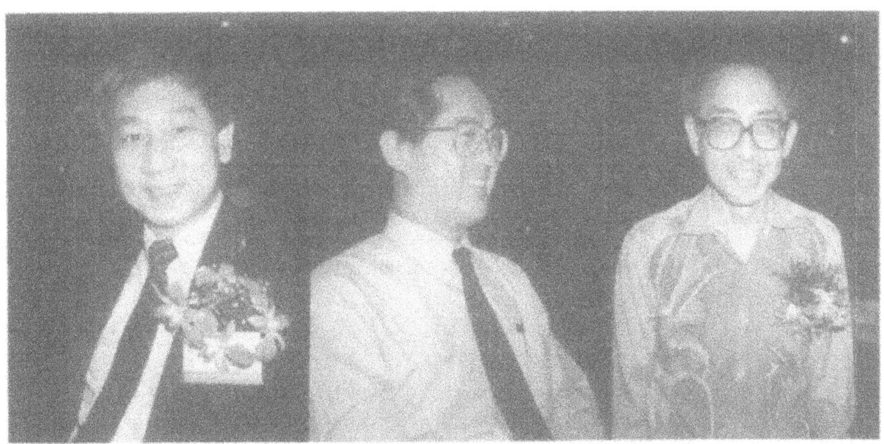

FIGURE 1. ***Left:*** **Dr. P. J.** ***Center:*** **Dr. D. R. N.** ***Right:*** **Dr. Oon Chong Hau.**

cific Symposium on Cardiac Rehabilitation organized by Dr. Oon Chong Hau (Figure 1). The trip, my third to Singapore, provided an opportunity to see more of the gracious Singaporeans and to learn more of their enormously impressive city-state.

Singapore consists of a relatively flat (most former hills have been used to fill in swamps and to reclaim land from the sea), formerly swampy island 42 km in length from east to west and 23 km from north to south with an area of 570 km^2 (225 square miles) and approximately 56 smaller islands, half of which are tiny. The total land area is 636 km^2, which is smaller than New York City, but 55 km^2 of that is from landfill. Singapore is located at the southern tip of the Malay peninsula 80 miles north of the equator (Figure 2). The average maximum and minimum temperatures are 31 and 24°C, respectively. The relative humidity in the early morning usually exceeds 90% and rain falls all year round.

Although inhabited since the 1300's, when Sir Thomas Stamford Raffles (1781–1826), an official of the English East India Company, landed on January 18, 1819, less than 1,000 persons inhabited the island, nearly all of which was covered with dense lowland tropical rain forest, where tigers, leopards, wild boars and mustang roamed.[1] Solid rock underlay the jungle. Raffles anchored his 8 small ships with 130 men, including 100 Indians, at the mouth of the Singapore River and the next day signed an agreement with the local Malay chieftain to permit the British to set up a trading post. To establish Singapore as a thriving trading port that would secure British interests in the Orient, Raffles, a visionary intellectual and a humanitarian, saw Singapore as a well-sheltered harbor and from the beginning made her a free port with open immigration. As a consequence, immigrants, particularly from China but also from Malay and India and elsewhere, flocked to the island, intent on saving money and then returning to their homelands.

From its beginning, Singapore flourished; it was a natural center for southeastern Asian trade. By 1821, Singapore had 5,000 inhabitants, by 1824, 11,000, and it was becoming a cosmopolitan town.[1] In 1824, Raffles negotiated a new treaty with the local sultans, who ceded the entire island to the British in return for increased pensions and cash payments. In 1826, Singapore became part of the British Straits Settlements together with Penang and Malacca and by 1832 was the center of government of these settlements, which became a Crown Colony in 1867. In 1869 the Suez Canal opened and steamships began replacing sailing ships and therefore needed coaling stations. Singapore's key location as the major waterway between Europe and the far east, the expansion of colonial rule in southeast Asia, and its deep water harbor made it flourish even more rapidly. When rubber and tin production started flourishing in the Malay peninsula by about 1900, Singapore became the major exporting center of the world for both products. Today, Singapore is Asia's busiest port and ranks with New York and Rotterdam as the busiest in the world.

Singapore's rapidly expanding economy attracted ever-increasing numbers of immigrants. By 1911 the population was >185,000, and men outnumbered women by 8 to 1![1] About 75% were Chinese. The predominantly young adult male population consisting primarily of transients, who did not regard Singapore as home, made Singapore a relatively violent place. Prostitution prospered. Taverns were everywhere. Opium smoking was rampant. By about 1850 it was estimated that 20% of the entire population and 50% of the Chinese population were opium addicts.[1] Addicts became beggars living on rotten fish and decaying vegetables and ended up in

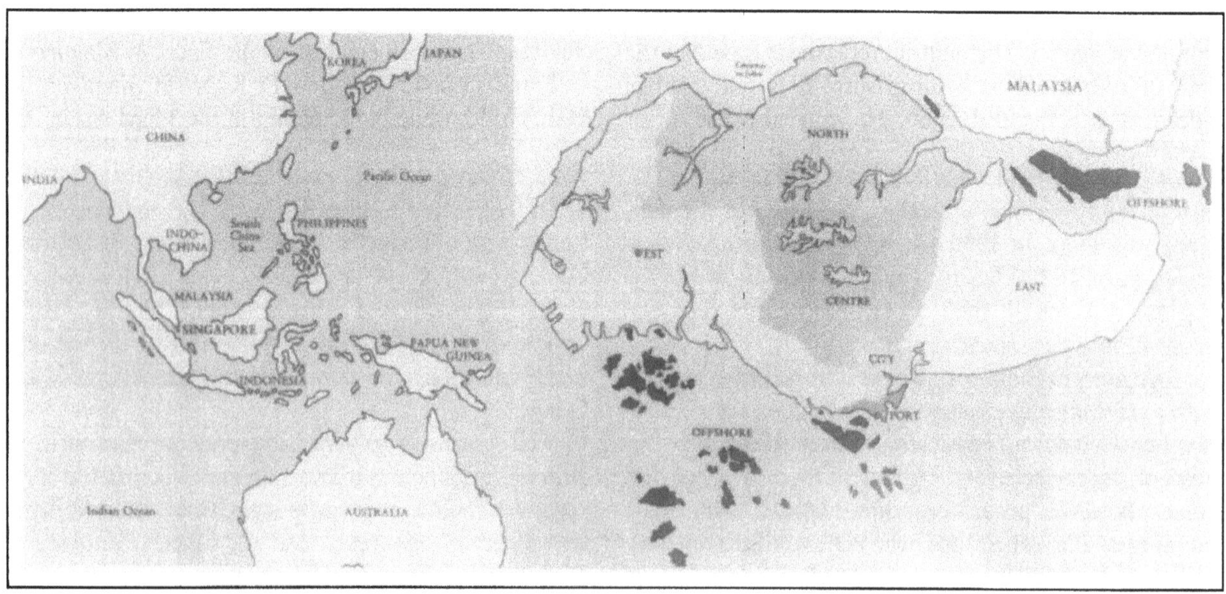

FIGURE 2. Map of Southeast Asia (*left*) and of Singapore (*right*).

prison or in the pauper hospital or were driven to suicide. The opium trade was the mainstay of the government's revenue up to the twentieth century. Poverty, malnutrition, overcrowding and heavy opium smoking devastated the immigrants during the first 75 or so years of Singapore. The island was the prison for the convicts of the Asian British empire for the first 50 years of its existence and, therefore, many derelicts were shipped to Singapore. Most of the still-present impressive government buildings and infrastructure were built by convict labor, including Fort Canning, St. Andrew's Cathedral, a town hall, a court house, a general hospital, a lunatic asylum, Government House, Istana, various bridges across the Singapore River, etc. The Chinese gradually lost their control over immigration, labor, prostitution, and for a period switched their interest to gambling, which was widespread. It was not until 1890 or after that the government was able to control the band of thugs who extorted "protection money" from shops, gambling dens, opium dens, brothels and hawkers. The final banishment of the secret Chinese societies, which controlled crime, was not until the 1890's, when law and order finally became part of the Singaporean society.

The disparity between the numbers of men and women was obviously a major social problem. The ruling class wanted to promote Chinese female immigration to encourage permanent settlement, to divert shifting rootless youths from crime, to curb the secret societies' hold over prostitution, and to stem the drain to China of family remittances that could have been used to develop Singapore. It was not until 1933 that the Aliens Ordinance imposed for the first time a monthly quota on male immigration. Shortly thereafter there was a free flow of female immigration and, as a result, a population that had always been transient sank roots as more women arrived and families were formed.

World War II changed Singapore forever. The island fell to the Japanese forces on February 15, 1942, and remained under their control for 3.5 years. After the war the British never really recovered the prestige they had enjoyed earlier. Singapore became a separate Crown Colony in April 1946 while Penang and Malacca became part of the Federation of Malaya in 1948. But this existence was short. In 1959 Singapore became a self-governing state. In 1963, Singapore became part of Malaysia, but on August 4, 1965, broke this brief marriage and became an independent country.

Independent Singapore was established as a republic with a parliamentary system of government. Its constitution provided for a ceremonial, figurehead president as head of state, elected by Parliament every 4 years. The power, however, lay in the prime minister, who was a member of Parliament and who commanded the confidence of the elected members (initially 58, later 81) of the single-chamber Parliament. The Cabinet, formed by the prime minister, consists of 14 other ministers who also are members of Parliament. Voting in elections by Singaporeans is compulsory.

The priorities of the new government after independence were industrialization, elimination of unemployment, higher income levels and decent housing for all. Many multinational companies were attracted to Singapore and they brought not only technology and skills but also worldwide markets for their products. The work force was hardworking, the unions cooperative, and the rest is history.

Today, Singapore is a bustling, modern, clean, safe, prosperous, comfortable, green, noisy, and friendly metropolis containing 2.7 million people (12,000 per square mile), 77% of whom are Chinese, 15% Malays and 6% Indians, and 365,000 cars, trucks and buses and maybe as many motorcycles.[2] Singapore is a major port, a major shopping center, the transport hub of the Orient, and the most advanced city in Southeast Asia. Everything works, the country is super rich, and the parks and greenery make it look like a campus. Modern, air-conditioned skyscrapers abound and from one 73-story hotel (Westin Stamford) the entire island, i.e., country, can be seen on a clear day.[3] About half of the island is built up and the other half contains forest, marsh and tidal waste, and still a few farms. About 85% of the population live in the abundant high-rise apartment buildings built by the government, which encourages the occupants to buy their 2-, 3- and 4-bedroom living quarters.[4] The majority do. Households now average 3.8 persons, down from 5.1 only 16 years ago.[5] For many years the government encouraged only 2 children per family, but because of a labor shortage 3 children per family have been encouraged in recent years. Its subway (42-km tract) is one of the best in the world.

Free enterprise flourishes in Singapore. Shipbuilding, oil refining, electronics, banking, textiles, food, rubber, lumber processing and tourism are its industries.[2] Singapore is the strongest of the 3 pacific dragons (Hong Kong and Republic of China [Taiwan] being the other 2).[6] Its economy has expanded by 8 to 10% during most of its years of independence, and its unemployment (<2%) and inflation (±3%) rates are low.[6] The newspapers are loaded with advertisements of job openings. Manufacturing is gradually being replaced by research and development, banking and other services.[6] The per capita income of Singaporeans is $14,000 yearly, second only to Japan among the non-oil-producing nations of the Orient.[4]

The success of modern Singapore is reflected in its airline—Singapore Airlines (SIA)—which is the most profitable (a 24% after-tax margin)[7] and the most popular carrier in the world,[8] and the biggest company in Singapore.[7] Compared with other international carriers, SIA has the highest percentage of filled seats (79%), the youngest plane fleet (average 4.6 years), it spends the most on meals, and it has the youngest flight attendants. (The women comprise 40% of the attendants and they must retire by age 40; the male attendants do not have to retire until age 55.[7]) The government currently owns 54% of SIA but plans to reduce this stake to 30%.[7] The modern and beautiful Changi Airport in Singapore is one of the world's finest and it is used by 54 international carriers.

To keep Singapore clean and its citizens safe and healthy, the government under Cambridge-educated Lee Kuan Yew, its prime minister who served from 1956 to 1990, passed many laws. Jaywalkers are fined $50, littering of any kind costs $1,000, and anyone caught smoking indoors in any public building must part with $500. Possession, consumption or trafficking of drugs in small amounts (10 to 15 g) will result in 10 to 30 years in prison, a $20,000 fine and 5 to 15 lashes; larger amounts (>15 g) result in the death penalty (hanging).[9] Not flushing a public toilet is against the law.[10] A local bromide goes: "Singapore is a fine city; there's a fine for everything."[10] Mr. Lee has carried on national campaigns to exhort citizens to smile more, to act more polite. When the high-rise apartments were first introduced, a drive was initiated to stop men, who had previously lived in slums, from urinating in the elevators.[11] The government ordered the landlords to install devices that sounded alarms and jammed the doors as soon as urine hit the elevator's floor.[11] The government with relative little resistance has maintained public morality. No strip joints, no adult book stores and no "girlie" magazines are available in Singapore.

Although Singapore has 21 political parties, the government since 1959 has been run by one political party and, for its first 31 years, by the same prime minister. Although young Singaporeans joke about their authoritarian government, no one seriously proposes change—even though the domestic press is stringently controlled and the foreign media are increasingly suppressed. Satellite dishes that can receive broadcasts of the Cable News Network are banned and both the respected *Far East Economic Review* and the *Asian Wall Street Journal* are no longer available in Singapore because these media have criticized the Singaporean bureaucrats.[10] Nevertheless, the same strong-willed, intolerant, puritanical government is a graft-free one and this government is responsible for providing the high standard of living of its citizens, its safe streets and the excellent housing. To prevent graft, the higher government officials are extremely well paid. The prime minister is said to be the highest paid in the world and his cabinet officers also are well compensated.

Historically, despite its constant damp heat, marsh and swamp, rotting vegetation, filth and stench, Singaporeans have always been relatively healthy.[1] Malaria and leprosy were always uncommon and cholera and smallpox occurred only in the most overcrowded nineteenth century slums.[1] In the 1950s, the major causes of death in Singapore were tuberculosis, gastroenteritis, pneumonia, and various childhood infections. By the 1980s coronary artery disease and cancer were the 2 major killers of Singaporeans, each accounting for approximately 25% of deaths.[5] The mortality rate from coronary artery disease is greatest among their Indian population, their rate being about twice that of the Malays and Chinese in Singapore. From 1960 until 1985, the percentage of calories from fat of the Singaporeans increased enormously, consumption of meat and offal increased 135%, and egg consumption increased 80%. Physical activity from 1960 to 1985 decreased in women (not men), obesity frequency increased, and smoking from 1960 to 1977 increased but since has decreased. Singapore aims to be a smoke-free nation.[12] The heart disease rate per 100,000 Singaporeans now is 120.[5] Singapore has overtaken Australia in having the highest mortality rate from coronary artery disease in Asia. Eating and food are the first items of conversation among Singaporeans. (They rarely talk about the weather because it is always the same—hot and humid.) McDonald's and most of the fast-food chains flourish in Singapore. They have eaten well over 14 million hamburgers, an average of about 14,000 per day. It has the second fastest growing aging society in the world and this fact worsens its heart disease problem. The average lifespan of Singaporean women is 77 years, and men, 73 years.

It is no surprise that heart disease is now so rampant in Singapore. Coronary artery disease has increased roughly in proportion to its per capita income. The average serum total cholesterol level in adult Singaporeans without clinical evidence of myocardial ischemia is now 228 mg/dl (5.9 mmol/liter) and among those with clinical evidence of myocardial ischemia, 239 mg/dl (6.2 mmol/liter).[13,14] These levels rank Singaporeans fifth highest in the world; only Finland, Norway, the United Kingdom and Germany have higher levels. Among Singaporean adults, 55% have serum total cholesterol levels >200 mg/dl (5.2 mmol/liter),[14] and 27% of Singaporeans have levels >250 mg/dl (6.5 mm/liter).[13] The low-density lipoprotein and high-density lipoprotein cholesterol levels among the adult Singaporeans with and without clinical evidence of myocardial ischemia average 163 and 39 mg/dl, respectively, and the total to high-density lipoprotein cholesterol ratio, 6.3. The serum triglyceride levels usually are <160 mg/dl (2.1 mm/liter).

Medicine in Singapore compares with the best in the world. Its 20 hospitals (7 government, 3 government being restructured to private, and 10 private), with nearly 10,000 beds, provide modern equipment and facilities for treatment and rehabilitation.[5] In 1990, approximately 3,300 physicians provided care for the 2.7-million population, a doctor-population ratio of 1:825.[15] Singapore, therefore, in contrast to Europe and probably the USA, does not have too many physicians. A higher percentage of their physicians each year are specialists.[16]

Its one medical school graduates 150 physicians yearly but graduates abroad also enter Singapore each year. For many years the medical school was attracting the best students and their admission was based purely on meritocracy, the results of a written examination. The University/Government believed that this occurrence prevented other disciplines from obtaining their fair share of talent and that this state of affairs could have serious consequences for the country. Consequently, now only 15% of the top 10% of students can get into medical school and the other 85% are selected from the pool of students just under the top 10% of the pre-medical school classes.[15] Although women's rights are entrenched in Singapore's constitution, women can constitute no more than a third of the medical school classes (because "many married women doctors are not as economically productive as their male counterparts and the country cannot afford the luxury of giving women an education in Medicine.").[15]

Cardiology in Singapore is now high-tech, as in most other developed countries. Coronary angioplasty and bypass flourish. There are only 12 cardiologists doing angioplasty and only 12 cardiac surgeons in Singapore. About half of the cardiac operations are coronary bypass, about 25% are valve operations, and about 25% are for congenital cardiovascular anomalies. The cardiac surgeons, of course, are financially secure in Singapore as in most other parts of the world. There is considerable emphasis on preventive cardiology in Singapore, more so, I suspect, than in the USA.

Health care accounts for 2.7% of the gross national product in Singapore (in the USA and Germany it is 11 to 12%), but the percentage is rising.[5] Costs of medical care are paid for primarily by the patient.[17,18] In hospitals, the type of bed occupied by a patient determines the cost: 80% of the C class beds are subsidized by the government; the class B1, B2 and A beds are not government supported and are more expensive. To help people pay for the type of bed they choose, the government introduced *Medisave* in 1989. With this plan, individuals can use up to a sixth of their retirement savings (contributed to by their employer) to pay for approved medical bills, but only up to a maximum of $15,000. In 1990, *MediShield*, a low-cost medical insurance plan, was introduced to provide further help in meeting individual health costs.

Thus, as skyscrapers rise, as traffic increases, as subways are introduced, as per capita income rises, and as modern medicine becomes available, atherosclerotic plaques increase in number and size. Singapore is another example of how "progress" is equated with coronary artery disease. A major challenge is to provide "progress" without providing atherosclerotic plaques. The answer simply is not to spend the increased monies on FAT.

William C. Roberts

William Clifford Roberts, MD
Editor in Chief

1. Turnball CM. A History of Singapore 1819–1988. Second edition. Oxford: Oxford University Press, 1989:388.
2. Hoffman MS, ed. World Almanac and Books of Facts 1991. New York: Pharos Books, 1991:960.
3. Lloyd I, Hoe I. Singapore from the Air. Second edition. Singapore: Times Editions, 1990:125.
4. Tan Han Hoe. Singapore 1988. Singapore: Information Division of the Ministry of Communications and Information, 1988:324.
5. Khoo Chian Kim, ed. Yearbook of Statistics Singapore 1989. Singapore: Department of Statistics, 1990:366.
6. Weinburger CW. Three strong pacific dragons. *Forbes* 1991; (April 1) 147:35.
7. Tanzer A. The prime minister is a demanding shareholder. *Forbes* 1990;(April 2)145:152–153.
8. Trick DR. Air travel is the pits, fliers say. *USA Today* 7 September 1990.
9. Kelsey IH. From under the rubble Singapore rises, again. *The Globe and Mail* Toronto, 20 October 1990:A9–A10.
10. Sklarwitz N. Singapore. "Switzerland of the East." *Frequent Flyer* February 1991:31–33.
11. Hammes S. An insider's guide to seven cities. *Fortune* (Special Issue on Asia-Mega-Market of the 1990s) Fall 1990;122:69–77.
12. Lee JP. Patterns of smoking among Singaporeans. *Ann Acad Med Singapore* 1989;18:286–288.
13. Hughes K, Yeo PPB, Lun KC, Sothy SP, Thai AC, Wang KW, Cheah JS. Ischemic heart disease and its risk factors in Singapore in comparison with other countries. *Ann Acad Med Singapore* 1989;18:245–249.
14. Ng ASH, Chee TS, Wong WM, Aw TC, Quek SSS, Tan ATH, Arulanandan S. Coronary risk profile screening during National Heart Week—1986. *Ann Acad Med Singapore* 1990;1930–1933.
15. Pillay VK. Towards excellence in medicine. *Singapore Med J* 986;27: 369–373.
16. Mah GK. The doctor in the future. 1987;28:547–551.
17. Delamothe T. Singapore restructured. *Br Med J* 1990;300:1223.
18. Anonymous. Round the world—Singapore. *Lancet* 1990;335:1208–1209.

Day-to-Day Cardiology in Bombay, India

Dr. Venkata Ram, Professor of Internal Medicine, The University of Texas Southwestern Medical Center, Dallas, organized a cardiology meeting held in Goa, India, in October 1995 and invited me to participate. It was my third trip to India, and I would have to be sick or dead not to accept an invitation to that subcontinent, a third the size in land area of the USA but containing nearly 4 times as many people. During a stopover in Bombay, I dined with Doctor Satyavan Sharma and his wife Meeta and Doctor Bharat Dalvi. Our discussions gave me some insight into day-to-day cardiology in Bombay, where I had visited briefly on 2 previous occasions.[1,2]

Dr. Sharma is in the private practice of cardiology in Bombay. Until nearly 3 years earlier he was Professor and Chief of the Department of Cardiology in 1 of 4 of Bombay's medical schools, and in that position he became prominent as an interventionalist, having performed the first mitral valve balloon angioplasty in Bombay. Although he loved the academic environs, he left so that he could better support his young family.

He arises each day about 6:30 A.M. He leaves home at about 8:15 for the 45-minute ride in his chauffeured small Renault, arriving about 9:00 A.M. at his hospital where his office also is located. Two days a week he goes directly to the catheterization laboratory where he does several diagnostic and therapeutic procedures including coronary angioplasty and balloon valvuloplasty. He now uses stents frequently in his coronary patients.

The other 5 days of the week, Dr. Sharma goes directly to the wards to see his 35 or so patients, his usual hospital census. From there he goes to his hospital office where he works until about 10 P.M. The ride home is shorter at this hour than the ride to the hospital—about 30 minutes. Home at 10:30 P.M., he usually has one "whiskey" or beer, eats dinner prepared by his lovely wife, and then to bed at about midnight. Sleep comes quickly. On Saturdays, hospital and office work lasts from 8:30 A.M. to 6 P.M., when he returns home for an evening with family and friends. Sunday it's back to the hospital for 2 hours to see his hospitalized patients and then home to devote all his remaining energies to his wife and 2 girls aged 7 and 5 years. His wife calls him "a splendid daddy." The Sharmas married when he was 35 and she 26, about average today for Bombay's professionals. Their girls go to private schools where kindergarten begins at age 4. Meeta is a homemaker and vigorous supporter of her husband's activities.

Time off is a bit difficult for Dr. Sharma. He, like all private cardiologists in Bombay (there are about 75 of them and about 30 cardiovascular surgeons in Bombay), is in solo practice. During 6 weeks of the year he is on "holiday"—these are usually arranged around cardiologic meetings—a fellow private cardiologist covers his practice and vice versa when his fellow cardiologist is away. Reading of medical journals is done in the automobile, a bonus of being chauffeured.

Few people in India have insurance and thus his patients, with few exceptions, pay from their own pockets. Most of his patients, therefore, are wealthy or at least relatively well-to-do. The diagnostic and therapeutic procedures in India, however, cost considerably less than in the USA. The total cost to the patient for a coronary angioplasty in a private hospital in Bombay is only $3,000 (US dollars) and $2,000 for a patient with lesser income. Stents, however, are extra, adding about $2,000 to each angioplasty. The total cost to the patient of coronary artery bypass grafting in India is only $5,000 (US dollars). In the public sector hospitals, in contrast to the private ones, coronary angiography costs $80, coronary angioplasty $1,000, and coronary bypass $1,000, and those who cannot afford these prices are granted further concessions. In India, there is not a particular rush to get the patient out of the hospital. Coronary angioplasty patients usually stay 3 days after the procedure and coronary bypass patients stay about 12 days in the hospital after the operation.

Dr. Dalvi is an Associate Professor in the Department of Cardiology in the K.E.M. Hospital and Medical School, and in this position he earns $350 per month. Aged 37, he arrives at the hospital about 8:30 A.M., but his drive is only 15 minutes and, therefore, he can sleep later. His work day ends at about 8:15 P.M., so he is home by 8:30 pm. His patients are mainly the indigent and poor with essentially no money of their own for medical care. (The public hospitals in India take care of almost 99% of the population.) His weekends are not as

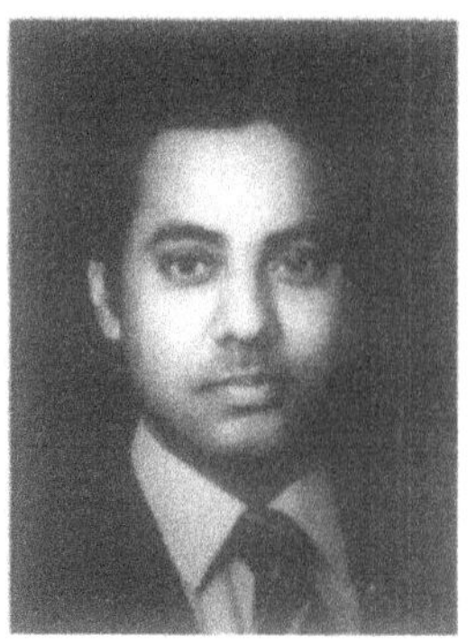
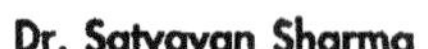
Dr. Satyavan Sharma

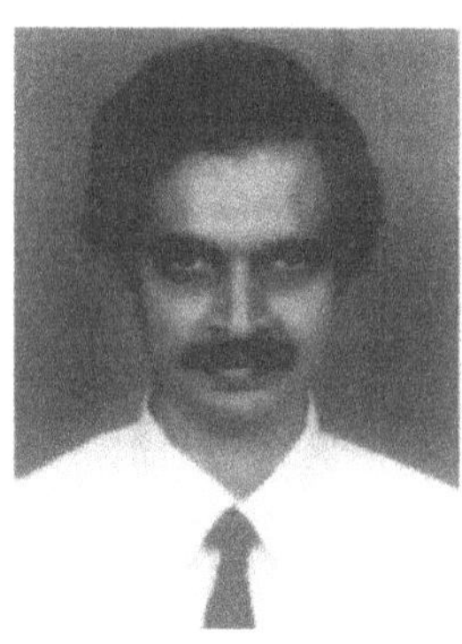
Dr. Bharat Dalvi

busy as his counterpart in private practice. Although he is rapidly becoming well known in Bombay and in other portions of India—he tries to focus on pediatric cardiology—his salary is a small fraction of that of Dr. Sharma. Dr. Dalvi's small salary makes living rather difficult in terms of necessities of life, leave alone luxuries. He, too, has a wife and 6-year-old twin daughters who also are in private school. Private practice is not permitted by medical school professors in Bombay. He may eventually be forced to move to private practice to support his family adequately.

Both Drs. Sharma and Dalvi are major cardiologic leaders in their communities. Their lives in Bombay are not easy but no one's life is easy in Bombay, a city of an estimated 11 million—no one knows for sure how many. The roads in Bombay were built, for the most part, when the city was <1 million. The traffic is so horrendous that sometimes it may take an hour to go a few blocks. An estimated 2,000 Indians arrive in Bombay to settle permanently each day, mainly coming from the rural regions where still about 75% of India's population reside. Housing is totally inadequate. There are no private homes anymore. The value of land in Bombay is as high as in Tokyo, the highest in the world. Professionals such as Drs. Sharma and Dalvi live in apartment houses. About 8 million Bombayites live in heart-rending slums and the poorest live on sidewalks.

Other features of Indian society I learned on this visit include: 1. *Low crime rate:* Only 136 murders were committed in Bombay in 1994, and that in a city of over 11 million inhabitants. Few citizens have guns. To possess a handgun or a long gun, personal protection purposes must be demonstrated to the governmental authorities, and that is difficult. Furthermore, all guns are very expensive. Only 1 in 10,000 owns a handgun and 1 in 50,000, I was told, owns a long gun. Hunting is not permitted in India. Murder and rape, both extremely rare in Bombay, are essentially limited to the slums. Indians respect each other, others' property, and animals.

2. *Low illegitimate birth rate:* It is <1%. The reason is that sex before marriage is taboo. About 80% of marriages are arranged by parents and agreed to by other family members and the 2 participants. Only 20% of marriages are "love marriages" and decided exclusively by the participants. My guide told me that he was marrying 2 months hence, that his marriage was an arranged one, that he had been engaged for 2 years, that he had not seen his fiance during this period more than once every 6 months, that at this point, he was not "in love" with his fiance, that he and she would live with his parents until his wife had a baby, that he wanted only one child irrespective of its sex, that he had never dated and neither had his fiance before their engagement, and that "character" was the important ingredient in a mate, not sexual attraction or other attributes. Neither males nor females date in India before their prearranged marriages. For a partner of a prearranged marriage to break an engagement is a fatal blow to the bride. She will never again be asked for marriage and the groom can recover completely only about 20% of the time. A commitment is a commitment in India.

3. *Low divorce rate:* It is <5% but beginning to climb. Not only is the divorce rate low but extramarital affairs are comparatively uncommon—about 25% of marriages.

4. *Low alcoholism rate:* Most alcohol in India is drunk in the home because alcohol purchased at a store is much less expensive than that bought at bars and restaurants. Except in Goa, where wine is produced locally, most alcohol consumed in India is in the form of beer or whiskey (scotch). There is simply not enough money in enough Indian hands to make alcohol a problem in India.

5. *Low accident rate:* Despite inadequate roads, fast drivers, and far too many old motorized vehicles, the accident rate in Bombay is low. The reason may be due to the fact that nearly all drivers are professional drivers. Most individuals in Bombay do not own motorized vehicles. Those who drive are chauffeurs for the well-to-do or are taxi, bus, or truck drivers, and that is their occupation. Although I was told that 10% of drivers are women, I did not see any women driving motorized vehicles. Those who can afford an automobile simply pay a professional driver (chauffeur) to do the driving.

Although I enjoyed the visit to India, I nevertheless was happy to be home again. India in general is too poor to be bothered by atherosclerosis. But as the numbers of vehicles increase, so will the frequency of coronary narrowing. The latter, however, still affects a relatively small percent of their population.

William C. Roberts

William Clifford Roberts, MD
Editor in Chief
Baylor University Medical Center
Dallas, Texas 75246

1. Roberts WC. India and Indian cardiology. *Am J Cardiol* 1988;62:1326–1329.
2. Roberts WC. Bombay and a congress on coronary artery disease. *Am J Cardiol* 1990;65:824–825.

Singapore

I visited Singapore for 3 days in March 2003. My 2 favorite places in Asia are Hong Kong and Singapore, so if I get an invitation to either, I try to accept. Hong Kong has 7 million people and Singapore, 4 million. Singapore is not quite as bustling as Hong Kong, but that's not always readily perceivable. Singapore is only about 60 miles from the equator, and, as a consequence, its temperature ranges all year long from 78° to 88° Fahrenheit, and its humidity is 90%. Virtually every building is air conditioned. It takes a long time to get to Singapore from Dallas. The flight from Dallas to Tokyo is >13 hours, and the flight from Tokyo to Singapore is nearly 8 hours. Nevertheless, it's well worth the ride. Singapore is the only place in the world where every flight is an international one.

Singapore consists of just over 60 islands, most of which are uninhabited. The main island is shaped like a flattened diamond and is 26 miles long from east to west and 14 miles long from north to south. Near the northern peak is the causeway leading to the Malaysia Peninsula, and at the southern foot is Singapore city. To the east is Changi International Airport, which is connected to the city by a beautiful parkway. The airport may be the most magnificent one in the world. Of the islands' total land area, more than half is built up, and the balance is made up of parkland, farmland, plantations, swamp areas, and forests.

Although it may no longer be the richly exotic and romantic city so vividly documented by *Conrad* and *Kipling*, Singapore, nevertheless is a unique city where the gentle manners of the East peacefully coexist with the comforts, conveniences, and efficiency of the West. It contains some of the world's most luxurious hotels, offering incomparable service and all the amenities. Most major ones are located on or near Orchard Road, where smartly dressed shoppers browse among glittering shop windows, which are so attractive it's almost like wandering in a museum. Unfortunately, the merchandise is no longer inexpensive. The prices in most shops are about the same as in New York City or London or Paris, and the prices of the hotels are also about the same as in these other cities. But Singapore, in contrast, is easy to explore, and that can be done on foot. It's difficult to get lost in this city. Every street has signposts in English and most Singaporeans speak English.

In contrast to Hong Kong, where about 97% of its citizens are Chinese, Singapore is more multicultural. The Chinese make up about 77% of the population, Malays about 14%, Indians about 12%, and others the remainder. The city itself is divided roughly into 4 or 5 sections, including Colonial Singapore, Chinatown, the Arab District, and a Little India, among others. That division was initiated in 1819, when *Sir Thomas Stamford Raffles* founded and laid out the city for the East Indian Company. When he arrived in the early part of the 19th century, Singupura, as it was called then, consisted of jungle and marshes and contained many tigers. Until approximately 1850 or 1860, at least 5 humans each year were killed by the tigers that roamed the islands.

Singapore is a nation of contradictions. Except for Japan, it has the best educated, most knowledgeable, and most worldwide society in Asia, but nevertheless the government in many ways regulates its citizens' lives. Although its relations with its immediate neighbors, Malaysia and Indonesia, have improved dramatically over the years, Singapore maintains one of the largest armies in the world proportionate to population and has a ruthlessly efficient and intrusive intelligence agency, the Internal Security Department, which is tireless in its pursuit of dissent. Nevertheless, Singapore is a bastion of capitalism, and the government owns many of the largest local companies. The government is so conservative that it bans *Cosmopolitan*, as well as *Playboy*, yet the national airline promotes itself with slogans on the order of "Singapore Girl, you're a great way to fly." Although Singapore has many of what are called "hawker centers," each with an ethnic mélange of food stalls, which offer some of the best street food in the world, young Singaporeans flock to American fast food restaurants.

The city is spotlessly clean, traffic jams are infrequent, and pollution is nearly nonexistent. The airport is so efficient, the taxis are so numerous, and the roads are so good that a visitor arriving at the airport on the eastern tip of the island 12 miles from downtown can reach the hotel within 30 minutes after stepping off the plane. When arriving at the airport, a driver was waiting for me, and on our way into the city, he called the front desk of The Four Seasons Hotel, so that when we arrived I was already checked in. Tap water is clean. An international phone call can be direct-dialed as quickly in Singapore as in the USA.

Although 4 languages are spoken in Singapore, the most common one publically spoken is English. All business is conducted in English and that is the language used in the schools. (Only 1 of 5 Singaporeans, however, speaks English at home. Mandarin is the most common language spoken at home.)

Most Singaporeans live in high-rise flats, over 80% of which were built by the government. Most of these are 10 to 20 stories high and are subsidized by the government, namely the Housing Board. The flats can be anywhere from 1 to 5 rooms in size. The occupants buy a 99-year lease. The 1-room flats cost $100,000 and 5-room flats, approximately $500,000. The lease is actually renewed every 10 years and the person has to either renew it or evacuate the flat. The flats in the public housing facilities are owned by the occupants and the high-rises are well maintained by the government. The taxi driver told me that each complex is painted every 5 years.

Despite the high-rise buildings nearly everywhere, Singapore has retained enough greenery to make it a very pleasant city for walking. Every block has trees and flowers. The entire east coast facing the South China Sea is a string of parks and beaches, and only a half hour from downtown Singapore City are nature preserves and some semi-rural areas with farms. No litter mars a walk through Singapore streets. A litterbug pays a fine, and cigarette butts are counted as litter. Singapore has nearly 50,000 litter baskets throughout the city. Everything in Singapore is clean and everything works.

In a nation known for efficiency, the government is the most efficient of all. When someone calls to report a pothole, the Public Works Department fills it within 48 hours. The Telecommunication Authority will install a new phone the day after the order is received. Secretaries are so conscientious that a journalist gets unsolicited wake-up calls to make sure he or she will be on time for early morning interviews with their bosses. There is no bribing in Singapore. A bribe, whether a small tip to an employee or a large payoff to a high-ranking minister, represents a ticket to jail. Thus, corruption is nonexistent.

The government makes many rules. The walls of buildings are plastered with rules, telling people what they can't do and how much they have to pay if they try to do it. The fines represent considerably more than a slap on the wrist, and they are enforced often enough to make most potential violators think twice. Violations do not always depend on a passing policeman for discovery. Trucks and commercial vans are required to install a yellow roof light that flashes when the vehicle exceeds the speed limit. When a taxi exceeds the maximum speed on a freeway of 48 miles an hour, loud chimes go off inside. The chimes are so annoying that the driver is likely to slow down. At some intersections, cameras photograph the license plates of cars that pass through as the light is changing to red. The drivers receive bills for that offense in the mail.

Today, Singapore is a city with almost no poverty. In Hong Kong, the gap between rich and poor is visible everywhere. In Singapore, there are no shabbily dressed citizens, and everyone appears to have at least a passable place to live. Food is relatively cheap and plentiful. All have access to high quality medical care.

Singapore was not always so prosperous or so tidy. When Lee Qwan Yew, prime minister from 1959 to 1990, took power, Singapore represented a mosquito-infested swamp dotted with pig and chicken farms, fishing villages, and squatter colonies of tin-roofed shacks. The streets of the central city were lined with shop houses, mostly 2-story buildings with ornate facades. A family would operate a business on the ground floor and live on the second floor, often without plumbing and electricity, and housing as many as 10 people to a room. The shop houses may have represented a picturesque sight for tourists, but they were not very agreeable for their occupants. Living conditions, in other words, were utter filth, and the occupants were poverty stricken. In not much more than a decade, Singaporeans passed from poverty to affluence and the nation's economy from a basket case to the powerhouse of southern Asia. The explanation for this transition, as for nearly everything else that happens in Singapore, rests with Lee Qwan Yew. Lee put his stamp on Singapore to an extent that few political leaders anywhere in the world have ever matched. He was tough and authoritarian, but uninterested in personal wealth among a people who devote their lives to financial gain, and often rude and contemptuous in a country that runs annual campaigns promoting the virtues of courtesy. Lee embodied as many contraindications as does Singapore itself.

I spoke at the Singapore General Hospital, which is the largest hospital among the 11 in Singapore. It has 1,400 beds. Singapore has only 1 medical school, the National University of Singapore. The school's primary hospital is the National University Hospital, but many medical students also rotate through Singapore General Hospital, which also has a very large housestaff. Medical students in Singapore, after finishing 12 years of school, take 2 years of preuniversity and then enroll in medical school, which is 5 years. The National University of Singapore has about 215 students in each class. Thus, 215 new physicians each year come out of this medical school. A number of Singapore students go to medical schools in other countries, however, and then return to Singapore to practice. Until this year (2003), the percent of women in the National University of Singapore Medical School was limited to 20%. In 2003, the quota was lifted.

Training of physicians in Singapore is similar to that in the USA. After medical school they are medical officers and then registrars. For those going into cardiology, there are 3 years of postgraduate training and then 3 years of a cardiology fellowship. I was told that there are approximately 70 cardiologists in Singapore and about 20 cardiovascular surgeons.

Of the 11 hospitals in Singapore, 7 are considered "restructured" or government subsidized hospitals, and the other 4 are private hospitals. The specialists practice at either the restructured or private hospitals. Those practicing at the restructured hospitals are on salary, although a few of them are allowed private practice. At the private hospitals, all of the staff have income entirely from their private practices. The private hospitals are entirely specialty hospitals. The general practitioners practice mainly at what are called "polyclinics" that are subsidized by the government for the less well to do. General practitioners have no hospital connections and do not spend time in the hospitals. The Singapore General Hospital has a heart center that includes cardiologists, cardiac surgeons, cardiac radiologists, and cardiac anesthesiologists. The restructured or government subsidized hospital pharmacies have a formulary that limits drugs the physician can use. The private hospitals have an open formulary.

Patients in Singapore are divided into 3 categories: A, B, and C. Patients in category A pay their entire physician and hospital bills; patients in category C (with incomes <24,000 Singapore dollars) are 100% subsidized by the government, and those in category B are partially subsidized by the government. I was surprised to learn that the 3 top drugs prescribed in Singapore are Viagra (sildenafil citrate), Xenical (orlistat), and Lipitor (atorvastatin).

Atherosclerotic disease is very common in Singapore. Coronary heart disease used to be the number 1 killer, but their preventive programs have reduced it to number 3; now cancer is the leading cause of death. Obesity and the metabolic syndrome are becoming more prevalent in Singapore, just like in the western world.

William C. Roberts

William Clifford Roberts, MD
Editor in Chief
Baylor Heart & Vascular Institute
Baylor University Medical Center
Dallas, Texas

Miscellaneous Topics

Animal Behavior—Human Behavior—Cardiac Behavior

Considerable study has been made through the years of behavioral characteristics of nonhuman animals—how they communicate, court, mate, fight, care for their young, acquire food, care for their bodies, and so on. Similar studies of humans, of course, are being performed constantly. In contrast to studying general features of one species or another, the pages of this journal focus on how the heart behaves under natural and unnatural conditions, primarily in humans, but in 10% or so of its pages, in nonhuman animals. Our methods of studying the heart change with the changing of our "instruments of precision," our pharmacopia and our ideas, but all the while the heart remains more or less unchanged. Despite the enormous amount of information gained about the heart in the last 75 years, in some respects we have not begun. Our knowledge of the *causes* of cardiac diseases remains poor. Our diagnostic and therapeutic abilities far exceed our knowledge of why the diseases occur in the first place. Despite not knowing precisely why most heart diseases occur, we do know how to prevent many of them. If our total serum cholesterol remains <150 mg/dl, our chances of developing atherosclerosis severe enough to obstruct or aneurysmally dilate an artery are extremely small. If we totally discard salt from the diet, our chances of developing systemic hypertension and all of its consequences, including stroke, are virtually nonexistent. If we live in sanitary, uncrowded and nonpromiscuous environments, our chances of developing rheumatic and syphilitic heart disease are minimal. If alcohol intake is not abused, our chances of developing our most common primary myocardial disease—dilated cardiomyopathy—are relatively small. Thus, most of our present-day common cardiologic conditions are acquired, man-made, of our own doing. The congenital cardiac conditions—holes in cardiac septa, obstructions to flow into or out of a cardiac chamber, improperly connected arteries and veins, malformed valves (bicuspid), which are prone to degenerate (calcific) or to become infected, floppy mitral valves and hypertrophic cardiomyopathy—will remain despite our alterations in dietary and living habits. As we continue to learn more about, and do more for, heart disease, it is humbling to reflect that the heart is only one of the bodies' many organs and that our major subjects of study are only one of the many species on this earth.

William C. Roberts

William C. Roberts, MD
Editor-in-Chief

Can Rest and Relaxation Be Obtained by Combining a "Vacation" with a Medical Meeting or a Medical Meeting with a "Vacation"?

No medical group appears to have more meetings than cardiologists. From October 1960 until December 1983, I participated in 577 medical meetings, all but a few of which were cardiologic meetings, and 450 (78%) were located in cities outside the Washington, D.C. area. Medical meetings often are located at sites that are vacation attractions. These meetings often include the opportunity to increase medical knowledge and, at the same time, obtain "a vacation" at a price less costly than if unconnected with a medical meeting because of the tax deductibility. But can both a vacation and increased medical knowledge really be obtained simultaneously? I think the answer is more often "no" than "yes."

All of us obviously need *rest* and *relaxation*. Because each is different, each is usually obtained by different means. Rest is always passive and includes activities such as sitting in an easy chair, lying on a beach or rocking in a hammock or sleeping. Rest allows tired muscles time to recover so that they can work efficiently again. It permits the rejuvenation of the physical being.

Relaxation, in contrast, may be either active or passive and includes such diverse activities as playing tennis, collecting stamps, lying on a beach, talking with another person, walking or picnicking. Relaxation rejuvenates the emotional being so that we can cope better with pressures, challenges and responsibilities of work and daily living. Relaxation helps prevent or relieve a general pessimism, diminished ability to cope, loss of enthusiasm, anger or irritability, a sense of personal isolation, and a utilization of tremendous amounts of energy to get very little accomplished. Relaxation, then, depends on how we experience an activity, not on what our body is doing or where we are during the activity. True relaxation is any satisfying involvement in any activity in which the primary reward is the experience itself. Therefore, absent from the relaxation experience is a win-lose goal orientation, an ego enhancement or creation of "products" for later evaluation and justification of the time spent. Active relaxation is actually play, which is active involvement in an activity that one enjoys for the experience itself rather than for a payoff. Passive relaxation involves withdrawing into "inner space" to shut out the distractions and concerns of the surroundings. Thus, rest primarily relieves physical fatigue, and relaxation, primarily emotional fatigue.

By knowing exactly what rest and relaxation are, it is clear that it can be difficult combining a true vacation with a medical meeting or vice versa. One might argue that the physician is not required to spend the entire day at the medical meeting. The problem with this position is the element of *guilt* (also Uncle Sam). For each of the last 11 years I have directed a 3-day course in cardiology in Williamsburg, Virginia. The medical program lasts from 8 AM to about 5:30 PM each day. A number of enrollees have complained to me that there is no time off during the daylight hours to enjoy the lovely Williamsburg setting and that at least 1 or 2 of the afternoons should be free to browse and savor the atmosphere. My position has been that enrollees are free to "take off" from the meeting at any time and by having the meeting continuously through the day those enrollees desiring entirely medical refreshment have the opportunity of obtaining it in concentrated form. This view sets poorly with the enrollees who want both medical and emotional refreshment, because guilt from "skipping the meeting" prevents full enjoyment of the sight-seeing or vacation portion of the trip. I have finally come to realize that the only way to prevent the "professional" guilt in many enrollees and allow the obtainment of at least some relaxation for the enrollees is to recess the meeting for some of the daylight hours.

To obtain rest and relaxation in conjunction with a medical meeting, I believe that thorough premeeting planning is essential. If the meeting is to run continuously and "guilt" is a problem with the attendee, that person must plan for 1 or 2 days off before or after the meeting for concentrated physical and emotional rebuilding. If the additional days are not possible, missing some portion of the meeting is necessary.

Attending a medical meeting in one's home town prevents the problem of trying to attend a medical meeting and have a vacation simultaneously, but then the medical meeting often is interrupted by practice obligations. One could also argue that not all pure vacations provide full rest and relaxation, but certainly the odds of obtaining them without interruption by a professional meeting clearly greatly increases the chances.

In conclusion, I find it difficult to infuse leisure time with work, and obtain either good rest or full relaxation. Although a medical meeting in a vacation spot produces a change and a break from the "dailyness" of medical practice and in itself may provide some rest and relaxation, the medical meeting itself generally prevents the obtainment of either full rest or full relaxation. The latter 2, in my opinion, are better obtained by completely separating the medical meeting from the vacation and vice versa.

William C. Roberts

William C. Roberts, MD
Editor-in-Chief

Forces Changing America

In the March 19, 1984, issue of the *U.S. News & World Report* appeared an article entitled, "10 Forces Reshaping America." A summary of these forces, which obviously will impact our nation's health and health providers well into the next century, may be appropriate.

(1) *More older persons.* For the first time in USA history, there are more people older than 65 years than below 20 years. By 1990 it is projected that >31 million Americans will be older than 65 years and 23 million younger than 20 years. The reason, of course, is the relatively stagnant birth rate combined with an increase in life expectancy. Persons older than 85 years are expected to number 3.5 million by 1990.

(2) *Movement to the South and the West.* The Northeast and Midwest are shrinking in population and the South and West are rapidly increasing. During the next 6 years alone, populations of 10 sunbelt states are predicted to increase by ≥20%. At the same time, movement of families from cities to suburbs or exurbia (areas just beyond the rims of suburbs) continues.

(3) *Computers.* The development of tiny electronic chips with computing power once available only in room-size machines is revolutionizing our society. From the 1940s until 1977, an estimated 0.5 million computers were installed in the USA. In 1983 alone, 6.7 million personal and home computers were sold in the USA. Of course, their ability to collect, analyze and disseminate information is having an enormous impact on medicine.

(4) *Foreign competition.* Progressively more of our major products are being made abroad. Our once consistent trade surplus is now a trade deficit; an imbalance of more than $100 billion is predicted for 1984. For the first time in 70 years, more foreign investment will come to America this year than American investment overseas.

(5) *Women gaining power.* In 1950, only a third of women held jobs outside the home. Today, >67% of women aged 25 to 44 years are employed and 57% of married women with children work outside the home—a 31% increase in 20 years. In 6 million USA homes, wives earn more money than their husbands. More women than men now are undergraduate students in colleges (52% vs 48%). About 25% of USA medical students are women. In my 1958 medical school class, only 1 of the 66 graduates was a woman. More women now vote than do men (53% vs 47%). Fewer women are marrying and those who do marry do so at a later age. The incidence of depression in women aged 35 to 55 years apparently has declined dramatically. Women outlive men in the USA by more than 7 years.

(6) *Minorities gaining power.* A black man is running for President. A black woman is Miss America. The birthday of a black man is now a national holiday. The nearly 27 million blacks account for 12% of the USA population. The number of Americans of Spanish origin increased by 61% in the 1970s, to 16 million. They are expected to overtake blacks and become the second largest minority in another decade. The number of Asian Americans increased 128%, to nearly 4 million, in the 1970s. Problems remain. In 1982, the median income of black families was $13,600; that of Hispanic families, $16,230; and that of white families, $24,600.

(7) *Declining superpowers.* World events are now less influenced by the USA and the Soviet Union. The 157 individual nations and the 1,000 different tongues each contend for their "piece of the pie."

(8) *Declining influence of government.* Fewer elected politicians have safe seats. The era of 2-term Presidents has passed. The Internal Revenue Service is having a

harder time collecting all the taxes. Voter turnout is down to 53%, from 63% a decade ago. Public trust is clearly on the decline.

(9) *Education boom.* One million persons earned college degrees in 1980, a 50% increase from 1960. More doctoral degrees were conferred from 1970 to 1981 than had been conferred in the previous 109 years since Yale granted the first such degree in 1861. Too many MDs are being graduated from the 129 USA medical schools. (Every big city in America already has enough physicians.) The percentage of minority students graduating from high school in 1981 was 79%, up from 23% in 1950. But college degrees and even advanced degrees are no longer guarantees of finding jobs. Continuing education programs now enroll 23 million Americans, 10 million more than 15 years ago.

(10) *Improving health.* Mumps, measles, polio and rheumatic fever have almost vanished in America. More cancers are being cured. Coronary heart disease is on the decline. The blood cholesterol level of Americans continues to fall. The mean total plasma cholesterol in American men aged 39 to 65 years is down to 211 mg/dl. Blood pressure is lower. Cigarette smoking is on the decline. Average body weight is probably on the decline. Alcohol consumption is on the decline. The level of fitness is improving. The number of organ transplants being performed is increasing. There are more nonsurgical solutions to former surgical problems. The expense of the advances, however, may eventually produce the situation of more rationing of medical care.

William C. Roberts

William C. Roberts, MD
Editor-in-Chief

Enticing Real and Potential Cardiovascular Researchers Away from Research

The number of physicians increases each year. Every city in America probably has too many physicians. For the first time in decades, several medical schools in 1984 decreased the number of students admitted to the freshman medical school class.

It appears that there are now too many cardiologists—both adult and pediatric—and cardiovascular surgeons in the USA. Certainly there are too many in the major cities. Competition is getting stiff, but nevertheless the financial reward continues to be good, particularly for those doing invasive procedures. I understand that the cardiologist's fee for coronary angioplasty is usually about $2,500, but that it can be twice that amount. A number of surgeons have told me that their fee for coronary artery bypass surgery usually is about $5,000, with sometimes $2,000 more for the surgical assistant; of course, the anesthesiologist's fee is separate. A cardiac-surgeon friend told me 5 years ago (February 1980) that a cardiac surgeon not making "half a million dollars a year was simply not a good cardiac surgeon." A half million, of course, is derived from 100 bypass operations or an average of only 2 a week. A few valve replacement operations additionally each year take care of the office expenses and malpractice insurance. Although most cardiac surgeons do coronary bypass operations and, therefore, most in private practice receive these high incomes, most cardiologists (however that might be defined[1]) do not do invasive procedures, and furthermore most who do invasive procedures do not do angioplasty. But the noninvasive procedures are also large financial generators in cardiology. Compared with other subspecialties of internal medicine, the income of adult cardiologists is usually substantial. The division of cardiology is the largest generator of income of any subdivision of internal medicine. Thus, both cardiology and cardiovascular surgery are financially rewarding, the most rewarding in these terms of any subspeciality of surgery or any subspeciality of medicine or pediatrics.

Is this high financial reward today in cardiologic practice (either medicine, pediatrics or surgery) too enticing to the creative mind which a decade or so ago would have relished a career in cardiovascular research? I think the answer is yes. Of course, there may be other factors. The young potential investigators observe the difficulty of their senior faculty in obtaining and retaining research grants. They observe the frustration of the senior faculty in trying to do research while managing large clinical responsibilities to generate their incomes. They observe the difficulty of their superiors in getting their research papers published, the near "harrassment" from reviewers and editors, neither of whom "really understand their papers." They observe in surprise the actual energy—both physical and mental—required to create and to generate the data to prove or disprove the idea and the discipline it takes to "package" the product once the results of the investigation are clear.

Although available clinical positions in cardiovascular medicine and surgery are decreasing, positions for cardiovascular researchers are plentiful and good candidates are few[2]. Despite the relative decrease in federal monies for cardiovascular research, pharmaceutical and other private monies are increasing. Money is and will be available to support the good ideas and the good research, but more resourcefulness is now required of the investigator. Cardiovascular disease will not be conquered by doing more coronary angioplasties or bypasses or performing more echocardiograms or nuclear angiograms. But successful research is a selfish and demanding mistress. She never lets up. She disdains fancy cars, elaborate boats, long vacations, too many long weekends, season tickets for this or that, and so on. But, opportunity to utilize one's potential to the fullest is sufficient reward.

William C. Roberts, MD
Editor-in-Chief

1. **Conti CR.** What is a clinical cardiologist in 1984? Am J Cardiol 1984;54: 229–230.
2. **Burns TW.** Physician investigators for academic medicine. Ann Intern Med 1984;101:708–709.

How Long Do Physicians Live?

In the USA today (1980 life tables), life expectancy from birth for white females is 78.1 years, for black females, 72.3 years, for white males, 70.7 years, and for black males, 63.7 years.[1] For persons who have reached age 25 years in the USA, an age reached by >95% of persons at the time of graduation from medical school, life expectancy is even greater. Thus, of persons reaching age 25 years, 54.5 additional years (to age 79.5) can be expected for white women and 49.5 additional years (to age 74.5) for black women, 47.8 additional years for white men (to age 72.8) and 41.7 additional years for black men (to age 66.7).[1]

Although physicians, of course, are included in these 1980 statistics, these expected ages are not reached by most USA graduates of USA medical schools. In the *Journal of the American Medical Association* each week is a column entitled "Obituaries." Included in it are the names of recently deceased physicians, their ages at death, the name of the medical school from which they graduated, frequently the American specialty board by which they were certified, and the date of their death. Their race is not included. For the 3 years 1981, 1982 and 1983 the age at death of the male and female physicians according to speciality was determined and the results of these tabulations are summarized in the accompanying table.

The table discloses 3 clear findings: (1) the average age at death of both the male and female physicians was below the national average for persons who had reached age 25 years; (2) the mean age of death of the female physicians was younger than that of their male counterparts; and (3) the mean age at death varied among the various subspecialties. The 9,705 male physicians lived a total of 689,184 years, an average of 71.0 years each; the 365 female physicians lived a total of 25,495 years, an average of 69.9 years each. Among the various subspecialties, those surviving the shortest periods on the average were neurosurgeons (58.9 years), anesthesiologists (58.9 years), family practitioners (62.4 years) and pathologists (63.9 years). The longest survivors on the average were those classified as both ophthalmologists and otolaryngologists (79.3 years), next those classified as otolaryngologists (76.7 years), and then those boarded in preventive medicine (74.4 years). The pediatricians survived on an average longer than did the internists (69.2 years vs 66.7 years). The specific numbers on survival for adult cardiologists, pediatric cardiologists, and cardiovascular surgeons are not available.

William C. Roberts, MD
Editor in Chief

1. National Center for Health Statistics. Vital Statistics of the United States, 1980, Vol. II, Sec. 6, Life Tables, DHHS Pub. No. (PHS) 84-1104. Public Health Service, Washington, D.C., U.S. Govt. Print. Off., 1984, 16 pp.

Mean Length of Survival of Physicians Listed in the Obituaries Section of the Journal of the American Medical Association, 1981, 1982 and 1983

	Men		Women		Totals		
Speciality	No.	Mean Age at Death (year)	No.	Mean Age at Death (year)	No.	Total Years	Mean Age at Death (year)
Unspecified	6,182	72.7	254	70.9	6,436	467,667	72.7
Internal medicine	514	66.8	13	61.0	527	35,149	66.7
Surgery	409	67.0	4	72.0	413	27,706	67.1
Obstetrics & gynecology	355	68.6	8	73.9	363	24,943	68.7
Psychiatry & neurology	303	68.7	20	72.7	323	22,259	68.9
Pediatrics	267	69.5	12	63.0	279	19,305	69.2
Radiology	216	67.1	6	82.8	222	14,988	67.5
Pathology	200	64.1	7	58.7	207	13,230	63.9
Opthalmology (Op)	182	70.1	3	80.7	185	13,007	70.3
Otolaryngology (Ot)	176	76.6	2	82.0	178	13,643	76.7
Orthopedic surgery	159	67.0	0	...	159	10,656	67.0
Urology	152	71.5	0	...	152	10,871	71.5
Family practice	151	62.7	6	54.8	157	9,800	62.4
Anesthesiology	107	59.2	10	55.8	117	6,891	58.9
Dermatology	82	71.2	6	81.0	88	6,323	71.9
Preventive medicine	72	74.5	6	73.0	78	5,801	74.4
Thoracic surgery	40	66.0	2	65.5	42	2,769	65.9
Neurosurgery	17	58.9	0	...	17	1,001	58.9
Op + Ot	15	79.3	0	...	15	1,190	79.3
Plastic surgery	7	64.0	0	...	7	448	64.0
All Others	99	67.6	6	56.8	105	7,032	67.0
Totals	9,705	71.0	365	69.9	10,070	714,679	71.0

The Most Powerful Cause of Sudden Death

In December 1982 at a cardiology course, I gave a talk on "sudden cardiac death" and described its many causes.[1] One that I did not mention was nuclear explosion. On the same program was Dr. Bernard Lown, who spoke on "physicians, nuclear weapons, and nuclear war."[1] The insignificance of my earlier talk on sudden cardiac death was dramatically exposed by Lown's description of the "litany of horrors resulting from blast, fire, and radiation" were a nuclear war to occur.[2] Since the dropping of the "small" (only 13 kilotons) nuclear bombs on Hiroshima and Nagasaki just over 40 years ago, world arsenals of nuclear weapons have increased to 15,000 megatons, the equivalent of 1 million Hiroshimas, and now nuclear weapons are "the greatest threat to health that human kind has ever known." [3] As so eloquently described by Cassel and associates[3]:

> . . . The arms race has progressed to such a point that even to think of nuclear weapons as 'weapons' rather as instruments of terror and mass destruction is to be dangerously misled about their physical and biologic effects. Physicians have become increasingly involved in speaking out about the medical consequences of the use of nuclear weapons. This involvement has been based on the following precepts: (1) nuclear war cannot be won, limited, or survived in any meaningful sense of the term; (2) there is no effective treatment once nuclear war has occurred—the only appropriate response is prevention; (3) the use of nuclear weapons would result in death, disease, and global environmental damage on a scale that cannot be justified by any ideological differences; (4) the nuclear arms race itself is attended by unacceptable social, psychological, and ecological costs; (5) the halt and reversal of the nuclear arms race and the reduction of international tensions are the first, most effective steps toward prevention of nuclear war; (6) it is only through education of the public that these steps will be achieved; and (7) physicians, as part of their responsibilities for the health of their individual patients and for the community, have a responsibility to further this education and to advance the steps that must be taken to prevent nuclear war.
>
> The prevention of nuclear war is not a partisan issue. It is something on which American and Soviet physicians can agree. It is a simple scientific truth that nuclear war would bring unimaginable disaster of proportions that cannot even be clearly estimated. Our undeniable cultural and political differences with the Soviet Union cannot be resolved or even 'managed' by the buildup of nuclear arsenals. The only ethical conclusion is that nuclear weapons should never be used and that international diplomacy must take other, more effective avenues.

The International Physicians for the Prevention of Nuclear War (IPPNW), an organization started by Cardiologists Bernard Lown and Eugene Chazov and which was awarded the Nobel Peace Prize in 1985, gathered in Budapest in June 1985 under the slogan, "Cooperation not confrontation is the imperative of a nuclear age." Since its inception 5 years ago, this organization has grown to 145,000 members from 45 countries. It has established a broad-based, free-flowing dialog between physicians of the 2 major power blocs—the USA and the USSR—and it now calls for a moratorium on all nuclear explosions.[2] It has previously urged freezing, reducing and eliminating nuclear weapons and a commitment to no first use as the best means of eradicating the greatest public health threat of all time.[2]

Cardiologist E. Greg Diamond has suggested an exchange program of university students between the USA and the USSR as a means of preventing nuclear confrontation.[4] Earlier, Diamond had stated that the 10,000 Chinese scholars in American universities today serve as virtual guarantors of peace with China.[5] Diamond now advocates exchange of 250,000 university students between the USA and USSR to act as agents of security for both sides because "people are unlikely to bomb their children."[4] George Lundberg, the editor of the *Journal of American Medical Association*, added 4 other prescriptions[6]: "1) extensive international travel at all times because people are unlikely to bomb their friends; 2) further development of global economy because people are unlikely to bomb their own companies; 3) extensive scientific and cultural exchanges because people are unlikely to bomb their colleagues, and 4) widespread intermarriage across countries because people are unlikely to bomb their own families and progeny."

William C. Roberts

William C. Roberts, MD
Editor in Chief

1. December 1982 Program in Williamsburg, Virginia, entitled "Coronary, Hypertensive, Valvular and Myocardial Heart Diseases and Peripheral Vascular Diseases: The Multidisciplinary Approach" sponsored by The American College of Cardiology.
2. Lown B, Chazov E. Cooperation not confrontation: the imperative of a nuclear age. JAMA 1985;254:655–657.
3. Cassel CK, Jameton AL, Sidel VW, Storey PB. The physician's oath and the prevention of nuclear war. JAMA 1985;254:652–654.
4. Diamond EG. The logic of a university student USSR-US exchange program. JAMA 1985;254:658–659.
5. Diamond EG. A fundamental unit of peace. JAMA 1984;251:512.
6. Lundberg GD. Prescriptions for peace in a nuclear age. JAMA 1985; 254:660–661.

Justifying a Cardiac Catheterization Laboratory

Recently I was asked to write a letter to a state commissioner on the usefulness of a cardiac catheterization laboratory in a large hospital in a populous community. I emphasized that the cardiac catheterization laboratory was no longer simply a diagnostic laboratory, but that the advent of thrombolytic therapy and percutaneous transluminal coronary angioplasty had added a therapeutic component to the catheterization laboratory.

Shortly after outlining my own views,[1] David E. Rogers, MD,* President of The Robert Wood Johnson Foundation, which has funded many studies on the costs of medical care and the means to decrease the costs, wrote a piece describing his own acute myocardial infarction and the treatment he received.[2] His description of his own experience is, in my view, a convincing justification for a cardiac catheterization laboratory in a large hospital in a large community:

> ... As a doctor who has spent much of his professional lifetime trying to listen very carefully to patients and to treat them appropriately, and then to teach others who are becoming doctors how to do it well, I now wish to try to describe a recent personal experience—to convey what one very common disease feels like "from the inside" when it starts.
>
> The disease is myocardial infarction, the commonplace heart attack.
>
> I have often told medical students that most people I have queried who were having genuine cardiac pain seemed instinctively to wish to remain very quiet, even when their pain was not particularly severe. Thus, I have generally felt that when patients told me they had to keep "wiggling about" to find a comfortable position or were "writhing with pain" and the like, their chest pain was probably noncardiac.
>
> My own experience would certainly confirm this. After the first fifteen to twenty minutes, when the pain was waxing and waning, and I was pretending it was esophageal and was popping a few Tums and drinking a glass of milk, the sensation certainly told me just what it seems to have told other patients. I felt I must sit down *very, very* quietly. Although I did so, the pain became a steadily expanding, deep, penetrating ache, spreading from beneath mid-breastbone, around the sides of my chest, up my neck into my lower jaw, and down the inner aspect of my left arm into my fourth and fifth fingers. It cycled a bit. Sometimes it seemed most dreadful in my chest, then in my jaw and lower teeth, then in my left arm. But it conveyed one clear message. What I felt from the outset and continued to feel through about two hours of what seemed absolutely intolerable pain was that if I remained *absolutely* immobile, not moving even an eyelash, perhaps it would let go of me. I would guess it took about ten to twelve minutes to build to maximal intensity, and there it stayed. During the entire period I sat absolutely still with my eyes closed, conscious of the fact that I was sweating profusely and that I probably looked very pale and lousy. Although my wife was bustling cheerfully about in the kitchen, not fifteen feet away, I said absolutely nothing, feeling that even moving my tongue or vocal chords was simply too much. I had no inclination to groan or cry out.
>
> There was another aspect of the pain that is frequently alluded to by others. There was absolutely no doubt in my mind that I was about to die. As the pain remained, I simply wished exodus would go ahead and happen. The emotion I can recapture regarding this certainty was not one of great fear, but rather of anger mixed with sadness. I felt angry because this goddamned thing was happening to me, and because I knew that some things I had done—smoking for years, and handling some recent episodes of stress rather poorly—had provoked it. I was sad because I was not going to be able to say goodbye to anybody—particularly my family and close friends and colleagues—or tell them what they had meant to me.
>
> The quality of the pain is as difficult for me to describe as it seems to have been for other observers over the last seventy-plus years. It was not the bright, or burning, or well-localized pain one feels with a cut, a puncture, or a burn, from which one instinctively and swiftly retreats. A very different set of nerve endings are involved. It was a dreadful, deep, nauseating ache. If you could multiply one hundred-fold the kind of ache in your arms you experience after working too long trying to

*Dr. Rogers was born in New York City in 1926, graduated from Cornell University Medical College in 1948, did postgraduate training in medicine at The John Hopkins Hospital and The New York Hospital, and in 1955 became Chief of the Division of Infectious Diseases, The New York Hospital–Cornell Medical Center. In 1959, he became Professor and Chairman of the Department of Medicine, Vanderbilt University School of Medicine, and in 1968, Dean of the Medical Faculty, The John Hopkins University School of Medicine and Vice-President (Medicine), The Johns Hopkins University. In 1974, he became President of The Robert Wood Johnson Foundation, Princeton, New Jersey. He is the recipient of 5 honorary doctorate degrees.
His article entitled, "Some Observations on Having a Coronary," is reprinted here with permission of Dr. Rogers and the publisher of *The Pharos*.

screw a recalcitrant light bulb into a ceiling socket that is a little too high over your head for you to reach decently, you would be close. The stunt I tried many years ago—putting a blood pressure cuff on my own leg above the knee and blowing it up to occlude arterial circulation, to feel the kind of pain that develops in one's calf—is yet closer. (At the time, I was trying to see if I could mimic heart pain.) What was exquisitely different about that experiment was that I could release the cuff when I felt I could not stand further intensity of pain. In this real instance, there was no such let up.

As to intensity, I keep wanting to use the word *unbearable*. Obviously, this word is not really appropriate, as I did manage somehow to bear the pain. But it was an absolutely, monstrously, awful sensation, and it was totally untouched by 20 or 30 or 40 milligrams of morphine, administered to me over the next two hours in the hospital. That morphine gave me so little relief has made me empathize deeply with the hundreds of patients with the same disease whom I have treated with this drug over the years.

So that is what it felt like. Now, let me add a few other comments about my treatment, which led to the nice ending that makes this introspection possible.

First, having a cardiac catheterization via the femoral artery and vein during an infarction is a piece of cake—almost no discomfort. Further, having frequent squirts of dye into one's coronary arteries, a procedure I could watch on a monitor, is totally painless. It did not improve my morale to see absolutely no dye going into my left anterior descending coronary artery, which appeared completely blocked, but I already knew that this was probably going to be the case, and all other arteries looked splendid.

One further episode was impressive and of profound relief to me. My cardiologist catheter artisans had maneuvered their catheter into the stump-like orifice of the left anterior descending coronary and had begun dripping in streptokinase (an ancient streptococcal enzyme that I had first used in crude form in 1950 to dissolve clots in patients' pleural spaces). Quite suddenly, and after only modest amounts of enzyme, I said—and I think these were some of my first words after onset of the episode—"I think you've dissolved it; I've lost my pain." The cardiologists were quite surprised, but they shot in some more dye, which confirmed part of what I was saying. A thin threadlike squirt of dye could be seen going through a very tight centimeter-long obstruction close to the origin of the coronary vessel. But the whole artery below the block looked fat and filled. They continued to profuse the streptokinase, but five to ten minutes later I said, "And now it's clotted off again," for my pain had just then returned, in its original intensity. More pictures showed that this indeed was true—there was no more filling beyond the stump.

Then followed the use of the latest in modern medical miracle technologies. My physicians skillfully threaded a tiny wire through the obstruction, guided a collapsed balloon over it and positioned it within the obstruction. This procedure I watched on the monitor with fascination. Then they expanded the balloon, forcing arterial wall, clot, and atheroma outwards. Again, I experienced swift and blissful relief of pain. The cardiologists measured pressures, gradients, fooled around, and inflated the balloon again a few times over the next thirty to forty minutes to make sure the gradient had been eliminated and that a clot did not form again. I have been pain-free ever since, and subsequent pictures of the coronary have looked virtually normal.

Let me add just one other thing that my physicians did for me later, for I have felt, in retrospect, that it was a vital factor in speeding my return to full function. Although I had been agitating to get home, I now confess that I did have some feelings of apprehension about being discharged. Being hooked up to all that gadgetry makes one feel surprisingly dependent and fragile and emotionally uncertain about one's ability to function adequately outside of the hospitals' technologic womb. Thus, I had doubts about how I would feel walking up the stairs or up the driveway, and the like.

But the night before discharging me, my cardiologists asked if I would like them to run a modified stress test on me before I left, and I agreed with enthusiasm. Consequently, the next morning they hooked me up, stuck me on the treadmill, and proceeded to work me until I thought I would drop. My legs were crying for relief, and I was puffing like an aging bull, but my electrocardiogram remained totally unchanged, my blood pressure behaved responsibly, and I had absolutely no chest pain. Afterwards, I felt that this test was perhaps the greatest gift they could have bestowed upon me as a going-away present. Although I was intellectually sure my heart was functioning splendidly, to have objective proof that it could handle vastly more effort than I was planning for it during the next month or so made me feel totally comfortable about cutting the umbilical cord and striking out on my own again.

So: I have had an experience unheard of until very recently—that of knowing first-hand what having a massive myocardial infarction feels like, but without having the full-blown event actually occur, and without having to live with its crippling aftermath. The residual myocardial damage looks modest and should repair rapidly. My coronaries now all resemble good-looking garden hoses, without obstruction. Perhaps of equal long-term significance—my priorities have been abruptly, but quite appropriately, reordered...

...As we continue to struggle to make medical care less expensive without lousing it up, I am obviously going to be thinking hard about the implications of what I have just experienced. I would guess that within a very few years it may be viewed as close to medical malpractice to hospitalize a patient with an acute evolving myocardial infarction anywhere but in a hospital with a cardiac unit with catheterization, angioplasty, and backup surgical capabilities, unless such a unit is more than two hours away. That practice surely will not reduce acute costs.

As some of my vintage colleagues and I have since said to each other, we used to care for people like me by slugging them with morphine until their blood-starved heart muscle died and their pain stopped. We would watch fairly helplessly when they developed fatal arrhythmias. We agonized about giving them digitalis when they went into congestive heart failure because of its propensity to produce fatal arrhythmias. Our patients stayed in the hospital for a minimum of six weeks (I stayed ten days), and we created a dreadful number of cardiac cripples, who never worked productively again.

One of my colleagues is fond of saying, "Sometimes the best medicine is the most expensive medicine." All I can say in this instance is, "Amen," but over the long haul, it seems pretty "cost beneficial" to me!

William C. Roberts

William C. Roberts, MD
Editor in Chief

References

1. Roberts WC. *When I have an acute myocardial infarction, take me to the hospital that has a cardiac catheterization laboratory and open cardiac surgical facilities. Am J Cardiol 1984;53:1410.*
2. Rogers DE. *Some observations on having a coronary.* The Pharos *1986;49: 12–14.*

Characteristics of Long-Term Successful Physician Researchers

About 2 years ago my physician son asked me, "What makes a good researcher?" The question has intrigued me. This piece attempts to answer the question by describing predictable characteristics observed in long-term, productive physician researchers whom I have known or studied during the past 30 years:

(1) *Absolute commitment (determination) to do research.* Research is priority number 1 for the successful physician researcher. Patient care, teaching, administration, travels for lectures, etc., are performed around the research work. Energies for nonresearch activities are carefully allocated so that enough energy is left for creating, collecting and writing. I have found that the energies required for research surpass those required for teaching, speaking, editing and patient service. The ability to refuse requests for one's time is vital. A commitment to research is incompatible with full development of nonmedical interests. Beach and mountain houses, country clubs and heavy social schedules rarely are compatible with successful long-term productive research.

(2) *Industriousness.* To say that chronic hard work is mandatory for success in research is almost trite. A week consists of 168 hours, not 40. Most writing is done before 8 AM after 5 PM or during weekends and holidays. Spending the long hours necessary for success requires love and enthusiasm for one's work. Research is both avocation and vocation.

(3) *Talent.* This characteristic includes an ability to generate ideas, to formulate good questions, and to design studies capable of converting ideas into facts and questions into answers. New ideas and good questions exhilarate researchers. Good instincts are useful in asking the most pertinent questions. Skepticism is common—"Convince me, show me the data." The researcher possesses the ability to spot "holes" in accepted knowledge.

(4) *Effective and efficient generator of data to answer questions.* The effective researcher is well organized and task oriented. The words *effective* and *efficient* are crucial. Results are measured not in terms of the number of hours worked, but in terms of accomplishment. Long hours of labor do not substitute for well planned and conceived experiments. Data are collected, not in a vacuum, but with an eye always seeking proper relations, underlying principles and proper conclusions. Answers are pursued in a planned logical fashion. Daily, weekly, monthly and yearly objectives are delineated and achieved.

(5) *Absolute honesty.* This attribute includes accuracy in collecting and collating data, and also acknowledgment of predecessors who previously contributed information on the subject under investigation. Dishonest researchers are short-term survivors. Unintentional errors, however, are far more common than intentional (dishonest) ones. Whether the error is intentional or unintentional does not negate an error's being an error. The long-term researcher interprets data as they are, not as he/she wishes them to be.

(6) *Pursuer of the highest standards of excellence.* Sloppy work, "the easy way" rather than "the right way," prevents long-term survival. "Getting it right" before "getting it out" requires much effort. Because errors are commonly found in manuscripts, all collected data is cross-checked. Standards of excellence rise with experience.

(7) *Resourcefulness.* This characteristic is essential in finding answers to questions, in acquiring funds to support the research, and in finding appropriate patients for the various studies.

(8) *Flexibility.* Ability to change course quickly is essential. The rigid, commander type personality is out of place in a research laboratory.

(9) *Perseverance.* Strength and patience are essential, for the researcher's life, like others, has its disappointments. Not all research endeavors are successful, manuscripts are rejected, research grants are not approved or funded, personnel bring disappointment, and unpredictable and/or uncontrollable factors prevent completion of projects. The successful researcher, however, anticipates obstacles and overcomes them.

(10) *Confidence.* The long-term researcher believes in

his/her abilities, judgments and instincts, but nevertheless, welcomes criticism at anytime from anyone (including manuscript reviewers) for he/she wants the product to be the best it can be. Hypersensitivity is the price of keen perceptiveness, but it is a small price to pay.

(11) *A recognizer and developer of opportunities.* Opportunities for research are not equally divided among individuals or among medical institutions. An opportunity once available is grasped and held. A move to another institution is made primarily for better opportunities in research, not for better titles, unless, of course, a change from a research career to another type of challenge is desired. The true researcher often converts non-research centers into research ones.

(12) *Congeniality.* Long-term investigators work well and "deal straight" with all associates, both those above and below on the hierarchical scale. They are neither selfish nor greedy. They have good negotiating skills, possess humility, and provide a pleasant and stimulating atmosphere in which to work.

(13) *Competitiveness.* Although not often discussed, the medical research community is competitive and the successful physician researcher finds the competitive element fun, challenging, and stimulating, knowing that it enhances efficiency in completing projects. Researchers can be compared to ducks moving on a pond—on the surface things are calm, the rapidly moving legs beneath the water's surface are invisible. Researchers do not withhold information from colleagues because of this characteristic.

(14) *A good writer.* Good writing requires good thinking and clear writing indicates clear thinking. Ability to describe observations clearly and concisely on paper is essential for long-term success in medical research.

William C. Roberts

William C. Roberts, MD
Editor in Chief

A Malpractice Dream

I had a dream the other night about going into private practice and about declining the opportunity to purchase malpractice insurance. In addition to the usual office-opening procedures, I did 2 unorthodox things:

(1) Hung a large sign in the waiting room that read:

> WILLIAM C. ROBERTS, MD, POSSESSES NO MALPRACTICE INSURANCE AND ALL HIS MATERIAL POSSESSIONS ARE IN HIS WIFE'S NAME

(2) Developed a letter to be presented to each new patient visiting my office. The letter, addressed to "Dear Potential Patient," contained the above announcement and reasons why this policy might be advantageous to patients. The savings incurred from not paying malpractice premiums would be passed on to patients in the form of lower physician bills. The type of medicine practiced would not be so-called "defensive medicine," whereby numerous laboratory tests, including radiographic, electrocardiographic, echocardiographic and exercise stressing, and even invasive procedures, would be obtained often simply to protect the physician, but they would be ordered only if considered useful to the patient. The nonphysician patient costs consequently should be substantially reduced compared to these costs when "physician-protection" rather than "patient-benefit" medicine was a major concern. The letter also indicated that this physician—like all persons—was not perfect and, therefore, was not free of occasional erroneous reasoning or judgment on a particular problem raised by a patient or by that patient's illness. In an attempt to hold inappropriate or potentially harmful recommendations concerning a patient to a minimum, the patient was informed in the letter that this physician had obtained medical training considered by colleagues to be of high quality. Furthermore, I pledged to my patients that I would keep abreast of medical advances by reading regularly leading medical journals in my field and by attending postgraduate medical courses and other study sessions on a regular basis. Additionally, consultations for my patients would be sought often. The letter also indicated that if any patient considered the above statements and pledges to be inappropriate that other physicians would be recommended. Persons seeking care by this physician, however, would be asked to sign a statement indicating that they understood the letter's contents. The signed copy would be given to the receptionist, who would provide a copy for the patient. Those patients wishing to discuss the letter with me before signing it certainly would be given that opportunity.

After the cardiology office opened, the receptionist received several comments from patients to the effect that the ideas discussed in the letter appeared reasonable. During the first 2 years of practice, only 2 patients did not sign the letter and they were referred elsewhere. The practice grew and the patients seemed to like their "patient-physician agreement."

After 4 years of practice, however, I was sued by a patient. The case involved a man who had had an acute myocardial infarction, had an early uncomplicated course, by day 6 was advised to begin walking about his room and in the hall outside his room, and on day 8, he suddenly collapsed and had cardiac arrest while drinking water at a fountain near the nurse's station. The suit brought by the patient's wife maintained that I had encouraged too rapid an ambulation program and had rehabilitation been slower the cardiac arrest, which was secondary to cardiac rupture, would not have occurred.

I considered the ambulation program even in retrospect to be a sound recommendation and, in my dream, informed all my patients by letter that the suit was pending. Numerous calls came to the office from patients who wanted the address of the spouse bringing suit. Of course, this information was withheld, but another letter was sent later to all my patients informing them of the time and location of the upcoming trial. When the trial began, the court room was packed with my patients. In the trial, I served as my own lawyer, and several other specialists gratefully served as expert witnesses for me, without cost. The jury's verdict was "not guilty." No other suits were brought against me during my subsequent 20 years in practice.

William C. Roberts

William C. Roberts, MD
Editor in Chief

Drug Developers and Drug Dispensers: Their Dependency on One Another

Several pharmaceutical company representatives have told me that the single group of specialists most difficult to visit are cardiologists. Many cardiologists refuse to see pharmaceutical representatives. For cardiologists this is not a good reputation to have. It is important that the relations between physicians and pharmaceutical representatives be good. Both parties want effective, safe and tolerable drugs.

Although some pharmaceutical companies are better than others and some physicians are better than others, both groups are obviously highly dependent on each other and both groups need to be sensitive to the contributions and problems of the other. I feel at times that we physicians forget who comes up with the drugs. It is the pharmaceutical industry, not physicians, who both develop and manufacture the drugs. Drug development today, of course, is enormously expensive, enormously risky and once the new drug is developed, the patent on it is already partially expired. Development of a new drug is somewhat analogous to drilling for oil—only a rare well actually hits the black gold.

Although less recognized, another contribution of the pharmaceutical industry to the medical profession is their generous support of postgraduate medical education. Many medical meetings are funded entirely by a single pharmaceutical company. In meetings sponsored by medical societies or by medical centers, the honoraria and expenses of speakers are often provided by pharmaceutical companies. The expenses and honoraria of visiting professorships often are provide by a pharmaceutical company.

A possibly overlooked or underappreciated support of postgraduate medical education provided by the pharmaceutica industry is their role in the publishing of medical journals. Nearly al clinical journals are dependent o advertising revenues from th pharmaceutical and medical instrument industries for survival. I *The American Journal of Cardiology* had no ads, the subscription cost would be approximately twice its present cost, and later, as the number of subscribers diminished because of the journal's high price, even more. Although few physicians pick up medical journals to read ads, there would be few journals to pick up were ads not present.

Thus, a belated salute to the pharmaceutical industry. Thanks for the splendid drugs and thanks for the generous support of our continued medical education.

William C. Roberts

William C. Roberts, MD
Editor in Chief

The Medical Book with the Most Information for the Price

My favorite general medicine textbook is the 2,258-page eleventh edition of Harrison's *Principles of Internal Medicine* edited by Eugene Braunwald and 5 others and published in 1987. The book costs $89.00 ($110.00 in the 2-volume version), it weighs 3,380 g and it contains more information than any single physician could learn in a lifetime. When I need it, however, it's not there: I'm at home and the book is at the office or vice versa, and I do not have the energy to move it from 1 place to the other.

I recently acquired the 2,696-page fifteenth edition of *The Merck Manual of Diagnosis and Therapy*, also published in 1987, under the editorship of Robert Berkow of Merck Sharp & Dohme Research Laboratories (Figure). This book sells for $21.50 (the softcover version comes in 2 volumes and it sells for $20.00), and it weighs 1,063 g. Examining this splendid edition of *The Merck Manual* stimulated my curiosity about its development and its impact.

The Merck Manual first appeared in English in 1899 (having been translated from German) as a 262-page text titled *Merck's Manual of the Materia Medica.* It was designed to meet the needs of general practitioners in selecting medications, noting that "memory is treacherous" and even the most thoroughly informed physician needs a reminder "to make him at once master of the situation and enable him to prescribe exactly what his judgment tells him is needed for the occasion." The subject material was arranged in 3 sections: materia medica, therapeutic indications, and classification of medicaments according to their physiologic actions. Over 900 items were listed in the materia medica. The drugs mentioned in the 1899 edition and in the present one were nitroglycerin, codeine, atropine, chloral hydrate, digitalis and quinidine. In the therapeutic indications section the various diseases were listed as well as the drugs useful for them. Arsenic was listed under 105 diseases according to Morowitz.[1] Other widely used drugs included belladonna, cannabis indica, eucalyptol, iodine and mineral acids. Bloodletting was still indicated for acute bronchitis, headache, insomnia, intermittent fever, pericarditis, pleurisy, puerperal convulsions, pyemia, spinal concussion and sunstroke. For diphtheria and gonorrhea, bacterial diseases for which no cure existed in 1899, there were 75 and 96 possible treatments listed.[1] By the twelfth edition of *The Merck Manual* in 1972, only 1 treatment was listed for each of these diseases. As Morowitz pointed out,[1] "the less a disease was understood, the larger the number of treatments available." A surprisingly large fraction of the book was devoted to sexual disorders including chordee, emissions and erections, exhaustion-sexual, impotence, nymphomania, satyriasis and spermatorrhea. The "classification of medicaments . . ." section listed 10 aphrodisiacs and 16 anaphrodisiacs.[1] Among the cures for nymphomania was "tobacco: so as to cause nausea: effectual but depressing." [1]

The 1899 edition, which was priced at $1.00, was distributed free to physicians and it contained the trade names of drugs manufactured by Merck; drugs of other companies were listed generically.[2] It also carried a full-page ad for the company.[2] In nearly all subsequent editions "The Manual" has been completely free from all promotion of Merck products, all drugs have been listed by generic name or by both generic and trade names and all editorial board members have been entirely free of pharmaceutical company influence. The company does not even tell editor-in-chief Berkow when to bring out a new edition. The book is published at no profit to Merck, and the company loses money on some editions.

The first *Merck Manual* was an instant success. It was followed by a second edition in 1901, and a third in 1905. The fourth edition in 1911 had nearly doubled in size and was far more fact-packed than the preceding editions. The fifth edition appeared in 1923, and the sixth, a completely new book with a new title and 1,200 pages, appeared in 1934. The seventh edition came in 1940, and the eighth edition, bearing today's title, appeared in 1950. Editions since the eighth for the most part have retained the Manual's successful format, each one containing new developments in science and medicine. These multiple editions contain the pragmatic history of medical practice during this century. *The Merck Manual* is the oldest continuously published medical textbook known by the same name in American history.

The fifteenth edition of *The Merck Manual* is a remarkable book. Editor-in-chief Berkow, who also headed the thirteenth and fourteenth editions, has a physician editorial board and consultant board of 20 (only 1 cardiologist), a Merck editorial staff of 5 and 269 outside authors, which include approximately 20 cardiologists. Of its 2,576 text pages (there are an additional 120 pages of index), 240 (9%) concern cardiovascular disorders. All manuscripts are edited repeatedly (an average of 10 revisions for each manuscript) in-house so that the whole book appears as if it is written by the same individual.

FIFTEENTH EDITION

THE MERCK MANUAL

OF

DIAGNOSIS AND THERAPY

Robert Berkow, M.D., *Editor-in-Chief*

Andrew J. Fletcher, M.B., B.Chir., *Assistant Editor*

Editorial Board

Philip K. Bondy, M.D.
L. Jack Faling, M.D.
Alvan R. Feinstein, M.D.
Eugene P. Frenkel, M.D.
Robert A. Hoekelman, M.D.
Robert G. Petersdorf, M.D.
Fred Plum, M.D.
John Romano, M.D.
G. Victor Rossi, Ph.D.
John H. Talbott, M.D.
Paul H. Tanser, M.D.

Published by
MERCK SHARP & DOHME RESEARCH LABORATORIES
Division of
MERCK & CO., INC.
Rahway, N.J.
1987

FIGURE. Title page of the fifteenth edition of *The Merck Manual.*

Every mention of a drug or its dosage is reviewed by a separate outside consultant. No other medical text undergoes as many reviews and revisions as *The Merck Manual.* Discussions of various diseases and their treatments tend to be succinct, clear and surprisingly complete. The book is devoid of references. The fifteenth edition is published on extremely fine (19 pound) Bible paper with a rich maroon, gold stamped cover, and the 24 chapters are thumb indexed for rapid use.

The fifteenth edition is expected to sell over 1,000,000 copies, mostly to physicians and nurses but since 1975 Merck has permitted sales to the public. No other medical book in history has sold this many. (Medical books that sell 5,000 generally are considered quite successful, and 20,000 or more is considered sensational.) The fifteenth edition also will be translated into Spanish, German, Italian, French, Portuguese and probably Chinese.

The $21.50 price for the fifteenth edition makes it the best buy of any medical book in the world. I have briefly reviewed 89 cardiology books published in the years 1986,[3] 1987[4] and 1988[5] and only 6 of them sold for a lower price. The average cost of the 31 cardiologic books published in 1987 and reviewed by me was $63.00.[4]

Thus, for the medical book with the most information for the lowest price, *The Merck Manual* is the winner. If a physician could have only 1 medical book, *The Merck Manual* should be it.

William C. Roberts, MD
Editor in Chief

1. Morowitz HJ. The Merck of time. *Hospital Practice 1976 (December);11:107–108.*

2. Forman M. For medicinal purposes. *American Way March 1984;160–162.*

3. Roberts WC. Some good cardiologic books published in 1986. *Am J Cardiol 1986;58:1271–1272.*

4. Roberts WC. Some good cardiologic books published in 1987. *Am J Cardiol 1987;60:1423–1424.*

5. Roberts WC. Some good cardiologic books published in 1988. *Am J Cardiol 1989;63:153–154.*

Sensitive Areas Between Physicians and Pharmaceutical Companies

A representative of a pharmaceutical company recently told me that a physician, whom he visits regularly, says "How are we doing?" when he enters the doctor's office. The physician owns stock in the representative's company. I have heard of physicians involved in clinical trials owning large amounts of stock in the company whose drug they are investigating. Some particularly prominent physicians occasionally advise pharmaceutical companies, and are paid large fees for doing so, and large lecture fees for speaking publicly on the drug(s) produced by the company they advise. Many physicians, including myself, give lectures, and both the honoraria and expenses occasionally are paid by pharmaceutical companies.

Although investors tend to buy stocks in industries of which they are knowledgeable and physicians have some knowledge of the pharmaceutical industry, physicians who prescribe drugs to patients must be sensitive to the potential conflict of owning stock, or their families owning stock, in pharmaceutical companies. I own a few shares of Exxon and no shares of Texaco and when buying gasoline I nearly always favor the Exxon station. If I owned similar numbers of shares of both Exxon and Texaco, I presumably would not favor one over the other. There are potential conflicts when a physician owns stock in only 1 or 2 pharmaceutical companies. Probably there would be no potential or real conflicts if a physician owned similar amounts of stock in as many as 10 pharmaceutical companies. If more than 1 pharmaceutical company produces a single class of drug and a physician owns stock in only 1 of the producing companies, it is reasonable to believe that the physician would prescribe the drug produced by the company of which he or she is an owner. If a physician owned stock in a company which produced, for example, a calcium antagonist, but not in a company which produced an angiotensin converting enzyme inhibitor, the physician might use the former drug more often than the latter drug for hypertensive patients.

Physicians involved in clinical trials also must be sensitive to the potential conflict of owning shares in the pharmaceutical company whose drug they are investigating or in a company producing a similar drug or in one producing a drug useful for the condition although of another class. It is appropriate that investigators reporting results of drug trials mention in their publication if they or their families own stock in the company whose drug they are investigating.

Many pharmaceutical companies seek advice periodically from physicians and certainly the physician should be compensated for his or her time. When these physicians speak in public on the value of the drugs produced by companies to which they have a special relation, this relation, in my view, should be openly acknowledged.

A large part of postgraduate medical education today is funded by the pharmaceutical industry. Many medical meetings are funded entirely by a single pharmaceutical company. Not only are speakers paid honoraria and their expenses, but occasionally the expenses of listeners also are covered. In meetings sponsored by local medical societies, often the honoraria and expenses of speakers are provided by pharmaceutical companies. The expenses and honoraria for visiting professorships often are provided by a pharmaceutical company. Most pharmaceutical companies have "their faculties" and their names are often suggested by pharmaceutical representatives to education directors and/or division and department directors of medical centers as potential speakers for their conferences and meetings. When new drugs are approved many pharmaceutical companies sponsor numerous talks by investigators in the drug's clinical trials and also others as a way of disseminating knowledge on the new agents.

I am not opposed to pharmaceutical companies' sponsoring lectures by physicians. Indeed, I have often been the recipient of these sponsorships. Whenever a pharmaceutical company sponsors a lecture, it is appropriate that this be acknowledged from the podium. It is also appropriate that a speaker who accepts pharmaceutical company support for a lecture not be sponsored each time by the same company. It of course is essential that the views of the speaker not be altered by the sponsor.

Editors of medical journals and their families, in my view, should not own stock in pharmaceutical companies or in manufacturers of medical equipment. Most manuscripts submitted to medical journals are pretty good. A few are outstanding and obviously should be accepted, a few are poor and obviously should be rejected, but most are neither outstanding nor poor. It is in this latter group that an editor could easily accept or reject a manuscript. If a manuscript in the latter group was favorable toward a drug produced by a company in which the editor owned stock, the tilt might be more toward acceptance than toward rejection, and vice versa.

In summary, prescription-writing physicians, clinical investigators of drugs, and editors of medical journals need to be sensitive to the potential or real conflict of owning stock, or their families owning stock, in pharmaceutical companies. If a physician owns pharmaceutical stock it appears advisable to own shares in several pharmaceutical companies to avoid the appearance of favoritism. Editors of medical journals and their immediate family should not, in my view, own stock in a pharmaceutical or in a medical-device company.

William C. Roberts

William C. Roberts, MD
Editor in Chief

Clogged Arteries and Clogged Roads

In the USA all adults have 1 heart and nearly all have 1 car. Sometimes I wonder which one is the more important. With each beat blood leaves the heart to enter the superhighway of the vascular system—the aorta—and from there multiple arteries carry the blood to the various organs and tissues and through them the erythrocytes march single file though the capillaries. From them the organs and tissues are supplied with oxygen and the blood returns via the venules, small veins and finally vena cava to the heart once again. Each day most physicians leave their homes in their automobiles, and probably most who are in large cities enter a highway from which they exit to the smaller roads winding through cities and they eventually return home each evening. As the organs and tissues of our bodies are dependent on our heart's pumping blood to them, our practices are dependent on our automobiles' transporting us to our offices and hospitals. Medicine in America is automobile dependent just as our organs and tissues are heart dependent. But, just as our hearts are killing us from clogged coronary arteries, our automobiles are killing us by clogging our roads and destroying our environment.

Andrew Kimbrell, an environmental-law attorney with the Foundation on Economic Trends and policy director of the Greenhouse Crisis Foundation, has provided some facts:

1. *The death and injury* consequences of automobiles are enormous. The more than 2.5 million Americans who have died violent deaths on our highways represent more than 4 times the 641,691 Americans killed in World War I, World War II, and the Korean and Vietnam wars combined. The 1.8 million Americans who sustained disabling injuries in traffic accidents during 1987 alone represent over a half-million more injuries than the number sustained by Americans in all twentieth century wars. In the USA the automobile killed its first million by 1952, its second million by 1975, and its third million is likely by 1994. Additionally, some 90 million Americans have sustained disabling injuries in automobile accidents. In 1988, 46,644 people were killed in traffic accidents in the USA, an increase of 13,000 from 1987.

Automobile accidents are not limited to the USA. In Europe close to 60,000 people are killed each year in car accidents and 2 million are injured. In some Third World countries the fatality/mile-travelled rates are 20 times higher than those of industrialized nations. An estimated 350,000 people are killed each year worldwide in automobile accidents with another 10 million suffering disabling injuries. These estimates, moreover, may be too low because fatalities occurring several days after accidents or off-road are not included in motor-vehicle death reports in most countries.

Human beings are not the only animals killed by automobiles. It is estimated that 1 million nonhuman animals are killed each day on US roads. Only the meat industry kills more animals everyday in the USA than do motorized vehicles.

2. *The environmental consequences* of the automobile are enormous. In the USA, transportation sources are responsible for 69% of lead, 70% of carbon monoxide, 45% of nitrous oxides, and 35% of hydrocarbons released into the air. These emissions cause tens of thousands of deaths a year by contributing to lung cancer and to various noncancerous respiratory disorders. These gases also harm terrestrial and aquatic ecosystems. Car emissions result in $2.0 to 4.5 billion losses each year in our wheat, corn, soybean and peanut crops. Cars, trucks and buses also are the largest single contributor to the buildup of carbon dioxide, a major component of the global-warming threat. Each vehicle emits an average of 5 tons of carbon dioxide into the atmosphere each year—a total of about 600 million tons a year for US cars alone.

Automobiles also contribute to the destruction of the ozone layer. While ozone at the ground level—created primarily by car pollution—can kill us, ozone in the upper atmosphere provides a vital shield that prevents hazardous ultraviolent radiation from reaching the earth. Increasingly, release of chlorofluorocarbons is destroying that layer of protecting ozone. The largest single source in the USA of chlorofluorocarbons is automobile air conditioners, and there are about 95 million auto air conditioners in use in the USA. The installation of each one releases about 2.5 pounds of chlorofluorocarbons, annual recharges add another pound, and these chlorofluorocarbons remain in the atmosphere for >100 years.

3. *Too many automobiles*. In 1950, only 50 million automobiles were in operation on the planet and 75% were in the USA. Today, 400 million automobiles are in operation worldwide, 35% of them in the USA. Including commercial vehicles, the worldwide number of motor vehicles is about 500 million. Each year 38 million new automobiles are produced worldwide, and the number is expected to rise to 60 million by the year 2000. From 1900 to 1984 US factories produced 846,198,000 cars, trucks and buses and now >650,000,000 lie in landfills. In the USA we have 135 million privately owned cars and trucks: 1 car in 36% of households, 2 cars in 35%, and 20% of households have 3 or more cars.

4. *Car time is excessive, wasteful and energy depleting*. American drivers put in the equivalent of 10, forty-hour weeks behind the wheel each year while driving a total of 1.25 trillion miles. Men average 11 hours a week, and women 9 hours a week in total travel time. More than 80% of Americans commute to work in automobiles, and most cars have only the driver as passenger. Travel hours per week in the auto increase with income and education. The private car is the overwhelming transportation of choice of Americans. About 80% of all trips are made by cars, 13% by air, and 7% by all other forms of transporta-

tion. Since 1976 there has been a 30% increase in US car travel (a 45% increase in Japan). This increase in auto use, especially in the post-World War II period, has taken place at the expense of public transport. In 1950, the nation's transit system provided more than 17 billion rides, by 1987 it was down to 8 billion, a number about equal to the riders in 1900.

5. *Automobile transportation is the most expensive form of transportation.* In addition to the enormous costs of the automobiles themselves, the federal, state and local governments annually spend $300 billion to subsidize automobile use in the form of road building and maintenance, municipal services, tax losses from land lost to highways, and health care services. It has been estimated that each passenger car is subsidized at about $2,400, not including the untold environmental costs. Additionally, the average household spends about 1 of every 5 dollars earned to support "automobility"—not counting parking, and 1 of every 6 Americans are employed in an auto-related industry. The Federal Highway Act of 1956 has cost the USA tens of billions of dollars, and now much of the 3,600,000 miles of road in the USA is in need of repair. Although the USA continues to be the largest oil-producing nation, 1989 was the first year where our imports of oil exceeded our own production. Oil imports are the largest contributor to our import bill, and the major reason why our imports exceed our exports.

Thus, just as we must decrease our intake of fat and cholesterol to prevent our arteries from becoming obstructed, we must decrease both the number and size and energy source of our automobiles to prevent our planet and its inhabitants from being suffocated. Driving gasoline-powered automobiles has become an addiction potentially much more dangerous than our addiction to fat and cholesterol (or to any illicit drug).

What can we do? There are no ready solutions, of course, but we must begin:

1. *We must drive less.* We need to live closer to our offices and hospitals. Ideally, we need our offices adjacent to hospitals, so that we park our cars only once during the day. Putting more passengers in a car is difficult for physicians, less so for others. We need higher fuel costs. The average cost for a gallon of gasoline in the USA is only about $1.25. If the government subsidies to the automobile were passed along in gas prices, as happens in many non-USA countries, the cost of a gallon of gasoline would be $4.50. This cost excludes costs of environmental cleanup and research. If we paid more for gasoline many of us would drive less.

2. *We must drive more fuel-efficient automobiles.* Our low oil prices also discourage the production and use of more fuel-efficient automobiles. European prototypes of fuel-efficient vehicles are getting >80 miles/gallon on highways.

3. *We need to improve our mass-transit systems* both in and out of core urban areas and between suburban areas. Monies for these systems need massive expansion.

4. *We must work toward the elimination of the gasoline-powered automobile.* Solar-powered cars and electric cars run on renewable fuels need top priority research.

5. *We must greatly reduce or eliminate the use of car air conditioners.*

Cardiac disease is a major problem in the world, but in comparison to many others it is hardly in the top 10.

William C. Roberts

William Clifford Roberts, MD
Editor in Chief

Limited Research Funds and Cardiac Medicine Without Cardiac Surgery

Bad times have befallen the National Institutes of Health (NIH). Although NIH's total budget rose steadily during the 1980s (in constant dollars it increased by 50% between 1981 and 1990), the number of new and renewable grants funded dropped sharply in 1989 and will plunge again in 1990 (Figure 1). Although some of the new monies have been allocated to national priorities such as AIDS ($300 million in 1990) and the human genome project ($59 million in 1990), the major explanations for the drop in funding of new and renewable grants are the increased number of grants awarded in previous recent years, the increase in average cost of each grant, and the increase in average length of each research project. The number of new and renewable grants that received funding went from 5,493 to 6,477 from 1984 to 1987 and the average length of each project went from 3.3 to 4.1 years from 1983 to 1988. Thus, research projects approved in previous years are soaking up most of the available grant money, and little is left to launch new ones.

Federal medical research monies are not being allocated in proportion to the magnitude of the problems. According to the National Center for Health Statistics, in the USA in 1989 AIDS will cause about 34,400 deaths, cancer about 494,400, and heart disease 777,630 deaths. In contrast to these death totals, federal spending in fiscal 1989 for research and education in AIDS will amount to $1.3 billion, for cancer $1.4 billion, and heart disease, $1.0 billion.

The National Heart, Lung, and Blood Institute (NHLBI) has been hard hit. Only 13% of its approved grants will be funded this year and of those funded, the numbers of dollars allocated will be 13% less than the amount approved. The intramural program (the on-campus research program) of the NHLBI also is being hard hit. A big item in the intramural budget is that spent for patient care, and nearly 60% of the $17 million so spent is for cardiac surgery. Thus, the elimination of cardiac surgery would free up a sizable amount of money for research in other NHLBI laboratories. And that's what was done. The Surgery Branch will discontinue clinical activities in June 1990 and research activities in June 1991.

But can a broad clinical research program in heart disease exist without cardiac surgery? Can cardiology be strong in the absence of cardiac surgery? I think not. Unfortunately, with certain notable exceptions like systemic hypertension, most symptomatic heart diseases are best treated by surgery because most heart diseases produce mechanical blood flow problems. Congenital heart disease (with its defects in cardiac septa or abnormal communications or connections between vessels or cardiac chambers or obstruction at, below or above cardiac

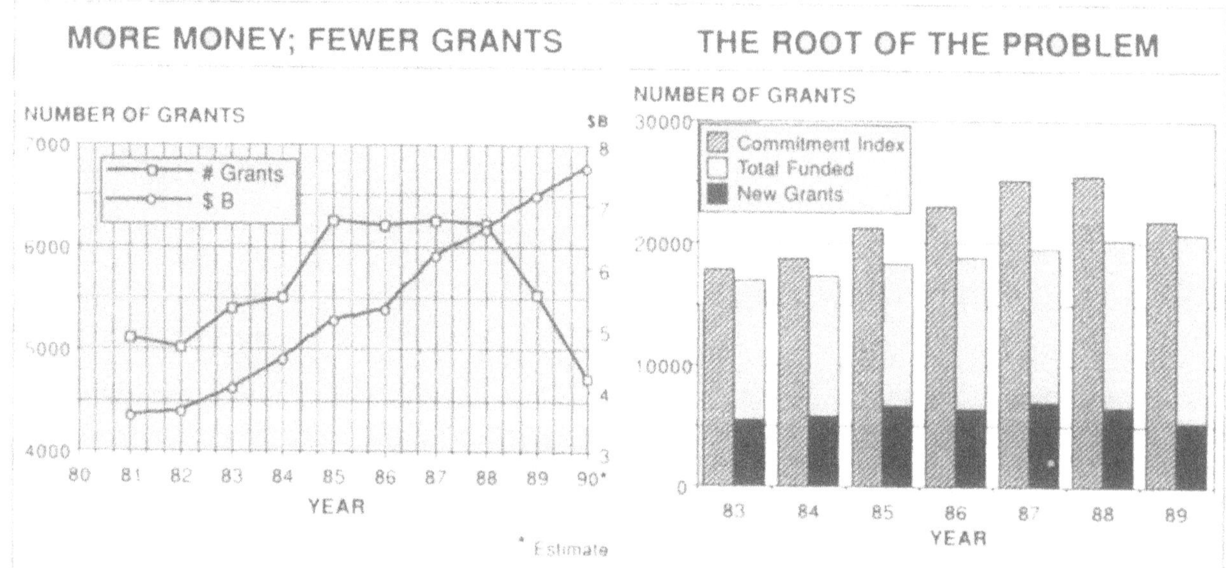

FIGURE 1. NIH's total budget rose steadily during the 1980s, but the number of new and competing grants dropped sharply in 1989 and it will plunge again in 1990. The budget figures are in current dollars. In constant dollars, NIH's budget increased by 50% between 1981 and 1990.

As the number of new grants increased in the mid-1980s, NIH took on a commitment that it could not keep. Until 1988, the commitment index, calculated by multiplying the number of new grants by their average length, rose much faster than the total number of grants NIH could support. Reproduced with permission from Palca J, *Science 1989(November 24);246:988.*

valves) is definitively treated only by surgery. Valvular heart disease (with its obstructions and leaks) is definitively treated only by surgery. Coronary artery disease today is more definitively treated by surgery than by other means. Pericardial disorders often require surgery. The cardiac catheterization laboratory is purely a diagnostic one—not a therapeutic one—without cardiac surgery readily available. Treatment of heart disease today requires both cardiology and surgery and centers without both will, in my view, not be major centers for long. The intermingling of specialists in cardiac medicine and in cardiac surgery under the same roof is essential for the proper development of each.

So Surgery at the National Heart, Lung, and Blood Institute is going because the money is needed elsewhere for more "high-risk research." (Other reasons given for its demise also include the "changing nature of the cardiology research programs," the "inability to recruit and maintain a permanent cadre of qualified surgeons," and "program priorities.") The entire NIH budget in 1990 is about $7.5 billion. In contrast, the Defense Department's budget currently is $302 billion—nearly 30% of the entire federal budget. By contrast, $249 billion is spend on Social Security, $181 billion on interest payments, and $99 billion on Medicare. Of the $302 billion defense budget, $86 billion is spent for operations and maintenance—the cost of keeping troops in the field and maintaining weapons; $85 billion for procurement—the cost of weapons and other supplies; $79 billion for payroll and retirement benefits, and $38 billion (5 times the NIH budget) for research and development on new weapons systems. The cost of the M-1 battle tanks ($1.9 billion) is nearly twice that of the entire NHLBI budget. The cost of the F/A-18 A Hornet jet fighter planes ($2.2 billion) is over twice the NHLBI budget. The cost of the F-16 Falcon jet fighter planes ($3.3 billion) is over 3 times the NHLBI annual budget. The United States share of NATO costs is now $130 billion, over a third of the entire Defense Department budget, and some estimate that 60¢ of every dollar in our $302 billion defense budget is devoted to the defense of Europe. Over 50 years after the end of World War II the USA still has 305,000 troops in Europe. And now after the crumbling of the Berlin Wall and of the Communist regimes in Eastern Europe, the cold war is over. Troops must come home. Resources must be reallocated.

To discontinue cardiac surgery and its potential research arm in the largest cardiac research center in the world because 11 million dollars could better be used elsewhere is a statement to cardiac surgeons the world over that surgeons are no longer players in the cardiac investigative world. In actuality, there is no better research laboratory for human beings than the operating room. When cardiac surgery goes, cardiac medicine will soon follow for obstructed coronary arteries or cardiac valves or intracardiac defects or maldirected blood flow usually require operative therapy. Mr. President, a few less M-1 battle tanks every year and a major cardiac research center will prosper, not fade away.

William C. Roberts

William Clifford Roberts, MD
Editor in Chief

"Anything To Be Done Right Has Got To Be Done By People That Make Their Living At It"

While waiting for an eye examination recently, I picked up a golf magazine and found in it a 1931 syndicated column on professional golf by the great American humorist Will Rogers. What follows are observations by Rogers on this subject, and a few comments* discussing golf and medicine.

Well all I know is just what I read in the papers.

We have had a lot of Golf Players out here in California with us lately, they are just playing a regular circuit of Tournaments. Why it's like show business in vaudeville. All the good ones are out here. By that I mean the Professionals, men who make a living at it, and a mighty good living too. They are about as fine a lot of fellows as you ever met, and fine bunch of sportsmen.

You know it's a kind of funny business at that. You see these fellows don't get anything at these Tournaments unless they win it. The prizes generally run to about the first ten. Well sometimes there is sixty or eighty that start, so you can see somebody has got to have some other visible means of support than his "Putter." They pay their railroad fare and all their living expenses and if they can't find that Gopher Hole in less knocks than the other sixty why, it's just too bad.

I saw 'em all playing in the $10,000 Professional Championship, where the winner got I think $3500. Now Golf is no joke when it gets into jack like that, I have done my fair share of kidding about it, but when there is $3500 bucks strung along on the green and you have to project a little Gutapercha missle into the empty end of a sardine can twenty feet away to get your clutches onto any part of that dough, I want to tell you neighbors the humor of the game immediately vanishes into cold prespiration . . . .

You are shooting for your marmalade on every shot, on every hole, on every day, the thing lasts. There is no three strikes here . . . . Every move is the big one. When one is sliced out into the forest reserve nothing goes with it but your week's board bill, and fare to the next Niblick Rodeo. There is not only a story, but a meal hanging on every putt. You just get the worry of one hole out of your system and onto your handkerchief, then all you have to do is walk up to a nearby executioneer's stand, and look from there down across a beautiful valley . . . and by exact geometrical survey just 543 yards and ⅞th inches is located another of these cunning little resepticles in the ground with a mouth no bigger than a Higlander's heart, and to give aid and comfort to you in distress there is a well painted sign staring you in the face with the information that if you are any kind of a Golfer whatever that four swipes at this little cascaret is all that "Should" be required. That any you take over that, you are simply deducting from your own Bank account.

Then there is a pardner, or accomplice, who plays along with you. You are not sent out for company but to annoy each other, if it wasent for watching what he was doing you could do pretty good. Sometimes it's (what I think) is called a match play that is all you have to beat is the Guy with you. But generally it's medal play, (I think that's it) then all you have to beat is eighty professionals (that you know in your own heart are better than you) and Bobby Jones, and Par, and O.B. Keelers Typewriter . . . .

---

*I was not particularly pleased with the "comments" I initially developed and asked my brother, Dr. Stewart R. Roberts, Jr. (Emory Clinic), for help. The resulting "comments" therefore are those of both of us.

Then there is wives. Yes Sir these fellows actually have wives, and they are following around. What must those poor creatures go through. They all look young. I guess there never was an old woman Golfer's wife, either the strain or starvation get 'em along before middle life. I would think one tough season of tournament would wear out about three wives on a fellow. Think of the prospects of a new dress hanging on every approach. If he goes in the bunker she goes back to last years "Cerise." Just think of having to see your husband's every mistake. Other wives know of them, but they don't see 'em happen. Not only you seeing what a fool he has made of himself by missing a ten inch putt, "But it was right before everybody. What must they think?" Then when you get through the game, the strain is not over, you have to wait till the last Guy comes in at sundown to find out what happened to you. Oh, It's a game, don't kid yourself about that. I don't mean this Junk these old fat Birds go out and call Golf, I mean it's a game when you have to do it right, or you don't eat. Anything to be done right has got to be done by people that make their living at it, like football, look what it has done since it's for the old ham and eggs.

But these Golfers are a cheerful lot, win or lose, wives and all. They laugh it off, take the husband home, dress him up and send him back for another beating on the morrow. But don't kid yourself Comrades that there is nothing to this game. Put $3500 smackers down and tell us we had one putt to win it. I think I would be so nervous I would pick up the caddy and swing him at it.

It is true for both the golfer and the physician that the best work is done by those who earn their living at it. The best scores are not shot by the weekend golfer or the part-time physician. The full-time physician is more available and usually more experienced than the part-time physician. The physician-clinical researcher is being replaced by the full-time physician and the full-time researcher, now often a PhD rather than an MD. Whether practice, research, or administration, "doctoring" increasingly requires the single-minded purpose and quality of work provided by those who "make their living at it."

Back in Will Rogers' day, the gutta-percha golf ball was in play. That golf ball has undergone about as much change as has medicine in the past 60 years. But although the course and tools (clubs) of both golf and medicine continue to change, the stance and swing of both the golfer and the physician remain the same. Compared to yesterday the golf courses today are tougher, but the professional golfers of today are better. Medicine today is much more complex and difficult, of course, than yesterday. Third-party intervention and waiting lawyers are like being in the rough most of the time. The patients in hospitals in the USA today are required to be sicker than those of yesterday, their length of stay is shorter, and their discharge sooner. Hospitalization for a diagnostic workup is a thing of the past. Today's golf course of medicine is longer, contains more sandtraps, more "dog-legs," and less flat greens than the one of yesterday, but physicians—as have the professional golfers—have risen to the challenge. The present day ones are better and provide better care than those of the past.

William C. Roberts

William Clifford Roberts, MD
Editor in Chief

Portions of "Golf is Good—When There's Dough in It!" are reprinted courtesy of the Will Rogers Memorial, Claremore, Oklahoma.

The Government is in *Your* Office and Listening to *Their* Script

Pharmaceutical representatives for some time have been limited in the USA in what they can say about their products to physicians. The government — and rightly so — has decreed that they must limit their statements concerning indications for their products to those described in the package insert included with their product. Now physicians can be told what they can say to their patients.

Some background. In 1970, Congress enacted the family planning program known as Title X of the Public Health Service Act. It provided federal grants to some family-planning clinics, including Planned Parenthood, and now costs $144 million annually. In the 2 decades since then, the federal government has interpreted the law first to *permit* (1971), then to *require* (1976), and finally to *forbid* (1988) clinic workers to discuss the abortion option with their patients. On 23 May 1991 the Supreme Court ruled in the case *Rust v. Sullivan* to uphold the 1988 interpretation of the 1970 family planning law. The Supreme Court thus approved the following regulations:

"A Title X project may not provide counseling concerning the use of abortion as a method of family planning or provide referral for abortion as a method of family planning.

"Once a client is diagnosed as pregnant, she must be referred for appropriate prenatal and/or social services by furnishing a list of available providers that promote the welfare of mother and unborn child."

"A Title X project may not use referrals as an indirect means of encouraging or promoting abortion by including on the list of referral providers health care providers whose principal business is the provision of abortions or by 'steering' clients to providers who offer abortion.

"A Title X project must be organized so that it is physically and financially separate from (abortion) activities."

Dr. Irving Rust, who brought the case through the courts, is the medical director of a Planned Parenthood family-planning clinic in the South Bronx. A Harlem-raised physician, Dr. Rust had worked since 1981 with the guidelines that forbid the use of federal funds to perform abortions. But in 1988, when the Reagan administration wrote the regulations for Title X that banned even talking about abortion, he balked. As Dr. Rust said in 1990, what was at stake was the relationship between a physician and a patient, the ability to talk freely and honestly. "If a woman came in with cancer of the ovary and there were three methods of treatment," he explained as an analogy, "could I tell her the government says that chemotherapy is *the* treatment, no matter what I think?" In other words, as the new Justice David Souter remarked, the government in effect may preclude professional speech.

The Supreme Court's 5-4 decision forbids anyone who works in one of the 4,000 federally funded clinics that provide family planning to 4 million poor American women from using the word "abortion." If a patient asks about abortion, he or she must read from the federal script: "The project does not consider abortion an appropriate method of family planning." If the patient then asks for referral, there are more scripts. Her physician or provider has to refer her for prenatal care to those who "do not perform abortions." Thus, as Ellen Goodman has put it: "a concrete crisis in the life of a poor woman becomes an abstraction in the words of the justices."

The *Rust v. Sullivan* case is not a case about whether abortion should be legal. Like it or not, it is legal. This is rather a case about whether it is permissible to talk about abortion in a federally funded clinic. Thus, for the first time in history, the Supreme Court has prohibited the expression of a certain viewpoint in a government-sponsored setting. This edict is clearly wrong and even scary. As Michael Gartner has expressed it: "We are all dependent on the government for economic support. Farmers get subsidies. Will they be told they can't talk about the dangers of chemicals or complain about the weather? Bankers get deposit insurance. Will they be told they can't criticize the Fed or talk about a recession? Newspapers get a break on postage. Will they be told they can't write about the Pentagon or editorialize about the Supreme Court?" Clearly our cherished freedom of speech is being affected by this court decision.

Possibly some of the regulations will change. Congress is now moving with unusual speed to act on legislation that will reverse this recent Supreme Court decision upholding the government's ban on abortion counseling at federally funded family planning clinics. According to a recent Washington Post-ABC News Poll, 63% of Americans favor allowing the staff of federally funded family planning clinics to mention abortion as an option to pregnant women.

Tomorrow it may be cardiologists, not obstetricians, who are told what they may say to their patients.

William C. Roberts

William Clifford Roberts, MD
Editor in Chief

Goodman E. Abortion: the government in the doctor's office...*The Washington Post*, May 25, 1991.
Cole D. Get government out of the doctor's office. *The Washington Post*, May 28, 1991.
McCarthy C. The courts' consistency. *The Washington Post*, May 30, 1991.
Gartner M. Don't breathe a word; freedom of speech has been suspended. *USA Today*, May 31, 1991.
Marcus R. Court steers through conflicting precedents. *The Washington Post*, June 3, 1991.
Dewar H. Hill moves briskly on abortion bills. *The Washington Post*, June 4, 1991.

Human Records and a Tribute to the *Guinness Book of World Records*

In 1953 or 1954, Sir Hugh Beaver, the managing director of United Kingdom's largest brewery, Guinness, Ltd, while at a grouse shoot at the Guinness estate, missed a golden plover with his shot. At dinner that evening Beaver initiated a discussion on the fastest game birds and observed that none in attendance had any idea of their flying speed. Beaver recognized an opportunity and approached the Guinness board of directors about producing a record book. Lord Iveach, the company's chief executive officer, liked the idea and the McWhirter twins, Norris and Robert, were recommended as potential authors. The first edition of the *Guinness Book of World Records* appeared in the United Kingdom in 1955 and subsequently 262 editions in 35 languages have appeared. By 1974, the *Guinness Book of World Records* became the top-selling copyright book in publishing history. By 1989, global sales surpassed 60 million. The present book[1] is the 29th US edition, the first of which appeared in 1956. The book has become *the* authoritative source of records in nearly all fields of human and non-human endeavor, and now the Guinness company publishes about 40 books of various sorts each year.

Tallest human being: Robert Pershing Wadlow (1918–1940) was measured in 1940 by Doctors C.M. Charles and Cyril MacBryde of the Washington University School of Medicine to be 8 feet 11.1 inches (272 cm) tall and to have an arm span of 9 feet 5.75 inches (289 cm). At age 21 he reached his maximal weight (491 pounds [223 kg]). Because he was still growing, he probably would have reached a height of >9 feet (>274 cm) had he lived longer than 22 years. His shoes were size 37AA (18.5 inches [47 cm]), and his hands measured 12.75 inches (32 cm) from the wrist to the tip of the middle finger. At least 10 other human beings, 9 men, were known to be >8 feet (>244 cm) tall and their life spans ranged from 18 to 56 years (mean 37); only 2 were over 50 years of age and only 4, over 40 years of age. At least 7 of the 11 humans >8 feet tall had acromegaly. Thus, tall bodies, just like large hearts, are not associated with long survival.

Shortest adult human being: Pauline Masters (1876–1895), who died at age 19 years, reached a height of only 23.2 inches (59 cm) and her peak weight was 9 pounds (4.1 kg). The shortest recorded adult male dwarf was Calvin Phillips (1791–1812) who lived 21 years and at age 19 he was only 26.5 inches (67 cm) tall and weighed slightly less than 12 pounds (5.4 kg). For comparison, the average length of newborn babies is about 19 inches (48 cm). The most famous midget was Charles Sherwood Stratton, alias "General Tom Thumb" (1838–1885) who toured with the P.T. Barnum circus. He grew to a height of 40 inches (102 cm) and weighed 70 pounds (32 kg). At age 25, he married Lavinia Warren, 32 inches (81 cm) tall. At their wedding reception, the bridal couple stood on top of a piano to greet the 2,000 guests, and then cut the wedding cake that weighed more than they did together.

Heaviest human being: Jon Brower Minnoch (1941–1983) weighed approximately 1,400 pounds (635 kg) when in congestive heart failure at age 37 years. When not in heart failure the 73-inch (185 cm) tall man usually weighed 800 to 900 pounds. His wife weighed 110 pounds (50 kg) when he weighed 1,300 pounds (590 kg), a 12-fold difference. At least 5 other men have been reported to weigh >1,000 pounds (>454 kg). The heaviest woman was Percy Pearl Washington (__-1972) who weighed approximately 880 pounds (399 kg) and she was 72 inches (183 cm) tall. The largest waist measured 119 inches (302 cm) in a 1,200-pound man.

Lightest human being: The thinnest recorded adults of normal height are those with anorexia nervosa. One such person was Emma Shaller (1868–1890) who weighed 45 pounds (20 kg) and she was 62 inches (157 cm) tall. Edward C. Hagner (1892–1962), alias Eddie Masher ("Skeleton Dude"), was 67 inches (170 cm) tall and weighed 48 pounds (22 kg). The smallest adult waist among women of normal stature measured 13 inches (33 cm) and belonged to the French actress Mlle. Polaire (1881–1939).

Heaviest organ: The *skin* is the heaviest, averaging about 2,675 g. The heaviest internal organ is the *liver* which normally weighs about 1,700 g. The adult male *brain* averages about 1,425 g, and the adult female's, about 1,265 g. There is no correlation between intelligence and brain size. Human brains appear to be getting bigger. The heaviest brain weight recorded was 2,050 g in a 50-year-old man. The normal adult *heart* weighs <400 g. The largest reported was >1,800 g but I suspect the weight was inaccurate.[2] I have seen approximately 35 hearts weighing >1,000 g. Most had aortic regurgitation. Only 1 patient was a woman and she had the largest heart I have seen — 1,260 g and she weighed 123 pounds

(56 kg), stood 63 inches (160 cm) tall, and had hypertrophic cardiomyopathy.[3]

Births and babies: The most children born to one mother is 69. In 27 confinements she gave birth to 16 pairs of twins, 7 sets of triplets and 4 sets of quadruplets. At least 67 who survived infancy were born in the USSR from 1725 to 1765. The oldest medically verified mother was Ruth Alice Kistler (1899–1982) who was 57 years and 129 days old when she gave birth to a daughter. Dr. E. Derasse in 1891 reported in a French medical journal a 59-year and 5-month-old mother who birthed a healthy baby. The woman already had a married daughter aged 40 years. Long pregnancies of 14, 16 and 36 months have been reported. In 1961 a Burmese woman aged 54 years was delivered by Cesarean section of a 3 pound (1.4 kg) calcified fetus after 25 years' gestation. She had gone into labor in 1936, but no child was born. The most premature surviving newborn was 128 days premature and weighed 1.4 pounds (0.6 kg).

The biggest surviving baby weighed 22.5 pounds (10 kg). Babies surviving <24 hours have had recorded weights of 24 pounds (11 kg), 25 pounds (11 kg) and 29 pounds (13 kg). The lowest birth weight recorded for a surviving infant is 0.6 pound (0.28 kg). The highest number of infants reported at a single birth was 10 (decaplets). The highest number surviving was 6 of 6. The heaviest quadruplets together weighed 22.8 pounds (10.3 kg); the heaviest triplets 26.4 pounds (12 kg); and the heaviest twins together, 27.75 pounds (12.6 kg).

Longevity: No subject is more obscured by vanity, deceit, falsehood and fraud than human longevity. Claims apparently are generally made on behalf of the very aged rather than *by* them. The greatest *authenticated* age to which any human has ever lived is 120 years and 237 days. He was born in Japan in June 1865 and died of pneumonia in February 1986. Thirty other persons have had authenticated life spans of 105 to 115 years.

Hands, feet and hair: *Fingernails*, which grow about 0.05 cm a week, in an Indian man in aggregate in one hand measured 173 inches (439 cm): 102 cm thumb, 77 cm first finger, 86 cm second and third fingers, and 88 cm fourth finger. He did not cut his fingernails from 1952 to 1990. The largest *feet* have required size 22 sandals. Human *hair*, which grows at a rate of 1.3 cm a month, if left uncut will usually grow to a maximum of 2 to 3 feet. Hair measuring 12 feet (3.7 meters) long has been reported. The longest *beard* measured 17.5 feet (5.3 meters). The longest *mustache* reached 9.5 feet (2.9 meters).

Best memory: A man recited 16,000 pages of the Buddhist canonical texts; another man memorized >15,000 telephone numbers; another man memorized on a single sighting a random sequence of 30 separate packs of cards (1,560) that had been shuffled together.

Body temperature: The highest body temperature recorded with survival was 116°F, and the lowest, 61°F.

Most common diseases: The most common noncontagious disease is gingivitis, which afflicts 80% of the US population; the commonest contagious disease is acute nasopharyngitis.

Medical extremes: The heart of a Norwegian fisherman, who fell overboard into icy waters, stopped for 4 hours while his temperature fell to 77°F. He made a full recovery. A woman was in coma for the last 44 years of her life. A woman was in an "iron lung" for the last 37 years of her life. A man hiccupped 20 to 40 times a minute for 68 years without a cure. A woman sneezed for 978 days; she sneezed an estimated 1 million times during the first 365 days of the attack. (The highest speed at which expelled sneezed particles have ever been measured to travel is 104 miles/hour.) The highest sound level recorded by any chronic snorer is a peak of 90 decibels. (A city traffic bylaw for acceptable noise where the snorer resided was 80 decibels.) The longest recorded period for which a person has voluntarily gone without sleep is nearly 454 hours in a man who sat in a rocking chair during the sleeplessness period. Some persons have been found to have not slept for years (total insomnia — chronic colestites). The longest period for a person to remain motionless continuously is 24 hours — he sat on a motorcycle. The worst reported case of compulsive swallowing involved a woman who was found to have 2,533 objects in her stomach, including 947 bent pins. The longest period for which anyone has gone without food is 382 days. Most well-nourished individuals can survive without medical consequences on a diet of sugar and water for about 30 days. The longest recorded survival without food *and* water is 18 days. The longest stay in a hospital is >99 years. The highest recorded number of total pills swallowed by a patient is 565,939 during a 21-year period. The most injections was by a woman with diabetes mellitus who gave herself an estimated 61,123 insulin injections over a 59-year period.

This is enough. You get the idea.

William Clifford Roberts, MD
Editor in Chief

1. McFarlan D, editor (McWhirter ND, founding editor). The Guinness Book of World Records 1991. New York: Bantam Books, 1991:820.

2. Roberts WC, Podolak MJ. The king of hearts: analysis of 23 patients with hearts weighing 1000 grams or more. *Am J Cardiol* 1985;55:485–494.

3. Roberts CS, Roberts WC. Hypertrophic cardiomyopathy as a cause of massive cardiomegaly (>1000 g). *Am J Cardiol* 1989;64:1209–1210.

What Medical Students Are Asking

In April 1990 at the invitation of Dr. Howard R. Horn, I spoke at an initiation banquet of the incoming members of the Alpha Omega Alpha (AOA) Honor Medical Society at the University of Tennessee College of Medicine in Memphis. When asked what topic I would speak about, I asked Dr. Horn to ask the AOA inductees to provide me with some questions to discuss. The following request was sent to each of the 25 AOA recipients: "During your 3+ years in medical school have there been some questions that have continued to recur in your mind and that you have had difficulty in answering? For example, when I was in medical school I had a terribly difficult time in deciding which subspecialty to choose. How does one decide? Can you provide 3 questions that keep recurring in your mind?" Fourteen of the 25 students responded and 42 questions were submitted. Similar questions were submitted by several students. An attempt was made to retain the wording of the questions as submitted. They are arranged under 7 general topics.

Choosing the appropriate professional career path: Should that path be the academic or the purely practice one? What are the rewards and shortcomings of the various career paths? Should I be a specialist or a generalist? Does primary care really have a future? If a specialist, which specialty? What are the important factors to consider in selecting a specialty? How can I select a specialty that requires prolonged training or pursue an academic position when I have so many loans (for schooling) to repay? Should I compromise my career goals for the sake of "my significant other"? Which professional path will allow me adequate time to pursue my nonmedical interests? Does the prestigious AOA honor obligate me to pursue a career that might fulfill the expectations of others (friends, family and advisors) rather than one that would make me most happy?

Balancing family and professional life: Can I be both an excellent physician and an excellent parent? How much of one's life should be devoted to medicine and does it make one a lesser physician to consider family more important than medicine? How does one best balance family life and professional life? How does one prevent professional "burn out"?

Public image of physicians: How do physicians improve the deteriorating image held of them by the community? Are physicians responsible for their declining reputations? How do we mend the dwindling trust that patients once had in their physicians?

Role of government in medicine: What will be the future role of government in medicine with regard to physician compensation? Is socialized medicine (if administered by medical personnel) such a bad idea? How should physicians address the problem of increasing numbers of indigent patients?

Medical ethics: What are ethically acceptable reasons for a physician to refuse to treat a patient? How can the conflicts between expensive new technology, cost-effective medicine and quality of life be resolved? As technology to prolong life becomes more abundant, how will the distribution of this technology to individual patients be decided? How do we "ration" health care dollars? With ever increasing malpractice premiums, what future legal/medical changes will occur to ensure both plentiful and competent prenatal care?

Medical education: Is present medical education successful enough in developing traits such as patience, compassion and understanding of human behavior or is too much emphasis put on attempting to expose students to the entire breadth of the ever-expanding medical science data base? How often do I or my classmates trade places in our mind's eye even for an instant with those whom we are treating? Should we make an effort to do more of this or is this emotionally self-destructive and counterproductive to the job we must perform? Will drastic changes in the way medical students are trained occur in the future? How are students going to be able to afford medical education in the future considering increasing tuition, more difficulty in obtaining student loans, stricter loan repayment schedules, etc.? How can the traditional medical student education be made a more progressive and less harmfully rigorous experience? Will computers play an ever widening role in medical education? Should basic research be a requirement of students in medical school?

Miscellaneous: How successful are marriages between 2 physicians? How does one maintain the "to-serve-humanity" idealism in the face of long hours, hard work and, at times, an atmosphere of cynicism? Are the long hours expended by house officers in internship and residency training programs detrimental or necessary to excellent training? Why do certain groups of physicians (i.e., surgeons vs internists) continually "backbite and bad-mouth" each other? What areas of medicine will make the most significant advances over the next 20 years?

Many good questions. Few good answers.

William C. Roberts

William Clifford Roberts, MD
Editor in Chief

Doctors, Save Your Money Because There Will Be Less in the Future

The November 1991 issue of *The Annals of Thoracic Surgery* published the first Ralph D. Alley lectureship which was given by Dr. Harry Schwartz and entitled "The future of American thoracic surgery."[1] Dr. Schwartz, trained as an economist, is a writer whose pieces have appeared in such publications as the *Wall Street Journal*, *New York Times*, and *USA Today* and most commonly in *The American Medical News*. His address was so "right on the mark" that I believe his comments deserve a wider audience, and that they are applicable to all branches of medicine and to all our citizenry. His major points:

1. *American medicine today is more effective than ever in history, is doing more good things for more Americans than ever in history, and is responsible both for many of the good things in the United States and many of the problems.*

Example: Despite acquired immunodeficiency syndrome (AIDS) and the relative higher mortality in the black population, total *infant mortality* has declined steadily each year in the USA for at least 30 years so that every year it is the lowest in history. In 1991, the infant mortality in the USA was about 9.5 deaths/1,000 live births, which means that less than 1 baby in 100 in the USA will die early. Several decades ago the infant mortality was 90 deaths/1,000 live births. Thus, the infant mortality has decreased 90% in my lifetime and in the lifetime of Dr. Schwartz. In contrast, in Russia the infant mortality rate is about 25 deaths/1,000 births, 2.5 times the rate in the USA. That more babies now survive in the USA creates the problem of more babies and eventually more adults to take care of.

Example: Life expectancy, i.e., the average length of life of people who die this year, continues to increase except for that of the black male which is declining, mainly because of homicides. The proliferation of the elderly — a success of medicine — in turn creates enormous problems and costs.

2. *Physicians as a group are not liked by the American public because doctors are regarded as too rich and they got rich by profiteering on human misery.* Although most individuals like their own physicians, doctors as a group are liked by few individuals. The median income of physicians in the USA is about $130,000 and most Americans consider that too much. Over 20% of cardiovascular surgeons earned over $600,000 in 1989 and their median income was $300,000. Again, figures considered "too much" by most Americans. Moreover, there is a widespread impression that much of what physicians do, and particularly what surgeons do, is unnecessary. Thus, the public (including politicians), which means the payers, is going to do everything possible to compress the earnings of physicians (also those of the hospitals, the pharmaceutical makers, etc.).

3. *Health-care costs are exploding because most Americans get "free" or "almost free" care and the demand for it is unrestrained.* Although about 15% of the US population (roughly 37 million persons) has no health insurance, about 85% of the population (roughly 212 million persons) has health insurance and it is pretty good health insurance. Because the potential demand for free medical care is *infinite*, those 212 million, whose care is not coming directly from their pocket, want the very best care available and they want it when they want it. The problem, of course, is that human resources are limited, i.e., *finite*, but the demand for them is out of control. In 1991, health care in the USA cost nearly $700 billion, which means about $2,800 for every person in the USA. And the US government is bankrupt. The national debt is now in excess of $3 trillion (A trillion dollars has 12 zeros in it, a million dollars, 6 zeros.). In 1991 alone, the US government increased its debt by $400 billion, which means 400,000 million dollars! Thus, the deficit for 1991 alone was 57% of the health care costs in 1991. And the only reason the USA can finance such a huge shortfall each year is because foreigners have been willing to buy our debt and buy it, amazingly enough, in US dollars whose value continues to decrease. The consequence of this debt will be that fees paid to and incomes earned by physicians will be more and more set by third-party payers. In 1992, the government will no longer pay fees for "routine electrocardiogram readings" which are being folded into the office visit. The following year, it may be the echocardiogram. The pressure on the US government is now so enormous that it will continue to cut what it pays for medical care.

4. *What physicians can do.* Probably very little but Schwartz recommends *better communication with patients.* It worked for the British Medical Association when the British government tried to revolutionize the British National Health Service and turn it, in effect, into one great big HMO. The British doctors communicated with British patients who made the Thatcher reform so unpopular that she lost her job. The handwriting is getting clearer — physicians in the foreseeable future will not be allowed to do everything to their patients that they are scientifically able to do. We must all communicate better.

William Clifford Roberts, MD
Editor in Chief

1. Schwartz H. The future of American Thoracic Surgery. *Ann Thorac Surg* 1991;52:1039–1043.

The Best Hospitals in the USA for Patients with Heart Disease

The July 12, 1993, issue of the *U.S. News & World Report* contained an article entitled "America's Best Hospitals." The 41 "best" hospitals for patients with heart disease are listed in the accompanying table.

Evaluating quality among hospitals, of course, has been done in the past. The 3 previous hospital quality evaluations by the *U.S. News & World Report* (in 1990, 1991 and 1992) were based purely on reputation of hospitals by physicians. The method chosen to identify the best hospitals in 1993, more objective than that used for previous surveys, was developed for *U.S. News* by the National Opinion Research Center, a much respected social-science research arm of the University of Chicago. The Research Center examined 1,488 tertiary care hospitals utilizing the following categories of information: (1) *reputational score* — the percentage of specialists, surveyed in 1991, 1992 and 1993, who nominated the hospital; (2) *mortality rate* — the ratio of actual deaths to those expected from all procedures and causes in 1988, 1989 and 1990, as reported by the Health Care Financing Administration (HCFA), which administers Medicare; (3) *membership in the Council of Teaching Hospitals (COTH)* — which includes 25% of the 1,488 tertiary hospitals in the USA; (4) *ratio of interns and residents to beds* (About 230 USA medical centers have ratios of at least 0.25.); (5) *ratio of full-time registered nurses to beds;* (6) *ratio of board certified M.D.'s to beds;* (7) *ratio of annual inpatient numbers of operations to the hospital's size* (Higher is better because quality generally rises with volume.); (8) *technology score* — number of 19 possible in-house services, like magnetic resonance imaging, provided (The higher the number [maximal = 19], the less likely a patient would need transfer to receive needed diagnostic or therapeutic care.); (9) *availability of organized social work and patient representative services to plan discharge from the hospital* (One point for each of the 2 services.); (10) *ratio of full-time registered nurses to full-time licensed practical nurses;* (11) *availability of outpatient and community services,* such as substance abuse programs, home health services, etc; and (12) *availability of geriatric services* (a possible 9 services available).

The *overall* score represents the total measure of quality of care, one third of which is based on reputation, one third on mortality rate, and one third on the above "objective" measures. The top ranking hospital in each of the 16 specialties analyzed (AIDS, cancer, cardiology, endocrinology, gastroenterology, geriatrics, gynecology, neurology, orthopedics, otolaryngology, rheumatology, urology, ophthalmology, pediatrics, psychiatry, and rehabilitation) was assigned an overall score of 100. The cutoff for 12 of the 16 specialties was the top 3% of the number of hospitals in a given specialty, yielding 41 or 42 per list.

The list of 41 best hospitals for treatment of patients with heart disease may be useful to both physicians and patients.

William C. Roberts

William Clifford Roberts, MD
Editor in Chief

Rank	Hospital	Overall Score	Reputational Score	Mortality Rate	COTH Member	Residents to Beds	Technology Score	R.N.'s to Beds	Board-Certified M.D.'s to Beds	Inpatient Operations to Beds
1	Mayo Clinic, Rochester, MN	100.0	43.4%	0.65	+	NA	16	0.86	1.40	21.9
2	Cleveland Clinic	88.8	36.4%	0.75	+	0.50	14	1.44	0.36	20.4
3	Massachusetts General Hospital, Boston	88.5	36.2%	0.78	+	0.47	19	1.20	1.06	19.3
4	Stanford University Hospital, Stanford	60.8	21.1%	0.94	+	0.72	14	0.85	1.56	15.8
5	Johns Hopkins Hospital, Baltimore	60.4	19.1%	0.76	+	0.44	16	1.28	0.97	14.7
6	Duke University Medical Center, Durham	57.3	18.0%	0.85	+	0.38	19	1.37	0.59	13.6
7	Brigham and Women's Hospital, Boston	56.4	16.4%	0.74	+	0.62	17	0.77	1.20	20.1
8	Texas Heart Institute (St. Luke's Episcopal Hospital), Houston	52.9	19.9%	1.22	+	0.17	10	1.03	0.57	17.2
9	Emory University Hospital, Atlanta	51.0	16.0%	0.88	+	0.29	10	1.12	0.54	14.9
10	University of California, San Francisco Medical Center	42.1	7.0%	0.76	+	0.32	17	1.85	1.59	19.0
11	Cedars-Sinai Medical Center, Los Angeles	41.4	9.1%	0.83	+	0.24	15	0.99	1.13	17.7
12	UCLA Medical Center, Los Angeles	41.2	4.6%	0.78	+	1.29	17	1.61	1.64	16.8
13	University of Michigan Medical Center, Ann Arbor	39.7	7.3%	0.84	+	0.41	17	1.26	0.62	18.5
14	Mount Sinai Medical Center, New York	37.2	4.4%	0.78	+	0.52	16	1.58	1.18	12.8
15	Barnes Hospital, St. Louis	36.8	6.4%	0.74	+	0.41	5	0.79	0.85	11.2
16	New York University Medical Center, New York	36.5	3.8%	0.64	+	0.20	12	1.15	1.15	13.6
17	Hospital of the University of Pennsylvania, Philadelphia	35.2	3.0%	0.83	+	1.06	15	1.18	0.94	15.0
18	Indiana University Medical Center, Indianapolis	34.9	1.0%	0.64	+	0.37	17	1.82	0.90	17.6
19	Thomas Jefferson University Hospital, Philadelphia	34.9	1.2%	0.68	+	0.71	17	1.41	1.11	16.5
20	New York Hospital–Cornell Medical Center, New York	34.4	3.4%	0.72	+	0.36	15	0.88	0.95	11.0
21	University of Alabama Hospital, Birmingham	34.3	7.1%	1.03	+	0.21	15	0.67	0.52	17.1
22	Columbia-Presbyterian Medical Center, New York	34.0	3.6%	0.75	+	0.30	16	1.01	0.63	7.6
23	Methodist Hospital, Houston	34.0	6.1%	1.00	+	0.14	15	1.24	0.58	17.3
24	Baylor University Medical Center, Dallas	33.9	5.8%	0.94	+	0.14	14	1.23	0.49	18.7
25	New England Medical Center, Boston	33.7	1.9%	0.75	+	0.58	13	1.66	1.70	15.9
26	Beth Israel Hospital, Boston	33.3	3.7%	0.75	+	0.01	13	1.36	0.83	14.1
27	University of Chicago Hospitals	32.7	2.3%	0.90	+	0.77	17	1.53	0.74	17.5
28	University of Illinois Hospital and Clinics, Chicago	32.6	0.6%	0.75	+	1.23	12	1.06	0.54	13.7
29	University of Wisconsin Hospital and Clinics, Madison	32.0	0.0%	0.68	+	0.65	16	1.25	0.67	18.2
30	University of Iowa Hospitals and Clinics, Iowa City	31.8	1.7%	0.89	+	0.78	18	1.31	0.49	24.6
31	Presbyterian University Hospital, Pittsburgh	31.7	1.1%	0.83	+	0.66	11	2.12	1.20	17.7
32	University of Washington Medical Center, Seattle	31.7	0.6%	0.74	+	0.31	15	1.88	1.86	15.0
33	Rush-Presbyterian-St.Luke's Medical Center, Chicago	31.5	0.9%	0.75	+	0.61	16	1.18	0.84	13.4
34	Montefiore Medical Center, New York	31.0	2.4%	0.83	+	0.53	14	0.91	0.40	11.2
35	University of Virginia Medical Center, Charlottesville	30.9	0.6%	0.85	+	0.78	17	1.70	0.44	16.4
36	Deaconess Hospital, Boston	30.9	0.4%	0.71	+	0.59	13	1.14	0.78	14.2
37	University of California, San Diego Medical Center	30.7	1.2%	0.89	+	0.27	17	2.66	0.91	18.7
38	University Hospitals of Cleveland	30.6	0.6%	0.87	+	0.61	18	1.72	1.16	14.4
39	Green Hospital of Scripps Clinic, La Jolla	30.3	0.0%	0.61	0	0.00	11	0.82	0.58	23.3
40	University of California, Davis Medical Center, Sacramento	30.1	1.9%	0.94	+	0.63	18	2.59	0.60	16.1
41	University of Minnesota Hospital and Clinic, Minneapolis	30.0	0.6%	0.75	+	NA	15	2.05	0.76	16.2

Reputational Score = the percentage of doctors surveyed who named the hospital; Mortality Rate = ratio of actual to expected deaths (lower is better); COTH Member = member of Council of Teaching Hospitals; Residents to Beds = ratio of interns and residents to beds; Technology Score = index from 0 to 19; R.N.'s to Beds = ratio of registered nurses to beds; Board-Certified M.D.'s to Beds = ratio of doctors certified in a specialty to beds; Inpatient Operations to Beds = ratio of annual inpatient operations to beds; NA = not available.
Adapted with permission from *U.S. News & World Report,* July 12, 1993.

Personal Finances

The financially secure physician is usually a better physician than the financially insecure one. Indeed, the hungry physician may be a dangerous physician. Although the cost of medical care almost surely will not decrease in coming years, the percent of the medical care dollar going to physicians almost certainly will decrease.[1] Thus, becoming financially secure such that physicians can devote their energies fully to providing the best of care to their patients without worry of financial compensation will become more difficult. Management of their money, therefore, will become more important than ever before.

Mr. Boone Powell, Jr., President and Chief Executive Officer of Baylor University Medical Center, in May 1995, spoke to Baylor's medical house staff on how to manage money. His talk was the best I have heard on the subject and the sound principles he espoused can serve us all well:

1) *Have an integrated financial plan:* This includes summarizing one's current financial situation (living expenses, debt retirement, taxes and contributions); establishing financial goals; establishing means of increasing cash-flow margin, and controlling cash flow.

2) *Save money and save regularly:* The average savings rate of US citizens is about 4.5%. In contrast, the Japanese save at about 14%, and families in Singapore save at 41%. We need to change back to being savers and not just spenders. The reason for this is that, according to the Social Security Administration, only 2% of Americans at age 65 are financially independent, and only 5% of professionals at age 65 are financially independent. Becoming financially secure requires time (determined externally) and self-discipline (determined internally). Every dollar spent is a dollar lost for saving. Saving $2.74 each day amounts to $1,000 saved in a year, and $1,000 compounded annually at 10% amounts to $57,275 in 20 years. Mr. Powell quoted Albert Einstein who called "compound interest the world's greatest invention." Easy access to money makes saving in the USA difficult.

3) *Avoid the consumptive lifestyle:* This type of lifestyle, of course, means spending more than one can afford, or spending more than one should, given the other goals and priorities. Financial freedom and success come from spending less than one earns and doing it over a long period of time. Diminishing consumption requires delaying gratification. Defer purchases until they can be purchased with cash. Most debt problems are spending problems, not income problems. The borrower is a slave to the lender. If one increases his/her indebtedness by only $1,000/year at 12% interest, compounded annually, the interest after 15 years will be $26,754, and total indebtedness will be $41,754! If you should then attempt to get out of debt by repaying the loan at $6,000/year, it will take almost 16 more years and cost an additional $53,696 in interest. Thus, debt accumulation of $1,000/year for 15 years has cost a total of $80,454 in interest, an average of $2,595/year for the 31-year period.

4) *Prepare a monthly budget and live by it:* The budget is a short-term plan that guides one (like a roadmap when driving in an unfamiliar area) and tells one that he/she is on course. Without a budget one lives as a responder. Thus, a budget can be a financially freeing endeavor.

5) *Retain automobiles longer:* The most economical car to own is the one currently owned. The longer a car is driven, the less expensive it is to operate. The time to sell a car is when its annual repair expenses exceed the car's value or when a problem of safety arises. Defer the purchase of a more expensive automobile until cash is available to buy it without borrowing money. If, for example, you desire a $15,000 car but do not have the money, but do have a car that still runs, save $484.00/month for 3 years and then $17,424 will have been saved (not including compound interest) and then the car can be bought with cash. But continue the saving process so that the next car also can be bought with cash. Try never to borrow money for any item that is depreciable.

6) *Pay off a home mortgage early and/or make the length of the mortgage relatively short:* A $100,000 mortgage at 10% for 30 years costs $878/month or $315,925 in total. A $100,000 mortgage at 10% for 20 years costs $965/month or $231,605 in total, so that $87/month more saves $84,320, a 27% savings. A $100,000 mortgage at 10% for 15 years costs $1,075/month or $193,428 in total, so that an extra payment of $197/month saves $122,497 or 38% compared with the 30-year mortgage.

7) *Six steps to investing:* Before even considering this option, eliminate ALL high-interest short-term debt (credit cards, automobiles, small debts) (Step 1), and place in an interest-bearing checking account one month's living expenses (determined from the monthly budget) (Step 2). Keep 3- to 6-months' living expenses in a money-market fund or a savings account, reserved to protect in case of disability, accident, or any emergency (Step 3). Put money for major purchases (automobile, furniture, down payment on a home) in a money-market fund, certificate of deposit, or treasury bill (possibly in a mutual fund) (Step 4). Invest to meet long-term goals in equities, bonds, real estate, treasury bills, and/or money-market funds or certificates of deposit (Step 5). Then speculate to save more, spend more, and give more (Step 6). Try to place savings in a tax-deferred account; compounding in this manner further increases interest or dividends. When steps 5 and 6 are reached, a financial advisor or consultant is recommended; use one whose fee is for advice, not one whose fee is dependent on buying a product. The advisor should take some of the tension out of finances so the acquirer of the money is freer to do what he/she wants to do. Financial peace of mind is the goal.

Mr. Powell emphasized that money can both help and harm, and that we can be smart or dumb with it. If we follow the above advice, our mony worries will not be great ones.

William C. Roberts

William Clifford Roberts, MD
Editor in Chief
Baylor University Medical Center
Dallas, Texas 75246

1. Roberts WC. Doctors, save your money because there will be less in the future. *Am J Cardiol* 1992;69:432.

The Best Hospitals in the USA for Patients With Heart Disease

During each of the past 6 years the *U.S. News & World Report* has published an article entitled "America's Best Hospitals." The latest survey appeared in its August 12, 1996, issue. The report surveyed 1,961 tertiary-care facilities (i.e., the major teaching and research centers) utilizing the following categories of information: 1) *reputational score*: the percentage of specialists, surveyed in 1994, 1995, and 1996, who then nominated the hospital; 2) *mortality rate:* the ratio of actual deaths to those expected overall as reported by the Health Care Financing Administration (HCFA), which administers Medicare; 3) *ratio of interns and residents to beds:* about 230 United States medical centers have ratios of at least 0.25; 4) *ratio of full-time registered nurses to beds*; 5) *ratio of board certified MD's to beds;* 6) *ratio of annual in-patient numbers of operations to the hospital's size;* 7) *technology score:* number of 19 possible in-house services (e.g., magnetic resonance imaging) provided (the higher the number [maximal = 19], the less likely a patient would need transfer to receive needed diagnostic or therapeutic care.); 8) *availability of organized social work and patient representative services to plan discharge from the hospital* (1 point for each of the 2 services.); 9) *ratio of full-time registered nurses to full-time licensed practical nurses;* 10) *availability of outpatient and community services:* such as substance abuse programs, home health services, etc; and 11) *availability of geriatric services* (a possible 9 services available).

The *overall* score represents the total measure of quality of care, one third of which is based on reputation, one third on the mortality rate, and one third on the above "objective" measures. The top ranking hospital in each of the 16 specialties analyzed (AIDS, cancer, cardiology, endocrinology, gastroenterology, geriatrics, gynecology, neurology, ophthalmology, orthopedics, otolaryngology, pediatrics, psychiatry, rehabilitation, rheumatology, and urology) was assigned an overall score of 100. The cutoff for 12 of the 16 specialties was the top 3% of the number of hospitals in a given specialty, yielding 42 per list.

William Clifford Roberts, MD
Editor in Chief
Baylor University Medical Center
Dallas, Texas 75246

TABLE 1 Top-Ranked Hospitals for Cardiology in the United States

Rank	Hospital	U.S. News Index	Reputational score	Cardiology mortality rate	Technology score (of 9)	RN's to beds	Procedures to beds
1	Cleveland Clinic	100.0	54.6%	0.65	8.5	1.10	9.10
2	Mayo Clinic, Rochester, Minn.	92.3	52.9%	0.75	8.0	0.83	10.43
3	Massachusetts General Hospital, Boston	67.6	30.6%	0.64	9.0	1.40	8.68
4	Duke University Medical Center, Durham, N.C.	58.2	23.7%	0.74	9.0	1.73	7.09
5	Texas Heart Institute-St. Luke's Episcopal, Houston	53.6	28.0%	1.22	8.0	1.31	11.20
6	Emory University Hospital, Atlanta	49.3	21.7%	0.88	9.0	0.87	9.39
7	Brigham and Women's Hospital, Boston	48.3	23.7%	0.94	7.0	0.76	5.92
8	Stanford University Hospital, Stanford, Calif.	44.9	18.3%	0.87	8.0	1.18	7.20
9	Johns Hopkins Hospital, Baltimore	35.2	13.8%	1.16	9.0	1.36	5.01
10	University of California, San Francisco Medical Center	33.2	6.5%	0.76	9.0	1.41	2.77
11	Barnes-Jewish Hospital, St. Louis	30.0	8.4%	0.92	9.0	1.00	5.35
12	Cedars-Sinai Medical Center, Los Angeles	29.6	7.9%	0.87	8.0	1.04	7.90
13	Columbia-Presbyterian Medical Center, New York	29.1	9.7%	1.12	9.0	1.17	4.72
14	Methodist Hospital, Houston	28.9	10.9%	1.13	8.0	1.03	7.15
15	Beth Israel Hospital, Boston	28.9	4.0%	0.77	8.0	1.53	11.60
16	Mount Sinai Medical Center, New York	27.5	3.3%	0.78	8.5	1.39	3.74
17	UCLA Medical Center, Los Angeles	26.8	3.2%	0.68	9.0	1.03	4.55
18	University of Alabama Hospital at Birmingham	26.7	9.4%	1.19	7.0	1.42	7.76
19	Hospital of the University of Pennsylvania, Philadelphia	26.6	1.7%	0.76	9.0	1.52	4.95
20	University of Chicago Hospitals	26.3	1.6%	0.77	9.0	1.63	4.46
21	William Beaumont Hospital, Royal Oak, Mich.	25.6	2.5%	0.85	9.0	1.51	10.65
22	New York Hospital-Cornell Medical Center	25.2	4.6%	0.88	9.0	0.93	3.85
23	University of Washington Medical Center, Seattle	25.0	0.4%	0.70	9.0	1.88	4.29
24	University Hospitals of Cleveland	24.3	0.5%	0.79	9.0	1.84	4.99
25	Baylor University Medical Center, Dallas	23.9	4.2%	0.91	8.0	1.19	6.89
26	Fairfax Hospital, Falls Church, Va.	23.9	0.9%	0.75	8.0	1.33	8.48
27	Ochsner Foundation Hospital, New Orleans	23.9	1.4%	0.75	8.0	1.17	11.12
28	Rush-Presbyterian-St. Luke's Medical Center, Chicago	23.8	1.0%	0.74	9.0	1.07	4.55
29	New England Medical Center, Boston	23.4	0.0%	0.66	8.0	2.16	6.72
30	California Pacific Medical Center, San Francisco	23.4	0.4%	0.75	8.0	1.41	3.55
31	UCSD Medical Center, San Diego	23.3	0.0%	0.72	8.0	1.73	3.30
32	Maimonides Medical Center, Brooklyn, N.Y.	23.0	0.7%	0.74	8.0	1.22	4.04
33	Sinai Samaritan Medical Center, Milwaukee	23.0	0.0%	0.76	8.5	1.33	12.60
34	New York University Medical Center	22.8	2.3%	0.81	8.5	0.91	4.14
35	Washington Hospital Center, Washington, D.C.	22.8	7.7%	0.98	8.0	0.12	9.52
36	University of Louisville Hospital, Louisville, Ky.	22.8	0.0%	0.70	8.0	1.39	3.00
37	Thomas Jefferson University Hospital, Philadelphia	22.7	0.0%	0.75	8.0	1.38	3.03
38	University of Miami, Jackson Memorial Hospital	22.4	1.0%	0.78	6.5	1.49	1.06
39	Albany Medical Center Hospital, Albany, N.Y.	22.4	0.0%	0.79	8.0	1.63	7.23
40	Georgetown University Hospital, Washington, D.C.	22.3	0.0%	0.68	7.0	1.63	5.34
41	University Hospital, Portland, Ore.	22.3	0.0%	0.68	7.0	1.88	3.02
42	Cook County Hospital, Chicago	22.1	0.0%	0.63	7.0	1.49	2.84

"Reputational score" is the average percentage of board certified heart specialists surveyed in 1994, 1995, and 1996 who named the hospital. "Cardiology mortality rate" is the ratio of actual to expected cardiac deaths; lower is better. "Technology score" reflects available technology in cardiology. "RN's to beds" is the hospital wide ratio of full-time registered nurses to beds. "Procedures to beds" is the ratio of cardiac-related procedures to beds.

*Adapted by permission from: America's best hospitals. *US News & World Report.* August 12, 1996.

Longitude, The Longitude Act, Scurvy, and the Beginning of Government-Supported Research

In May 1997, my son Cliff and I visited Greenwich, United Kingdom, observed the prime meridian, and read Dava Sobel's book entitled *Longitude, The True Story of a Lone Genius Who Solved the Greatest Scientific Problem of His Time.*[1] As we all know, the *latitude lines,* the parallels, stay parallel to each other as they girdle the globe from the Equator to the poles in a series of shrinking concentric rings. The Equator, of course, marks the zero degree parallel of latitude, and on this line, the sun, moon, and planets pass almost directly overhead. The Tropic of Cancer and the Tropic of Capricorn, 2 other famous parallels, mark the northern and southern boundaries of the sun's apparent motion over the course of the year. The *longitude meridians* loop from the North to the South Pole and back again in great circles of the same size such that they all converge at the north and south ends of the earth. The zero degree parallel of latitude is fixed by laws of nature, and is relatively easily and accurately determined. In contrast, the zero degree meridian of longitude is determined by political decision. The zero prime meridian has been Greenwich, England, since 1767.

Measurement of longitude meridians, in contrast to latitude lines, is difficult. At sea, it is necessary to know what time it is aboard ship and also the time at the home port or another place of known longitude at the very same moment. The 2 clock times enable the navigator to convert the hour difference into a geographical separation. Because the earth takes 24 hours to complete 1 full revolution of 360 degrees, 1 hour marks 1/24th of a spin or 15 degrees. Thus, each hour time difference between the ship and the starting point indicates 15 degrees of longitude to the east or the west. Everyday at sea, when the navigator resets his ship's clock to local noon when the sun reaches its highest point in the sky, and then consults the home port clock, every hour discrepancy between them translates into another 15 degrees of longitude. Those same 15 degrees of longitude also correspond to a distance traveled. At the Equator, where the girth of the earth is greatest, 15 degrees equal 1,000 miles. North or south of that line the mileage value of each degree decreases. One degree of longitude equals 4 minutes of time the world over, but in terms of distance one degree shrinks from 68 miles at the Equator to virtually zero at the poles.

Precise knowledge of the hour in 2 different places at once, a longitude prerequisite, was simply unobtainable until the late 18th century. On rolling ships, pendulum clocks slowed or sped up or stopped. Changes in temperature from a cold country of origin to a tropical country or vice versa thinned or thickened a clock's lubricating oil and made its metal parts expand or contract with equally disastrous results. A rise or fall in barometric pressure or a change in the earth's gravity from 1 latitude to another also could cause a clock to gain or lose time.

Despite the lack of a practical method to determine longitude and therefore a reliable means to establish a ship's whereabouts, more and more sailing vessels set out in the 16th, 17th, and 18th centuries to conquer or explore new territories, to wage war, or to carry gold and commodities between foreign lands. Ship captains relied on "dead reckoning" to gage their distance east or west of home port. The captain would throw a log overboard and observe how quickly the ship receded from this temporary guide post. The crude speedometer reading in his ship's log book was noted along with the direction of travel, which he took from the stars or a compass, and the length of time on a particular course, counted with a sandglass or a pocketwatch. Factoring in the effects of ocean currents, fickle winds, and errors of judgment, longitude was then determined. But too often the technique of dead reckoning meant death to many of the crew because voyages were prolonged and the extra time at sea condemned sailors to scurvy, thirst and occasionally starvation. The ocean going diet of the day, devoid of fresh fruits and vegetables, deprived them of vitamin C, and their bodies' connective tissues deteriorated. The blood vessels leaked, wounds failed to heal, legs swelled, blood extravasated into muscles and joints, gums bled, teeth loosened, breathing became labored, intracerebral blood vessels ruptured, and they died.

The global ignorance of longitude also wreacked economic havoc on the grandest scale. By the end of the 17th century, nearly 300 ships a year sailed between the British isles and the West Indies. The sinking of a single cargo vessel caused terrible losses. The magnitude of the problem of longitude came to a head on October 22, 1707, at the Scilly Isles when 4 homebound British warships ran aground and 2,000 men lost their lives.*

The disastrous wreck on the Scillies catapulted the longitude question to the forefront of national affairs. The sudden loss of so many lives, so many ships, and so much honor all at once underscored the folly of ocean navigation without a means for finding longitude. Thus, was born the Longitude Act of 1714 in England, in which Parliament promised a prize of 20,000 pounds (a sum equal to at least 20,000,000 pounds today) for a solution to the longitude problem. In addition, the Longitude Act allowed the Board of Longitude to give incentive awards to help impoverished inventors bring ideas to fruition. This control over purse strings made the Board of Longitude the world's first official research and development agency. (The Board of Longitude remained in existence until 1828, and by then it had dispersed funds in excess of 100,000 pounds or in today's terms, over 100,000,000 pounds.)

From 1714 until 1760 a number of astronomers and a single watchmaker struggled to find a practical solution to determining longitude at sea. During these investigations, scientists, mainly astronomers, made other discoveries that changed their views of the universe, including the first accurate determination of the weight of the earth, the distance to the stars, and the speed of light. Although a number of world-renowned astronomers devoted their lives to the solution of the longitude problem, the answer came from an English clockmaker named *John Harrison,* a mechanical genius who pioneered the science of precision clock making. He devoted his life to inventing a clock that would carry the true time from the home port, like an eternal flame, to any remote part of the world. Harrison, a man of simple birth and high intelligence, had no formal education or apprenticeship to any watchmaker. Nevertheless, he constructed a series of virtually friction-free clocks that required no lubrication and no cleaning, that were made from materials impervious to rust, and that kept their moving parts perfectly balanced in relation to one another, regardless of how the world pitched or tossed about them. He did away with the pendulum, and he combined different metals inside his works in such a way that when one component expanded or contracted with changes in temperature, the other counteracted the change and kept the clock's rate constant.

His every success was parried by members of the scientific elite, who distrusted Harrison's "magic box." The commissioners charged with awarding the longitude prize changed the contest rules whenever they saw fit, so as to favor the chances of astronomers over the likes of Harrison, considered simply a "mechanic." But the utility and accuracy of Harrison's approach triumphed in the end. His followers shepherded Harrison's intricate exquisite invention through the design modifications that enabled it to be mass produced and enjoy wide use. An aged, exhausted Harrison, taken under the wing of King George III, ultimately claimed his rightful monetary reward in 1773 after 40 struggling years of political intrigue, international warfare, academic back biting, scientific revolution, and economic upheaval. With reliable clocks on board, scurvy virtually vanished; although sauerkraut, lemons, and limes helped, shipwrecks became less frequent, and the world became more prosperous and smaller.

I wonder sometimes if we are not a bit off course occasionally in managing patients with heart disease. Cardiology, of course, is not as exact a science as is longitude and latitude, but nevertheless, we should continually strive to make it so.

William C. Roberts

William C. Roberts, MD
Editor in Chief
Baylor Cardiovascular Institute
Baylor University Medical Center
Dallas, Texas 75246

* One of the sailors of Admiral Sir Clowdisley Shovell's ship earlier had approached the Admiral claiming to have kept his own reckoning of the fleet's location during the foggy night of October 22. Such navigation by an inferior was forbidden and considered subversive in the Royal Navy and Admiral Shovell had the man hanged for mutiny on the spot. It turned out, of course, that the sailor's calculations were correct and those of the Admiral, incorrect.

1. Sobel D. Longitude. The True Story of a Lone Genius Who Solved the Greatest Scientific Problem of His Time. London: Fourth Estate, 1995:184.

The Best Hospitals in the USA for Heart Disease—1997

Each of the last 8 years the U. S. NEWS & WORLD REPORT has published a list of the best hospitals in the USA for various medical specialties. The results of the 1997 evaluation, appearing in the July 28, 1997 issue, are shown in the table. The evaluation score has 3 equal components: 1) reputation with board-certified specialists, 2) predicted mortality by specialty, and 3) various factors such as use of advanced medical technology and the availability for services for patients with specific needs. The results of this analysis for patients with heart disease is included in the accompanying table.

William Clifford Roberts, MD
Editor in Chief
Baylor Cardiovascular Institute
Baylor University Medical Center
Dallas, Texas 75246

TABLE I Top-Ranked Hospitals for Cardiology in the United States – 1997

Rank	Hospital	U.S. NEWS INDEX	Reputational score	Cardiology mortality rate	Technology score (of 9)	Cardiology surgical discharges	R.N.'s to beds	Trauma center
1	Cleveland Clinic	100.0	53.1%	0.70	9.0	5,401	1.06	0
2	Mayo Clinic, Rochester	97.8	50.4%	0.79	8.0	4,265	1.52	+
3	Massachusetts General Hospital, Boston	72.4	34.2%	0.90	9.0	3,403	1.66	+
4	Duke University Medical Center, Durham	54.2	22.4%	0.84	9.0	3,466	1.60	0
5	Brigham and Women's Hospital, Boston	53.1	22.0%	0.88	8.5	1,981	1.28	+
6	Texas Heart Institute-St. Luke's Episcopal, Houston	51.1	25.2%	1.14	8.0	3,217	1.24	0
7	Stanford University Hospital, Stanford	45.7	17.6%	0.86	8.0	1,839	1.09	+
8	Johns Hopkins Hospital, Baltimore	40.2	14.0%	0.95	9.0	2,328	1.32	+
9	University of Washington Medical Center, Seattle	33.1	8.3%	0.69	9.0	733	2.00	0
10	Cedars-Sinai Medical Center, Los Angeles	32.2	9.1%	0.91	8.0	2,114	1.05	+
11	Barnes-Jewish Hospital, St. Louis	28.5	7.4%	0.88	9.0	1,815	0.77	0
12	University of Alabama Hospital at Birmingham	27.8	8.3%	1.11	7.0	3,309	1.56	+
13	Beth Israel Hospital, Boston	27.0	5.4%	0.92	8.0	1,789	1.41	+
14	Baylor University Medical Center, Dallas	26.8	4.0%	0.86	8.0	3,281	1.52	+
15	Hospital of the University of Pennsylvania, Philadelphia	24.7	2.4%	0.86	9.0	1,234	1.66	+
16	Columbia-Presbyterian Medical Center, New York	24.7	7.2%	1.17	9.0	1,720	1.30	0
17	University of Chicago Hospitals	24.5	2.3%	0.83	9.0	830	1.51	+
18	University Medical Center, Tucson	24.2	2.5%	0.79	8.0	595	1.34	+
19	William Beaumont Hospital, Royal Oak	24.2	2.1%	0.83	9.0	4,745	1.59	0
20	University of Michigan Medical Center, Ann Arbor	23.8	4.2%	1.07	9.0	1,867	1.43	+
21	UCLA Medical Center, Los Angeles	23.7	3.2%	0.90	9.0	1,004	1.25	+
22	University of California, San Francisco Med. Ctr.	23.7	3.6%	0.86	9.0	692	1.40	0
23	North Carolina Baptist Hospital, Winston-Salem	23.3	1.5%	0.81	9.0	2,260	1.42	0
24	University Hospitals of Cleveland	22.9	0.5%	0.82	9.0	1,256	1.83	+
25	Indiana University Medical Center, Indianapolis	22.9	1.7%	0.80	9.0	816	1.65	0
26	Mount Sinai Medical Center, New York	22.3	2.7%	0.93	8.5	2,095	1.57	0
27	University of Iowa Hospitals and Clinics, Iowa City	22.2	0.9%	0.82	9.0	922	1.26	+
28	St. Louis University Hospital	21.9	0.4%	0.82	9.0	1,100	1.36	+
29	Henry Ford Hospital, Detroit	21.9	1.1%	0.85	8.0	1,225	1.58	+
30	Ochsner Foundation Hospital, New Orleans	21.6	1.5%	0.67	7.0	1,235	2.02	0
31	UCSD Medical Center, San Diego	21.4	0.7%	0.73	7.0	625	1.73	+
32	Methodist Hospital, Houston	21.3	7.1%	1.33	8.0	3,441	0.98	0
33	Fairfax Hospital, Falls Church	21.1	0.9%	0.87	8.0	2,125	1.24	+
34	Medical Center of Delaware, Wilmington	21.0	0.0%	0.87	8.0	2,203	1.80	+
35	Temple University Hospital, Philadelphia	21.0	0.4%	0.85	8.0	1,185	1.65	+
36	Medical University of South Carolina, Charleston	21.0	0.0%	0.86	8.5	1,456	1.78	+
37	Yale-New Haven Hospital, New Haven	20.9	2.8%	1.01	8.5	2,759	0.87	+
38	Rush-Presbyterian-St. Luke's Medical Center, Chicago	0.9	1.0%	0.80	9.0	1,199	1.06	0
39	Mary Hitchcock Memorial Hospital, Lebanon	20.7	0.5%	0.84	9.0	1,314	1.59	0
40	University of Cincinnati Hospital	20.6	0.0%	0.80	7.5	915	1.61	+
41	University of Utah Hospitals and Clinics, Salt Lake City	20.5	0.7%	0.67	7.0	293	1.48	+
42	Winthrop-University Hospital, Mineola	20.5	0.4%	0.85	7.0	1,753	1.57	+

"U.S. News Index" scores have been rounded, which may produce apparent ties. "Reputational score" is percentage of heart specialists in 1995, 1996, and 1997 who named the hospital. "Cardiology mortality rate" is the ratio of actual to expected cardiac deaths. "Technology score" reflects cardiology-related technology available. "Cardiology surgical discharges" is number of specialty-related surgical discharges. "R.N.'s to beds" is hospital-wide ratio of full-time registered nurses to beds. "Trauma center" indicates whether on-site trauma services are offered.

Adapted with permission from *U.S. NEWS & WORLD REPORT.*

Measuring the Meter and Using the Metric System

The metric system changed the world! It was a radical innovation. It made possible free trade, the open market, and globalization. Before the metric system, a pint in one community was quite different than a pint in another community, and therefore, trade among communities was a bit hazardous. Ken Alder has written a book entitled *The Measure of All Things. The Seven-Year Odyssey and Hidden Error That Transformed the World.*[1] In the midst of the French Revolution, 2 astronomers set out in opposite directions from Paris, 1 going north to Dunkirk, the other south to Barcelona, for the purpose of measuring a portion of the north–south meridian to define the meter as one ten-millionth of the distance between the pole and the equator so that all countries would have a specific unit of measure. Jean-Baptiste-Joseph Delambre led the northern portion and Pierre-Francois-André Méchain led the southern portion of the meridian expedition. Ken Alder located the long-lost correspondence between these 2 men, along with their mission logbooks, and he stumbled upon a 200-year-old secret, and that is that the meter is in error! Méchain, 1 of the 2 astronomers, made contradictory measurements from Barcelona and, in a panic, covered up the discrepancy. The guilty knowledge of his misdeed drove him to the brink of madness and ultimately to his death. Only then, after the meter had already been publicly announced, did his partner, Delambre, discover the truth and face a fateful choice: to disclose the error or cover it up.

The measurement brought back by Delambre and Méchain not only made science into a global enterprise and made possible our global economy, but it also revolutionized our understanding of error. Their error, interestingly, was the equivalent of the thickness of 2 sheets of paper. These 2 astronomers measured out a meter in platinum and that platinum bar stills resides in Paris. Today, 95% of the people on the earth live in countries that use the metric system. The only countries today that do not use the metric system are Myanmar (Burma), Liberia, and the United States of America (USA). Interestingly, Napoleon banned the metric system in 1812 because his people got annoyed with the measurements. It was not until 1920 that the metric system returned to France! Thomas Jefferson in 1790, when Secretary of State, first proposed that the USA adap't the metric system but was unable to do so. He did persuade Congress to do so with decimal coinage rather than pounds, shillings, and pence. Measuring the meridian from Dunkirk to Barcelona was the first state sponsorship of science! These 2 astronomers were the first to be called "scientists." Before that "scientists" were called "natural philosophers."

These 2 astronomers worked at a time when scientists believed they could redefine the foundations of space and time. The French Revolution created the 30-day month, the 10-day week, and the 10-hour day with each hour measured at 100 minutes and each minute 100 seconds. Of all the changes associated with the metric system, the date and time changes were the most unpopular and this change was quickly rescinded.

The November 25, 2002, issue of *BARRON'S* had a piece by Thomas G. Dolan entitled "Measure for Measure. It's Time for the United States to Join the World in Using the Metric System."[2] Americans buy liquor, wine, and soda pop by the liter, but beer by the fluid ounce. We buy medicines by the milligram, but meat by the pound. In some ways, the USA has been officially on the metric system for more than a century. Using metric measurements has been legal in the USA since 1866. The USA signed an international metrification treaty in 1875. In 1890, the National Bureau of Standards took delivery of the official national kilogram, a precise duplicate of the world's standard kilogram enshrined in Paris. In 1893, the US pound was officially defined as 0.4535924277 kg, and the yard as 3,600/3937th of a meter. In 1906, Congress rejected a bill to put the metric system into general use. A metrification law enacted in 1975 required the federal government to use the system wherever "practical," and many reasons have been found to declare it impractical to buy things in metric sizes.

Things "scientific" have gone metric with occasionally mixed results: food packages are usually in the antique system; nutrition labels are in metric. Thus, the nutrition label on a 1.5-ounce bag of potato chips reveals that the contents include 12 mg of fat. A footnote offers a conversion table for grams to calories, but not grams to ounces. The US Metric Association claims that by not going metric, US industry loses billions of dollars in lost export business annually.

However, metrification has not been easy anywhere. The European Union still permits dual labeling in the metric and the antique system. Canada went metric in 1971 putting its speed limit signs in kilometers per hour along with nearly all measurements the government uses. However, in 1984, a new government made further metrification optional, leaving the process in a state of suspended animation. Frozen turkeys, for example, in Canada are sold by the kilogram and fresh turkeys by the pound, even in the same store.

The United Kingdom, formally the land of the 20-ounce Imperial pint, went the other way, ending the shilly-shallying of a voluntary system and imposing metrification in concert with the European Union. Freeborn Englishmen rebelled, and in a test case last year a grocer was fined for selling bananas by the pound, but otherwise enforcement has ground nearly to a halt.

Having both the metric system and the antique system in simultaneous use has its drawbacks. One disaster occurred in 1999 when National Aeronautic Space Administration (NASA) lost a spacecraft intended to orbit Mars. Some data on rocket thrust that the Jet Propulsion Laboratory (JPL) believed was in the metric system was actually in pounds, so a rocket burned for orbital insertion was drastically mistimed. An Air Canada jetliner ran out of fuel in 1983 because it was loaded with thousands of pounds of fuel instead of thousands of kilograms. Fortunately, the pilot was able to glide to an emergency landing strip.

In the USA, the blame must go to Congress. Fixing the standard of weights and measures is one of its enumerated powers in the Constitution. Since 1975, however, Congress has only attempted a conversion to the metric system. Government buys and builds in the metric system, hoping to jump-start the free market. All it has done is raise the cost of doing business with the government! There are few places in the economy where the government can actually legislate American efficiency. The system of weights and measures is one of them. Congress can and should convert the country to the metric system!

Most cardiac measurements are metric. In the USA we weigh the heart in grams, but the body in pounds and the height in inches. Volumes are in milliliters and pressures in mm Hg. Percentages probably produce the least accurate of all cardiac measurements. Ejection fractions vary with the estimator. At least cardiology is ahead of most other areas in the USA in using the metric system.

William C. Roberts

William Clifford Roberts, MD,
Editor in Chief
Baylor Heart & Vascular Institute
Baylor University Medical Center
Dallas, Texas

1. Alder K. The Measure of All Things. The Seven-Year Odyssey and Hidden Error That Transformed the World. New York: The Free Press 2002:400.
2. Dolan TG. Measure for Measure. It's time for the United States to join the world in using the metric system. *BARRON'S*, November 25, 2002:35.

Infections

If you want to be frightened I suggest Madeline Drexler's new book, *Secret Agents. The Menace of Emerging Infections.*[1] She begins this way: "Infection is an inescapable part of life. All creatures feast on other creatures and in time are feasted upon in a kind of Escheresque food chain. When humans are the meal, we call it infectious disease." The book is about today's new and emerging infections—those that have increased in attack rate or geographic range or threatened to do so. It explores why these infections are materializing now and why they will never go away. Each chapter looks at a different threat: animal- and insect-borne diseases, food-borne pathogens, antibiotic resistance, pandemic influenza, infectious causes of chronic disease, and bioterrorism.

Early on she quotes the famous bacteriologist and historian, *Hans Zinsser*, who wrote in 1934: "However secure and well-regulated civilized life may become, bacteria, protozoa, viruses, infected fleas, lice, ticks, mosquitoes, and bedbugs will always lurk in the shadows ready to pounce when neglect, poverty, famine, or war lets down the defenses. And even in normal times they pray on the weak, the very young, and the very old, living along with us, in mysterious obscurity waiting their opportunities."

Drexler describes the swine food debacle of February 1976, when the U.S. government pulled out all stops preparing for a repeat—which never occurred—of the deadly 1918 influenza pandemic. The summer of 1976 brought Legionnaires' disease, which struck in Philadelphia, killed 34 people, and stumped the infectious disease experts for nearly 6 months. Other outbreaks followed and a new vocabulary arose: Lyme disease, toxic shock syndrome, *Escherichia coli* O157:H7, sexually transmitted diseases, Ebola virus. In June 1981 came the now landmark report from the Centers for Disease Control and Prevention (CDC). Nine brief paragraphs described a strange cluster of fatal symptoms among 5 gay men in Los Angeles: acquired immune deficiency syndrome (AIDS), which has already infected 250,000 persons in the United States. Before the recent headline accounts of avian flu, a silent hepatitis C epidemic, parasite-contaminated water slides, new-variant Creutzfeldt-Jakob disease, and anthrax, we had smallpox, typhus, polio, cholera, rabies, and the Black Death. We still have them. None have been consigned to history. Small human populations suffer the oldest diseases of humankind: either chronic, such as leprosy or herpes, or those that have reservoirs in animals or in soil, such as yellow fever, the virus of which circulates in monkeys. Only when a community is dense and filthy enough to keep spreading germs and big enough to keep supplying new susceptibles do such infections such as measles, smallpox, typhoid, and influenza—crowd diseases or "zymotics"—stay in circulation.

The "plagues" of history are still with us. In 79 A.D., an outbreak believed to be malaria contributed to the Roman Empire's fall. The plague of Antoninus (166 to 180 C.E.), probably smallpox, killed about 30% of Italy's population. The plague of Justinian (542 to 543 C.E.), one of the first documented cases of rat-borne bubonic plague, killed 10,000 people daily in Constantinople and eventually spread as far north as Denmark, annihilating much of the human race in its path. Between 1346 and 1350, 1/3 of Europe's population died of bubonic plague, spread from Asia to Europe by Mongol armies, whose retinues of rodents carried infected fleas that subsequently bit humans. In the sixteenth and seventeenth centuries, slave ships from West Africa brought yellow fever and its mosquito vector to the New World. Smallpox, transported to the Americas by Spanish conquistadors, killed 1/3 of the relatively disease-free native population and was followed by a similar lethal onslaught of measles. Diseases introduced from Europe killed an estimated 95% of the pre-Columbian Native American population, and exotic infections attacked the other direction also. European colonials succumbed to malaria, yellow fever, and other endemic infections in tropical Africa, India, Southeast Asia, and New Guinea. Syphilis appeared in 1494, perhaps with Columbus' returning soldiers. The industrial revolution of the nineteenth century amplified such diseases as tuberculosis, an ancient bacterial infection that thrives in squalid close quarters. Illnesses from contaminated food and water, such as typhoid fever and cholera, also went on a spree.

Beginning in the late 1870s, the new discipline of bacteriology found the agents that caused cholera, tuberculosis, gonorrhea, typhoid, and scarlet fever. By 1900, most scientists agreed that microorganisms—spread by casual contact, food and water contamination, insects, and even (in the cases of typhoid and tuberculosis) healthy human carriers—caused communicable diseases. These discoveries spurred expansion of government health initiatives such as water purification, food inspection, and rodent control, as well as more awareness of individual hygiene measures such as covering a cough or washing hands before eating.

In the later 1930s and 1940s came specific antimicrobial therapies such as sulfa compounds and penicillin, and by the mid 1960s numerous antibiotics were available to treat such infections as gonorrhea, syphilis, pneumonia, tuberculosis, bacterial meningitis, typhoid fever, and even bubonic plague, whereas new vaccines prevented epidemics of measles, rubella, and polio. The study of infectious disease became unfashionable between 1970 and 1975. The National Institutes of Health's budget increased 100%, but the budget for infectious diseases increased only 30%. Cancer and heart disease got most of the money. When human immunodeficiency virus (HIV) came along in the early 1980s, the government initially looked the other way. Public health agencies had already stopped surveillance for drug-resistant tuberculosis just as the disease started to rise. In the 1980s and 1990s, the U.S. infectious disease mortality rate jumped 58% even after removing AIDS from the tally during that period, and infectious disease deaths in the United States rose 22%. In 1998, the CDC issued a detailed 5-year plan to prepare the nation for emerging infections, but congressional funding has lagged.

Microorganisms (viruses, bacteria, fungi, protozoa) play the survival game exceedingly well. They adapt far more quickly than humans do as the environment changes. Humans produce a new generation every 20 years or so; bacteria do it every 30 minutes, and viruses even faster. Natural selection, whereby genetically better adapted individuals leave more progeny and thus transmit those desirable characteristics, operate far more efficiently in the microbial world. Because they assemble in enormous numbers, viruses and bacteria can support considerable variety in their communities, including mutated oddballs that further proliferate when circumstances change. When an enterovirus like polio goes through the human intestinal tract in 3 days, its genome mutates about 2%. That level of mutation—2% of the genome—takes the human species 8 million years to accomplish!

Compared with humans, microorganisms are relatively simple. A virus (the word comes from a Latin term for "poisonous substance") is nothing more than nucleic acid, DNA or RNA, surrounded by a shell of protein and sometimes lipids. Viruses range in size from about 20 to 400 nm in diameter such that millions can fit in a period at the end of a sentence. Outside a living cell a virus is a dormant particle, lacking the raw materials for synthesis. Only when it enters a congenial host cell does it explode into action, hijacking the cell's metabolic machinery to produce copies of itself that may burst out of infected cells or simply bud off a cell membrane. Viruses cannot be cultured in artificial media. They can only be propagated in live cells, fertilized eggs, tissue cultures, or bacteria. Viruses hurt us by killing the host cells. Viral infections are harder to fight once the process is underway because our immune responses usually kick in too late to subdue them.

Bacteria: One-celled organisms that are more self-sufficient, are about 1,000 times larger than viruses, and are generally visible under a light microscope. Bacteria are known as prokaryotic—so primitive they lack a membrane-bound nucleus with neatly linear chromosomes inside. Instead, bacteria usually carry a tangled necklace of DNA joined at the ends and sometimes smaller rings of DNA known as plasmids, which contain genes that enable them to manufacture proteins. Bacteria carry only 1 set of chromosomes instead of 2, an arrangement that means that every gene counts and every selected advantage must be conserved.

Over eons, bacteria have learned tricks to help them cleave to cells, make paralyzing poisons, allude or suppress our bodies' defenses, and shrug off drugs and antibodies. They pick up genes from almost everywhere: from other bacteria, viruses, plants, and even from yeast. When a virus picked up a toxic gene from a deadly *Shiegella dysenteriae* and inserted into a harmless *E. coli*, it created *E. coli* O157:H7, a bacterial hybrid that clings to mucosal surfaces in the intestine and produces toxins that trigger hemolytic uremic syndrome, the most common cause of acute kidney failure in children. Bacteria inflict damage in a different way than viruses. Sometimes they multiply so rapidly they crowd out host tissues and disrupt normal function. Sometimes they kill cells and tissues outright. Sometimes they manufacture toxins that can paralyze, destroy metabolic pathways, or generate a massive immune reaction that is itself toxic. Drug-resistant bacteria often make an enzyme that destroys antibiotics or spits them out. Bacteria do not attack until their numbers are high enough to establish an infection ("quorum sensing"). Nevertheless, bacteria remain easier to treat than viruses. Because they are free living and because their structure differs from that of mammalian cells, they are more susceptible to drugs delivered by way of the bloodstream.

The newly discovered infectious agents such as bovine spongiform encephalopathy (BSE or mad cow disease)—and its human counterpart new-variant Creutzfeldt-Jakob disease—apparently repealed the laws of biology. Called prions, these proteins are folded in an unusual way; when they come in contact with other proteins, they turn them into prions, setting off a chain reaction that eventually riddles the brain with holes. A cow can contract BSE by eating 1 g of prion-infected tissue—the size of a peppercorn—from another cow. Unlike virus or bacteria, prions cannot reproduce and evoke no immune response. More frightening, they resist heat, ultraviolet light, radiation, and sterilization.

A traditional wisdom about emerging pathogens is that they are noxious because they are new and, therefore, ill adapted to a human host. Animal viruses, such as the Ebola virus or the Sin Nombre virus that causes hantavirus pulmonary syndrome, can trigger unusual symptoms because our immune response has not evolved with the virus. Over the long haul, microorganisms in humans usually reach a subtle accommodation. Humans acquire resistance to the infectious agent whereas the parasite becomes milder, permitting us to survive its assault and permitting it to transmit its genes to someone else. Microorganisms need their host to survive; a dead host is a dead end. The reason the lethal spore-forming bacillus *Clostridium botulinum*—the cause of botulism—has not leveled our species is because when it kills us with its toxins, it kills its prospect for spreading.

In the case of emerging infections, the collision is between pathogens and people. Emerging infections come because change is everywhere—not only for humans but also for non-human animals, plants, seeds, and insects. Virtually every aspect of American culture—from where we live to where we play, from how we raise livestock to how we raise children—is changing, and change creates new markets, so to speak, for pathogens, which have a knack for leveraging the slimmest advantage. Every day, >2 million people worldwide cross national borders; every year >1.5 billion people travel by air. The United States hosts 47 million visitors yearly. With air travel today, people in India are like neighbors. Just as in the nineteenth century when cholera traveled on steamships to Europe and Africa, so in the early 1990s cholera reached the oyster beds of Mobile Bay by stowing away in the bilge water of ships from Latin America. Trucks, freighters, and airplanes have replaced caravans and steamships. Our stores are now filled with foods from all over the world. Any pathogen, not just those present in food, can be virtually anywhere in the world within 48 hours. Lyme disease came to us courtesy of nineteenth-century deforestation in the Northeast, followed by patchy and less diversified second-growth forests. Coastal population growth has led to contamination of shellfish beds with human waste, fostering the transmission of viral and bacterial pathogens. Human encroachment on the tropical rain forest may open the way for hemorrhagic fever viruses and perhaps even HIV's mysterious retroviral cousins.

Communing with nature is not the only path to pathogens—microbes also love crowds. In 1900, only 5% of the world's population lived in cities with >100,000 residents. By 2025, 65% of the population in developing regions will inhabit cities. Dense urban enclaves are magnets for infections from isolated rural areas and launch pads that allow pathogens to reach other fast-growing populations. Overwhelmed by unsafe water, poor sanitation, and widespread poverty, tomorrow's mega cities will become cauldrons for new infections. The devastating 1998 to 1999 Nipah virus outbreak in Malaysia that killed nearly 1/3 of infected people probably sprang from intensive pig raising, which permitted a novel virus (probably carried by fruit bats) to propagate and then jump to farmers. Thus, pig farms acted as mega cities for the deadly agent, and pig farmers became sentinel cases. In industrialized countries, daycare centers are notably noxious settings in which the combination of frequent infections, susceptible children, poor hygiene, and high antimicrobial use breeds diarrheal diseases and antibiotic-resistant microbes.

Keeping ourselves alive longer also increases our susceptibility to infection. In 1900, only 4% of the U.S. population was over the age of 65 years—in 2040, it will reach almost 25%. Elderly individuals, with their fading immunity, are at the mercy of microorganisms that are normally benign. Although chemotherapy and other immunosuppressive treatments have enabled people to live with cancer and other illnesses, they of course also increase our susceptibility to ubiquitous pathogens such as cytomegalovirus and West Nile virus. Modern technologies intended to make our lives easier may also make life easier for microbes. The bacterium of Legionnaires' disease, which is normally a habitué of moist soil in lakes, not only thrives in water of narrowly warm temperature ranges, but also must be misted into tiny particles to penetrate deep into human lungs—and so is neatly accommodated by cooling towers, whirlpool spas, and even hot water pipes. One major worry about organ transplant from pigs is that these organs could infect humans with porcine endogenous retroviruses, which are in the same class as HIV. These viruses, which are insinuated in the donor pig's DNA, could interact with human viruses to create new, potentially dangerous species that might spread to the general population.

Bugs themselves are changing. In 1954, the United States produced 2 million pounds of antibiotics. Today it makes tens of millions of pounds per year, 1/2 or more administered to livestock. As a result, 70% of bacteria that cause the infections patients acquire in hospitals are resistant to at least 1 antibiotic, and the animals we eat have become favorites for drug-resistant microbes. If vancomycin-intermediate *Staphylococcus aureus,* or VISA, defies our most powerful antibiotic, simple scrapes could become mortal wounds and surgery could be as dangerous as it was 100 years ago. It takes 17 years to produce a new antibiotic, but a bacterium can develop resistance in minutes!

What many biologists fear most is a new deadly virus. Viruses, of course, are harder to fight with drugs and intimately entangled with the genes and metabolic machinery in our cells. Viruses also seem to stimulate our immune systems more violently and self destructively than do bacteria. And, unlike with bacteria, it's harder to predict whether a particular virus will radiate quickly or will be especially savage. In the 1930s during the "Great Depression," Hans Zinsser wrote, "Infectious disease is one of the few genuine adventures left in the world." Even the most extreme sports would not produce the adrenaline of a race against pandemic influenza or a cloud of anthrax at the Super Bowl. In the field of infectious disease, reality is stranger than anything a writer could dream up. The most menacing bioterrorist is Mother Nature herself!

Madeline Drexler has written a splendid book!

William C. Roberts

William Clifford Roberts, MD
Editor in Chief
Baylor Heart & Vascular Institute
Baylor University Medical Center
Dallas, Texas

1. Drexler M. Secret Agents. The Menace of Emerging Infections. Washington, DC: Joseph Henry Press, 2002:295.

Krakatoa—The Ultimate Heart Attack

Individuals when first developing chest pain that leads to cardiac arrest and/or acute myocardial infarction might describe the sudden initial cardiac event as *Krakatoa*, a name that has become a byword for cataclysmic disaster. In 1883, a volcano exploded on the island of Krakatoa, causing an immense tsunami that killed nearly 36,000 people! The waves were felt as far away as France. Barometers in Bogotá and Washington, DC, went haywire. The sound of the island's destruction was heard on islands thousands of miles away.

The author of *The Professor and the Madman* and *The Map that Changed the World* has now written *Krakatoa*. Most volcanoes, of course, continue to exist after erupting. Rarely is an eruption so great that it destroys an entire mountain. Such was the case with Krakatoa and a few others—Mount Mazana (leaving behind Crater Lake in Oregon), Santorini (which may have taken out the Minoan civilization and left a great hole in the Agean), and Yellowstone (in Montana).

Krakatoa was located in the Sundra Strait between the large islands of Sumatra and Java and was composed of 3 peaks: Rakata, at 2,600 ft; Danan, at nearly 1,500 ft; and Perboewatan, at 400 ft. The volcano began violent earthquakes in May 1883. After 3 months of earth tremors, the island blew up. (If Pike's Peak in Colorado had exploded with the same force, every person in the continental United States would have heard it!) There were 4 detonations over 5 hours. The last one occurred on Monday morning August 27, 1883; it was one of the largest explosions in recorded history.

At Krakatoa when cold sea water contacted the red-hot magma, the steam exploded with catastrophic violence, and 6 cubic miles of rock and ash were hurled >20 miles into the stratosphere. An hour after the explosion, as lightning lit up the blackening skies, a thick muddy rain fell on Batavia (now Jakarta). Boiling-hot debris from the blast, some chunks 3 feet around, fell over hundreds of square miles. Because the island was uninhabited at the time, nobody on Krakatoa was killed, but giant tsunamis rolled out in all directions, flooding the coast of Java and Sumatra, submerging nearly 300 towns and villages, and killing >36,000 people. It was as if a mountain-sized red-hot rock had been dropped into the ocean.

A 72-ft-high wave engulfed and totally destroyed the town of Telokbetong at the head of Sumatra's Lampong Bay, killing 2,200 people. Water cascaded into the town of Tangerang, and when it swept out again, it carried people, animals, houses, and trees. No one expected the waves to return after they had receded. It is likely that many people believed the worst was over and returned to their shore-side villages, only to experience another, more catastrophic inundation. The town of Merak, which had suffered little damage from the first wave, was destroyed by the second. The huge wave, after traveling at hundreds of miles per hour, entered the narrow bay, and as the shoaling beach slowed down the leading edge of the wave, millions of gallons of water began piling up behind until the wave reached the height of 135 ft, as tall as a 10-story building. This mountain of water rolled over Merak, obliterating everything in its path and drowning all but 2 of 2,700 inhabitants. Anjer was drowned by a 33-ft wave and Tyringin, 24 miles from the volcano, was smashed by 70-ft-high locomotive of rolling water. It was not the lava, noxious gases, flame, smoke, or volcanic bombs that destroyed those unfortunate thousands, it was the power of the water. In most instances death came at the hands of seismic sea waves.

Accompanied by thunderous explosions, the waves swept around St. Nicholas Point on Java and headed for Batavia, 94 miles from the epicenter. At approximately 12:15 P.M., 2 hours after the final explosion, the sea roared into the capital city. It receded and then came back. Thousands of ships, ranging in size from steamships to small proas, were destroyed in Batavia's harbor. Nine hours after the eruption, many riverboats were swamped and sunk in Calcutta, 2,000 miles away, and ships strained at their anchors in Port Elizabeth, South Africa, 5,000 miles from the blast.

What did not remain was the volcano that had caused it all. Krakatoa, after the final concatenation of seismic and tectonic climaxes that occurred just after 10:00 on that Monday morning, had simply and finally exploded itself out of existence. Where once there had been a tropical peak that was 2,600 ft tall, there was now a hole in the ocean floor that was 1,000 ft deep. Krakatoa's explosion generated a climate-altering ash cloud that produced lurid red, blue, green, and copper colored sunsets and lowered temperatures around the world.

Krakatoa (the volcano) was not the largest or deadliest of recent Indonesian volcanic eruptions. That dubious distinction goes to Tambora, which erupted with more than twice the power of Krakatoa, killed 10,000 people outright, and caused the deaths of another 82,000 by starvation and disease. *Krakatoa* (the book) must be one of the best books ever written about the history and significance of a natural disaster. And Simon Winchester, its author is a trained geologist.

William C. Roberts

William Clifford Roberts, MD
Editor in Chief
Baylor Heart & Vascular Institute
Baylor University Medical Center
Dallas, Texas

1. Winchester S. Krakatoa. The Day the World Exploded: August 27, 1883. New York: HarperCollins, 2003.

Sudden Death in Chicago

The phrase "sudden death" sometimes is used to describe the extended play when certain football games or golf matches end regular play with a tied score. Most of the time the phrase is used to describe a mode of death, and it commonly is the result of accidents, natural disasters, war, homicide and suicide, as well as nontraumatic events. Among the latter, the most common, of course, is cardiovascular disease and among them, atherosclerotic coronary artery disease is the most common. Occasionally, sudden death is iatrogenic in nature in that it results from an arrhythmia produced by a drug prescribed by a physician or from uncontrolled bleeding when a physician inadvertently pierces the wall of a blood vessel or cardiac chamber. Recently, I encountered a book describing a physician who was responsible for numerous sudden deaths in one of the great cities in the United States.

Erik Larson, who authored *Isaac's Storm*, has now written a frightening book entitled *Devil in the White City. Murder, Magic, and Madness at the Fair that Changed America.*[1] This new book is about 2 men, one a great architect, and the other a psychopath physician. The architect, Daniel Hudson Burnham, built some of America's most important structures, among them the Flatiron building in New York City and Union Station in Washington, DC, and he designed and built the Chicago World's Fair of 1893, officially called "The World's Columbian Exposition," its official purpose being to commemorate the 400th anniversary of Columbus' discovery of America. Burnham made the fair something enchanting; it was known throughout the world as the "White City." The fair lasted just 6 months, yet during that time it had 27.5 million visits at a time when the country's total population was only 65 million. On its best day, the fair drew >700,000 visitors.

That the fair had occurred at all was something of a miracle. To build it, Burnham confronted a legion of obstacles, any one of which could have and should have killed it long before opening day. Together he and his architectural and construction colleagues built a dream city whose grandeur and beauty exceeded anything anyone could have imagined. The fair occupied over 1 square mile and filled >200 buildings. A single exhibit hall had enough interior space to have housed the U.S. Capitol, the Great Pyramid, Westminster Cathedral, Madison Square Garden, and St. Paul's Cathedral, all at the same time. The Ferris wheel became the fair's emblem, a machine so huge and terrifying that it instantly eclipsed the tower of Alexandre Eiffel that had so wounded Americans' pride 5 years earlier.

That something magical had occurred in that summer of the World's Fair was beyond doubt. But darkness too had touched the fair. Scores of workers had been hurt or killed in building the dream, their families consigned to poverty. Fire had killed 15 more, and an assassin had transformed the closing ceremony from what was to have been the century's greatest celebration to a vast funeral. Worse had occurred too, although these revelations emerged only slowly. A murderer had moved among the beautiful things Burnham had created. Young women were drawn to Chicago by the fair and by the prospect of living on their own. Only after the exposition had Burnham and his colleagues learned of the anguished letters describing daughters who had come to the city and then fallen silent. Amid so much turmoil, it was understandable that the work of a young and handsome doctor would go unnoticed.

Chicago in 1893 was a dark city. A thousand trains a day entered or left Chicago. Many of these trains brought single young women who had never even seen a city but now hoped to make one of the biggest and toughest their home. Anonymous death came early and often. Each of the thousand trains that entered and left the city did so at grade level. You could step from a curb and be killed by the Chicago Limited. Every day, on average, 2 people were destroyed at the city's rail crossings. Their injuries were grotesque. There were other hazards. Streetcars fell from drawbridges. Horses bolted and dragged carriages into the crowds. Fires took a dozen lives a day. There was diphtheria, typhus, cholera, and influenza, and there was murder. In the time of the fair, the rate at which men and women killed one another rose sharply throughout the nation, but especially in Chicago, where police found themselves without the human power or expertise to manage the volume. In the first 6 months of 1892, the city experienced nearly 800 violent deaths—4 a day. Jack the Ripper's 5-murder spree in 1888 in London had defied explanation and captivated readers throughout America, who believed such a thing could not happen in their own home towns.

In August 1886, a man calling himself H.H. Holmes walked into one of Chicago's train stations and there he acquired a ticket to a village called Englewood in the town of Lake, a municipality of 200,000 people that abutted Chicago's southernmost boundary and encompassed the Union Stock Yards (which employed 25,000 men, women, and children and each year slaughtered 14 million animals) and 2 large parks: Washington Park and Jackson Park (where the fair was located). Holmes conjured an impression of wealth and achievement. He was 26 years old, 68 inches tall, and weighed 155 lbs. He had dark hair and striking blue eyes.

When he resolved to move to Chicago, he was still using his given name, Herman Webster Mudgett. At 16, Mudgett had graduated school and then taught in New Hampshire. At 19, he enrolled in the medicine program at the University of Vermont in Burlington but found the school too small. After 1 year, he moved to the University of Michigan School of Medicine in Ann Arbor. He graduated in June 1884 with a lackluster record and set out to find some favorable location in which to launch a practice. He initially settled in Mooers Forks, New York, where he remained for 1 year. There were rumors that a boy seen in his company had disappeared, but no one could imagine charming Dr. Mudgett causing harm to anyone, let alone a child. After other brief periods in Philadelphia and New York, he arrived in Chicago having passed his license examination to be a druggist in the state capital of Springfield. He registered under the name H.H. Holmes.

It was not long before Holmes had acquired property at 63rd Street and Wallace, on which he built a hotel that catered only to young women. In the basement of his hotel he built an incinerator to dispose of bodies. At trial in the fall of 1895, Holmes admitted killing 27 people, but exactly how many people he killed will never be known. Estimates ranged as high as 200. If it had not been for a single persistent detective named Frank Geyer, the numerous murders by Holmes, almost all young women, would have never been confirmed nor Holmes ever prosecuted. Herman Webster Mudgett, alias H.H. Holmes, was hung on the gallows May 7, 1896.

In 1997, police in Chicago arrested another physician named Michael Swango at O'Hare Airport. The initial charge was fraud, but Swango was suspected of being a serial killer who murdered hospital patients through the administration of lethal doses of drugs. Eventually, Dr. Swango pled guilty to 4 murders, but investigators believe that he had committed many more. During the airport arrest, police found a notebook in Swango's possession in which he had copied passages from certain books. One passage was from a book about H.H. Holmes called *The Torture Doctor*, by David Franke. The copied passage sought to put the reader into Holmes' mind: "He could look at himself in a mirror and tell himself that he was the most powerful and dangerous man in the world." Swango's notebook read, "He could feel that he was a god in the skies."

William C. Roberts

William Clifford Roberts, MD
Editor in Chief
Baylor Heart & Vascular Institute
Baylor University Medical Center
Dallas, Texas

1. Larsen E. The Devil in the White City. Murder, Magic, and Madness at the Fair that Changed America. New York: Crown Publishers, 2003.

Saving Money and Investing Money: Advice from a Cardiologist

There are 125 medical schools in the USA, and to my knowledge only 1 of them has a single class having anything to do with saving money and investing money. There has just appeared (2005) a superb book by cardiologist Robert M. Doroghazi entitled *The Physicians Guide to Investing. A Practical Approach to Building Wealth* (Figure 1),[1] and I strongly recommend it to anyone interested in preserving and growing a dollar bill.

But first, something about the author, Bob Doroghazi. His grandparents came to the USA from Hungary and settled in Granite City, Illinois, a suburb of St. Louis, Missouri. He paid his own way through college (University of Illinois, Champaign/Urbana), graduating with high honors (Phi Beta Kappa) and through the University of Chicago Pritzker School of Medicine with honors (Alpha Omega Alpha). His internship and residency in internal medicine was at the Massachusetts General Hospital in Boston, and his cardiology training was at Barnes Hospital in St. Louis. In 1983, 1 year after completing his cardiology fellowship, he and Dr. Eve E. Slater coauthored *Aortic Dissection,* a book published by McGraw-Hill. Dr. Doroghazi has been in practice since 1982 with the Missouri Cardiovascular Specialists in Columbia. He has given greatly of his time and his money to his community: past president of the Great Rivers Council of Boy Scouts of America, past president of the Columbia Northwest Rotary, past president of Advent Enterprises, and he has served on the boards of Columbia United Way, Great Rivers Council of the Boy Scouts of America, The Boone Hospital Center Foundation, The Museum of Art and Archeology at the University of Missouri-Columbia, and University of Chicago Medical Alumni Association. He also plays in the first clarinet section in the Columbia Community Band. He and his wife have endowed the Susan Case Doroghazi Faculty Excellence Awards at the College of Nursing of Texas Women's University and the Robert and Susan Doroghazi Outstanding Clinical Teacher Award at the University of Chicago-Pritzker School of Medicine. His library numbers >700 volumes.

Now to his book. His observations are too numerous to summarize here but some of them are as follows.

Financial goals: For the long term, physician investors should anticipate a 10% annual return on noncash investments. With some work, common sense, and knowledge of where mistakes may arise, a 15% annual return on annual investments may be realized. Dividends are important. The best investors are the best savers. Being a physician does not make one necessarily smart at investing. Compound interest is the most valuable investment tool. Even seemingly small amounts of money have amazing potential. The younger the person, the more valuable the money. Lost money can never be recouped. The goal should not be to be rich but to have financial security. He suggests that more money is lost in the hospital doctor's lounge or other similar settings, where physicians tend to congregate and talk, such as at a party or the country club, than anywhere else. It is in such situations, he emphasizes that, arrogance, ego, and greed overwhelm sanity. The best investment one can make is not making a stupid investment that was motivated by arrogance, ego, greed, desire to impress others, or being concerned about being left out.

Financial needs and goals must be identified before appropriate plans to achieve them can be made. Investing is a 3-step process: earn money, save money, invest money. Doroghazi states that the most important item to remember from his book is the following: learn to say, "This is too expensive. I cannot afford this." This is the first step toward a lifetime of financial security.

Another important statement: "I married a gold mine. My spouse is thrifty." The essence of thrift is not to waste any resource. Do not buy things you do not make adequate use of, and use to the fullest things you purchase. A purchase at any price is not a bargain if you do not make use of the product. Do not allow your spending to increase more rapidly than your income. Physicians should be able to save 25% to 50% of their after tax income.

The mark: He tells of a cartoon showing 2 deer in the woods. One has a huge red symbol on its chest that looks like a bull's eye. The other deer says, "Bummer of a birth mark, Hal. " Many business people view physicians as having "The Mark" on their chests. He advises to accept we physicians are considered "The Mark. " Physicians are notorious for being poor negotiators, often because of dealing in an area outside of their expertise. He advises hiring someone to negotiate for you. To be referred to as a "rich doctor" is a sign of disrespect.

Identifying and managing risk: Avoid long shots. They rarely pay. There is no reason to "risk" any amount of money.

Invest in what you know and like: Knowledge equals money. Being a successful investor requires hard work. Great investment ideas frequently come from daily life.

Make your own investment decisions: Allowing someone else to make your investment decisions has the potential for financial devastation and ruin. Never invest in anything just because someone else does. Do not allow your name to be used to induce others to invest. No one else should ever know that you are even interested in any investment. Financial information is as private as medical information. You

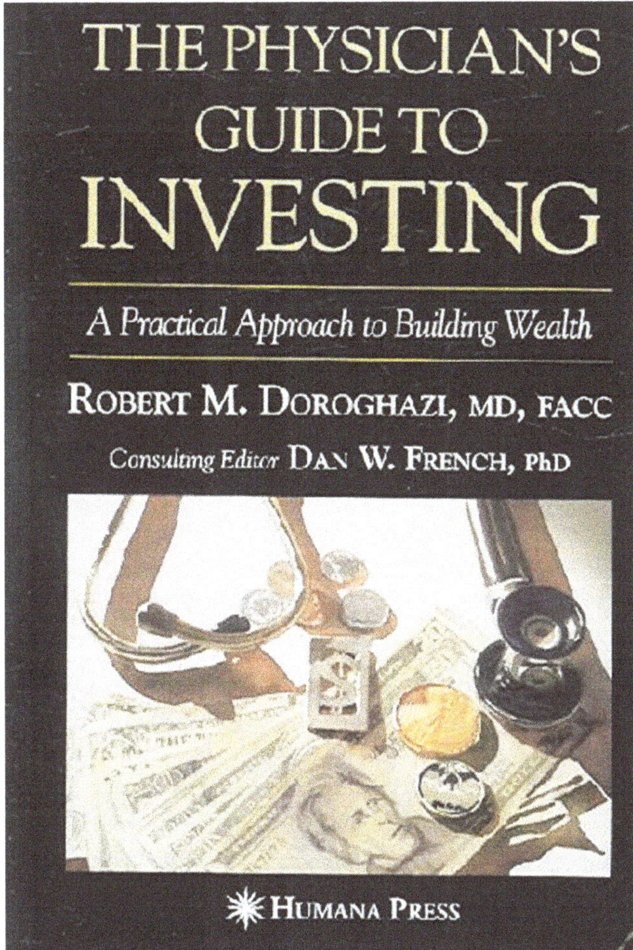

Figure 1. The cover of *The Physicians Guide to Investing. A Practical Approach to Building Wealth* (from Doroghazi RM,[1] with permission).

may seek the advice of others but, in the end, you must make your own investment decisions. The goal of investing is to make money.

Keep a budget: Be a good record keeper. Have a will. Keep a personal financial statement and update it yearly. Be conservative when estimating the value of assets.

Pay your bills in full and on time: Purchase a home that is financially within your budget at the earliest possible time. Resist the temptation to buy a home as large as your parents or your senior associates. Control ego when buying a home. Real estate is illiquid. If you do not have a 20% down payment that you have saved, you cannot afford a home. Do not take an interest-only loan. Take a 10 (or at most 15) year mortgage. Have your home paid for by age 45. Insist on no prepayment penalties when buying a home. The early pay off of a home can be the equivalent of a lifetime of successful investing. Pay cash for remodeling or additions. Limit the number of times you move.

Funding children's education: Encourage your children to pay for as much of their own educational expenses as possible. Take complete advantage of all financial aid. Take advantage of tax options to fund your children's education.

Insurance: Disability insurance is the most important type of insurance a physician can have. A physician's most valuable asset is not their home, car or any other piece of personal property. A physician's most valuable financial asset is his/her capacity to work and produce income. The average person is almost 5 times more likely to become disabled as to die prematurely. Purchase term life insurance; avoid whole life insurance. Have a long-term care insurance policy, but consult a tax professional before purchasing it. No life insurance should be required after age 60. Get medical insurance. Avoid extended warranties. Consider an umbrella policy.

Funding retirement: The most expensive part of everyone's retirement will be medical bills. The average senior citizen currently pays $175,000 for *out of pocket* medical charges. Doroghazi's advice is:

> 1. Stay healthy, don't smoke, exercise regularly, monitor your blood pressure, watch your diet, maintain ideal weight, keep you LDL <100 (preferably 60 to 70), have a colonoscopy preformed at appropriate intervals, buckle your seatbelt, use sunscreen, obtain appropriate female and male tests and examinations, keep your vaccinations up to date, brush your teeth and floss as instructed...
>
> 2. Save as much money as possible, and intend to spend it on your health.

Have all major obligations funded before retirement. An investment that does not match inflation is a loss. Have sufficient savings such that you can live off of 5% of your total assets per year. Make full use of every tax advantaged opportunity and contribute the maximum. Do not purchase an annuity.

Debt: The less debt the better. Debt is seductive and it can ruin your life. Do not lease a car. Never purchase stock on margin. The longer the repayment period, the greater the burden of debt. Debt is compound interest in reverse, working to the detriment of the borrower. Use unanticipated financial windfalls to pay off debt. There are few better investments than the early repayment of debt.

Fees: Fees can drain your financial health. Even small fees can represent large amounts of money over time. Do not invest in any mutual fund that charges a "load." Core investment positions for all physician investors should include index mutual funds and no-load actively managed funds with a long-term record of superior performance. Full service brokers rarely justify their higher fees. If you make your own investment decisions, execute your trades as cheaply as possible. All fees are negotiable. Anything added to the basic cost of an item is a fee. Never buy anything from a cold-call telemarketer. Physicians are preferred customers. Use this advantage to minimize fees and obtain perks. Fees are either money in your pocket or money in someone else's pocket.

Investment areas to avoid: Avoid tax shelters. Forget about owning a restaurant or any store front business. Avoid direct foreign investments. Art or any collectible is rarely profitable. Avoid hedge funds. Avoid penny stocks. Don't worry about "getting in on the ground floor." Completely avoid anything where all the potential investors are physicians. Avoid limited partnerships sold by a broker or salesman or where the general partner has not invested any of his money.

Bankers and loans: Deal with bankers on your terms, not theirs. Every word in a loan document is important. Read it closely. Do not sign a "callable" loan. Loaning money to a family member only to "help" them is actually doing them and you a terrible disservice. Only trust people you know well and have earned your trust and respect.

Asset allocation and diversification: The first rule in investing is suffering no huge loss. A reasonable asset allocation would be 65% stocks, 10% cash, and 25% fixed income. Doroghazi loves Certificates of Deposit (CD), and he believes that they should represent most or even all of the money allocated to fixed income investments. Have CDs at several banks in town. There is no commission charges to purchase or redeem a CD. CDs are not "callable." Most are insured by the government for up to $100,000 at each institution. He considers CDs cash and fixed income investment. Doroghazi views diversification with caution because it mandates investing outside your area of expertise. He suggests that diversification will increase not decrease your investment losses. Doroghazi notes that this advice is different from almost all standard investment texts. Invest in what you know and stay with it.

Identifying real investment opportunities: These occur approximately once a year. Keep your eyes open. Real opportunities should be so obvious that you never have to talk yourself into them.

When to buy: Money is made when an asset is purchased. It is impossible to make money when overpaying for an asset. Never buy just because the price is down. A sure way to be wiped out is to add to losing positions. Try to buy assets for less than they are worth. Buy when there is "blood in the streets," but this requires tremendous personal confidence.

When to sell: Take profits "too early." An asset must be sold to lock in a profit. When you are congratulating yourself on your investment genius—sell. There are no 1 decision investments. Do not fall in love with an investment. Aggressively sell nonperforming assets.

Miscellaneous: Donate at least 3% to 5% of your income to charity each year. Medical schools should implement courses providing instruction to assist physicians in handling and investing their money. Realize the financial consequences of changing practices. The most expensive part of a vacation is not the travel, logging, meals, and entertainment, but the income lost from not working. Avoid gambling. The odds of winning are too great, and it can be addictive and destroy one's life. Doroghazi donates any honoraria received from speaking for pharmaceutical companies and for reviewing malpractice cases (only for the defense) to charity. This avoids being "beholden" to them. Cut your own grass. It is illogical to go out jogging while paying someone else to cut one's grass. It helps a high income professional such as a physician maintain perspective.

His concluding advice as to the most important factors for obtaining financial security are thrift, compound interest, patience, discipline and investing in what you know, and the 5 most important factors that destroy wealth are greed, debt, fees, trusting everyone, and not making your own decisions.

I highly recommend this book! Bob Doroghazi is a wise man who will retire from practice in 3 months at age 54!

William Clifford Roberts, MD
Editor in Chief
Baylor Heart and Vascular Institute
Baylor University Medical Center
Dallas, Texas
13 October 2005

1. Doroghazi RM, consulting editor French DW. The Physicans's Guide to Investing. A Practical Approach to Building Wealth. Humana Press: New Jersey 2006: 228, $59.50 (hardback), $34.95 (softback).

Board Certification Scams

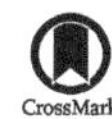

In May 2014 I received the letter printed below with the caption American Board of Cardiology Committee on Honors and Awards, dated May 9, 2014, and signed by A.J. Alaa Windsor, MD. I was a bit surprised and transiently honored when I read the letter until I got to the second page which indicated that there were actually 3 engraved award plaques: one stated *The American Board of Cardiology Award of Honor for 2014*; another *The Distinguished*

AMERICAN BOARD OF CARDIOLOGY
COMMITTEE ON HONORS AND AWARDS
304 NEWBURY STREET
SUITE 309
BOSTON, MA 02115

May 9, 2014

Dear Doctor Roberts,

On the basis of your outstanding record as a Cardiologist and Educator, Distinguished Member of the Association of University Professors of Cardiology, Master Educator at one of America's finest medical schools, and as a physician respected for excellence of knowledge and experience and willingness to share knowledge with future cardiologists and medical students, we wish to honor you for the excellence and humanitarian work that has been your life's accomplishment to the benefit of mankind.

After decisions at meetings in Las Vegas, Nevada, this week, we wish to bestow the 2014 Award of Honor. It is a very great pleasure and honor for me to notify you of the award and to express our deep respect for the excellence that you bring to the medical specialty of Cardiology. We are pleased to designate you as a Distinguished Master Laureate of the American Board of Cardiology.

The American Board of Cardiology considers the designation as Laureate to be a higher level than Diplomate. The Laureate has the distinction of being exemplary as a humanitarian, as well as being excellent in knowledge and professional excellence in the specialty of Cardiology. Designation as Master Laureate is our very highest designation. Master Laureates are named Senior Consultant to the American Board of Cardiology.

Awarding is based on outstanding dedication as a medical educator, profound excellence in the specialty of Cardiology, and humanitarian aspects of medical practice including highest ethics, compassion, and the most noble qualities of a true healer.

At your earliest convenience, please send written acknowledgement of your acceptance of the award of the American Board of Cardiology, and indicate preferred exact spelling of your name and degree for proper engraving of certificates and for plaque engraving.

Very Truly,

A. J. Alaa Windsor, M.D
Acting Director, Committee on Honors and Awards

Founded as Not For Profit NV Corporation

Master Laureate of the American Board of Cardiology, and the third one as *Senior Consultant to the American Board of Cardiology*. Under each of these was the option to order a number of plaques. Near the bottom of the second page was the following: "Please assist in the funding of this program of recommendation of excellence. Please enclose registration fee of $300 made to: American Board of Cardiology. Please enclose engraving and preparation fee of $70 for each 10″ × 8″ engraved plaque and $15 for shipping and handling of each plaque." Also at the top of this second page was the following titled: ACCEPTANCE OF AWARD – "I hereby accept the American Board of Cardiology Award of Honor and the designation as Master Laureate and Senior Consultant of the American Board of Cardiology. I promise to continue to uphold the centuries old traditions of excellence and humanitarianism in medicine and shall continue to practice medicine in accordance with the Oath of Hippocrates, the Ten Commandments, and the Golden Rule to treat others as I would have others treat me. And I will continue to always faithfully work to support and promote excellence, education, compassion, kindness and truest humanitarianism in medicine."

I thought about this particular document overnight and became leery and the next day searched for A.J. Alaa Windsor, MD, on Google and could not find one thing on him. My assistant, Becky Banks, then searched Google for *The American Board of Cardiology*. The search included the American Board of Internal Medicine which had the following scam warning (The link to this warning is *abim.org/news/scam-certification-boards.aspx*.): "The American Board of Internal Medicine has received reports from several regarding letters and solicitations from their members from groups offering "certification" in geriatric medicine, cardiology and hospital medicine, among other specialties. The American Board of Internal Medicine of course is concerned about the welfare of patients who may choose doctors representing themselves as "board certified" based on their possession of a certificate from unaccredited "boards" that awards certificates but require no accredited training, testing or medical background review. If contacted by any of the listed "phony" certification boards, the American Board of Internal Medicine would like to hear about it."

Beware!

William Clifford Roberts, MD
Baylor Heart and Vascular Institute
Baylor University Medical Center
Dallas, Texas
May 21, 2014

Medical History

Oslerian Advice

In 1959 I purchased from Old Hickory Bookshop in Brinklow, Maryland, a book entitled *Sir William Osler, Bart., Brief Tributes to His Personality, Influence and Public Service Written by His Friends, Associates and Former Pupils, In Honor of His Seventieth Birthday and First Published in The Bulletin of The Johns Hopkins Hospital for July, 1919.* This 167-page book, which also contains Osler's bibliography, has since been a steady companion of mine. My favorite chapter was written by his former Johns Hopkins' Chief Resident, William S. Thayer, who described the third heart sound, and is entitled "Osler, The Teacher." In it, Thayer paraphrases comments of Osler apparently reiterated many times during rounds and other discussions. The comments are as appropriate 64 years later as when they were recorded by Thayer:

> Observe, record, tabulate, communicate.
>
> Use your five senses. The art of the practice of medicine is to be learned only by experience; 'tis not an inheritance; it cannot be revealed. Learn to see, learn to hear, learn to feel, learn to smell, and know that by practice alone can you become expert. Medicine is learned by the bedside and not in the classroom. Let not your conceptions of the manifestations of disease come from words heard in the lecture room or read from the book. See, and then reason and compare and control. But see first. No two eyes see the same thing. No two mirrors give forth the same reflection. Let the word be your slave and not your master.
>
> Live in the ward. Do not waste the hours of daylight in listening to that which you may read by night. But when you have seen, read. And when you can, read the original descriptions of the masters who, with crude methods of study, saw so clearly.
>
> Record that which you have seen; make a note at the time; do not wait. "The flighty purpose never is o'ertook, unless the deed go with it."
>
> Memory plays strange pranks with facts. The rocks and fissures and gullies of the mountain-side melt quickly into the smooth, blue outlines of the distant panorama. Viewed through the perspective of memory, an unrecorded observation, the vital details long since lost, easily changes its countenance and sinks obediently into the frame fashioned by the fancy of the moment.
>
> Always note and record the unusual. Keep and compare your observations. Communicate or publish short notes on anything that is striking or new. Do not waste your time in compilations, but when your observations are sufficient, do not let them die with you. Study them, tabulate them, seek the points of contact which may reveal the underlying law. Some things can be learned only by statistical comparison. If you have the good fortune to command a large clinic, remember that one of your chief duties is the tabulation and analysis of the carefully recorded experience.
>
> The collection and study of your own observations is much, but he who works in his own small compartment leads, after all, a restricted and circumscribed life. Go out among your fellows, and learn of them. The good observer is not limited to the large hospital. The modest country doctor may furnish you the vital link in your chain, and the simple rural practitioner is often a very wise man.
>
> Respect your colleagues. Know that there is no more high-minded body of men than the medical profession. Do not judge your confrères by the reports of patients, well meaning, perhaps, but often strangely and sadly misrepresenting. Never let your tongue say a slighting word of a colleage [sic]. It is not for you to judge. Let not your ear hear the sound of your voice raised in unkind criticism or ridicule or condemnation of a brother physician. If you do, you can never again meet that man face to face. Wait. Try to believe the best. Time will generally show that the words you might have spoken would have been unjust, would have injured a good man, and lost you a friend, and then—silence is a powerful weapon.
>
> When you have made and recorded the unusual or original observation, or when you have accomplished a piece of research in laboratory or ward; do not be satisfied with a verbal communication at a medical society. Publish it. Place it on permanent record as a short, concise note. Such communications are always of value.
>
> Mix with your colleagues; learn to know them. But in your relations with the profession and with the public, in everything that pertains to medicine, consider the virtues of taciturnity. Look out. Speak only when you have something to say. Commit yourself only when you can and must. And when you speak, assert only that of which you know. Beware of

words—they are dangerous things. They change color like the chameleon, and they return like a boomerang. Do you know the story of the young physician, about to enter practice, who was sent by his father to his old friend, Sir William Stokes, for advice? A pleasant conversation, and, at the doorway, a last word: "Charley, don't say too much." Then, at the gate, a voice: "Charley, come back a minute; I'm very fond of you, my boy; don't *do* too much."

"Don't do too much." Remember how much you do not know. Do not pour strange medicines into your patients. Our greatest assistance is given by simple physical and mental means, and by the careful employment of such drugs as have been adequately studied, with regard to the action of which we have real information. Do not rashly use every new product of which the peripatetic siren sings. Consider what surprising reactions may occur in the laboratory from the careless mixing of unknown substances. Be as considerate of your patient and yourself as you are of the test-tube.

Familiarize yourself with the work of others and never fail to give credit to the precursor. Let every student have full recognition for his work. Never hide the work of others under your own name. Should your assistant make an important observation, let him publish it. Through your students and your disciples will come your greatest honor.

Be prompt at your appointments; that is always possible. Many are always late at a consultation; few miss a train. There is no excuse for tardiness.

Live a simple and a temperate life, that you may give all your powers to your profession. Medicine is a jealous mistress; she will be satisfied with no less.

Save the fleeting minute; do not stop by the way. Learn gracefully to dodge the bore. Strike first and quickly, and before he has recovered from the blow, be gone; 'tis the only way. . . .

If you can practice consistently all this, . . . and then, if you can bring into corridor and ward a light, springing step, a kindly glance, a bright word to every one you meet, arm passed within arm or thrown over the shoulder of the happy student or colleague; a quick, droll, epigrammatic question, observation or appellation that puts the patient at his ease or brings a pleased blush to the face of the nurse; an apprehension that grasps in a minute the kernel of the situation, and a memory teeming with instances and examples that throw light on the question; an unusual power of succinct statement and picturesque expression, exercised quietly, modestly and wholely without sensation; if you can bring into the lecture room an air of perfect simplicity and directness, and, behind it all, have an ever-ready store of the most apt and sometimes surprising interjections that so light up and emphasize that which you are setting forth that no one in the room can forget it; if you can enter the sick-room with a song and an epigram, an air of gaiety, an atmosphere that lifts the invalid instantly out of his ills, that produces in the waiting hypochondriac so pleasing a confusion of thought that the written list of questions and complaints, carefully compiled and treasured for the moment of the visit, is almost invariably forgotten; if the joy of your visit can make half a ward forget the symptoms that it *fancied* were important, until you are gone; if you can truly love your fellow, and, having said evil of no man, be loved by all; if you can select a wife with a heart as big as your own, whose generous welcome makes your tea-table a Mecca; . . . if you can do all this, you may begin to be to others the teacher that "the chief" is to us!

William C. Roberts

William C. Roberts, MD
Editor-in-Chief

Reprinted from the May 15 issue of **The American Journal of Cardiology**, A Yorke Medical Journal. Published by Technical Publishing, a Division of Dun-Donnelly Publishing Corporation, a Company of The Dun & Bradstreet Corporation, 875 Third Avenue, New York, N.Y., 10022.

Who Was Holter?

Several months ago at our weekly conference, we examined a Holter Monitor that had been in place at the time of a patient's sudden death. I asked my colleagues at the conference, "Who is Holter?" and no one knew. I then asked my young associate, Dr. Marc Silver, to "bring us the scoop" on Holter. Marc initially went to the library to round up some of Holter's publications, learned that Holter lived in Helena, Montana, and a telephone dialog with Holter began. We asked Holter to send us his curriculum vitae, copies of his most important publications and any other bits and pieces of information that might be useful in writing an article on him and his contributions to medicine. Shortly after Holter, his wife (Joan) and assistant (Karma Alfredson) had gathered these materials together, Holter died (on July 21, 1983) of prostatic cancer. We received the package of Holter information 2 weeks later.

In collaboration with his life-long friend and former teacher, Joseph A. Gengerelli, PhD, Holter first demonstrated the effectiveness of radiotelemetry in broadcasting and recording an electrocardiogram in a person while active. Subsequently, nearly 7,000 articles have been published on Holter Monitoring (which Holter always preferred to call *Holter electrocardiography*) and a medical journal (*Biotelemetry and Patient Monitoring*) was started solely for publications on this subject. Holter's invention of continuous electrocardiographic recording on magnetic tape with accelerated interpretation was to conventional electrocardiography what motion-picture photography was to still photography—not a bad accomplishment for a man who had neither an MD nor a PhD degree, funded his own research, and had his own laboratory in a former train station in a town with a population of <30,000, and was unassociated with a medical center and indeed located far away from any medical research center.

The article that introduced the concept of recording an electrocardiogram "at a distance" appeared in the *Rocky Mountain Medical Journal* in September 1949, when Holter was 35 years old. Holter was proud that he did not receive personal financial gain from the monitoring equipment that today is a $200 million industry. "Its name is the only return I have in the system," he remarked.

It is clear from reading the writings of Holter and from examining his varied activities that this man was a force to be reckoned with. His family was among the original settlers of Montana and his grandfather and father were involved in a number of business enterprises, which "Jeff" Holter inherited and expanded. He was elected to numerous boards of directors of major companies in Montana and elsewhere. He was an artist and among his creations were sculptures called "Geometry in Steel," a 40-piece collection displayed at the Helena Poindexter gallery of contemporary art. His involvement in the evaluation of nuclear weapons shortly after World War II made him an active spokesman about the dangers of nuclear weapons. Holter reiterated often that ". . . if statesmen fail to prevent atomic war, the war after that will be fought with sticks and stones." He foresaw in 1947, however, that atomic research could create major advances in medicine and biology and he was one of the organizers and later president of the Society of Nuclear Medicine.

It is good that the word "Holter" as used in present-day cardiology stands for a man of such distinction.

William C. Roberts

William C. Roberts, MD
Editor-in-Chief

Reprinted from the October 1 issue of **The American Journal of Cardiology,** A Yorke Medical Journal. Published by Technical Publishing, a Division of Dun-Donnelley Publishing Corporation, a Company of The Dun & Bradstreet Corporation, 875 Third Avenue, New York, N Y. 10022.

Benjamin Franklin's *Poor Richard's Almanack* and Its Maxims on Physicians, Medicine and Nutrition

As a boy one of my favorite books was Benjamin Franklin's autobiography.* Only recently did I read his *Poor Richard's Almanack*, the most popular publication of the American colonies. This piece will present some of Poor Richard's maxims on health and its providers. But first some facts on Poor Richard's author, one of our greatest Americans and probably the first world citizen.[2-5]

Benjamin Franklin was born in Boston on January 6, 1706, and died in Philadelphia on April 17, 1790. He was the fifteenth of 17 children, and the youngest of 10 sons. He never remembered when he could not read. At age 8 he started school but by 10, for financial reasons, his father pulled him out to work in his shop making candles and soap. At age 12 he became a journeyman in a brother's printing business. By 16 he was writing pieces in his brother's newspaper under the name "Silence Dogood." At 17 he became a vegetarian so that he could have more money to buy books. (Years later at a fish fry, he saw little fish removed from the stomachs of the larger ones and thought, "If you eat one another, I do not see why we may not eat you. It was then easy to return to an omnivorous diet.") At 18 he left Boston for New York City, but when unable to find employment he sailed for Philadelphia where he became a journeyman printer the day after arriving in October 1723. A year later he went to London to acquire materials to set up his own printing company but he was unable to find financing. He worked in London as a printer for 18 months before returning to Philadelphia in October 1726. At age 22 he formed the *Junto*, a self-improvement and mutual aid society for ambitious young men, and it later became the American Philosophical Society. At age 23 (1728) he began his own printing business (initially with a partner) and the next year purchased the failing *Pennsylvania Gazette* which, during the next 10 years, became the most widely read newspaper in the colonies, inhabited by about 3,000,000 persons. In 1730 his son William was born out of wedlock to an unidentified mother, and later that year he formed a common-law union with Deborah Read Rogers, whose husband had run away, and to whom he was "married" for 44 years. At age 26, Franklin started the first American subscription library, formed the first of several printer partnerships in other colonies, and wrote and published the first of the 25 annual issues of *Poor Richard's Almanack*, which ceased in 1757 when Franklin left for a near 20-year sojourn in London. At age 32 (1737) he became Postmaster of the Pennsylvania colony and at age 48, Postmaster General of North America. Another son was born in 1737 (he died 4 years later) and his daughter was born in 1743.

At age 43 (1748) Franklin, now a man of means, retired from the day-to-day activities of his printing company by bringing in a partner. For the remaining half of his life (42 years) he devoted himself primarily to scientific research, civic affairs, and statesmanship. In Philadelphia, he organized the first police force and the first fire company in the colonies, initiated the lighting and paving of streets, co-founded the first hospital (later called the University of Pennsylvania Hospital)[6,7] and an academy (later to be the University of Pennsylvania), and he became president of the first abolition society (although at one time he owned slaves).

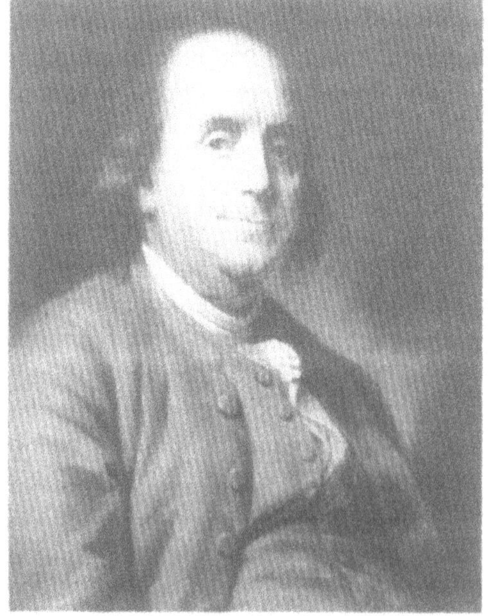

FIGURE 1. Benjamin Franklin at age 78 (1783) while in Paris.

*My father in 1925 also wrote a piece on Benjamin Franklin.[1] The first sentence of his article was better than mine: "Two hundred and fourteen years after Columbus discovered America and seventy before the Declaration of Independence, there was born in the bleak Boston in the early eighteenth century a boy by the name of Benjamin Franklin. . . "

Shortly after retirement from business, Franklin began his experiments on electricity. He proved that lightning was electricity, and invented the lightning rod ("Franklin's rod").[8,9] He was recognized as the leading American scientist of that day and the authority on electricity.[8,9] His studies made him immensely famous, a member of the important learned societies in Europe, and the best known American by Europeans. He also invented the Franklin Stove (This was the first stove—also called the Pennsylvania fireplace—that made a cold room warm and comfortable and free from smoke.[1]), a rolling press for making copies of letters, an artificial hand and arm for placing books on high shelves, bifocal eyeglasses, the water-glass harmonica, and a flexible urinary catheter made of silver. His contributions to medicine were many.[10–18] In 1759 at age 54 he received 2 honorary doctorate degrees (St. Andrews and Oxford) and thereafter he was called "Doctor Franklin."

In 1757 (age 52), Franklin was appointed agent to England from the Pennsylvania Colony (later also from 3 other colonies), and he returned to North America only once until 1775 (age 70). His wife, who refused to cross the Atlantic, died in 1774 at age 69. He was well equipped to be America's "agent" to London (or later to Paris). As Postmaster General, Franklin read most newspapers in the colonies and he had visited most post offices so he knew America well. Franklin was one of the early backers of independence for the American colonies. Upon returning from England, he headed the delegation from the Pennsylvania Colony to the Congress which wrote the Declaration of Independence (1776). Later that year he was elected Commissioner to France to seek their support for the American side during the Revolutionary War. He did not return to North America until 1785. In 1787 he was a delegate to the Constitutional Convention.[19] Three years later, at age 85, he died.

In France, Franklin was regarded as a friend of humankind. John Adams said he was better known than Frederick the Great or Voltaire. His phrase *ca ira*—it will all come right in the end—became the song of the French Revolution. He was full of witticisms, jokes, memories, knowledge and keen observations, and these, with his charity and gentleness, made him a charming and available social asset. He was represented in France in busts and prints, in statuettes, on snuffboxes, on rings, and in miniatures, on handkerchiefs and dishes, and in medallions. All these images showed him as patriarchal, old and wise, and his face became as familiar as that of the moon.[2]

Poor Richard's Almanack, like other almanacs of the time, contained calendars and road-books with lists of places to stay and descriptions of the highways, the names of British kings and rulers of Europe, dates of eclipses, days for courts and fairs, a chronicle of "remarkable things," prognostications about the weather, recipes, jokes, maxims and cautionary rhymes.[2] Peddlers carried them in their packs with needles and pins and china bowls, worsted stockings, gloves and looking glasses. They were strung on a stick and hung by the fireplace, often with records of the family written in for many years. They were sometimes paid for in wheat and potatoes, a handful of nails or a bottle of rum.

The maxims of *Poor Richard's Almanack* were not all Franklin's own. They were, he said, "the wisdom of many ages and nations," and he borrowed them freely from Dryden, Pope, La Rochefoucauld and Rabelais, changing the words, reworking them, and including popular adages.[2] His rule for writing, he once said, was to be "smooth, clear, and short." His sayings soon passed into everyday speech and were quoted in sermons, on title pages of pamphlets, or as mottoes in newspapers. In the twenty-fifth almanac in 1758—the last one—Franklin presented "Father Abraham's Speech" or "The Way to Wealth" composed of a string of adages from previous almanacs. Most colonists, Franklin said, were "middling people" who were obliged to work and save to prosper and survive, and the popularity of the proverbs was due to this fact. They also were immensely popular in Europe.

In 1990, 200 years after Franklin's death, Peter Baida[20] pointed out that Franklin was the first writer of success literature. In all his work, Franklin talked about character as the source of success, citing industry, frugality, sobriety, honesty, perseverance, loyalty and reliability. Both his autobiography and the maxims in *Poor Richard's Almanack* have exerted a considerable influence for over 200 years. We can all profit from Franklin's ideas of success, whether in business or in health. The remainder of this piece lists some of Poor Richard's comments on physicians, medical wisdom, medical advice, eating, foods, alcohol and heart:

PHYSICIANS

He's a Fool that makes his Doctor his Heir.

Beware of the young Doctor & the old Barber.

God heals, and the Doctor takes the Fees.

He's the best physician that knows the worthlessness of the most medicines.

Don't misinform your Doctor nor your Lawyer.

It is ill Jesting with the Joiner's Tools, worse with the Doctor's.

MEDICAL WISDOM

Early to bed, and early to rise, makes a Man healthy, wealthy and wise.

A good Wife & Health, is a Man's best Wealth.

A good Man is seldom uneasy, an ill one never easie.

The Tongue is ever turning to the aching Tooth.

An ill Wound, but not an ill Name, may be healed.

Love, Cough, & a Smoke, can't well be hid.

Changing Countries or Beds, cures neither a bad Manager, nor a Fever.

Pride and the Gout, are seldom cur'd throughout.

We are not so sensible of the greatest Health as of the least Sickness.

If thou dost ill, the joy fades, not the pains; If well, the pain doth fade, the joy remains.

Pain wastes the Body, Pleasures the Understanding.

A long Life may not be good enough, but a good Life is long enough.

Watch the disease in time: For when, within The dropsy rages, and extends the skin, In vain for helebore the patient cries, And sees the doctor, but too late is wise: Too late for cure, he proffers half his wealth; Ten thousand doctors cannot give him health.

Death takes no bribes.

MEDICAL ADVICE

Would you live with ease, Do what you ought, and not what you please.

Keep your mouth wet, feet dry.

Hot things, sharp things, sweet things, cold things All rot the teeth, and make them look like old things.

Be temperate in wine, in eating, girls, & sloth; Or the Gout will seize you and plague you both.

Be not sick too late, nor well too soon.

He that can take rest is greater than he that can take cities.

Don't go to the doctor with every distemper, nor to the lawyer with every quarrel, nor to the pot for every thirst.

To Friend, Lawyer, Doctor, tell plain your whole Case. . . .

Time is an herb that cures all Diseases.

EATING

Eat to live, and not live to eat.

To lengthen thy Life, lessen thy Meals.

Three good meals a day is bad living.

Eat few Suppers, and you'll need few Medicines.

Dine with little, sup with less: Do better still; sleep supperless.

Sleep without Supping, and you'll rise without owing for it.

He that lives carnally, won't live eternally.

Many dishes many diseases, Many medicines few cures.

I saw few die of Hunger, of Eating 100000.

A full Belly is the Mother of all Evil.

A full Belly makes a dull Brain: The Muses starve in a Cook's Shop.

Hold your Council before Dinner; the full Belly hates Thinking as well as Acting.

If it were not for the Belly, the Back might wear Gold.

No wonder Tom grows fat, th' unwiedly Sinner, Makes his whole Life but one continual Dinner.

9 Men in 10 are suicides.

He that never eats too much, will never by lazy.

Hunger is the best Pickle.

Too much plenty makes Mouth dainty.

Where there is Hunger, Law is not regarded; and where Law is not regarded, there will be Hunger.

He that would travel much, should eat little.

Fools make feasts and wise men eat them.

A fat kitchin, a lean Will.

Give me yesterday's Bread, this Day's Flesh, and last Year's Cyder.

Many a Meal is lost for want of meat.

Eat to please thyself, but dress to please others.

How happy is he, who can satisfy his hunger with any food, quench his thirst with any drink, please his ear with any musick, delight his eye with any painting, any sculpture, any architecture, and divert his mind with any book or any company! How many mortifications must he suffer, that cannot bear anything but beauty, order, elegance & perfection! *Your man of taste, is nothing but a man of distaste.*

On the 18th of this month, anno 1546 died that famous reformer, LUTHER: who struck the great blow to papal tyranny in Europe. He was remarkably temperate in meat and drink, sometimes fasting four days together; and at other times, for many days eating only a little bread and a herring. Cicero says, There was never any great man who was not an industrious man; to which may, perhaps, be added, There was never any industrious man who was not a temperate man: For intemperance in diet, abates the vigour and dulls the action both of the mind and body.

. . . eat for Necessity, not Pleasure, for Lust knows not where Necessity ends. . . .

If thou art dull and heavy after Meat, it's a sign thou hast exceeded the due Measure; for Meat and Drink ought to refresh the Body, and make it cheerful, and not to dull and oppress it. . . .

Keep out of the Sight of Feasts and Banquets as much as may be; for 'tis more difficult to refrain good Cheer, when it's present, than from the Desire of it when it is away. . . .

If a Man casually exceeds, let him fast the next Meal, and all may be well again, provided it be not too often done; as if he exceed at Dinner, let him refrain a Supper, . . .

A temperate Diet frees from Diseases; such are seldom ill, but if they are surprised with Sickness, they bear it better, and recover sooner . . .

Use now and then a little Exercise a quarter of an Hour before Meals, as to swing a Weight, or swing your Arms about with a small Weight in each Hand; to leap, or the like, for that stirs the Muscles of the Breast.

A temperate Diet arms the body against all external Accidents; so that they are not so easily hurt by Heat, Cold or Labour; if they at any time should be prejudiced, they are more easily cured, either of Wounds, Dislocations or Bruises.

But when malignant Fevers are rife in the Country or City where thou dwelst, 'tis adviseable to eat and drink more freely, by Way of Prevention; for those are Diseases that are not caused by Repletion, and seldom attack Full-feeders. . . .

FOODS

Much Virtue in Herbs, little in Men.

When you taste Honey, remember Gall.

Cheese and salt meat, should be sparingly eat.

The misers cheese is wholesomest.

After Fish, Milk do not wish.

An Egg to day is better than a Hen to-morrow.

Pray don't burn my House to roast your Eggs.

Onions can make ev'n Heirs and Widows weep.

ALCOHOL

There's more old Drunkards than old Doctors.

Nothing more like a Fool, than a drunken Man.

Life with Fools consists in Drinking . . .

He that drinks fast, pays slow.

Poor Dick, eats like a well man, and drinks like a sick.

Against Diseases here, the strongest Fence, Is the defensive Virtue, Abstinence.

He that drinks his Cyder alone, let him catch his Horse alone.

He that spills the Rum, loses that only; He that drinks it, often loses both that and himself.

When the Wine enters, out goes the Truth.

Take counsel in wine, but resolve afterwards in water.

Drink Water, Put the Money in your Pocket, and leave the Dry-bellyach in the Punchbowl.

HEART

Light purse heavy heart.

The heart of a fool is in his mouth, but the mouth of a wise man is in his heart.

When Man and Woman die, as Poets sung, His Heart's the last part moves, her last, the tongue.

Great Beauty, great strength, & great Riches, are really & truly of no great Use; a right Heart exceeds all.

William C. Roberts

William Clifford Roberts, MD
Editor in Chief

1. Roberts SR. Benjamin Franklin, Patron of Medicine, *Ann Clin Med* 1925;3:501–507.

2. Brooks VW (writer of introduction) and Rockwell N (artist of illustrations). Poor Richard: The Almanacks for the Years 1733–1758. New York: Bonanza Books 1979:300.

3. Leo Lemay JA, editor, Benjamin Franklin's Writings, New York: The Library of America, 1987:1605.

4. Van Doren C. Benjamin Franklin. New York: The Viking Press, 1938:845.

5. Morgan ES. Secrets of Benjamin Franklin. *The New York Review* 1991 (January 31);38:41–46.

6.Malcolm RL. Benjamin Franklin and the founding of Pennsylvania Hospital. *J Michigan State Med Soc* 1931;30:525–532.

7. Hunter RJ. Benjamin Franklin and the rise of free treatment of the poor by the medical profession of Philadelphia. *Bull History Med* 1957;31:137–146.

8. Mitchell SW. Pioneers of science in America: Benjamin Franklin. *Popular Science Monthly* 1907;10:291–292.

9. Cohen IB, editor. Benjamin Franklin's Experiments. Cambridge, MA:Harvard University Press, 1941:273.

10. Cushing HK. Notes suggested by the Franklin-Heberden pamphlet of 1759. *Johns Hopkins Hospital Bulletin* 1904;15:276–285.

11. Cumston CG. Benjamin Franklin from the medical viewpoint. *New York Med J* 1909;89:3–12.

12. Diller T. The writings of Benjamin Franklin pertaining to medicine and the medical profession. *The Aesculapian* 1909;1:65–84 and 156–197.

13. Diller T. Ben Franklin's views [on alcohol]. *JAMA* 1915;65:189–191.

14. McKenzie RT. Benjamin Franklin. Illustrious pioneer in physical education. *J Health Phys Educ* 1936;7:67–71.

15. Wright RD. Benjamin Franklin. *JAMA* 1939;112:2224–2228.

16. Willius FA, Keys TE. The medical history of Benjamin Franklin (1706–1790). I and II. *Proc Staff Meet Mayo Clinic* 1942;17:391–397,410–416.

17. Vincent EH. "Poor Richard." *Surg Gynecol Obstet* 1952;94:630–634.

18. Pepper W. The Medical Side of Benjamin Franklin. New York: Argosy-Antiquarian Ltd 1970:137.

19. Bowen CD. Miracle at Philadelphia. The Story of the Constitutional Convention May to September 1787. Boston: Little, Brown and Company, 1966:346.

20. Baida P. Poor Richard's Legacy. American Business Values from Benjamin Franklin to Donald Trump. New York: William Morrow and Company, 1990:360.

A Son's Book on His Father's Father

I guess that one must be careful in trying to review a book on one's father written by one's son. I'm proud of both of them, however, and since I did not take part in the writing of the book or the choosing of my father, maybe a few comments on each are not inappropriate.

My father, Stewart Ralph Roberts (SRR), was born October 2, 1878, only 13 years after the end of the Civil War, in Oxford, Georgia, a small college town about 40 miles from Atlanta. SRR's grandfather, a member of the Confederate Army, died in 1861, and 4 years later SRR's father, at age 13, watched from a basement window as Sherman's soldiers marched down his street in Atlanta. Shortly afterward, SRR's father was adopted by a family with 6 children in Oxford. In 1877 SRR's father married one of the 5 daughters in that family and the same year graduated with first honors from Emory College in Oxford. He became a minister and later was president of a women's college.

SRR was the first of 5 children. In 1900, he graduated from the Atlanta College of Physicians and Surgeons and then returned to Emory College in Oxford where, like his father, he graduated with first honors in 1902 and also delivered the Valedictory Address. He then went to The University of Chicago, Department of Zoology, where he received a Master of Science degree in 1904. His dissertation was entitled "A Comparison of the Cervical and Brachial Plexuses in Certain Reptiles." In 1905 he settled in Atlanta where he remained until his death on April 14, 1941, at the age of 61.

During those last 36 years he practiced internal medicine with a focus in the last 20 years on heart disease; he taught medicine to hundreds of students, house officers, and colleagues, serving as Professor of Clinical Medicine at Emory University School of Medicine from 1915 to 1941; he read much and wrote much, publishing 100 medical articles including a book on pellagra (1912); he served his medical societies as President of the Fulton County Medical Society (Atlanta, 1915), of the Southern Medical Association (1925), and of the American Heart Association (1933–1934); he lectured on medicine to many audiences in many cities; he fathered 3 boys (the 2 healthy ones became physicians) and he vigorously supported his family, his friends, his institutions, his hospital, his region, and his country.

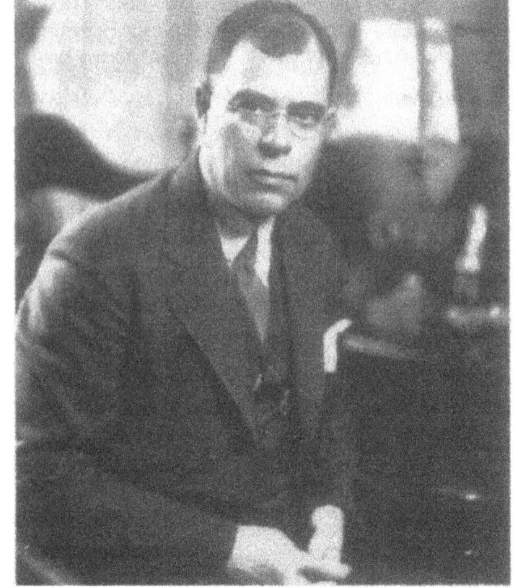

Stewart R. Roberts, MD, at age 53 years in 1932.

The book[1] entitled *Life and Writings of Stewart R. Roberts, M.D., Georgia's First Heart Specialist* was written by my son, Charles Stewart Roberts, M.D., presently a fellow in cardiothoracic surgery at the University of North Carolina, Chapel Hill. In addition to the description of SRR's life with accompanying photographs, Chuck reproduced 310 passages from SRR's writings and 137 of them are presented in the remainder of this piece.

LIFE AND HUMAN NATURE

The value of a man's life depends upon his contribution to his day and generation. To do the day's work with a poise that admits of no yesterday and no tomorrow, no surprise and no disappointment, no regret and no preference,—just the work of today; a little play, a little love, a little worship,—these make up the joy of living.[2]

•

Modern life is so intense and striving, the struggle for existence so sharp, human rivalry and jealousy so frequent, social relations so delicate, domestic relations so often conductive to emotional strain and temperamental friction, life so changed from the jog trot gait of forty years ago, and the same nervous system to bear it and the mind to manage one's relations to it all. Motion is an elementary quality of matter impossible to define and American life is nearly all motion, very little of stasis or meditation or relaxation. We know how to rush but we know little of how to rest.[3]

•

We hear much of one's duty to make a living, but it is far more one's duty to make a life,—and a well rounded life at that, which includes the cultivation of the financial, the physical, the cultural, the spiritual and the mental.[4]

•

When one remembers how great a thing is knowledge, greater than space or time, greater than woman unless her price be above rubies, greater than a king unless he be first of all a man. Socrates and Solomon knew it, and every pioneer mind that has thrown any of his life sincerely into school or university to touch the higher things offered, he too knew how great a thing is knowledge. It is that that makes libraries and classes and graduations. Every empty mind knows it. Every private soldier in the ranks is silent before the far seeing eye of him who wears the star and issues the orders. He is a private because he lacks the knowledge to command, the knowledge that gives power.[5]

There is more of doing nothing than of doing anything else in the world. For the price, one selects the best coat, picks it out with energy. One's time is much more valuable than a mere coat. There are many coats but one's mind shall not pass this way again. One's leisure is far more important and dangerous for that matter than the time one spends at his work. What one does at his work depends on his gifts or lack of them, on his leanness or fulness of training, on his energy and enthusiasm, on his strength and endurance. But what he does with his leisure, that is what kind of man he is, that labels him truly with the signs of that group to which he belongs, and gives promise of whether there be in him hope of development or power of greater gifts.[5]

•

Great lives are apt to be quiet lives; hurried lives are worried lives.[6]

•

Old ideas died because better ideas became true and active. It holds for all civilization whether it be Church or State, machines or farming or business, profession or society. Socrates talked to Plato and Jesus to Peter face to face. The Indians talked with distant moving objects and smoke, Morse with his telegraph wire, Bell with his telephone wire, Marconi with his wireless, and television now sends pictures. Talk has grown from face to face to next to nothing though heard around the world.[7]

•

Loyalty is a beautiful word. It appeals to the royal in human nature. Its foundation stone is honesty; stones of truth, courage and character follow as the monument of the single life rises; and Loyalty and Love are the highest, pointing stones. What differences exist between Love and Loyalty I do not know; they are so closely related. Men judge each other more by their Honesty and their Loyalty than in any other way.[8]

•

Jealousy is probably the most ruining and devastating of human qualities for the personality and for the happiness of those around. The jealousy of those in power certainly spurred Judas Iscariot to the triumph of his betrayal kiss and the avarice for his silver. He could live neither with his Disloyalty nor with the Weight of his silver, and he hung himself to get rid of both. Disloyalty and Ingratitude differ in degree only, and both are incompatible with Loyalty. They are the snakes of the soul, and we should avoid them as quickly and as accurately as we do snakes on the ground. We are all unworthy of these soul snakes. Even those on the ground are far preferable. Loyalty in its deepest sense runs out all snakes of the spirit.[8]

PEOPLE

Caesar seemed to have lost all of his friends, at the critical moment but Mark Antony, and he was absent. Job had his three friends and they consistently gave him the wrong advice. Even his wife advised him to "curse God and die." It is doubtful if Napoleon had intimate friends in the usual acceptance of the term. Lee and Lincoln had great numbers. Wells claimed only five in all his life. This five-fold friendship was the rare joy of his lonely life, and has conferred a degree of fame and tenderness on his friends, and through his short memoir there runs the recurring strain of intimate association with each of them.[6]

•

By fate or an unfortunate conjunction of circumstances I have never seen this man Osler. I have studied his methods from his students.[9]

•

I know he has always been the wise friend of my clinical life, the unseen consultant with my patients, the Abou Ben Adam of my spirit (Osler).[10]

•

He wrote more than six hundred medical papers, the premier textbook of medicine in the English tongue, edited an encyclopedia of medicine, was the world's choicest medical bibliophile, and was ranked as the world's premier teacher of internal medicine. He was clinical observer, research student, world citizen and moulder of better thinking and nobler living, and yet his own estimation of himself was expressed in the simple words, "If I am anything, I am a clinician" (Osler).[11]

•

There is more in the man than in the land. Beaumont used his mind in an Indian fort, Sims on a cotton plantation and McDowell in a country village.[12]

•

Two hundred and fourteen years after Columbus discovered America, and seventy before the Declaration of Independence, there was born in the bleak Boston of the early eighteenth century a boy by the name of Benjamin Franklin. An increasing glamor gathering about his name and the drama of his life make him the first great American.[13]

•

It seems rather strange that he was not a public speaker. He relied rather on the facility of his pen, the soundness of his opinions and the magnetism of his private conversation. Jefferson declared that he never heard either Washington or Franklin speak as long as ten minutes on any subject, but always to the point (Franklin).[13]

•

His patronage of medicine includes three lines of activity: (1) his research work and inventions; (2) his medical observations and scientific papers; and (3) his medical friendships. And yet these do not accent sufficiently his wide interest and enthusiasm for the profession (Franklin).[13]

•

He was an intellectual with an almost impermeable personality to the common run of men. His great mind and his genius for research carried him beyond the clinical into the realm of physics and chemistry. He was a great physician without patients, a great scientist without a university to nurture him, and a great soul without tact. Had there been in him a quick and surprising touch of humor and some real rubber in his disposition, he might have reached to the heights of a Newton or a Darwin or a Sydenham (Wells).[6]

•

Then came the Civil War. This six-year-old child sat in the open window of the Old Armory at Charleston and saw Beauregard open on Fort Sumter and said, "Mother, isn't it solemn?" It became more solemn later and it has been solemn to the Nation ever since. The Northern father became Brigadier-General Gorgas, Chief Ordinance Officer of the Confederacy, stationed at Richmond. His eldest son saw the pomp and felt the poverty of war, went with his little hand in his father's to see the dead Stonewall Jackson lying in state in the Virginia Capitol, sat on the knee of General Lee on one of his visits to Richmond, heard the guns at Yellow Tavern that cost the Confederacy the life of General Stuart, saw the smoke from the battles of the Wilderness, was in Richmond when it was shelled and burned, and turned up in Baltimore after Appomatox with his mother and the five younger children, "a ragged, barefoot little rebel with empty pockets and an empty stomach" (Gorgas).[14]

•

The problem before him was this: Panama was unhealthy because of an excessive rainfall, much fresh water and a continual warm temperature and in these conditions mosquitoes breed the year round. Introduce into such an environment the non-immune white race, and yellow fever and malignant malaria are the natural results. These two diseases with plague, amebic dysentery, hookworm disease, and beriberi formed the six chief tropical diseases (Gorgas).[14]

•

It is difficult to separate a great man from his labors and to view him as a personality. Gorgas was a great man and he had a personality of distinct quality. His great mind worked simply by the obliteration of details and the vision of the main road. He was neither a great clinician nor a great laboratory worker, but he was the outstanding sanitarian of all time.[14]

•

Mere words spoken of him are as empty as echoes, for veneration is the requiem of his sleep (Washington).[14]

•

But he left us a legacy of character that we can never outgrow. Were he among us today he would bring to the problems of this new time that clarity of thought which he brought to those of his own day; that self-discipline which would prevent his mind being clouded by passion; that sense of justice for all; that desire that his country should be honorable and honored; that honesty and integrity which colored every act; and above all that utter disregard of every thought of self when the call came for service to his fellow men (Washington).[14]

•

That vast soul, triply opposed to war, to slavery, and to secession, stepped outside the path of human progress in his loyalty to his native state, and went home the only defeated general in human history a defeated people cheered. Ranked in war with Caesar, Hannibal and Napoleon, his mastery of himself was above his mastery of war (Lee).[14]

•

Frail of body and fierce in the flame of his ideal, careless of human friendship and careful of human destiny, he woke the dull, slumbering peoples of the earth to the realization that organized peace on earth among the nations is no idle dream (Wilson).[14]

•

A dreamer, awkward and tender, gentle even in the severities of life, he put the poetry of his soul into prose and the Gettysburg address is the anthem of the Nation (Lincoln).[14]

•

One of president Von Hindenburg's associates noted day after day the amazing and placid nervous system of the old General, and asked,

"What do you do when you are nervous?"

"I whistle."

"But I have never heard you whistle."

"I never whistle."[6]

•

James Mackenzie relates that during his medical course at Edinburgh one of his teachers sent for him and told him he was a dunce. The boy had a great mind with great reasoning powers and a relatively poor memory. In the present day medical school in America he would probably meet an academic mortality by the close of the first semester.[15]

•

And yet since Galen had appeared in medicine no outstanding figure who was born with energy, gifted with personality, blessed with blood and family, of wide education and culture, powerful with the beauty, accuracy, and execution of his work, resentful of authority, forceful enough to issue his work, provided it conformed to the proof of nature, against all the organized beliefs, customs, and traditions of his art, medicine; of the jealousies of his colleagues; of the authority and dogma of his church; of the power to give and to take and to bind of his state. This man appeared in the person of one Andrew Wesel, called (in Latin) Andreas Vesalius; of whom Senac said he discovered a new world before he was twenty-eight; and of whom Garrison said, "the most commanding figure in European medicine after Galen, and before Harvey."[16]

•

The good start he had from a medical and famous family, the bent to dissection even as a boy, the hard study and classical training at Louvain, Paris, and Padua had borne fruit in this full Professorship. We can imagine with what a shaking of heads and surprise the youthful genius was received. He started as a full professor. Genius knows no grades of lesser promotions. It is either genius, or if compared with genius, something mediocre (Vesalius).[16]

•

Vesalius made medicine a free science, the medical mind a free mind, the medical world a free world. He showed how a genius who concentrated could work. He had sat at the feet of many Gamaliels before students sat at his feet. He shows what training will do for the medical mind. Familiar with the classics, he added German and French, Italian, Hebrew, and Arabic, made the body the true Bible of anatomy, foreshadowed embryology and physiology and added to the training of every medical student since his day. What might he not have done for medicine had he not burned his notes and papers and quit his studies at 28? He was young and sensitive, but even a genius cannot get mad and destroy his papers and notes. The gods destroy those who first get mad. And then his success as a court physician was but the natural result of his general culture, his training in anatomy, and an illustration of how intensive training in any one branch of medicine may make one an improved clinician. Poise, analysis, and proportion are choice traits of the clinical mind.[16]

•

Few of us can stand very much mortality. Marion Sims lost his first two patients, two babies, and went from South Carolina across Georgia to the woods of Alabama, to escape his failures.[6]

GEORGIA

One is not without honor save in his own country and among his own people, and one also may be neglectful of his own state, so that his own state is without honor among its own people. One of my distinguished medical friends this morning said that if he had had charge of his borning, he would have been born in one of the old families of Virginia; I believe he thought he would prefer to have been born in the valley of the Shenandoah; but if I had had my borning in my own hands, I would have been born, as I was, in Georgia.[17]

•

And then sometimes the layman forgets that the Bible is not a scientific text-book, but a spiritual guide, and in his thoughtless devotion to a divine religion fails to realize that "it is futile to attempt to curb science, and that the Bible does not need to be bolstered up by legislation." There is room for a minister and a doctor and a teacher under every roof that the things of the spirit and the things of the body and the things of the mind may keep step. What we need in Georgia is to get away from the domination of cotton and politics, from the negation of ignorance and intolerance, that the mind of Georgia may have a new birth of freedom and a real practical vision of science and service.[18]

•

If one walks through one of the older cemeteries, as the Colonial Cemetery in Savannah, which dates back to the time shortly after Oglethorpe came, the early average age of the dead is around 25 years, which is not only surprising but in the light of modern medicine is a real waste of life.[4]

•

In all these problems dealing with public health we return ever and again to the center of the circle and there alternate with the apparently ever present conditions of apathy and poverty. Apathy, which is the world and the lack of interest and sometimes ignorance and custom and tradition and the inherent abhorrence to change. Apathy is neither laziness nor ignorance but both and more. Conservatism is too often a polite name for being in a rut, worn too deep by habit to see over the edges into the promised land of progress. Then, the other enemy, poverty, either real, acquired, or imagined. Is there any reason for poverty? Is not poverty a plastered and passing excuse for laziness and ignorance and individual or civic inertia? How many farmers in Georgia read? It is said that only 10 per cent read even about farming. How many of them work the year round? It is estimated the average farmer does not work more than three months during the year. Are these merely sayings or are these facts? We have talked so long in Georgia of the boll weevil, of poverty and hard times that as a state are we becoming anesthetized and immunized to progress?[4]

EMORY UNIVERSITY

Funds left to a University are safer and of more lasting value and influence than to any other institution. What greater opportunity than for men and women with ample financial reserve to send a youth every year through the University. One can live in the youth he educates as well as in his own children or in his writings.[19]

•

It is the friction of bright minds that causes the spark of truth to scintillate and civilization to advance. There can be no advance unless there be freedom of the mind. The mind of the ancient Greeks and the mind of the Elizabethan English were free to roam in search of truth and beauty, and what a harvest. The mind that lends itself to invention and research necessarily wanders free. The University stands for this freedom.[19]

•

Remember that a university is the most permanent of all earthly institutions. Oxford and Cambridge are the oldest corporations in England, that most stable of countries. Harvard, Yale, and Columbia are older than the Government of the United States. The University of Vienna was far older than Emory is today long before Columbus discovered America. Banks merge, fail and liquidate, churches unite and dismantle, only one business in twenty lives long enough to reach lasting success, governments change their form and cease to exist, but the university outlasts them all. Let the University do the day's work and all will be well. Let us think about the University in terms of decades and centuries and not in terms of days and weeks.[19]

•

I remember even the color of the books I studied at Emory. Virgil was bound in green, Economics in brown. The words of my teachers still live. Emory gave me within a cool and gentle fountain of unforgettable and pleasant things. One should stand by Emory.[8]

•

I like to think, too, that we are growing some ivy here on the Campus. I want its roots to reach deep into the old red clay of Georgia, its climbing tendrils to take clutching hold on the Georgia marble of the buildings, the rich dark green of its leaves to soften every outline, and then at last for the fresh lighter green of its tips to peep timidly over the edge of the red tiled roofs to the blue of a Georgia sky.[19]

MEDICAL PHILOSOPHY

Sometimes the stress of nearness to his race, the fangs of pain, the despotism of death, make one year seem two years, a decade a score, and life a century of breathing.[20]

•

With the spirit of hospitality there is unconsciously developed tone; what in physical diagnosis is called pitch; in college, spirit; in battle, the *esprit de corps*. It made the little French Lieutenant at Mons shine his sabre and don his white gloves for the charge; and later dead, with his red blood across his white glove, what mattered it—was he not a Lieutenant in the French Army, an officer of Joffre? This same tone made Lee wear a new and full-dress uniform of the Commanding General when he met Grant in surrender at Appomattox.[21]

In regard to Dr. Davis' patient, when a patient presents himself and begins to dictate what food he shall eat, what rest he shall take, what medicine he shall take, I think perhaps the best thing the medical man can do in this instance is to resign before he begins, because I think with two doctors on the case, one of them being the patient, is one too many doctors. I do not think one is justified in taking on such a case, because he would neither be thanked for it, nor be paid for it, nor do any good to the patient.[22]

•

Men will stand nearly everything in their colleagues but laziness. There must be efficiency and not one whit of slackness, indifference or carelessness or a failure to use one's personal gifts and put over one's personal part of the work to the limit of one's ability; the using of one's gifts, the hypnotizing of obstacles, the initiative that develops energy and envelopes accomplishment.[23]

•

In medicine if one makes training, service and efficiency his triple aim, his financial reward is certain. Only this: the financial reward must not be the primary aim and ambition; otherwise, in the long run money is above medicine and as Osler wrote, "the patient becomes a chattel and a mortgage."[23]

•

No official notice is taken of the fitness or unfitness of personality among medical students; it is only a question of class standing, whereas in life it is the Person who is a Doctor who attracts patients. Hence it is that a young man must take stock of himself, for what doth it profit a man to spend and toil and hope if a petty vice, discourtesy to custom or carelessness in the careful ways of life mar his mastery over men and medicine? Personality is the insistent force in medicine, and its possession and cultivation assures power and service.[12]

•

Can he tell in good English and with good address what happened on the ward? Are his enunciation and pronunciation good or is he all modulation? Does he mumble his paper or discussion or does he take a verbal stance and drive to the point?[12]

•

He either spiritualizes and ennobles his medicine, or materializes and coins it. Medicine and mammon are usually incompatible.[12]

•

Wherever two or more are gathered together in the name of a patient, a medical society is in session, and the friction of bright minds causes the spark of truth to scintillate to the benefit of the patient and the learning of medicine.[24]

•

Interpretation permitted Hippocrates to write his Aphorisms, Galen his text-book that lasted 1500 years, made Osler what he was, is the keen secret of English medicine, the ranking factor in the service of every clinician and clinical institution and in reality is but a clinical vision, which joins the science with the art. Any man can see a lot of facts, but fortunate indeed is the man who knows an important fact when he sees it, and gifted is he who can interpret the many facts about one patient.[25]

Those students and scholars of medicine in whom burns the insatiate lure for more and more knowledge of their art are the pearls of great price to the Hospital. What John B. Murphy meant to the Mercy Hospital in Chicago, what Crile meant to the Lakeside Hospital in Cleveland, and what Osler meant to the Johns Hopkins Hospital—we hope more than one man will mean to the Wesley.[26]

•

The study of the combination of qualities that makes a great clinician is interesting. Man unwell is the problem of clinical medicine, the clinician is the artist, and clinistry the science and art. It is a science of fact and probability and an art of tact and experience.[10]

•

We are more than doctors of the body and the clergy has no monopoly on things of the spirit. Our patients may be in body protoplasm like a worm of the dust, but in mood and manner they are "created a little lower than the Angels." The larger diagnosis considers the whole of man and ministers to his every need, remembering that the ideal is

"The flawless symmetry of man,
The poise of heart and mind."[25]

•

I often wondered when I really knew what I thought I knew. The patient's condition at times was like a bulb that one had planted the previous autumn. Spring was here and the first shoots were green above ground, but the name had been forgotten. As soon as the flower came, we could tell its name and all about it. I learned to wait until nature unfolded the case after I had done all I could to hurry the unfolding along. Great old nature was my best friend, and the patient's, too.[6]

•

I had to watch my tongue. It functioned more easily than my mind. I had to learn not always to talk about what I was talking about. I learned too, that when a patient or his family were irritated, he and they were not always mad about what he thought he was mad about. On such occasions the less I said, the more quickly the unpleasantness was over and the better they liked me, later. Woe came to me when I did my thinking aloud. It would not do to say that it might be this and it might be that. The patient was entitled to my conclusions, not to my psychic mechanisms.[6]

•

No man ever made very many clinical mistakes by keeping his clinical mouth under cautious control. Patients have a way of remembering what the doctor said long after he has forgotten it.[6]

•

The human touch of the clinical artist in the sick-room is usually proportionate to the human experience of the artist outside the sick-room.[6]

•

A man of sixty goes to his physician. What did he bring? A great deal more than a body born sixty years ago.[6]

•

The prizes go not always to him who climbs the fastest or has the better mind, but to the patience endured of many patients, the lesson learned of many lives. Let him read and interview many distant minds; he will see Shakespeare in his patients and his patients in Shakespeare, and the Proverbs of Solomon illustrate their wisdom and folly.[6]

•

Primarily I am an artist, and mainly a scientist for my art's sake. I acquire my science by study and experiment and my art by experience. My field is the life of my patient from body to mind, and into my patients' lives do I enter. I am a scientist and more, I am an artist.[11]

•

The whole man is your problem. However much technique is necessary, it is but a part of the clinical life. The super-technician and nothing more is one of the banes of our profession.[11]

•

You will quickly learn to get to a patient and perhaps never learn to get away from some of them. It is an art in itself.[11]

•

Keep close to a microscope. Look through it once a day at something. It promotes accuracy and prevents your clinical mind taking too many theoretical and vertical ascents. Do not expect too much of the microscope or even of the laboratory. Do some thinking yourself. Spend less money for an automobile and more for a microscope.[11]

•

Stay in your class and select the best class. Capitulate to no clique, faction or political group. When you join the herd you run with it. Courtesy does not mean the surrender of your own individuality. Keep step with progress, otherwise unfeeling engine that she is, she will step on you and crush you. Imitate the great and not the small. Never argue. That function is one of the vocal attributes of the politician, the lawyer, and the hair-splitting theologian. Never fuss. At such temptations the greatest argument is silence.[11]

•

An Ideal of Modern Medicine

Whenever and wherever my work, by day or night, in peace or war, on land or sea, in laboratory or office, home or hospital, classroom or open field, may I be patient, poised, and thorough; loyal to science and to men, unselfish in labor and pure in life. May I hold that science is better than gold, and men than greed, that service is proportionate to preparation, and reward to labor. May I use drugs only when indicated, diagnose before I treat or operate, clean before I deliver, use my laboratory, preserve a sense of proportion, respect but not worship my own opinion, seek consultation often, be slow to judgment and cautious in word and deed, and mingle in mind and touch with medical men. In the laboratory may I keep my records, in clinical cases my histories, and between them and me preserve the accuracy of truth. May I be strong with the weak, righteous with the wicked, wise with the foolish, honest with myself and kind to all men. May I avoid professional comparisons and sensitiveness, speak well of those of the household of medical faith, shun jealousy and eschew envy, follow progress, beware lest the demands of life chill my enthusiasm for study and knowledge, play sometimes and wander when I may. May I take injustice gracefully, disappointment easily, fight disease cheerfully, death hopefully, believe victory and defeat equally a part of the larger plan, and rise from both fresh for repeated conflicts. May I remember that I am heir to the same diseases as my patients, must meet the same death, pass with them beyond the River, and may I go with a smile.[21,27]

•

The gathered traditions, entrenched customs, and meticulous ethics of the profession are hardly safe unless they meet the social and economic demands of a progressive day. There was an ostrich who hid his head in the sand. The medical profession needs the glare of publicity and the glow of dignified advertising, that its problems, trials, and triumphs as well as its service may be known of all men. The best way to rid civilization of quacks and incompetents is to tell of the service of the competents.[28]

•

Medicine is of greatest value when it prevents or cures sickness in all the people within their economic ability to pay promptly. The doctor can best serve at lowest cost in an atmosphere of professional life, liberty, and competition peculiar to his own people. Therefore, write first these things: Preserve his private status, encompass him with no entangling government control of private practice, avoid the strings of the bureau of authority that would come between him and the patient, do nothing by law or force that would lessen his initiative, blur his enthusiasm for his art, or reduce him to a clinical cog in a medical machine. Write these things at the top—and then under them write the newer things demanded by a newer time, and he will be first on the field for service, prevention, and cure.[28]

•

The panic has irrigated our social concepts and made our social relations grow and assume a greater importance. Social relations are mutual relations. In the Declaration of Independence Jefferson wrote "of certain inalienable rights," that "among these are Life, Liberty, and the pursuit of Happiness." "Among these"—but he mentioned but three of them. We are beginning to see others. Many of us believe that economic security for the individual and health security for the individual are also inalienable rights. There is not much liberty without some economic safety and not much happiness without some health, and not much life without both.[7]

•

What does all this mean? It means that the average family in the low income group can no longer pay for adequate medical and dental care on the old fee-for-service basis. It means that any serious illness in the middle classes drains the family income to the uttermost. It means that medical services must compete with every other form of salesmanship known, radios, movies, recreation, automobiles, education, insurance, clothes and food. "Bear ye one another's burdens" is an economic command applied in fire, light, accident, and all other forms of insurance in this country except health insurance. Forty-one countries of the world have such health insurance. Indeed, the United States is the only one of the leading countries in the world without it. There is practically no important opposition to the principles of health insurance in any of these countries. There are efforts to improve the service and change the details but no effort to repeal the law. Health insurance for the low-income classes is a necessity, if they are to receive adequate medical care and if the physicians and dentists who practice for them are to be paid. For this large group of our population, the present situation is a social and economic wilderness.[7]

•

The Negro plowing in the river bottom is as much entitled to adequate medical care as an inalienable right as any of us. The expectant mother in a two-room cabin has an inalienable right to adequate medical care. The opposition to it will be ultimately as helpless as a small canoe in a great storm on the open sea. What is best for everybody is best for medicine. When the time of a great idea and the time of a great social service unite, progress is inevitable and opposition helpless.[7]

MEDICAL RESEARCH AND STATISTICS

Treatment is largely empirical and is based on clinical judgment and clinical results when we face a new disease whose cause we do not know. Added to this therapeutic difficulty is the limited number of cases any of us have seen and the briefness of observation thus far. However, we can all make better progress if a treatment that seems wise is used by different men in different areas, and receives the benefit of their combined trials, criticisms, and suggestions. Therapeutics is still an essential in clinical medicine.[29]

•

No man in medicine today can think with the larger vision and the higher bird's-eye view unless one phase of this thinking is in figures and statistics.[30]

•

The history of medicine is largely the history of the discoveries of this intellect. Witness Sydenham, Harvey, Heberden, Laennec, Louis, Romberg, Erb, Withering, Graves, Trudeau, and Mackenzie with their clinical medicine, Jenner with his vaccination, Hunter, Sims, McDowell, Kocher, the Mayos, Horsley, Halsted, Cushing, Murphy and Crile with their surgery, Virchow with his pathology, Pasteur with his bacteriology, Lister with his asepsis and antisepsis, Koch, Laveran, Schaudinn and Wassermann. Nothing in medicine just happens. Nature guards her secrets and yields them tediously to the toiling thinker.[12]

•

Indeed probability is the real rule of diagnosis and the true guide of the medical life.[25]

•

Of discoveries in medicine, like books, there is no end. Each one is a blessing to man. Each makes the parable of Lazarus or the good Samaritan insignificant in comparison. Each of them is given to the world by the Discoverer. There is neither price nor patent asked, whether it be Koch's discovery of the germ of tuberculosis, Lister's discovery of aseptic surgery, Banting's discovery of insulin for the relief of diabetes, Behring's antitoxin for diphtheria, Jenner's vaccination for smallpox, Pasteur's serum of rabies, the vaccine for typhoid fever, quinine for malaria, serum for meningitis, liver for pernicious anemia. Each discovery is given freely and without restriction for the cure of disease or its prevention. It is a gift from medicine to mankind. Such gifts in their application constitute what Osler called "man's redemption of man."[4]

TEACHING

Many are called and few are chosen, and teachers of medicine are born, not made; they are the wand-bearers and torch-holders to many, and in knowledge and in character, not in riches, they should rank high among their fellows. A clinical teacher will in the future limit his work to his subject; teacher and specialist should be one and the same. These teachers in the future will be poor men, spending themselves during the school year in teaching and practice, and in the summer in travel and ward-walking in other centers. No provincialist can be a great teacher of medicine.[21]

•

In the selection of teachers and faculties much consideration is given to the training and research ability of a man, and but little to his real teaching ability, or his personal power to impart his training and knowledge.[31]

•

Students and teacher are together teachers and student, and their teacher is simply an older student, or in the beautiful word of the Japanese for teacher, *sensi*, one born before, or one who has experience.[31]

•

Briefly the plan was a round table idea for didactic teaching. Each student was given a subject which he studied, handed in as a medical paper, presented the subject orally to the class, and remained the authority on that subject for the year in the class. The sum total of these subjects constituted the outline for the course and the papers with their discussions the course itself. By this method responsibility was thrown upon the student; his ability to think, write, and express himself developed with the gain of his voluntary interest and enthusiasm.[9]

•

The man who just lectures to his students will not accomplish very much. I remember asking a graduate of one of our best schools what he got out of his senior work and he answered: "Well, I don't know." I asked him who he thought his best teachers were, and he mentioned two or three. In reference to the teaching methods of Dr. Osler, this same graduate said that he did not remember everything that Dr. Osler told him, but that he did remember everything Dr. Osler told him *to look up*, and particularly those things that he *looked up* and *reported* to him. A clinic is something more than opportunity to give vent to one's opinions. In the clinical methods that I have outlined I often take time to outline briefly a point, to emphasize an important matter, and to assist the student to distinguish between the essentials and the non-essentials. If the student is on the wrong track, it is promptly shown him. And this method of throwing the burden upon the student seems to reach his understanding better and to leave him better off medically.[9]

•

Certain tendencies are therefore apparent. The teacher tends to over-accent his subject and teach too much. Detail is substituted for perspective and memory for wisdom. The personal relation and development of the student is largely eliminated. Even whole time teachers often do not know the name of their students. "I will ask you that," he says, nodding to a certain student.[15]

•

That section of my mind devoted to medical teaching and medical school experience has long been under three distinct impressions. (1) We are attempting to teach the medical student too much. (2) The academic mortality among freshmen students is too high. (3) The textbooks for the students are too big.[15]

•

In five short years he [Vesalius] revolutionized the teaching of anatomy because he taught from his own dissections on the dead body rather than read from a book. He showed that anatomy was to be learned from dissection and not from a book alone. He popularized dissection and the teaching of science. He made, until recently at least, anatomy the foundation stone in a medical course, introduced laboratory work into medicine and demonstrated what he taught as he taught it. By his work he showed that a teacher must work on the same ground as his students and learn with them. By his example and method of teaching he destroyed forever the authority of Galen, the high platform of his own teacher Sylvius, and more than any other man made Padua the successor of Paris as a medical center and flung far the fame of his subject, his teaching and his university (Vesalius).[16]

READING

To whom I give my mind is very important. He will influence me to a degree and I would be wise in the choice of authors, safe in their thoughts, and secure in their influences.[5]

•

He adds thinking to reading and reading to thinking and comes gradually to the full mind of the mental aristocrat.[5]

•

If you do not read you will be relatively ignorant at fifty and will probably not know it. Everybody else will. Remember the Bible, Shakespeare and his creatures, all of whom are among your patients, some of the Ancients, the jewels in the Harvard Classics, and include Carrel's "Man, the Unknown." Read enough to learn to talk to your patients and not about them. And think a little.[11]

WRITING AND EDITING

We men of the South should go to writing, not words, but real scientific papers; until we do, we shall remain unrecognized. We have a wealth of pathology not possessed by any other region, and we owe it to the world, as well as to ourselves, to put it on paper.[21]

•

Can you read his writing or did the canary step that way from the ink bottle? Can he write good English or is he waiting until he is older to accumulate data and begin to write? The only way to learn how to write is to write.[12]

•

With this Volume 1, Number 1, *The Emory Medical Review* begins its periodic printed life. It will be a welcome visitor to the hand and mind of every Alumnus of the Medical School. For sixty-six years these Alumni have been sent forth as the clinical assets of their Alma Mater, and it is time for the touch of memory to awaken afresh the relations of their student days and kindle anew their interest in the Institution whose growth and power honors them and who in turn with their interest and enthusiasm will honor it. Years of clinical experience and scientific accuracy and soothing therapy find their source in the "precept on precept" of the Medical School. Here the science of clinistry and surgery and obstetrics is born again in the mind and technique of every plodding but persistent student and flowers in the full maturity of his active practice.

The Review aims to serve many purposes. It aims in time to be a scientific journal of rank and to do its part in raising the level of southern medicine. To this end its pages are open to the Alumni, the Faculty, the students and representative medical men as a mouthpiece for articles of scientific value. It therefore aims to stimulate medical writing in the Southeast. It is well to dip the medical pen in medical ink and promote a medical literature. It aims to promote observation and research and the spirit of research—all three invaluable practices of every medical center. It aims to be a graphic opportunity in medicine to every Alumnus from the day of his graduation. It aims to discuss medical pedagogy and the problems of medical education. It aims to promote organization and reunion among the Alumni. It aims above all to keep the Alumni in living touch with the University and the University in living touch with the Alumni. It will take a generation to accomplish all these aims. So easy are they to state, so difficult and gradual perhaps in their realization, but thereby are they all the more certain and valuable to the life and the time and the section of every Alumnus who enters gladly into the association and upbuilding of the Medical School of his University. The seal of the University carries the motto "Lex-Lux," or "Law and Light," or "Science and Vision."[32]

•

Future medical progress is dependent to no small degree on keeping alive and encouraging the spirit of medical writing. How little of the accomplishments of the past would be available for the present day practice of medicine, had the pioneers been content to let their knowledge and discoveries go unpublished and perish with them. How much more recognized would be Crawford W. Long's priority for the discovery of anesthesia had he relied upon the written rather than the spoken word.[33]

•

It has been well said that medical literature is already overburdened with volumes of writing that have little of value to merit their preservation. It is therefore fitting that medical publications should enforce upon authors a strict adherence to the necessity of not only having something worth while to say, but to say it in terse, well-chosen language which will at once impress the reader's mind and not leave him groping for the idea, in a maze of verbosity. The present age leaves little time to the busy physician and it behooves the writer who wishes to hold his reader's attention, to conserve the latter's time.[33]

•

A well written interesting case report or original investigation not only serves an educational purpose to its readers but is a great factor in developing in its author keener powers of clinical or scientific observation and encourages the keeping of case records, thereby making him a better physician. It naturally follows, therefore, that medical writing is a great factor in developing medical authorities, and medical authorities in turn lead to the development of medical centers.[33]

•

The Emory Medical Review aims first to strive to inoculate the "Sons of Emory" with the virus of medical authorship to such an extent that there will gradually be developed an immunity to the present apparent aversion to writing.[33]

BOOKS

Lastly, I want to pay a passing compliment to the work of Dr. Harvey Cushing for his monumental monograph on the pituitary. It is possibly the acme of American research and a real contribution to the medicine of our time. It is a training in medical science to read the book, whether one gets anything out of his patient investigation or not.[34]

•

During his life he wrote more than twelve hundred separate papers. His textbook, used everywhere and translated into other languages, is as much a classic as a textbook and is in its tenth edition. His *Modern Medicine* is in seven volumes and has had two editions. There are several monographs with the titles of *Angina Pectoris, Chorea, Abdominal Tumors*, and *The Evolution of Modern Medicine*. His two addresses on *The Growth of Truth* and a *Way of Life* have been widely read. The *Alabama Student* contains thirteen biographical essays. The twenty-two essays in *Equanimitas* constitute probably in time to come the most lasting of all his writings, and in power for good outdoes the *Religio Medici* of his beloved Sir Thomas Browne. Every medical student should read it before graduation and then reread it in his medical life and all of us should try to live it.[10]

•

Senac, the Frenchman, published his book on the heart in 1749. This was the first treatise on heart disease. He first emphasized the fact that heart disease is more common in middle and old age, showed that the whole heart could be inflamed, accented diet in heart disease and used squills for dropsy. He first recognized heart murmurs and precordial bulging and called attention to the accumulation of fat on the heart. Senac broke away from vague notions and marked a distinct advance. Auenbrugger, of Vienna, in his *Inventum Novum*, published in 1761, described percussion of the heart and was able to demonstrate cardiac enlargement in the patient. This was the beginning of physical diagnosis. His discovery was forgotten until Corvisart, physician to Napoleon I, in his book on *Maladies of the Heart*, published in 1808, gave rebirth to percussion and for the first time accented disease of the heart muscle, as distinguished from diseases of the pericardium and the endocardium.[35]

•

Allan Burns published at Edinburgh in 1809 the first book in English on diseases of the heart.[35]

•

James Hope, the Englishman, in 1832 by direct experiment on the aortic valve segments showed that the second sound disappeared when these were hooked aside, and the first sound was shown to depend on the vibration of the auriculo-ventricular valves and the contracting ventricular muscle. The Frenchman, Bouillaud, in 1835, showed the true causes and proper explanation of the heart sounds, accented the great importance of inflammation of the valves, and first used the term "endocarditis." Hope's book was published in England in 1831 and Bouillaud's in France in 1835, and these two books really revolutionized cardiology.[35]

•

Mackenzie published his *Study of the Pulse* in 1902; his *Diseases of the Heart* in 1908, his *Principles of Diagnosis and Treatment of Heart Disease* in 1916; his *Heart Disease in Pregnancy* in 1921; and his *Angina Pectoris* in 1923. Thomas Lewis wrote his *Mechanism of the Heart Beat* in 1910, though his most valuable clinical contribution is the *Clinical Disorders of the Heart Beat*. Gross' *Blood Supply to the Heart* is valuable. W. S. Thayer's *Study of Endocarditis*, published this year, is the great contribution to the subject, and clinically, Cabot's *Facts on the Heart*, also just published, certainly revises some views from the standpoint of 1906 autopsies.[35]

•

The first edition of Gray's *Anatomy* published about 1860, is the beginning of big books, as textbooks. Big Books represent an easier task for the author. Restricted to a smaller book he must condense, simplify, conclude; in the large book, he can amplify, enlarge, reiterate.[15]

•

Even good teaching fades from the memory except that its principles and influence may survive in the individual and through him with less impress upon others. Children die or too often disappoint the hope of parents; monuments erode and shallow unreadably their chiselled praises or time cracks and scatters them; but the printed page, alive with genius, accuracy, and fact, carries on to the mind of the generations. The precious printed page is a greater promise of mortal perpetuity than is child or marble or gift. In 1543 at Basel, Vesalius issued his *Fabrica*, the first and greatest book of modern medicine, the keystone of the arch of the art, "one of the greatest books of the world, and would come in any century of volumes which embraced the richest harvest of the human mind." Without it Vesalius would be but a ghost of memory. It was copied, pirated and plagiarized, translated in many languages, a second edition issued in 1555, an immortal book as books go, and it made Vesalius immortal as men go. All other anatomies find their primal source in it; paper, print, and art of drawing are here joined. The greatest of all anatomists had finished his professorship and published his book at 28. This book is the richest bloom of the medicine of the Renaissance.[16]

SEX AND VENEREAL DISEASE

The ascendency of man is a direct result of sexual reproduction, and in the making of an offspring the parent is under a twofold responsibility. He is under obligation to produce another like himself; this is a duty to himself as an individual of the human species. He is under obligation to produce another better than himself; this is his promise and contribution to racial progress.[36]

The human race has wondered at and admired the human mind. It is mysterious in its slow development, marvelous in its cunning, great in its accomplishment, and strange in its going. More mysterious and stranger still are the insane, the body left and the mind gone somewhere. Therefore it is no wonder we are late in coming to view the insane man as the definite effect of a definite cause, and the causes in one-fourth of all cases of insanity are syphilis and alcohol.[37]

NEUROLOGY AND PSYCHIATRY

The human animal does not get nervous until he gets civilized, and the neurotic child, as well as the neurotic adult, in the last analysis, may rightly be regarded as the product of civilization, or indoor living and mental work.[38]

•

Individuals who are not nervous are not aware that they have a nervous system.[38]

•

The nerve centers tire and may be renewed; strain and rest are the opposing forces that work on the plastic nerve system; and rest, air, exercise, sleep, are the greatest therapeutic agent in any neurosis.[38]

•

Nature abhors inbreeding, and the usual result in the human family is a blow at the nervous system of the offspring. Two cousins may produce a good liver or spleen, but nature balks at a brain. I have in mind two cousins of ordinary strength, health, and mentality, whose three children were all deaf and dumb, one blind, one choreic. This was a passion that moaned itself to sleep in protoplasm but could not produce a mind.[38]

•

Next to the minor ailments, such as constipation and headache, the psychoneurosis is the most frequent clinical problem that the internist faces in the day's work.[39]

•

There is no substitute, therapeutically, for the overwhelming personality of the physician. The neurotic who wrote out long series of questions for Wm. Osler to answer usually forgot where the paper was when he was in the consulting room. So genial was Osler's personality, so great was the faith in him, why discuss egotistical nonessentials! Leave it to him. Here was the power of an unconscious psychotherapy. Here, too, Weir Mitchell was at his best. Negation, passivity, and mere professional formality are of no service to the neurotic. He needs positive force, positive statements, positive honesty, a genial warmth, and a firm sympathy. The same faith that has carried the human race for all time is his great need. Doubt of himself is his boon companion. He looks for everything from his physician, to whom he has told everything. Psychotherapy is just the agent of personality.[39]

•

One would be convicted of clinical folly who would belittle the laboratory or any of its fields, but the wise clinician yearns for proportion and perspective and believes the personality to be just as scientific a field as the urine or the fluoroscope, and far more neglected. A real diagnostic study investigates the whole of this psychophysical totality and believes every function equally the domain of science. It is a duty of science to find what is the matter with the patient, and one cannot do this in many cases by merely studying the body, the soma, the flesh, unless he would emasculate his opportunities for service.[40]

•

Nothing is more different in practice than the routine papers of a medical society and the conduct of a medical ward; the paper is likely to omit the art and the ward to submerge the science in the art. Any clinician might do well to read the conversation between Christ, the prostitute Mary Magdalene, and Simon. He might catch a glimpse of the genius in psychotherapy that might relight his waning faith in his more narrow medical therapeutics.[40]

•

The great problem is to decide whether we are dealing with a cellular pathology, a functional pathology, or a personality pathology, or variations and combinations of two or three.[40]

•

Probably in no calling is there as much opportunity afforded for the study of psychology as in medicine; nowhere is psychology more needed and nowhere is it more neglected.[40]

PELLAGRA

The history of pellagra is a romance of clinical medicine. The disease originated in the Asturias of northern Spain, and was first described there in 1735, when it was called *mal de la rosa*, or sickness of the rose, referring to the reddish eruptions of the hands and face. It next appeared in northern Italy about 1750, and now is disappearing from that country. In 1911, I searched northern Italy for a case of pellagra as severe as we had then in the south, and as we still have in the south. There was not a case of acute, severe, malignant typhoid pellagra to be found. It appeared in France in 1828, and was reported in Egypt in 1847. In America it was first reported in 1864.[41]

•

So variable is pellagra in its onset, signs, symptoms, course and effects, so changeable, shifting and clinically amoeboid in its varying degrees and types that, next to syphilis, it is probably the most bizarre of all human diseases.[42]

CARDIOVASCULAR DISEASE

The diagnosis of every case of heart disease should include the known or probable cause of the lesion. It is not enough to say that one has an aortitis, or a mitral lesion. There is a cause for every heart lesion, and the cause influences the treatment and the prognosis.[43]

•

After forty the circulation is the largest gate to death. Arterial failure and cerebral hemorrhage, renal failure and uremia, and cardiac failure with edema or anginal states are the three great paths to the end.[44]

•

We are living in the age of noise and lights; the result is lessened sleep and nerves; the myocardium bears the brunt of the wear.[45]

•

The returning cardiac is an old story. Often he returns to the same hospital many times for rest, digitalis and comfort. The return to activity is the danger. The circle of activity must be made very small. Shortness of breath on exertion means stop and rest and do less. Short rules impress the patient if he be taken into full pathological confidence. Avoid stairs, the broom, alcohol, tobacco, and overeating. Sidetrack into easy living. Quit pushing and begin to saunter along. We can do so much so easily if the patient only gets the reason and the mental outlook, and he usually obeys and cooperates for the sake of comfort and results.[45]

•

We have come to the period in which heart disease is the chief cause of death in civilization and I am very anxious to know how to prevent so much heart disease in the next generation.[46]

•

The chief hope is preventive medicine and the chief problem before us now is the prevention of organic heart disease.[46]

•

Digitalis will repay a life-time study. It is not to be used merely because there is a murmur or because there is a cardiac neurosis; a false cardiopath, the French call it. It is to be used first and above all as a drug of power in auricular fibrillation and secondly in heart muscle failure whether associated with fibrillation or not.[35]

•

The chief point in the diagnosis of heart disease is to evaluate accurately the efficiency of the heart muscle.[35]

•

Pneumonia now is a mere captain in the ranks, but heart disease is a general of the men of death. It seems that the evidence from city, state, and insurance statistics points to a still rising mortality, while pneumonia and tuberculosis statistics point to a decreasing mortality. The practice of the internist and the general practitioner bear evidence to the steady increase. Here is "main street" in internal medicine today.[35]

•

The physician has no right as a medical leader in his community, to live contrary to the dictates of preventive medicine. Example is greater than precept, and self-denial than self indulgence. Obesity, tobacco, alcohol, muscle laziness, overeating, worry, strain, loss of sleep, and irregular hours are bad medicines for the myocardium that needs the "by reason of strength" to carry it even to, much less by, the seventieth year.[35]

•

We have tried to find *the one cause* of angina pectoris, but there is probably no more one cause of angina pectoris than there is one cause of meningitis.[47]

•

A crude axiom that "if the diastolic be 90 mm. or below, it makes no difference what the systolic is," is largely true. The systolic represents largely peripheral resistance but it is nevertheless a vague expression of heart muscle power. Better than the axiom that "a man is as old as his arteries," is this: "The lower the diastolic, the longer the life, other conditions being normal." No heart can stand long against a diastolic of 120 mm. A diastolic of 130 mm. or over usually means death within two years, more or less. Variations in pulse pressure are relatively unimportant. An individual with a diastolic and a pulse pressure below the average is apt to live long and that without cardiac hypertrophy. The greatest cause of cardiac hypertrophy is a high diastolic pressure. Mortality increases rapidly as blood pressure figures are raised above the normal. A diastolic blood pressure reading is of more value than a single urine examination as a measurement both of heart work and arterial strain.[48]

•

We have thought of heart disease at different periods in such different terms and in such varying points of view. In the time of Senac, Corvisart, and Burns we thought in terms of enlargement and dilatation and dropsy; in the time of Withering, in terms of dropsy and digitalis and just a little of heart strength; in the time of Laennec chiefly in terms of murmurs, and then not until in the time of Mackenzie did we apparently begin to accent heart disease in terms of muscle and muscle strength and muscle failure, as it deserves to be. Lewis and Mackenzie and Wenckeback explained the arrhythmias, but probably not even yet do we think of heart disease adequately in the larger accents of its etiological criteria.[47]

•

One who fears death, dies many times before he dies. Moreover, the patient realizes that he is helpless unless the doctor can help him. The doctor may tell him what the disease is, may give him medicines and accent what to do when the attack comes, but after all this is but treating the pain of the attack. It is a hypodermic for pain and nothing more. Only the anginous have angina. To have angina is to be more anginous. Merely to treat the attack is to view the patient bodily, not as a personality, and does not in the least lessen the drive of life that perhaps more than any other factor, causes the angina.[49]

•

The cerebral eye of the internist and the retinal eye of the surgeon together add to the safety of the patient. The one hears and observes clinically, purrs over his patients, sagaciously observes and pliably and keenly concludes. The other comes with powers, technic and courage and an amazing execution in the field of his particular operation. Recovery depends upon the functional capacity of the circulation and the organism as a whole. It is rest, safety and conservation versus risk, pain, and danger. And no one of us can stand very much mortality.[50]

•

It is relatively easy to tell a good heart. It is more difficult to prove a bad heart and still more difficult to state how bad it is. Not every normal heart meets every strain. Not every good heart is a normal heart and not every bad heart is a dangerous heart. The primary question is not whether the heart is anatomically normal, but rather whether it is functionally capable. The physical examination of the heart is important but it does not permit conclusions regarding its power to do work or to stand strain. One wishes to know the size of the heart, its sounds and murmurs, its rate, rhythm, and peripheral blood pressure. This is the more objective and anatomic examination and has failed as a chief basis of thought in heart disease.[50]

•

Coronary artery sclerosis without angina is probably the most overlooked disease of the circulation after 50.[50]

ABDOMINAL DISEASES

The word abdomen is from *abdo*, I conceal, and abdominal complaints are the key and clue to a concealed pathology and disease somewhere, but not necessarily in the abdomen, much less in the stomach.[51]

•

The average patient with "yellow jaundice" knows no more about his liver or his bile than the average Greek did in the time of Hippocrates or the average Roman in the time of Galen. The average student at graduation can seldom give the four sources of the portal blood or the anatomical boundaries of the liver itself. To the average surgeon the liver is relatively uninteresting, but the small bile pouch that hangs beneath it is a veritable haven of activity. To the average physician the gall bladder is relatively uninteresting unless he be a biased devotee of tubing and drainage, but the liver is a large organ of many functions, much mystery, and few facts.

For twenty-five years internal medicine has focussed itself upon the heart, and largely left the abdomen, apart from a few organic conditions, to those who call themselves gastroenterologists, and to that braver group, the abdominal surgeons. But the liver is as important as it is large, and the time is at hand when we are beginning to think in terms of liver problems and to develop a liver mind.[52]

GRANULOPENIA

But the main question is this: Is there a separate disease in which there is first of all an unaccountable physiologic paralysis of the bone marrow that stops quickly and completely, or nearly completely, the manufacture of the polymorphonuclear leukocytes?[53]

•

We have had nothing like it before either in biology or in medicine. In the beginning there is as yet no demonstrable infection, but only a selective hypoplasia or aplasia of the myelocytic cells of the bone marrow. The myelocytic series of cells either completely or nearly completely disappears. About four days after this event, the granulocytes are either absent or nearly absent from the blood stream. About two days after they disappear from the blood stream, the clinical onset begins, often in severe cases with dramatic suddenness, with collapse, chills, fever, red throat or ulceration of the mucosa, and stupor and death unless the granulocytes quickly reappear in the blood stream, because the marrow has begun to make myelocytes. If, and when, sepsis develops, it is a result and complication of the disease rather than a cause.[54]

Thanks Dad. Thanks Son.

William C. Roberts

William Clifford Roberts, MD
Editor in Chief
Baylor University Medical Center
Dallas, Texas

1. Roberts CS. *Life and Writings of Stewart R. Roberts, M.D., Georgia's First Heart Specialist.* Spartanburg, South Carolina: Reprint Co. Publishers 1993:138.
2. Roberts SR. The care of success. *High School Quarterly* 1920.
3. Roberts SR. The personality of the patient. *Chicago Med Rec* 1923;45:575–582.
4. Roberts SR. Health conditions in Georgia. *Bull Univ Georgia* 1929;30:3–16.
5. Roberts SR. Reading. *The Pulse* [Emory University Hospital] 1931;3:1–2.
6. Roberts SR. The art and human nature. *Boston Med Surg J* 1932;20:670–676.
7. Roberts SR. The social trends underlying health and hospital insurance. *N Engl J Med* 1935;212:1123–1129.
8. Roberts SR. Emory: a place of loyalty. *Emory Alumnus* 1940;16:10–11.
9. Roberts SR. The senior student. *Southern Med J* 1918;11:395–399.
10. Roberts SR. William Osler. Clinician–teacher. *Southern Med J* 1924;17:40–42.
11. Roberts SR. The doctor's visit. *Texas State J Med* 1936;32:266–271.
12. Roberts SR. The young men in medicine. *Kentucky Med J* 1922;20:43–46.
13. Roberts SR. Benjamin Franklin, patron of medicine. *Ann Clin Med* 1925;3:501–507.
14. Roberts SR. William C. Gorgas of Alabama. *Southern Med J* 1925;18:859–864.
15. Roberts SR. Big books and much teaching. *Southern Med J* 1928;21:548–553.
16. Roberts SR. The influence of Versalius. *J Med Assoc Georgia* 1930;19:324–329.
17. Roberts SR. Response to addresses of welcome. *J Med Assoc Georgia* 1917;7:25–27.
18. Roberts SR. Health. *High School Quarterly* 1927;16:182–192.
19. Roberts SR. Emory after twenty-five years. *Emory Alumnus* 1927:7–10,20.
20. Roberts SR. The doctor. *The Aesculapian, Year Book of Atlanta Med Coll* 1915.
21. Roberts SR. A medical center. Retiring address of the President of the Fulton County Medical Society, Atlanta, Georgia (pamphlet). 1915.
22. Roberts SR. Hyperpressure. *J Med Assoc Georgia* 1917;7:159–165.
23. Roberts SR. The principles of organization in group medicine. *Southern Med J* 1921;14:910–912.
24. Roberts SR. Association vs. isolation for a young man in private practice. *Southern Med J* 1922;15:411–415.
25. Roberts SR. The larger diagnosis. *Kentucky State Med J* 1929;27:94–100.
26. Roberts SR. The responsibilities of us all. *Emory Med Rev* 1923;2:5–7.
27. Roberts WC. Dr. Stewart R. Roberts' "An ideal of modern medicine." *Ann Intern Med* 1969;70:1016–1017.
28. Roberts SR. The multiple care and costs of medicine. *Bull Am Hosp Assoc* 1931;5:7–22.
29. Roberts SR. The treatment of encephalitis lethargica. *J Med Assoc Georgia* 1920;10:164–166.
30. Roberts SR. Vital statistics and medicine. *J Med Assoc Georgia* 1921;10:637–639.
31. Roberts SR. Teaching internal medicine. Each student a teacher. *J Am Med Assoc* 1917;68:392–399.
32. Roberts SR. Foreword. *Emory Med Rev* 1922;1:1.
33. Roberts SR. Medical writing—an index of medical progress. *Emory Med Rev* 1925;3:48–49.
34. Roberts SR. The signs and symptoms of hypopituitarism. *Southern Med J* 1920;13:549–553.
35. Roberts SR. Heart disease and life. *Ann Clin Med* 1926;4:535–540.
36. Roberts SR. The battle of sex. The white life vs. the red light. *Southern Students Conf, Y.M.C.A.* (pamphlet). 1908.
37. Roberts SR. Syphilis and the paretic group. *Atlanta J-Rec Med* 1910;56:226–230.
38. Roberts SR. Conditions producing the nervous child. *St. Louis Med Rev* 1911; January:10–12.
39. Roberts SR. The problem of the neuroses. *Ann Clin Med* 1924;2:416–420.
40. Roberts SR. Personality pathology. *Southern Med J* 1932;25:628–636.
41. Roberts SR. Pellagra: its symptoms and treatment. *Am J Nursing* 1920;20:885–890.
42. Roberts SR. Pellagra of today. *Int Clin* 1929;1:65–76.
43. Roberts SR. Syphilis of the heart. *Southern Med J* 1915;8:447–450.
44. Roberts SR. The diagnosis of the arterial group. *Arch Diagnosis* 1917;10:129–139.
45. Roberts SR. The failing heart. *J Florida Med Assoc* 1921;8:66.
46. Roberts SR. The larger view of heart disease. *Southern Med J* 1925;18:391–395.
47. Roberts SR. The diagnostic relations between the gallbladder and the heart. *Illinois Med J* 1929;56:317–321.
48. Roberts SR. Functional pressure versus structural sclerosis. *Ohio State Med J* 1926;22:1021–1025.
49. Roberts SR. Nervous and mental influences in angina pectoris. *Am Heart J* 1931;7:21–35.
50. Roberts SR. The relation of the heart to surgery. *Southern Surgeon* 1935;4:85–100.
51. Roberts SR. An alphabet of abdominal diagnosis. *Southern Med J* 1919;12:655–660.
52. Roberts SR. The liver. *J Tennessee State Med Assoc* 1928;21:1–5.
53. Roberts SR, Kracke RR. Agranulocytosis. Report of a case. *J Am Med Assoc* 1930;95:780–786.
54. Roberts SR, Kracke RR. Agranulocytosis: its classification. Cases and comments illustrating the granulopenic trend from 8,000 blood counts in the South. *Ann Intern Med* 1931;5:40–51.

Ruby Viola Holbrook Roberts (1903–1994)

She was the fifth of 11 children, 10 girls and 1 boy, plus 2 older stepsisters and 1 older stepbrother. She was the sickly one as a child, but the longest survivor thus far. Her father died when she was 9. He was sick periodically and I think he had little effect on her life. She had great admiration for her mother and for her oldest stepsister and loved all her siblings. Growing up was pleasant; there wasn't much money, but she had a warm, loving family. The city (Atlanta) was safe; a movie cost 5¢, and the streetcar to Technical High School, where she learned to type and take dictation, also cost 5¢. She always thought that there was plenty of time for English and History even in a technical high school, and she was disappointed when more was not offered. Her dream was to go to Agnes Scott College and become an English teacher, but she had to go to work immediately after high school. Only the youngest 4 siblings were able to go to college (Georgia College, Milledgeville).

In her early 20s, she became secretary to her future husband, a prominent physician in Atlanta.[1,2] They married in December 1929, when she was 26 and he 51. This was a second marriage for him, with no children by the first. In September 1929, he had borrowed much money to invest in the stock market to "take care" of his alimony responsibility. The market crash occurred the next month. Their marriage lasted a short 11 years, ending in 1941 with his death, and in 1945 she finished paying off her husband's debt.

The marriage was a good but unusual one. All her life she referred to her husband as "Dr. Roberts." The marriage yielded 3 boys. One was mentally retarded, and sending him away to a care facility was the hardest decision of her life, but, in my view, one of her many good decisions.

Within a year of her husband's death, their country house near Atlanta burned, and she and her 2 boys moved to the Woodcrest Avenue home in Atlanta where she lived for 47 years. In 1942 she began working again, this time as Executive Secretary for the Fulton County Medical Society. In 1946 she started her own business, Medical Placement and Mailing Service, which she sold 27 years later. She didn't enjoy retirement. She always felt a bit guilty for not accomplishing more each day. When her energies became diminished over these last several years, she did not want to delay the inevitable. Sarah, her only surviving sister, and Stewart, her first son, were her caretakers during these energyless years.

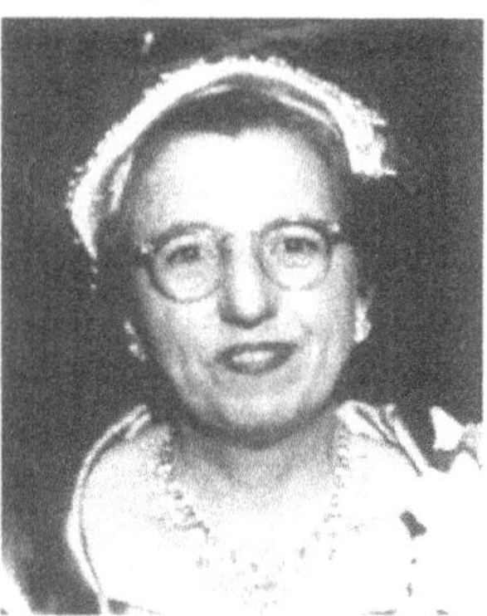

Ruby Viola Holbrook Roberts

Who was this Ruby Viola Holbrook Roberts? She was accepting, caring, curious, friendly, generous, gracious, hardworking, honorable, independent, kind, likable, optimistic, pleasing, resourceful, straightforward, trusting, and unselfish. In her makeup there was no element of arrogance, cynicism, deviousness, dishonesty, falseness, greed, or manipulativeness. She rarely complained. She accepted disappointments and heartaches as a part of life, and she rebounded from them quickly. She never expected things to be perfect and she felt fortunate to have the hand of cards that had been dealt to her. She never uttered curse words, smoked cigarettes, or drank alcohol, and she never judged harshly those who did.

When I was a teenager she shared her business problems with me. She instilled a kind of confidence in me from those many discussions by indicating in various ways that my opinions as a teenager were useful in some way to her. She was a self-reliant person, and, I believe, passed on these qualities to her 2 healthy sons at an early age. By age 11, Stewart and I were responsible for buying our clothes and doing our share around the house. She encouraged my going 850 miles away from home to college, knowing full well that I would never really come home again and that those friendly and meaningful conversations after dinner would essentially come to an end. She supported her sons' endeavors extremely generously in light of her financial state, and never would accept any monetary gift from me, despite my attempts to make things a bit easier for her. She would never scold me on the occasions when several weeks would go by and I wouldn't call. Whenever I apologized, the answer predictably was "The idea!" I have never subsequently encountered such a forgiving soul. I learned of her respect for honorableness when the manager of a movie theater called her to say that he had just caught me trying to sneak into the theater. Seeing her face when arriving home that night convinced me that I could not again hurt this near-pure lady with that type of conduct.

I will miss her smiles, her laughs, her warmth, her eternal optimism. Simply being in her presence made me a better person, or at least gave me the desire to become a better person. I hope that in the new world she's entered that she won't work so hard, that she will learn more about play and take the time to play more. I hope that she will be able to finish all those books she started, and that she will rest in peace, knowing that she was such a loved woman.

William C. Roberts

William Clifford Roberts, MD
Editor in Chief
Baylor University Medical Center
Dallas, Texas 75246

1. Roberts CS. Life and Writings of Stewart R. Roberts, M.D., Georgia's First Heart Specialist. Spartanburg, South Carolina: Reprint Co. Publishers 1993:138.
2. Roberts WC. A Son's Book on his Father's Father. *Am J Cardiol* 1994;74:518–529.

Life's Master Molecule and James Watson

The year 2003 represents the 50th anniversary of the discovery of the structure—the fabled double helix—of deoxyribonucleic acid or DNA by Watson and Crick.[1,2] Earlier experiments by others had shown that DNA from 1 strain of bacteria could permanently alter another, and this observation convinced Watson and Crick that it may hold the secret of heredity. They had also seen some x-ray pictures done by Rosalind Franklin. On February 28, 1953, Watson cleared off his desk and began fiddling with cardboard models of 4 key parts of DNA: adenine, guanine, cytosine, and thymine. Suddenly, the puzzle pieces fit into place: *a* linked with *t* and *c* with *g*. The 2 pairs looked identical and Watson realized they could form the steps of a spiral staircase. This double helix could duplicate itself by unzipping into 2 strands, each a template for building another helix with the same sequence of letters. DNA has achieved superstar status, and its lovely double spiral is an icon of science. DNA has cured deadly diseases and allowed labs to create animals with new features. It has freed the innocent from death row and caught a president in a tawdry lie. Now, 50 years later, the finishing touches are being put on the full 3–billion-letter sequence of our DNA.

Many scientists believe that DNA evolved from another long-chain molecule, namely RNA. Like DNA, RNA has 4 "letters" that store information, but it has an extra oxygen unit that makes it highly reactive. That oxygen unit even attacks RNA itself, making it unreliable for long-term information storage.

Watson and DNA is the title of Victor K. McElheny's new book on James Watson.[3] In 1968, James Dewey Watson published a book called *The Double Helix*. The book presented a picture of science as something thrilling, even obsessive, undertaken by persons who were perfectly capable of spite, vanity, and folly but who raced to be the first to offer the world a picture of the universal machinery of conception, growth, and procreation. Reviewers both loved and hated the book. It caused huge offense in the scientific community. Chapter 1 opened with, "I have never seen Francis Crick in a modest mood." Others have supposed that few people have seen Watson in a modest mood either. But Victor McElheny's life of Watson, published to mark the 50th anniversary of the discovery of the double helix structure, confirms a suspicion surely held by anyone who ever met Watson: he rarely believed he had a lot to be modest about.

The book is the story of a thin, bookish, birdwatching boy, the son of a bill collector, who entered the University of Chicago at the age of 15 years and left 4 years later with 3 questions in his head: What is the gene? How is the gene copied? How does the gene function? It was his capacity for putting questions as simply and sometimes as annoyingly as possible that kept Watson in science and in trouble for the next 55 years.

After he, Crick, and Maurice Wilkins won the Nobel Prize in 1962, Watson went on not to do science as such, but to make it happen: at Harvard, at Cold Spring Harbor, New York, and in the power structures of Washington. Watson was at the heart of the first genetic engineering debates. He was one of a handful who made the human genome project happen. He was one of an even smaller handful who then insisted that the data must be freely available to every researcher in the world rather than patented and sold. That stance—along with his capacity to exasperate—cost him the leadership of the human genome project. But Watson went on saying what he thought, in a manner that was almost the antithesis of diplomacy. The book tells the Watson story well and warmly. Watson refused to be interviewed by McElheny at any time.

I recently saw Watson interviewed on television. He used "you know" in every sentence, often times more than once per sentence. I guess I should not be annoyed when hearing "you know" by teenagers and athletes when Nobel Prize winners copy them.

William C. Roberts

William Clifford Roberts, MD
Editor in Chief
Baylor Heart & Vascular Institute
Baylor University Medical Center
Dallas, Texas

1. Boyce N. Triumph of the helix. *US News & World Report*, February 24/March 3, 2003:38–41.
2. Senior K. From the standing start to human genome sequence in 50 years. What was biology really like before Watson and Crick discovered the DNA double helix 50 years ago? *Lancet* 2003;361:580–581.
3. McElheny VK. Watson and DNA. Making a Scientific Revolution. Cambridge, MA: Perseus, 2003.

Life Lessons from Modern-Day Greats in Cardiovascular Disease

In July 1996, interviews of prominent cardiovascular specialists began appearing in *The American Journal of Cardiology* (*AJC*). Listed in Table 1 are the names of the 62 cardiovascular internists whose interviews have been published in the *AJC*. One interview was done by Dr. Mark Silverman, 2 by Dr. J. Willis Hurst, 1 by Dr. Charles Stewart Roberts, 1 by Dr. Colin Ku Lo Phoon, and the others by me. Three interviews focused on medical topics rather than on the interviewees, and they are not further considered in this presentation.

Interviews of 8 cardiovascular surgeons also have appeared in the *AJC*, and their names are listed in Table 2.

In addition to the 70 interviews in the *AJC*, 74 others (with me as the interviewer) have been published in the *Baylor University Medical Center Proceedings* (Table 3), but they are not further considered in this piece.

Certain data on the 59 cardiovascular internists and on the 8 cardiovascular surgeons (a total of 67 interviews) are listed in Table 4. Their ages when interviewed averaged 65 and 74 years, respectively. Most were born from 1926 to 1950. Eleven (17%) were born outside the United States. Of the 52 internists who grew up in the United States (1 was born abroad), 26 (50%) grew up in the Northeast, mostly in New York City (15 of 26); 11 grew up in the middle portion of the United States, 15% in the Southeast, and 14% in the West. Seven of these 67 had no siblings. Of those with siblings, the interviewees were most often the first children (>50%). Ten of the 67 interviewees (15%) had lost parents when the interviewees were <20 years of age. More than 1/2 played on ≥1 high school athletic team and >20% on college varsity teams. The interviewees had averages of 2.7 and 3.1 children, respectively. Ten of the 59 cardiovascular internists (16%) and none of the 8 cardiovascular surgeons were divorced. The interviewees' first publications came at relatively early ages (mean 29 years, range 23 to 36). (That finding is of interest, because the present average age of a recipient of his or her first National Institutes of Health research grant is 42 years.) All of these interviewees were highly productive, and 41% had >500 publications in medical journals. A number were presidents of the American Heart Association or the American College of Cardiology, and 7 of the surgeons were presidents of ≥1 national surgical organization. About 1/3 of the interviewees' mothers worked, and also 1/3 of the interviewees' spouses worked. Seven were married to physicians, but only 2 practiced. Fewer than 1/3 were overweight. Six had PhDs in addition to their MDs. Of the 59 cardiovascular internists, 24 (41%) were Jewish, as was 1 of the 8 cardiovascular surgeons. Of the 54 cardiovascular internists who attended college or medical school or did training in the United States, just over half had some training at an Ivy League university or medical center (not including, however, such institutions as New York University, Johns Hopkins University, or any school in the South, Midwest, or West). None of these 67 interviewees could be considered heavy alcohol users: 1+ represents drinking wine at a social event, 2+ usually daily wine, and 3+ includes spirits.

Some characteristics of the parents of the 67 interviewees are listed in Table 5. One or both members of the 25 couples (37%) were born outside the United States. In 42 couples (63%), 1 or both parents attended college; in 8 of the 67 couples, 1 or both were physicians; only 2 (3%) were divorced; the average number of children was 2.8; and the interviewees were the only children of 8 couples (12%).

The major commonalities among these 67 interviewees are listed in Table 6. Without exception, their parents were devoted to their children, love was abundant in their homes, education was heavily stressed by their parents, the home atmosphere provided an enormous curiosity to learn, nearly all were superb students, all had a passion for medicine, and all worked exceedingly hard. Most slept <6 hours per night, and all were incredibly focused on their goals. Writing was a major priority, and they all worked hard at it. Most were good teachers and good mentors. In my view, all were very competitive. They had strong character. Most had a good capacity for friendship, alcohol played little to no major role in their lives, and most maintained healthfulness.

I have selected to reproduce small portions from 2 interviews: those of Dr. Eugene Braunwald,[1] the most renowned cardiologist of the 20th century, and Dr. Michael E. DeBakey,[2] the most renowned cardiovascular surgeon of the past century.

Eugene Braunwald, MD (1929-)

Dr. Braunwald was born on August 15, 1929, in Vienna, Austria, and lived his first 9 years there.

Roberts: *Can you discuss your life in Vienna?*

Braunwald: My memory of that period falls into 2 very distinct phases: before and after March 13, 1938. On that date the Nazis occupied Austria in the so-called *Anschluss*. My childhood was idyllic before that. We lived in one of the elegant areas of Vienna, I went to an excellent school and had private tutors in English and piano. My parents were very interested in opera, and by the time I was 6 they had begun taking me to the Vienna State Opera. Vienna was a gracious city in the 1930s, the cultural capital of central Europe. Then, suddenly, on March 13, 1938, everything changed. I recall vividly the enthusiastic crowds welcoming Hitler and his troops marching into Vienna. My father's and other Jews' businesses were taken over several days later and their liquidation was begun. We lived in constant terror

Table 1
Interviews of cardiovascular medicine specialists published in *The American Journal of Cardiology*, 1996 to 2008 (n = 62)

Eric Jeffrey Topol	Carl John Pepine
James Thornton Willerson	Kenneth Hardy Cooper
Joseph Stephan Alpert	Watkins Proctor Harvey
John Willis Hurst*	Joseph Kayle Perloff
Jesse Efrem Edwards	Charles Richard Conti
Howard Bertram Burchell	William Watts Parmley
William Howard Frishman	Dean Michael Ornish
Robert Ogdon Bonow	Dean Towle Mason
Eugene Braunwald	George Allan Beller
Joseph Cholmondeley Greenfield	Leslie David Hillis
Norman Mayer Kaplan	Douglas Peter Zipes
Robert McKinnon Califf	Nanette Kass Wenger
Bernard John Gersh	Andrew Peter Selwyn
Dean James Keriakes	Arthur Garson, Jr.
Jeffrey Michael Isner	Edward David Frolich
Scott Montgomery Grundy	Robert Alan Vogel
Burton Elias Sobel	Ferid Murad
Robert Anthony O'Rourke	Steven Evan Nissen
Spencer Bidwell King III	William Peter Castelli
Robert Roberts	Wallace Bruce Fye III
Eugene Austin Stead, Jr.†	Anthony Nicolas DeMaria
Bertram Pitt	Barry Lewis Zaret
Christopher John Dillon Packard‖	Franz H. Messerli
Terje Rolf Pedersen‖	Joseph Loscalzo
Valentin Fuster	Donald Carey Harrison
Henry Arthur Solomon	Hollis Bryan Brewer
Harvey Stanley Hecht‖	Barry Joel Maron
Myrvin Harold Ellestad	William Clifford Roberts§
Richard John Bing†	Jean Schlatter Kan‡
Melvin Mayer Scheinman	Robert William ("Bobby") Brown
James Stuart Forrester III	Lawrence Cohen

* Interviewed by Mark Silverman.
† Interviewed by John Willis Hurst.
‡ Interviewed by Colin K.L. Phoon.
§ Interviewed by Charles S. Roberts.
‖ Topic interviews.

Table 2
Interviews of cardiovascular surgeons published in *The American Journal of Cardiology*, 1997 to 2006 (n = 8)

Michael Ellis DeBakey
Denton Arthur Cooley
John Webster Kirklin
David Coston Sabiston, Jr.
David Kempton Cartwright Cooper
Francis Robicsek
Magdi Habib Yacoub
Lawrence Harvey Cohn

Table 3
Interviews by William Clifford Roberts published in the *Baylor University Medical Center Proceedings*

Baylor physicians	Robert Peter Perrillo
Lloyd Wade Kitchens, Jr.	David Wesley Barnett
David Joseph Ballard	William Clifford Roberts
Adrian Ede Flatt	George Kennedy Hempel, Jr.
J.B. Howell	Joseph Allen Kuhn
George Justice Race	Virginia Pascual
Michael Emmett	William Mark Armstrong
Marvin Jules Stone	William Levin Sutker
Ronald Coy Jones	Perry Edward Gross
Jimmie Harold Cheek	Barry Wayne Uhr
Robert Wilson Jackson	Carolyn Michele Matthews
George Marion Boswell, Jr.	**Baylor nonphysicians**
Göran Bo Gustaf Kintmalm	Luz Remedios Tolentino
Robert Pickett Scruggs, III	Boone Powell, Jr.
Wilson Weatherford	Joel Tribble Allison
Fred David Winter, Jr.	Mark Timothy Parris
Gary L. Davis	Gary Dale Brock
Peter Allen Dysert, II	Julie Michelle O'Bryan
Zelig ("Zeck") Lieberman	Herman Grant Lappin
Martin Alan Menter	Albert Julio Alvarez
Harold Clifton Urschel, Jr.	**Visiting professors**
John Flake Anderson	Gerald Bernard Appel
John W. Hyland	Robert William Schrier
Joyce Ann O'Shaughnessy	Larry Harold Hollier
Daniel Earl Polter	Charles Stone Bryan
Jonathan Martin Whitfield	Richard Vaille Lee
Andrew Zolton Fenves	Gregory Gordon Dimijian
Glenn Weldon Tillery	Peter Emanuel Dans
Clement Richard Boland, Jr.	Donald Wayne Seldin
Elmer Russell Hayes	Ellen Taylor Seldin
Robert Lee Fine	Thomas John (Jock) Murray
Jay Donald Mabrey	Matthew Whitfield Ridley
Donald Alan Kennerly	Robert Ogden Bonow
Barry Cooper	David Westfall Bates
Robert Gary Mennel	Robert Steven Galvin
Paul Bernard Convery	Carolyn Maureen Clancy
Irving David Prengler	Lynne Anne Marcum Kirk
Zaven Hogop Chakmakjian	Lee Marshall Nadler
Priscilla Larson Hollander	

from March until the end of July 1938, when we escaped from Austria. Many people in our situation, of course, did not escape.

Roberts: *Before March 13, 1938, you lived next to your father's business? What was your father like? Your mother? What were your day-to-day activities, not only at school, but at home in those more pleasant moments?*

Braunwald: Our apartment was just off the Schottenrink, Vienna's major thoroughfare, close to the University and to the State opera. I saw a good deal of my father because the proximity of our apartment to his business allowed him to have lunch with us quite frequently. In childhood, both of my parents had been too poor to receive an education beyond high school. My father was fifth generation Viennese, and my mother was born in a small town in the east of what was then the Austro-Hungarian empire. Her family fled to Vienna at the end of World War I because of an anti-Jewish pogrom in her town. My father had built a successful wholesale clothing business by the time I was born, and we enjoyed a very pleasant life. The 3 most important things that I learned from those early years were: a central focus on the well being of the nuclear family; a reverence for learning; and an interest in classical music. As I just mentioned, we lived not far from the University of Vienna, and when I was 6 or 7 years old my mother took me for walks in the Stadtpark adjacent to the University. She would point to the University and say to me, "You will be a professor there someday." Because my parents had been deprived of an education themselves, they made my education their highest priority.

Table 4
Data on the interviewees

Variable	Internists (n = 59)	Cardiovascular Surgeons (n = 8)
Age (yrs)	41–91 (mean 65)	59–88 (mean 74)
Years of birth		
1901–1925	9 (15%)	5 (63%)
1926–1950	45 (76%)	3 (37%)
1951–1954	5 (8%)	0
Country of birth		
United States	53 (90%)	5 (63%)
Outside the United States	6 (10%)	3 (37%)
State of childhood residence		
Northeast (26/52 [50%])		
New York	15*	
Pennsylvania	4	
Connecticut	1	
New Jersey	4	
Massachusetts	1	
Maryland	1	
Middle United States (11/52 [21%])		
Indiana	1	
Ohio	4	
Minnesota	0	1
Oklahoma	2	
Texas	4	1
Southeast (8/52 [15%])		
Virginia	1	
Georgia	4	
South Carolina	1	
North Carolina	0	1
Louisiana	1	1
Alabama	1	
West (7/52 [14%])		
California	5	1
Wyoming	1	
Utah	1	
No. of siblings		
None	5 (8%)	2 (25%)
1–5	54 (92%)	6 (75%)
Hierarchy of interviewees in the families with >1 child		
First child	29/54 (54%)	3/6 (50%)
Last child	12/54 (22%)	2/6 (33%)
Middle child	12/54 (22%)	1/6 (17%)
A parent died when interviewee was aged ≤20 years	8 (14%)	2 (25%)
Competitive athlete		
High school only	31 (53%)	7 (88%)
College also	13 (22%)	5 (63%)
Children	157 (2.7%)	25 (3.1%)
0	2 (3%)	1 (12%)
1	2 (3%)	0
2	23 (39%)	1 (12%)
3	21 (36%)	3 (38%)
4	9 (15%)	1 (12%)
5	2 (3%)	2 (25%)
Divorced	10 (17%)	0
Age (yrs) at first publication	24–36 (mean 29)	23–34 (mean 29)
Publications in medical journals¶		
<250	15/58 (26%)	1 (12%)
251–500	19/58 (33%)	2 (25%)
>500	24/58 (41%)	5 (63%)
President of the American Heart Association, the American College of Cardiology, or a major surgical society	21 (36%)	7 (88%)
Mother worked	21 (36%)	2 (25%)
Spouse worked	19 (32%)	2 (25%)
Married a physician	5† (8%)	2† (25%)
Overweight	19 (33%)	2 (25%)
PhD	5 (8%)	1 (12%)
Jewish	24 (41%)	1 (12%)
Ivy League education‡		
College	13/54§ (24%)	0
Medical School	12/54 (22%)	1/5‖ (20%)
Houseofficership	11/54 (20%)	1/5 (20%)
Fellowship	15/54 (28%)	0
At least 1 of the 4	28/54 (52%)	2/5 (40%)
Drinks alcohol (0–3+)		
None	6 (10%)	1 (12%)
1+	16 (27%)	0
2+	24 (41%)	0
3+	7 (12%)	6 (75%)
Uncertain	6 (10%)	1 (12%)

* One interviewee was born outside the United States but grew up in New York City.

† Only 1 practiced.

‡ Brown University, Columbia University, Cornell University, Dartmouth University, Harvard University, Princeton University, the University of Pennsylvania, and Yale University; does not include New York University, Johns Hopkins University, or any school in the South, Midwest, or West.

§ The other 5 had all their training abroad.

‖ The other 3 had all their training abroad.

¶ One interviewee who was not in academic medium was excluded.

Table 5
Data on parents of interviewees

Variable	Value
One or both born outside the United States	25 (37%)
Attended college (1 or both)	42 (63%)
Were physicians (1 or both)	8 (12%)
Divorced (after interviewee was born)	2 (3%)
No. of children	185 (mean 2.8)
1	8 (12%)
2	24 (36%)
3	18 (27%)
4	9 (13%)
5	6 (9%)
6	2 (3%)

Roberts: *Did you have intellectual discussions at the dinner table at night or at lunch time?*

Braunwald: I remember discussions of history, economics and politics at the dinner table. My parents probably did emphasize such discussions because of their own lack of higher education. Of course, there was much talk about music. Actually, my parents had met in the standing room area at the Vienna State Opera!

Table 6
Commonalities among interviewees

Parents devoted to children
Abundant love from parents
Education stressed by parents
Enormous curiosity to learn
Superb students
Passion for medicine
Worked exceedingly hard
Slept little (<6 h)
Incredibly focused on goals
Good writers
Good teachers and mentors
Competitive
Strong character
Good capacity for friendship
Consumed little or no alcohol
Maintained healthfulness

Roberts: *Although your parents were poor initially, your father became quite successful?*

Braunwald: Yes. By the time of the *Anschluss* he had a prosperous business, but the Nazis quickly sent SS officers to liquidate all Jewish businesses. The officer who was assigned to my father's business had, I believe, been imprisoned for the assassination of Chancellor Dolfuss of Austria several years earlier. I got to know this SS officer because sometimes he came over to the apartment for lunch or coffee.

Roberts: *What was he like?*

Braunwald: He was cold and businesslike but always polite, as he went about destroying our livelihood. The liquidators themselves were able to make off with most everything, and therefore he wanted the process to be rapid and complete.

Roberts: *How did it come about that your father was arrested by the Nazis within a couple of months of their invading Austria?*

Braunwald: It was the proverbial knock on the door in the middle of a night in May 1938. I remember being awakened by my parents at about 3:00 A.M. My mother was hysterical, screaming, "They are taking your father away." He had 15 minutes to get dressed and to say goodbye to us. I now recall that he was remarkably stoic about it. Then my mother, my younger brother and I ran to the window and saw him herded into an open truck with 15 or 20 other men. They were then driven off to the railroad station.

Roberts: *How did your mother get him back? I gather he came back the next day?*

Braunwald: Yes. It is incredible what life can hinge on. When "our" S.S. officer came to the business the next morning, he asked for my father. My very upset mother said he had been taken away, presumably to a work camp. He shrugged his shoulders. (My mother and I subsequently talked about this event innumerable times.) Then came the pivotal moment, she said something along the following: "You need him back because you have liquidated only half of the business, and if you get him back you can liquidate the rest. Look how much richer you would be." He replied, "You might be right." He then phoned the depot to find that my father was about to board the train. My mother only overheard his side of this conversation in which he pulled rank on the officer at the depot, saying, "I don't care if you are a full colonel in the German army, I am a captain in the SS and I want this Jew returned!" So it ultimately became a matter of authority. By 11 A.M. my father was returned to us. He had been gone for only 8 hours, but it was a very close call. If my mother had not acted at that moment, none of our family would have survived, and of course, we wouldn't be having this interview.

Roberts: *From that point it was about 2 months before you escaped? What happened in the interim?*

Braunwald: My father had actually begun preparations for our escape in March immediately after the occupation, but he redoubled his efforts after his brief arrest. There were several opportunities for him to leave Vienna alone and to try to bring us along later, but he refused to allow the family to be separated. He insisted that we stay together even though that made escape more difficult. But he obviously calculated correctly. We left at the end of July 1938, in something that resembled the *Sound of Music* story, except that there was no music. We ended up in London, totally destitute, literally with only the shirts on our backs. We were taken care of by a relief agency. I spoke a little English because of the special tutoring I had received, but my parents did not then speak a word of English. (They later learned English in night school.). . .

Michael Ellis Debakey, MD (1908–2008)

Roberts: *What was it like growing up in your family and in Lake Charles, Louisiana?*

DeBakey: First, Bill, I was blessed with parents who were both highly intelligent and exceedingly kind and generous in their temperament and psyche. They lived almost exclusively for their children. They wanted to give us the best of everything, and they believed education was crucial. They were both first generation immigrants, having come to this country as children. Because they believed that a good education was essential to prepare us for a fulfilling life, they always encouraged us to excel in our studies. For example, they urged us to go to the local library once a week and choose any book we wanted to read. We had a small but very good library in Lake Charles. I came home from the library one day and told my Father that there was a wonderful set of books there, but you could not borrow them; you had to read them in the library. He asked me the name of the book, and I responded, *The Encyclopaedia Britannica*. He said, "Well, we will get it." I don't remember how many volumes there were at that time—not as many as there are today—but he purchased the complete set. All of us, my brother, sisters, and I, before we went to college, had each read that whole set of *The Encyclopaedia Britannica.* That is how important it was to us, not only from an educational standpoint, but mainly because we enjoyed reading. All of us excelled at school; we all led our classes. My sisters all led their classes. They were smarter than I was; at least they were a little more studious. My brother and I wanted to play and do other things. The one thing that I never got an "A" in was deportment. In those days we had a deportment grade, and I had great difficulty with it because I would finish all my studies and would get bored because the teacher was dealing with material I had already mastered. In what we then called grammar school or elementary school—I think I was in the fifth or sixth grade—the classes were divided into 2 sections—A and B—and the same teacher taught both classes. While she was teaching one class, she would give the other class a study period of 30 minutes, after which she would go back to the other side. She noticed I was sitting in the center, paying attention to what she was doing, whether she was in my class or the other one. So near the end of the class, she said to me one day, "I notice that you are paying attention to both classes, would you like to take the exam for both of them?" I said, "Sure." I took both exams and was permitted to skip a grade because I passed the exam. School was fun for me because I enjoyed learning new things. My parents had always emphasized to all of us the joy of learning. I studied, learned, and earned good grades, and I think that became a habit.

Roberts: *Did your parents go to college?*

DeBakey: No, but they were self-educated, read widely, and had remarkably critical minds and retentive memories.

Roberts: *And they pushed education to the hilt.*

DeBakey: Yes, absolutely.

Roberts: *I presume you read the book or books that you got from the library once a week?*

DeBakey: Yes, regularly.

Roberts: *From age 6 through age 17, I calculate that you must have read over 600 books outside of school.*

DeBakey: Yes, at least, plus the encyclopedia. I was a voracious reader. In fact, we had to go to bed at a certain time. We would do our lessons—our parents would make sure we had done our lessons—and then if we had time, we would read the library book or sections of *The Encyclopaedia Britannica*. Often, we were all going to *The Encyclopaedia Britannica* at the same time. Of course we would not read the same thing. Usually by 10:00 o'clock, our parents wanted us in bed, because we had to get up early. Our Father was a very early riser, and we all had assigned chores, to encourage self-discipline and responsibility, even though my parents had a house staff. By 5:00 A.M. we were up. I guess I got habituated to the early rising. That came in handy, because when I first started as a freshman in college, I lived in a dormitory, and the boys were raising cane all night. I wanted to study, but couldn't because of the commotion. I would just go on to bed, and get up at 3:00 or 4:00 in the morning and do all my studying while it was quiet. So I got into the habit of getting up early, and it does not matter what time I go to bed now; I still arise at 5:00 A.M. I read *The New York Times* and *The Wall Street Journal* in about 30 minutes. After that I can get some of the things done that I may not be able to do during the day—work on a manuscript or attend to some other paper work. Getting up early has been of great value not only in my surgical practice, but also in allowing me an additional couple of hours beyond that of the average person. Fortunately, I manage well on 5 or 6 hours of sleep a night, just as my Father did.

Roberts: *So if you get 5 hours sleep a night, and you are 88 years old, you have slept only 14 of your last 68 years?*

DeBakey: You are probably right about that. If you sleep 8 hours a night (one-third of every day) and you live 60 years, you have really lived only two-thirds of that time or 40 years. So whatever you can take from your sleep extends your conscious living.

Roberts: *So you are 88 years and a maximum of one-fifth of your life has been spent sleeping.*

DeBakey: That is about right. And that gives me a tremendous advantage. People ask me, "How in the world could you write nearly 1,500 articles in that period of time?" If you live your life long enough and you have enough time, you can do it.

Roberts: *Yes, but you don't waste a minute. You spend very little time commuting. You live 5 minutes from the hospital.*

DeBakey: In fact, I deliberately chose to live near the College. When I first came to Houston, I rented a house that was also only about 10 minutes from here. . . .

William Clifford Roberts, MD
Baylor Heart and Vascular Institute
Baylor University Medical Center
Dallas, Texas

1. Braunwald E, Roberts WC. Eugene Braunwald, MD: a conversation with the editor. *Am J Cardiol* 1998;82:93–108.
2. DeBakey ME, Roberts WC. Michael Ellis Debakey, MD: a conversation with the editor. *Am J Cardiol* 1997;79:929–950.

Editing and Writing

A Few Words From the *Journal*'s Second Editor

I am pleased and at the same time humbled to be the *Journal*'s new editor.* I am well aware of the enormous responsibility of an editor of a major journal today, and will do my best not to abuse or misuse that power. Editors, of course, play major roles in governing the fate of ideas and of their creators. I intend to seek advice and counsel from many quarters.

The *Journal* seeks your finest manuscripts. I pledge to those so submitting that their manuscript will be processed and reviewed expeditiously, that the authors will be treated respectfully, courteously and fairly, and that the interval from submission to acceptance or rejection will be held to a minimum. I have 2 suggestions for authors submitting papers: (1) that they include a *letter* to me stating precisely and concisely the significance and uniqueness of the work in their view, and (2) that they provide several *names* of nonlocal experts who they believe could give objective and informed reviews of their work. These suggested reviewers will be carefully considered along with other experts in the field. Additionally, I would listen if authors occasionally provided the name of an investigator they consider unlikely to give an objective or fair review of their work.

The focus of the *Journal* will remain strongly clinical. I welcome suggestions from readers at any time.

William C. Roberts, MD
Editor-in-Chief

* *A tribute to the former editor from the new one appeared in the July 1978 issue of the* Journal (*Roberts WC. SIMON DACK and the American Journal of Cardiology. Am J Cardiol 1978;42:14–6*).

Reprinted from the July issue of **The American Journal of Cardiology.**
A Yorke Medical Journal. Published by Technical Publishing Company, A Division of Dun-Donnelley Publishing Corporation, a Dun & Bradstreet Co., 875 Third Avenue, New York, N.Y., 10022.

Blind Reviews

Revised "Instructions to Authors" appear in this issue of the *Journal.* I urge authors to study these instructions before the final typing of their manuscripts for submission. Let me call attention to one new item in these instructions, namely the submission of two title pages, one that includes the article's title plus the authors' names and institution from which the work originated, and the second, including only the article's title. The omission of the authors' names and institution in the second title page will allow the editor to send the manuscript for review without the reviewer's knowledge of the authors or their institution. The authors of course must be careful not to refer to their institution or to previous work (by personal pronoun) in the text.

There has been much debate over the years about the advantages and disadvantages of reviewing manuscripts without knowledge of the authors or their institutions. Reasonable arguments can be made for both sides of this question. Many authors believe, I think, that their papers are unfairly reviewed because of bias on the part of the reviewer. Having two title pages will allow the editor the option of acquiring either blinded or nonblinded reviews or both. I welcome requests (in the covering letter) from submitting authors to have their paper reviewed in a blinded or nonblinded fashion or both, and I will try to honor that request. Comments on this question are welcomed.

William C. Roberts

William C. Roberts, MD
Editor-in-Chief

Brief Reports

Few major medical journals today have room for lengthy case reports. "Doctoring," however, comes down to a single patient, and often principles of disease and ideas for large studies come from ideas conceived from study of only 1 patient. Therefore, I am instituting a "Brief Reports" section in the *Journal* which will include case studies of only 1, 2, or 3 patients (see page 658 in this issue).*

Usually case studies have only 1 point, and information not pertinent to that point is unnecessary. Indeed, unnecessary words and nonessential details actually prevent clear focus on the point. Thus, these "Brief Reports" must be brief—no more than 2 or 3 double-spaced typed pages with few references. Reports only 1 page long probably will be favored over those 3 pages long. Pertinent illustrations may be the dominant element in conveying the message.

Brief Reports require clear thinking. Each word must count. I recall in medical school the dean's mention of a 4 page letter he had received with the following PS: "Sorry I did not have time to write a shorter one." Space in medical journals is enormously expensive (hundreds of dollars per printed page for the paper, ink, and printing, and hundreds more per page to cover personnel, overhead, and so on). Four double-spaced typewritten pages form 1 printed page in the *AJC*, and 4 figures generally form 1 printed page. The shorter these Brief Reports, the larger the number of reports that can be published. I envision publication of about 2 or 3 Brief Reports each month, and I welcome your contribution.

William C. Roberts

William C. Roberts, MD
Editor-in-Chief

* *The originator of the brief case report was Dr. Jesse Edwards, who provided a nice justification of its usefulness in an editorial 20 years ago (Edwards JE. A new look for the case report. Circulation 1972; 25:277).*

The Editorial Board

Shortly after becoming Editor of the *AJC*, I began reflecting on physicians who I would ask to serve as editorial board members. I realized immediately that a *large board* would be essential if the board members, rather than outside consultants, were to be the primary reviewers of manuscripts submitted to the *Journal*. Each major and minor subspecialty of cardiology needed to be represented by several respected investigators. I was particularly anxious to increase the representation of cardiovascular surgeons because their role is a vital one in the present-day management of patients with cardiovascular disease, and because in the past they have been underrepresented on the boards of cardiology journals.

I also realized immediately that many individuals I would want on the new editorial board would already be members of one or more other editorial boards. In the past I have had the privilege of serving simultaneously on the editorial boards of 6 different medical journals, and as a reviewer I have paid little attention to the name of the journal for which I was reviewing a manuscript. An editorial board member's expertise is not the monopoly of a single medical journal. The board member's charge is to evaluate promptly the scientific quality of a manuscript and the means to improve that manuscript. Board-member reviewers, as do nonboard reviewers, serve the entire medical community by providing expert opinions to any editor who asks them to do so. They do not and should not take a loyalty oath to a specific journal—their loyalty is to the writer and the reader. Placing a reviewer on an editorial board gives him public recognition as a superb manuscript reviewer and is the means by which the editor says "thanks" for his help. If one editor rewards a reviewer by placing him on his editorial board, that action should not prevent another editor from rewarding the same reviewer similarly. Indeed, membership on more than one editorial board is further acknowledgment of a reviewer's sought-after expertise. Just as the medical writer (investigator) is free to submit his manuscript to any journal he chooses, the expert reviewer is free to provide his expertise to any journal so requesting. If an *AJC* board member is a member of another editorial board, that is the business of the editorial board member and the other journal, and of no concern to the present Editor of the *AJC*.

After establishing the principle that a large editorial board would be necessary, I prepared lists of adult and pediatric cardiologists, cardiac surgeons, and related specialists such as radiologists, pathologists, and pharmacologists, and in July 1982 I began dialing the telephone. I initially contacted 110 potential editorial board members, 103 of whom accepted the invitation. I am grateful and indeed the entire cardiovascular community must be grateful to these expert manuscript reviewers who devote their time freely to improving the quality of articles published in our medical journals.

William C. Roberts, MD
Editor-in-Chief

Reviewing Manuscripts: Occasionally a Test of Character

One of the least appreciated tasks performed by members of the medical academic community is their objective review of manuscripts submitted to them by the editors of medical journals. Although occasionally a reviewer may be able to evaluate a manuscript in only a few minutes, most reviews require much longer.

Reviewing a manuscript can sometimes be a test of character. A manuscript sent to a reviewer often concerns a subject about which the reviewer himself has contributed information previously, or a subject he is currently investigating or planning to investigate. Thus, the reviewer may be asked to evaluate work done by someone else on a subject of personal interest to himself. In this situation the reviewer and reviewee might well be described as competitors. Furthermore, the reviewer is asked not only to evaluate the author's work but also to provide suggestions for improving it free of charge. Medicine and science appear to be the only areas in which competitors consult one another for free advice. Can you imagine Ford Motor Company asking General Motors Corporation to provide suggestions for improving the quality of a newly designed automobile—without remuneration? Occasionally a reviewer may be asked to evaluate the manuscript of an author for whom he has no fondness, either for professional or personal reasons, or conversely, to evaluate the manuscript of an author for whom he has a high personal regard. In either of these cases the reviewer may be less than objective and the review less than ideal.

Detecting prejudice (conscious or otherwise) in a review is a continuing challenge for an editor. To help meet this challenge, I have requested that authors submitting manuscripts to the *AJC* (see the *From the Editor* column, July 1982 issue, page A3) provide in the covering letter names of potentially objective and nonobjective reviewers so that predictable or possible conflicts might be avoided.

In this professionally competitive and human atmosphere in which we all reside, the consistently objective reviewer deserves our appreciation and admiration.

William C. Roberts

William C. Roberts, MD
Editor-in-Chief

Speeding Up the Manuscript-Reviewing Process

All reviewers for the *AJC* are asked to send their reviews to the Editor within 3 weeks. When this time period is met by each reviewer, authors can be notified that their manuscript is accepted or rejected within a month. Although this time sequence operates well for most manuscripts submitted to the *AJC*, some reviewers fail to return their reviews to the Editor for several additional weeks. Indeed, I have been surprised by the length of time some reviewers retain a manuscript before returning it, with or without their opinion, to the Editor.

The "frequent" author is usually a "frequent" reviewer, but the 2 hats are worn at different times. When authors submit manuscripts to a journal, their patience for delay in receiving the "acceptance" or "rejection" decision is generally short; however, when these same authors become reviewers, their patience for delay appears much longer. Reviewers should treat authors as they would like to be treated when they are authors—*this might be the golden rule of reviewing.*

How can a reviewer decrease the length of time between receipt of a manuscript and its return to the Editor? One procedure which has proved useful to me is to *examine the manuscript briefly the day it arrives.* In this way, the subject of the manuscript can be reflected upon for several days before the review is actually prepared. If the manuscript concerns a subject of considerable interest to a colleague, the colleague can be presented with the manuscript the day it arrives. Some reviewers do not look at a manuscript received for 3 or 4 weeks, then pass it along to a colleague who delays another 3 or 4 weeks before providing a review. If a manuscript is particularly poor, cursory examination on the day it arrives is often sufficient to make the decision to advise rejection. It surely makes the Editor's job easier when there is little delay in providing a negative decision to an author. And, finally, if an editorial board member is going to be away from his office for an extended period, notification of the Editor's office can prevent the delay produced by having the manuscript returned a month later marked "not reviewed, out of town."

In summary, let us try to review other authors' manuscripts as promptly as we want our own manuscripts reviewed.

William C. Roberts, MD
Editor-in-Chief

Getting the Manuscript Accepted: Think Like a Lawyer and Cover the Flanks

A manuscript might be viewed as a legal brief in which an author presents logical arguments supporting the contention that he has created and proven a new concept. Reviewers, in a way, are like defense lawyers who attempt to find a flaw in the author's contention. Finding such flaws often casts doubt on other claims of the author or claimant. Indeed, the finding by reviewers or the Editor of *omissions of mention* can be a major stumbling block preventing the acceptance of a manuscript.

A manuscript's quality may be compared to the game of tic-tac-toe, in which 2 players, in turn, fill in 9 compartments, 1 at a time, with X's and O's. The *best paper* fills in all the blocks—covers all the bases—and in addition lines up 3 X's in a row (see the figure below), signifying focus and clarity. A row of zeros indicates that the manuscript provides an essentially negative observation. A manuscript also can have all the blocks filled in but no symbols lined up in a row, indicating a lack of clarity and focus. The *worst paper* fails to fill in 1 or more compartments with either symbol (omissions of mention) and none line up in a row, an indication that the author has failed to mention all the points necessary to prove his case and to focus the points properly.

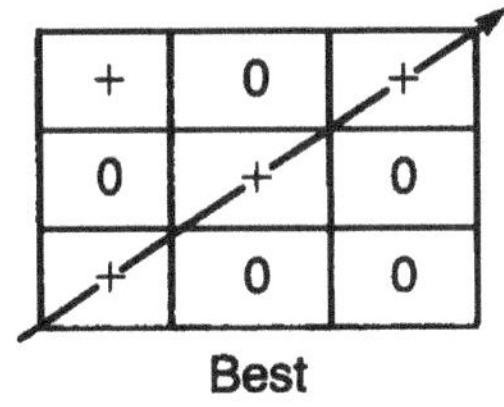

Best

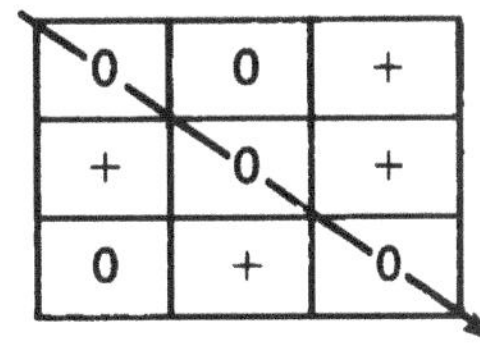

+	0	0
0	0	+
+	+	0

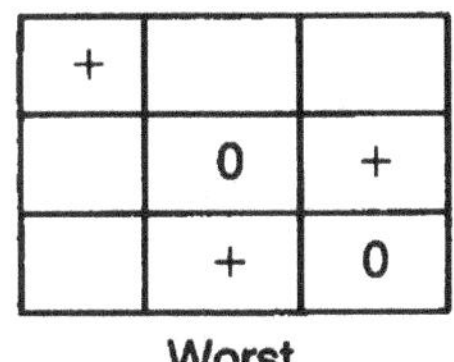

Worst

William C. Roberts

William C. Roberts, MD
Editor-in-Chief

Reprinted from the January issue of **The American Journal of Cardiology.**
A Yorke Medical Journal. Published by Technical Publishing
Company, A Division of Dun-Donnelley Publishing Corporation,
a Dun & Bradstreet Co., 875 Third Avenue, New York, N Y , 10022

Paper Accepted/Abstract Rejected or Vice Versa: Differences In the Grading of Abstracts and the Reviewing of Manuscripts

Through the years I often have been amazed that an abstract I considered excellent was rejected, and yet when the subject of that abstract was submitted later in manuscript form, it was rapidly accepted. The grading of abstracts and the reviewing of manuscripts are 2 entirely different processes.

I have had the privilege of serving on program committees of both The American Heart Association and The American College of Cardiology, and this responsibility included grading abstracts for presentation at the annual scientific sessions. An abstract from either society is graded similarly—by a score of 0 to 10, with a 10 representing the highest quality. Each abstract is graded by about 7 to 10 reviewers, and the final grade given is the average of the multiple grades. The most common grade given is a 7; very few abstracts receive grades <5. The average grade of abstracts accepted for presentation—either from the podium or by poster—is about 7.7. If the grader happens to be an author of an abstract, he or she is instructed to use the letter *P* for "prejudiced," and if the grader is "unqualified"—that is, does not have sufficient knowledge of the subject of the abstract—the letter *X* is used. Although a single line is provided for it, no explanation or justification for the grade is required. On one program committee of which I was a member, 50% of the abstracts were graded 1 by one committee member, whereas another member on the same committee registered a 7 or 8 on all abstracts he graded. Few graders give many 10's, and some rarely give a 9. Of course, the most useful grader is the one who clearly differentiates the good abstracts from the bad ones. In the 1960s, only the members of the program committee graded the abstracts for 1 of the 2 national cardiology societies, and that meant that each member graded a large number—about 300. During recent years both organizations have used non-committee member experts as graders, so that no grader is asked to review more than about 100 abstracts; the period of time allowed, however, remains short—about 2 weeks.

In contrast, when a reviewer recommends to an editor that he or she accept or reject a manuscript, that recommendation must be substantiated by criticisms or the lack of them. Although one could argue that because abstracts have far more graders than manuscripts have reviewers, the selection process for abstracts is a just one. I have no constructive suggestions for how to improve the abstract grading process. My enthusiasm, however, for abstracts is far weaker than that for manuscripts; in fact, my enthusiasm is roughly proportional to the amount of space occupied by a published abstract compared with that occupied by an average published manuscript.

Several years ago 3 of my abstracts were rejected for presentation at the annual meeting of one of the 2 cardiology societies, and all 3 were accepted without change of a single word for the annual meeting of the other society. I have about reached the point where for me abstracts simply provide a specified date for submission of an investigation, whereas original manuscripts have no deadline for submission.

An abstract should be viewed as a preliminary report on an investigation. (Incidentally, the use of abstracts as references should be avoided, except in unusual circumstances.) Thus, give me the manuscript—this is the final forum.

William C. Roberts

William C. Roberts, MD
Editor in Chief

Reprinted from the February Issue of **The American Journal of Cardiology,** A Yorke Medical Journal, Published by Technical Publishing, a Division of Dun-Donnelley Publishing Corporation, a Company of the Dun & Bradstreet Corporation, 875 Third Avenue, New York, N.Y. 10022.

Author-Editor-Reviewer: How the Triumvirate Is Working at the AJC

An author submitting a manuscript to be considered for publication in a medical journal deserves to know how the manuscript will be evaluated by that journal. This piece describes the process as it now works at the AJC.

Early decision by editor only or thorough evaluation by out-of-office reviewers: Once logged and given a number, each manuscript is given to the Editor-in-Chief, who asks 4 basic questions as he reads it: (1) Is the subject of the manuscript appropriate at this time for the AJC? (2) Would the manuscript have wide or narrow appeal to the readers of the Journal? (3) Does the manuscript represent scientific quality? (4) Is the subject of the manuscript presented clearly and succinctly?

If the manuscript is considered inappropriate for the Journal, of insufficient interest to its readers, of obviously poor scientific quality, or poorly presented, it is returned immediately to the author with a statement that it is unacceptable for publication in the AJC. For manuscripts rejected solely on the basis of poor presentation, a request for reconsideration might be granted provided the manuscript is thoroughly revised. During my 9-month tenure as Editor, about 10% of submitted manuscripts have fallen into this immediate-reject category. This prompt decision allows the author to send his manuscript elsewhere or revise it without delay. Furthermore, it prevents having reviewers provide reviews simply to justify an editor's decision that already had been made. Although such an early decision by the editor may not engender friendship from the submitting author, it conserves the time and energy of all parties involved.

About 5% of manuscripts submitted are reviewed solely by the Editor; a rare one is accepted virtually without change, and his suggestions for improving the other manuscripts are returned to the authors immediately. If appropriate changes are made or if appropriate explanations are provided as to why changes were not made, the revised manuscript is accepted.

The remaining approximately 85% of manuscripts are sent out of office to be reviewed by 2 or more editorial board members or nonboard consultants. Some manuscripts, particularly potentially controversial ones, may be sent immediately to 3 rather than 2 reviewers.

Selection of reviewers: A major editorial decision in the manuscript-evaluation process is the selection of the most appropriate reviewers. Many submitting authors now participate in this decision (see the From-the-Editor column, July 1982, page A3), but the final selection is made by the Editor. When submitting authors request that their manuscript not be reviewed by a particular consultant or editorial board member or group of investigators, this request is honored by the Editor. If authors suggest 1 or more nonbiased, nonlocal reviewers for their manuscript, usually 1 author-suggested reviewer and 1 editor-selected reviewer are chosen. The Editor, of course, seeks the most objective reviewers, recognizing that this selection can predetermine the final decision regarding a manuscript.

Evaluation of reviews by the Editor: After reviews are returned to the Editor, the manuscript is reevaluated in light of the criticisms and recommendations of the reviewers. When both reviews are favorable, the Editor's decision is usually simple. When both reviews are negative, the Editor's decision also is usually easy. In these 2 situations the Editor's initial reaction to the manuscript is usually compatible with the reviewer's recommendations.

When 1 reviewer's recommendation is unequivocal rejection and that of the other is unequivocal acceptance, the manuscript is often sent out for a third review. Many times, however, the third reviewer is not necessary. One of the 2 reviewers may have made a far stronger case for his point of view than the other reviewer, or the Editor may feel comfortable with the subject of the manuscript and therefore can make the decision without the delay produced by seeking another out-of-office opinion. When 1 of 2 reviewers returns a manuscript unreviewed (he may be out of town, sick, or too busy), the Editor must then decide whether to seek another review or to make a decision based on only 1 outside review and his own analysis. This decision generally depends on the quality of the single out-of-office review.

After the manuscript has been returned to the Editor after having been reviewed by 1 or more outside consultants or editorial board members and the decision is made to probably accept the manuscript, the Editor at this stage carefully examines the manuscript to suggest other alterations and to make sure that the authors have adhered to the style of the Journal. If certain changes are to be required in the manuscript for its acceptance, the authors are so informed at this stage. When a manuscript is tentatively accepted, the Editor often makes editorial changes on a xerographic copy of the manuscript containing his initials on the title page so that these changes can be considered for incorporation into the revision by the author. The Editor spends more time on a manuscript at this point than at any other stage, excluding manuscripts accepted without outside review.

Return of the manuscript and reviews to the author: When a manuscript is tentatively accepted pending either major or minor revision, the manuscript must be revised appropriately or the suggestions of the reviewers and the Editor must be rebutted appropriately. Authors must be careful not to be offended by criticisms of their manuscripts. Such criticism is provided by both outside reviewers and by the Editor in an attitude of genuine helpfulness. The author should evaluate critical comments carefully before discounting them as inappropriate. The revised manuscript must be retyped and resubmitted. The author also is asked to return the original version of the manuscript containing the Editor's handwritten suggestions.

Evaluation of the revised manuscript: The Editor evaluates the revised manuscript in light of the comments of the reviewers and the changes or rebuttals of the authors. If the changes made by the authors are considered appropriate, the manuscript at this stage is accepted without delay. Occasionally, however, the Editor considers the changes by the author inadequate or inappropriate and returns the manuscript for further changes. At times, the revised manuscript is returned to an earlier reviewer for reexamination. When this reexamination by an earlier reviewer is done, the authors usually are so advised when their manuscript was initially returned to them.

Manuscript to the publisher: After a final review by the Editor, the manuscript is sent to the publisher for copy editing and printing. Both the Editor and the Publisher have made strenuous efforts to diminish the lag time from acceptance to publication in the AJC. This time period is now *4 months*, and it is my intent to keep this short interval in the future. This means that manuscripts accepted in March 1983 will be scheduled for publication in July 1983.

William C. Roberts

William C. Roberts, MD
Editor-in-Chief

Reprinted from the March 1 issue of **The American Journal of Cardiology**, A Yorke Medical Journal. Published by Technical Publishing, a Division of Dun-Donnelly Publishing Corporation, a Company of The Dun & Bradstreet Corporation, 875 Third Avenue, New York, N.Y., 10022.

Author-Advertiser: Their Dependency on One Another

Occasionally I hear a physician complain about the number of advertising pages in medical journals. The number of medical journals, however, would be few and very expensive were it not for the ads. If there were no advertisements, a year's subscription to the AJC instantly would be approximately twice its present cost and later, as the number of subscribers diminished because of the journal's high price, even more. Although few physicians pick up a medical journal to read ads, there would be few journals to pick up were ads not present. Thus, physicians must appreciate the enormous contribution of advertisers to their education.

All elements of a medical journal (see figure) focus on providing the reader the best available information in the most presentable form. The 2 key elements in publishing medical articles are the authors (investigators) and advertisers. Among his many responsibilities, the publisher acquires the ads; the more ads acquired, the more text pages are provided. The publisher provides the editor with text pages based on several factors, a major one being the projected number of ads to be acquired over a specified period. During the first 6 months of 1983, each monthly issue of the AJC will average 228 text pages. Three additional issues, published during this period (in January, March, and May) will average 116 pages. All 9 issues consist of original articles; symposia sponsored by pharmaceutical companies are published separately and are not included in these figures. Thus, excluding symposia, 1,716 text pages will be published during the first 6 months of 1983. Without the advertisements, the number of text pages would diminish enormously and the patient would be the ultimate loser.

William C. Roberts

William C. Roberts, MD
Editor-in-Chief

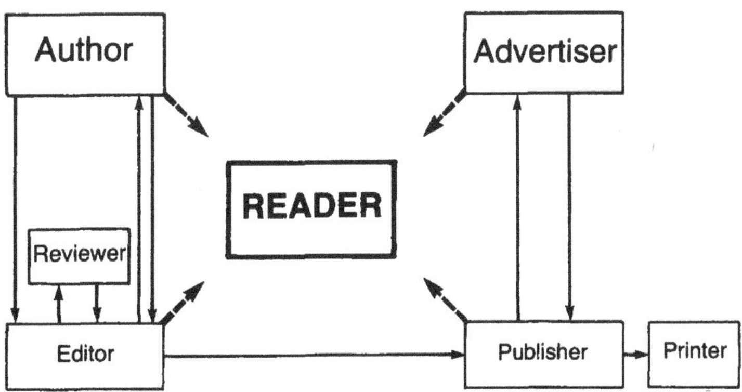

Reprinted from the March 15 issue of **The American Journal of Cardiology**, A Yorke Medical Journal. Published by Technical Publishing, a Division of Dun-Donnelly Publishing Corporation, a Company of The Dun & Bradstreet Corporation, 875 Third Avenue, New York, N.Y., 10022.

Abbreviations in the AJC

Some editors of medical journals allow abbreviations and others do not. I favor *limited numbers* of *appropriate abbreviations for commonly used terms* in articles submitted to the AJC for 2 reasons: (1) abbreviations save space and, therefore, permit more articles to be published, and (2) abbreviations, if limited to commonly used terms, decrease rather than increase reading time. In general, I prefer to limit abbreviations to 3 per manuscript and to the terms appearing in the manuscript's title.

An upcoming paper in the AJC was entitled "*Left ventricular* response to isometric exercise and its value in predicting the change in ventricular function after *mitral valve replacement* for *mitral regurgitation.*" The phrase "left ventricular" (occupying 16 spaces) appeared 38 times, "mitral regurgitation" (20 spaces) 28 times, and "mitral valve replacement" (24 spaces) 12 times. Spelling out these 3 phrases would have occupied 1,456 spaces, but by abbreviating each (LV, MVR, MR), only 168 spaces were used and 24 single-column lines were saved—an average of nearly 8 column lines per printed page. (Each column in the AJC contains 62 lines and each line, 54 spaces.) Another paper entitled "Relation between the site of origin of *ventricular tachycardia* and relative *left ventricular* myocardial perfusion and wall motion" used the phrase "ventricular tachycardia" (23 spaces) 57 times and the phrase "left ventricular" 42 times. Spelling out these 2 phrases would have occupied 1,983 spaces, but the abbreviations occupied only 198 spaces and 33 single-column lines were saved, an average of >8 column lines per printed page. Another recent paper entitled "Effect of *atrial fibrillation* on atrial blood flow in conscious dogs" used the phrase "atrial fibrillation" (19 spaces) at least 78 times and the single abbreviation "AF" saved 1,326 spaces or >24 lines. Because >40 articles appear now in each regular monthly AJC, averaging 228 text pages per issue, the savings in text pages each month by use of a few abbreviations is enormous, and this saving allows more articles to be published!

Abbreviations must be limited to *commonly recognized terms* (see later). Recently, I reviewed a manuscript which used the abbreviation "LVT," indicating "left ventricular thrombus." "LVT" is not a commonly recognized abbreviation and therefore I changed it to "LV thrombus," abbreviating "left ventricular" throughout but not "thrombus." Incidentally, the most commonly used phrase in cardiologic journals is "left ventricular"; hence, the abbreviation "LV" is highly useful. It should be noted that "LV" most commonly signifies "left ventricular," not "left ventricle," which is far less commonly used.

Not only must abbreviations be limited and of commonly used terms, but they must be *appropriate* in that *each letter of the abbreviation must stand for a single word.* It is inappropriate to use a letter for 1 word in a phrase, then use >1 letter for a second word in the same phrase. Specifically, it is inappropriate to abbreviate "hypertrophic cardiomyopathy" as "HCM"—this abbreviation breaks the rule of parallelism—1 letter stands for 1 word and a separate letter stands for each of 2 major syllables in the second word. The proper abbreviation is "HC." The commonly used abbreviations for the coronary arteries, namely, "RCA," "LAD," and "LCx" are not consistent. If "CA," the abbreviation for "coronary artery," is used after the "right" to read "RCA," then it should be used after the "left anterior descending" to read "LADCA" and after the "left circumflex" to read "LCCA." It is inappropriate to abbreviate 2 syllables in "circumflex" and not follow the same principle for the "anterior descending." It is best to abbreviate "left anterior descending" as "LAD" and "left circumflex" as "LC" (omitting the "x"), but not to abbreviate the "right coronary artery"; simply let it be known as "right."

Occasionally, it is warranted to make exception to the

abbreviation principle of 1 letter per word. The commonly used abbreviations for "electrocardiogram" (ECG), "atrioventricular" (AV), and "radionuclide angiography or angiocardiography" (RNA) are really inappropriate, but each is so ingrained that they have become appropriate. To abbreviate "electrocardiogram" as "E" or "atrioventricular" as "A" or "radionuclide angiography" as "RA" is confusing. An abbreviation for "echocardiogram" or "echocardiography" is another exception; probably "echo" is the most appropriate abbreviation for either word.

It is best to use certain terms universally to prevent confusion when abbreviating. The term "mitral regurgitation" is better than the term "mitral insufficiency" for several reasons; one is that it allows the abbreviation "MR," which prevents its confusion with "MI," which best stands for "myocardial infarction" or "infarct." Although obviously it would be consistent with the rule of parallelism to abbreviate "coronary heart disease" as "CHD," this might produce confusion with "congenital heart disease" and, therefore, it is preferable to allow "CAD" to signify both "coronary heart disease" and "coronary artery disease." To use the terms "*inter*atrial septal defect" and "*inter*ventricular septal defect" is undesirable because each implies that *extra*atrial or *extra*ventricular septal defects also exist. The prefix "inter" should be discarded. Of course, only 1 atrial septum and only 1 ventricular septum exist. Therefore, the proper terms are "atrial septal defect" (ASD) and "ventricular septal defect" (VSD), not "IASD" and "IVSD." On echocardiograms, the ventricular septum should be labeled "VS," not "IVS."

Finally, once initiated it is important to use abbreviations consistently throughout each page of a paper. When first appearing in both summary and introduction, the phrase to be abbreviated should be spelled out and thereafter abbreviated elsewhere in the manuscript.

Although abbreviations save enormous space, their use results in more time expended by authors, editors, and copy editors to ensure uniformity and appropriateness. It would save all 3 much time and effort if abbreviations were not allowed; but in our era of enormous expense for each published page and limited time to read each page, it is only proper that limited numbers of appropriately used abbreviations be permitted in manuscripts.

Some of the most commonly used standard cardiologic abbreviations are listed at right.

TERMS COMMONLY ABBREVIATED

AF = atrial fibrillation
AR = aortic regurgitation
AS = aortic stenosis
ASD = atrial septal defect
AV = atrioventricular
AVR = aortic valve replacement
BBB = bundle branch block
BP = blood pressure
CABG = coronary artery bypass grafting
CAD = coronary heart disease
CHF = congestive heart failure
Coronary arteries:
- LAD = left anterior descending
- LC = left circumflex
- LM = left main

ECG = electrocardiogram
echo = echocardiogram or echocardiography
EF = ejection fraction
HC = hypertrophic cardiomyopathy
LV = left ventricular
MI = myocardial infarct or infarction
MR = mitral regurgitation
MS = mitral stenosis
MVP = mitral valve prolapse
MVR = mitral valve replacement
PA = pulmonary artery
PDA = patent ductus arteriosus
RNA = radionuclide angiocardiography
RV = right ventricular
TF = tetralogy of Fallot
TGA = complete transposition of the great arteries
TR = tricuspid regurgitation
VF = ventricular fibrillation
VPC = ventricular premature complexes
VSD = ventricular septal defect
VT = ventricular tachycardia
WPW = Wolff-Parkinson-White syndrome

William C. Roberts

William C. Roberts, MD
Editor-in-Chief

References: A Clue to Scholarship

References are an important part of a manuscript. Their selection is an indicator of the author's knowledge of and regard for work preceding his own, and their accuracy of recording is a clue to the quality of the author's own work. Indeed, their selection and the accuracy of their recording is a clue to the scholarship of the manuscript. This piece examines the process of selecting references, suggests a procedure to record them accurately, and describes the reasons why references are listed as they are in the AJC.

The Selection Process: Some authors tend to support statements in their manuscripts by multiple references, but often when this is done, some references do not support the statement for which they are being used. Other authors provide few references and open themselves to criticism for not giving sufficient credit to their predecessors. Should the initial or latest work on the subject be cited, or simply the present author's previous work on the subject? A clear answer to this question is lacking. A middle course between "too many" and "too few" references appears most reasonable.

A frequent criticism by reviewers of manuscripts is that their work was not cited. Accordingly, the reviewer may feel slighted and may react by being overcritical. Reference to an individual increases the chance, however, that that person will review the manuscript in question. I certainly look at the references cited when deciding to whom I will send a manuscript for review. When reading a published or unpublished paper on which they too have contributed information, many author-readers review the list of references cited. I am reminded of a story regarding 2 prominent present-day authors. William Buckley sent his most recent book to John Kenneth Galbraith, who, upon receiving it, immediately turned to the title page, anticipating a note from his friend Buckley. Finding none, Galbraith turned to the list of references and beside the first citation of one of Galbraith's books, Buckley had written, "Hi, John, Bill."

Manuscripts containing innumerable references are more likely a sign of insecurity than a mark of scholarship. It requires enormous confidence to submit a manuscript devoid of references, but references may not be necessary if the data presented is entirely new. I sometimes see manuscripts with too many references and too little data. That a publication has been read during the preparation of a manuscript is not justification for its being cited as a reference. References, in other words, should not represent a list of publications read by the author—"how much work he (she) did," so to speak. In my own manuscripts, I tend to cite about one-half to two-thirds of the publications I read in preparing the manuscript. References should be carefully selected, the references cited should in general be for quality papers, they should clearly support the statement or comment to which they are attributed; and, just as a good paragraph should have no unnecessary sentences and a good sentence no unnecessary words, a manuscript should have no unnecessary references. Each reference, like each paragraph or sentence, should have a meaningful purpose.

In the Brief Reports section of the AJC, the number of references should be limited to 6 or fewer; in Letters to the Editor, usually to 3 or fewer.

Accuracy of Recording References: Many errors are made in recording references in manuscripts. Examine any 10 references in any medical journal and usually at least 1, often more, will contain an error. Errors in references represent inadequate regard for the work of previous researchers, and I suspect that inaccurately recorded references are found most frequently in manuscripts containing inadequately recorded data. Therefore, as an editor, as well as reader, I carefully examine all references in manuscripts submitted to the AJC. Names are frequently misspelled, initials preceding the last name are often wrong, and "Junior" or "III" occasionally are omitted. Titles often are recorded inaccurately and subtitles frequently are omitted. Volume numbers, page numbers, and year of publication often are erroneously recorded. A major source of error in citing a reference is recording a reference listed in another publication. In this situation, the error recorded in the first listing is propagated in the subsequent publication. The same careful attention should be given to references as is given to other aspects of a manuscript.

The following procedures have proved useful to me in diminishing errors in recording references for my own manuscripts.

1. Each reference initially is recorded on a 3- by 5-inch card and the writing is print rather than script to prevent subsequent misinterpretation when typed. All authors, full title with subtitle, volume, inclusive page numbers, and month and year of publication are recorded on these cards. If a reference is obtained from a previous author's reference list, a notation is made on the card that the original needs to be reviewed. The reason for recording the month of publication is that this ensures review of the original report because month of publication, of course, is not listed in published reference lists. Additionally, recording both the month and year of publication allows chronologic listing of references published in the same year on the same subject.

2. The senior or established author must check references recorded by young or relatively new investigators to ensure accuracy. Some medical institutions have librarians who check the accuracy of recorded references, but this is a luxury afforded by few medical centers or research institutions.

3. References are recorded only from the original publication. To cite a reference from a previously published reference list without checking the original publication is poor research. A medical publication should never be referenced without reading it!

4. References are *typed only once* and that is in final form in the final manuscript directly from the 3- by 5-inch cards on which they were originally recorded. The cards are numbered in pencil in the order in which they will appear. Having each reference on a separate card allows the author to change the order without altering the entire typed format.

5. The typed list of references is carefully proofed from the original 3- by 5-inch reference cards by the recorder of the references on the cards. This person can read his or her own handwriting better than anyone else. More typographical errors are made in typing references than in any other portion of a manuscript. Therefore, the single typing of references from the original reference cards prevents errors which occur from multiple typings.

6. The references in the galley proofs are again checked against the original 3- by 5-inch reference cards.

Listing of References in the AJC: References listed in the AJC are complete in that the names of *all authors*, *subtitles* as well as primary titles, and *inclusive page numbers* are required. Manuscripts submitted to the AJC with references in another format suggest that the paper has been submitted previously to another journal which rejected it, or that the authors are not sensitive students of medical publications. With text pages at a premium, why are all authors, all titles, and inclusive page numbers required in the AJC? By listing all authors, all titles, and inclusive page numbers (rather than just the first page number of the article), the authors of the manuscript are virtually required to check the original article, and this checking increases the likelihood that the entire reference is recorded accurately. Supplying all authors' names allows better identification of the investigators because the last author is more often better recognized than the first author, and by having all authors listed the editor is assisted in the selection of possible manuscript reviewers. (The last author is more likely to be a member of the journal's editorial board than is the first author.) The subtitle might provide more information regarding the actual substance of a publication than the primary title. Listing inclusive page numbers prevents the confusion of a reference to a previously published manuscript with a reference to an abstract, which is never more than 1 page. To diminish the space occupied by references without diminishing their accuracy or usefulness, the type size utilized for printing references in the AJC was significantly reduced beginning in the October 1982 issue.

In summary, references are a reflection of a manuscript's quality and should be selected carefully and recorded accurately.

William C. Roberts

William C. Roberts, MD
Editor-in-Chief

Changes in The AJC Since June 1982

This piece will describe certain visible and nonvisible changes in the AJC during the first 12 months (since June 1982) of the present editorship.

1. Alteration of the *Instructions-to-Authors* page came first. This page is an extremely important one and I encourage all authors submitting manuscripts to the AJC to read these Instructions carefully before the final typing of their manuscripts. I include a reprint of the Instructions page when returning a manuscript to an author requesting revision of his or her manuscript. In addition to the required stylistic changes delineated in the Instructions, authors are encouraged, as stated in this page, to suggest 1 or more nonlocal potentially objective reviewers and also potentially biased reviewers for their manuscripts. These suggestions have been quite useful to me, and, I hope, to the authors. I generally send a manuscript to 1 reviewer suggested by the authors and to 1 reviewer of my choosing. I never send a manuscript to a potentially biased reviewer if so requested by an author. The Instructions page also describes the method of having a manuscript reviewed blindly. This method of review is available to the submitting authors on request and this request is always honored by the editor.

2. The next change made was on the *Editorial Board* page. The board members were separated according to subspeciality.

3. The format of the *Title Page* was changed in October 1982 to make the content of this page more compact and the layout more attractive. Initially, both the title and authors' names were "flush left" but now each is centered.

4. The style and type size of the *References* was changed in October 1982. Although all authors as well as inclusive pages are now listed, the space occupied by each reference is considerably less than previously.

5. The *Table of Contents* page was changed in January 1982. The articles are now grouped by the various disease categories—Coronary, Valvular, Myocardial, Congenital, Arrhythmias and Conduction Disturbances, Systemic Hypertension, Congestive Heart Failure, etc. Exceptions to these categories include Methods, Cardiac Pharmacology, Experimental Studies, Brief Reports, Editorials, Point of View, Historical Studies, Letters, and The AJC 25 Years Ago.

6. The bottom half of the *Cover* was changed in January 1983 to include the general categories of the table of contents.

7. The Letters to the Editor were retitled simply *Letters* and in March 1983 they were laid out in 3-column rather than 2-column format to add variation. The layout of this section was made more compact, and a request was inserted on the initial "letter page" of each issue indicating that a letter concerning an article published in the AJC must be received from USA readers within 2 months of the article's publication.

8. A *Brief Report* section was added in September 1982. These are primarily single case reports and they now average about 1.4 printed pages apiece, including figures.

9. The *Point-of-View* section was added in March 1983. This section is intended to provide a medium for brief presentation of a concept or idea. The idea may or may not be provable and references are not required. The section may be considered in the category of a "capsule editorial." The editorial, in contrast, is a well-developed thesis.

10. *Quotations*, inserted on empty spaces of pages at the end of individual articles, began appearing in February 1983. These will focus primarily, but not entirely, on scientific matters. I would be pleased to receive quotations from any reader and if the quotation appears, appropriate credit will be given to the submitter.

11. The *From-the-Editor* page began in July 1982, initially to emphasize some items described in the Instructions to Authors page, and has continued with discussions of the manuscript review process, relations between authors, editors, reviewers, publishers, and advertisers, and viewpoints on various portions of a manuscript. It is my intent to continue these columns for awhile.

12. A new section entitled "The AJC 25 Years Ago" was added in May 1983 and will be a monthly feature hereafter.

As the foregoing changes were being implemented, a number of other changes also were taking place. A strenuous attempt has been made to make each manuscript more compact so that there is more content per page for the reader without an increase in the *Journal*'s size or price. During this first year, the average content per page has increased by slightly over 20%. The means by which this increased content per page was made possible are the following: (1) The title page is more compact. (2) The references are smaller than previously, and in recent months, fewer in number. (3) More figures and tables occupy only a half column rather than portions of 2 columns. (4) Less space is now (last 2 months only) retained between figures and/or tables and the text. (5) An additional line in each column was acquired by deleting the Journal's title at the bottom of each page. (6) The use of abbreviations, numbers (<10 as well as >10) and symbols has saved many lines per page. I prefer no more than 3 abbreviations per manuscript and that they be limited to commonly recognized cardiologic terms, preferably those appearing in the article's title. The symbols for percent (%), less than (<) and greater than (>) save space and decrease reading time. It takes 36 spaces to spell out the first 9 numbers (1 to 9), but only 9 spaces are utilized when numbers are used, a 4-fold savings of space.

Moreover, the publisher is providing more pages per issue than a year ago. Comparison of 4 items in the last 2 months of the previous editorship (May to June 1982) with the 2 latest months (before this piece went to press) under the present editorship is illustrated in the table. The number of articles published between these 2 periods increased 52% while the number of pages published increased only 8%. The average number of pages per article decreased 29%. Although the number of lines per page

COMPARISON OF MAY-JUNE 1982 AJC TO FEBRUARY-MARCH 1, 1983 AJC

	Combined 5/82 + 6/82	Combined 2/83 + 3/83	Percent Change
Number of papers	64	97	+52
Average number of pages per paper	7.5	5.3	−29
Number of pages	480	519	+ 8
Number of lines per column	61	62	+ 2

(2 columns per page) increased by nearly 2%, the utilization of a single additional line per page potentially provides 4 additional full pages per issue and 48 additional pages per year.

In addition to the visible changes made in the *Journal* in the past 12 months, several visible changes have been made in the processing of manuscripts: (1) The *reviewer forms* have been changed so that 1 entire page is for "confidential comments to the editor" and another for "comments to the authors." The editor has requested all reviewers to answer the following question on the "confidential" page: "Would you grant the editor permission to make the authors aware of who reviewed their manuscript?" (2) All manuscripts now are sent to reviewers in thick blue-and-white *container folders* which help in the organization of the text, figures, tables, and review forms. (3) New blue-and-white *mailing envelopes* have been provided. (4) *Personal letters* from the editor now accompany all manuscripts returned to authors and to nonboard reviewers when requesting a review.

The intent of most of these changes in the *Journal* is to increase content per page and this translates into increased content per issue. Suggestions for further improvements to the *Journal* are always welcomed by the editor.

William C. Roberts

William C. Roberts, MD
Editor-in-Chief

The Summary: The Manuscript's Bottom Line

Through the years I have asked numerous readers of medical journals which journal they read monthly and how they select which articles to read in a particular journal. The responses to the latter question indicate that the most frequent portion of a manuscript read is the manuscript's title, and next the manuscript's summary. If the latter is unappealing, most readers do not pursue other portions of the manuscript. But is the summary given the same attention by the author as it is given by the reader? I think not.

When writing medical papers with young associates, rarely have I been presented with a rough draft of a manuscript containing a summary. The summary, I suspect, tends to be written by many authors just before the final typing of the manuscript. Thus, when written last, the summary tends to be disjointed as it attempts to tie together the important points of the paper. When written first, the summary serves as an outline, focusing the thrust of the manuscript. Moreover, by being done last, the summary may not receive the thoughtful deliberation given other portions of the manuscript.

Because the summary is so important to a manuscript, I suggest that an author write this portion *first* (after the title) rather than last. By so doing, one may focus better on the number of points the particular manuscript is trying to make. If the manuscript has essentially only 1 point, the summary can be particularly crisp and short; if more than 1 point, the summary provides an outline of the points to be made. After the point or points of the manuscript are clearly in focus, the remainder of the paper can more readily build the case demonstrating the validity of each point. The summary then needs to be given the same emphasis and importance by authors as it receives from readers.

William C. Roberts

William C. Roberts, MD
Editor-in-Chief

Season's Greeting and the Best for 1984

This Journal owes much to its readers, its contributors, its reviewers and its advertisers. In 1983 the Journal published more pages, more issues and more articles than any cardiovascular journal in the world. The authors contribute their articles without compensation; the reviewers contribute their time and expertise without compensation, and the non-board reviewers do so without any overt recognition. Thus, to the *readers*, thanks for your support; to the *authors*, thanks for your manuscripts; to the *reviewers*, thanks for your unselfish and invaluable recommendations and suggestions, and to the *advertisers*, thanks for the support which makes all this possible. Thanks also to my assistant, Ann K. Bradley, who superbly manages the editorial office in Bethesda, to Maggie Ann Inman, the Managing Editor in New York, and her staff for a job well done, and to Robert T. Brawn, the Publisher, for his strong support through the year. The nicest gifts the Journal receives are a new subscriber and a renewing subscriber, a superb manuscript, an excellent review of a manuscript, a quality ad, and, of course, a satisfied reader and a satisfied author. The best from all of us to all of you for a most satisfying 1984.

William C. Roberts

William C. Roberts, MD
Editor-in-Chief

Studying the "Instructions to Authors" Before Final Typing of a Manuscript for Submission to a Medical Journal

In this issue appears a revised (since 18 months ago) "Instructions to Authors." These instructions, when followed, save much time for authors and editors. Since becoming editor of the AJC, I have become acutely aware of the importance of the items mentioned in these instructions. The first change instituted after becoming editor 19 months ago was to revamp these instructions. Manuscripts that have followed the instructions to the letter are processed more expeditiously than are those that have ignored the instructions. I must confess, however, that before becoming editor of the AJC, I seldom spent much time on the instructions of a particular medical journal to which I was submitting a manuscript. Since becoming editor, however, I now give close scrutiny to these instructions because following them immediately attracts an editor's friendly eye and, most importantly, speeds up the manuscript's processing time. Study of the instructions is especially important when a manuscript is submitted to a medical journal with a short "lag time," and this period between acceptance and publication of a manuscript now averages 3.5 months in the AJC.

The following are the most common technical errors in manuscripts submitted to the AJC and all could be prevented if the instructions were carefully read and followed:

1. *References are not in the format of the AJC:* The names of authors are incomplete. (All names are required, not just the first 3.) Inclusive pages are omitted. Subtitles are omitted.

2. *Numbers are spelled out.* Numerals should be used, even for numbers less than 10.

3. *"Percent", "less than" and "greater than"* are spelled out. Symbols should be used (%, <, >).

4. *Abbreviations are inappropriate, inconsistent and excessive.* Only commonly recognized cardiologic phrases should be abbreviated after their initial spelled-out appearance followed by the abbreviation in both abstract and introduction, and the abbreviation should be used on every page of the manuscript, not just the article's abstract. The number of abbreviations should be limited to 3 or 4 and usually only to terms appearing in the title (See From-the-Editor column, April 1983).

5. *The miniabstract for the table of contents is omitted.* The AJC requires a full abstract for the manuscript proper and a miniabstract for the table of contents page. The latter should appear on a separate but unnumbered page and should include at its top the article's full title with the names of all authors.

6. *A running title of 3 to 6 words is omitted.*

7. *Key words for indexing are omitted.*

8. *Tables are too busy.* In most articles, only a single line should be used for individual patient or nonhuman animal data. The symbols "+" or "0" or "−" (no information available) should be used rather than "yes" or "no" or "positive" or "negative" or "none." The units of measurement should be stated at the top of a column and not after each item. Abbreviations used in tables should be so stated alphabetically at the bottom of the table.

9. *Figures are uncropped, not combined and mounted.* Multiple-part figures should be cropped, combined (if >1 in a figure) and taped together (unmounted) on their back.

William C. Roberts

William C. Roberts, MD
Editor-in-Chief

The AJC in '83

Elsewhere in this issue (page 862) appears an article comparing *quantitatively* the editorial contents of 7 cardiology journals for the year 1983. Although it throws favorable light on the AJC, the article's intent was not to bolster the AJC, but to examine in a scientific fashion the amount of space available in each of 7 English-language cardiology journals for publication of medical information and also to examine how that space was utilized. The article in no way examines the *quality* of the content in any of the 7 journals. During the past 18 months of the present editorship, an attempt has been made to increase the amount of content on each page of the AJC. In 1983, the AJC published at least 20% more content per page and an average of 44% more articles in its regular issues than did the other 3 cardiologic journals published in the U.S.A. The increase in the number of articles published and content per page was produced by (1) requiring authors to abide by certain length limitations in their manuscripts, (2) cropping figures and reducing the space they occupied (fitting them as often as possible into 1 rather than 2 columns), (3) "tightening" of tables so that the space they occupied was diminished, (4) using appropriate abbreviations, (5) using numerals at all times (except when they began sentences), and (6) increasing the number of lines per column. Excluding symposia sponsored by grants from pharmaceutical companies, 643 articles (average of 4.9 pages per article) were published in the AJC in 1983, and 389 articles (average 7.6 pages per article) were published in 1982, a 40% increase in the number of articles published.

The amount of content published in most medical journals increases with time. In 1958, the first year of the AJC, only 117 articles occupying 778 pages appeared. In 1983, 643 articles were published in its 15 regular issues, occupying 3,250 pages, and in addition, 60 articles occupying 341 pages were published in its 5 supplemental symposia. In 1958, each article was written by an average of 1.8 authors; by 1983, this average had increased to 4.7 authors per article. The cost of an individual U.S.A. subscription to the AJC in 1958 was $12.00, and in 1983, $52.00, a 4-fold increase in cost; but a 4.6-fold increase in number of pages published (778 to 3,591) and a 6-fold increase in the number of articles published offset this cost increase. Compared with 1958, the number of figures and tables published in the AJC in 1983 had increased 7-fold (from 292 to 2,033) and 5-fold (from 161 to 1,154), respectively. The indexes in 1958 occupied only 10 pages; in 1983, they occupied 79 pages, nearly an 8-fold increase.

But is this intent to increase the amount of content in the AJC a proper one? The new editor of CIRCULATION has gone the other direction. Which viewpoint is correct? My view is that cardiology has become so specialized that only a few articles in each issue of any cardiology journal appeal to a particular reader. The articles on arrhythmias and conduction disturbances appeal to a highly specialized group of cardiologists. The reader interested in the articles concerning coronary heart disease probably has little interest in the articles concerning congenital heart disease, but both deserve their space. The AJC in 1983 had 79 articles on congenital heart disease, whereas the other 3 major USA cardiology journals combined had only 63. Thus, to satisfy the diversity of cardiologic readership, many articles on varied subjects are necessary, and the AJC attempts to satisfy these varied interests.

William C. Roberts

William C. Roberts, MD
Editor-in-Chief

Further Comments on the "Instructions to Authors"

Every scientific journal has its "Instructions to Authors" (or "Information for Contributors"), a description of the requirements and specifications expected in a manuscript submitted to that journal for consideration of publication. The "Instructions" most often occupies a single page, occasionally 2 pages, in each issue of the journal. Occasionally, the "Instructions" appear only once per volume, usually the volume's initial issue. The "Instructions" page is important to submitting authors because it provides a clue to certain items considered important by the editor, who, of course, is responsible for providing the "accept" or "reject" verdict on every manuscript. When I became editor of *The American Journal of Cardiology* 2 years ago, the first alteration I made was to revamp the "Instructions to Authors" page. After 18 months in the Editor's chair, I made further alterations in the "Instructions" to include additional specifications for submitted manuscripts. I also send a copy of these "Instructions" to each author to whom a manuscript is returned for revision after review. Thus, these "Instructions" are important to editors, to managing editors and to copyeditors, for much time is saved for all of them when the "Instructions" are followed by authors. Preparation of manuscripts according to the "Instructions" is particularly important when a manuscript is submitted to a scientific journal with a short "lag time," the period between acceptance of and publication of a manuscript, and this period in the AJC averages 3.5 months.

But why is complying with a particular journal's "Instructions" important to authors? *Because this compliance by an author improves the possibility that the manuscript wil be accepted for publication*! Technical excellence is a clue to scientific excellence. The 2 tend to go together. The best manuscripts submitted to the AJC from a scientific standpoint nearly always have been prepared in accordance with the specifications delineated in the "Instructions to Authors," and the scientifically inferior manuscripts are rarely prepared in accordance with the "Instructions." Because scientific editors are not experts in the subject matter of all submitted manuscripts, final decisions on some scientifically borderline manuscripts hinge on their technical and craftsmanship features. Furthermore, compliance to the "Instructions" demonstrates sensitivity on the part of authors to items viewed important to editors; therefore, those manuscripts prepared according to the journals' specifications immediately attract the editor's friendly eye. Conversely, a submitted manuscript that has obviously not been prepared according to the journal's "Instructions" may evoke immediate annoyance on the part of the editor and suggest carelessness, insensitivity and amateurism on the part of the author.

Authors also should be aware that editors are careful students of the "Instructions to Authors" of their competing journals. References, for example, prepared according to the style of a competitor's journal suggest that the manuscript has already been rejected, which is of no consequence to me, but, more importantly, suggests that no revisions have been made in the manuscript before submission to another journal. Thus, when a manuscript is prepared for submission to 1 journal and is rejected, the manuscript will usually need retyping before submission to another journal so that it complies with the specifications of the new journal, because no 2 journals have identical "Instructions." Because the acceptance rate today in most major scientific journals is relatively low, or, to state differently, far more manuscripts are submitted to the major scientific journals than can possibly be accepted and published in them, retyping of manuscripts according to the "Instructions" often must be done more than once.

Finally, compliance to the "Instructions" must be done eventually in all manuscripts before they can be accepted. Manuscripts prepared not in accordance with the journal's "Instructions" have to be returned to the authors for correction. Because the manuscript must be technically correct before it is published, it adds little additional effort to make it technically correct when it is submitted initially. Compliance, in other words, cannot be avoided if the manuscript is to be published. Initial compliance is a sign of respect for both the journal and the journal's editor and this respect is returned to authors by increasing the chance of acceptance of their manuscript.

William C. Roberts

William C. Roberts, MD
Editor-in-Chief

Editorial Board Changes

The manuscript reviewers for the AJC as of September 1984 number 1,120 scientists; of them, 127 (11%) are members of the AJC's editorial board. This month, 22 members left the editorial board because their services were underutilized, for varying reasons, by the editor and because certain non-board, frequent reviewers deserved recognition, namely board status, for their unselfish efforts. Of the 31 new board members added this month, all but 1 had reviewed for the AJC during the preceding 18 months 4 to 14 manuscripts (mean 7.5). The reviews were of excellent quality and they were prepared promptly.

The following letter was sent to the retiring board members:

Dear ________________:

As of July 1984, you will have served for 2 years as a member of the AJC. I have decided to make some changes of board members beginning September 1984, and wish to thank you for having served this 2-year term as a board member. A number of previously non-board reviewers also have helped me considerably during these past 2 years and it is only fair to provide them board status in recognition of their perceptive and prompt reviews during this time. I hope, however, that I may continue to ask you to review an occasional manuscript for the AJC, and I hope also that you will continue to submit fine manuscripts to the AJC. Again, thanks.

Best regards,

The letter sent to 32 reviewers inviting them to be board members was the following (31 accepted):

Dear ________________:

During the past 2 years you have helped the AJC considerably by your fine and prompt reviews of manuscripts. As a token of recognition of your past efforts and for expected similar efforts in the future, I invite you to become a member of the editorial board of the AJC beginning September 1984. Your acceptance of this invitation carries with it the obligation to continue to review manuscripts submitted to the AJC and to review them within the allotted time frame. Board members of the AJC review a maximum of 1 manuscript each month. Of the 118 board members in 1983, however, only 10 (9%) reviewed more than 10 manuscripts. It is essential that reviews by board members be prompt. From the time the manuscript leaves the editor's office until it is due back in the editor's office, a period of 3 weeks is allocated. The mails, however, being what they are, require that the manuscript be retained by the reviewer no more than about 7–10 days. If you will not be able to fulfill this time requirement, please do not accept this offer to become a board member. If you can, however, the AJC would be honored to have you as a member of the board. Please let me hear from you promptly on your willingness or unwillingness to serve. If you wish to discuss any item with me, please give me a call (301/496-5203 or 301/656-3923). Thanks so much.

Best regards,

In addition to the changes made in the editorial board last month, I am pleased to announce the appointment of 2 Associate Editors. I have delayed the appointment of Associate Editors for 28 months because I was uncertain how best to utilize their talents and because I was a bit uncertain what talents I was seeking. Editorship of the AJC has progressively taken more of my time because of the steady increase in the number of new manuscripts received each month. It is now unwise to be away from the editor's desk for longer than 2 days because upon return, the accumulated stacks of newly received manuscripts, of those back from reviewers, and of revised manuscripts back from authors require such extended effort that it is not worth the pleasure derived from the absence. Thus, the initial task of the 2 Associate Editors will be to "run the ship" when I'm away. Gradually, I expect both Associate Editors, however, to play widened, but as yet less defined, editorial roles when I am in town. I am confident that both reader and author will be pleased with their performance.

One Associate Editor is *William P. Baker, MD, PhD*, a 57-year-old native of Albion, Illinois, a cum laude MD graduate of the University of Michigan, the husband of Gwen Baker, the father of 3 daughters, and Chief of the Cardiology Division at the Naval Hospital, Bethesda, Maryland. Bill is Professor of Medicine at both the Uniformed Services University of the Health Sciences and at George Washington University. Presently, Bill is a member of the Advisory Council of the National Heart, Lung, and Blood Institute (NHLBI), and in the past was a member of the NHLBI Subcommittee of the Multiple Risk Factor Intervention Trial (MRFIT), the NHLBI Circulatory Assistance and Artificial Heart Working Group, and the Federal Health Resources Sharing Committee.

The other Associate Editor is *Paul A. Tibbits, MD*, a 38-year-old native of New Orleans, Louisiana, a graduate of Tulane Medical School, the husband of Dr. (PhD) Mercedes Tibbits, the father of a boy and a girl, and for the past 5 years, a member of the Cardiology Division of the Naval Hospital, Bethesda, Maryland. Paul received (1976) the Surgeon General's Award for Scholastic Achievement in 1976. He is Assistant Professor of Medicine of the Uniformed Services University of the Health Sciences, a member of the Scientific Review Committee of the Naval Hospital, and a member of the Tri-Service Medical Information System Committee.

William C. Roberts

William C. Roberts, MD
Editor-in-Chief

Writing Versus Editing

For nearly 25 years my professional fate was determined by what I wrote and had published in medical journals. One of the hardest lessons for me to learn during that long period was that creating, "packaging," and publishing of new ideas really never got easier. Although the focusing and writing got easier, standards continued to improve, and therefore, the amount of time and energy—both physical and mental—expended continued to be about the same for each major published investigation. This period of trying to go to work every day with a new idea was obviously challenging, but enormously rewarding and fulfilling. To have a position that stretches one's potential to the fullest and to be paid for this work is certainly one of life's greatest blessings.

After this near 25-year production period, the editorship of a major cardiovascular journal was offered. Again, a mentally and physically "stretching" position, but, unlike writing, one that involves not creating new ideas, but determining which ones of those created, and to some extent in what form, reach the cardiovascular community. Editing, however, is quite different from writing. Writing is relatively lonely and selfish. One's time must be enormously protected to create new ideas and publish them. Editing, in contrast, is relatively social and unselfish in that it requires much communication with authors, publishers and readers. But after nearly 25 years in the other role, the change to editorship is surprisingly easy to make. Of the 2, however, editing is much easier than writing, judging is much easier than creating; it is the creator who will provide the significant change, and deservedly so, not the judger of the creator's work.

William C. Roberts

William C. Roberts, MD
Editor-in-Chief

A Good Year—1984

This month completes an upbeat year in America. A feeling of optimism abounds. More Americans have jobs than ever before, incomes are highest in history, the dollar is strong; inflation rates, interest rates, cigarette sales, and hospital admissions are down, and stock prices are up. The Olympics made us all athletes for 2 weeks.

It was a good year for the AJC also. Compared with 1983, the number of articles published in its 15 regular issues increased 16% (643 to 747), despite a 2% decrease in the number of pages published; the number of manuscripts submitted in the 6 months preceding October 1, 1984, increased 27% compared to the same period in 1983; the number of symposia published increased from 5 to 11; the number of subscribers increased 6%, and the number of ad pages increased 2%. Despite the increase in number of manuscripts submitted, the interval from acceptance to publication has remained short (average <4 months). The high quality of most submitted manuscripts, however, is making the accept-reject decision increasingly difficult. Far more manuscripts receive favorable review than can be published. The quality of the reviews and the promptness of their completion continue to improve. Fewer late reviews are received now than a year ago. The Journal is now received by USA subscribers on or near the first day of the month, an improvement by several days from a year ago.

Thus, the AJC owes much to many. Thanks to the readers who inspire us to do better. Thanks to the authors for sending us their superb manuscripts. Thanks to the reviewers who devote their time unselfishly to assure the high standards for which we all strive. Thanks to Ann Bradley for managing the Bethesda editorial office so effectively and efficiently and to Maggie Inman for managing the AJC New York operation similarly. Thanks to the advertisers for making all this possible, and thanks to Paul Carnese, our new publisher whom I already consider a friend after his being at the helm only a few months, for making all our work a little easier.

Best wishes to all for the New Year.

William C. Roberts

William C. Roberts, MD
Editor-in-Chief

A Suggestion to Lighten the Load of Manuscript Reviewing

One of the most unselfish acts performed by productive members of the medical academic community is the reviewing of manuscripts submitted for publication by others. The time devoted to this task can be considerable, particularly so for the more prominent members of academia. Many leaders of academia are on the boards of several medical journals simultaneously—not because their names add prestige to the journal, but because they are wise and prompt reviewers whose counsel is widely sought. But reviewing manuscripts takes time away from their own tasks and too much energy expended on others subtracts time devoted to their own creative efforts.

An unfortunate principle of the peer-review process is that the best manuscripts receive the fewest reviews and the worst manuscripts receive the most reviews. The best manuscripts are usually accepted by the first journal to which they are sent. Therefore, they receive 1 to 3 reviews, depending on the policy of the particular journal; the manuscript usually is revised to varying degrees, and then accepted. The process for the less-than-superb or the inferior manuscript is not so rapid. The first journal to which the manuscript is sent may acquire 2 reviews for it, and when neither reviewer recommends acceptance and the editor agrees, the manuscript with the reviews is returned to the submitting author. Then the latter usually submits the manuscript to another journal, ideally after having revised the manuscript as suggested by the reviewers from the first submission. The editor of the journal receiving the previously rejected manuscript then sends it to 2 more reviewers—on occasion, to one who happened to have reviewed the manuscript for the first journal. These reviewers in turn often also provide unfavorable recommendations for the manuscript. The editor then returns the rejected manuscript to the authors, who in turn send it to another journal with or without additional revisions. The duplication process continues.

To prevent this depletion of reviewers' energies and also to prevent further publication delay, I suggest to authors who submit a manuscript rejected by another journal to the AJC that the authors enclose copies of all reviews from the previous journal, a copy of the original manuscript, 3 copies of the revised manuscript, and a response to all items raised by all reviewers from the previous journal. In other words, the response to the reviews from the previous journal should be identical to the response given reviews had they been sent from the AJC. This procedure might allow the AJC editor to make a rapid accept or reject decision on the manuscript, or it might allow him to send the manuscript for reexamination to only 1 reviewer rather than 2. The editor may choose to enclose the reviews from the previous journals' reviewers with the revised manuscript for the new reviewer.

I would welcome a thorough evaluation of this time-saving process and I will do my best not to be offended because the manuscript had not been sent initially to the AJC. I also urge other editors of cardiovascular journals to adopt the same procedure, because all 4 major USA cardiovascular journals essentially use the same pool of reviewers. The concept needs full testing so that the energies for reviewing will be conserved and those energies expended will be utilized more effectively and efficiently.

William C. Roberts

William C. Roberts, MD
Editor-in-Chief

Brief Reports in the AJC in 1984

The September 1982 From-the-Editor column in the AJC was entitled "Brief Reports." In this column, I naively envisioned publication of about 2 or 3 Brief Reports each month thereafter. Two or 3 a month, of course, would amount to 24 to 36 each year. In 1984 a total of 204 Brief Reports were published in the AJC, an average of 17 each month. The 204 Brief Reports occupied 308 published pages, an average of 26 pages each month or 1.5 published pages for each Brief Report. Included in the 204 Brief Reports were 432 figures, an average of 2.12 figures per Brief Report or 1.40 figures per Brief Report page, and 56 tables, an average of 0.27 tables per Brief Report or 0.18 tables per Brief Report page. The 204 Brief Reports accounted for 27% of the 747 articles published in the AJC in 1984, but the 308 pages utilized for Brief Reports accounted for only 10% of the 3,077 pages for articles.

Although Brief Reports are often thought of as "Case Reports," the 2 actually are not synonyms. Of the 204 Brief Reports published in 1984, only 122 (60%) involved 1 patient; 33 (16%) involved 2 patients; 12 (6%), 3 patients; 8 (4%), 4 patients; 5 (2%), 5 patients; 4 (2%), 6 to 10 patients; 9 (4%), 11 to 25 patients; 3 (1.5%), 26 to 50 patients, and 7, over 50 patients. One of the latter reports involved 2,418 patients. The 1 feature characterizing all Brief Reports in the AJC is brevity—not the number of patients described.

The percentage of cardiac diseases discussed in the Brief Reports was a bit different from that of the major articles appearing in the same year. The types of cardiac diseases discussed in the 204 Brief Reports compared with those discussed in the 489 *major* articles (excludes 15 From-the-Editor columns, 11 historical articles and 28 editorials or points or view) were: coronary heart disease, 16% (Brief Reports) vs 29% (full-length articles); arrhythmias and conduction disturbances, 22% vs 15%; systemic hypertension, 0.5% vs 4%; congestive heart failure, 1% vs 2%; valvular heart disease, 8% vs 8%; cardiomyopathy, 7% vs 4%; congenital heart disease, 21% vs 10%; methods, 2% vs 6%; cardiovascular pharmacology, 1% vs 2%; pericardial heart disease, 2.5% vs 0.5%; miscellaneous, 19% vs 6%; and experimental studies (non-human animals), 0% vs 13%. Thus, the largest number of Brief Reports concerned arrhythmias and conduction disturbances (n = 45), followed by congenital heart disease (n = 43), miscellaneous topics (n = 38), coronary heart disease (n = 32), valvular heart disease (n = 16), cardiomyopathy (n = 15), and all others (n = 15).

I believe the Brief Reports are useful and popular, and I welcome comments from readers on their usefulness.

William C. Roberts

William C. Roberts, MD
Editor-in-Chief

The "Hot Eye" and the "Cold Eye"

For many years I submitted manuscripts to medical journals for publication immediately after the final draft had been typed. Before the final typing I would check the manuscript carefully for accuracy, clarity and precision of meaning, conciseness of expression and for errors in grammar, punctuation and spelling. Then, when the manuscript was returned from the journal's editor for revision after the 1- to 3-month review process, I was always surprised on reexamining the manuscript that I was almost always able to detect some minor inaccuracy or able to delete 1 or more paragraphs that now did not seem so pertinent, or more concisely describe a method, result or idea. Why could these improvements not have been accomplished before the initial submission of the manuscript?

The answer, I believe, has to do with the "hot-eye"–"cold-eye" concept. Before initial submission of the manuscript, 1 draft was followed by another without essentially any cooling-off period between the various manuscript drafts. The manuscript in this circumstance may be thought of as being examined with a "hot eye" (Figure). Return of the manuscript to the author after the 1- to 3-month review process provides a needed cooling-off period for the authors so that now the manuscript can be reexamined with a "cold eye" (Figure). This first reexamination allows authors to identify previously unrecognized errors, unwarranted conclusions, flawed reasonings, exaggerated statements, redundancies, needless words, sentences and paragraphs, and grammatical and spelling errors. I am convinced that this cooling-off period provides such an opportunity for manuscript improvement that even manuscripts in which both reviewers and editor have found few or no faults usually are returned to the authors for reexamination.

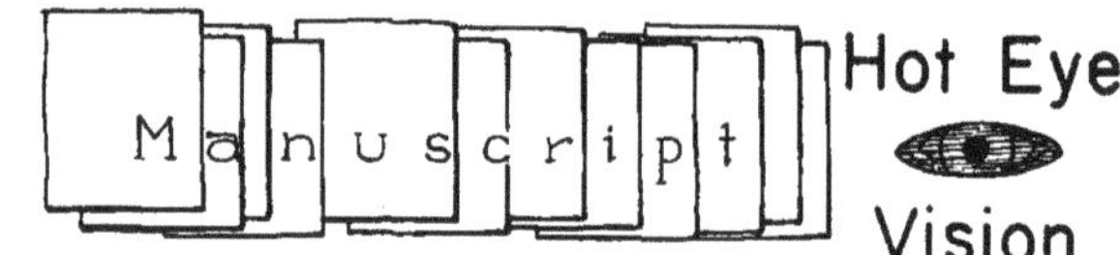

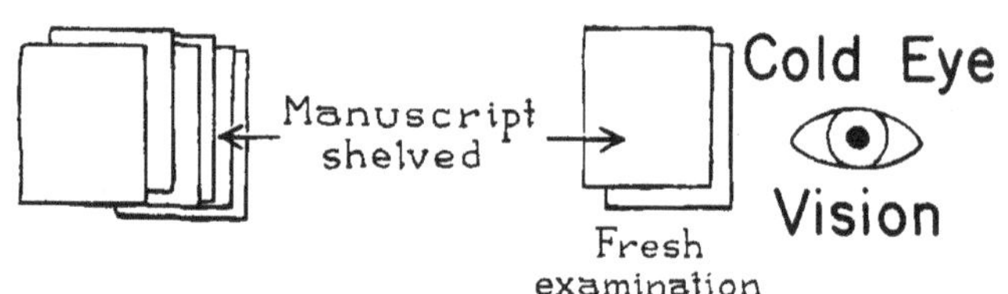

One reason almost any editor or reviewer can find defects in the work of almost any writer, however talented, is that they view the manuscript with a "cold eye" because they have not seen it before. The cooling-off period provided for authors by the review process allows the author to review his manuscript more like an editor or reviewer—with a "cold eye." I suspect that all of our manuscripts would be improved if we shelved them for a week or so before our final check preceding the final typing for initial submission to a medical journal.

William C. Roberts

William C. Roberts, MD
Editor in Chief

The Article's Title

The only part of an article read by most readers is the title. Much new medical information can be acquired, however, simply by reading the article's title, if it is a good one. Although it is the most frequently read part of a manuscript, the title is given too little attention by most authors. Indeed, the last thing written by many authors, just before the final typing of their manuscript, is the manuscript's title. The title, if done in this manner, may be more of an afterthought and not of the same standards as other portions of the manuscript.

Whenever I write an article the first words put on paper are those of the article's title. Then with each revision of the manuscript the title is carefully reexamined and usually reworded. Usually the article's title is changed several times before the final typing of the manuscript. Focusing on the title requires careful focusing on the actual contents of the manuscript because the title should be a precise description of those contents. Often I have read manuscripts and was surprised that their titles did not portray what was actually in the article's contents. As Fishbein has stated, "Thousands of papers lie buried in medical literature because their titles did not designate the subject." [1] I change the titles of most articles accepted for publication in the AJC. The change in some may be the deletion or addition of only 1 or 2 words. In others, the change may be extensive. My title changes are made before the manuscript is returned to the authors for revision so that they can approve the changes. If the changes are made on the revised manuscript, the authors are always informed of these changes so that they have an opportunity to approve or disapprove of them.

What constitutes a good title? Above all, as already mentioned, the title should be descriptive of the manuscript's contents. This description should not be in general terms but in as specific and precise terms as possible. The title should be devoid of excessive words but sufficient in words to adequately describe the manuscript's contents. The title should have a smooth flow. Although one could readily argue otherwise, in my view, the message of the manuscript should not be the manuscript's title. The title ideally should arouse the reader's curiosity so that he or she will go past the title into the manuscript's contents. If the manuscript's message is in the title, the curiosity may be immediately satisfied and the next article is then sought. Subtitles, in my view, should be avoided. Subtitles often are more specific than the main title and, therefore, they deserve to be the main title or at least incorporated into the main title. A minor factor against use of subtitles is that often when articles containing subtitles are referenced, the subtitle is omitted from the reference. This practice, of course, is wrong. Titles of experimental studies should include the animal species on which the studies are done so that the reader knows before beginning the article that the study is an experimental one. Titles as questions generally should be avoided. Abbreviations in titles should be avoided. Occasionally, use of italics for 1 or 2 words in a title provides useful emphasis.

Cardiologic titles are of many types, but common recurring ones can be identified. The first 2 words of these common ones immediately characterize the type of manuscript and include the following: Analysis of . . . , Association of . . . , Comparison of . . . , Effect of . . . , Efficacy of . . . , Evaluation of . . . , Importance of . . . , Influence of . . . , Limitations of . . . , Relation of . . . , Results of . . . , Usefulness of . . . , and Value of . . . . The remainder of this piece will provide specific examples of some of my changes in titles in a 3-month period in 1985 in manuscripts submitted to the AJC.

Excessive Words

(1) "*Effects of Coenzyme Q10 on Exercise Tolerance in Chronic Stable Angina: A Double Blind Randomized, Placebo-Controlled Crossover Trial.*" The last 8 words were deleted.

(2) "*Interhospital Transport of Patients With Ongoing Intraaortic Balloon Pumping: A Five-Year Experience.*" The last 4 words were deleted.

(3) "*The Clinical Utility of Two-Dimensional Echocardiography in Patients With Suspected Aortic Root Dissection*" to "*Utility of 2-Dimensional Echocardiography in Suspected Ascending Aortic Dissection.*" The phrases "in patients," "in a case of" and "in man" usually can be deleted.

Insufficient Wording

(1) *"Unrecognized Myocardial Infarction Detected in Geriatric Patients"* to *"Unrecognized Q-Wave Myocardial Infarction in Patients Over 64 Years of Age in a Long-Term Health-Care Facility."*

(2) *"Extravascular Lung Water in Children With Atrial Septal Defect"* to *"Extravascular Lung Water in Children Immediately After Operative Closure of Either Atrial Septal Defect or Ventricular Septal Defect."*

(3) *"Echocardiographic Assessment of Right Ventricular and Pulmonary Artery Size in Children With Atrial Septal Defect"* to *"Usefulness of Echocardiographic Assessment of Right Ventricular and Pulmonary Trunk Size For Estimating Magnitude of Left-to-Right Shunt in Children With Atrial Septal Defect."*

Imprecise Description of Manuscript's Contents

(1) *"Cardiac Rehabilitation of Children After Surgical Repair of Cyanotic Congenital Heart Disease"* to *"Effect of Intense Aerobic Training on Exercise Performance in Children After Surgical Repair of Either Tetralogy of Fallot or Complete Transposition of the Great Arteries."*

(2) *"Effects of Hydralazine on Pressure-Volume and Stress-Volume Relationships in Ventricular Failure"* to *"Effects of Hydralazine on Pressure-Volume and Stress-Volume Relations in Congestive Heart Failure Secondary to Idiopathic Dilated Cardiomyopathy."*

(3) *"Intracoronary Thrombolysis Long After Myocardial Infarction: Therapy For Post-Infarction Angina"* to *"Intracoronary Thrombolysis 3 to 13 Days After Acute Myocardial Infarction For Post-Infarction Angina Pectoris."*

(4) *"Doppler Diagnosis of Aortic Stenosis in the Elderly"* to *"Doppler Diagnosis of Valvular Aortic Stenosis in Patients Over 60 Years of Age."* This title is one in which the phrase "in patients" is better present than absent.

(5) *"Quantitative Assessment of Semilunar Insufficiency By Doppler Echocardiography"* to *"Quantitative Assessment by Doppler Echocardiography of Pulmonic or Aortic Regurgitation."*

(6) *"Incidence of Intracoronary Thrombus in Unstable Angina"* to *"Frequency of Intracoronary Filling Defects (Presumably Thrombus) by Angiography in Angina Pectoris At Rest."*

Avoiding Subtitles

(1) *"Prediction of One-Year Mortality After Myocardial Infarction: Value of Programmed Stimulation and Exercise Testing"* to *"Value of Programmed Stimulation and Exercise Testing in Predicting 1-Year Mortality After Acute Myocardial Infarction."*

(2) *"Fick Versus Indicator Dilution Measurements of Cardiac Output: An Analysis of Factors Affecting the Variability of the Technique"* to *"Analysis of Factors Affecting the Variability of Fick Versus Indicator Dilution Measurements of Cardiac Output."*

(3) *Hemodynamic Improvement With Intravenous Verapamil in Hypertrophic Obstructive Cardiomyopathy: Cardiac Catheterization and Simultaneous Continuous Wave Doppler Findings"* to *"Usefulness of Doppler Echocardiography For Determining Hymodynamic Improvement With Intravenous Verapamil in Hypertrophic Cardiomyopathy."*

(4) *"False Tendons: Association With Left Ventricular Aneurysm"* to *"Association of False Tendons With Left Ventricular Aneurysm."*

(5) *"Magnetic Resonance Imaging of The Left Ventricle: The Importance of Image Plane"* to *"Importance of the Imaging Plane For Magnetic Resonance Imaging of the Normal Left Ventricle."*

(6) *"Complex Coronary Angioplasty: A New Technique For Safe, Effective Dilation of Bifurcation Stenosis"* to *"Angioplasty For Dilatation of Complex Coronary Artery Bifurcation Stenosis."*

(7) *"Aortic to Mitral Valve Opening Area Ratio: A Parameter For the Presence and Severity of Mitral Regurgitation"* to *"Echocardiographic Aortic-to-Mitral-Opening-Area Ratio for Determining The Presence and Severity of Mitral Regurgitation."*

(8) *"Disturbances of the Cardiac Conduction System and Its Autonomic Regulation in Patients With Familial Amyloid Polyneuropathy. Electrophysiological Evaluation and Pharmacological Intervention"* to *"Electrophysiological Evaluation of the Cardiac Conducting System and Its Autonomic Regulation in Familial Amyloid Polyneuropathy."*

(9) *"Coronary Vasomotion in a Patient with Angina at Rest: Augmentation of Coronary Blood Flow by Sublingual Nitroglycerin"* to *"Coronary Vasomotion in Rest Angina and Effect of Sublingual Nitroglycerin on Coronary Blood Flow."*

(10) *"Coronary Revascularization With The Internal Mammary Artery: The Other Bypass Graft"* to *"Coronary Bypass Using the Internal Mammary Artery."*

Avoid Placing the Manuscript's Message in the Title

(1) *"Inhibition of Epinephrine and Norepinephrine Release During Exercise Stress by a Benzodiazepine in Man"* to *"Effect of a Benzodiazepine (Alprazolam) on Epinephrine and Norepinephrine Release During Exercise Stress."*

(2) *"The High Prevalence of Brown Adipose Tissue in Chronic Heart Failure Patients: A Potential Role in Thermoregulation"* to *"Prevalence of Brown Adipose Tissue in Chronic Congestive Heart Failure Secondary to Coronary Heart Disease."*

(3) *"Doxorubicin-Induced Heart Failure: Failure of Prevention By a Free Radical Scavenger"* to *"Usefulness of a Free-Radical Scavenger in Preventing Doxorubicin-Induced Heart Failure in Dogs."*

(4) *"Prevention of Left Ventricular Thrombosis By High Dossage Anticoagulants in Acute Myocardial Infarction"* to *"Usefulness of High-Dose Anticoagulants in Preventing Left Ventricular Thrombus in Acute Myocardial Infarction."*

(5) *"Changes in the Intensity of Heart Sounds With Age"* to *"Relation of Intensity of Cardiac Sounds to Age."*

(6) *"Attenuation of the Cardiovascular Responses to Early Exercise in Patients With Inferior Wall ST Infarction"* to *"Cardiovascular Responses to Early Exercise in Inferior Wall ST Acute Myocardial Infarction."*

(7) *"The Beneficial Effect of Atenolol on Exercise Capacity in Patients With Mitral Stenosis in Sinus Rhythm"* to *"Effects of Atenolol on Exercise Capacity in Mitral Stenosis With Sinus Rhythm."*

(8) *"Intraoperative Left Ventricular Microbubbles Do Not Predict Poor Neurologic Outcome"* to *"Usefulness of Intraoperative Left Ventricular Microbubbles Detected By Transesophageal 2-Dimensional Echocardiography in Predicting Neurologic Outcome After Cardiac Operations."*

(9) *"Reduction of Right Ventricular Hypertrophy in an Experimental Model Hypoxic Pulmonary Hypertension With Diltiazem and Ibuprofen"* to *"Effect of Diltiazem and Ibuprofen on Right Ventricular Hypertrophy in an Experimental Model of Hypoxic Pulmonary Hypertension."* In retrospect, the name of the animal, rat or dog, etc., rather than "an experimental animal" is preferred.

Clearly Identify Nonhuman Experimental Articles by Identifying the Animal Species

(1) *"The Protective Effect of Intact Endothelium Against Platelet-Induced Coronary Artery Spasm In A Supported Isolated Heart Preparation"* to *"Effect of Intact Endothelium Against Platelet-Induced Coronary Artery Spasm in Isolated Rabbit Hearts."*

Avoid Abbreviations in Titles

(1) *"Relationship of the Occlusion Pressure During PTCA to Collaterals"* to *"Relation of the Coronary Arterial Occlusion Pressure During Percutaneous Transluminal Coronary Angioplasty to Presence of Collaterals."*

(2) *"Case Report: Uncommon A-V Node SVT"* to *"Atrioventricular Nodal Supraventricular Tachycardia."*

(3) *"AV Fistula: An Infrequently Recognized Complication of Cardiac Catheterization"* to *"Arteriovenous Fistula: A Rare Complication of Arterial Puncture For Cardiac Catheterization."*

(4) *"Accidental Death Immediately After Technically Successful PTCA: Pathological Findings"* to *"Coronary Arterial Findings Following Accidental Death Immediately After Successful Percutaneous Transluminal Coronary Angioplasty."*

Avoid Questions in Titles

(1) *"Outpatient Cardiac Catheterizations—Are They Safe?"* to *"Safety of Outpatient Cardiac Catheterizations."*

(2) *"Nonsustained Ventricular Tachycardia During Programmed Ventricular Stimulation: What Constitutes a Positive Test Result?"* to *"Nonsustained Ventricular Tachycardia During Programmed Ventricular Stimulation: Criteria For a Positive Test."*

Poor Flow of Words

(1) *"The Left Ventricular Volume For the Indication of Total Correction of Fallot's Tetralogy"* to *"Usefulness of Left Ventricular Volume in Assessing Tetralogy of Fallot for Total Correction."*

(2) *"Left Ventricular Thrombus Complicating Acute Reversible Cardiomyopathy Following Natural Gas Poisoning"* to *"Acute Left Ventricular Dysfunction and Thrombosis Following Natural Gas Poisoning."*

Conclusion

None of the suggestions provided above are absolute. On many occasions subtitles *are* useful. A question as a title sometimes is useful. I often have used the abbreviation AJC in titles of From-the-Editor columns in this Journal. On occasion, the manuscript's message in the title is useful. The title *"Left Atrial Hemorrhage After Balloon Atrial Septostomy: A Technique for Successful Resuscitation"* was changed to *"Infusion of Blood From Pericardial Sac Into Femoral Vein: A Technique For Survival Until Operative Closure of a Cardiac Perforation During Balloon Septostomy."* Nevertheless, general principles for titles of medical articles are useful. Because the title is the most frequent and often the only portion of an article read, more attention needs to be given to its development.

William C. Roberts

William C. Roberts, MD
Editor in Chief

1. **Fishbein M.** Medical Writing. The Technique and the Art. 4th Ed. Springfield, IL: Charles C Thomas, 1972:39.

Country of Origin of Articles in the AJC in 1984

Although the "A" in the AJC stands for American, the "A" actually means "published in America," not necessarily "authored in America." As the accompanying table indicates, nearly 30% of all long reports, brief reports, editorials and letters published in the AJC in 1984 were produced by authors living in a country other than the USA. Of the 826 articles and letters published in the AJC in 1984, 582 (70.5%) came from the USA and 244 (29.5%) came from 30 other countries. Of the 244 non-USA contributed articles, 26 (3.1% of the total) came from Canada and 26 (3.1%) came from Japan; 24 (2.9%) from the Federal Republic of Germany; 22 (2.7%) from Italy; 20 (2.4%) from England; 19 (2.3%) from Israel; 7 (0.8%) from Australia; 7 (0.8%) from France; and 6 (0.7%) from Belgium, 6 (0.7%) from Spain, and 6 (0.7%) from Switzerland. Fifteen countries each contributed 1 or 2 articles or letters. The United Kingdom (England, Scotland, Northern Ireland and Wales) contributed 25 articles, a number placing it third behind Canada and Japan, which tied for first among non-USA contributors. No article was contributed by the 3 most populous countries (People's Republic of China, Union of Soviet Socialist Republics, or India).

Excluding the 30 articles which originated from more than 1 country (the USA was 1 of the countries in 22), the continent of origin of the 796 single-country-of-origin articles or letters was: North America, 609 (76.5%); Europe, 120 (15.1%); Asia, 51 (6.4%); Australia, 9 (1.1%); South America, 5 (0.6%); and Africa, 2 (0.3%).

William C. Roberts

William C. Roberts, MD
Editor in Chief

		Long Reports No. (%)	Brief Reports No. (%)	Editorials No. (%)	Letters No. (%)	From the Editor	AJC 25 Years Ago	Totals No. (%)
1	USA	346 (70.8)	134 (65.7)	25 (89.3)	52 (65.0)	15	10	582 (70.5)
2	Canada	16 (3.3)	6(2.9)		4 (5.0)			26 (3.1)
2	Japan	18 (3.7)	7 (3.4)		1 (1.3)			26 (3.1)
4	Federal Republic of Germany	18 (3.7)	5 (2.5)		1 (1.3)			24 (2.9)
5	Italy	12 (2.5)	9 (4.4)		1 (1.2)			22 (2.7)
5	USA + ≥ 1 other country	14 (2.9)	4 (2.0)	3 (10.7)	1 (1.3)			20 (2.7)
7	England	12 (2.5)	4 (2.0)		4 (5.0)			20 (2.4)
8	Israel	9 (1.8)	6 (2.9)		4 (5.0)			19 (2.3)
9	Netherlands	8 (1.6)	5 (2.5)		0			13 (1.6)
10	≥ 2 countries excluding USA	4 (0.8)	0		4 (5.0)			8 (1.0)
11	Australia	2 (0.4)	4 (2.0)		1 (1.3)			7 (0.8)
11	France	4 (0.8)	2 (1.0)		1 (1.2)			7 (0.8)
13	Belgium	5 (1.0)	0		1 (1.2)			6 (0.7)
13	Spain	5 (1.0)	1 (0.5)		0			6 (0.7)
13	Switzerland	3 (0.6)	3 (1.5)		0			6 (0.7)
16	Republic of China	1 (0.2)	4 (2.0)		0			5 (0.6)
17	Scotland	1 (0.2)	2 (1.0)		1 (1.2)			4 (0.5)
18	Finland	2 (0.4)	1 (0.5)		0			3 (0.4)
19	Argentina	1 (0.2)	1 (0.5)		0			2 (0.2)
19	New Zealand	1 (0.2)	0		1 (1.3)			2 (0.2)
19	Norway	1 (0.2)	1 (0.5)		0			2 (0.2)
19	South Africa	1 (0.2)	1 (0.5)		0			2 (0.2)
19	Sweden	1 (0.2)	1 (0.5)		0			2 (0.2)
24	Austria	1 (0.2)	0		0			1 (0.1)
24	Brazil	0	1 (0.5)		0			1 (0.1)
24	Chile	1 (0.2)	0		0			1 (0.1)
24	Denmark	1 (0.2)	0		0			1 (0.1)
24	Greece	0	0		1 (1.3)			1 (0.1)
24	Hungary	0	1 (0.5)		0			1 (0.1)
24	Mexico	0	0		1 (1.2)			1 (0.1)
24	Northern Ireland	0	1 (0.5)		0			1 (0.1)
24	Singapore	0	0		1 (1.2)			1 (0.1)
24	Venezuela	1 (0.2)	0		0			1 (0.1)
Totals		489 (100)	204 (100)	28 (100)	80 (100)	15	10	826 (100)

The AJC in 1985

Shown in Table I are the numbers of editorial (non-advertising) pages and how they were used in the regular issues of the AJC in 1985 compared to the 2 previous years. Of the 3,014 editorial pages in the 16 regular issues, 2,623 (87%) were used for articles, 207 (7%) were used for the tables of contents with abstracts, and 70 pages (2%) were used for volume indexes.

Of the 645 articles published in the 16 regular issues in 1985 (Table I), 138 (21.4%) concerned coronary artery disease; 71 (11.0%) arrhythmias and conduction distur-

TABLE I Number of Pages and Types of Articles Published in the Regular Issues of the AJC in 1983, 1984 and 1985

	1983	1984	1985
No. of pages (avg/month)	3,435 (286)	3,403 (284)	3,014 (251)
For articles (pages/article)	3,130 (4.87)	3,077 (4.12)	2,623 (4.07)
For letters (number) [No. with replys]	27 (53)[40]	36 (80)[38]	21 (40)[16]
For staff, editorial board	15	15	17
For contents in brief	28	31	44
For contents with abstracts	142 (4.1%)	145 (4.3%)	207 (6.9%)
For volume indexes	79	69	70
For information for authors	12	15	17
For other	2	15	15
No. of articles (avg/month)	643 (54)	747 (62)	645 (54)
Coronary artery disease	132 (20.5%)	140 (18.7%)	138 (21.4%)
Arrhythmias and conduction dist.	74 (11.5%)	76 (10.2%)	71 (11.0%)
Systemic hypertension	18 (2.9%)	19 (2.5%)	15 (2.3%)
Congestive heart failure	22 (3.4%)	16 (2.1%)	18 (2.8%)
Valvular heart disease	47 (7.3%)	37 (5.0%)	29 (4.5%)
Cardiomyopathy	22 (3.4%)	18 (2.4%)	9 (1.4%)
Pericardial heart disease	3 (0.5%)	3 (0.4%)	3 (0.5%)
Congenital heart disease	79 (12.3%)	47 (6.3%)	38 (5.9%)
Cardiovascular pharmacology	5 (0.8%)	10 (1.3%)	10 (1.6%)
Miscellaneous	36 (5.6%)	28 (3.8%)	28 (4.3%)
Methods	29 (4.5%)	31 (4.2%)	21 (3.3%)
Experimental studies	52 (8.1%)	64 (8.6%)	49 (7.6%)
Editorials	19 (2.9%)	28 (3.7%)	16 (2.5%)
Brief reports	81 (12.6%)	204 (27.3%)	172 (26.7%)
Historical studies	2 (0.3%)	0	3 (0.5%)
AJC 25 years ago	8 (1.2%)	11 (1.5%)	13 (2.0%)
From-the-editor columns	14 (2.2%)	15 (2.0%)	12 (1.9%)

TABLE II Brief Reports in the AJC in 1985

No. of reports	172	
No. of pages	278/2623	(10.6%)
No of patients in each report		
0	7	
1	93	(54.1%)
2	18	(18.6%)
3	5	
4	3	
5	6	
6–10	12	(7.0%)
11–25	13	(7.6%)
26–50	6	(3.5%)
>50	9	(5.2%)
No. of figures	302	(1.76/BR)
No. of tables	57	(0.33/BR)

TABLE III Subjects of Brief Reports in the AJC in 1985

Coronary artery disease	39 (22.7%)
Arrhythmias and conduction dist.	26 (15.1%)
Systemic hypertension	0
Congestive heart failure	2
Valvular heart disease	17 (9.9%)
Cardiomyopathy	11 (6.4%)
Pericardial heart disease	3
Congenital heart disease	34 (19.8%)
Cardiovascular pharmacology	1
Miscellaneous	33 (19.2%)
Methods	4
Experimental studies	2
Historical studies	0
Totals	172

TABLE IV Symposia in the AJC in 1985

Number	Month of Publication	Subject of Symposium	Guest Editor	No. Articles	No. Pages	Industry Sponsor
1	January 11	Congestive heart failure	Jay N. Cohn	9	56	MS&D
2	January 25	Calcium-channel blockers	Stephen E. Epstein	29	232	Searle
3	March 15	Bepridil	Jay N. Cohn	12	72	McNeil and Wallace
4	April 26	Beta blockers	Donald C. Harrison	31	176	Stuart
5	May 17	Antianginal medicines	William W. Parmley	7	40	Pfizer
6	July 10	Nitrates for CHF	Jay N. Cohn	5	32	Ives
7	July 22	Amrinone for CHF	Eugene Braunwald	9	48	Winthrop-Breon
8	August 23	Cost containment in cardiology	Donald C. Harrison	15	80	MS&D and Hewlett Packard
9	August 30	Potassium, catecholamines and β blockade	David P. Lauler	10	64	Ayerst
10	September 18	Coronary vasoconstriction	Eugene Braunwald	7	48	Pfizer
11	October 23	Esmolol	Edmund H. Sonnenblick	9	64	American Critical Care
12	November 22	Metropolol in AMI	Åke Hjalmarson	10	68	A. B. Hässle
13	December 6	Calcium-channel blockers for systemic hypertension	Edward D. Frohlich	19	118	Marion
14	December 27	Transdermal nitroglycerin	William H. Frishman	8	33	Key
15	December 31	Lipid values	Scott M. Grundy	12	30	Merrell Dow

AMI = acute myocardial infarction; CHF = congestive heart failure; MS&D = Merck Sharp & Dohme.

bances; 38 (5.9%) congenital heart disease; 49 (8%) experimental studies, and only 15 (2.3%) systemic hypertension.

Brief reports in 1985 numbered 172 or 26.7% of the total articles. As shown in Table II, only 93 (54%) concerned a single patient and the other 79 (46%), more than 1 patient. The subjects of the Brief Reports are summarized in Table III.

In addition to the 16 regular issues published in 1985, 15 symposia also were published in the AJC in 1985. The topics and numbers of articles and pages published in them are summarized in Table IV.

William C. Roberts

William C. Roberts, MD
Editor in Chief

The AJC in 1986

This piece contains 4 tables that summarize how the editorial (nonadvertising) pages were utilized in the regular issues of the AJC in 1986 compared to the 3 previous years of the present editorship (Tables I, II and III), and also a listing of the symposia published in the AJC in 1986 (Table IV). Of the 3,004 editorial pages published in the 16 regular issues in 1986, 2,644 (88%) were for articles (2,627 pages) and letters to the editor (17 pages). The remaining 360 pages were used for contents with abstracts (179 pages), volume indexes (86 pages), contents in brief (44 pages), listings of editorial board and staff (16 pages), information for authors (15 pages) and "continuing medical education" questions and answers and "books received." The types of articles in both the long (Table I) and brief reports (Table III) were similar to previous years except for the near elimination of full-length experimental (nonhuman) articles in 1986. The number of articles published in the regular issues in 1986 was down 5% compared to 1985 (616 vs 645), but the average number of published pages of each article was up 5% (4.26 vs 4.07) (Table I).

I am pleased that the number of brief reports involving a single patient continues to decline. In 1983, the first full year of the present brief-report format, 65 (80%) of 81 brief reports published concerned a single patient. In 1984, this percentage had dropped to 60% (122 of 204), and by 1986 to 52% (83 of 160). In addition, the numbers of tables in the brief reports section has continued to increase: from 0.18 table per brief report in 1983; to 0.27 in 1984; to 0.33 in 1985, and to 0.48 table per brief report in 1986. Thus, now 1 in 2 brief reports contains a data table. Each brief report averages just over 1.5 figures.

In addition to the 16 regular issues published in 1986, 13 symposia were published, and these included 143 articles and 823 editorial pages. None of the 13 symposia contained an advertising page, although all were sponsored by a pharmaceutical company.

Annual analysis of how the editorial pages of the AJC are used is useful in selecting manuscripts for publication and in attempting to provide maximal information per editorial page.

William C. Roberts

William C. Roberts, MD
Editor in Chief

TABLE I Number of Pages and Types of Articles Published in the Regular Issues of the AJC in 1983–1986

	1983	1984	1985	1986
No. of pages (mean/month)	3,435 (286)	3,403 (284)	3,014 (251)	3,004
Articles (pages/article)	3,130 (4.87)	3,077 (4.12)	2,623 (4.07)	2,627 (4.26)
Letters (number) [no. with replies]	27 (53)[40]	36 (80)[38]	21 (40)[16]	17 (40)[8]
Staff, editorial board	15	15	17	16
Contents in brief	28	31	44	44
Contents with abstracts	142 (4%)	145 (4%)	207 (7%)	179 (6%)
Volume indexes	79	69	70	86
Information for authors	12	15	17	15
Other	2	15	15	20
No. of articles (mean/month)	643 (54)	747 (62)	645 (54)	616 (51)
Coronary artery disease	132 (21%)	140 (19%)	138 (21%)	153 (25%)
Arrhythmias and conduction defects	74 (12%)	76 (10%)	71 (11%)	86 (14%)
Systemic hypertension	18 (3%)	19 (3%)	15 (2%)	10 (2%)
Congestive heart failure	22 (3%)	16 (2%)	18 (3%)	21 (3%)
Valvular heart disease	47 (7%)	37 (5%)	29 (5%)	39 (6%)
Cardiomyopathy	22 (3%)	18 (2%)	9 (1%)	7 (1%)
Congenital heart disease	79 (12%)	47 (6%)	38 (6%)	34 (6%)
Cardiovascular pharmacology	5 (1%)	10 (1%)	10 (2%)	11 (2%)
Miscellaneous	39 (6%)	31 (4%)	31 (5%)	33 (5%)
Methods	29 (5%)	31 (4%)	21 (3%)	9 (1%)
Experimental studies	52 (8%)	64 (9%)	49 (8%)	4 (1%)
Editorials	19 (3%)	28 (4%)	16 (3%)	21 (3%)
Brief reports	81 (13%)	204 (27%)	172 (27%)	160 (26%)
Historical studies	2 (<1%)	0	3 (1%)	5 (1%)
AJC 25 Years Ago	8 (1%)	11 (2%)	13 (2%)	11 (2%)
From-the-Editor columns	14 (2%)	15 (2%)	12 (2%)	12 (2%)

TABLE II Brief Reports in the AJC, 1983–1986

	1983	1984	1985	1986
No. of reports (no./month) (% of total)	81 (7) (13%)	204 (17) (27%)	172 (14) (27%)	160 (13) (26%)
No. of pages (no./month) (% of total)	123 (10) (4%)	308 (26) (10%)	278 (23) (11%)	276 (23) (11%)
No. of patients in each report				
0	1 (1%)	0	7 (4%)	1 (<1%)
1	65 (80%)	122 (60%)	93 (54%)	83 (52%)
2	9 (11%)	33 (16%)	18 (10%)	11 (7%)
3	5 (6%)	12 (6%)	5 (3%)	8 (5%)
4	0	8 (4%)	3 (2%)	8 (5%)
5	0	5 (2%)	6 (3%)	6 (4%)
6–10	1 (1%)	4 (2%)	12 (7%)	16 (10%)
11–25	0	9 (4%)	13 (8%)	12 (7%)
26–50	0	3 (1.5%)	6 (4%)	4 (2%)
>50	0	7 (3%)	9 (5%)	11 (7%)
No. of figures (no./report)	183 (1.49)	432 (1.40)	302 (1.76)	254 (1.59)
No. of tables (no./report)	22 (0.18)	56 (0.27)	57 (0.33)	76 (0.48)

TABLE III Subjects of Brief Reports in the AJC, 1983–1986

	1983	1984	1985	1986
Coronary artery disease	19 (23%)	33 (16%)	39 (23%)	25 (16%)
Arrhythmias and conduction defects	15 (19%)	45 (22%)	26 (15%)	39 (24%)
Systemic hypertension	0	1 (<1%)	0	2 (1%)
Congestive heart failure	0	2 (1%)	2 (1%)	3 (2%)
Valvular heart disease	7 (9%)	16 (8%)	17 (10%)	22 (14%)
Cardiomyopathy	7 (9%)	14 (7%)	11 (6%)	7 (4%)
Miscellaneous topics	19 (23%)	44 (22%)	36 (21%)	28 (18%)
Congenital heart disease	13 (16%)	43 (21%)	34 (20%)	27 (17%)
Cardiovascular pharmacology	0	2 (1%)	1 (1%)	1 (<1%)
Methods	0	4 (2%)	4 (2%)	0
Experimental studies	1 (1%)	0	2 (1%)	3 (2%)
Historical studies	0	0	0	3 (2%)
Totals	81	204	172	160

TABLE IV Symposia in the AJC in 1986

No.	Publication Date	Subject	Guest Editor	No. Articles	No. Pages	Sponsor
A	Jan 24	Diuretics	Andrew Whelton	9	56	Hoffman-LaRoche
B	Jan 31	Ventricular arrthythmias in congestive heart failure	J. Thomas Bigger, Jr.	8	48	Mead Johnson
C	Feb 12	Lipids and hypertension	Walter M. Kirkendall Paul Samuel	12	72	Sandoz
D	Feb 26	Calcium anatagonists in hypertension	John H. Laragh	21	112	Knoll AG
E	Mar 28	*Guanfacine* for hypertension	Donald G. Vidt Peter A. Van Zwelten	13	73	A.H. Robins
F	Apr 25	Nonselective β blockers	Stephen E. Epstein Robert J. Lefkowitz	10	56	Merck, Sharp & Dohme
G	May 30	Hyperlipidemia	Antonio M. Gotto, Jr.	8	48	Warner-Lambert
H	Jun 27	*Probucol* for hypercholesterolemia	Howard A. Eder	9	56	Merrell Dow
A	Jul 31	Diuretics	James C. Melby	5	24	Merck, Sharp & Dohme
B	Aug 15	Silent myocardial ischemia	Bramah N. Singh	10	64	Key
C	Aug 29	*Encainide*	Donald C. Harrison Joel Morganroth	18	120	Mead Johnson
D	Sep 30	Calcium antagonists in hypertension	William W. Parmley Henry A. Solomon	11	46	Miles
E	Nov 26	*Bevantolol*	Stanley H. Taylor	9	48	Warner-Lambert
13				143	823	

Reviews of Classic Books and Ineptness of Reviewers: Lessons for Judges of Medical Manuscripts

A manuscript submitted to the AJC generally receives 2 reviews. On the review form the recommendations available to the reviewer are "definitely accept," "probably accept," "definitely reject," and "probably reject." The most frequent recommendations from 2 reviewers of the same manuscript are "probably accept" from 1 and "probably reject" from the other. It is rare for both reviewers of the same manuscript to recommend "definitely accept" or "definitely reject." For both to recommend "probably accept" or for both to recommend "probably reject" is common. On occasion, the same manuscript receives a "definitely accept" recommendation from 1 reviewer and "definitely reject" from the other reviewer. When this situation occurs the reputation and experience of both reviewers are carefully weighed and the reasons for their respective recommendations are analyzed. Unfortunately, when this situation exists both reviewers may be major forces in their particular areas of expertise. Thus, when a manuscript reviewed by 2 leaders receives completely opposite recommendations, the reviewer recommending "definitely reject" may be upset if the manuscript is accepted, and the reviewer who recommended "definitely accept" may be upset if the manuscript is rejected. Obviously, the same manuscript cannot be both "terrible" and "excellent." Does this particular example illustrate more about the reviewer than it does about the manuscript? How can 2 experts have such opposite reactions to the same subject matter? If 2 experts disagree so sharply, how meaningful are recommendations, similar or divergent, from reviewers who are not major forces or leaders in their area of expertise?

It is clear to me that no one—including editors—has a monopoly on correct decisions when it comes to degrees of quality of our manuscripts. With these conflicting recommendations from experts in mind, I was delighted to acquire the recently published book *Rotten Reviews: A Literary Companion*, edited by Bill Henderson (Pushcart Press, 93 pages, 1986). The book contains excerpts from 175 scathing notices about a number of famous books and poems published up to 1961. While researching for his book, Henderson was impressed by the balance, intelligence and fairness of most reviews and emphasized that truly malicious reviews were rare. He found, however, striking examples of inability of reviewers to appreciate quality or the lack thereof in the books they were evaluating. Often reviewers went into spasms of appreciation for books of slight value: "Martin Tupper (1810–1889) has won for himself the vacant throne waiting for him amidst the immortals, and has been adopted by the suffrage of mankind and the final decrees of publishers into the same rank with Wordsworth, Tennyson and Browning." (*The Spectator*—1866). Even bad reviews sometimes were appreciated. When the Concord, Massachusetts public library banned *Huckleberry Finn*, Mark Twain exulted: "That will sell 25,000 books for sure!".

Rotten Reviews is filled with examples of how great writers can be wrong about other great writers, a reason for some humility in those of us passing judgments on works of others. It was Henry James who called *Wuthering Heights* (1847) by Emily Bronte "a crude and morbid story" and said of Charles Dickens' great novel, *Our Mutual Friend*, that "We are convinced that it is one of the chief conditions of his genius not to see beneath the surface of things. . . We are aware that this definition confines him to an inferior rank." It was Emile Zola who said of Charles Baudelaire's *Les Fleurs Du Mal* (1857), "In a hundred years the histories of the French literature will only mention (this work) as a curio." It was Gertrude Stein who called Ezra Pound "A village explainer, excellent if you were a village, but if you were not, not." It was Ralph Waldo Emerson who said of Jane Austen: "I am at a loss to understand why people hold Miss Austen's novels at so high a rate, which seem to me vulgar in tone, sterile in artistic invention, imprisoned in the wretched conventions of English society, without genius, wit, or knowledge of the world. Never was life so pinched and narrow. The one problem in the mind of the writer. . .is marriageableness. . . Suicide is more respectable." And Edmund Wilson on W.H. Auden: "Mr. Auden himself has presented the curious case of a poet who writes an original poetic language in the most robust English tradition but who seems to have been arrested in the mentality of an adolescent schoolboy."

And virtually every reviewer had a field day with Walt Whitman and Herman Melville. On Walt Whitman's *Drum-Taps* (1865), Henry James wrote: "Mr. Whitman's attitude seems monstrous. It is monstrous because it pretends to persuade the soul while it slights the intellect; because it pretends to gratify the feelings while it outrages the taste. . . Our hearts are often touched through a compromise with the artistic sense, but never in direct violation of it." Robert Louis Stevenson: "Whitman, like a shaggy dog, just unchained, scouring the beaches of the world and baying at the moon." Peter Bayne: "Incapable of true poetical originality, Whitman had the cleverness to invent a literary trick, and the shrewdness to stick to it." And Francis Fisher Browne: Whitman's ". . .lack of a sense of poetic fitness, his failure to understand the business of a poet, is clearly astounding."

A few reviewers' comments on Herman Melville: "*Redburn* was a stupid failure, *Mardi* was hopelessly dull, *White Jacket* was worse than either; and, in fact was such a very bad book,

The Search For The Masterful Figure

I enjoy examining a new manuscript (or a published article). After reading the title, authors' names, and summary, I immediately go to the figures, seeking the 1 figure that provides the message of the manuscript. I have a better chance of remembering the manuscript's message if I can visually recall the figure that most clearly provides that message. With my own publications, I spend considerably more time in developing the figures and tables than I do in writing the manuscripts. I believe that the graphic or tabular presentations of the data carry more impact than the written text, which in essence simply describes the findings in the graphs and tables.

Because of my interest in and search for beautifully prepared graphic materials, I was pleased 4 years ago to acquire Edward R. Tufte's *The Visual Display of Quantitative Information* (Graphics Press, Cheshire, Connecticut, 1983). Contained in this 187-page book are numerous data graphics that, of course, display measured quantities by combined use of points, lines, coordinates, numbers, symbols, shading, sometimes color, and a few words. As pointed out by Tufte, the use of abstract pictures to show numbers is a surprisingly recent invention. Statistical graphics—length and area to show quantity, time series, scatterplots and multivariate displays—were not invented until 1750–1800, long after such mathematic triumphs as logarithms, Cartesian coordinates, calculus and the basics of probability theory. As Tufte emphasized, modern data graphics do much more than simply substitute for statistical tables. They serve as instruments for reasoning about quantitative information. Often the most effective way to describe, explore and summarize a set of numbers is to look at pictures of those numbers. Of methods for analyzing and communicating statistical information, well designed data graphics usually are the simplest and the most powerful. According to Tufte, who presently is Professor of Political Science and Statistics at Yale University, each year somewhere between 900 billion and 2,000 billion images of statistical graphics are printed, and some of them appear in cardiology journals. Therefore, most cardiologic authors can profit from this book about the design of statistical graphs.

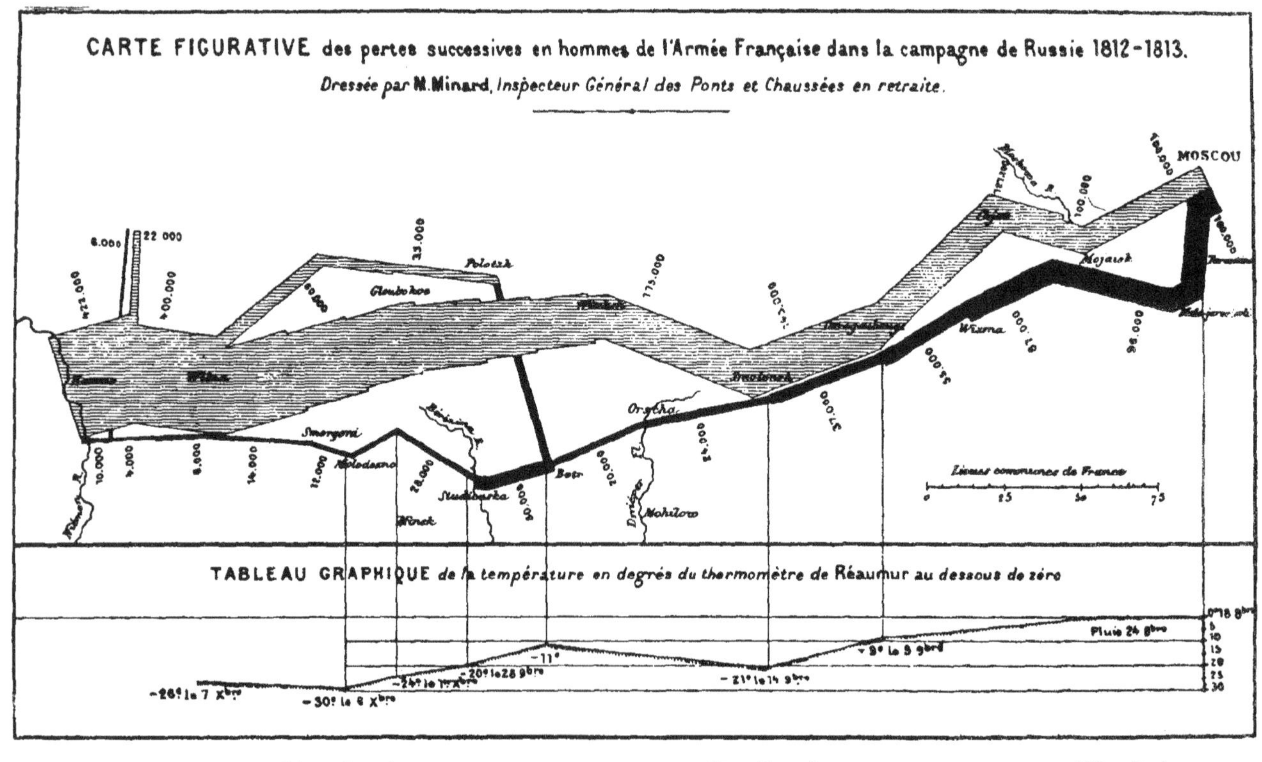

FIGURE 1. See text.

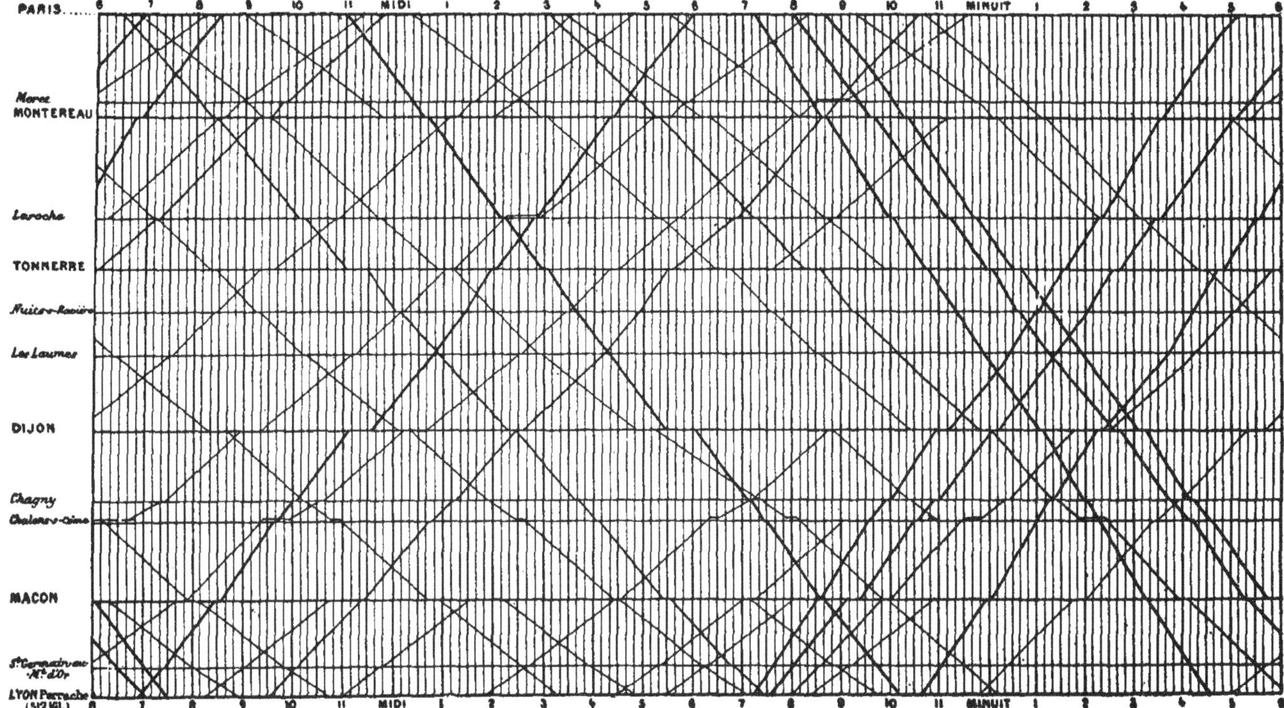

FIGURE 2. See text.

I particularly like 2 graphs in Tufte's book. The first **(Figure 1)** is the classic of Charles J. Minard (1781–1870), the French engineer, and it protrays the devastating losses suffered in Napoleon's Russian campaign in 1812. Beginning at the left on the Polish-Russian border near the Niemen River, the thick band shows the size of the army (422,000 men) as it invaded Russia in June 1812. The width of the band indicates the size of the army at each place on the map. In September, the army reached Moscow, by then sacked and deserted, with 100,000 men. The path of Napoleon's retreat from Moscow is depicted by the darker, lower band linked to a temperature scale and dates. In the bitterly cold winter, many froze on the march back. The crossing of the Berezina River was a disaster. When the returning army finally reached Poland, only 10,000 men remained. Also shown are the movements of auxiliary troops to protect the rear and the flank of the advancing army. Minard's graph plots the size of the army, its location on a 2-dimensional surface, the direction of the army's movement, the distance between geographic sites, and the temperature on various dates during the retreat from Moscow. Tufte believes that this statistical graph may be the best ever drawn.

The second **(Figure 2)** is a graphic train schedule from Paris to Lyon in the 1880s, and it was drawn by E.J. Marey, also a French engineer. Arrivals and departures from a station are located along the horizontal; length of stop at a station is indicated by the length of the horizontal line. The stations are separated by their distances from one another. The slope of the line reflects the speed of the train: the more vertical the line the faster the train. The intersection of 2 lines locates the time and place that trains going in opposite directions pass each other.

Neither of the above 2 graphs needs many words to describe them. Our cardiologic articles, in my view, need better graphics and fewer words.

William C. Roberts

William C. Roberts, MD
Editor in Chief

Publishing Manuscripts Faster Than Abstracts

Recently, I received 2 letters from authors asking that their manuscripts originally scheduled for publication in the November 1, 1987, AJC be moved forward so that they would be published instead in the December 1, 1987, AJC. These requests were made because abstracts on the topic of the manuscripts had just been accepted for presentation at the Annual Scientific Sessions of the American Heart Association (AHA) and abstracts are not eligible for presentation if a manuscript on the same subject is published before the presentation. In both cases, the manuscripts had been submitted to the AJC just after the abstracts had been submitted to the AHA. Specifically, both manuscripts and abstracts were submitted in May 1987. The manuscripts were reviewed and revised in a 6-week period, accepted for publication in June 1987, and scheduled for publication in the November 1, 1987, AJC. Notification of acceptance of the abstracts by the AHA was in August 1987 and the abstracts were scheduled for publication in the October abstract supplement and for presentation at the November 1987 meeting. Thus, the manuscripts were reviewed, revised and accepted for publication before the authors were notified of acceptance of their abstracts.

The same scenario holds true for the Annual Scientific Sessions of the American College of Cardiology (ACC). Abstracts for this meeting are due by early September and, if accepted, the abstracts are published in their February abstract supplement the following year and presented at their annual meeting in March of that year. Because the interval between acceptance and publication of a manuscript in some cardiology journals is only 4 months, a manuscript would be published before an abstract would be presented if both were submitted simultaneously or nearly so and this manuscript-publication efficiency would, therefore, conflict with the policy that "Abstracts are not eligible for consideration if the manuscript has been published prior to the ACC meeting."

Publication of manuscripts should not be delayed, in my view, because of slow processing of abstracts on the same topics. The authors cited above performed their research in the ideal fashion; i.e., their research endeavor was completed by the time the abstract was submitted, and, therefore, they were able to submit both abstract for presentation and manuscript for publication nearly simultaneously. If all investigators were as efficient, the accuracy of the abstracts would improve.

There are at least 2 solutions to the problem: (1) change the rules of abstract submissions to both the AHA and the ACC so that abstracts would still be eligible for consideration so long as the abstract was submitted to a meeting before the manuscript on the same topic was submitted to a journal; and/or (2) speed up the processing time and publication date of abstracts. Efficient research should not be penalized. If a manuscript is submitted to a journal the same time that an abstract on the same subject is submitted to a meeting, the authors should not be penalized by the meeting if the manuscript happens to be published a month or two before the abstract data are presented. If the manuscript is submitted to a journal, however, before the abstract on the same subject is submitted to a meeting, the abstract should neither be published nor presented.

I hope that both the AHA and the ACC will change their present abstract-submitting policy so that efficient researchers will not be penalized.

William C. Roberts

William C. Roberts, MD
Editor-in-Chief

The AJC in 1987

The year 1987 was a good one for the AJC. A total of 2,833 pages for articles (2,810 pages) and letters (23 pages) was published in the 16 regular issues of the AJC in 1987 (Table I). This number represents an increase of 189 pages (7%) for articles and letters compared to 1986. In addition to these 2,833 pages, 395 other editorial (i.e., nonadvertising) pages were published in the regular issues in 1987. Of this number, 202 were used for the "contents with abstracts," and I am pleased to report that the publisher is considering discontinuing this section in July 1988. The publisher also will change the layout of the "contents in brief" in July 1988.

The number of articles published in the regular issues in 1987 was 695, an average of 58 each month, and an increase of 79 articles (11%) compared to 1986 (Table I). Each of the 695 articles averaged 4.04 pages in length, a 5% decrease in average article length compared to the preceding year. Although the percent of articles in each of the various categories in 1987 was roughly similar to what it had been in 1986, the number of articles on systemic hypertension increased to 28 from 10 in the preceding year (Table I). Because systemic hypertension is such a common condition (60 million Americans have it), articles on this subject should, in my view, occupy more than 4% of the articles published. No experimental articles were published in 1987 (except those which could fit into the Brief Report format).

I am enormously pleased about how the *Brief Reports* section of the AJC has developed during the past 5.5 years. This section was initiated in September 1982. In 1983, 65 (80%) of the 81 brief reports published were single-case studies (Table II); in 1984, 122 (60%) of the 204 brief reports published were single-case studies; in 1985, 54% were single-case studies and in 1987 only 34% of the 203 brief reports published were single-case studies. In 1987, 33% of the brief reports involved >10 patients and many involved >100 patients. It is clear that the Brief Reports section of the *Journal* is no longer a case-report section. To emphasize this change, beginning in April 1988 the reports which include case descriptions will be placed in a new section to be called simply *Case Reports*. The Brief

TABLE I Number of Pages and Types of Articles Published in the Regular Issues of the AJC in 1983 to 1986

	1983	1984	1985	1986	1987
Number of pages (mean/month)	3,435 (286)	3,403 (284)	3,014 (251)	3,004	3,228
For articles (pages/article)	3,130 (4.87)	3,077 (4.12)	2,623 (4.07)	2,627 (4.26)	2,810 (4.04)
For letters (number) [no. with replies]	27 (53) [40]	36 (80) [38]	21 (40) [16]	17 (40) [8]	23 (45) [18]
For staff, editorial board	15	15	17	16	16
For contents in brief	28	31	44	44	50
For contents with abstracts	142	145	207	179	202
For volume indexes	79	69	70	86	101
For information for authors	12	15	17	15	16
For other	2	15	15	20	10
Number of articles (mean/month)	643 (54)	747 (62)	645 (54)	616 (51)	695 (58)
Coronary artery disease	132 (21%)	140 (19%)	138 (21%)	153 (25%)	180 (27%)
Arrhythmias and conduction defects	74 (12%)	76 (10%)	71 (11%)	86 (14%)	83 (12%)
Systemic hypertension	18 (3%)	19 (3%)	15 (2%)	10 (2%)	28 (4%)
Congestive heart failure	22 (3%)	16 (2%)	18 (3%)	21 (3%)	25 (3%)
Valvular heart disease	47 (7%)	37 (5%)	29 (5%)	39 (6%)	30 (4%)
Cardiomyopathy	22 (3%)	18 (2%)	9 (1%)	7 (1%)	14 (2%)
Congenital heart disease	79 (12%)	47 (6%)	38 (6%)	34 (6%)	31 (4%)
Miscellaneous	44 (7%)	41 (5%)	41 (7%)	44 (7%)	26 (4%)
Methods	29 (5%)	31 (4%)	21 (3%)	9 (1%)	24 (3%)
Experimental studies	52 (8%)	64 (9%)	49 (8%)	4 (1%)	0
Editorials	19 (3%)	28 (4%)	16 (3%)	21 (3%)	26 (4%)
Brief reports	81 (13%)	204 (27%)	172 (27%)	160 (26%)	203 (29%)
Historical studies	2 (<1%)	0	3 (1%)	5 (1%)	7 (1%)
AJC 25 years ago	8 (1%)	11 (2%)	13 (2%)	11 (2%)	6 (1%)
From-the-editor columns	14 (2%)	15 (2%)	12 (2%)	12 (2%)	12 (2%)

TABLE II Brief Reports in the AJC 1983 to 1987

	1983	1984	1985	1986	1987
No. of reports (no./month) (% of total)	81 (7) (13%)	204 (17) (27%)	172 (14) (27%)	160 (13) (26%)	203 (17) (29%)
No. of pages (no./month) (% of total)	123 (10) (4%)	308 (26) (10%)	278 (23) (11%)	276 (23) (11%)	367 (31) (13%)
No. of patients in each report					
0	1 (1%)	0	7 (4%)	1 (<1%)	7 (3%)
1	65 (80%)	122 (60%)	93 (54%)	83 (52%)	68 (34%)
2	9 (11%)	33 (16%)	18 (10%)	11 (7%)	18 (9%)
3	5 (6%)	12 (6%)	5 (3%)	8 (5%)	10 (5%)
4	0	8 (4%)	3 (2%)	8 (5%)	9 (4%)
5	0	5 (2%)	6 (3%)	6 (4%)	3 (2%)
6–10	1 (1%)	4 (2%)	12 (7%)	16 (10%)	21 (10%)
11–25	0	9 (4%)	13 (8%)	12 (7%)	23 (11%)
26–50	0	3 (1.5%)	6 (4%)	4 (2%)	15 (8%)
>50	0	7 (3%)	9 (5%)	11 (7%)	29 (14%)
No. of figures (no./report)	183 (1.49)	432 (1.40)	302 (1.76)	254 (1.59)	336 (1.66)
No. of tables (no./report)	22 (0.18)	56 (0.27)	57 (0.33)	76 (0.48)	142 (0.70)

TABLE III Subjects of Brief Reports in the AJC 1983 to 1987

	1983	1984	1985	1986	1987
Coronary artery disease	19 (23%)	33 (16%)	39 (23%)	25 (16%)	57 (28%)
Arrhythmias and conduction defects	15 (19%)	45 (22%)	26 (15%)	39 (24%)	34 (17%)
Systemic hypertension	0	1 (<1%)	0	2 (1%)	2 (1%)
Congestive heart failure	0	2 (1%)	2 (1%)	3 (2%)	4 (2%)
Valvular heart disease	7 (9%)	16 (8%)	17 (10%)	22 (14%)	33 (16%)
Cardiomyopathy	7 (9%)	14 (7%)	11 (6%)	7 (4%)	8 (4%)
Miscellaneous topics	19 (23%)	46 (23%)	37 (22%)	29 (18%)	28 (14%)
Congenital heart disease	13 (16%)	43 (21%)	34 (20%)	27 (17%)	29 (14%)
Methods	0	4 (2%)	4 (2%)	0	2 (1%)
Experimental studies	1 (1%)	0	2 (1%)	3 (2%)	6 (3%)
Historical studies	0	0	0	3 (2%)	0
Totals	81	204	172	160	203

TABLE IV Symposia Published in the *American Journal of Cardiology* in 1987

Number	Month, Day	Title	Guest Editor(s)	Articles	Pages	Sponsor	Date of Symposium	Interval (months) Symposium to Publication
A	January 23	Calcium Ion, Cardiac Myocyte, Vascular Smooth Muscle in Hypertension	Edward D. Frohlich	19	121	Marion Laboratories	March 27–29, 1986	10
B	January 30	Calcium Antagonists	Eugene Braunwald	25	187	Sandoz Pharmaceuticals	Sept. 11–12, 1986	4
C	March 9	Total Ischemic Burden	Attilio Maseri	7	38	Pfizer Laboratories	September 14, 1986	5
D	April 24	Ramipril—A New Angiotensin Converting Enzyme Inhibitor	J. Ian S. Robertson	31	177	Hoechst AG	May 2–4, 1986	11
E	April 30	Proarrhythmia	Leonard N. Horowitz Douglas P. Zipes	10	56	Berlex Laboratories	March 9, 1986	14
F	May 15	Betablockade, Cardioselectivity and Intrinsic Sympathomimetic Activity	Aram V. Chobanian Stanley H. Taylor	12	54	Wyeth Laboratories	Sept. 28–29, 1986	8
G	May 29	Doxazosin	Klaus Starke	18	104	Pfizer International	June 7, 1986	11
H	June 15	Pirmenol	H. Just	12	57	Warner-Lambert	December 2, 1985	19
J	June 30	Nicardipine	William W. Parmley	8	37	Syntex International	September 13, 1986	9
A	July 15	Cardioprotection in Ischemic Heart Disease	Desmond Julian	8	41	ICI Pharmaceuticals	January 18, 1986	18
B	July 31	Restenosis After PTCA	Spencer B. King, III	16	69	USCI, Division of C.R. Bard	June 7, 1986	14
C	August 14	Enoximone for Heart Failure	Karl T. Weber	18	90	Merrell Dow Research Institute	September 14, 1986	11

TABLE IV Symposia Published in the *American Journal of Cardiology* in 1987 (*cont'd.*)

Number	Month, Day	Title	Guest Editor(s)	Articles	Pages	Sponsor	Date of Symposium	Interval (months) Symposium to Publication
D	August 31	Beta blockers as Anti-Arrhythmic Agents	Joel Morganroth	12	67	Princeton Pharmaceutical Products (Squibb)	December 12–13, 1986	8
E	September 18	Beta Blocker with ISA for Hypertension	William C. Roberts	7	37	Rhône-Poulenc Santé	June 23–27, 1986	15
F	October 16	Moricizine HCl	Bernard Lown	14	89	Du Pont	April 20, 1985	28
G	October 30	New Approaches to Cardiovascular Therapy	George L. Blackburn	15	93	Sandoz Pharmaceuticals	March 5–8, 1987	8
H	November 16	Nitroglycerin	Jonathan Abrams	10	48	W. H. Rorer	September 13, 1986	14
I	December 14	Hypertension—The Heart and Kidney	Edward D. Frolich	24	132	Marion Laboratories	April 9–11, 1987	8
J	December 28	Behavioral Disorders in Heart Disease	Sheldon H. Gottlieb Rudolf Hoehn-Saric	13	79	Upjohn	April 3–4, 1987	9

Reports will be reserved for major studies that are concise and have only 1 or 2 major points. At least a third of the articles published as Brief Reports were initially submitted as regular length articles but converted to the shorter format. I urge the readership to examine the brief reports more carefully because these reports provide the most information per page of any section in the *Journal*. The topics of the Brief Reports in 1987 were roughly similar to what they had been in 1986 (Table III). The editor particularly welcomes reader reaction to the Brief Reports.

And 1987 also was a good year for supplements. A total of 19 supplements was published in the AJC, and they included 279 articles occupying 1,576 pages (Table IV). Some of the more prominent cardiovascular investigators in the world served as guest editors of these supplements. The average interval between the symposium meeting and the publication of the proceedings of the symposium was 12 months. Supplements are published, however, within 3 months of receipt of all the manuscripts by the editor.

Thus, including both regular issues and supplements a total of 974 articles occupying 4,412 pages was published in the AJC in 1987. At a yearly subscription cost of $66.00, each article in 1987 cost a subscriber <7 pennies and each page for articles and letters, <2 pennies. The subscription cost throughout 1988 will remain the same as in 1987, so the *Journal* in 1988 should be an even better bargain.

William C. Roberts, MD
Editor-in-Chief

Making Clinical Studies Involving Many Patients Useful to the Single Patient

"Doctoring" centers on the single patient, the 1-to-1 relationship. Yet most clinical studies published in medical journals involve many patients. How can articles in medical journals be presented such that practitioners can fit their single patient into a large clinical study? Two suggestions:

1. Keep patient populations as homogenous as possible: I was surprised when becoming a medical journal editor 8 years ago how heterogenous were some patient populations included in various studies. An example: a manuscript on the effects of 1 or more drugs on ventricular tachycardia typically might include 80 patients in whom the ventricular tachycardia was associated with atherosclerotic coronary artery disease, 25 patients in whom it was associated with idiopathic dilated cardiomyopathy, 5 patients with mitral valve prolapse, 4 patients who earlier had had valve replacement for aortic valve disease, 3 patients with "hypertensive heart disease," 5 patients who earlier had had tetralogy of Fallot repaired, and 10 patients without structural heart disease. The results of the study were pooled together so that it was impossible to know whether or not the results were similar in the various conditions associated with the ventricular tachycardia. In these circumstances I have asked authors to limit their study to the 80 patients with ventricular tachycardia associated with coronary artery disease, often with the comment that when the numbers of patients with the other conditions were large enough that another manuscript focusing on that group would be welcomed.

Another example: another area where a heterogenous population is likely to be found are studies describing the effects of 1 or more drugs in patients with congestive heart failure. A study might include 20 patients in whom the chronic congestive heart failure was associated with coronary artery disease (ischemic cardiomyopathy), 10 patients with idiopathic dilated cardiomyopathy, 3 patients with pure mitral regurgitation, 2 patients who earlier had had aortic valve replacement for reasons unspecified, 4 patients with "hypertensive heart disease" and 2 patients in whom the etiology of the heart failure was not determined. In this circumstance I ask the authors to limit their study to the patients with congestive heart failure associated with coronary artery disease and with idiopathic dilated cardiomyopathy and to separate the data by these 2 etiologic groups.

Another "trap" may occur in manuscripts reporting results of valve replacement of 1 or more cardiac valves or results using a particular type of mechanical prosthesis or bioprostheses. In these circumstances, it is important of course not to intermix results of replacement of 1 cardiac valve (e.g., mitral) with that of another cardiac valve (e.g., aortic). Additionally, it is useful to be able to determine results when valve replacement was performed for pure valvular regurgitation as opposed to that performed for valve stenosis (with or without associated regurgitation) because the etiologies of the stenotic lesions are usually entirely different from those of the purely regurgitant lesions.[1]

2. Provide individual patient data rather than pooled data: Many manuscripts submitted to medical journals report on 10 or so patients, and, surprisingly, despite the small numbers, the data are pooled. In studies involving up to 30 patients it is preferable to present the pertinent data in each patient. To present individual patient data in studies involving 30 patients, however, much care must be exerted in formulating a table. With rare exception, no patient should occupy more than 1 line across. Each column must ask a precise question that is answerable by either a number or by a "+" (positive or present), a "0" (negative or absent) or by a "—" (no information available). Writing within the body of a table usually indicates that a precise question has not been formulated and that the table needs additional work. In my own manuscripts I spend far more time on the tables and figures than I do on the writing of the text.

Another important aspect of tables presenting individual patient data is that in this way data points ("holes") that are missing are readily discernible. When data are pooled, missing data points usually cannot be detected. I have been surprised on occasion when returning a manuscript to an author requesting an individual patient table rather than a pooled data table to find many pertinent data items in some patients to be unavailable. Thus, presenting individual patient data tables allows the reader to insert his/her single patient more readily into a study, and it also provides a good means for detecting missing data. Of course, individual patient variability is more readily detected by presentation of individual patient data.

Thus, study populations should be as homogenous as possible, and tables displaying individual patient data are preferable to those showing pooled data.

William C. Roberts

William Clifford Roberts, MD
Editor in Chief

1. Roberts WC. Morphologic features of the normal and abnormal valve. *Am J Cardiol 1983;51:1005–1028.*

Comparison of the Four Major USA Cardiology Journals in 1990: A Look at 51 Kilograms (112 Pounds) of Journals and Over 15,000 Editorial Pages

In 1984, an article appeared comparing 7 English language cardiology journals for the year 1983 in terms of numbers of editorial (non-advertising) pages, articles, types of articles, figures and tables.[1] An article comparing the 4 major USA cardiology journals also appeared in 1985.[2] A single table comparing the numbers of pages and articles and types of articles in 3 of the 4 major USA cardiology journals the previous year was published in 1988, 1989, and 1990.[3-5] This piece summarizes the results of counting the numbers of editorial pages published and the types of articles published in 1990 in the *American Heart Journal* (AHJ), *The American Journal of Cardiology* (AJC), *Circulation*, and the *Journal of the American College of Cardiology* (JACC).

Table I summarizes the numbers of pages and numbers of articles published in both the regular issues and in the symposia (or supplements) in each of the 4 journals. In the regular issues, 13,488 editorial pages *for articles* were published and in the symposia issues, 2,483 pages; 2,219 articles appeared in the regular issues and 417 articles in the symposia issues.

Table II provides data on utilization of all editorial pages—not just those for articles—in each of the 4 journals and also the types of articles published. Each journal has distinctive features. The AHJ published the most case reports (actual case descriptions), 168 or 34% of the articles published in it, whereas *Circulation* published none, JACC published only 6 and the AJC published only 23. The unique feature of the AJC is the brief reports, which are short articles with only 1 or 2 major points. They numbered 158 or 24% of the articles in the AJC, whereas only 12 were published in the AHJ and none in either *Circulation* or JACC. A major feature of *Circulation* is the large number of studies involving non-human animals (Experimental Studies). They numbered 132 or 25% of its articles, whereas 50 (9%) appeared in JACC, 29 (6%) in the AHJ and none in the AJC. The numbers of editorials were large in JACC (141 [26%]) and in *Circulation* (109 [21%]) and few in the AHJ (9 [2%]) and the AJC (33 [5%]). Reviews made up about 4% of the articles in the AHJ, *Circulation* and JACC and none appeared in the AJC. The AJC published almost as many "letters" (called Readers' Comments) as the other 3 journals combined (40 vs 46).

The symposia published in the AHJ in 1990 are listed in Table III (n = 4), those in the AJC in Table IV (n = 20), and those in *Circulation* in Table V (n = 7). None were published in JACC.

The numbers of words per page in the 4 journals are presented in Table VI. The AJC published approximately 34% more words per page than did the AHJ, 19% more than JACC, and 12% more than *Circulation.*

The numbers of subscribers of each of the 4 journals are shown in Table VII.

The regular issues of the 4 journals in 1990, including all ads and covers, weighed 43.25 kg, the symposia issues for these 4 journals weighed 5.25 kg, and the 2 abstract issues (JACC in February and *Circulation* in October) weighed 2.17 kg. The total for the regular issues, symposia issues and abstracts for 1990 was 50.67 kg (112 pounds). The 15,971 pages of articles in the regular and symposia issues averaged 1,331 pages a month, and the 2,636 articles averaged 220 a month. Happy reading.

William C. Roberts

William Clifford Roberts, MD
Editor in Chief

1. Roberts WC. Comparison of 7 English-language cardiology journals for 1983. *Am J Cardiol* 1983;53:862–869.
2. Roberts WC. Analysis of page utilization and types of articles published in four major American cardiology journals in 1984. *Int J Cardiol* 1985;8:353–360.
3. Roberts WC. AJC Editorial Board Meeting — March 1988. *Am J Cardiol* 1988;61:1161–1164.
4. Roberts WC. Editorial board meeting of The American Journal of Cardiology — March 1989. *Am J Cardiol* 1989;63:1159–1165.
5. Roberts WC. Editorial board meeting of The American Journal of Cardiology — March 1990. *Am J Cardiol* 1990;65:1162–1168.

TABLE I Numbers of Pages for Articles and Numbers of Articles in All Issues of the Four USA Cardiology Journals in 1990

	Numbers of Pages			Numbers of Articles		
	Regular Issues	Symposia	Totals	Regular Issues	Symposia	Totals
AHJ	2,715	202	2,971	489	37	526
AJC	3,001	1,169	4,170	662	226	888
Circulation	4,346	1,112	5,458	528	154	682
JACC	3,426	0	3,426	540	0	540
Totals	13,488	2,483	15,971	2,219	417	2,636

TABLE II Numbers of Editorial (non-advertising) Pages and Articles Published in the Regular Issues (excludes symposia issues) of the Four Major USA Cardiology Journals in 1990

	American Heart Journal	American Journal of Cardiology	Circulation	Journal of the American College of Cardiology	Totals
Numbers of pages	2,911	3,498	4,967	3,753	15,129
For articles	2,715 (93.27%)	3,001 (85.79%)	4,346 (87.50%)	3,426 (91.21%)	13, 488 (89.15%)
For "letters"	17	20	33	12	82
For staff, editorial board	12	24	24	42	102
For contents in brief	59 (2.03%)	83 (2.37%)	46 (0.93%)	28 (0.75%)	216 (1.43%)
For contents with abstracts	0	233 (6.66%)	120 (2.42%)	121 (3.22%)	474 (3.13%)
For boxed abstracts	0	0	137 (2.76%)	0	137 (0.91%)
For information for authors	24	24	24	42[g]	114 (0.75%)
For meeting abstracts	0	10[b]	19[d]	0	29 (0.19%)
For erratum	0	0	4	0	4
For miscellaneous	10[a] (0.34%)	0	150[e] (3.02%)	18[h] (0.48%)	178 (1.18%)
For volume indexes	74 (2.54%)	103 (2.94%)	64 (1.29%)	64 (1.70%)	305 (2.02%)
Numbers of articles	489 (41/month)	662 (55/month)	528 (44/month)	540 (45/month)	2,219
Long reports	277	448	388	373	1,486
Concerning humans	248 (50.72%)	448 (67.67%)	256 (48.48%)	323 (59.81%)	1,275 (57.46%)
Concerning non-humans	29 (5.93%)	0	132 (25.00%)	50 (9.26%)	211 (9.51%)
Brief reports	12 (2.45%)	158 (23.87%)	0	0	170 (7.66%)
Case reports	168 (34.36%)	23 (3.47%)	0	6 (1.11%)	197 (8.88%)
Reviews	23 (4.70%)	0	31[f] (5.87%)	20 (3.70%)	74 (3.33%)
Editorials	9 (1.84%)	25 (3.78%)	109 (20.64%)	141 (26.11%)	284 (12.80%)
From the editor	0	8 (1.21%)	0	0	8 (0.36%)
Numbers of "letters" (replies)	17 (9)	40 (11)[c]	17 (12)	12 (5)	86 (37)
Annual subscription cost in USA	$65.00	$66.00	$84.00	$82.00	$297.00
Individual journals/year	12	24	12	14	62
Weight of journals/year in kg (lbs)[i]	7.65 (16.86)	10.20 (22.49)	12.26 (27.03)	13.14 (28.97)	43.25 (95.35)

[a] Includes "Bookshelf" and "Acknowledgment to Reviewers."
[b] Includes 38 abstracts of the annual meeting of the Section on Cardiology of the American Academy of Pediatrics.
[c] Letters to the Editor are called "Readers' Comments" in this journal.
[d] Includes abstracts of the 30th Annual Conference on Cardiovascular Disease Epidemiology.
[e] Includes "News from the American Heart Association," "Meetings Calendar" (domestic and abroad), and table of contents of 4 other American Heart Association journals (*Arteriosclerosis, Circulation Research, Hypertension* and *Stroke*), and "In Appreciation" to non-board reviewers.
[f] Includes American Heart Association Medical/Scientific Statements.
[g] Fourteen of the pages (The reference format one. . .) is included among the numbered editorial pages; the other 28, among the "A" (advertising) pages.
[h] Includes "newly elected members of the College, Board of Governors, Books Received, American College of Cardiology News, Committee appointments, and Participants in Bethesda Conference.
[i] Includes journal as received from the printer. Therefore, it includes the advertisements, covers, etc.

TABLE III Symposia Published in the *American Heart Journal* in 1990

1990 Date of Publication	Subject of Symposium	Guest Editor(s)	Sponsor	Number of Articles	Number of Discussions	Number of Pages	Interval (months) Symposium to Publication
February	Nicardipine	Joel A. Kaplan Michael A. Weber	DuPont Pharmaceuticals Syntex Laboratories	10	0	54	11
March	Costs and benefits of coronary risk factor reduction	C. Mancia	Pfizer International	13	4	66	8
August*	Metoprolol OROS	—	CIBA-GEIGY	5	0	28	—
September*	Nitrates for myocardial ischemia	Jonathan Abrams	CIBA-GEIGY	9	2	54	9
Totals				37	6	202	9 (mean)

* Included within the regular issues of these months.

TABLE IV Symposia Published in *The American Journal of Cardiology* in 1990

	1990 Date of Publication	Subject of Symposium	Guest Editor(s)	Sponsor	Number of Articles	Number of Discussions	Number of Pages	Interval (months) Symposium to Publication
A	January 2	Sotalol	Bramah N. Singh	Bristol-Myers	12	4	88	13
B	January 16	Cardiac arrhythmia suppression trial	Craig M. Pratt	Parke-Davis	7	0	42	5
C	February 2	Thrombosis and anti-thrombotic therapy	Valentin Fuster William C. Roberts	DuPont Pharmaceuticals	11	0	54	9
D	February 20	Moricizine HCl	Joel Morganroth J. Thomas Bigger, Jr	DuPont Pharmaceuticals	12	1	71	4
E	March 6	Hypokalemia in congestive heart failure	Milton Packer	Key Pharmaceuticals	8	2	52	—
F	March 20	Hypercholesterolemia and lovastatin	William C. Roberts Gerd Assmann	Merck Sharp & Dohme	10	0	43	9
G	April 3	Systemic hypertension	Bodo E. Strauer	Bayer AG Schwarz Pharma GmbH Merck Sharp & Dohme GmbH	16	0	88	9
H	May 2	Indapamide	Helios Pardell Paul M. Vanhoutte	Institut de Recherches Internationales Servier	16	0	80	12
I	May 22	Angiotensin-converting enzyme inhibitors	William W. Parmley	Merck Sharp & Dohme	10	0	53	14
J	June 4	Nitrate therapy	Adam Schneeweiss Marija Weiss	C.V.R.F. and Schwarz Pharma	13	0	56	—
K	June 19	Aldosteronism and aldosterone antagonism	David P. Lauler	G.D. Searle	19	0	57	—
A	September 4	High-density lipoprotein cholesterol	Antonio M. Gotto, Jr	Parke-Davis	7	1	31	12
B	September 18	Lovastatin	Scott M. Grundy	Merck Sharp & Dohme	7	0	55	10
C	September 25	Acebutolol after acute myocardial infarction	William H. Frishman Stanley H. Taylor	Rhône-Poulenc Sante	11	0	55	6
D	October 2	Angiotensin-converting enzyme inhibitors for heart failure	Jay N. Cohn	Merck Sharp & Dohme	7	0	45	8
E	October 16	Technetium-99 m myocardial perfusion imaging agents	Daniel S. Berman	DuPont Company	16	0	96	8
F	October 26	Cardiac imaging	Jeffrey A. Brinker Gerald L. Wolf	Winthrop Pharmaceuticals, Diagnostic Imaging Division	12	0	62	6
G	November 6	Factors triggering conversion from chronic to acute coronary syndromes	James E. Muller Geoffrey H. Tofler	Bristol-Myers Squibb	18	0	70	18
H	November 20	Managing ischemic myocardium	Robert A. Kloner	Pfizer Laboratories	6	0	31	12
I	December 18	Antiatherosclerotic effects of verapamil	William W. Parmley	GD Searle and Knoll Pharmaceuticals	8	0	40	9
20	Totals				226	8	1,169	10 (mean)

TABLE V Supplements* to *Circulation* Published in 1990

	1990 Date of Publication	Subject of Symposium	Guest Editor(s)	Industry Sponsor	No. of Articles	No. of Discussions	No. of Pages	Interval (mo) Symposium to Publication
I	January	Thromboxane A_2 antagonism in acute coronary syndromes	Attilio Maseri	Glaxo Pharmaceuticals	17	1	82	24
II	January	Measuring functional capacity in heart failure	Karlman Wasserman	Merck & Co.	7	0	64	—
III	February	Diastolic function in heart failure	Hubert Pouleur	ICI Pharmaceuticals Merck Sharp & Dohme Syntex Research	21	0	158	16
IV	March	Interventional cardiology	Kenneth M. Kent	Alpha Therapeutic Corp.	16	0	116	16
I	August	Sympathetic nervous system in heart failure	Milton Packer	ICI Pharmaceuticals	13	0	113	—
II	September	New concepts in heart failure	Richard Gorlin	ICI Pharmaceuticals Stuart Pharmaceuticals	19	0	160	20
IV	November	Cardiovascular surgery	D. Craig Miller	0	61	0	419	12
	Totals				154	1	1,112	18 (mean)

* Excludes the abstracts from the 63rd Scientific Sessions of the American Heart Association.

TABLE VI Number of Lines/Column and Words/Page in the Four Major Cardiology Journals in 1990

Journal	No. of Columns per Page	Lines per Column	Average Words per Column Line	Words per Page
AHJ	2	54	6.8	740
AJC	2	62	9.0	1,115
Circulation	2	61	8.0	980
JACC	2	53	8.5	900

TABLE VII Statement of Ownership, Management and Circulation of the Four Major USA Cardiology Journals in 1990

Journal	Filing Date	Mean No. of Copies Printed Each Month	Mean No. of Copies Distributed Each Month	Mean Paid Circulation Each Month
AHJ	10/1/90	13,200	12,500	11,800
AJC	9/20/90	32,000	30,000	22,100
Circulation	10/1/90	27,200	23,600	22,400
JACC	10/1/90	29,800	25,500	24,700

Oft-Repeated Requests to Authors from an Editor of a Cardiology Journal

During each of the past 9 years, *The American Journal of Cardiology* (AJC) has published from 650 to 750 articles in its regular issues (excludes symposia issues where costs are underwritten usually by one or more pharmaceutical companies). Before each article was published the originally submitted manuscript had been reviewed by 2 outside consultants (including board members) and then by me. After examining manuscripts which will eventually be accepted for publication I write (by hand) a tentative acceptance letter to the authors. (The letter is typed in the editorial office usually the next day.) This letter lays down the conditions which, if carried out, assures acceptance of the manuscript. Thus, I write 650 to 750 conditional acceptance letters yearly. Many conditional acceptance letters contain oft-repeated requests to authors and 9 of these oft-repeated requests are listed in this piece. Manuscript alterations which fulfill these requests make manuscripts more understandable, more readable, and more scientifically sound.

1. Limit the study to the patients whose heart disease was caused by only 1 or 2 conditions and eliminate the small numbers of patients in whom multiple different disease states caused the heart disease.[1] This circumstance is most commonly observed in manuscripts on congestive heart failure or arrhythmias. The study typically concerns the effects of 1 or more drugs on the failure or on the arrhythmia and let's say 80% of the patients have coronary artery disease, 10% have idiopathic dilated cardiomyopathy, 3% have valvular heart disease (type undefined), 2% have prosthetic or bioprosthetic cardiac valves, and 5% have no structural heart disease. It is best in this circumstance to limit the study to the patients in whom the failure or arrhythmia was associated with the same underlying condition, namely coronary artery disease, and to eliminate the other patients.

2. Eliminate the present tables displaying pooled data and in their place provide a single table listing the pertinent data in each study patient but no more than one line (at most 2 lines) across for any patient. Individual patient data are preferable to pooled data for studies involving no more than 30 patients. List the patients in some logical order, such as by age, etiology of disease, etc. The order in which the patients were seen or studied is usually a random order on a table, not a logical one. The headings at the top of each column should be precise phrases which can be answered by a plus, a zero, or a hyphen (indicating no information available or not applicable), or by a number, or, occasionally only, by a short phrase such as the etiology of a disease.

3. Decrease the length of the manuscript, particularly the discussion and/or introduction portions. Most manuscripts accepted for publication in the AJC are shorter than the originally submitted manuscripts. Thus, during the revision process most originally submitted manuscripts are shortened. Excessively lengthy manuscripts are most commonly caused by excessively long discussions. The length of the discussion is sometimes longer than the rest of the manuscript. In general, the discussion should be no more than a third of the manuscripts' text pages (those before the references and including the title page), and often can be much less.

Long introductions are rarely necessary. I favor single paragraph half-page introductions. Many authors repeat in the first paragraph of the discussion what was stated in the introduction. This duplication is unnecessary. A summary paragraph at the end of the discussion portion of the manuscript is usually redundant.

4. Try not to repeat data in the tables again in the text. Data clearly presented in a table need not be repeated in the text which is better used for commenting on unusual features about the data or for emphasizing particular features.

5. Limit the number of abbreviations to 3, to commonly recognized cardiologic phrases, and preferably to those phrases appearing in the manuscript's title.[2] If the subject of the manuscript concerns the frequency of atrial fibrillation (AF) in mitral stenosis (MS), limit the number of abbreviations to 2, namely MS and AF, and use them throughout the manuscript (not just in the abstract). The largest number of abbreviations I have seen in a manuscript submitted to the AJC is 26 but many have been in the low 20's. A manuscript containing this number of abbreviations indicates that the authors have not read the Instructions to Authors and that they are not students of the journal to which they have submitted the manuscript. More important, such technical insensitivities suggest that the manuscript's scientific worth is probably not high. I suspect I spend an hour a week getting abbreviations out of manuscripts. One journal (*Journal of the American College of Cardiology*) does not permit abbreviations other than the use of "AV" for atrioventricular and "ECG" for electrocardiogram. I try to avoid the use of abbreviations for single words. Authors use "ECG" sometimes to indicate "electrocardiogram," and, at other times, "electrocardiographic." I try to avoid its use. Abbreviations must be logical and appropriate. The proper abbreviation of "hypertrophic cardiomyopathy" is "HC," not "HCM." It is improper to abbreviate a syllable in one word and not in another. Abbreviations should not be used in titles of articles, in subheadings within articles, and in titles of figures and tables. Sentences should not begin with abbreviations (or with numerals). Only standard cardiologic abbreviations should be used. TAM (Tricuspid Annular Motion), ICA (enteric coated aspirin) and PPP (platelet poor plasma), for example, are not standard cardiologic abbreviations and they and similar ones should be avoided.

6. Limit the number of references to no more than 30 and eliminate references to abstracts. Scholarship is indicated by which references are selected, not by the number selected.[3] I prefer not to reference abstracts because too many errors occur in them and because they do not receive the type of careful peer review received by most manuscripts. The AJC publishes manuscripts faster than abstracts are published for the annual scientific sessions of the American Heart Association and the American College of Cardiology.[4] The barring of abstracts as references might in a small way serve to stimulate publication of data presented at meetings. The product that lives and the one that receives official peer review is the manuscript for the journal, not the abstract for the meeting.

7. Prepare the references in the style of the AJC. The form must conform to that of the *Journal*. The names of all authors are required, not just the first 3. The phrase "et al" is not used in any reference list in the AJC. No periods are used after the initials of the authors or after the abbreviations of the journals. The abbreviations of the names of journals are those used in the Index Medicus. The name of the journal is in italics. (Underlying the name is the proper substitute for italics when the latter is not available.) The year of publication comes after the name of the journal, not after the volume number. Inclusive pages are required. References are typed double spaced, not single spaced.

8. Crop the figures. Eliminating the nonessential parts of a photograph will allow larger sized reproduction of the important elements and therefore easier viewing. I crop figures when authors fail to do so. So take your choice--you or me. Few authors, I am afraid, really understand what figure-cropping is all about.

9. Read the Instructions to Authors and study the journal for style before resubmitting the manuscript. (This request should be standard before submitting the manuscript initially.)[5] When becoming editor of the AJC in June 1982 the first task I performed was picking the editorial board and the second was writing the Instructions to Authors, which appears in each issue of the AJC. When these Instructions are carried out to the letter an author provides a clear sign that he/she is sensitive to an editors' biases and the display of that sensitivity is heartwarming, I believe, to any editor. More important, manuscripts that are technically correct are usually scientifically sound.

William C. Roberts

William Clifford Roberts, MD
Editor in Chief

1. Roberts WC. Making clinical studies involving many patients useful to the single patient. *Am J Cardiol* 1990;65:1408.

2. Roberts WC. Abbreviations in the AJC. *Am J Cardiol* 1983;51:A9 A10.

3. Roberts WC. References: a clue to scholarship. *Am J Cardiol* 1983;51: A9–A10.

4. Roberts WC. Publishing manuscripts faster than abstracts. *Am J Cardiol* 1987;60:1133.

5. Roberts WC. Further comments on the "Instructions to Authors." *Am J Cardiol* 1984;54:470.

Alkaline Paper and Preserving the Record

The paper used for articles published in many of our major medical journals including *The New England Journal of Medicine, The Journal of the American Medical Association, Circulation, The American Heart Journal*, and *The American Journal of Cardiology* is acidic, and, therefore, these pages will crumble and blow away as dust within 50 years.[1-4] * In contrast, if these journals had been published on acid-free (alkaline) paper, the articles would be preserved for 500 years, maybe longer, depending on how they were stored. So why do these journals which record our scientific record use the non-permanent paper?

Magnitude of the problem: Nearly 80 million books in North American research libraries and an estimated 1,000 million books in libraries worldwide are threatened with destruction because they were printed on acidic paper.[1-4] In most university libraries in the USA about 30% of the volumes are brittle such that just 1 reading or 1 xerographing or 1 microfilming of the pages causes them to shatter irreparably. At the New York Public Library over 35 of 88 miles of bookshelves contain over 2.5 million dying books.[4,5] An estimated 25% of the 24 million books in the Library of Congress are not circulated because the pages crack when folded, and every year 77,000 more books in the collection become equally brittle.[4] It is estimated that 97% of the volumes in the federal government's premier library—which not only houses the largest collection of our English language heritage but also that of Latin America and the Arab world—will eventually disintegrate. The collection of the National Library of Medicine, the world's largest research library in a single scientific and professional field, contains 4.5 million items—books, journals, technical reports, manuscripts, microfilms and pictorial materials—and about 158,000 (12%) print volumes are brittle.[2,3,4,6] It is estimated that 92% of the post-1800 holdings of the library were printed on acidic paper. Seventy percent of books and journals printed in the twentieth century will be unusable by the year 2000.[4]

Origin of the acid in the paper: The oldest materials in libraries and archives are not the most endangered ones because acid was not introduced into the paper-making process until about 1850. Before that time linen and cotton rags were beaten by hand in water and the separated fibers collected on wire frame molds to make individual sheets of paper which were virtually devoid of acid.[7,8] With the coming of the industrial revolution and the increase in literacy in the mid-nineteenth century, the demand for paper skyrocketed. The result was that the hand-processed rag stock was largely abandoned in favor of wood pulp churned out by newly perfected machines. The wood pulp was of 2 types. *Mechanical* wood pulp is that produced by grinding up logs or shredding and grinding wood chips.[4] This type of pulp contains lignin, which is the primary non-cellulosic component in trees, and it causes paper to darken upon exposure to light and to degrade relatively quickly by oxidation and hydrolysis. (Newsprint has a high lignin content.) Because mechanical wood pulp contains lignin and other impurities, paper containing it has a relatively short lifespan. *Chemical* wood pulp is pulp produced by cooking wood chips in chemicals (to remove impurities).[4] Depending on what chemicals are added in subsequent processing, the resulting paper can be either acidic and have a relatively short shelf life, or alkaline and have a long shelf life. Unfortunately, until recent years, the most common chemical added was aluminum sulfate, an acid salt. Not until the late 1930s was it discovered that it was the acid, primarily sulfuric acid derived from the aluminum sulfate or alum, in the paper that caused it to be unstable and to degenerate. Already by 1910, however, it was learned that papers containing alkaline fillers, calcium carbonate for example, were quite stable and therefore permanent.[4]

Preservation of the deteriorating acidic publications: Preservation of the present print heritage is the major problem facing most libraries today.[1-3] During the next 10 years The National Library of Medicine is expected to invest the equivalent of one third of its acquisition budget to "clean up" the backlog of embrittled material. Microfilming of the brittle books, which costs about $70 a volume, is about the only currently available recourse but this process does not save the book. Currently, The National Library of Medicine is microfilming 20,000 to 25,000 volumes a year as part of its preservation program. Another preservation technique, which also treats one book at a time, consists of placing the book in a water-based solution, but this technique requires removal of the book's binding and is even more expensive than microfilming. In yet another process, which takes

**The Annals of Internal Medicine* switched to alkaline paper on November 1, 1991. The printer of the journal switched from acid to alkaline paper at no additional charge to the journal.

hours, each page is sprayed by hand with a base that neutralizes the acid. Several companies are trying to develop affordable techniques that rely on either a liquid or a vapor to treat hundreds of books at a time.[4,9,10] The books are immersed in a bath of magnesium butoxytriglycolate or some like substance, then drained, rinsed with a solvent, and dried again. The process theoretically neutralizes the acid and then the paper is treated with a buffering agent that bonds broken fibers and, therefore, strengthens the brittle pages. Books may be impregnated in a large chamber using gases such as diethyl zinc or ethylene oxide as deacidifying agents. So far, the Library of Congress has not been convinced that these "dry cleaning" processes for books are reliable or effective. Electronic document storage and retrieval using digital optical discs as the storage medium is being developed, but thus far this method of preserving the record is not ideal. Most discs have a lifetime of about 10 years, shorter than that of acid paper![11]

Prevention of deterioration of future print publications: The prevention of future paper embrittlement is actually easy. The answer is simply to use acid-free (alkaline) paper for all future publications.[1–4] In actuality, tremendous progress is being made rapidly toward that goal. In January 1987 the first meeting took place of The National Library of Medicine's Permanent Paper Task Force consisting of 34 members representing publishers, paper manufacturers, printers, editors, writers, and librarians. I was pleased to be the only physician on that task force. In January 1987 only 4% of the 3,050 titles of *Index Medicus* were published on acid-free paper. By October 1991, the time of the most recent meeting of the Permanent Paper Task Force, 48% of the titles of *Index Medicus* were known to be published on acid-free paper! In 1987 acid-free paper was in short supply and 2 manufacturers had a virtual monopoly on it in North America. Now, an estimated 35 paper manufacturers provide acid-free paper, such that today it is probably easier to purchase acid-free paper than acid paper. It is estimated that slightly over 50% of the paper produced for US print is now on alkaline paper. The expense of lost production is the biggest cost in conversion from acid to acid-free paper making. Conversion can vary from days to weeks among paper producers. Once the conversion is made it is cheaper to produce the alkaline paper than the acid paper. The reason is because calcium carbonate is cheap and larger quantities of this type of filler can be used than the more expensive filler used in acid paper. The alkaline papermaking process also requires considerably less water than does the process for acidic paper, and therefore the amount and need for treatment of discharge from mills into streams and rivers is drastically reduced. Alkaline paper making also is cleaner and less corrosive to machinery than acid-based paper making. Alkaline paper is an important marketing tool for both paper manufacturers and publishers. Alkaline paper is smoother and stronger than acidic paper, and type printed on it is usually sharper and easier to read than type on acidic paper. And shattering a commonly held belief, acid-free paper is price comparable in quality weights and grades to acidic paper.

Another factor pushing conversion toward alkaline paper is the increased sensitivity or awareness of the problem by paper producers, publishers, and authors. About 3 years ago I was asked to serve as a consultant to a new publishing company of medical books. I mentioned to the publisher that I would be glad to serve as a consultant but only if the books were to be published on acid-free paper. He asked "what was acid-free paper?" and what were its advantages over other paper? I was surprised to learn that he had never heard of acid-free paper. Four years ago I was talking to a publishing executive of the only USA cardiology journal published on acid-free paper. He had become aware only a month or so earlier that his journal was published on alkaline paper. It so happened that all journals published by that particular publisher used acid-free paper.

Authors are becoming progressively more sensitive to the problem. In March 1989 nearly 100 distinguished authors and major publishing figures gathered at the New York Public Library to pledge their commitment to the preservation of the printed word.[12] They signed a landmark declaration of book preservation calling for the use of acid-free paper for all first printings of quality hard-cover trade books. The declaration was signed at a special program entitled "Commitment Day" which was spearheaded by author and library trustee Barbara Goldsmith who has been galvanizing the literary community for this national preservation effort.

A major impetus toward conversion to acid-free paper has come from the federal government of the USA. In October 1990 the 101st Congress passed Public Law 101-423, which requires "the use of acid free permanent papers for publications of enduring value produced by the Government Printing Office or produced by Federal grant or contract. . . ."[4] This law has had a rapid impact on paper producers in North America because of the enormity of the USA's governmental printer. The Government Printing Office publishes 60,000 titles a year, a total valued at 1 billion dollars. The government's printer uses 500,000 tons of paper annually, an amount equivalent to 2.2% of all printed paper in the USA. In 1991, 77% of the paper used by the Government Printing Office will be alkaline and by 1996, 100% of the paper it uses will be alkaline. A good portion of this paper is of the recycled type and recycled and new alkaline paper is indistinguishable.

One item in Public Law 101-423 was the following[4]: "The Congress of the United States urgently recommends that American publishers and state and local governments use acid-free permanent papers for publications of enduring value. . ." Since passage of the federal law at least 21 states in the USA have passed similar laws or resolutions in their state houses, a move further pushing paper manufacturers in the USA to rapidly move from producing acid paper to alkaline paper. It is expected that most of the remaining states will pass similar laws or resolutions in the next few years.

Another item in Public Law 101-423 was the following[4]: "The Congress of the United States urgently recommends that the Secretary of State, Librarian of Congress, Archivist of the United States and other officials make known the national policy regarding acid free permanent papers to foreign governments and appropriate international agencies since the acid paper problem is worldwide and essential foreign materials being imported by our libraries are printed on acid paper." Europe began the move toward using alkaline paper about 20 years ago and thus is far ahead of the USA in publishing on alkaline paper. Virtually all paper produced in the 5 Scandinavian countries is now alkaline. Several other European countries as well as Canada and Australia are developing permanent paper standards.

Identifying publications using permanent paper: It is important that the use of permanent paper for a publication be identified by a notice on the verso of the title page of a book or in the masthead or copyright area of a periodical.[4] Such identification attests to the concern of the publisher and the author(s) for the preservation of the material published. Without it, libraries would have to test each publication and may in the future inadvertently apply time-consuming and expensive preservation treatments to publications that do not need them. The National Information Standards Organization (NISO) was selected by the American National Standards Institute (ANSI) and it approved and published in 1984 permanent paper standards for non-coated paper. The standards included (1) a minimum pH of 7.5; (2) tear resistance; (3) fold endurance; (4) minimum alkaline reserve equivalent to 2% calcium carbonate, and (5) absence of groundwood pulp. The infinity symbol within a circle was chosen to indicate that paper in the publication meets all 5 requirements of the permanent paper standard (Figure 1). For publications on coated paper and on uncoated paper that have not been demonstrated to meet all 5 requirements of the standard, but are known to be at least acid-free and free of groundwood, the phrase "Printed on acid-free paper" would appear in the publications. The permanent paper standard of 1984 (NISO/ANSI Z39.48) is now being revised and the revised standard, which is scheduled to appear in 1992, is being expanded to apply to both coated and uncoated papers.

Electronic publishing versus print publishing: There is a view that publishing in the foreseeable future will be by electronic means rather than by print means,

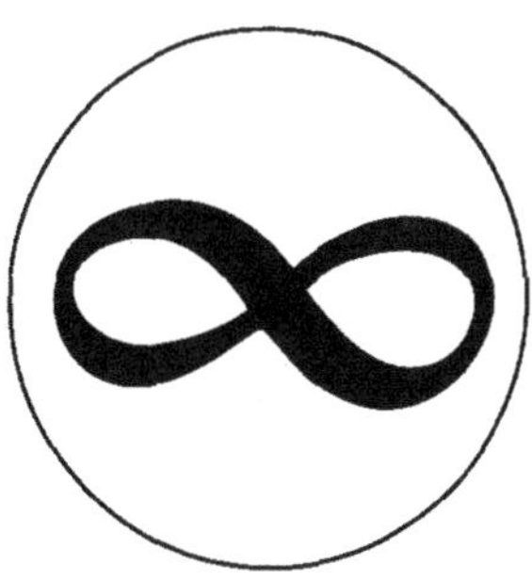

FIGURE 1. The infinity symbol within a circle should appear in all publications using alkaline paper and fulfilling 4 other criteria (see text).

and, therefore, it will not be necessary to preserve our previous print record or to prevent deterioration of our future print publications. Although electronics someday may be dominant, most experts today believe that paper publishing will remain the dominant type for many decades to come. The reasons are many. Paper publications are easy to read; they are highly portable; they are very comfortable to read; they are well accepted legally, and socially; they are durable (if published on alkaline paper); they can be published in a wide range of sizes, and they can accept advertising. In contrast, it is difficult to read to a grandchild from a screen. The electronic equipment is expensive. Advertising is difficult by electronic means. Databases are costly. There are legal problems in protecting the copyright because electronic publications are easy to copy. The quality of most electronic displays is not nearly as good as that of print publications. The user of electronic publications must be well trained in the use of the electronic equipment which rapidly becomes obsolete. So many people now use computers at work that it is nice to pick up a print publication when getting home. Thus, it is unlikely that electronic publishing will replace print publishing for years to come. Indeed, print publishing is increasing rather than the reverse. In 1990, an average of 320 pounds (145 kg) of printing and writing paper was used by each citizen in the USA, an increase from 308 pounds (140 kg) used in 1989, up again from the 294 (134 kg) pounds used in 1988.[6] At least 95% of all organizational records are estimated to reside on paper.[6]

Summary: The most productive period of human beings on planet earth has been the last 140 years (since 1850), and most publications during that period have been on acid paper and therefore they have or soon will vanish into dust. The next 140 years surely will be an even more productive period for humankind, and that record of accomplishment must be prevented from slowly burning into ashes. It is easy to prevent such an outcome. Simply printing our records on alkaline paper will allow our writings to remain permanently for future generations. A good quantity of toilet paper and paper towels now consists of acid-free paper. Surely if some of our toilet paper can be alkaline, most of our medical publications, including all our peer-reviewed journals, can use a paper of at least similar quality.

William Clifford Roberts, MD
Editor in Chief

1. Hafner AW, Whitely WP. The crisis facing printed medical literature. Acid paper. *Arch Intern Med* 1988;148:1439–1440.

2. DeBakey L. Book-burning in our medical libraries: prevention or palliation? *Am J Cardiol* 1988;62:458–461.

3. Debakey L, DeBakey S. Our silent enemy: ashes in our libraries. *Bull Med Libr Assoc* 1989;77:258–268.

4. Association of Research Libraries, *in collaboration with* American Library Association, Commission on Preservation and Access, and National Humanities Alliance. Preserving Knowledge: The Case for Alkaline Paper. Washington, DC: Association of Research Libraries 1990 (revised): 128.

5. Goldsmith B. Time to make books last longer. *Publishers Weekly*, January 22, 1988.

6. Kalina C. A tale of two papers: now at last the best of times. Among Friends. Newsletter of the Friends of the National Library of Medicine 1991;6(2):4–5.

7. McMurtrie DC. The Book. The Story of Printing & Bookmaking. New York: Dorset Press 1971:676.

8. Chappell W. A Short History of the Printed Word. New York: Dorset Press 1989:259.

9. Rensberger B. Acid test: stalling self-destruction in the stacks. *Washington Post*, August 29, 1988.

10. Harris J. Dry cleaning. *Forbes*, March 4, 1991, page 128.

11. Zachary G. Compact disks for data aren't forever, it turns out. *The Wall Street Journal*, October 16, 1991.

12. Declaration of Book Preservation. The New York Public Library Commitment Day, March 7, 1989, *The New York Times*, March 16, 1989.

FROM THE EDITOR and PUBLISHER

Design Changes in the AJC

In early 2005, Elsevier assembled 3 focus groups in 3 different US cities to discuss several medical journals, with particular focus on *The American Journal of Cardiology* (AJC). Each focus group included 8 cardiologists, most of whom were not presently AJC subscribers, but all of whom periodically examined the AJC. The discussions were witnessed via 1-way windows by 3 Elsevier publishers, including 1 of us (DHD) in 2 out of 3 and 1 of us (WCR) in 1. Although many of the recommendations had value, 3 items, in particular, emerged in all 3 focus groups that provided the stimulus for the changes appearing in this July 1, 2005, issue.

One suggestion was to display all or at least some of the contents on the journal's cover so that articles of interest were easier to find. This first suggestion was readily introduced by decreasing the amount of space on the cover to print the name of the journal, which, in turn, opened up space for the contents.

The second was to organize the "Brief Reports" in a format similar to those of the "Long Reports." This second suggestion was acted on by including those reports previously included under the heading of Brief Reports in the same section as the Long Reports on the same topic. (This latter suggestion was actually made by a member of the editorial board—Dr. John Kastor—several years ago.) One of us (WCR) has felt for many years that Brief Reports in the AJC have not received their proper recognition. Including them with the Long Reports and starting each report on a separate page, rather than "back-to-back" as previously published, will give them the same weight as the Long Reports. The new format, for example, will allow at times the insertion of a Brief Report before a Long Report in a particular disease category, such as coronary artery disease, cardiomyopathy, etc. The length of an article does not determine its value. Watson and Crick won the Nobel prize for a 1-page article! The major difference between a Long Report and a Brief Report is that the former makes >1 point and the latter, mainly 1 point.

The third suggestion of the focus group participants was to create a more reader-friendly interior layout design, so that readers would not have to struggle visually with the dominant boldface and large type throughout the articles. To this end, we have created a more user-friendly look without sacrificing the editorial integrity of the articles.

Another major AJC change occurred in April 2005, namely, the implementation of an Internet-based online submission system for the journal. The system provides online submission for authors with a faster more efficient seamless link from submission through the editorial and peer-review process, including swifter processes at the production stage. In short, this Internet submission system reduces the transfer time of the entire editorial workflow process—from author to editorial office, from editorial office to reviewer and back, and ultimately to transmitting final, accepted manuscripts to the publisher. The online processing of manuscripts makes the workflow process speedier and more efficient, and it also saves on editorial office postage costs.

Galleys, too, are currently being sent to the authors electronically, via a PDF page proofing process, which expedites the production and manufacturing processes.

Online editing is more of a challenge (at least for one of us—WCR) but, overall, we are convinced that this Internet process will facilitate the submission of more quality manuscripts both from here and abroad. We are thrilled with the potential the system offers authors, reviewers and readers, but the editor will continue to wield his pen on those manuscripts in need of adjustments.

We hope that you are happy with the changes. We are always open to suggestions for improvements (wc.roberts@baylorhealth.edu).

William C. Roberts, MD
Editor in Chief, AJC

David H. Dionne
Executive Publisher, AJC

Revising Manuscripts After Studying Reviewers' Comments

When reviewing manuscripts submitted to *The American Journal of Cardiology (AJC)*, I often sense that a manuscript had earlier been sent to another journal that had declined it. This suspicion is usually prompted by observing that the submitted manuscript was not formatted according to the AJC's Instructions to Authors (e.g., the abstract is structured rather than nonstructured; names of all authors and full inclusive pages are not provided for every reference, etc.) Not infrequently, a reviewer will indicate to me that "I earlier reviewed this manuscript for another journal and the authors made no attempts to alter their manuscript in response to my suggestions." Such behavior on the part of authors is an affront to the review process. A rejection by one journal is not a ticket to ignore the comments of the reviewers or to refrain from revising the manuscript appropriately before sending it to another journal. Reviewers serve authors unselfishly, and authors must respect their objective comments by revising their manuscripts accordingly before sending their manuscripts to other journals.

I have on several occasions reacted inappropriately to reviews of *my own* manuscripts, thinking "The reviewers didn't really understand my manuscript or appreciate its quality" or "The reviewers didn't really read the manuscript," or "Their comments were not appropriate or applicable to my manuscript." Nearly always after further reflection on the comments of reviewers, I have realized that their criticisms, although not always stated in a beautifully articulate manner, were in actuality quite useful. Many reviewers, especially our best investigators, today are burdened with too many manuscripts to review. The busier the potential reviewers, the less time he/she has to spend on a review. Most, I suspect, dictate their reviews and spend little time editing the reviews once prepared. Thus, reviews are not like manuscripts. They are not edited multiple times but are performed relatively quickly and, as a consequence, sentence structure is not always the best and paragraphs are not always well developed. As a result, it is important for authors after receiving reviewers' comments to try to "smell out" what the reviewer is really getting at by his/her words. It's the intent of the reviewer, not his/her actual words, which is important for an author to perceive. That might take several readings of the reviews to sense what the reviewer feels is wrong or inappropriate or unsupported in another's manuscript.

In conclusion, we all need to be grateful for reviews of our manuscripts and more appreciative of those who spent time reviewing our work. We must respond to reviewers' comments by revising our manuscripts appropriately, whether they are returned to the journal where the manuscript was originally submitted or submitted to an entirely different journal for the first time.

William Clifford Roberts, MD
Baylor Heart & Vascular Institute
Baylor University Medical Center
Dallas, Texas

Present-Day Challenges of Managing Successfully a Non-Society Owned Cardiovascular Journal

There are 2 basic types of medical journals: those in which the journal's title is owned by a society and those in which the journal's title is owned by the publisher. Subscriptions to the societies' publications are usually included in the societies' dues. Subscriptions to journals owned by publishers are paid by the subscribers directly to the publishers of the journals. Several current publisher-owned journals initially were the official journals of societies, but later, the societies broke the relationships and started their own journals (i.e., owned the journals' titles). *The American Heart Journal* (begun in 1926) and *The American Journal of Cardiology* (*AJC*) (begun in 1958), for example, began as the official publications of their societies, but the journal titles were owned by the publishers. Later, the societies and publishers dissolved their relationships, but each journal continued independent of the society. *Circulation* and *The Journal of the American College of Cardiology* were the first journals owned by the American Heart Association and the American College of Cardiology, respectively, and the publishers of their journals are under contract with the societies.

The publisher-owned journals also are of 2 types: (1) those with *uncontrolled* circulations, in which subscribers pay publishers directly for their subscriptions, and (2) those with *controlled* circulations, in which publishers send the journals free of charge to recipients of their choice.[1] These latter journals are entirely dependent on advertisers for support. *Clinical Cardiology* is an example of these journals, but it has peer review of its manuscripts. Most purely advertiser dependent journals, referred to as "throwaway" journals, however, are not peer reviewed. Most publisher-owned journals, whether with uncontrolled or controlled circulations, are entirely clinically oriented. Virtually all of the basic science cardiovascular journals are society owned.

A major challenge today for all clinical cardiovascular journals—and even more so for general medical and multispecialty journals—is the *decreasing advertising revenue for medical journals*. The shift by pharmaceutical companies of sizable portions of their advertising budgets directly to consumers via television, radio, newspapers, and magazines and the slowing of growth rates for the pharmaceutical companies diminish advertising monies available for medical journals. As the number of ads in medical journals decreases, subscription costs increase, which in turn causes the number of subscribers to decrease. As a consequence, subscriptions to non-society-owned medical journals have either leveled off or are decreasing. In contrast, because the numbers of cardiologists increase each year over the number retiring or dying, the number of subscribers to society-owned journals continues to increase. Thus, the reduction in advertising revenue potentially hurts the publisher-owned cardiovascular journals more than the society-owned cardiovascular journals. The publisher-owned journals also do not have the leverage of some society-owned journals, which can promise prime exhibition space at their annual scientific sessions to pharmaceutical and device companies, for example, if a certain number of ads are placed in their journal or journals in a particular year.

In 2008, 8 *new American society-owned cardiovascular journals* appeared, all in a single year and all society owned! All are presently bimonthly. The long-term effect on publisher-owned cardiovascular journals is so far unclear, but certainly this enormous influx of society-owned journals in a single year cannot be beneficial to the publisher-owned journals. The number of manuscripts submitted to *AJC* in 2008 is running only slightly less than in 2007 (about 3,000), but the percentage of total manuscripts submitted from outside the United States has increased.

The more recently certified American cardiologists, nearly all of whom become members of the American Heart Association and the American College of Cardiology, are accustomed to *getting their medical journals free*, which is not the case after fellowship, and having to pay for non-society-owned journals is a habit not acquired by many of the younger cardiologists. Furthermore, many of the younger cardiologists get their information online, a habit not as frequent among older cardiologists.

The *process of selecting editors-in-chief* is much different for a society-owned journal compared with a publisher-owned journal. Societies have publication committees, and they are the ones who select editors-in-chief for their particular journals. The editor-in-chief of a publisher-owned cardiovascular journal serves at the pleasure of the publisher and is selected by the publisher. An independent publisher may have less access to the leaders of the cardiovascular community than do society publishing committees. (In my opinion, few society publishing committees or publishers, however, have thoughtfully developed criteria for potential editors-in-chief. Whether specified criteria would be useful in the selection process, however, is unclear.)

There is *competition among the better clinical cardiovascular journals for the better cardiovascular manuscripts*. Editors of publisher-owned journals need to be proactive in recruiting manuscripts, particularly reviews and editorials, especially from the elite in the cardiovascular community. Another means by which publisher-owned cardiovascular journals can compete effectively with society-owned cardiovascular journals is to publish manuscripts that are as clinically useful as possible, ideally applicable to the next patient seen. Manuscripts involving nonhuman animals are rarely helpful when seeing the next patient, and therefore, they were eliminated when the *AJC* became a publisher-run journal rather than a society-run journal. Publisher-owned journals also need features that are unique to them. The *AJC*, for example, publishes *interviews* of prominent cardiovascular specialists, informal *roundtables* on particular topics discussed by experts, and symposia from meetings.

Publisher-owned cardiovascular journals also must operate as efficiently as possible and deal with authors as pleasantly as possible. Manuscripts submitted to the *AJC* are sent out usually the next day to 2 potential reviewers, each of whom was asked if he or she was willing to review the manuscripts in question. Most manuscript decisions are made within a month of receipt. Revised manuscripts are usually accepted promptly. Manuscripts declined by other journals can be submitted to the *AJC* along with reviews from the other journals and the authors' responses to them, and an "accept (with further revision)" or "reject" decision can then be made promptly.

Another means by which publisher-owned cardiovascular journals can compete effectively with society-owned journals is to *publish symposia* under separate cover. These are sponsored by ≥1 pharmaceutical or device company, and they are welcomed, for example, in the *AJC*. These are all organized by ≥1 guest editor. In 2008, Dr. Clyde Yancy began serving as the overall editor of all symposia submitted to the *AJC*. Readership surveys have shown very favorable responses to the published symposia, all of which are published under separate cover, with a different color from the regular issues. No advertisements appear in the supplement issues. Symposia are profitable to the publisher and help support the regular issues.

In the past, sales of reprints have been a prominent profit source for publishers of medical journals, but now authors order far fewer reprints than they did in the past.

As have newspapers, the publishers of multiple medical journals now sell Internet packages that include not only access to their particular journals but to other journals published by the same publisher. These Internet packages are becoming important revenue sources for publishers of multiple medical journals. Electronic editions of the journals and the advertisements in them, on the journals' Web sites and in the tables of contents, also are sources of revenue.

And the *open access of publishing* model pioneered by BioMed Central (*http://www.biomedicentral.com*) and the Public Library of Science (*http://www.plos.org*) are made freely and permanently accessible online immediately upon publication. Bentham Open is another open-access journal devoted to various disciplines in science and technology (*http://www.oa.cardiovascular-med.org*). This type of competition almost surely will increase with time.

In summary, there are too many cardiovascular journals! Because of inadequate advertising revenue, many controlled (throwaway), publisher-owned cardiovascular journals have disappeared in recent times, and others will follow. This is not all bad. In 2008, the American Heart Association started 6 new cardiovascular journals, and the American College of Cardiology started 2 new journals, all bimonthly. The long-term effect on the remaining uncontrolled publisher-owned cardiovascular journals is as yet unclear, but there will be an effect. The new journals and the enormous amount of cardiovascular information provided online, however, will surely put pressure on the publisher-owned journals to be as clinically useful as possible and to provide unique features, such as interviews, roundtables, and symposia, not available in most society-owned cardiovascular journals.

William Clifford Roberts, MD
Baylor Heart and Vascular Institute
Baylor University Medical Center
Dallas, Texas

1. Roberts WC. Some realities of present-day cardiologic journal publishing in the USA. *Cardiology* 1987;74:254–262.

The *AJC* and the World Wide Web

Vincent E. Friedewald, MD[a,*] and William C. Roberts, MD[b]

There is nothing wrong with change, if it is in the right direction.

—Sir Winston Churchill

Since its first issue in 1958, *The American Journal of Cardiology* (*AJC*) has been dedicated to current, clinically relevant, and scientifically sound information. Dramatic advances in communications, led by the Internet, have fundamentally altered the exchange of information, however, and now challenge the role of traditional print media. The *AJC* is a committed participant in this electronic and digital revolution, as it has been since its full-text electronic posting for institutional customers on ScienceDirect (*http://www.sciencedirect.com*) in 1997 and for individual customers at *http://www.AJConline.org* since 2000.

As Sir Winston implied, change is not inherently good, and it is often detrimental to good causes. We guarantee that *AJC*'s changes "in the right direction" will not compromise a half century of publishing excellence. Traditional criteria for publication will be preserved, because scientific rigor and editorial excellence are just as important when they reside on the Internet. Furthermore, we do not embrace new technologies for the sake of novelty; rather, every new "e" feature will truly enhance our mission of providing the best possible services to contributors and readers of the *AJC*.

Here are some features currently available at *http://www.AJConline.org*:

Full-text Articles: All articles published in regular and supplemental issues of the *AJC* since 1995.

"Push" Tables of Contents: Registration for bimonthly e-mail notification of the table of contents of every upcoming *AJC* issue.

Forthcoming Tables of Contents: Article titles and their authors in forthcoming issues of the *AJC* at least 3 to 4 months in advance of the print publication.

Articles in Press: Full corrected author page proofs, available on-line 4 to 8 weeks before print publication.

Interviews Collection: All published interviews from 1997 onward by Dr. William Roberts of notable specialists in cardiovascular medicine.

The Editor's Roundtable: In-depth discussions by opinion leaders on topics of particular importance in clinical cardiology, offered for free on-line continuing medical education credit by Baylor University Medical Center.

The Editor's Consensus: Evidenced-based clinical guidelines authored by opinion leaders on select topics, also offered for free continuing medical education by Baylor University Medical Center.

Multimedia Library: A multimedia collection of video, audio, and animation complementing certain published articles, enhancing their value and providing subscribers high-quality, free materials for their personal education and research.

Internet Submissions: Article submissions at the "Submit Manuscript" button/link or at the *AJC* Elsevier Editorial System link (*http://ees.elsevier.com/ajc/*).

In addition to these features of *AJConline*, the *AJC* now offers Medline advance transmission: corrected author proofs transmitted at least 6 weeks before print publication, accelerating Medline citations.

Finally, new features are on the way, beginning on June 9, 2009, with the *AJC* "Case of the Month." Each month, a patient with special diagnostic and treatment challenges will be presented in the *AJC*, solvable only by going to *http://www.AJConline*, selecting "Case of the Month," and figuring out the answers using the Argus1 Medical Decision Support System.

Thus, our changes are all "in the right direction." If you have not already done so, please go to *http://www.AJConline*, and you will agree.

[a]University of Notre Dame, Notre Dame, Indiana; and [b]Baylor Heart and Vascular Institute, Baylor University Medical Center, Dallas, Texas.
Manuscript received February 11, 2009; revised manuscript received and accepted February 11, 2009.

*Corresponding author: Tel: 574-631-6675; fax: 574-631-4505.

E-mail address: vfriedew@nd.edu (V.E. Friedewald).

Reducing Flaws in the Review Process of Manuscripts Submitted to Medical Journals for Publication*

Before addressing the assigned topic, let me briefly provide my qualifications for doing so. I became editor of *The American Journal of Cardiology* (AJC) in June 1982. From 1983 through 2008, 58,282 manuscripts passed across my desk, and 17,979 were accepted. In 1982, a little more than 1,100 manuscripts were submitted; in 2007, a little more than 3,200. Additionally, I have authored >1,000 publications in peer-reviewed journals. Being on the author's end has taught me more than being on the editor's end.

Before providing suggestions to reduce flaws in the review process, let me mention some advantages and disadvantages of the process. First, some *advantages:* Clearly, the review process improves the reporting of medical science and in this way is useful to authors, to editors, to reviewers themselves, and consequently to patients. Most reviewers are impartial, and most are good at detecting inconsistencies, incongruities, omissions, commissions, and inadvertent errors; inadequate descriptions or characterizations of the populations studied; improper study designs; outdated methods; poor figures and tables; inappropriate or exaggerated conclusions; and poor syntax. The correction of these deficiencies obviously improves manuscripts. Reviewing a manuscript makes a reviewer read more critically than he or she might do otherwise; it thus improves his or her own database and theoretically makes for a better investigator, teacher, and physician. Another infrequently mentioned advantage of the review process is that it makes authors more careful in their preparation of manuscripts, because they need to "cover their flanks," so to speak, to persuade reviewers and editors that their manuscripts are of high quality. And reviewers also provide "ammunition" for editors, making the rejection of manuscripts, particularly ones from very prominent investigators or friends, a bit easier.

Now to *disadvantages:* The review process, of course, is time-consuming and expensive; delays publication; is often biased; is relatively poor at detecting plagiarism, deceit, and intentional errors (fraud); and, on occasion, the suggestions provided (if carried out) do not improve the scientific quality or readability of a manuscript. Manuscripts tend to be reviewed by investigators involved in the same type of research presented in the manuscripts they are asked to review. The reviewers, in other words, are often scientific competitors. (The process is like asking Ford to review plans for a new car design by General Motors without compensation.) Not all reviewers are experts in the subjects of the manuscripts they are asked to review. The process also can exhaust the better reviewers. And the worst manuscripts usually get the most reviews because they move from 1 rejection to another until they are finally accepted by some journal for publication.

Now to *suggestions*, directed mostly to editors, *for reducing flaws in the review process*:

1. *Give careful thought to who would be the best reviewers of a manuscript.* The expertise of the review is dependent on the expertise of the reviewer.
2. *Request that authors give names of potential out-of-city reviewers who they believe will provide* **nonbiased** *critical reviews of their work.* Editors have no monopoly on the correct picking of reviewers! Reviews and recommendations of reviewers recommended by authors are usually relatively similar to those recommended by editors.
3. *Request of authors also the names of potential out-of-city reviewers who they believe will provide* **biased** *(unfair) reviews of their work, and honor those requests.*
4. *Refrain from sending many manuscripts to hypercritical potential reviewers to whom no manuscript or work (other than their own) is quite good enough.* Likewise, reviewers with obvious conflicts of interest or those who abuse the review process (acquiring ideas or protecting their own investigations) should be avoided.
5. *Do not overwork exceptional reviewers.* These particularly helpful reviewers tend to review for multiple journals, and their energies can be depleted by excessive reviewing. Consider saving them for the most controversial or potentially controversial manuscripts.
6. *Refrain from regularly sending manuscripts that initially receive mixed recommendations to third reviewers.* At times, I have exchanged the positive and negative reviews between initial reviewers with advantage to all parties before returning manuscripts to their authors. Discussion of these manuscripts with associate editors also saves additional reviews.
7. *Compose the editorial board in a meritorious fashion, including individuals proved to be conscientious*

Manuscript received December 5, 2008; revised manuscript received and accepted December 11, 2008.

* An address given at the 69th Congress of the Italian Society of Cardiology, December 14, 2008.

and prompt reviewers, not just prominent investigators or chiefs of prominent departments or divisions.

8. *Refrain from sending some types of manuscripts for review,* or at least have no requirement that all submissions be sent for outside review, for example, editorials, readers' comments (letters to the editor), reviews, debates, pros-and-cons, symposia, and case reports.
9. *Do not substitute reviewers for editors.* All manuscripts need the editor-in-chief's opinion. Authors deserve it. I edit originally submitted manuscripts before returning them to authors for their revisions.
10. *Refrain, except in unusual circumstances, from sending revised manuscripts back to 1 or more reviewers of the originally submitted manuscript for reevaluation.* If this is to be done, I inform authors when returning to them the originally submitted manuscripts.
11. *Decline extremely poor manuscripts without outside review, thus saving the time and energy of reviewers for more worthwhile manuscripts.*
12. *Reduce the reviewing of previously rejected manuscripts by other journals by sending the previous reviews and responses to them, the manuscripts originally sent to the other journals that rejected them, and the revised manuscripts to the new journal.* This option has been used by *AJC* since 1982 and it usually prevents the necessity of starting the review process anew.
13. *Remember the golden rule of reviewing. Frequent* authors are usually *frequent* reviewers, but the 2 hats are worn at different times. When authors submit manuscripts to a journal, their patience for delay in receiving the "acceptance" or "rejection" decision often is short. When these same authors, however, become reviewers, their patience for delay often appears to be much longer. Reviewers need to treat authors as they would like to be treated when they are authors.
14. *Do the reviewing process online or, if not, convert accordingly.* Online reviewing improves efficiency: reviews are returned much more quickly, authors receive decisions more quickly, and so on, than when transferring paper.
15. *Forget blind reviewing, whereby the names and institutions of the authors are not supplied to the reviewers.* This system was tried at *AJC* for 6 months, and a few reviewers resented not knowing for sure the names of the authors of the manuscripts they were asked to review. Giving authors, however, the option of requesting blind reviews and giving reviewers the option of signing their reviews are reasonable and improve the transparency of the process.
16. *Keep the final decision on manuscripts in the hands of the editor-in-chief.* Reviewers serve to provide suggestions to authors and editors on means to improve the quality of manuscripts. Reviewers should not replace editors, whose charge is to decide, among other things, which manuscripts to accept and which to reject and, if acceptable, in what form.
17. *Continuously update the reviewer files.* Periodically ask editorial board members, among others, for names to be added to the journal's reviewer file. Get investigators involved in the reviewing of manuscripts of others early in their careers. The young are often more critical than the old, and they generally have more time to do reviews.
18. *Emphasize to authors the importance of following the journal's instructions to authors.* Study the journal's format before submitting a manuscript. An editor's patience can be tested by not doing so. And if a manuscript is rejected by 1 journal, make sure that the previous reviewers' comments are responded to by altering the manuscript before sending it to the next journal. Not doing so is an insult to the review process.
19. *Befriend the publisher.* Work in parallel as much as possible. Minimize surprises on both sides. The process works more smoothly when there exists a friendly relationship between editor and publisher.
20. *Before sending a manuscript to a journal, have a local fellow investigator—a friend—examine the work.* Others can see oversights in our manuscripts that can be corrected before submission to a journal.
21. *Peer review also follows publication by the publication of readers' comments (letters to the editor) and other discussions* (such as journal clubs, medical meetings, media).
22. *Thank reviewers for particularly outstanding reviews.* Occasionally publish their reviews alongside the manuscripts reviewed. Recognize them in the journal.

In summary, as many have pointed out, peer review is imperfect, being subjective, frequently biased, and not reliable at detecting many imperfections or even fraud, but nevertheless, the review process improves most manuscripts, and there is no substitute for it. Reviewing manuscripts of others is unselfish, honorable, altruistic, and poorly rewarded, but it is absolutely essential to keep the reporting of scientific investigations to high standards. All of us benefit by having others make suggestions for improving our manuscripts.

William Clifford Roberts, MD
Baylor Heart and Vascular Institute
Baylor University Medical Center,
Dallas, Texas 75246

Piercing the Impact Factor and Promoting the Eigenfactor™

The publisher of *The American Journal of Cardiology* (*AJC*), Jane Grochowski, in late June 2011 shared with me a copy of the most recently released *Journal Citation Reports*, 2010 Science Edition, which ranks among others the "Cardiac and Cardiovascular System" journals by their Impact Factors (IFs). The list included the names of 114 cardiovascular journals, their International Standard Serial Numbers, their total citations in 2010, their latest IFs, their 5-year average IFs, their Immediacy Indexes, the number of articles published in each journal in 2010, the cited half-life, the Eigenfactor™ Score, and the Article Influence Score.

Numbers of articles published in 2010 in each journal: The numbers of articles published in the 114 journals in 2010 ranged from 0 (*The American Journal of Geriatric Cardiology*) to 608 (*Annals of Thoracic Surgery*): 59 journals (52%) published ≤100 articles in 2010, 31 (27%) published 101 to 200, 11 (10%) published 201 to 300, 5 (4%) published 301 to 400, and 6 journals (5%) published >400 articles. Thus, 90 (79%) of the 114 journals (79%) published <200 articles in 2010. The 6 journals publishing >400 articles in 2010 were the following: *Annals of Thoracic Surgery*, 608; *AJC*, 604; *Circulation*, 549; the *Journal of Thoracic and Cardiovascular Surgery*, 492; the *American Journal of Physiology—Heart and Circulatory Physiology*, 490, and the *Journal of the American College of Cardiology* (*JACC*), 456.

Numbers of citations in 2010 in each journal: The numbers of citations for each of the 114 journals are listed in the *Journal Citation Reports*, 2010 Science Edition, as "2010 Total Cites." What does "2010 Total Cites" mean? These are total numbers of citations for each journal from the time the journal started through 2010. The numbers of citations in the 114 journals ranged from 1 (the *Russian Journal of Cardiology*) to 151,020 (*Circulation*): 51 journals (45%) had ≤100 citations, 28 (25%) had 1,001 to 2,000, 10 (9%) had 2,001 to 3,000, 11 (10%) had 3,001 to 10,000, 6 (5%) had 10,001 to 20,000, and 7 (6%) had >20,000 citations. The latter 7 journals included *Circulation*, 151,020; *JACC*, 69,405; *Circulation Research*, 42,343; *AJC*, 36,401; the *American Journal of Physiology—Heart and Circulatory Physiology*, 29,457, and the *European Heart Journal* (*EHJ*), 26,311. The length of time a journal has been in existence does not necessarily correlate with its number of total citations. The *American Heart Journal* started in 1926 (total citations 19,976), *Circulation* began in 1952 (total citations 151,020), the *AJC* began in 1958 (total citations 36,401), the *JACC* began in 1983 (total citations 69,405), and the *EHJ* started in 1980 (total citations 26,311). Obviously, being a major cardiologic society's official journal plays a huge role, indeed the dominant role, in determining the number of citations a journal receives.

IF calculation: The IF is calculated as follows: citations to "citable articles" (excludes editorials and letters to the editor [called Readers' Comments in the *AJC*]) in a single year of articles published in the previous 2 years divided by the number of citable articles published in the same 2-year period. For example, if a journal has an IF of 3 in 2010, then its articles published in 2008 and 2009 each received an average of 3 citations. Some published articles, however, in a small number of publications receive an enormous number of citations, and others receive hardly any. Thus, the IF for a particular journal can be based almost entirely on relatively few of its articles.

IFs for cardiovascular system journals in 2010: The IFs in 2010 for the 114 journals ranged from 0 (the *Russian Journal of Cardiology* and *Cardiovascular Therapeutics Preview*) to 14.43 (*Circulation*). IFs in 2010 were <1.0 in 25 journals (22%), 1.0 to 2.0 in 32 (28%), >2.0 to 3.0 in 18 (16%), >3.0 to 4.0 in 15 (13%), >4.0 to 5.0 in 11 (10%), >5.0 to ≤10.0 in 10 (9%), and >10.0 in 3 (3%).

IF of the *AJC* in 2010: Despite the AJC's publishing the largest number of articles of any cardiology journal and being the fourth most cited cardiovascular journal, the *AJC* ranked only 27th in the IF category. The IF for the *AJC* in 2010 was 3.68, whereas that for *Circulation* was 14.43, for *JACC* was 14.29, and for *EHJ* was 10.05.

The *AJC* published 623 articles in 2008 and 623 in 2009. The *AJC*'s IF for 2010 was derived by dividing the number of citations from these 2 previous years (total 4,854) by the number of articles published in the 2 previous years (total 1,319), the result being 3.68. Examination of the 26 journals with higher IFs than the *AJC* in 2010 discloses that none published as many articles as did the *AJC*, and only 3 had more citations. Indeed, of the 26 journals with higher IFs, 11 (42%) published <100 articles in 2010, 9 (35%) published 101 to 300, and only 4 (15%) published >300 articles (*Circulation*, 549; the *American Journal of Physiology — Heart and Circulatory Physiology*, 490; *JACC*, 456; and *Circulatory Research*, 322).

Methods to improve a journal's IF: First, publish as many guidelines, surely the most frequently referenced type of article, as possible. Essentially, only journals owned by major societies now publish guidelines. Thus, *Circulation* (the official journal of the American Heart Association), *JACC* (the official journal of the American College of Cardiology Foundation), and the *EHJ* (the official journal of the European Society of Cardiology)

Manuscript received and accepted April 8, 2011.

are the only journals publishing guidelines, and these 3 have the highest IFs of all cardiovascular journals. Generally, guidelines are published simultaneously in both *Circulation* and *JACC*, thus benefiting both journals from the citations.

Second, publish as many reviews, another frequently referenced type of article, as possible. For example, *Nature Reviews Cardiology* published only 57 articles in 2010 and had only 440 citations the 2 previous years, and its 2010 IF was 7.47; *Progress in Cardiovascular Disease* published only 53 articles in 2010 and had 1,883 citations, for a resulting IF of 4.84; and *Current Problems in Cardiology* published only 12 articles in 2010 and had 413 citations, yielding an IF of 3.44, not much different from the IF of the *AJC* (3.68), which published 50 times as many articles! The *AJC* in 2010 published 21 reviews. Only in recent years has the *AJC* published reviews, each of which of course diminishes the number of editorial pages available for original investigations, which generally do not get as many citations as do reviews.

Third, publish relatively few articles each year. The larger the number of articles published, the larger the denominator, which lessens the IF. The *EHJ*, the journal with the third highest IF, published 275 articles in 2010, 329 (55%) fewer than published in the *AJC*. At the same time, the *EHJ* had 10,000 fewer total citations through 2010 than the *AJC* (26,311 vs 36,401). *Heart* published 287 articles in 2010, 317 fewer than in the *AJC* the same year, and *Heart* has had a third of the number of total citations as the *AJC* (12,289 vs 36,401). Nevertheless, *Heart*'s IF (4.71) ranked 22% higher than that of the *AJC*. And the most overt example of all is *Current Problems in Cardiology*, which published only 12 articles in 2010; despite its low citation number of 413, its IF is relatively good (3.44).

Fourth, do not limit the number of references in articles. The larger the number of references published, the greater the likelihood that one's own journal will be referenced. The *AJC* generally limits the number of references in articles to no more than 30.

Fifth, require authors to reference generously the journal to which their manuscripts are submitted. I recently received a cover letter in which the author indicated that most of the references in his manuscript were to articles previously published in the *AJC*. I presume that his mentioning that fact was to increase the possibility of acceptance of his manuscript. (I do not check which journals are referenced in manuscripts submitted to the *AJC*.) I understand, however, that some editors do encourage authors to reference generously the journals they edit. Self-citations among the largest cardiology journals as a percentage of their total citations (to 2010) are as follows: *Circulation*, 5% of its 151,020 total citations; *JACC*, 5% of its 69,405; *EHJ*, 3% of its 26,311; and *AJC*, 3% of its 36,401 total citations).

Sixth, have a large readership audience. There are far more cardiologists than cardiac surgeons. The latter group I would think gets far more information from cardiovascular surgical journals, which have relatively small circulations, than from the cardiology journals, which, for the most part, have much larger potential audiences. The society-owned *Journal of Thoracic and Cardiovascular Surgery* and *Annals of Thoracic Surgery* had IFs in 2010 of 3.61 and 3.56, respectively, they published 492 and 608 articles, respectively, and they had 19,274 and 27,678 total citations, respectively. The 3 large society-owned cardiology journals (*Circulation*, *JACC*, and *EHJ*) each published fewer articles in 2010 than did either of the 2 aforementioned cardiovascular surgical journals and had far more total citations (151,020, 69,405, and 26,311) and the highest IFs (14.43, 14.29, and 10.05). Some of the general medical journals (the *New England Journal of Medicine*, *The Lancet*, and *JAMA*) have huge audiences and huge IFs (53.48, 33.63, and 33.01, respectively). (One could argue, of course, that the reason they have huge audiences is because they have high IFs.)

Ranking scientific journals by the Eigenfactor™: The Eigenfactor™ Score and Article Influence Scores rank journals much as Google ranks Web sites. The Eigenfactor™ algorithms use the structure of the entire network, not just citation information, to evaluate the importance of each journal. Eigenfactor.org reports both journal prices and citation influence. Although the Eigenfactor™ Score and Article Influence Score do not incorporate price information directly, the Cost-Effectiveness Search ranks journals by a measure of the value per dollar that they provide. The Eigenfactor™ Score and Article Influence Score rely on citation data over a 5-year period, not a 2-year period. And the Eigenfactor™ Score and Article Influence Score are free and searchable.

Eigenfactor.org rankings of cardiovascular journals: The latest Cost-Effectiveness Search results list 60 cardiovascular journals. The top 10 with their prices per Eigenfactor™ were the following: (1) *Circulation* ($1,373), (2) *JACC* ($2,118), (3) *AJC* ($3,883), (4) *Circulation Research* ($6,198), (5) the *American Heart Journal* ($9,734), (6) the *Journal of Thoracic and Cardiovascular Surgery* ($9,939), (7) the *American Journal of Physiology — Heart and Circulatory Physiology* ($11,836), (8) the *Journal of Heart and Lung Transplantation* ($13,804), (9) *Cardiovascular Research* ($20,753), and (10) the *EHJ* ($20,753). The lower the price per Eigenfactor™, the higher the ranking.

In summary, the IF obviously has value, but its importance, in my view, is not great enough to alter the operation of any scientific journal. The IF can be spuriously manipulated, and doing so diminishes considerably its value and also that of its manipulators. The IF in a way is like unadjusted versus adjusted data. A factor such as the number of original articles published yearly in a journal is underrated, whereas reviews are overrated. Whether or not a journal publishes guidelines is not included in the analysis. The potential size of the readership for a journal seems underrated in some instances and overrated in others. And whether a journal is an official organ of a major society or not is a nonfactor for calculating the IF, while at the same time, it is probably the most important variable of all. Metrics, putting a number on things, is a tough and complicated business. The IF is a major attempt to measure the quality of scientific journals by a single number, and that is a useful endeavor.

I have become intrigued by the Eigenfactor™. It ranks cardiovascular journals in a much more logical fashion, in my view, than does the IF. It provides a 5-year analysis of articles published and citations rather than a 2-year evaluation, and it does not include self-citations in its analyses. Although the method of calculating the Eigenfactor™ has been well described and is available to all, one needs to be a mathematician to understand it, and I am not that. Nevertheless, I suspect that the Eigenfactor™ will be the major metric in the future for evaluating the quality of scientific journals.

William Clifford Roberts, MD
Baylor Heart and Vascular Institute of
Baylor University Medical Center
Dallas, Texas

From-the-Editor Columns by William C. Roberts, MD, in *The American Journal of Cardiology* 1982–2011

When I became editor of *The American Journal of Cardiology* in June 1982, I thought that it might be useful for the readers and authors to have some idea of the thoughts of the new editor. The result was the initiation of the "From the Editor" columns beginning in July 1982. During the first 1.5 years, the publisher placed these columns among the advertising pages with an "A" page number, which excluded them from indexing and binding. In 1984, these columns began appearing in the regular editorial pages of the journal. During the first 5 years, the columns appeared in each issue, and during that time, there were 15 issues a year. We now publish 24 issues a year, and the "From the Editor" columns appear about 5 times yearly. Through the years, some colleagues have suggested to me that the columns, or at least some of them, be collected in a single volume. That suggestion has not been carried out, but publication of the titles of the columns may serve as a substitute for that suggestion.

I have been honored to serve and to continue to serve as the *AJC*'s editor-in-chief, and that position has allowed the smooth publication of these columns, only a few of which have gone through the strenuous manuscript review process. My hope is that a few *AJC* readers will find some of these 188 columns interesting, and all possibly a useful record. Your comments are welcomed.

Preventive Cardiology

1. An agent with lipid-lowering, antihypertensive, positive inotropic, negative chronotropic, vasodilating, diuretic, anorexigenic, weight-reducing, cathartic, hypoglycemic, tranquilizing, hypnotic and antidepressive qualities. (53:261–262) January 1, 1984.
2. Reducing the blood cholesterol level reduces the risk of heart attack. (53:649) February 1, 1984.
3. Extreme hypercholesterolemia = malignant atherosclerosis. (54:242–243) July 1, 1984.
4. Cardiac rupture, abdominal aneurysmal rupture and dissecting aortic rupture: a preventive trio. (57:892–893) April 1, 1986.
5. In one day in the USA. (58:193–194) July 1, 1986.
6. Fast foods and quick plaques. (59:721–723) March 1, 1987.
7. Stone agers in the atomic age: lessons from the Paleolithic life-style for modern man. (61:1365–1366) June 1, 1988.
8. The Friedewald-Levy-Frederickson formula for calculating low-density lipoprotein cholesterol, the basis for lipid-lowering therapy. (62:345–346) August 1, 1988.
9. Factors linking cholesterol to atherosclerotic plaques. (62:495–499) September 1, 1988.
10. Atherosclerotic risk factors: are there ten or is there only one? (64:552–554) September 1, 1989.
11. Lipid-lowering therapy after an atherosclerotic event. (64:693–695) September 15, 1989.
12. We think we are one, we act as if we are one, but we are not one. (66:896) October 1, 1990.
13. The best antiarrhythmic agent will be a lipid-lowering agent. (66:1402) December 1, 1990.
14. More on fast foods and quick plaques. (70:268–270) July 15, 1992.
15. Getting cardiologists interested in lipids. (72:744–745) September 15, 1993.
16. The ineffectiveness of a commonly recommended lipid-lowering diet in significantly lowering the serum total and low-density lipoprotein cholesterol levels. (73:623–624) March 15, 1994.
17. Calculating the percentage of calories from fat and the grams of fat consumed daily to maintain an ideal body weight. (73:719–720) April 1, 1994.
18. Mexican food: oilé. (74:974–975) November 1, 1994.
19. Retail costs of the statin lipid-lowering drugs. (74:1181) December 1, 1994.
20. The underused miracle drugs: the statin drugs are to atherosclerosis what penicillin was to infectious disease. (78:377–378) August 1, 1996.
21. Tobacco. (78:1084–1085) November 1, 1996.
22. The rule of 5 and the rule of 7 in lipid-lowering by statin drugs. (80:106–107) July 1, 1997.
23. Floating in fat: fat kids and fat adults. (80:1117–1119) October 15, 1997.
24. Obtaining and maintaining an ideal body weight. (83:639) February 15, 1999.
25. Shifting from decreasing risk to actually preventing and arresting atherosclerosis. (83:816–817) March 1, 1999.
26. An address to the Dallas, Texas, Rotary Club on 19 May 1999. (84:493–495) August 15, 1999.
27. High salt intake, its origins, its economic impact, and its effect on blood pressure. (88:1338–1346) December 1, 2001.
28. Evaluating lipid-lowering trials in the twenty-first century. (103:1325–1328) May 1, 2009.
29. It's the cholesterol, stupid! (106:1364–1366) November 1, 2010.

Cardiovascular Disease

1. Mitral commissurotomy—still a good operation. (52:A9-A10) August 1983.

Manuscript received April 8, 2011; revised manuscript received and accepted April 8, 2011.

2. The "blessing" of angina pectoris. (52:1154) November 1, 1983.
3. The 2 most common congenital heart diseases. (53: 1198) April 1, 1984.
4. When I have an acute myocardial infarction take me to the hospital that has a cardiac catheterization laboratory and open cardiac surgical facilities. (53: 1410) May 1, 1984.
5. The worst heart disease. (54:935) November 1984.
6. I still prefer ventricular premature complex. (55: 1117) April 1, 1985.
7. The silver anniversary of cardiac valve replacement. (56:503–506) September 1985.
8. Mitral valve prolapse and systemic hypertension. (56:703) October 1, 1985.
9. Effects of antihypertensive therapy on blood lipid levels. (57:379–380) February 1, 1986.
10. Sudden cardiac death: definitions and causes. (57: 1410–1413) May 1, 1986.
11. A simple histologic classification of pulmonary arterial hypertension. (58:385–386) August 1, 1986.
12. The senile cardiac calcification syndrome. (58:572–574) September 1, 1986.
13. Good-bye to thoracotomy for cardiac valvulotomy. (59:198–202) January 1, 1987.
14. Examining operatively excised cardiac valves. (59: 1434–1436) June 1, 1987.
15. The logic of using either two mechanical valves or two bioprosthetic valves for replacement of both mitral and aortic valves. (61:871) April 1, 1988.
16. Defining idiopathic dilated cardiomyopathy. A courtroom discussion. (63:893–896) April 1, 1989.
17. The echocardiographic diseases. (64:1084) November 1, 1989.
18. Living with a congenitally bicuspid aortic valve. (64:1408–1409) December 1, 1989.
19. Coronary "lesion," coronary "disease," "single-vessel disease"—"two-vessel disease": word and phrase misnomers providing false impressions of the extent of coronary atherosclerosis in symptomatic myocardial ischemia. (66:121–123) July 1, 1990.
20. The best anti-heart failure agent will be a lipid-lowering agent. (71:628) March 1, 1993.
21. A unique heart disease associated with a unique cancer: carcinoid heart disease. (80:251–256) July 15, 1997.
22. Primary and secondary neoplasms of the heart. (80: 671–682) September 1, 1997.
23. Papillary fibroelastomas of the heart. (80:973–975) October 1, 1997.
24. Fewer hearts than earlier predicted. (81:660–661) March 1, 1998.
25. Fifty years of hypertrophic cardiomyopathy. (103: 431–434) February 1, 2000.
26. Forty-five years in the cardiovascular arena. (103: 752–753) March 1, 2009.
27. So you want to see your heart. (106:1520) November 15, 2010.
28. Prophylactic replacement of the dilated ascending aorta at the time of replacement of a dysfunctioning congenitally unicuspid or bicuspid aortic valve. (108:1371–1372) October 2011.

International Cardiology

1. China and Chinese cardiology. (60:201–202) July 1, 1987.
2. Japan and Japanese medicine. (60:427–429) August 1, 1987.
3. The Kingdom of Saudi Arabia, oil, money and cardiology. (61:410–412) February 1, 1988.
4. Argentina and Argentine cardiology. (62:167–169) July 1, 1988.
5. Brazil and Brazilian cardiology. (62:991–993) November 1, 1988.
6. India and Indian cardiology. (62:1326–1329) December 1, 1988.
7. Bombay and a congress on coronary artery disease. (65:824–825) March 15, 1990.
8. Singapore and Singaporean cardiology. (67:1298–1302) June 1, 1991.
9. Day-to-day cardiology in Bombay, India. (76:3019–3020) December 15, 1995.

Miscellaneous Topics

1. Animal behavior-human behavior-cardiac behavior. (52:A14) September 1983.
2. Can rest and relaxation be obtained by combining a "vacation" with a medical meeting or a medical meeting with a "vacation"? (53:987) March 15, 1984.
3. Forces changing America. (52:1737–1738) June 1, 1984.
4. Enticing real and potential cardiovascular researchers away from research. (55:503) February 1, 1985.
5. The most powerful cause of sudden death. (57:190) January 1, 1986.
6. Justifying a cardiac catheterization laboratory. (58: 860–862) October 1, 1986.
7. Characteristics of long-term successful physician researchers. (58:1052–1053) November 1, 1986.
8. The malpractice dream. (60:938) October 1, 1987.
9. Drug developers and drug dispensers: their dependency on one another. (62:840) October 1, 1988.
10. The medical book with the most information for the price. (63:390–391) February 1, 1989.
11. Sensitive areas between physicians and pharmaceutical companies. (63:1421) June 1, 1989.
12. Clogged arteries and clogged roads (64:959–960) October 15, 1989.
13. Limited research funds and cardiac medicine without cardiac surgery. (65:536–537) February 15, 1990.
14. "Anything to be done right has got to be done by people that make their living at it" (67:445–446) February 15, 1991.
15. The government is in your office and listening to their script. (68:143–144) July 1, 1991.
16. Human records and a tribute to the Guinness Book of World Records. (68:288–289) July 15, 1991.
17. What medical students are asking. (68:1260–1261) November 1, 1991.

18. Doctors, save your money because there will be less in the future. (69:432) February 1, 1992.
19. The best hospitals in the USA for patients with heart disease. (72:626–627) September 1, 1993.
20. Personal finances (76:427) August 15, 1995.
21. The best hospitals in the USA for patients with heart disease. (78:1188–1189) November 15, 1996.
22. Longitude, the Longitude Act, scurvy, and the beginning of government-supported research. (80: 540–541) August 15, 1997.
23. The best hospitals in the USA for heart disease—1997. (80:1258–1259) November 1, 1997.

Medical History

1. Oslerian advice. (51:A10-A11) May 15, 1983.
2. Who was Holter? (52:A17) October 1983.
3. Benjamin Franklin's Poor Richard's Almanack and its maxims on physicians, medicine and nutrition. (68:703–706) September 1, 1991.
4. A son's book on his father's father. (74:518–529) September 1, 1994.
5. Ruby Viola Holbrook Roberts. (74:1078) November 15, 1994.
6. Life lessons from modern-day greats in cardiovascular disease. (103:287–291) January 15, 2009.

Editing and Writing

1. A few words from the Journal's second editor. (50: A3) July 1982.
2. Blind reviews. (50:A45) August 1982.
3. Brief reports. (50:A3) September 1982.
4. The editorial board. (50:A3) October 1982.
5. Reviewing manuscripts: occasionally a test of character. (50:A3) November 1982.
6. Speeding up the manuscript-review process. (50:A3) December 1982.
7. Getting the manuscript accepted: think like a lawyer and cover the flanks. (51:A3) January 1983.
8. Paper accepted/abstract rejected or vice versa: differences in the grading of abstracts and the reviewing of manuscripts. (51:A3) February 1983.
9. Author-editor-reviewer: how the triumvirate is working at the AJC. (51:A9-A10) March 1, 1983.
10. Author-advertiser: their dependency on one another. (51:A3) March 15, 1983.
11. Abbreviations in the AJC. (51:A9-A10) April 1983.
12. References: a clue to scholarship. (51:A9-A10) May 1, 1983.
13. Changes in the AJC since June 1982. (1:A9-A10) June 1983.
14. The summary: the manuscript's bottom line. (52:A3) July 19, 1983.
15. Season's greetings and the best for 1984. (52:1356) December 1, 1983.
16. Studying the "instructions to authors" before final typing of a manuscript for submission to a medical journal. (53:398) January 15, 1984.
17. The AJC in '83. (53:729) March 1, 1984.
18. Further comments on the "instructions to authors." (54:470) August 1, 1984.
19. Editorial board changes. (54:704) September 1, 1984.
20. Writing versus editing. (54:934) October 1984.
21. A good year—1984. (54:1395) December 1, 1984.
22. A suggestion to lighten the load of manuscript reviewing. (55:247) January 1, 1985.
23. Brief reports in the AJC in 1984. (55:870) March 1, 1985.
24. The "hot eye" and the "cold eye." (55:1663) June 1, 1985.
25. The article's title. (56:210–212) July 1985.
26. Country of origin of articles in the AJC in 1984. (56:380) August 1, 1985.
27. The AJC in 1985. (57:711–712) March 1, 1986.
28. The AJC in 1986. (59:391–392) February 1, 1987.
29. Reviews of classic books and ineptness of reviewers: lessons for judges of medical manuscripts. (59:922–923) April 1, 1987.
30. The search for the masterful figure. (60:633–634) September 1, 1987.
31. Publishing manuscripts faster than abstracts. (60: 1133) November 1, 1987.
32. The AJC in 1987. (61:672–674) March 1, 1988.
33. Making clinical studies involving many patients useful to the single patient. (65:1408) June 1, 1990.
34. Comparison of the four major USA cardiology journals in 1990: a look at 51 kilograms (112 pounds) of journals and over 15,000 editorial pages. (67:551–554) March 1, 1991.
35. Oft-repeated requests to authors from an editor of a cardiology journal. (68:1121–1122) October 15, 1991.
36. Alkaline paper and preserving the record. (68:1729–1732) December 15, 1991.
37. Reducing flaws in the review process of manuscripts submitted to medical journals for publication. (103: 891–892) March 15, 2011.
38. Piercing the impact factor and promoting the Eigenfactor™. (108:896–898) September 15, 2011.

Good Cardiologic Books (Good Books on Cardiology)

1. Some good cardiologic books. (56:1001–1002) December 1, 1985.
2. Some good cardiologic books published in 1986. (58:1271–1272) December 1, 1986.
3. Some good cardiologic books published in 1987. (60:1423–1424) December 1, 1987.
4. Some good cardiologic books published in 1988. (63:153–154) January 1, 1989.
5. Some good cardiologic books published in 1989. (65:116–118) January 1, 1990.
6. Some good cardiologic books published in 1990. (67:106–108) January 1, 1991.
7. Some good cardiologic books published in 1991. (69:141–144) January 1, 1992.
8. Cardiologic books published in 1992. (71:126–130) January 1, 1993.
9. Good cardiologic books appearing in 1993. (73:98–101) January 1, 1994.
10. Good cardiologic books appearing in 1994. (75: 106–109) January 1, 1995.

11. Good cardiologic books appearing in 1995. (77:111–114) January 1, 1996.
12. Good books on cardiovascular disease appearing in 1996. (79:248–252) January 15, 1997.
13. Good books on cardiovascular disease appearing in 1997. (81:524–529) February 15, 1998.
14. Good books on cardiovascular disease appearing in 1998. (83:470–474) February 1, 1999.
15. Good books in cardiovascular disease appearing in 1999. (85:275–279) January 15, 2000.
16. Good books in cardiovascular disease appearing in 2000. (87:251–255) January 15, 2001.
17. Good books in cardiovascular disease appearing in 2001. (89:785–790) March 15, 2002.
18. Good books in cardiovascular disease appearing in 2002. (91:649–653) March 1, 2003.
19. Good books in cardiology appearing in 2003. (93: 520–523) February 15, 2004.
20. Good books in cardiovascular disease appearing in 2004. (95:814–816) March 15, 2005.
21. Good books in cardiology appearing in 2005. (97: 430–433) February 1, 2006.
22. Good books in cardiovascular disease appearing in 2006. (99:745–748) March 1, 2007.
23. Good books in cardiovascular diseases appearing in 2007 and in early 2008. (101:1066–1067) April 1, 2008.
24. Good books in cardiovascular disease appearing in 2008. (103:1180–1181) April 15, 2009.
25. Good books in cardiovascular disease appearing in 2009. (105:1200–1201) April 15, 2010.
26. Good books in cardiovascular diseases appearing in 2010. (107:1250–1251), April 15, 2011.

Editorial Board Meetings

1. The AJC editorial board meeting—1984. (53:1483–1485) May 15, 1984.
2. The AJC editorial meeting—1985. (55:1451–1452) May 1, 1985.
3. AJC editorial board meeting—1986. (57:1209–1211) May 1, 1986.
4. Annual AJC editorial board meeting—March 1987. (59:1226–1229) May 1, 1987.
5. AJC editorial board meeting—March 1988. (61: 1161–1164) May 1, 1988.
6. Editorial board meeting of The American Journal of Cardiology—March 1989. (63:1159–1165) May 1, 1989.
7. Editorial board meeting of The American Journal of Cardiology—March 1990. (65:1162–1168) May 1, 1990.
8. Editorial board meeting of The American Journal of Cardiology—5 March 1991. (67:1033–1037) May 1, 1991.
9. Editorial board meeting of The American Journal of Cardiology on 14 April 1992. (69:1645–1649) June 15, 1992.
10. Editorial board meeting of The American Journal of Cardiology in March 1993. (71:1500–1504) June 15, 1993.
11. Proceedings of the editorial board meeting of The American Journal of Cardiology on March 14, 1994. (73:926–931) May 1, 1994.
12. Proceedings of the editorial board meeting of The American Journal of Cardiology on March 21, 1995. (75:1075–1080) May 15, 1995.
13. Proceedings of the editorial board meeting of The American Journal of Cardiology on March 26, 1996. (77:1138–1144) May 15, 1996.
14. Proceedings of the editorial board meeting of The American Journal of Cardiology on 17 March 1997. (79:1716–1720) June 15, 1997.
15. Proceedings of the editorial board of The American Journal of Cardiology on 30 March 1998. (81:1512–1517) June 15, 1998.
16. Proceedings of the editorial board meeting of The American Journal of Cardiology on 9 March 1999 (83:1588–1591) June 1, 1999.
17. Proceedings of the editorial board meeting of The American Journal of Cardiology on 14 March 2000. (85:1507–1509) June 15, 2000.
18. Proceedings of the editorial board meeting of The American Journal of Cardiology on 19 March 2001. (87:1332–1334) June 1, 2001.
19. Proceedings of the editorial board meeting of The American Journal of Cardiology on 18 March 2002. (89:1145–1148) May 1, 2002.
20. Proceedings of the editorial board meeting of The American Journal of Cardiology on 31 March 2003. (91:1526–1531) June 15, 2003.
21. Proceedings of the editorial board meeting of The American Journal of Cardiology on 8 March 2004. (93:1328–1331) May 15, 2004.
22. Proceedings of the editorial board meeting of The American Journal of Cardiology on 7 March 2005. (95:1273–1276) May 15, 2005.
23. Proceedings of the editorial board meeting of The American Journal of Cardiology on 13 March 2006. (97:1670—1675) June 1, 2006.
24. Proceedings of the editorial board meeting of The American Journal of Cardiology on 26 March 2007. (99:1768–1774) June 15, 2007.
25. Proceedings of the editorial meeting of The American Journal of Cardiology on 30 March 2008. (102: 231–236) July 15, 2008.
26. Proceedings of the editorial board meeting of The American Journal of Cardiology on March 29, 2009. (104:453–457) August 2, 2009.
27. Proceedings of the editorial board meeting of the American Journal of Cardiology on March 14, 2010. (105:1645–1646) June 1, 2010.
28. Proceedings of the editorial board meeting of The American Journal of Cardiology, April 3, 2011. (107:1864–1865), June 15, 2011.

William C. Roberts, MD
Baylor Heart and Vascular Institute
Baylor University Medical Center, Dallas, Texas

Good Books on Cardiology

Some Good Cardiologic Books

Most publishers of medical books send recently published books to editors of medical journals in hopes that their books will be reviewed, and, of course, reviewed favorably. During my 42-month tenure as editor of AJC, no book reviews have appeared, although recently received books are listed in the *Journal* about every 3 months. Picking the best of the medical books each year obviously is difficult. What is "best" to one person is not necessarily "best" to another. This piece lists a few of the better books that have crossed my editor's desk in 1985.

1. Braunwald E, editor *Heart Disease. A Textbook of Cardiovascular Medicine.* 2nd ed., Philadelphia: WB Saunders Company, 1984:1943, $95.00.

2. Hurst JW, ed. *The Heart, Arteries and Veins.* 6th ed., New York: McGraw-Hill Book Company, 1986:2193, $92.00.

These are the 2 most important books that a cardiologist can own. Because the subject matter in each book is written by different authors and because the material in each book is organized and presented quite differently, it is advantageous to own both books. Since each has a new edition every 3 years, it would appear most reasonable to purchase 1 book 1 year and the other book when its new edition appears.

The magnitude of the information presented in these 2 books is astounding and a tribute to the writing and organizational skills of the 2 editors. The Braunwald book weighs 4,380 grams, contains 1,943 pages with a maximum of 1,050 words per page, 57 chapters (25 of which were authored or coauthored by Braunwald) written by 51 authors, 15,112 references, 1,193 figures and 252 tables. The Hurst book weighs 3,260 grams, contains 2,193 pages with a maximum of 850 words per page, 140 chapters (8 of which were authored or coauthored by Hurst) written by 183 authors, 11,083 references, 1,005 figures and 199 tables.

3. Kirklin JW, Barratt-Boyes BG. *Cardiac Surgery. Morphology, Diagnostic Criteria, Natural History, Techniques, Results, and Indications.* New York: John Wiley & Sons, 1986: 1572, $150.00.

Absolutely magnificent book! As Dwight McGoon says in the foreword: "Perhaps you are like me in having fancied at one time or another of someday being able to encompass the entire body of essential information of a selected specialty and then 'wrap it up' into a skillfully coordinated, comprehensive, concise compendium. Increasingly rare are the occasions when that fantasy can be transformed into reality. Indeed, for cardiac surgery, such an accomplishment may never again occur after this book. This is especially true if an aspiring author is also required to be a principal contributor to essentially every frontier of progress in the entire specialty. Thus, from its very inception, this book has been unique. . . . The entire expanse of cardiac surgery seems to be here, laid out in the same crisp, logical, fully documented style that we have all come to recognize and respect in the many other reports, lectures, and publications provided by these particular authors."

This book has only 2 authors and each chapter reflects their combined outstanding authority on that subject. This book is a must for all physicians and surgeons involved in caring for persons with cardiac disease. It is one of the very best medical books ever published! I confidently predict that another edition of it will never appear. It is a classic from the beginning.

4. Crawford ES, Crawford, JL. *Diseases of the Aorta Including an Atlas of Angiographic Pathology and Surgical Technique.* Baltimore: Williams & Wilkins, 1984: 401, $135.00.

It is ideal, of course, when *the* recognized authority in a field authors a book on his (her) area of expertise. Such is the case in the above book. "Diseases of the Aorta" is primarily an atlas with magnificent color drawings by Perrin Sparks Smith. The drawings depict most aortic diseases, their varying appearances, and the techniques available for their surgical treatment. Although the book lacks computed tomography and echocardiographic observations, it nevertheless is masterful and should be owned by all surgeons who operate on patients with aortic disease. What pride the senior author must feel for his son to be a coauthor.

5. Wilcox BR, Anderson RH. *Surgical Anatomy of the Heart.* New York: Raven Press (published by special arrangement with Gower Medical Publishing), 1985: 148, $55.00.

This book is a color atlas combining photographs of normal and congenitally malformed hearts with accompanying color and line diagrams with appropriate text. The book combines efforts of a cardiac surgeon (Ben Wilcox) and a cardiac morphologist (Bob Anderson). The result is a splendid book. It actually concerns only the normal and the congenitally malformed heart and therefore its title is not fully descriptive of its contents. This book should be in the library of surgeons who operate on patients with anomalies of the heart and great vessels.

6. King SB III, Douglas JS Jr. *Coronary Arteriography and Angioplasty.* New York: McGraw Hill Book Company, 1985:478, $70.00.

Spencer King and John Douglas have lived in the cardiac catheterization laboratory for a number of years, the last 5 of which were working with the late Andreas Gruentzig, and this book shows that they know what they were doing.

7. Cohn PF, editor. *Diagnosis and Therapy of Artery Disease.* 2nd ed. Boston: Martinus Nijhoff Publishing, 1985:517, $69.50.

8. Connor WE, Bristow JD, editors. *Coronary Heart Disease. Prevention, Complications and Treatment.* Philadelphia: J.B. Lippincott, 1985:461, $45.00.

9. Califf RM, Wagner GS, editors. *Acute Coronary Care, Principles and Practice.* Boston: Martinus Nijhoff Publishing, 1985:556, $52.50.

All 3 books are multiauthored with inherent advantages and disadvantages of each. None of these should be purchased until both the Braunwald and Hurst books have been bought.

10. Ellestad MH. *Stress Testing. Principles and Practice.* 3rd ed. Philadelphia: FA Davis Company, 1986: 564, $48.00.

Almost certainly the best book on this subject.

11. Feigenbaum H. *Echocardiography.* 4th ed. Philadelphia: Lea & Febiger, 1986:685, $55.00.

The first edition of this classic appeared in 1972 and a new edition has appeared every 4 or 5 years since. This new edition contains more 2-dimensional echocardiograms and also a good number of Doppler echocardiograms. This is the first echo book to buy.

12. Nanda NC, editor. *Doppler Echocardiography.* New York: Igaku-Shoin, 1985:522, $55.00.

An authoritative up-to-date book on a rapidly expanding subject.

13. Wenger NK, Hellerstein HK, editors. *Rehabilitation of the Coronary Patient.* 2nd ed. New York: John Wiley & Sons, 1984:563, $37.50.

14. Pollock ML, Schmidt DH, editors. *Heart Disease and Rehabilitation.* 2nd ed. New York: John Wiley & Sons, 1986:788, $47.50.

Two good and different multiauthored books on an important subject. I also like the book: Peterson LH. *Cardiovascular Rehabilitation. A Comprehensive Approach.* New York: MacMillan, 1983:363, $48.00.

15. Zipes DP, Jalife J, editors. *Cardiac Electrophysiology and Arrhythmias.* Orlando: Grune & Stratton, 1985:567, $98.50.

A book honoring Gordon K. Moe and having 174 contributors.

16. Freedom RM, Culham JAG, Moes CAF. *Angiocardiography of Congenital Heart Disease.* New York: MacMillan, 1984:691, $125.00.

Surely the best book on this subject.

William C. Roberts

William C. Roberts, MD
Editor-in-Chief

Some Good Cardiologic Books Published in 1986

This piece briefly mentions some of the better books that have crossed my desk in 1986.

1. Cheng TO, editor. *The International Textbook of Cardiology*. New York: Pergamon Press, 1986:1299, $125.00

The intent of this fine book is to give "serious students of international cardiology a source of reference in one single textbook." Cheng assembled 136 contributors, two-thirds of whom are from the USA, to produce 83 chapters occupying 1,272 pages. This book is about 35% smaller and it costs about 20% more than either the Braunwald or Hurst cardiologic textbooks.

2. Kaplan NM. *Clinical Hypertension*. 4th ed. Baltimore: Williams & Wilkins, 1986:492, $54.95.

This book, in my view, is the best of the clinical books on systemic hypertension. Although the book covers all forms of systemic hypertension, the most common forms receive the most attention. This is a very practical book by one of the best teachers in medicine.

3. Antman EM, Rutherford JD. *Coronary Care Medicine. A Practical Approach*. Boston: Martinus Nijhoff, 1986:384, $69.95.

This book covers virtually all aspects of management of patients with coronary problems necessitating hospitalization in a coronary care unit.

4. Conti CR, editor. *Coronary Artery Spasm. Pathophysiology, Diagnosis, and Treatment*. New York: Marcel Dekker, 1986:347, $59.75.

This book is the best one on this subject. It records what is known and pertinent about coronary artery spasm.

5. Grossman W, editor. *Cardiac Catheterization* and *Angiography*. 3rd ed. Philadelphia: Lea & Febiger, 1986:562, $49.50.

This book is a classic and a must possession of physicians who spend time in a cardiac catheterization laboratory.

6. Vlietstra RE, Holmes DR, Jr., editors. *PTCA Percutaneous Transluminal Coronary Angioplasty*. Philadelphia: FA Davis, 1986:268, $49.00.

A timely book.

7. Iskandrian AS. *Nuclear Cardiac Imaging: Principles and Applications*. Philadelphia: FA Davis, 1986:527, $75.00.

This fine book by a single author provides an in-depth analysis of the usefulness of the most commonly available cardiac imaging modalities: thallium-201 scintigraphy, myocardial infarct avid imaging, and radionuclide ventriculography. The emphasis is on the implications of these diagnostic procedures on patient management rather than on detailed technical considerations.

8. McArdle WD, Katch FI, Katch VL. *Exercise Physiology. Energy, Nutrition, and Human Performance*. 2nd ed. Philadelphia: Lea & Febiger, 1986:696, $32.50.

This is an excellent book combining information on nutrition, energy and exercise performance. The price is right.

9. Schneeweiss A. *Drug Therapy in Cardiovascular Diseases*. Philadelphia: Lea & Febiger, 1986:835, $84.50.

This is a drug-oriented scholarly book. The drugs are classified by their pharmacologic properties and each chapter deals with 1 drug. Three-fourths of the book is devoted to 4 major drug classes: beta blockers, calcium-channel blockers, converting-enzyme inhibitors and antiarrhythmic agents. The remainder of the book is devoted to 32 other drugs. The purpose of this book is not to suggest which drug to use but to supply information about available drugs.

10. Schneeweiss A. *Drug Therapy in Infants and Children with Cardiovascular Diseases*. Philadelphia: Lea & Febiger, 1986:398, $45.00.

This book is organized similarly to the one above by the same author, and it should be of great value to physicians who care for children with cardiovascular disease. A section on diuretics is not included in either book by Schneeweiss.

11. Opie LH, editor; Chatterjee K, Gersh BJ, Harrison DC, Kaplan NM, Marcus FI, Singh BN, Sonnenblick EH, Thadani U, collaborators. *Drugs for the Heart*. 2nd ed. Orlando, FL: Grune & Stratton, 1987:238 $18.95.

This pocket-sized compendium provides information on 10 kinds of cardiovascular drugs—beta blockers; nitrates; calcium antagonists; digitalis, sympathomimetics, and inotropic-dilators; diuretics; vasodilators; angiotensin-converting-enzyme inhibitors; antithrombotic agents; and lipid-lowering agents—their uses, doses and side effects. This is a wonderfully useful book.

12. Barlow JB. *Perspectives on the Mitral Valve*. Philadelphia: FA Davis, 1987:381, $49.00.

John Barlow's name, of course, is synonymous with mitral valve prolapse. This well-done book summarizes his

30-year experience with the Barlow syndrome and with the many other conditions that affect the mitral valve.

13. Furman S, Hayes DL, Holmes DR Jr. *A practice of Cardiac Pacing.* Mount Kisco, NY: Futura, 1986:480, $59.50.

A book on pacing co-authored by Seymour Furman is one to take note of. This text discusses and illustrates how pacemakers work and what telemetric, radiologic and electrocardiographic findings are associated with normal and abnormal function. The book provides a personal approach from 2 large cardiac pacing practices, the Montefiore Medical Center and the Mayo Clinic.

14. Benditt DG, Benson DW Jr., editors. *Cardiac Preexcitation Syndromes. Origins, Evaluation, and Treatment.* Boston: Martinus Nijhoff, 1986:556, $105.00.

I suspect that this book will be the gospel on preexcitation for some time to come.

15. Huhta JC. *Pediatric Imaging/Doppler Ultrasound of the Chest: Extracardiac Diagnosis.* Philadelphia: Lea & Febiger, 1986:225, $42.50.

16. Swischuk LE, Sapire DW. *Basic Imaging in Congenital Heart Disease.* 3rd ed. Baltimore: Williams & Wilkins 1986:312, $58.95.

17. Williams RG, Bierman FZ, Sanders SP. *Echocardiographic Diagnosis of Cardiac Malformations.* Boston: Little, Brown, 1986:237, $48.50.

I think No. 14 is the best of the 3.

18. Perloff JK. *The Clinical Recognition of Congenital Heart Disease.* 3rd ed. Philadelphia: WB Saunders, 1987: 705, $95.00.

This book, an update and expansion of the second edition appearing in 1978, focuses entirely on the clinical diagnosis of congenital heart disease. The 32 chapters contain 733 figures, 54 (7%) of which are echocardiograms (all cross-sectional except for 1 Doppler) and 3,539 references. This book by a master clinician has been a classic since its beginning.

19. Roberts WC, editor. *Adult Congenital Heart Disease.* Philadelphia: FA Davis, 1987:752, $75.00.

When an editor reviews his own handiwork the reader is at least clearly forewarned that the impartial judgments will be from the author's point of view. This book is an outgrowth of *Congenital Heart Disease in Adults* which FA Davis published in 1979 as part of their Cardiovascular Clinics Series. The 1979 book was the first ever published on congenital heart disease in adults. During these past 7 years, much new information on this subject has been accumulated, and although the present book is an outgrowth of the 1979 book, the new one is different. Five chapters have been added, 20 of the remaining 22 have been expanded, and several have additional or new authors. The publisher is to be complimented for the attractiveness of the book.

20. Roberts WC, editor: Mason DT, Rackley CE, Willerson JT, Graham TP Jr., Pacifico AD, Karp RB, contributors. *Cardiology 1986.* New York: Yorke Medical Books, 1986: 444, $55.00.

21. Harvey WP, Kirkendall WM, Laks H, Resnekov L, Rosenthal A, Sonnenblick EH, editors. *1986 Yearbook of Cardiology.* Chicago: Year Book Medical Publishers, 1986: 364, $44.95.

The 2 books are quite different. The Yorke book (no. 20), which appeared in June 1986, contains summaries of 771 articles, all published in 1985, plus 112 figures, 31 tables and 444 pages. The Yearbook (no. 21), published in August 1986, contains summaries of 309 articles, 42 (14%) of which were published in 1984 and only 21 (7%) of which were published in October–December 1985, plus 49 figures, 17 tables and 364 pages. All summaries in the Yorke book (no. 20) were selected by and written by the physician authors; all summaries in the Yearbook (no. 21) were selected by the physician editors who wrote brief comments, but the articles themselves were summarized by the publisher. Separation of the editors' comments from the summaries themselves is the unique feature of the Yearbook. The Yorke book costs 18% more than the Yearbook, but it contains 18% more pages, it summarizes 60% more articles, and it provides 56% more figures and 45% more tables.

22. Paul O. *Take Heart. The Life and Prescription For Living of Dr. Paul Dudley White.* Boston: Harvard University Press, 1986:315, $18.95.

23. Meijler FL, Burchell HB, editors. *Professor Dirk Durrer. 35 Years of Cardiology in Amsterdam. A Selection of Papers and Full Bibliography.* Amsterdam: North-Holland, 1986:678, $101.75.

24. Cournand AF with the collaboration of Meyer M. *From Roots to Late Budding. The Intellectual Adventures of a Medical Scientist.* New York: Gardner Press, 1986:232, $18.95.

Three good books for the cardiologic historian.

William C. Roberts

William C. Roberts, MD
Editor in Chief

Some Good Cardiologic Books Published in 1987

This piece briefly mentions some of the better books that crossed my desk in 1987.

1. Braunwald E, editor. *Heart Disease. A Textbook of Cardiovascular Medicine*, 3rd ed. Philadelphia: W.B. Saunders, 1988:2016, $99.00 (single volume), $115.00 (2-volume set).

The book is superb because it was done by Eugene Braunwald. He demands excellence in his own work and in the work of his contributors. The book contains 62 chapters, 25 (40%) of which were authored or coauthored by Braunwald. Of the more than 1,900 text pages, Braunwald authored or coauthored 725 (38%) of them and he clearly edited the other 1,175 pages. References were added to the galleys to make the book as timely as possible. This book cost Braunwald a bleeding peptic ulcer, but the product is worth it.

2. Parmley WW, Chatterjee K, editors. *Cardiology*. Philadelphia, J.B. Lippincott, 1987:2212, $175.00.

A looseleaf 2-volume textbook of cardiology containing 112 chapters. It is expected that about 10% of the book will be revised every year. The revision for the first year is included in the initial price but thereafter the additions will cost $50 a year. Although this is a fine book by leaders of cardiology, I favor the less expensive Braunwald book, which is completely revised every 3 years. The looseleaf feature, however, is innovative.

3. Page IH. *Hypertension Mechanisms*. Orlando, Florida: Grune & Stratton, 1987:1102, $69.50.

This is an extraordinary book by an extraordinary man, and it will be a classic. It contains 923 pages of text and 161 pages of references (9,000 in all, none after 1984 and all at the end of the book) and not a single figure or table. The book describes basic pathophysiologic mechanisms of systemic hypertension in both human and nonhuman animals, and it provides Page's perspectives after more than 50 years of research in hypertension.

4. Messerli FH, editor. *The Heart and Hypertension*. New York: Yorke Medical Books, 1987:482, $47.50.

A fine book on an important topic.

5. Froelicher VF. *Exercise and the Heart: Clinical Concepts*. 2nd ed. Chicago: Year Book Medical Publishers, 1987:508, $53.00.

May be the best book on this subject.

6. Maseri A, Sobel BE, Chierchia S, editors. *Hammersmith Cardiology Workshop Series*, volume 3. New York: Raven Press, 1987:293, $45.00.

Thirty-eight topics are presented by major leaders in world cardiology with few numbers and lots of discussion. Interesting reading.

7. Abrams J. *Essentials of Cardiac Physical Diagnosis*. Philadelphia: Lea & Febiger, 1987:482, $34.50.

A good book at a good price.

8. Heger JW, Niemann JT, Criley JM. *Cardiology for the House Officer*, 2nd ed. Baltimore: William & Wilkins, 1987:313, $13.95.

9. Alpert JS, Francis GS. *Manual of Coronary Care*. Fourth ed. Boston: Little, Brown & Company, 1987:221, $17.50.

Two little books for the doctor's bag.

10. Sobel BE, Collen D, Grossbard EB, editors. *Tissue Plasminogen Activator in Thrombolytic Therapy*. New York: Marcel Dekker, 1987:264, $55.00.

This agent was approved recently by the Food and Drug Administration. The book price is relatively high, but comparatively nothing compared to the price for TPA treatment (over $2,000).

11. Mandel WJ, editor. *Cardiac Arrhythmias: Their Mechanisms, Diagnosis, and Management*, 2nd ed. Philadelphia: J.B. Lippincott, 1987:861, $75.00.

This book with 66 contributors is comprehensive, easy to read and worthy of the price. The authors describe how to recognize the various arrhythmias, and they provide much information on the disordered cellular mechanisms responsible for them. Other subjects discussed are electrophysiologic testing, ablative techniques, new modes of pacemaker therapy, antiarrhythmic drugs and automatic implantable defibrillators.

12. Bayes de Luna A. *Textbook of Clinical Electrocardiography*. Dordrecht: Martinus Nijhoff, 1987:496, $180.00 (hardcover); $60.00 (paperback).

The first book on electrocardiography in English by Dr. Bayes de Luna, an astute scholar and gifted teacher of electrocardiography, but an outrageous hardcover price.

13. Ward DE, Camm AJ. *Clinical Electrophysiology of the Heart*. London: Edward Arnold, 1987:390, $75.00.

A useful book for those working in electrophysiologic laboratories.

14. Platia EV, editor. *Management of Cardiac Arrhythmias: The Nonpharmacologic Approach*. Philadelphia: J.B. Lippincott, 1987:420, $55.00.

About one-third of this book deals with assessment of arrhythmias, and the remainder with their nonpharmacologic management, including the use of pacemakers, electroshock, implantable defibrillators and cardioverters, catheter ablation and operative therapy.

15. Moses HW, Taylor GJ, Schneider JA, Dove JT. *A Practical Guide to Cardiac Pacing*, 2nd ed. Boston: Little, Brown & Company, 1987:147, $17.50.

This paperback is practical and easy to read. It contains only

21 references.

16. Steinberg D, Olefsky JM, editors. *Hypercholesterolemia and Atherosclerosis: Pathogenesis and Prevention* (Contemporary Issues in Endocrinology and Metabolism, Vol. 3). New York: Churchill Livingstone, 1987:270, $36.00 (Distributed by Longman, White Plains, New York).

Ten good chapters and 2 appendixes from National Institutes of Health conferences are included.

17. Meier B. *Coronary Angioplasty.* Orlando: Grune & Stratton, 1987:279. $49.50.

This single-authored monograph, by one who worked with Andreas R. Gruentzig for 7 years, is well done.

18. Dalen JE, Alpert JS, editors. *Valvular Heart Disease,* 2nd ed. Boston: Little, Brown & Company, 1987:600, $68.00.

19. Greenberg BH, Murphy E, editors. *Valvular Heart Disease.* Littleton, Massachusetts: PSG, 1987:278, $45.00.

I prefer the Dalen-Alpert book although all contributors are from the same medical center, namely Worcester, Massachusetts. Information on percutaneous valvuloplasty is lacking.

20. Omoto R, editor. *Color Atlas of Real-Time Two-Dimensional Doppler Echocardiography,* 2nd ed. Philadelphia: Lea & Febiger, 1987:214, $124.00.

Expensive, but a beautiful book.

21. Bruijn NP, Clements FM. *Transesophageal Echocardiography.* Boston: Martinus Nijhoff, 1987:133, $33.75.

For those interested in this topic this is probably the only book available.

22. Pierpont MEM, Moller JH, editors. *The Genetics of Cardiovascular Disease.* Boston: Martinus Nijhoff, 1987:374, $110.00.

A needed but overpriced book that provides much information on the genetic aspects of all forms of cardiovascular disease. About one-third of the text deals with cardiac malformations, whether isolated, syndromal or chromosomal.

23. Lock JE, Keane JF, Fellows KE. *Diagnostic and Interventional Catheterization in Congenital Heart Disease.* Boston: Martinus Nijhoff, 1987:189, $55.00.

For pediatric cardiologists spending time in a cardiac catheterization laboratory, this is a good book to own.

24. Anderson RH, Crupi G, Parenzan L, editors. *Double Inlet Ventricle. Anatomy, Diagnosis and Surgical Management.* New York: Elsevier, 1987:234, $59.00.

All one needs to know and then some on a single rare congenital anomaly.

25. Hallman GL, Cooley DA, Gutgesell HP. *Surgical Treatment of Congenital Heart Disease,* 3rd ed. Philadelphia: Lea & Febiger, 1987:235, $45.00.

This book provides illustrations and comments on operative therapy in 19 congenital anomalies of the heart and great vessels.

26. McGoon DC, editor. *Cardiac Surgery,* 2nd ed. (Cardiovascular Clinics, Vol. 17, number 3). Philadelphia: FA Davis, 1987:446, $75.00.

A product of Dwight McGoon is expected to be good and this book is no exception. His 2 essays "Prologue: From Whence?" and "Epilogue: To Where?" personalize cardiac surgical history and philosophize about its future, and they are particularly nice.

27. Cohn LH, Doty DB, McElvein RB. *Decision Making in Cardio-Thoracic Surgery.* Toronto: BC Decker, 1987:221, $40.00.

Over 100 clinical problems are presented in a decision-tree format. The authors do not advocate cardiac catheterization for valve replacement or repair in persons younger than 40 years of age. I disagree. The authors advocate immediate operation for acute aortic dissection beginning at the aortic isthmus or below. I agree, but most do not. In patients with combined severe narrowing of the carotid and coronary arteries, the authors advocate simultaneous repair of both vascular systems, a view in disagreement with many but maybe the right view. Good reading.

28. Webb WR, Kerstein MD, editors. *Cardiovascular Emergencies.* Rockville, Maryland: Aspen, 1987:223, $34.50.

The emergencies covered are acute myocardial infarction, hypertensive crises, aortic dissection, trauma to the heart, injuries to peripheral vessels, acute vascular occlusive disease, thrombophlebitis and pulmonary embolism. No discussions are provided on sudden cardiac death, life-threatening arrhythmias, acute valvular infection and regurgitation and acute pulmonary edema. The book is more useful to surgeons than to internists.

29. Texon M. *Can the Cardiac Stand Trial?* New York: Hemisphere Publishing, 1987:644, $37.00.

An analysis of 100 cardiac cases that went to trial.

30. Schlant RC, editor in chief, Collins JJ Jr., Engle MA, Frye RL, Gifford RW Jr., O'Rourke RA. *1987 Year Book of Cardiology.* Chicago:Year Book Medical Publishers, 1987:410, $44.95.

31. Roberts WC, editor, Rackley CE, Mason DT, Willerson JT, Pacifico AD, Graham TP Jr, Karp RB. *Cardiology 1987.* New York: Yorke Medical Books, Cahners Publishing, 1987:518. $55.00.

The *Year Book* contains a new group of editors but the format has not changed except for a brief introduction to each of the 6 major sections. The 311 articles summarized are from those published in November to December 1985 and January to October 1986.

The Yorke Medical book summarizes 858 publications, all published in 1986. I obviously prefer the latter book.

William C. Roberts

William C. Roberts, MD
Editor in Chief

Some Good Cardiologic Books Published in 1988

This piece briefly mentions some of the better cardiologic books published in 1988.

1. Eagle KA, Haber E, DeSanctis RW, Austen WG, editors. *The Practice of Cardiology, The Medical Surgical Cardiac Units at the Massachusetts General Hospital.* Second edition. Volumes I and II. Boston: Little, Brown and Company, 1989:1830, $125.00.

This nicely prepared book is authored by physicians from a single institution, and, as amazing as it may seem, the contributors number 70. A few have subsequently left "the MGH". Differences of opinion among colleagues are freely discussed. Because single-authored, comprehensive cardiology textbooks are essentially no longer available, a volume from a single institution is the closest thing to it. This book is a good one.

2. Kerber RE, editor. *Echocardiography in Coronary Artery Disease.* Mount Kisco, New York: Futura Publishing Company, 1988:541, $86.00.

This book puts in 1 place a large body of information on the use of echocardiography in coronary artery disease. The book, which includes nearly all forms of echocardiography (transthoracic, Doppler, transesophageal, epicardial, etc.), is highly recommended.

3. Califf RM, Mark DB, Wagner GS. *Acute Coronary Care in the Thrombolytic Era.* Chicago: Year Book Medical Publishers, Inc., 1988:771, $49.95.

4. Holmes DR Jr, Vlietstra RE, editors. *Interventional Cardiology.* Philadelphia: FA Davis Company, 1989: 400, $70.00.

5. Angelini P. *Balloon Catheter Coronary Angioplasty.* Mount Kisco, New York: Futura Publishing Company, 1988:414, $98.00.

6. Topol EJ, editor. *Acute Coronary Intervention,* New York: Alan R. Liss, Inc., 1988:302, $49.50.

These 4 books are all good. The Califf one is the best for the money.

7. Singh BN, editor. *Silent Myocardial Ischemia and Angina. Prevalence, Prognostic, and Therapeutic Significance.* New York: Pergamon Press, 1988:311, $33.60.

A fine update on this subject.

8. Higgins MW, Luepker RV, editors. *Trends in Coronary Heart Disease Mortality. The Influence of Medical Care.* New York: Oxford University Press, 1988:302, $39.95.

A useful book describing time trends and regional patterns of coronary artery disease and medical care, determinants of coronary mortality, influence of medical care on risk factors, out-of-hospital and in-hospital management of acute coronary syndromes and influence of medical care on chronic coronary artery disease.

9. Wollam GL, Hall WD, editors. *Hypertension Management. Clinical Practice and Therapeutic Dilemmas.* Chicago: Year Book Medical Publishers, Inc., 1988:541, $55.00.

A clearly written practical book and reasonably priced.

10. Boudoulas H, Wooley CF, editors. *Mitral Valve Prolapse and the Mitral Valve Prolapse Syndrome.* Mount Kisco, New York: Futura Publishing Company, 1988:673, $80.00.

This book, which contains 34 chapters covering nearly all aspects of mitral valve prolapse, is the best yet on this subject.

11. Konstam MA, Isner JM, editors. *The Right Ventricle.* Boston: Kluwer Academic Publishers, 1988:342, $125.00.

An all-inclusive, expensive book on a portion of the heart.

12. Virmani R, Forman MB, editors. *Nonatherosclerotic Ischemic Heart Disease.* New York: Raven Press, 1989:428, $89.00.

This fine but expensive book discusses causes of myocardial ischemia in the absence of significant atherosclerosis.

13. Douglas PS, editor. *Heart Disease in Women.* Philadelphia: FA Davis Company, 1989:316, $75.00.

Birth control pills, cigarettes, estrogen replacement, 2 jobs and delayed childbirth make heart disease in this half of our population a bit different than in the other half. This book, written mainly by women, is the first on heart disease in women, and, therefore, it will be useful.

14. Fardy PS, Yanowitz FG, Wilson PK. *Cardiac Rehabilitation, Adult Fitness, and Exercise Testing.* Philadelphia: Lea & Febiger, 1988:402, $42.50.

A new player. It looks good.

15. Fletcher GF, editor. *Exercise in the Practice of Medicine.* Second revised edition. Mount Kisco, New York: Futura Publishing Company, Inc., 1988:513, $62.00.

Myrvin H. Ellestad calls this book "a classic," and ". . . a must for the serious student of exercise physiology and cardiac rehabilitation . . ." It contains contributions from only 12 authors.

16. Marriott HJL. *Practical Electrocardiography.* Eighth edition. 1988:556, $27.95.

My favorite book on standard electrocardiography.

17. Singh BN, editor. *Control of Cardiac Arrhythmias by Lengthening Repolarization.* Mount Kisco, New York: Futura Publishing Company, 1988:596, $80.00.

This book focuses on class III antiarrhythmic agents (sotalol, N-acetylprocainamide, bretylium, melperone, and amiodarone), i.e., those which prolong the refractory period by selectively lengthening cardiac repolarization. This text of 24 chapters by multiple authors reviews much information on controlling arrhythmias by lengthening repolarization. The presence of Bramah Singh as editor assures superb quality.

18. Goldberg SJ, Allen HD, Marx GR, Donnerstein RL. *Doppler Echocardiography.* Second edition. Philadelphia: Lea & Febiger, 1988:314, $45.00.

19. Duncan WJ. *Color Doppler in Clinical Cardiology.* Philadelphia: WB Saunders Company, 1988:163, $95.00.

20. Kisslo J, Adams DB, Belkin RN. *Doppler Color Flow Imaging.* New York: Churchill Livingstone, 1988: 183, $59.00.

21. Redel DA. *Color Blood Flow Imaging of the Heart.* Berlin: Springer-Verlag, 1988:130, $169.50.

The Duncan and Redel books are very expensive. Each page in the Redel book costs $1.30. The Kisslo book, which contains 163 color illustrations, is the best of the color books.

22. Reed KL, Anderson CF, Shenker L. *Fetal Echocardiography. An Atlas.* New York: Alan R. Liss, Inc., 1988:138, $62.50.

This atlas is a guide to examination of the fetal heart by ultrasound.

23. Yang SS, Bentivoglio LG, Maranhão V, Goldberg H. *From Cardiac Catheterization Data to Hemodynamic Parameters.* Third edition. Philadelphia: FA Davis Company, 1988:430, $52.00.

This book provides some competition to the Grossman book on this subject. The title could be better.

24. Dunn JM, editor. *Cardiac Valve Disease in Children.* New York: Elsevier, 1988:370, $67.50.

An expensive but good book.

25. Mullins CE, Mayer DC. *Congenital Heart Disease. A Diagrammatic Atlas.* New York: Alan R. Liss, Inc., 1988:352, $72.50.

This atlas presents a diagram on virtually every possible combination and permutation of congenital cardiac anomalies. Included are 167 diagrams, which evolved from a collection of line drawings of congenital heart anomalies over 27 years by the senior author.

26. Grillo HC, Austen WG, Wilkins EW Jr, Mathisen DJ, Vlahakes GJ, editors. *Current Therapy in Cardiothoracic Surgery.* Toronto: BC Decker Inc., 1989:590, $84.50.

This practical book offers an up-to-date guide to treatment of cardiac and general thoracic surgical problems by 226 contributors.

27. Symbas PN. *Cardiothoracic Trauma.* Philadelphia: WB Saunders Company, 1989:390, $89.00.

Dr. Symbas has focused on this subject for many years and his extensive experience is obvious.

28. Wallwork J, editor. *Heart and Heart-Lung Transplantation.* Philadelphia: WB Saunders, 1989:576, $99.00.

A comprehensive book.

29. Yankah AC, Hetzer R, Miller DC, Ross DN, Somerville J, Yacoub MH, editors. *Cardiac Valve Allografts 1962–1987. Current Concepts on the Use of Aortic and Pulmonary Allografts for Heart Valve Substitutes.* New York: Springer-Verlag, 1988:394, $86.00.

These editors are the pioneers in this subject, and they have put in 1 place a great deal of information on cardiac valve allografts.

30. Isner JM, Clarke RH, editors. *Cardiovascular Laser Therapy.* New York: Raven Press, 1989:300, $65.00.

The laser light is here and it may prove to be beneficial in opening or widening atherosclerotic obstructions. Much information on this evolving topic is provided here.

31. Schlant RC, Collins JJ Jr, Engle MA, Fry RL, Kaplan NM, O'Rourke RA. *The Year Book of Cardiology 1988.* Chicago: Year Book Medical Publishers, Inc., 1988:378, $47.00.

32. Roberts WC, editor, Rackley CE, Mason DT, Willerson JT, Pacifico AD, Graham TP Jr, Karp RB. *Cardiology 1988.* Boston: Butterworths, 1988:505, $60.00.

The Schlant book is the twenty-eighth in the cardiology series by Year Book, and it summarizes 296 articles published in either 1987 or 1986. Most summaries of articles—provided by the publisher but chosen by the editors—receive editorial comments by an editor.

The Roberts book summarizes 837 articles, all published in 1987. Additionally, 159 figures and 32 tables are included. Of course, this is my favorite of the annual review books.

33. Griffin JC, Mandel WJ, editors. *Clinical Concepts in Arrhythmias: An Annual Review—1988.* Mount Kisco, New York: Futura Publishing Company, 1988: 341, $38.00.

This book is the first of what is planned to be a series of books reproducing abstracts of what are considered by the 2 editors to be the best articles on arrhythmias and conduction disorders published the previous year. The present book contains exactly 400 reproduced abstracts of articles published in 1987 plus a few titles of articles without summaries. For electrophysiologists this book should be a useful one.

34. Zollinger RM, editor. *Elliott Carr Cutler and The Cloning of Surgeons.* Mount Kisco, New York: Futura Publishing Company, 1988:235, $35.00.

This book is about the man who performed the first mitral valvulotomy. The year was 1923 and the place was the Peter Bent Brigham Hospital in Boston. In 1932 he succeeded Harvey Cushing as chief of surgery at "the Brigham". Cutler died at age 59 but by this time he had trained and stimulated many surgeons including the author of this book. Brief biographies of Cutler-appointed residents elected to The American Surgical Association are included.

William C. Roberts

William C. Roberts, MD
Editor in Chief

Some Good Cardiologic Books Published in 1989

Books, books, books! Some of the nonmedical ones in 1989 included Nancy Reagan's *My Turn: The Memoirs of Nancy Reagan;* former attorney general Ed Meese's *Witness to History: Power and Politics in the Reagan White House;* Robert Bork's *The Tempting of America: The Political Seduction of the Law;* John Barry's *The Ambition and the Power: The Fall of Jim Wright;* Norman Cousins' *Head First: The Biology of Hope;* Bill McKibben's *The End of Nature;* Stephen Jay Gould's *Wonderful Life: The Burgess Shale and the Nature of History;* Gore Vidal's *Hollywood;* James Michener's *Caribbean;* Carey Roberts' *Touch a Cold Door;* 4 books on Richard Nixon; at least 12 new books on World War II; and of course many others. More cardiologic books appeared in 1989 than in 1988. The average cost of a cardiologic book in 1989 was $65.00. This piece will mention some good cardiologic books appearing in 1989.

1. Hurst JW, Editor in Chief, Schlant RC, Associate Editor. *The Heart, Arteries and Veins*. New York: McGraw-Hill Information Services Co., 1990:2,348, $99.00 (single volume), $115.00 (double volume).

2. Julian DG, Camm AJ, Fox KM, Hall RJC, and Poole-Wilson PA, editors. *Diseases of the Heart*. London: Bailliere Tindall, 1989:1,709, $125.00.

The Hurst book is a must for a cardiologic library. It actually complements the Braunwald book in that it has a bit more on therapy and a bit less on diagnosis and pathophysiology, the opposite of the Braunwald book. The Hurst book is less expensive and contains much more information than does the Julian book.

3. Long WA, editor. *Fetal and Neonatal Cardiology*. Philadelphia: WB Saunders Co., 1990:863, $195.00.

I suspect that this book will rapidly become the bible on this subject.

4. Adams FH, Emmanouilides GC, Riemenschneider TA, editors. *Moss' Heart Disease in Infants, Children, and Adolescents*, Fourth edition. Baltimore: Williams & Wilkins, 1989:1,066, $149.95.

This excellent book by 73 contributors includes nearly all forms of cardiac disease in the young. Exactly 50% of the text concerns congenital defects; the other 50% concerns acquired heart diseases, procedures and special problems.

5. Elkayam U, Gleicher N, editors. *Cardiac Problems in Pregnancy. Diagnosis and Management of Maternal and Fetal Disease*. New York: Alan R. Liss, Inc., 1990:809, $124.50.

A comprehensive book on this subject.

6. Gazes PC. *Clinical Cardiology*. Philadelphia: Lea & Febiger, 1990:594, $55.00.

This easily readable book presents in a simple, concise manner nonencyclopedic cardiologic information useful in everyday practice. This book is a good one for noncardiologists seeking cardiologic information.

7. Opie LH. *Clinical Use of Calcium Channel Antagonist Drugs*. Boston: Kluwer Academic Publishers, 1989:304, $80.00.

An excellent book.

8. Williams R. *The Trusting Heart. Great News About Type A Behavior*. New York: *Times* BOOKS, 1989:240, $17.95.

Dr. Williams is director of the Behavioral Medicine Research Center at Duke University. He has linked certain kinds of type A behavior, such as hostility and rage, with cardiac disease, and he maintains that these harmful traits can be separated from positive aspects of type A personality such as ambition, high energy and enthusiasm, thereby rendering the type A person even healthier than the placid type B counterpart.

9. Francis GS, Alpert JS, editors. *Modern Coronary Care*. Boston: Little, Brown and Co., 1990:797, $95.00.

This book by an array of distinguished cardiologists provides a huge amount of information on acute myocardial infarction and how to manage it.

10. Julian DG, Kubler W, Norris RM, Swan HJ, Collen D, Verstraete M, editors. *Thrombolysis in Cardiovascular Disease*. New York: Marcel Dekker, 1989:460, $79.75.

A fine update on a rapidly changing topic.

11. Franklin BA, Gordon S, Timmis GC, editors. *Exercise in Modern Medicine*. Baltimore: Williams & Wilkins, 1989:300, $42.95.

Although there are numerous books on exercise testing and training for presumably healthy adults and cardiac patients, this one is comprehensive and includes requirements of special patient populations such as those with peripheral vascular disease, diabetes mellitus, end-stage renal disease, severe obesity, chronic obstructive pulmonary disease, asthma, cystic fibrosis, healthy elderly subjects, wheel chair-dependent patients and pregnancy.

12. Pepine CJ, Hill JA, Lambert CR, editors. *Diagnostic and Therapeutic Cardiac Catheterization*. Baltimore: Williams & Wilkins, 1989:612, $69.50.

13. Miller G. *Invasive Investigation of the Heart. A Guide to Cardiac Cathertisation and Related Procedures*. Oxford: Blackwell Scientific Publications, 1989:496, $160.00.

14. Leachman DR, Leachman RD. *Coronary and Peripheral Angiography and Angioplasty*. Philadelphia: JB Lippincott, 1989:149, $34.50.

Although the Miller book is beautifully prepared, its cost is prohibitive (because it was published abroad). The Pepine book is superb, fully packed, and very reasonable in view of its 612 pages, 19% more than in the Miller book. It will give the Grossman book (1986, third edition) on this subject a run for its money. The Pepine book has 180 pages on specific clinical states, and their assessment and intervention by catheter techniques. The book discusses how noninvasive data and results of clinical trials may supplement or replace catheterization. One chapter deals with radiographic contrast agents. This book should be useful both to those who do catheterizations and to those who refer patients for these procedures. The Leachman father-and-son book is a handy practical guide.

15. Topol EJ, editor. *Textbook of Interventional Cardiology*. Philadelphia: WB Saunders Co., 1990:954, $95.00.

16. Kapoor AS, editor. *Interventional Cardiology*. New York: Springer-Verlag, 1989:415, $99.00.

Two books of nearly similar price but the Topol book contains over twice the amount of information as the Kapoor book. The Topol book is the best so far on this rapidly changing subject.

17. Schoen FJ. *Interventional and Surgical Cardiovascular Pathology. Clinical Correlations and Basic Principles*. Philadelphia: WB Saunders, 1989:410, $82.35.

This good book focuses on morphologic features of hearts that had been subjected to interventional (operative or nonoperative) procedures. It contains 3,267 references in its 9 chapters, all but 1 of which is written by Schoen.

18. Laragh JH, Brenner BM, editors. *Hypertension, Pathophysiology, Diagnosis, and Management*. Volumes I and II, New York: Raven Press, 1990:2,436, $295.00.

Almost surely this is the most comprehensive book published on systemic hypertension. If it is not in these 2 volumes, the information must not be available.

19. Schamroth L. *The 12 Lead Electrocardiogram*. In 2 books. Oxford: Blackwell Scientific Publications, 1989:848, $199.00.

20. Dunn MI, Lipman BS. *Lipman-Massie Clinical Electrocardiography*. Eighth edition. Chicago: Year Book Medical Publishers, Inc., 1989:620, $64.95.

21. Fisch C. *Electrocardiography of Arrhythmias*. Philadelphia: Lea & Febiger, 1990:451, $49.50.

Schamroth's comprehensive texts deal exclusively with 12-lead contour analysis and do not include abnormal heart rhythms. It is the magnum opus of the late Leo Schamroth. It is divided in 4 major divisions: genesis of the normal and abnormal electrocardiogram; acquired heart disease; congenital and hereditary heart disease; and electrocardiographic case studies. The latter constitute most of book 2.

The Dunn-Lipman book began in 1951 as *Clinical Unipolar Electrocardiography*. The present title is the fourth this book has carried. This edition is the first to have references after each chapter. This book reminds me of Grant's wonderful electrocardiography book published in the 1950s.

Charles Fisch has focused his professional life on the electrocardiography of arrhythmias, and taught this subject to literally thousands of physicians. His long overdue book, which encompasses nearly all arrhythmias, focuses on mechanisms and electrocardiographic concepts rather than definition and classification. It includes 451 figures, and nearly all are electrocardiographic tracings recorded from the body's surface. The tracings and their explanations are the essence of this fine book.

22. St. John Sutton M, Oldershaw PJ, editors. *Textbook of Adult and Pediatric Echocardiography and Doppler*. Boston: Blackwell Scientific Publications, 1989:880, $110.00.

23. Hagan AD, DeMaria AN. *Clinical Applications of Two-Dimensional Echocardiography and Cardiac Doppler*, Second edition. Boston: Little, Brown and Company, 1989:556, $75.00.

24. Schapira JN, Harold JG, editors. *Two-Dimensional Echocardiography and Cardiac Doppler*, Second edition. Baltimore: Williams & Wilkins, 1990:670, $99.50.

25. Atlee JL III. *Perioperative Cardiac Dysrhythmias: Mechanisms, Recognition, Management*, Second edition. Chicago: Year Book, 1990:443, $69.95.

The St. John Sutton book is comprehensive and contains much information for the money. On the other hand, it includes both congenital and acquired heart diseases, and those interested in one may not be so interested in the other. The Hagan and DeMaria book also is of high quality. The Atlee book, written by an anesthesiologist, focuses on cardiac arrhythmias occurring in the operating room or recovery room or in the surgical intensive care unit. This book could use more illustrations.

26. Nanda NC. *Atlas of Color Doppler Echocardiography*. Philadelphia: Lea & Febiger, 1989:544, $135.00.

27. Nanda NC, editor. *Textbook of Color Doppler Echocardiography*. Philadelphia: Lea & Febiger, 1989:359, $110.00.

28. Gura GM Jr. *Video Atlas of Two-Dimensional Color Flow Doppler Echocardiography*. Boston: Little, Brown and Co., 1989:180, $250.00.

29. Maurer G, Mohl W, editors. *Echocardiography and Doppler in Cardiac Surgery*. New York: Igaku-Shoin, 1989:355, $97.50.

The Nanda *Atlas* encompasses Nanda's experience with Doppler flow imaging for nearly 5 years. The various types of flow patterns seen in both acquired and congenital cardiac disease are seen in over 1,600 anatomic and color Doppler illustrations and they represent the most detailed, definitive and comprehensive work in this field to date. The *Textbook* is a companion to the *Atlas*. It includes 32 chapters and an appendix written by well-recognized authorities. A *Video Tape of Color Doppler Echocardiography* of about 2 hours length was also prepared by Nanda to supplement both the *Atlas* and the *Textbook*.

The Gura and accompanying 2 videos occupying 2.5 hours feature 50 case studies. The excellent color prints are shown in more detail in video.

30. Erbel R, Khandheria BK, Brennecke R, Meyer J, Seward JB, Tajik AJ, editors. *Transesophageal Echocardiography. A New Window to the Heart*. Berlin: Springler-Verlag, 1989:360, $112.50.

This book comprises proceedings of a symposium. Methods, technique, anatomic correlation and future applications are discussed by recognized experts. The book is overpriced and disappointing.

31. Gray RJ, Matloff JM, editors. *Medical Management of the Cardiac Surgical Patient*. Baltimore: Williams & Wilkins, 1990:378, $52.95.

32. Bojar RM with Murphy RE, Payne DD, Diehl JT. *Manual of Perioperative Care in Cardiac and Thoracic Surgery*. Boston: Blackwell Scientific Publications, 1989:381, $27.50.

Although both books are useful, I prefer the Gray and Matloff one. The price of the Bojar book is nice.

33. Edmunds LH Jr, Norwood WI, Low DW. *Atlas of Cardiothoracic Surgery*. Philadelphia: Lea & Febiger, 1990:287, $125.00.

One page of illustrations by Dr. Low are presented in apposition to a page of print.

34. Ebert PA. *Atlas of Congenital Cardiac Surgery*. New York: Churchill Livingstone, 1989:138, $125.00.

A great surgeon, Paul Ebert, and a great illustrator, Leon Schlossberg, combine to produce a beautiful book. The page space could have been better utilized.

35. Hopkins RA. *Cardiac Reconstructions with Allograft Valves*. New York: Springer-Verlag, 1989:194, $125.00.

Although allograft cardiovascular tissues have a number of applications, the focus of this volume is on valved ventricular outflow tract reconstructions. This book, which is beautifully illustrated, is a "how-to" guide for surgeons in using allograft valves and conduits in cardiac reconstructions. It will not be a big seller but it is nicely done.

36. Milnor WR. *Hemodynamics*, Second edition. Baltimore: Williams & Wilkins, 1989:419, $74.95.

This book is concerned with the forces generated by the heart and the resulting motion of blood through the cardiovascular system. This book is "heavy" for most cardiologists because physicists and mathematicians have contributed to it equally with physicians and physiologists.

37. Camilleri J-P, Berry CL, Fiessinger J-N, Bariety J, editors. *Diseases of the Arterial Wall*. London: Springer-Verlag, 1989 (English edition): 693, $370.50.

The French edition of this book was published in 1987, and the English translation in 1989. This English edition is a nice heavy book, but it should be. It is the most expensive newly published medical text I have ever seen.

38. Freedom RM. *Pulmonary Atresia with Intact Ventricular Septum*. Mount Kisco, New York: Futura, 1989:262, $55.00.

This book includes 19 chapters, 18 of which are written or cowritten by Bob Freedom. One can question whether a defect that makes up <1% of all major congenital cardiac anomalies deserves a separate book, but if information on this defect is desired, here it is.

39. Roberts WC, editor, Mason DT, Rackley CE, Willerson JT, Graham TP Jr, Karp RB. *Cardiology 1989*. Boston: Butterworths, 1989:523, $60.00.

Of course I could be biased but *Cardiology 1989* is really a good book. Articles on the same subject are placed together. A total of 824 articles are summarized and supplemented by 166 figures and 68 tables.

William C. Roberts

William Clifford Roberts, MD
Editor in Chief

Some Good Cardiologic Books Published in 1990

1. O'Rourke RA, Pohost GM, editors. *Principles and Practice of Cardiovascular Imaging.* Boston: Little, Brown and Company, 1991:880, $175.00.

O'Rourke and Pohost, as J. Willis Hurst states, know low technology, and as this book indicates, they also know high technology. The 2 editors call this "....a unique book providing comprehensive information on the sometimes confusing array of diagnostic methods for evaluation of the cardiovascular system." They may be right too.

2. Gersh BJ, Rahimtoola SH, editors. *Acute Myocardial Infarction.* New York: Elsevier, 1991:524, $84.00.

This multiauthored (49) book, the first of a new series entitled *Current Topics in Cardiology* and edited by Shahbudin H. Rahimtoola, is a comprehensive monograph on acute myocardial infarction. It is well done.

3. Gould KL. *Coronary Artery Stenosis.* New York: Elsevier, 1991:323, $99.00.

The title of this book provides little indication as to its contents. It describes pressure flow characteristics, physiologic behavior, and quantitative geometry of coronary stenoses experimentally in vivo and clinically using the most advanced invasive arteriographic analysis and noninvasive perfusion-metabolic imaging available. The first part of the book concerns anatomic and functional characteristics of coronary artery stenoses, and the second part, positron emission tomography of the heart. Although a scholarly book, it may be too "heavy" for most cardiologists.

4. Grossman W, Baim DS, editors. *Cardiac Catheterization, Angiography, and Intervention.* Fourth edition. Philadelphia: Lea & Febiger, 1991:698, $59.50.

5. Bashore TM, editor. *Invasive Cardiology: Principles and Techniques.* Toronto: B.C. Decker Inc., 1990:318, $65.00.

6. Serruys PW, Simon R, Beatt KJ, editors. *PTCA. An Investigational Tool and a Non-operative Treatment of Acute Ischemia.* Dordrecht: Kluwer Academic Publishers, 1990:404, $125.00.

7. Abela GS, editor. *Lasers in Cardiovascular Medicine and Surgery: Fundamentals and Techniques.* Boston: Kluwer Academic Publishers, 1990:480, $150.00.

The Grossman and Baim book has been the classic in this arena, but it is now getting some competition. It provides, as the editors state, "clear and concise descriptions of the major techniques currently used in cardiac catheterization...and the growing field of interventional cardiology."

The Bashore book is more expensive and contains far less information than the Grossman and Baim book.

The multiauthored Serruys et al book describes the effects of balloon-induced myocardial ischemia on the electrocardiogram, coronary blood flow dynamics, cardiac muscle metabolism, left ventricular function, and measures to counter these effects, including reperfusion, in unstable angina pectoris and acute myocardial infarction. The subject matter is of interest but the preparation of the product is not ideal. The word "Ischemia" is spelled on the title page as "Ischema."

The multiauthored Abela book describes the most up-to-date technology and procedural approaches of laser angioplasty using the various laser systems.

8. Messerli GH, editor. *Cardiovascular Drug Therapy.* Philadelphia: W.B. Saunders Company, 1990:1709, $84.00.

9. Antonaccio MJ, editor. *Cardiovascular Pharmacology.* Third edition. New York: Raven Press, 1990:556, $75.00.

The Messerli book discusses >100 cardiovascular agents and various therapeutic strategies by 184 authors. The Antonaccio book by 22 authors is a more basic pharmacologic book with less information and it costs nearly as much as the Messerli book. The Messerli book will be popular.

10. Kaplan NM. *Clinical Hypertension.* Fourth edition. Baltimore: Williams & Wilkins, 1990:466, $63.00.

11. McMahon FG. *Management of Essential Hypertension: The Once-A-Day Era.* Third edition. Mount Kisco, New York: Futura Publishing Company, Inc., 1990:684, $59.50.

The new edition of both the Kaplan and McMahon books are good. Both are single authored (which I like). The Kaplan one is my favorite despite the 220 more pages in the McMahon book for essentially the same price.

12. Grundy SM with illustrations by DuPrey LP. *Cholesterol and Atherosclerosis: Diagnosis and Treatment.* Philadelphia: J.B. Lippincott Company, and New York: Gower Medical Publishing, 1990:176, $55.00.

This book is outstanding. Its magnificent illustrations and beautiful layout make it unique and a most desirable addition to any personal or institutional cardiovascular library.

13. Davidson DM. *Preventive Cardiology.* Baltimore: Williams & Wilkins, 1991:300, $48.00.

14. Frohlich ED, editor. *Preventive Aspects of Coronary Heart Disease.* Philadelphia: F.A. Davis Company, 1990:239, $70.00. (Cardiovascular Clinics 20/3).

The Davidson book is single authored and easily readable. The Frohlich-editored book is a stronger one.

15. Gillette PC, Garson A Jr, editors. *Pediatric Arrhythmias: Electrophysiology and Pacing.* Philadelphia: W.B. Saunders Company, 1990:703, $195.00.

This textbook, by 31 authors, is probably the best thus far for diagnosis and treatment of arrhythmias in children and young adults.

16. Rosen MR, Janse MJ, Wit AL, editors. *Cardiac Electrophysiology: A Textbook Prepared in Honor of Brian F. Hoffman.* Mount Kisco, New York: Futura Publishing, Inc., 1990:1195, $160.00.

This book has contributions from 101 authors, including virtually all prominent investigators in this arena. Any book dedicated to Brian Hoffman must be a good one.

17. El-Sherif N, Samet P, editors. *Cardiac Pacing and Electrophysiology.* Third edition. Philadelphia: W.B. Saunders Company, 1991:784, $145.00.

The last edition of this book was 1980, and that book dealt only with cardiac pacing. This third edition has been much expanded by the 109 authors and is quite comprehensive.

18. Horowitz LN, editor. *Current Management of Arrhythmias.* Philadelphia: B.C. Decker, Inc., 1991:436, $75.00.

This multiauthored book summarizes recent developments in diagnosis and management of cardiac arrhythmias. Each chapter presents the views of the authors of that chapter rather than a compilation of many views.

19. Saksena S, Goldschlager N, editors. *Electrical Therapy for Cardiac Arrhythmias, Pacing, Antitachycardia Devices, Catheter Ablation.* Philadelphia: W.B. Saunders Company, 1990:731, $95.00.

This is mainly pacing but there is more. The 83 contributors represent viewpoints from 30 medical centers. A fine book.

20. Touboul P, Waldo AL, editors. *Atrial Arrhythmias. Current Concepts and Management.* St. Louis: Mosby Year Book, 1990:521, $75.00.

This book describes current concepts of the mechanisms responsible for atrial arrhythmias and their therapy by 108 contributors.

21. Hurst JW. *Ventricular Electrocardiography.* Philadelphia: J.B. Lippincott Company and New York: Gower Medical Publishing, 1991:312, $55.00.

A beautiful book stressing the vector method of interpretation of the 12-lead electrocardiogram by a masterful teacher.

22. Goldberger AL, Goldberger E. *Clinical Electrocardiography, A Simplified Approach.* Fourth edition. St. Louis: Mosby Year Book, 1990:348, $31.95.

One of the fine books from which to learn basic electrocardiography.

23. Jawad IA. *A Practical Guide to Echocardiography and Cardiac Doppler Ultrasound.* Boston: Little, Brown and Company, 1990:379, $40.00.

Another echo-Doppler book that physicians should buy, read, and then give to their echocardiography technicians.

24. Garson A Jr, Bricker JT, McNamara DG, editors. *The Science and Practice of Pediatric Cardiology.* Philadelphia: Lea & Febiger, 1990:1-668 (Volume I), 669-1616 (Volume II), and 1617-2557 (Volume III), $395.00.

These 3 volumes have it all. They require time and money. A big year for Tim Garson—2 major books in 1990.

25. Snider AR, Serwer GA. *Echocardiography in Pediatric Heart Disease.* Year Book Medical Publishers, Inc., 1990:379, $125.00.

A superb book.

26. Higgins CB, Silverman NH, Kersting-Sommerhoff BA, Schmidt K. *Congenital Heart Disease. Echocardiography and Magnetic Resonance Imaging.* New York: Raven Press, 1990:395, $135.00.

Two major diagnostic techniques from investigators in the forefront of their fields applied to a single type of cardiovascular disease—the result is an excellent product.

27. Soto B, Pacifico AD. *Angiography in Congenital Heart Malformations.* Mount Kisco, New York: Futura Publishing Company, Inc., 1990:669, $175.00.

This beautifully prepared book contains 37 chapters and 745 illustrations, most of which are angiograms, mainly axial views. This book may be the best thus far on this subject.

28. Clark EB, Takao A, editors. *Developmental Cardiology. Morphogenesis and Function.* Mount Kisco, New York: Futura Publishing Company, Inc., 1990:732, $135.00.

This monograph represents the Proceedings of the 3rd International Symposium on the Etiology and Morphogenesis of Congenital Heart Disease held in Tokyo in November 1989. The first symposium was held in 1978 and the second in 1983 and each also resulted in a book. The present book brings in "the disciplines of cellular and molecular biology, extracellular matrix, cell migration and interaction. . . ." into the morphogenesis of congenital heart disease.

29. Baumgartner WA, Reitz BA, and Achuff SE, editors, and illustrated by Schlossberg L. *Heart and Heart-Lung Transplantation.* Philadelphia: W.B. Saunders Company, 1990:406, $138.00.

30. Cooper DKC, Novitzky D, editors. *The Transplantation and Replacement of Thoracic Organs. The Present Status of Biological and Mechanical Replacement of the Heart and Lungs.* Dordrecht: Kluwer Academic Publishers, 1990:543, $225.00.

31. Thompson ME, editor. *Transplantation.* Philadelphia: F.A. Davis Company, 1990:271, $75.00.

Although the Baumgartner et al book is by 28 authors, most are from the same institution (The Johns Hopkins Medical Institutions). It is comprehensive and beautifully prepared. Some of Leon Schlossberg's drawings are in color. When a book cannot be written by a single author, a book from a single institution is advantageous. I like this book best of the cardiac transplant books thus far available. The Cooper et al and Thompson books also are good, but I prefer the book by the Baltimore group.

32. Gay WA Jr with illustrations by Roselius E. *Atlas of Adult Cardiac Surgery.* New York: Churchill Livingstone, 1990:189, $125.00.

This book contains 86 full-page drawings of various operative approaches to many *acquired* heart diseases for which surgical repair has been effective. The commentaries in the text accompanying the illustrations are brief and usually fill only a small portion of the page. The consequence is much wasted space.

33. Waldhausen JA, Orringer MB, editors. *Complications in Cardiothoracic Surgery.* St. Louis: Mosby Year Book, 1991:460, $110.00.

As Frank Spencer states in the foreword, this book is "a unique and valuable contribution in that no single book previously has concentrated in one source the available information about the numerous complications that can occur." The 86 contributors provide a valuable reference source.

34. Goldberger E. *Treatment of Cardiac Emergen-*

cies. Fifth edition. St. Louis: The C.V. Mosby Company, 1990:429, $44.95.

The topics include syncope, cardiac arrest, cardiogenic shock, arrhythmias, conduction disturbances, acute myocardial infarction, cardiopulmonary emergencies, hypertensive emergencies, aortic dissection, and cardiac tamponade, and apparatuses used for their treatment.

35. Soler-Soler J, Permanyer-Miralda G, Sagrista-Sauleda J, editors. *Pericardial Disease. New Insights and Old Dilemmas*. Dordrecht: Kluwer Academic Publishers, 1990:244, $102.50.

This book is not a comprehensive one on pericardial disease. Rather, it reviews several controversial aspects based on experiences primarily of the editors from Barcelona.

36. Bharati S, Lev M. *The Cardiac Conduction System in Unexplained Sudden Death*. Mount Kisco, New York: Futura Publishing Company, Inc., 1990:399, $115.00.

37. Rossi L, Matturri L. *Clinico-pathological Approach to Cardiac Arrhythmias—A Color Atlas*. Torino: Centro Scientifico Torinese Editore, 1990:325, $120.00.

Bharati and Lev discuss the findings in the conduction system in approximately 100 patients dying "suddenly and unexpectedly, instantaneously or within 24 hours after the onset of symptoms without any evidence of trauma" and they illustrate findings in 75 cases. These illustrations, which number 229, are almost entirely photomicrographs. The authors concluded that "the conduction system was abnormal in *all* (their italics) cases studied." The epicardial coronary arteries in their cases were "usually normal. The maximal changes were found in the bundle of His. . . ."

Rossi and Matturri also are recognized authorities on the morphologic aspects of arrhythmias and conduction disturbances. This book contains 248 color figures, also mainly photomicrographs of the conduction system. Neither book contains electrocardiograms or graphics from electrophysiologic studies. Although both are detailed anatomic descriptions of conduction tissue abnormalities, there is little in either book useful to clinical cardiologists.

38. Conti CR. *Introduction to Clinical Cardiology*. New York: Raven Press, 1991:288, $36.00.

39. Goldberger E. *Essentials of Clinical Cardiology*. Philadelphia: J.B. Lippincott Company, 1990:433, $49.95.

40. Sokolow M, McIlroy MB, Chetlin MD. *Clinical Cardiology*. Fifth edition. Norwalk, Connecticut: Appleton & Lange, 1990:659, $37.50.

41. Kloner RA, editor. *The Guide to Cardiology*. Second edition. New York: Le Jacq Communications, 1990:546, $44.00.

The Conti book is new and different. It is not intended to be as extensive as the other 3. It is quite personable, easy to read, and focuses on the appropriate approach by cardiologists to the 50 subjects under discussion. Although it is intended primarily for house officers and cardiology fellows, there are gems here for the clinical cardiologist. Chapter 2—"Communicating with Patients and Physicians"—is terrific. The usefulness or lack thereof of clinical trials is stressed. My only criticism of the Conti book would be the selection of references appearing at the end of each chapter under "Suggested Reading." More effort could have gone into selecting the most outstanding sources, including the classics, for each of the subjects under discussion.

The Goldberger book is a revision of the book, *Textbook of Clinical Cardiology*, which appeared in 1982 by the same author. The present book is half the size of the 1982 product. The Sokolow et al book is a revision of the one appearing in 1986. The Kloner-edited book is a revision of his 1984 first edition. For interns, residents, and cardiology fellows, the price of the Kloner book is $30.00. All 3 are intended primarily for non-cardiologists seeking cardiologic information.

42. Roberts WC, editor, Mason DT, Rackley CE, Willerson JT, Graham TP Jr, and Karp RB. *Cardiology 1990*. Boston: Butterworth, 1990:494, $75.00.

For some reason I continue to mention this annual book in this column every year. The book is not widely known because the publisher has few cardiology titles, the book is not presented on publishers' row at the 2 major cardiologic meetings in the USA, and maybe the authors have a few deficiencies. Nevertheless, take a peek and you will find 802 articles, each appearing in 1989, summarized, and those on the same subject are lumped together. To assist in the reading are 126 figures and 66 tables. Despite some biased views, I highly recommend this red book.

43. McDougall JA with recipes by McDougall M. *The McDougall Program. Twelve Days to Dynamic Health*. New York: NAL Books, 1990:436, $19.95.

44. Ornish D. *Dr. Dean Ornish's Program for Reversing Heart Disease*. New York: Random House, 1990:631, $24.95.

Dr. George Burch once said that "every doctor should read a diet book before he[she] retires." During the last few years I have sought out diet books and now have about 50 of them. The 2 titles above are among the better ones appearing in 1990. McDougall is the author of the 1985 book entitled *McDougall's Medicine. A Challenging Second Opinion* in which he provides the evidence for the role of dietary fat in certain cancers, osteoporosis, systemic hypertension, diabetes mellitus, certain types of arthritis, and some urinary disorders. His present book describes his 12-day plan for reversing some serious illnesses. This approach is not popular with some physicians but Dr. Nathan Pritikin was ahead of his time and persons like McDougall are similar advocates.

Ornish's 1-year study using a pure vegetarian diet plus other endeavors appeared in *Lancet* in 1990, and this book provides a step-by-step guide into his program for preventing and reversing heart disease. He is the author also of the 1982 book called *Stress, Diet & Your Heart*. McDougall and Ornish are on the right road and we need to get on it also.

William C Roberts

William Clifford Roberts, MD
Editor in Chief

Some Good Cardiologic Books Published in 1991

MAJOR TEXTBOOKS

1. Braunwald E, editor. *Heart Disease. A Textbook of Cardiovascular Medicine.* Philadelphia: WB Saunders Company, 1992:1918, $110.00 (single volume), $125.00 (double volume).

2. Chatterjee K, Cheitlin MD, Karliner J, Parmley WW, Rapaport E, Scheinman M, editors. *CARDIOLOGY. An Illustrated Text/Reference, Volume 1, Physiology, Pharmacology, Diagnosis* (approximately 1400 pages) and *Volume 2, Cardiovascular Disease* (approximately 1320 pages). Philadelphia: JB Lippincott, and New York: Gower Medical Publishing, 1991: approximately 2720 pages, $225.00 (both volumes).

3. Giuliani ER, Fuster V, Gersh BJ, McGoon MD, McGoon DC, editors. *Cardiology: Fundamentals and Practice*, Second Edition. St. Louis: Mosby Year Book, 1991:2261 (Volumes 1 and 2), $125.00.

All 3 are good. One originates from Boston (Harvard), 1 from San Francisco (University of California), and 1 from Rochester, Minnesota (Mayo Clinic). I prefer the Braunwald book because it contains the most information proportional to size and price. Each page is fully packed. Although it has 69 contributors, Braunwald is the author or coauthor of 23 (37%) of the 62 chapters, and he vigorously edited the other 39 (63%). Although the Braunwald book now has single-colored lines in illustrations, reddish background for tables, and red subheadings, the Chatterjee et al book has taken color much further to produce a beautiful 2-volume text on thick paper. The tradeoff, however, is that the Chatterjee text is twice the cost of the Braunwald book. The Chatterjee text actually represents a hardbound edition of the looseleaf *Cardiology* text edited by Drs. William Parmley and Kanu Chatterjee, published originally in 1987 and updated yearly since. The Giuliani book is a single institution one that is in the price range of the Braunwald book. All 3 texts are heavy, especially the Chatterjee one. If any of these volumes slip off a desk they can break a toe.

4. Fozzard HA, Haber E, Jennings RB, Katz AM, Morgan HE, editors. *The Heart and Cardiovascular System. Scientific Foundations.* Second Edition. Volumes I and II. New York: Raven Press, 1991:2335, $340.00.

These 2 volumes provide comprehensive reviews of principles and methods of cardiovascular research. The first edition was well received and this second edition looks even more comprehensive.

5. Flyer DC, editor. *Nadas' Pediatric Cardiology.* Philadelphia: Hanley & Belfus (also St. Louis: Mosby Year Book), 1992:784, $75.00.

Although it has Dr. Alexander S. Nadas' name in the title, this book represents a near complete new text and is written to honor Dr. Nadas who was chief to most of the contributors to this volume. The book remains easily readable. If one has a single textbook on pediatric cardiology, I would vote for this one, which is reasonably priced.

CARDIAC IMAGING

6. Marcus ML, Skorton DJ, Schelbert HR, Wolf GL, editors; Braunwald E, consulting editor. *Cardiac Imaging. A Companion to Braunwald's Heart Disease.* Philadelphia: WB Saunders Company, 1991:1318, $110.00.

7. Pohost GM, O'Rourke RA, editors. *Principles and Practice of Cardiovascular Imaging.* Boston: Little, Brown and Company, 1991:880, $175.00.

The Marcus book has 118 contributors and is published in the same format as the Braunwald book. Thus, each page is fully packed. The Pohost book, which costs 38% more and has 33% fewer pages, is also well-done. The best value here clearly is the Marcus book.

8. Elliott LP, editor. *Cardiac Imaging in Infants, Children, and Adults.* Philadelphia: JB Lippincott, 1991:927, $150.00.

This book focuses primarily on angiography and would appeal most to radiologists.

9. Gerson MC, editor. *Cardiac Nuclear Medicine.* Second Edition. New York: McGraw-Hill, Inc., 1991: 653, $100.00.

A good book by 37 contributors.

10. Gutierrez FR, Brown JJ, editors. *Cardiovascular Magnetic Resonance Imaging.* St. Louis: Mosby Year Book, 1992:233, $99.00.

Magnetic resonance imaging represents 1 of the most significant advances in diagnostic imaging in the last decade. This book from the Mallinckrodt Institute of Radiology summarizes current use and future applications of this technique to the cardiovascular system.

THROMBOSIS AND THROMBOLYSIS

11. Fuster V, Verstraete M, editors. *Thrombosis in Cardiovascular Disorders.* Philadelphia: WB Saunders Company, 1992:565, $95.00.

A superb and much needed book by 47 contributors. The best book so far on this subject.

12. Haber E, Braunwald E, editors. *Thrombolysis. Basic Contributions and Clinical Progress.* St. Louis: Mosby Year Book, 1991:357, $57.00.

Drs. Haber and Braunwald served as chairmen of a symposium on thrombolysis sponsored by the National Heart, Lung, and Blood Institute. The 25 chapters in this book are updates of presentations at that symposium. This book is loaded with information on thrombolysis, as one might expect from the editors and the sponsor.

CORONARY ARTERY DISEASE

13. Roberts R, editor. *Coronary Heart Disease and Risk Factors.* Mount Kisco: New York, 1991:346, $59.00.

A quick update book by 21 authors, 14 from Roberts' Baylor College of Medicine.

14. Redmond GP, editor. *Lipids and Women's Health*. New York: Springer-Verlag, 1991:260, $49.00.

A timely book with 14 contributors.

15. Rifkind BM, editor. *Drug Treatment of Hyperlipidemia*. New York: Marcel Dekkar, Inc., 1991:270, $79.75.

A timely book on lipid-lowering therapy by 11 experts in this field.

16. Goldberger AL. *Myocardial Infarction. Electrocardiographic Differential Diagnosis*. Fourth Edition with 210 illustrations. St. Louis: Mosby Year Book, 1991:386, $49.95.

This book focuses on the electrocardiogram in myocardial infarction and its electrocardiographic simulators. As such, it is comprehensive, authoritative and well-done.

17. Rutherford JD, editor. *Unstable Angina*. New York: Marcel Dekker, Inc., 1992:301, $89.75.

Dr. Eugene Braunwald in the foreword states that 750,000 patients are admitted to hospitals in the U.S. each year with unstable angina pectoris and that almost 100,000 each year develop acute myocardial infarction within 1 month after onset of unstable angina. Thus, a single book on a common problem is useful.

18. Abrams J, Pepine CJ, Thadani U, editors. *Medical Therapy of Ischemic Heart Disease. Nitrates, Beta Blockers, and Calcium Antagonists*. Boston: Little, Brown and Company, 1992:527, $75.00.

These 16 contributors and leaders in cardiovascular therapeutics provide a useful book.

19. Leier CV, editor. *Cardiotonic Drugs. A Clinical Review*. Second Edition. New York: Marcel Dekker, 1991:362, $115.00.

A good book on the positive inotropic agents, those that increase cardiac contractility.

20. Vlay SC, editor. *Medical Care of the Cardiac Surgical Patient*. Boston: Blackwell Scientific Publications, 1992:331, $29.95.

The least expensive book of quality in the present list. Very useful. Can be placed in the doctor's white coat.

21. Wenger NK, Hellerstein HK, editors. *Rehabilitation of the Coronary Patient*. Third Edition. New York: Churchill Livingstone, 1992:625, $74.95.

An excellent book with 44 contributors. Much expanded compared with the second edition.

ECHOCARDIOGRAPHY

22. Clements FM, de Bruijn NP. *Transesophageal Echocardiography*. Boston: Little, Brown and Company, 1991:163, $105.00.

23. Sutherland GR, Roelandt Jos RTC, Fraser AG, Anderson RH. *Transesophageal Echocardiography in Clinical Practice*. London: Gower Medical Publishing, 1991: approximately 120 pages, $167.00.

Clements and de Bruijn perform approximately 150 transesophageal echocardiographic studies yearly in awake patients and approximately 500 yearly in the operating room at Duke University. Their first book on this subject appeared in 1987, and at the time, I believe, their book was the first on the subject. This second one now has much competition, but it is still good. The Sutherland et al book is nicely prepared with lots of color illustrations, but its price is 38% more and it has 26% fewer pages than the Clements-de Bruijn book.

ELECTROCARDIOGRAPHY AND ELECTROPHYSIOLOGY

24. Rowlands DJ. *Clinical Electrocardiography*. London: Gower Medical Publishing, 1991:615, $109.00.

A beautifully prepared book in which nearly all of the many illustrations are in color.

25. Fisch C, Surawicz B, editors. *Cardiac Electrophysiology and Arrhythmias*. New York: Elsevier, 1991: 488, $84.00.

26. Naccarelli GV, editor. *Cardiac Arrhythmias: A Practical Approach*. Mount Kisco, New York: Futura Publishing Company, 1991:583, $70.00.

27. Dangman KH, Miura DS, editors. *Electrophysiology and Pharmacology of the Heart. A Clinical Guide*. New York: Marcel Dekker, Inc., 1991:756, $175.00.

The Fisch book is a comprehensive update of present knowledge in the broad field of investigative and practical electrocardiology by 69 contributors.

Dr. Douglas P. Zipes in the foreword of the Naccarelli book states, "While several texts have been published recently that encompass a wide area of cardiac electrophysiology, none have been devoted solely to a practical approach to arrhythmia management." Such is the edited book by Naccarelli and 43 experts in the field.

The Dangman-Miura book by 55 contributors is divided into 4 parts: Part I discusses the 4 major techniques used to investigate the electrical behavior of the heart; Part II discusses electrophysiology of the 5 major types of excitable tissue in the heart; Part III, the common laboratory models of cardiac arrhythmias; and Part IV, the positive inotropic agents and antiarrhythmic drugs. The price is outrageous.

28. Falk RH, Podrid PJ, editors. *Atrial Fibrillation. Mechanisms and Management*. New York: Raven Press, 1992:428, $95.00.

The authors estimate that 1 or 2 million persons living in the U.S. have atrial fibrillation of nonvalvular etiology. Thus, the subject is a very important one, and this entire book is devoted to various aspects of this arrhythmia. It is well done and will be useful.

29. El-Sherif N, Turitto G. *High-Resolution Electrocardiography*. Mount Kisco, New York: Futura Publishing Company, 1992:690, $98.00.

High-resolution electrocardiography (HRE) is a technique that allows detection and analysis of low-amplitude electrocardiographic signals that may not be detected on the body surface by routine measurements. The term "signal-energized electrocardiogram," which is frequently used synonymously with HRE, refers to 1 signal processing technique that enhances the detection of low-amplitude electrocardiographic signals. HRE began in the 1970s and the goal was to record the His-Purkinje signal noninvasively. In the mid-1970s, El-Sherif and associates observed that low-amplitude "fractionated" diastolic potentials—later called "late potentials"—are a potential marker for the anatomic electrophysiologic substrate of recurrent arrhythmias. This book provides a state-of-the art review of HRE.

30. Lüderitz B, Saksena S, editors. *Interventional*

Electrophysiology. Mount Kisco, New York: Futura, 1991:571, $95.00.

A good book.

INTERVENTIONAL CARDIOLOGY

31. Kulick DL, Rahimtoola SH, editors. *Techniques and Applications in Interventional Cardiology*. St. Louis: Mosby Year Book, 1991:527, $62.00.

32. White CJ, Ramee SR, editors. *Interventional Cardiology. Clinical Application of New Technologies*. New York: Raven Press, 1991:252, $75.00.

The Kulick-Rahimtoola book is a comprehensive, edited book divided into 4 parts: 10 chapters on intracoronary and peripheral vascular interventions; 3, on catheter valvuloplasty and dilatation of congenitally stenotic lesions; 5, on pacemakers, antitachycardia pacing, automatic implantable cardioverting and defibrillating devices, catheter ablation for tachyarrhythmias and transcoronary ablation of arrhythmogenic areas or pathways; and 2 on endomyocardial biopsy and pericardiocentesis. A fine book.

The White-Ramee book has 52% fewer pages and it costs 17% more. No comparison.

33. Clark DA. *Coronary Angioplasty*. Second Edition. New York: Wiley-Liss, 1991:302, $69.00 (with 5-hour videos, $495.00).

A fine book but the printer did not do justice to the many pictures. The price is very reasonable. Dr. Clark wrote 9 of the 13 chapters.

34. Black AJR, Anderson HV, Ellis SG, editors. *Complications of Coronary Angioplasty*. New York: Marcel Dekker, Inc., 1991:261, $99.75.

Of the many books on coronary angioplasty, relatively little attention has been given to its complications. This book is devoted exclusively to them and as such it is useful.

35. Shawl FA, editor. *Supported Complex and High Risk Coronary Angioplasty*. Boston: Kluwer Academic Publishers, 1991:261, $97.50.

Dr. Shawl has been a leader in the clinical application of percutaneous cardiopulmonary bypass support techniques, and this edited book provides to the interventionist the basic principles of cardiopulmonary bypass and other alternate support devices for myocardial protection. Dr. Shawl is joined by 15 other contributors, also leaders in this field.

36. Holmes DR Jr, Garratt KN, editors. *Atherectomy*. Boston: Blackwell Scientific Publications, 1992: 230, $59.95.

Twenty-two leaders in this field author this book that probably is the best so far on this subject.

37. Karsh KR, Haase KK, editors. *Coronary Laser Angioplasty. An Update*. New York: Springer-Verlag, 1991:178, $49.00.

This book focuses exclusively on laser techniques in coronary artery stenosis, and for those still interested it would be useful.

VALVULAR HEART DISEASE

38. Emery RW, Arom KV, editors. *The Aortic Valve*. Philadelphia: Hanley & Belfus, Inc. (St. Louis: Mosby Year Book), 1991:336, $65.00.

This book is edited by 2 cardiovascular surgeons. It is well done and I highly recommend it.

39. Bodnar E, Frater R, editors. *Replacement Cardiac Valves*. New York: Pergamon Press, 1991:482, $94.50.

This multiauthored book may be the best of the more recent books on this subject. It is very comprehensive.

40. Bashore TM, Davidson CJ, editors. *Percutaneous Balloon Valvuloplasty and Related Techniques*. Baltimore: Williams & Wilkins, 1991:351, $62.00.

Surely this book is the best one on this subject. Of the 19 chapters by the 29 contributors, 15 focus on the mitral and aortic valves.

ANNUAL CARDIOLOGY REVIEWS

41. Schlant RC (editor in chief), Collins JJ Jr, Engle MA, Frye RL, Kaplan NM, O'Rourke RA (editors). *1991 The Year Book of Cardiology*. St. Louis: Mosby Year Book, 1991:379, $57.95.

42. Roberts WC (editor), Willerson JT, Mason DT, Rackley CE, Graham TP Jr. *Cardiology 1991*. Boston: Butterworth-Heinemann, 1991:494, $80.00.

The Schlant book is the thirty-first in the series. It contains summaries and comments on 305 clinically relevant articles. The Roberts book is the eleventh in the series beginning in 1981. A total of 804 articles are summarized and all articles had appeared in 1990. Additionally, the book contains 120 figures and 61 tables. Each page is fully packed. Although obviously biased I prefer the Roberts book, which summarizes 63% more articles and costs only 28% more than the Schlant book.

MISCELLANEOUS

43. Fowler NO. *Diagnosis of Heart Disease*. New York: Springer-Verlag, 1991:429, $79.00.

It is nice to see a single-authored book. This one by a masterful clinician is a good one, too.

44. Perloff JK, Child JS, editors. *Congenital Heart Disease in Adults*. Philadelphia: WB Saunders, 1991: 342, $75.00.

I was fortunate to have edited in 1979 a book entitled *Congenital Heart Disease in Adults* and a new version in 1987 entitled *Adult Congenital Heart Disease*. Thus, I feel comfortable in evaluating the new book by Drs. Perloff and Child with 19 contributors, 14 of whom are at UCLA with the 2 editors. Dr. Perloff is the author or coauthor of 17 of the book's 20 chapters. This book is unique among textbooks on congenital heart disease in that it does not focus on the specific varieties of congenital anomalies, but rather on general concepts and problems in adults. For physicians seeing adults with congenital heart disease, this is the book to have.

45. Opie LH. *The Heart. Physiology and Metabolism*. Second Edition. New York: Raven Press, 1991:513, $72.00.

A single-authored book on the fundamentals of cardiac cellular physiology.

46. Wilcox BR, Anderson RH. *Surgical Anatomy of the Heart*. Second Edition. London: Gower Medical Publishing, 1992: approximately 120 pages, $125.00.

Dr. David C. Sabiston, Jr. states in the foreword: "The second edition embraces all the excellence of its predeces-

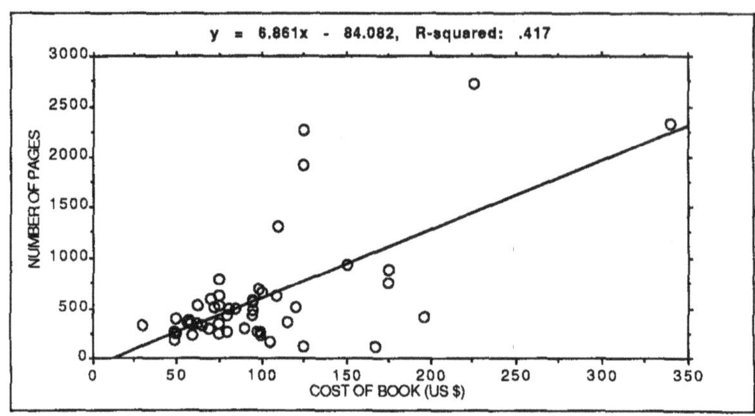

FIGURE 1. Diagram showing relation of number of pages in the 49 books to their cost.

sor and in addition contains new data on the previous subjects as well as the addition of detailed anatomy of the tricuspid, pulmonary, mitral and aortic valves and much new material on the surgical anatomy of the coronary circulation." The illustrations in this book are truly magnificent. I believe that Dr. Wilcox gets the best photographs in the operating room of any surgeon.

47. Kapoor AS, Laks H, Schroeder JS, Yacoub MH, editors. *Cardiomyopathies and Heart-Lung Transplantation.* New York: McGraw-Hill, 1991:511, $120.00.

This book provides up-to-date comprehensive coverage of developments in cardiomyopathies, cardiac assist devices and heart-lung transplantation. A fine book by 61 contributors.

48. O'Rourke MF, Kelly RP, Avolio AP. *The Arterial Pulse.* Philadelphia: Lea & Febiger, 1992:239, $49.95.

It's all here on this single topic.

49. Meester GT, Pinciroli F, editors. *Databases For Cardiology.* Dordrecht, the Netherlands: Kluwer Academic Publishers, 1991:418, $196.00.

The editors, 1 a cardiologist and 1 an information scientist, have provided "an extensive overview of the medical cardiological database field, with examples of design, construction and data-analysis, while not omitting possible problems and pitfalls."

COMMENTS

Of the 49 books reviewed here, 36 (73%) contained a 1991 publication date and 13 (27%), a 1992 publication date. The numbers of pages in these 49 books ranged from 120 to 2720 (mean 600), and the costs of the books ranged from $29.95 to $340.00 (mean $100.00). There was no relation between the number of pages a book contained and its cost (Figure 1) ($r = .42$, $p = 0.1$). Thirty-seven books (76%) were multiauthored (>10) and 12 (24%) had ≤6 authors; only 2 books had a single author.

Most books unfortunately continue to be published on acid paper.[1] Of the 49 books, only 11 (22%) (numbers 14, 15, 17, 19, 25, 27, 34, 37, 42, 43 and 49) were stated to have been published on acid-free paper, but only 1 (number 42) of them contained the permanent-paper insignia (infinity symbol within a circle) on the verso of the title page of the book indicating that the paper used was alkaline (i.e., permanent). None of the books published by American publishers were on acid-free paper! In contrast, all books published by Butterworth-Heinemann, Elsevier, Kluwer Academic, Marcel Dekker, and Springer-Verlag were on permanent (acid-free) paper. I encourage all authors to require in their book contracts that the paper used for their books be acid-free!

William C. Roberts

William Clifford Roberts, MD
Editor in Chief

1. Roberts WC. Alkaline paper and preserving the record. *Am J Cardiol* 1991;68:1729–1732.

Cardiologic Books Published in 1992

GENERAL CARDIOLOGY

*1. Willerson JT, editor, with 8 associate editors (Baim DS, Cooley DA, Frazier OH, Grundy SM, Kaplan NM, Packer M, Sweeney MS, Zipes DP). *Treatment of Heart Diseases*. New York: Gower Medical Publishing, 1992:528, $159.50.

Colorful and good.

*2. Loscalzo J, Creager MA, Dzau VJ, editors. *Vascular Medicine. A Textbook of Vascular Biology and Diseases*. Boston: Little, Brown and Company, 1992:1211, $165.00.

Excellent.

3. Cooke JP, Frohlich ED, editors. *Current Management of Hypertensive and Vascular Diseases*. St. Louis: B.C. Decker (An Imprint of Mosby Year Book), 1992:380, $79.00.

Good.

*4. Kapoor AS, Singh BN, editors. *Prognosis and Risk Assessment in Cardiovascular Disease*. New York: Churchill Livingstone, 1993:578, $79.95.

This book was designed to provide an authoritative source of current information for determining prognosis in major cardiovascular diseases. It appears to fulfill this mission. This is a very good book.

5. Marriott HJL. *Bedside Cardiac Diagnosis*. Philadelphia: JB Lippincott Company, 1993:291, $49.95.

Marriott makes the point in his preface that about 80% of cardiovascular diagnoses are made by history alone, another 10% require the physical examination, and only the remaining 10% are dependent on laboratory investigation. This good book of 40 relatively short chapters focuses on physical signs of cardiovascular disease. Good reading.

6. Chesler E. *Clinical Cardiology*. Fifth Edition. New York: Springer-Verlag, 1993:451, $89.00.

A bedside approach to cardiology. I would vote for the Marriott one.

7. Lilly LS, editor. *Pathophysiology of Heart Disease. A Collaborative Project of Medical Students and Faculty*. Philadelphia: Lea & Febiger, 1993:325, $24.50.

This book is a collaborative project of 38 Harvard Medical Students with faculty. The students, i.e., potential consumers, dissatisfied with currently available textbooks of cardiology, made their needs known. A useful book, particularly for the price.

8. Hillis LD, Lange RA, Wells PJ, Winniford MD. *Manual of Clinical Problems in Cardiology With Annotated Key References. Fourth Edition*. Boston: Little, Brown and Company, 1992:553, $28.00.

A useful book, particularly for house officers and cardiology fellows, and the price is right.

LIPIDS AND OTHER RISK FACTORS

9. Frishman WH, editor and coauthor. *Medical Management of Lipid Disorders: Focus on Prevention of Coronary Artery Disease*. Mount Kisco, NY: Futura Publishing Company, Inc., 1992:328, $60.00.

A very practical book.

10. Kreisberg RA, Segrest J, editors. *Plasma Lipoproteins and Coronary Artery Disease*. Boston: Blackwell Scientific Publications, 1992:390, $74.95.

Very good.

11. Thompson GR, Wilson PW. *Coronary Risk Factors and their Assessment*. London: Science Press, 1992: approximately 150, $60.00.

A colorful book. I prefer the Frishman one.

12. Goor R, Goor N. *Eater's Choice. A Food Lover's Guide to Lower Cholesterol. Third Edition*. Boston: Houghton Mifflin Company, 1992:571, $12.95.

This husband and wife team are cholesterol and nutrition experts. They have written several "best sellers" on this subject. I have liked all their books for adults (They have also written 7 childrens' books), and this one is no exception.

MEDICAL THERAPY

13. Ewy GA, Bressler R, editors. *Cardiovascular Drugs and the Management of Heart Disease. Second Edition*. New York: Raven Press, 1992:496, $105.00.

Fine book.

14. Taylor GJ. *Thrombolytic Therapy for Acute Myocardial Infarction*. Boston: Blackwell Scientific Publications, 1992:240, $24.95.

The price is right.

15. Opie LH. *Angiotensin-Converting Enzyme Inhibitors: Scientific Basis for Clinical Use*. New York: Wiley-Liss, 1992:266, $34.95.

Covers this topic well.

INTERVENTIONAL CARDIOLOGY

16. Vogel JHK, King SB III, editors. *The Practice of Interventional Cardiology, Second Edition*. St. Louis: Mosby Year Book, 1993:718, $95.00.

Good book.

17. Schwartz RS, editor. *Coronary Restenosis*. Boston: Blackwell Scientific Publications, 1993:387, $84.95.

Good book.

18. Serruys PW, Strauss BH, King SB III, editors. *Restenosis after Intervention with New Mechanical Devices*. Dordrecht: Kluwer Academic Publishers, 1992:504, $215.00.

A comprehensive assessment of restenosis from the perspective of new technologies including stenting, atherectomy, rotational abrasion, and lasers. At 42 cents a page, it is hardly worth it.

19. Ginsburg R, Geschwind HJ, editors. *Primer on Laser Angioplasty, Second Edition.* Mount Kisco, NY: Futura Publishing Company, Inc., 1992:520, $80.00.

For those interested in lasers, this is the book to have.

SYSTEMIC HYPERTENSION

20. Brunner HR, Waeber B, editors. *Ambulatory Blood Pressure Recording.* New York: Raven Press, 1992:192, $55.00.

Non-invasive ambulatory blood pressure recording is receiving progressively more attention since its beginning in about 1975. Over 300 publications on this subject appeared in 1990. This good small book nicely presents some of the problems and some benefits of ambulatory blood pressure monitoring.

*21. Loggie JMH, editor. *Pediatric and Adolescent Hypertension.* Boston: Blackwell Scientific Publications, 1992:416, $149.95.

Good.

22. Martinez-Maldonado M, editor. *Hypertension and Renal Disease in the Elderly.* Boston: Blackwell Scientific Publications, 1992:358, $79.95.

Nice book by outstanding contributors.

23. Cruickshank JM, Messerli FH. *Left Ventricular Hypertrophy and its Regression.* London: Science Press, 1992:107, $89.95.

In color. Not a lot of information. Almost a dollar a page!

CONGENITAL HEART DISEASE

*24. Freedom RM, Benson LN, Smallhorn JF, editors. *Neonatal Heart Disease.* London: Springer-Verlag, 1992:881, $180.00.

This book will probably be the bible for information on the newborn with heart disease. Although an edited book, one or more of the editors are authors of nearly all chapters.

25. Rao PS, editor. *Tricuspid Atresia. Second Edition.* Mount Kisco, NY: Futura Publishing Company, Inc., 1992:458, $98.00.

The first edition appeared just over 10 years ago. I like these comprehensive books on a single topic and that is what this one is.

26. Hess J, Sutherland GR, editors. *Congenital Heart Disease in Adolescents and Adults.* Dordrecht: Kluwer Academic Publishers, 1992:201, $100.00.

There are better ones on this subject.

ARRHYTHMIAS, ELECTROCARDIOGRAPHY, ELECTROPHYSIOLOGY, PACING, DEFIBRILLATORS

*27. Josephson ME, Second Edition. *Clinical Cardiac Electrophysiology: Techniques and Interpretations.* Philadelphia: Lea & Febiger, 1993:839, $95.00.

A must for students of this field. Josephson wrote every word. Outstanding.

28. Singer I, Kupersmith J, editors. *Clinical Manual of Electrophysiology.* Baltimore: Williams & Wilkins, 1993:453, $60.00.

Very few illustrations. Josephson a winner hands down.

29. Wit AL, Janse MJ. *The Ventricular Arrhythmias of Ischemia and Infarction. Electrophysiological Mechanisms.* Mount Kisco, NY: Futura Publishing Company, Inc., 1993:648, $150.00.

A fine book BUT the Josephson one is 37% less expensive and contains 23% more pages which are also larger.

30. Seelig CB. *Simplified EKG Analysis. A Sequential Guide to Interpretation and Diagnosis.* Philadelphia: Hanley & Belfus, Inc., 1992:119, $14.95.

31. Stein E. *Rapid Analysis of Electrocardiograms. A Self-Study Program. Second Edition.* Philadelphia: Lea & Febiger, 1992:404, $26.95.

32. Stein E. *Rapid Analysis of Arrhythmias. A Self-Study Program. Second Edition.* Philadelphia: Lea & Febiger, 1992:229, $24.95.

33. Kingma JH, van Hemel NM, Lie KI, editors. *Atrial Fibrillation, a Treatable Disease?* Dordrecht: Kluwer Academic Publishers, 1992:297, $99.00.

A hot topic. Content per page could have been more.

34. Luceri RM, editor. *Sudden Cardiac Death: Strategies for the 1990s.* Miami Lakes, Florida: Peritus Corporation, 1992:194, $60.00.

This book represents a collection of manuscripts concerning primarily implantable cardioverter-defibrillators and both the symposium and this publication are underwritten by Telectronics Pacing Systems. Not recommended.

35. Ellenbogen KA, editor. *Cardiac Pacing.* Boston: Blackwell Scientific Publications, 1992:464, $29.95.

A very good book for the money. Highly recommended.

ECHOCARDIOGRAPHY

*36. Silverman NH. *Pediatric Echocardiography.* Baltimore: Williams & Wilkins, 1993:628, $140.00.

Superb book. Loaded with fine illustrations.

37. Obeid AI. *Echocardiography in Clinical Practice.* Philadelphia: JB Lippincott Company, 1992:383, $125.00.

A large book loaded with 2-dimensional, Doppler, and transesophageal images. The images should have been cropped and then they could have been reproduced much larger. Nevertheless, the reproductions are excellent. A useful book.

*38. Nanda NC, editor. *Doppler Echocardiography. Second Edition.* Philadelphia: Lea & Febiger, 1993:466, $129.00.

Beautiful book. Illustrations are splendid. Probably the best so far on this subject.

39. Labovitz AJ, Williams GA. *Doppler Echocardiography. The Quantitative Approach. Third Edition.* Philadelphia: Lea & Febiger, 1992:131, $29.95.

This third edition appears only 5 years after the first edition. It incorporates real-time flow mapping techniques into the text. The illustrations are superb.

40. Oka Y, Goldiner PL, editors. *Transesophageal Echocardiography.* Philadelphia: JB Lippincott Compa-

ny, 1992:338, $150.00.

Nice book but a good bit of wasted space. Photographs could have been cropped.

41. Missri J. *Transesophageal Echocardiography. Clinical and Intraoperative Applications*. New York: Churchill Livingstone, 1993:248, $124.95.

Good.

42. Dittrich HC, editor. *Clinical Transesophageal Echocardiography*. St. Louis: Mosby Year Book, 1992:178, $95.00.

An edited book with 22 contributors.

43. Labovitz AJ, Pearson AC. *Transesophageal Echocardiography: Basic Principles and Clinical Applications*. Philadelphia: Lea & Febiger, 1993:157, $39.50.

Good.

INTRAVASCULAR ULTRASOUND IMAGING

44. Tobis JM, Yock PG, editors. *Intravascular Ultrasound Imaging*. New York: Churchill Livingstone, 1992:262, $89.95.

Probably the best so far on this subject.

45. Cavaye DM, White RA. *Intravascular Ultrasound Imaging*. New York: Raven Press, 1993:119, $59.00.

Good but short and relatively expensive. Good reproductions.

CARDIAC IMAGING

46. Jay ME. *Plain Film in Heart Disease*. Boston: Blackwell Scientific Publications, 1992:207, $34.95.

This book is loaded with chest roentgenograms with brief case presentations. The space on the pages is poorly utilized. The book which is already relatively small could have been much smaller.

47. van der Wall E, Sochor H, Righetti A, Niemeyer MG. *What's New in Cardiac Imaging? SPECT, PET, and MRI*. Dordrecht: Kluwer Academic Publishers, 1992:544, $149.00.

48. van der Wall EE. *Nuclear Cardiology and Cardiac Magnetic Resonance. Physiology, Techniques and Applications*. Leiden, The Netherlands: Hans Soto Productions, 1992:285, $115.00.

49. Wagner M, Lawson TL. *Atlas of Chest Imaging. Correlated Anatomy with MRI and CT*. New York: Raven Press, 1992:134, $80.00.

The use of abbreviations in titles is not ideal. Over half of the pages utilize only a half of the page. The book could have been much smaller and that would have made it better. The reader is not getting his/her money's worth here.

50. Stanford W, Rumberger JA, editors. *Ultrafast Computed Tomography in Cardiac Imaging: Principles and Practice*. Mount Kisco, NY: Futura Publishing Company, Inc., 1992:351, $80.00.

A useful book.

*51. Bregmann SR, Sobel BE, editors. *Positron Emission Tomography of the Heart*. Mount Kisco, NY: Futura Publishing Company, Inc., 1992:313, $98.00.

I suspect that this book is the best one on this subject.

CARDIOVASCULAR SURGERY

*52. Kirklin JW, Barratt-Boyes BG, with the collaboration of Blackstone EH, Jonas RA, Kouchoukos NT. *Cardiac Surgery. Morphology, Diagnostic Criteria, Natural History, Techniques, Results, and Indications. Second Edition. Volumes 1 and 2*. New York: Churchill Livingstone, 1993:1860, $250.00.

This book is by far the best on this subject.

53. Bojar RM. *Adult Cardiac Surgery*. Boston: Blackwell Scientific Publications, 1992:562, $99.95.

This book does not include congenital heart lesions except for the congenitally malformed aortic valve, mitral valve prolapse, hypertrophic cardiomyopathy, and the Marfan syndrome seen in adulthood. This book by a single author is both good and useful, but can hardly compete with the Kirklin-Barratt-Boyes one!

54. Bharati S, Lev M, Kirklin JW. *Cardiac Surgery and the Conduction System. Second Revised Edition*. Mount Kisco, NY: Futura Publishing Company, Inc., 1992:159, $75.00.

This book primarily presents drawings and some gross pictures of views of the heart as might be seen at operation with delineation of courses of the conduction system in various types of congenital anomalies of the heart. The text is brief. Much empty space is present on the pages. This book is important because of the authors.

55. Kotler MN, Alfieri A, editors. *Cardiac and Noncardiac Complications of Open Heart Surgery: Prevention, Diagnosis, and Treatment*. Mount Kisco, NY: Futura Publishing Company, Inc., 1992:418, $62.00.

A useful book, interestingly edited by 2 cardiologists. Very little emphasis is given to mechanical or anatomic complications of cardiac surgery. Certainly they are not as important in the 1990s as they were in the 1960s but they remain important.

56. Engelman RM, Levitsky S, editors. *A Textbook of Cardioplegia for Difficult Clinical Problems*. Mount Kisco, NY: Futura Publishing Company, Inc., 1992:334, $75.00.

As Frank C. Spencer states in the Preface: ". . . the book is an excellent description of the wide variety of methods of cardioplegia used for the most difficult clinical problems throughout the world. This wide variation indicates that no one method has evolved as superior to another."

57. Kay PH, editor. *Techniques in Extracorporeal Circulation, Third Edition*. Oxford, UK: Butterworth-Heinemann Ltd., 1992:336, $195.00.

The first edition of this book appeared 16 years ago, and the second edition 11 years ago. Thus, it is time for an update and this was nicely accomplished by 45 authors.

58. Ross DN, English TAH, McKay R. *Principles of Cardiac Diagnosis and Treatment. A Surgeons' Guide. Second Edition*. London: Springer-Verlag, 1992:269,

$129.00.

The first edition appeared in 1962, thirty years earlier. This book is pleasant reading but at nearly 50 cents a page, it's not worth it.

PERIPHERAL VASCULAR DISEASE

59. Polak JF. *Peripheral Vascular Sonography. A Practical Guide*. Baltimore: Williams & Wilkins, 1993:364, $78.00.

Good for this subject.

60. Dorros G. *Peripheral Vascular Interventions 1992. A Bibliographic Reference Manual*. Mount Kisco, NY: Futura Publishing Company, Inc., 1992:438, $80.00.

What it says it is, it is, a bibliography with some summaries. For those in this field, it may be useful.

61. Clement DL, Shepherd JT, editors. *Vascular Diseases in the Limbs. Mechanisms and Principles of Treatment*. St. Louis: Mosby Year Book, 1993:319, $79.00.

Well done.

MOLECULAR CARDIOLOGY

*62. Roberts R, editor. *Molecular Basis of Cardiology*. Boston: Blackwell Scientific Publications, 1993:518, $39.95.

As Eugene Braunwald states in the foreword, *Molecular Basis of Cardiology* is the best exposition of this new paradigm (the shift in cardiovascular science from organ physiology to molecular biology) currently available and will be of enormous value to cardiovascular scientists, scholarly cardiologists, and to new entrants in the field. The publisher provided the book in soft cover to keep the price reasonable.

63. Gotto AM, Jr, editor. *Cellular and Molecular Biology of Atherosclerosis*. London: Springer-Verlag, 1992:180, $83.00.

This book represents presentations at the 1991 Princess Lillian Symposium, which I attended. The presentations were good and their publication is better.

MISCELLANEOUS

*64. Katz AM. *Physiology of the Heart. Second Edition*. New York: Raven Press, 1992:687, $55.00.

The first edition was 1977. Thus, this second one is long overdue. This second edition is essentially an entirely new text.

65. Pashkow FJ, Dafoe WA, editors. *Clinical Cardiac Rehabilitation: A Cardiologist's Guide*. Baltimore: Williams & Wilkins, 1993:391, $59.00.

Good.

66. Anderson RH, Becker AE. *The Heart. Structure in Health and Disease*. London: Gower Medical Publishing, 1992:266, $165.00.

This book is a consolidation and expansion of their 2 previous books with Gower Medical Publishing, namely *Cardiac Anatomy* (1980) and *Cardiac Pathology* (1983). The pictures are in color. A beautiful book.

67. Yellon DM, Jennings RB, editors. *Myocardial Protection. The Pathophysiology of Reperfusion and Reperfusion Injury*. New York: Raven Press, 1992:214, $99.00.

This concise book on an important subject will be useful. The cost, however, is nearly 50 cents a page.

68. Fowles RE, editor. *Cardiac Biopsy*. Mount Kisco, NY: Futura Publishing Company, Inc., 1992:211, $47.00.

For anyone performing or examining biopsies of the heart, this is a good book to have.

69. Kaye D, editor. *Infective Endocarditis, Second Edition*. New York: Raven Press, 1992:497, $85.00.

This book is a follow-up of Kaye's first edition in 1976. The first edition emphasized the effects of antibiotics on infective endocarditis. The present edition, a considerable expansion from the first, continues to emphasize further changes in the disease including an older age of patients, less rheumatic heart disease, less pneumococcal and gonococcal endocarditis, more staphylococcal endocarditis, the increasing frequency in intravenous drug abusers, the problems of prosthetic and bioprosthetic endocarditis, the usefulness of echocardiography, and many management changes. This book is highly recommended.

CARDIOLOGIC ANNUALS

70. Roberts WC, Willerson JT, Mason DT, Rackley CE, Graham TP Jr. *Cardiology 1992*. Boston: Butterworth-Heinemann, 1992:480, $80.00.

71. Schlant RC (editor in chief), Collins JJ Jr, Engle MA, Frye RL, Kaplan NM, O'Rourke RA (editors). *Year Book of Cardiology 1992*. St. Louis: Mosby Year Book, 1992:441, $59.95.

The Schlant book, the thirty-second in the series, contains summaries and comments on 318 articles plus 111 figures and 5 tables. The Roberts book, the twelfth in the series, contains summaries of 740 articles plus 116 figures and 32 tables. The Roberts book provides 58% more summaries of articles than does the Schlant book on only 8% more pages because each page contains far more content. The cost of the Roberts book, however, is 30% higher than the Schlant book, and it lacks editorial comments from the editors on each article summarized.

COMMENTS

More and more cardiologic books! The first column I wrote on cardiologic books summarized those appearing in 1985 and it briefly discussed 16 books,[1] and the column in 1991 described 49 books.[2] The present piece discusses 71 books, 53 (75%) of which have a 1992 publication date and 18 (25%) of which have a 1993 publication date. The books marked with asterisks are those which I consider noteworthy either because of extremely high quality or uniqueness.

The costs of books continue to increase. The prices of the 71 books appearing in 1992 ranged from $12.95 to $250.00 (mean $88.39). The numbers of pages in the

71 books ranged from 119 to 1860 (mean 405). There was an insignificant relation between the number of pages a book contained and its cost. The total cost of the 71 books was $6,275.50 and the total numbers of pages in the 71 books was 28,835. Therefore, the average cost of each page was 22 cents.

Of the 71 books, 38 (55%) were edited with multiple contributors, and 33 (45%) were by 1 to 6 authors. Only 15 books (21%) had a single author.

Most books unfortunately continue to be published on acid paper.[3] Of the 71 books, only 9 (13%) were published on acid-free paper, i.e., permanent paper. The remaining 62 books (87%) will vanish into dust within 50 years. Congratulations to Butterworth-Heinemann, Kluwer Academic, and Springer-Verlag for publishing all of their books on acid-free paper, and to Futura for publishing some of their books on alkaline paper. I encourage all authors to require in their book contracts that the paper used for their books be acid-free. It is time for American book publishers to use permanent paper!

William Clifford Roberts, MD
Editor in Chief

REFERENCES

1. Roberts WC. Some good cardiologic books. *Am J Cardiol* 1985;56:1001–1002.
2. Roberts WC. Some good cardiologic books published in 1991. *Am J Cardiol* 1992;69:141–144.
3. Roberts WC. Alkaline paper and preserving the record. *Am J Cardiol* 1991; 68:1729–1732.

Good Cardiologic Books Appearing in 1993

MAJOR GENERAL CARDIOLOGIC TEXTBOOKS

1. Schlant RC, Alexander RW, editors; O'Rourke RA, Roberts R, Sonnenblick EH, associate editors. *Hurst's The Heart, Arteries and Veins. Eighth Edition.* New York: McGraw-Hill, Inc., 1994:2586, $125.00.

One hundred and 43 chapters by 203 contributors. Words describing this book might be authoritative, heavy, impressive, overwhelming, practical, useful. The Schlant-Alexander and Braunwald books are essential to a cardiovascular library.

2. Cheitlin MD, Sokolow M, and McIlroy MB. *Clinical Cardiology,* Sixth Edition. Norwalk, Connecticut: Appleton & Lange, 1993:741, $37.95.

Good general text. The cost of the Schlant-Alexander book is actually less in proportion to the information supplied.

CARDIOLOGIC TEXTS FOR THE NON-CARDIOLOGIST

3. Hurst JW. *Cardiovascular Diagnosis. The Initial Examination.* St. Louis: Mosby, 1993:556, $39.95.

4. Timmis AD, Nathan AW. *Essentials of Cardiology,* Second Edition. Oxford: Blackwell Scientific Publications, 1993:351, $36.95.

5. Harvey WP. *Cardiac Pearls.* Newton, New Jersey: Laennec Publishing, 1993:345, $74.00.

6. Carabello BA, Ballard WL, Gazes PC. *Cardiology Pearls.* Philadelphia: Hanley & Belfus, Inc., 1994: 223, $35.00.

7. Gessner IH, Victorica BE, editors. *Pediatric Cardiology.* Philadelphia: W.B. Saunders Company, 1993:283, $45.00.

Each of these 5 books is good reading. My teachers were Hurst and Harvey so naturally I am biased. The Harvey book, however, is expensive.

CARDIAC DISEASE IN WOMEN

8. Douglas PS, editor. *Cardiovascular Health and Disease in Women.* Philadelphia: W.B. Saunders Company, 1993:374, $65.00.

9. Wenger NK, Speroff L, Packard B, editors. *Cardiovascular Health and Disease in Women, Proceedings of an N.H.L.B.I. Conference.* Greenwich, Connecticut: LeJacq Communications, Inc., 1993:348, $66.00.

10. Pashkow FJ, Libov C. *The Woman's Heart Book. The Complete Guide to Keeping Your Heart Healthy and What to Do if Things Go Wrong.* New York: Dutton, 1993:358, $22.00.

Both the Douglas and the Wenger books are excellent. Obviously, the subject matter is a hot topic. The Pashkow-Libov book is intended for the non-physician.

HEART FAILURE

11. Hosenpud JD, Greenberg BH, editors. *Congestive Heart Failure. Pathophysiology, Diagnosis, and Comprehensive Approach to Management.* New York:Springer-Verlag, 1994:769, $180.00.

12. Gwathmey JK, Briggs GM, Allen PD, editors. *Heart Failure, Basic Science and Clinical Aspects.* New York: Marcel Dekker, Inc., 1993:715, $195.00.

13. Barnett DB, Pouleur H, Francis GS, editors. *Congestive Cardiac Failure. Pathophysiology and Treatment.* New York: Marcel Dekker, Inc., 1993:385, $135.00.

14. Gaasch WH, LeWinter MM, editors. *Left Ventricular Diastolic Dysfunction and Heart Failure.* Philadelphia: Lea & Febiger, 1994:498, $89.50.

It is difficult for me to choose the best of these 4 books. All appear to be good.

ELECTROCARDIOGRAPHY

15. Mirvis DM. *Electrocardiography. A Physiologic Approach.* St. Louis: Mosby, 1993:532, $34.95.

This interesting book on electrocardiography contains few electrocardiograms. It focuses more on underlying physiologic principles. Thus, this book is a different one on a subject that probably has produced more than 1000 books.

16. Gomes JA, editor. *Signal Averaged Electrocardiography. Concepts, Methods and Applications.* Dordrecht: Kluwer Academic Publications, 1993:583, $172.00.

For the wealthy physician interested in this topic, here it is.

ARRHYTHMIAS, CONDUCTION DEFECTS, PACEMAKERS, CARDIOVERTER-DEFIBRILLATORS

17. Kastor JA, editor. *Arrhythmias.* Philadelphia: W.B. Saunders Company, 1994:430, $85.00.

This comprehensive book was "specifically written for clinicians who are not now or plan to become clinical electrophysiologists." Good reading.

18. Josephson ME, editor. *Sudden Cardiac Death.* Boston: Blackwell Scientific Publications, 1993:432, $95.00.

You can count on Josephson to produce a good product.

19. Singh BN, Wellens HJJ, Hiraoka M, editors. *Electropharmacological Control of Cardiac Arrhythmias. To Delay Conduction or to Prolong Refractori-*

ness? Mount Kisco, New York: Futura Publishing Company, Inc., 1994:746, $97.00.

A major text.

20. Singer I, Kupersmith J, editors. *Clinical Manual of Electrophysiology.* Baltimore: Williams & Wilkins, 1993:453, $70.00.

As J. Thomas Bigger, Jr. states in the foreword, this book provides "an excellent introduction to electrophysiologic concepts and practice."

21. Shenasa M, Borggrefe M, Breithardt G, editors; Haverkamp W, Hindricks G, assistant editors. *Cardiac Mapping.* Mount Kisco, New York: Futura Publishing Company, Inc., 1993:711, $95.00.

I can only guess if this is a good book. It is the first full book I recall seeing on this subject.

22. Naccarelli GV, Veltri EP, editors. *Implantable Cardioverter-Defibrillators.* Boston: Blackwell Scientific Publications, 1993:443, $65.00.

ECHOCARDIOGRAPHY

23. Feigenbaum H. *Echocardiography.* 5th Edition. Philadelphia: Lea & Febiger, 1994:695, $95.00.

24. Weyman AE. *Principles and Practice of Echocardiography,* Second Edition. Philadelphia: Lea & Febiger, 1994:1335, $169.00.

Two major texts on the same subject published the same year by the same publisher! The Feigenbaum book is the 5th edition of this classic, written entirely by him. He has met his match, however, in the Weyman book which contains 41 chapters, 31 of which were written by Weyman. If I could afford the difference I would go for the Weyman book which is extremely comprehensive.

25. Roelandt JRTC, Sutherland GR, Iliceto S, Linker DT, editors. *Cardiac Ultrasound.* Edinburgh: Churchill Livingstone, 1993:1013, $275.00.

A major book containing 95 chapters by 149 contributors, virtually all from Europe. This book contains the full gamut of cardiac ultrasound.

26. Wilde P, editor. *Cardiac Ultrasound.* Edinburgh: Churchill Livingstone, 1993:552, $165.00.

27. Oh JK, Seward JB, Tajik AJ. *The Echo Manual From the Mayo Clinic.* Boston: Little, Brown and Company, 1994:252, $75.00.

I do not quite understand the purpose of this book. Twenty bucks more and one has the Feigenbaum book. No question where to go.

28. Goldman ME. *Clinical Atlas of Transesophageal Echocardiography.* Mount Kisco, New York: Futura Publishing Company, Inc., 1993:376, $149.00.

29. Maurer G, editor. *Transesophageal Echocardiography.* New York: McGraw-Hill, Inc., 1994:285, $149.00.

Both are good transesophageal books. The best value is the one by Goldman.

30. Hanrath P, Uebis R, Krebs W. *Cardiovascular Imaging by Ultrasound.* Dordrecht: Kluwer Academic Publishers, 1993:479, $237.50.

31. Hodgson J McB, Sheehan HM, editors. *Atlas of Intravascular Ultrasound.* New York: Raven Press, 1994:333, $115.00.

32. Roelandt J, Bom N, Gussenhoven EJ, editors. *Intravascular Ultrasound.* Dordrecht: Kluwer Academic Publishers, 1993:166, $45.00.

33. Nanda NC, Schlief R, editors. *Advances in Echo Imaging Using Contrast Enhancement.* Dordrecht: Kluwer Academic Publishers, 1993:405, $95.00.

NUCLEAR CARDIOLOGY

34. Zaret BL, Kaufman L, Berson AS, Dunn RA, editors. *Frontiers in Cardiovascular Imaging.* New York: Raven Press, 1993:362, $82.00.

This small book reviews imaging of myocardium using ultrafast computed tomography, positron emission tomography, single-photon emission computed tomography, nuclear magnetic resonance, ultrasound, magnetocardiography, digital subtraction angiography, synchrotran radiation, magnetic resonance angiography, echocardiography, radionuclides, and fluorescence spectroscopy in 362 pages! Four companies supported publication of this book.

35. Zaret BL, Beller GA, editors. *Nuclear Cardiology. State of the Art and Future Directions.* St. Louis: Mosby, 1993:347, $72.00.

This book of 31 chapters by 59 contributors is an outgrowth of the International Nuclear Cardiology Workshop held in Wintergreen, Virginia, in July 1991. The text is a state-of-the-art perspective of the field of nuclear cardiology.

INTERVENTIONAL CARDIOLOGY

36. Topol EJ, editor. *Textbook of Interventional Cardiology,* Volumes 1 and 2, Second Edition. Philadelphia: W.B. Saunders Company, 1994:1–684 (volume 1) and 685–1392 (volume 2), $179.00.

This book unquestionably is the tops in this area.

37. Faxon DP, editor. *Practical Angioplasty.* New York: Raven Press, 1994:273, $95.00.

Good but no comparison to the Topol book.

38. Topol EJ, Serruys PW, editors. *Current Review of Interventional Cardiology.* Philadelphia: Current Medicine, 1994:264, $149.00.

Not needed. Get the other Topol book.

39. Rao PS, editor. *Transcatheter Therapy in Pediatric Cardiology.* New York: Wiley-Liss, 1993:509, $124.95.

40. Kern MJ, editor. *Hemodynamic Rounds. Interpretation of Cardiac Pathophysiology from Pressure Waveform Analysis.* New York: Wiley-Liss, 1993:218, $38.95.

41. Herrmann HC, Hirshfeld JW Jr, editors. *Clinical Use of the Palmaz-Schatz Intracoronary Stent.* Mount Kisco, New York: Futura Publishing Company, Inc., 1993:196, $45.00.

If you are interested in this stent, here is the information.

42. Vetrovec GW, Goudreau E. *Coronary Angiography for the Interventionalist.* New York: Chapman & Hall, 1994:129, $99.00.

Beautiful angiograms but much wasted space on many pages.

43. Dyer R, editor. *Handbook of Basic Vascular and Interventional Radiology.* New York: Churchill Livingstone, 1993:275, $62.00.

PHARMACOLOGY AND DRUG THERAPY

44. Hurst JW, editor. *Current Therapy in Cardiovascular Disease.* Fourth Edition. St. Louis: Mosby, 1994: 454, $79.00.

45. Singh BN, Dzau VJ, Vanhoutte PM, Woosley RL, editors. *Cardiovascular Pharmacology and Therapeutics.* New York: Churchill Livingstone, 1994:1231, $149.95.

46. Frishman WH, Dollery CT, Cruickshank JM. *Current Cardiovascular Drugs.* Philadelphia: Current Medicine, 1994:297, $39.95.

These 3 books are all good. The Hurst book contains 97 chapters by 124 contributors, and it appears only 3 years after the previous edition. The Singh book has nearly as many contributors. The best buy is the Singh book.

47. O'Rourke MF, Safar ME, Dzau VJ, editors. *Arterial Vasodilation. Mechanisms and Therapy.* Philadelphia: Lea & Febiger, 1993:231, $89.50.

As the editors indicate, this book seeks to explain how and why vasodilator drugs are successful in treatment of stable, as well as variant, angina, and in treatment of cardiac failure and hypertension, and why some vasodilator agents are more effective than others.

48. Rezakovic DE, Alpert JS, editors. *Nitrate Therapy & Nitrate Tolerance. Current Concepts and Controversies.* Basel: Karger, 1993:547, $232.00.

49. Godfraind T, Govoni S, Paoletti R, Vanhoutte PM, editors. *Calcium Antagonists. Pharmacology and Clinical Research.* Dordrecht: Kluwer Academic Publishers, 1993:380, $132.00.

50. Escande D, Standen N, editors. *K^+ Channels in Cardiovascular Medicine.* Paris: Springer-Verlag, 1993: 332, $179.95.

GOOD CARDIOLOGIC NUTRITION

51. Piscatella JC, Piscatella B. *The Fat Tooth Fat Gram Counter.* New York: Workman Publishing, 1993: 299, $6.25.

52. Piscatella JC, Piscatella B. *The Fat Tooth Restaurant & Fast-Food Fat-Gram Counter.* New York: Workman Publishing, 1993:260, $6.25.

The 2 little Piscatella books together sell for $12.50. Every physician needs to know what is in these 2 books, and I highly recommend them. They are each pocket sized so they can go into the kitchen and restaurant easily.

53. Mogadam M. *Choosing Foods* for *a Healthy Heart.* Yonkers, New York: Consumer Reports Books, 1993:171, $19.95.

54. Chiavetta JM in collaboration with Barrett C and Chiavetta SV. *Eat, Drink and Be Healthy. A Guide to Healthful Eating and Weight Control.* Raleigh, North Carolina: Piedmont Publishers, 1993:419, $24.95.

This book is popular at the Duke University Medical Center. Every physician needs to own at least one good "healthful-eating" book.

CARDIAC FITNESS AND REHABILITATION

55. Fletcher GF, editor. *Cardiovascular Response to Exercise.* Mount Kisco, New York: Futura Publishing Company, Inc., 1994:446, $75.00.

56. Froelicher VF, Myers J, Follansbee WP, Labovitz AJ. *Exercise and the Heart,* Third Edition. St. Louis: Mosby, 1993:394, $59.00.

57. Franklin B. *Making Healthy Tomorrows. Cardiac Fitness and a Healthier Lifestyle.* Clarkston, Michigan: Glovebox Guidebooks Publishing Company, 1993:207, $12.95.

MISCELLANEOUS

58. Loscalzo J, Schafer AI, editors. *Thrombosis and Hemorrhage.* Boston, Blackwell Scientific Publications, 1994:1337, $225.00.

A major book consisting of 63 chapters by 93 contributors.

59. Kaplan JA, editor. *Cardiac Anesthesia,* Third Edition. Philadelphia: W.B. Saunders Company, 1993: 1353, $169.00.

The best on this subject.

60. Stark J, de Leval M, editors. *Surgery for Congenital Heart Defects,* Second Edition. Philadelphia: W.B. Saunders Company, 1994:712, $245.00.

A good book, but a stiff price. The foreword by Dr. John W. Kirklin is one of the best I have read. The emphasis in this book is on surgical techniques.

61. Salmasi A-M, Iskandrian AS, editors. *Cardiac Output and Regional Flow in Health and Disease.* Dordrecht: Kluwer Academic Publishers, 1993:555, $259.00.

62. Gravanis MB, editor. *Cardiovascular Disorders. Pathogenesis and Pathophysiology.* St. Louis: Mosby, 1993:576, $95.00.

63. Pohost GM, editor. *Cardiovascular Applications of Magnetic Resonance.* Mount Kisco, New York: Futura Publishing Company, Inc., 1993:459, $86.00.

64. Draznin B, Eckel RH, editors. *Diabetes and Atherosclerosis. Molecular Basis and Clinical Aspects.* New York: Elsevier, 1993:385, $85.00.

This book is divided into 3 parts: lipids, atherosclerosis and systemic hypertension in the diabetic patient. Although I know only 6 of the 41 contributors of the 20 chapters, the book appears to be excellent and is timely.

65. Sobel BE, Collen D, editors. *Coronary Thrombolysis in Perspective. Principles Underlying Conjunctive and Adjunctive Therapy.* New York: Marcel Dekker, Inc., 1993:338, $99.75.

66. Cohn PF. *Silent Myocardial Ischemia and Infarction,* Third Edition. New York: Marcel Dekker, Inc., 1993:268, $79.75.

67. Tresch DD, Aronow WS, editors. *Cardiovascular Disease in the Elderly Patient.* New York: Marcel Dekker, Inc., 1994:663, $125.00.

68. Wenger NK, editor. *Inclusion of Elderly Individuals in Clinical Trials. Cardiovascular Disease and Cardiovascular Therapy as a Model.* Kansas City, Missouri: Marion Merrell Dow, Inc., 1993:294, $0.00.

69. Waller BF, Harvey WP, editors. *Cardiovascular Evaluation of Athletes. Toward Recognizing Athletes at*

Risk of Sudden Death. Newton, New Jersey: Laennec Publishing, 1993:213, $75.00.

70. Nagano M, Takeda N, Dhalla NS, editors. *The Cardiomyopathic Heart.* New York: Raven Press, 1994: 464, $95.00.

Forty-four chapters by 183 contributors, 2 of whom are from the USA. Much experimental work is included. Not useful clinically.

71. Alpert JS, Francis GS. *Handbook of Coronary Care,* Fifth Edition. Boston: Little, Brown and Company, 1993:228, $27.00.

This neat little book fits nicely into the coat pocket.

72. Kapoor A, Laks H, editors. *Atlas of Heart-Lung Transplantation.* New York: McGraw-Hill, Inc., 1994: 212, $150.

A pictorial description of the operations currently performed for end-stage heart and lung failure. There is much unused space on too many pages in this expensive book.

PERIPHERAL VASCULAR DISEASE

73. Veith FJ, Hobson RW II, Williams RA, Wilson SE, editors. *Vascular Surgery. Principles and Practice,* Second Edition. New York: McGraw-Hill, Inc., 1994: 1250, $175.00.

74. Strandness DE Jr, van Breda A, editors. *Vascular Diseases. Surgical and Interventional Therapy.* New York: Churchill Livingstone, 1994:1–634 (volume 1) and 635–1270 (volume 2), $250.00.

Both the Veith and the Strandness-van Breda books are major ones, of similar length. One is priced better than the other.

75. Strandness DE Jr. *Duplex Scanning in Vascular Disorders,* Second Edition. New York: Raven Press, 1993:329, $95.00.

76. Lindsay J, Jr. *Diseases of the Aorta.* Philadelphia: Lea & Febiger, 1994:315, $75.00.

ANNUAL REVIEWS

77. Schlant RC, Editor-in-Chief; Collins JJ Jr, Engle MA, Gersh BJ, Kaplan NM, Waldo AL, editors. *1993 The Year Book of CARDIOLOGY®.* St. Louis: Mosby, 1993:502, $59.95.

78. Roberts WC, Willerson JT, Rackley CE, Graham TP Jr, Mason DT. *CARDIOLOGY 1993.* Boston: Butterworth-Heineman, 1993:490, $90.00.

The Schlant book is the 33rd in its series. It contains summaries of 337 articles, most published in 1992 but some in 1991, and an editor provides comments on the publisher-written summaries. Additionally, 11 tables and 97 figures are included. The Roberts book contains summaries of 758 articles all published in 1992 plus 122 figures and 34 tables. I obviously prefer the latter book.

79. Frohlich ED, Kotchen TA, editors. *Advances in Hypertension 1993.* Philadelphia: J.B. Lippincott Company, 1993:438, $65.00.

This book contains 475 abstracts of articles on systemic hypertension. Most of the articles were published in 1991. Each abstract is followed by comments from 1 of the 13 contributors.

CARDIOLOGIC HISTORY

80. Favaloro RG. *The Challenging Dream of Heart Surgery From the Pampas to Cleveland.* Boston: Little, Brown and Company, 1994:167, $24.95.

An autobiography by the surgeon who started the aorto-coronary bypass operation is most appropriate. A wonderful story.

81. Roberts CS. *Life and Writings of Stewart R. Roberts, M.D., Georgia's First Heart Specialist.* Spartanburg, South Carolina: The Reprint Company Publishers, 1993:138, $12.95.

This book on my father was written by my son. Obviously, I am proud of both of them.

COMMENTS

This annual book column first appeared in December 1985 and it briefly described 16 books,[1] 4 of which had a 1984 publication date, 7 a 1985 date and 5 a 1986 date: 9 were edited with multiple contributors, and 7 had only 1 to 3 authors; the costs of the books ranged from $37.50 to $150.00 (mean $77.00), and none were published on acid-free paper.[2] Of the 81 books appearing in 1993, 53 (65%) had a 1993 publication date and 28 (35%) a 1994 date; of the 73 non-historic books intended exclusively for physicians, 56 (77%) were multi-authored (>10 contributors), 9 (12%) had 2 to 5 authors, and only 8 (11%) had a single author; the costs of the 72 medical books (the 6 books [numbers 10, 51, 52, 53, 54 and 57] intended for the lay public were excluded, as was 1 book [number 68], which is free of charge, and the 2 historic books [numbers 80 and 81]) ranged from $27.00 to $275.00 (mean $111.00), and 24 (30%) (numbers 11, 12, 13, 19, 21, 28, 30, 32, 33, 39, 40, 41, 42, 48, 49, 55, 61, 63, 64, 65, 66, 67, 78 and 81) were published on acid-free paper. Of the 71 medical books briefly mentioned in this column 1 year ago,[3] only 9 (13%) were published on acid-free, i.e., permanent paper, so progress is being made. It is time for all American book publishers to use permanent paper. I encourage all authors to require in their book contracts that the paper used for their books be acid free.

William C. Roberts

William Clifford Roberts, MD
Editor in Chief

1. Roberts WC. Some good cardiologic books. *Am J Cardiol* 1985;56:1001–1002.
2. Roberts WC. Alkaline paper and preserving the record. *Am J Cardiol* 1991;68: 1729–1732.
3. Roberts WC. Cardiologic books published in 1992. *Am J Cardiol* 1993;71: 126–130.

Good Cardiologic Books Appearing In 1994

MAJOR GENERAL CARDIOLOGIC TEXTBOOKS

1. Willerson JT, Cohn JN, editors. *Cardiovascular Medicine*. New York: Churchill Livingstone, 1995:1,976, $125.00.

A major text by 131 contributors.

SMALLER CARDIOLOGIC TEXTS

2. Hollenberg NK, editor (Braunwald E, series editor). *Atlas of Heart Diseases. Hypertension: Mechanisms and Therapy.* Volume I. Philadelphia: Current Medicine, 1995:200 (approximately), $99.95.

Volume I is the first of a projected 12 volumes. It will be several years before all 12 are out. Beautiful picture books and the images are now available separately in print and slide form and also will soon be formatted for CD-ROM use.

3. Abelman WH, editor (Braunwald E, series editor). *Atlas of Heart Diseases. Cardiomyopathies, Myocarditis, and Pericardial Disease*. Volume II. Philadelphia: Current Medicine, 1995:200 (approximately), $99.95.

This is the second of the projected 12 volumes.

4. Hurst JW, Alpert JS (editors), Anderson RH, Becker AE, Wilcox BR (associate editors). *Diagnostic Atlas of the Heart*. New York: Raven Press, 1994:560, $150.00.

This book is mainly a picture book, and many of the illustrations are in color. Forty-four well-known physicians contributed to this beautiful book. It's a shame that this splendid product was not published on acid-free paper.

5. Dolgin M, editor. *Nomenclature and Criteria for Diagnosis of Diseases of the Heart and Great Vessels.* Ninth Edition. Boston: Little, Brown and Company, 1994:334, $29.95.

The first edition of this book appeared in 1928 with the primary objective of providing concise descriptions of the principal causes and manifestations of cardiovascular diseases and the specific criteria for their diagnosis. That objective has continued through the subsequent 8 editions, the last one appearing in 1979. Much has happened in cardiology in the last 15 years. The new edition replaces the old *Status and Prognosis with Functional Capacity and Objective Assessment*. A very handy handbook.

6. Gibler WB, Aufderheide TP, editors. *Emergency Cardiac Care*. St. Louis: Mosby, 1994:758, $89.95.

A large book by 28 contributors, none of whom I know.

7. Freed M, Grines C, editors. *Essentials of Cardiovascular Medicine*. Birmingham, Michigan: Physician's Press, 1994:628, $29.95 (spiral), $12.95 (shirt pocket companion).

This neat book for "the Doctor's bag" by 27 outstanding contributors is a patient care manual, a guide to electrocardiographic interpretation and to drug therapy, all in one. Recent clinical trials and controversies are reviewed. Some references date to only 6 weeks before publication.

8. Heger JW, Roth RF, Niemann JT, Criley JM. *Cardiology.* Third Edition. Baltimore: Williams & Wilkins, 1994:387, $20.00.

It fits into the pocket; it is the best book for the price in this review, and the graphics, particularly those on valvular heart disease, are magnificent, with Criley at his best.

9. Elefteriades JA, Geha AS, Cohen LS. *House Officer Guide To ICU Care. Fundamentals of Management of the Heart and Lungs*. Second Edition. New York: Raven Press, 1994:286, $39.95.

A good book for the white coat pocket.

GERIATRIC CARDIOLOGY

10. Martin A, Camm AJ, editors. *Geriatric Cardiology. Principles and Practice*. Chichester: John Wiley & Sons Ltd., 1994:813, $150.00.

The first book on this subject by the present 2 editors appeared several years ago. The present one is far more comprehensive and is considered a "new book" rather than a second edition. The definition of "elderly" appears to vary a bit in the various chapters by different contributors. Despite some careless technical errors, the book is needed and is useful.

11.* Chesler E, editor. *Clinical Cardiology in the Elderly.* Armonk, New York: Futura Publishing Company, Inc., 1994:598, $88.00.

I prefer the Martin–Camm book, but its price is also much higher.

PREVENTIVE CARDIOLOGY

12. Filer LJ Jr, Lauer RM, Luepker RV, editors. *Prevention of Atherosclerosis and Hypertension Beginning in Youth.* Philadelphia: Lea & Febiger, 1994:289, $48.50.

A summary of presentations at a conference held in July 1992. A nice collection of papers.

ACUTE MYOCARDIAL INFARCTION

13.* Julian DG, Braunwald E, editors. *Management of Acute Myocardial Infarction.* London: W.B. Saunders Company Ltd., 1994:433, $52.50.

Excellent.

REHABILITATION

14. Pollock ML, Schmidt DH, editors. *Heart Disease and Rehabilitation*. Third Edition. Champaign, Illinois: Human Kinetics, 1995:471, $59.00.

This large book sells for $59.00, which is 12¢/page. This is a splendid book for the cost.

SYSTEMIC HYPERTENSION

15. Swales JD, editor. *Textbook of Hypertension.* Oxford: Blackwell Scientific Publications, 1994:1328, $195.00.

A huge book by 185 contributors. It covers the whole field.

*Published on acid-free (permanent) paper.

16. Laragh JH, Brenner BM, editors. *Hypertension. Pathophysiology, Diagnosis, and Management.* Second Edition. Volumes One and Two. New York: Raven Press, 1995:3,260, $345.00.

The most comprehensive text on this subject.

17. Kaplan NM. *Clinical Hypertension.* Sixth Edition. Baltimore: Williams & Wilkins, 1994:482, $75.00.

A pleasurable book to read, and it's by a single author!

18. Messerli FH, editor. *The ABCs of Antihypertensive Therapy.* New York: Raven Press, 1994:266, $49.00.

An excellent little book by 30 contributors involving many of the best in the antihypertensive arena.

19. Krakoff LR. *Management of the Hypertensive Patient.* New York: Churchill Livingstone, 1995:298, $75.00.

20.* Kaplan NM, Ram CVS, editors. *Individualized Therapy of Hypertension.* New York: Marcel Dekker, Inc., 1995:282, $99.75.

The opinions and views are of the contributors, and they may differ considerably from those of the 2 editors. I'll take the earlier Kaplan book which is less expensive and more comprehensive.

HEART FAILURE

21.* Hosenpud JD, Greenberg BH, editors. *Congestive Heart Failure. Pathophysiology, Diagnosis, and Comprehensive Approach to Management.* New York: Springer-Verlag, 1994:769, $135.00.

A large book by 60 contributors, the leaders in the field. It has it all except for a chapter on how to prevent heart failure. Because atherosclerotic coronary artery disease is by far the most common cause of heart failure, its prevention is the prevention of atherosclerosis which means keeping or getting the serum total cholesterol level to the 150 mg/dl area.

ELECTROCARDIOGRAPHY

22. Wagner GS. *Marriott's Practical Electrocardiography.* Ninth Edition. Baltimore: Williams & Wilkins, 1994:434, $32.00.

I liked Barney Marriott's electrocardiography best, except for Robert Grant's book many years ago. Galen Wagner has continued the Marriott tradition. The Marriott electrocardiograms are the best cropped ones in any publication I know. To see a lot of wasted space in this book defeats the splendid trimming of the electrocardiograms.

23. Blake TM. *The Practice of Electrocardiography. A Problem-Solving Guide to Confident Interpretation.* Fifth Edition. Totowa, New Jersey: Humana Press, 1994:319, $49.50 (hard cover), $29.50 (paper back).

There are so many books on electrocardiography. This one is a bit different in that relatively few electrocardiograms are reproduced.

ECHOCARDIOGRAPHY

24. Freeman WK, Seward JB, Khandheria BK, Tajik AJ, editors. *Transesophageal Echocardiography.* Boston: Little, Brown and Company, 1994:599, $185.00.

A beautiful book. Probably the best so far on this topic.

25.* Marwick TH. *Stress Echocardiography. Its Role in the Diagnosis and Evaluation of Coronary Artery Disease.* Dordrecht: Kluwer Academic Publishers, 1994: 180, $145.00.

This book appears to cover this topic well, but 80¢ a page is a bit expensive.

26. Stümper O, Sutherland GR, editors. *Transesophageal Echocardiography in Congenital Heart Disease.* London: Edward Arnold, 1994:284, $165.00.

ARRHYTHMIAS, CONDUCTION DEFECTS, PACEMAKERS, CARDIOVERTER-DEFIBRILLATORS

27. Zipes DP, Jalife J, editors. *Cardiac Electrophysiology—From Cell to Bedside.* Second Edition. Philadelphia: W.B. Saunders Company, 1995:1,612, $235.00.

The most authoritative book on cardiac electrophysiology for the basic scientist and clinician by 273 contributors! No other volume serves both groups as well or as completely.

28. Podrid PJ, Koweg PR, editors. *Cardiac Arrhythmia. Mechanisms, Diagnosis, and Management.* Baltimore: Williams & Wilkins 1995:1,472 (approximately), $159.00.

A book by 168 contributors, most of them well-known.

29. Surawicz B. *Electrophysiologic Basis of ECG and Cardiac Arrhythmias.* Baltimore: Williams & Wilkins, 1995:622, $89.00.

The whole book by the same author. It's nice to see a single-authored book occasionally.

30. Prystowsky EN, Klein GJ. *Cardiac Arrhythmias. An Integrated Approach For the Clinician.* New York: McGraw-Hill, Inc., 1994:452, $60.00.

A good practical book by 2 clinicians with a similar clinical approach to arrhythmias.

31.* Huang SKS, editor. *Radiofrequency Catheter Ablation of Cardiac Arrhythmias. Basic Concepts and Clinical Applications.* Armonk, New York: Futura Publishing Company, Inc., 1995:594, $98.00.

Thirty-eight well-known contributors. Looks good.

32. Ellenbogen KA, Kay GN, Wilkoff BL, editors. *Clinical Cardiac Pacing.* Philadelphia: W.B. Saunders Company, 1995:838, $165.00.

I suspect that this is the best so far on pacemakers.

33.* Aubert AE, Ector H, Stroobandt R, editors. *Cardiac Pacing and Electrophysiology. A Bridge to the 21st Century.* Dordrecht: Kluwer Academic Publishers, 1994: 441, $175.00.

This book by 41 contributors, 37 of whom reside in Europe, appears to be well done, but it costs too much.

34.* Estes NAM III, Manolis AS, Wang PJ, editors. *Implantable Cardioverter-Defibrillators. A Comprehensive Textbook.* New York: Marcel Dekker, Inc., 1994: 929, $195.00.

It is "comprehensive."

35.* Camm AJ, Lindemans FW, editors. *Transvenous Defibrillation and Radiofrequency Ablation.* Armonk, New York: Futura Publishing Company, Inc., 1995:225, $48.00.

36. Akhtar M, Myerburg RJ, Ruskin JN, editors. *Sudden Cardiac Death: Prevalence, Mechanisms, and*

Approaches to Diagnosis and Management. Philadelphia: Williams & Wilkins, 1994:635, $98.50.

A fine book by 96 contributors.

37.* Goldstein S, Bayés-de-Luna A, Guindo-Soldevila J. *Sudden Cardiac Death.* Armonk, New York: Futura Publishing Company, Inc., 1994:343, $75.00.

PHARMACOLOGY AND DRUG THERAPY

38. Frishman WH, editor. *Current Cardiovascular Drugs.* Second Edition. Philadelphia: Current Medicine, 1995:317, $39.95.

A useful book.

39. Opie LH. *Angiotensin-Converting Enzyme Inhibitors: Scientific Basis for Clinical Use.* Second Edition. New York: Wiley-Liss, 1994:316, $34.95.

40. Opie LH, editor. *Myocardial Protection by Calcium Antagonists.* New York: Wiley-Liss, 1994:195, $34.95.

41. Starr JM, Whalley LJ. *ACE Inhibitors. Central Actions.* New York: Raven Press, 1994:254, $75.00.

NUCLEAR CARDIOLOGY

42. DePuey EG, Berman DS, Garcia EV, editors. *Cardiac SPECT Imaging.* New York: Raven Press, 1995: 290, $130.00.

This must be it in SPECT.

INTERVENTIONAL CARDIOLOGY

43. Pepine CJ, Hill JA, Lambert CR, editors. *Diagnostic and Therapeutic Cardiac Catheterization.* Second Edition. Baltimore: Williams & Wilkins, 1994:877, $95.00.

As the authors state in the preface, "this book is a complete text on all aspects of the practice of cardiac catheterization." The 3 editors and the 62 contributors produced a splendid book.

44. Surruys PW, Foley DP, de Feyter PJ, editors. *Quantitative Coronary Angiography in Clinical Practice.* Dordrecht: Kluwer Academic Publishers, 1994:719, $260.00.

A thorough book on this topic. Each page costs 36¢.

45. Popma JJ, Leon MB, Topol EJ. *Atlas of Interventional Cardiology.* Philadelphia: W.B. Saunders Company, 1994:359, $95.00.

Lots of angiograms—covers angioplasty, directional atherectomy, stents, and lasers. Although there is some wasted space, the angiograms are splendid. For the interventionalist I think this would be a very useful book.

46. Roubin GS, Califf RM, O'Neill WW, Phillips HR III, Stack RS, editors. *Interventional Cardiovascular Medicine: Principles and Practice.* New York: Churchill Livingstone, 1994:989, $179.95.

A major text for interventionalists.

CONGENITAL HEART DISEASE

47. Emmanouilides GC, Riemenschneider TA, Allen HD, Gutgesell HP, editors. *MOSS and ADAMS Heart Disease in Infants, Children, and Adolescents Including the Fetus and Young Adult.* Fifth Edition. Volumes I and II. Baltimore: Williams & Wilkins, 1995:1,912, $249.00.

Just splendid by 130 contributors, most of whom are leaders in heart disease in this age group.

48. Ho SY, Baker EJ, Rigby ML, Anderson RH. *Color Atlas of Congenital Heart Disease. Morphologic and Clinical Correlations.* London: Mosby-Wolfe, 1995:192, $100.00.

An attractive picture book. The morphologic pictures are some of the best I've seen by Anderson.

CARDIAC SURGERY

49. Baumgartner WA, Owens SG, Cameron DE, Reitz BA, editors. *The Johns Hopkins Manual of Cardiac Surgical Care.* St. Louis: Mosby, 1994:546, $39.00.

A neat little pocket book.

50.* Grooters RK, Nishida H, editors. *Alternative Bypass Conduits and Methods for Surgical Revascularization.* Armonk, New York: Futura Publishing Company, Inc., 1994:323, $65.00.

51.* Denber HCB. *Cardiac Surgery: Biological and Psychological Implications.* Armonk, New York: Futura Publishing Company, Inc., 1995:250, $35.00.

MISCELLANEOUS

52. Rapaport E, editor. *Cardiology and Co-existing Disease.* New York: Churchill Livingstone, 1994:391, $85.00.

What are the co-existing "diseases"? Pregnancy; autonomic dysfunction; pulmonary, neurologic, hepatic, endocrine, renal, hematologic, and oncologic disorders; and AIDS. Not worth $85.00.

53. Hurst JW, editor. *New Types of Cardiovascular Diseases.* New York: Igaku-Shoin, 1994:297, $69.50.

What are the "new types of cardiovascular diseases"? They include silent myocardial ischemia; stunned and hibernating myocardium; heart disease due to AIDS, ergot alkaloids, lyme disease, Kawasaki syndrome, noncardiac drugs, radiation, artificial heart valves, pacemakers, and the eosinophilia-myalgia syndrome; stroke due to patent foramen ovale; toxic oil syndrome and pulmonary hypertension; and narrow complex ventricular tachycardia.

54.* Ezekowitz MD, editor. *Systemic Cardiac Embolism.* New York: Marcel Dekker, Inc., 1994:393, $135.00.

An excellent book.

55. Lorell BH, Grossman W, editors. *Diastolic Relaxation of the Heart.* The Biology of Diastole in Health and Disease. Second Edition. Boston: Kluwer Academic Publishers, 1994:348, $125.00.

This book explores regulation of ventricular diastolic function at the levels of the gene, the myocyte, the intact heart, and the patient with heart failure. It summarizes presentations at an international symposium in January 1993.

56.* Gross DR. *Animal Models in Cardiovascular Research.* Second Revised Edition. Dordrecht: Kluwer Academic Publishers, 1994:494, $169.00.

57. Nagano M, Takeda N, Dhalla NS, editors. *The Adapted Heart.* New York: Raven Press, 1994:520, $99.00.

Each chapter describes the ability of the heart to adapt to a variety of stressful situations such as pressure overload (hypertension), volume overload (valvular disease), loss of myocardium (myocardial infarction), and primary cardiac muscle disease associated with changes in the circulating levels of various hormones and neuropeptides. An interesting book mainly by Japanese investigators.

58. Khaw B-A, Narula J, Strauss HW, editors. *Monoclonal Antibodies in Cardiovascular Diseases*. Philadelphia: Lea & Febiger, 1994:290, $115.00.

Looks good. My opinion is of little use here.

59.* Przyklenk K, Kloner RA, Yellon DM, editors. *Ischemic Preconditioning: The Concept of Endogenous Cardioprotection*. Boston: Kluwer Academic Publishers, 1994:196, $95.00.

60. Hurst JW. *Essays From the Heart*. New York: Raven Press, 1995:173, $65.00.

This book concerns "the emotional heart" and it is a pleasure to read. The price is 37¢ a page and some pages are half filled. Surely the publisher could reduce the price to a level where buyers would buy it.

PERIPHERAL VASCULAR DISEASE

61. Jamieson CW, Yao JST, editors. *Vascular Surgery*. Fifth Edition. London: Chapman & Hall Medical, 1994:676, $195.00.

A large book by 80 contributors.

62.* White RA, Hollier LH, editors. *Vascular Surgery. Basic Science and Clinical Correlations*. Philadelphia: J.B. Lippincott Company, 1994:657, $99.00.

Excellent, by 78 contributors.

63.* Comerota AJ, editor. *Thrombolytic Therapy for Peripheral Vascular Disease*. Philadelphia: J.B. Lippincott Company, 1995:553, $89.50.

A superb book by 47 contributors, a book dedicated to Sol Sherry, the father of thrombolytic therapy.

64.* Kazmers A, editor. *Cardiac Risk Assessment Before Vascular Surgery*. Armonk, New York: Futura Publishing Company, Inc., 1994:364, $52.00.

65.* Bunt TJ, editor. *Vascular Graft Infections*. Armonk, New York: Futura Publishing Company, Inc., 1994:408, $62.00.

CARDIOLOGIC HISTORY

66. Acierno LJ. *The History of Cardiology*. London: The Parthenon Publishing Group, 1994:758, $98.00.

Through the years I have collected several books on the history of cardiology. The present one is the largest—758 large-sized pages and all initially written in hand by the author—is also one of the best, maybe the best. The single author reviews most major cardiovascular diseases and techniques to diagnose and treat them from their very early descriptions to modern times. A book well worth having for any cardiologist.

ANNUAL REVIEWS

67.* Roberts WC, Rackley CE, Willerson JT, Mason DT, Parmley WW, Graham TP Jr. *Cardiology 1994*. Boston: Butterworth-Heinemann 1994:504, $95.00.

68. Schlant RC (editor in chief), Collins JJ Jr, Engle MA, Gersh BJ, Kaplan NM, Waldo AL (editors). *1994 Year Book of Cardiology*, St. Louis: Mosby-Year Book, Inc., 1994:511, $71.95.

The Roberts book summarizes 738 articles and the Schlant book, 330 articles. The Roberts book became available in July 1994, a bit late for it; the Schlant book is still unavailable for purchase as of November 1994.

GOOD MEDICAL AND NUTRITIONAL BOOKS INTENDED PRIMARILY FOR THE LAY PUBLIC

69. Silver MA. *Success With Heart Failure. Help and Hope for Those With Congestive Heart Failure*. New York: Insight Books, 1994:293, $23.95.

A most human book by a former fellow and a splendid physician.

70. Eliot RS. *From Stress to Strength. How to Lighten Your Load and Save Your Life*. New York: Bantam Books, 1994:276, $11.95.

71. Jacobson MF, Maxwell B. *What Are We Feeding Our Kids?* New York: Workman Publishing, 1994:309, $8.95.

72. Piscatella JC, Piscatella B. *Don't Eat Your Heart Out Cookbook*. Second Edition. New York: Workman Publishing, 1994:664, $17.95.

73. Chiavetta JM. *Eat, Drink and Be Healthy. A Guide to Healthful Eating and Weight Control*. Golden, Colorado: Fulcrum Publishing, 1995:414, $24.95.

COMMENTS

Of the 73 books mentioned herein, 21 (29%) have a 1995 publication date, which means that this piece, appearing January 1, 1995, is the first medical journal to mention the availability of these 21 books. The costs of the 68 books intended for a medical audience range from $20.00 to $345.00 (mean $106.00): 24 (35%) cost ≥$100.00. The mean cost for the 49 edited medical books (71% of total) is $117.00, for the 11 single-authored books, $79.00, and for the 8 books having 2 to 6 authors, $70.00. Unfortunately, only 20 of the 68 medical books (29%) (numbers 11, 13, 20, 21, 25, 31, 33, 34, 35, 37, 50, 51, 54, 56, 59, 62, 63, 64, 65, 67) were published on acid-free (permanent) paper, the same percent as last year.[1] Authors need to stipulate acid-free paper in their contracts with publishers. The year 1994 was a big year for books in systemic hypertension, arrhythmias, conduction disturbances, and peripheral vascular disease. What will next year bring?

William C. Roberts

William Clifford Roberts, MD
Editor in Chief
Baylor University Medical Center
Dallas, Texas 75246

1. Roberts WC. Good cardiologic books appearing in 1993. *Am J Cardiol* 1994; 73:98–101.

Good Cardiologic Books Appearing in 1995

MAJOR GENERAL TEXT

1. Chizner MA, editor. *Classic Teachings in Clinical Cardiology. A Tribute to W. Proctor Harvey, M.D.* Volume I and II. Cedar Grove, New Jersey: Laennec Publishing, Inc., 1996:1579, $145.00.

About 100 years ago it was not unusual for trainees of renowned professors of medicine, surgery, or pathology to compile a book in honor of their teacher. Not so in the last 50 years. Dr. Michael Chizner, however, has turned back the clock by gathering 52 of Dr. Proctor Harvey's former fellows to produce a well-rounded cardiology book in honor of their renowned teacher. The result is a fine book.

SMALLER GENERAL TEXTS

2. Kloner RA, editor. *The Guide to Cardiology.* Third Edition. Greenwich, Connecticut: Le Jacq Communications, Inc., 1995:752, $68.00.

This edition is a quarter larger than the second edition. Good book at a good price.

3. Hillis LD, Lange RA, Winniford MD, Page RL. *Manual of Clinical Problems in Cardiology with Annotated Key References.* Fifth Edition. Boston: Little, Brown and Company, 1995:579, $34.95.

Very useful. Can keep it in the pocket of the white coat.

4. Crawford MH, editor. *Diagnosis and Treatment in Cardiology.* Norwalk, Connecticut: Appleton & Lange, 1995:498, $41.95.

CORONARY ARTERY DISEASE AND ATHEROSCLEROSIS

5. Fuster V, Ross R, Topol EJ, editors. *Atherosclerosis and Coronary Artery Disease.* Volumes One and Two. Philadelphia: Lippincott-Raven Publishers, 1996: 1701, $275.00.

Beautiful book. The best book in cardiology appearing in 1995!

6. Califf RM, Mark DB, Wagner GS, editors. *Acute Coronary Care.* Second Edition. St. Louis: Mosby, 1995: 964, $95.00.

7. Francis GS, Alpert JS, editors. *Coronary Care.* Second Edition. Boston: Little, Brown and Company, 1995:804, $120.00.

Both the Califf and Francis-Alpert books are excellent. The Califf one is larger and less expensive.

8. Maseri A. *Ischemic Heart Disease. A Rational Basis for Clinical Practice and Clinical Research.* New York: Churchill Livingstone, 1995:713, $99.00.

Attillio Maseri, a major cardiologic investigator on the world scene for the last 2 decades, wrote every word of this fine book.

9. Ambrose JA, editor. *Complex Coronary Lesions in Acute Coronary Syndromes.* Armonk, New York: Futura Publishing Company, Inc., 1996:267, $65.00.

10. Koenig W, Hombach V, Bond MG, Kramsch DM, editors. *Progression and Regression of Atherosclerosis.* Vienna: Blackwell Wissenschaft, 1995:510, $80.00.

This book contains papers presented at an International Symposium in Ulm, Germany, in May 1993. Discussed are imaging techniques and their applications and limitations in epidemiological studies and in clinical trials.

INTERVENTIONAL CARDIOLOGY

11. Ellis SG, Holmes DR Jr, editors. *Strategic Approaches in Coronary Intervention.* Baltimore: Williams & Wilkins, 1996:763, $95.00.

12. Vetrovec GW, Carabello BA, editors. *Invasive Cardiology. Current Diagnostic and Therapeutic Issues.* Armonk, New York: Futura Publishing Company, Inc., 1996:618, $115.00.

13. White CJ, Ramee SR, editors. *Interventional Cardiology. New Techniques and Strategies for Diagnosis and Treatment.* New York: Marcel Dekker, Inc., 1995:353, $120.00.

14. Topol EJ, Serruys PW, editors. *Current Review of Interventional Cardiology.* Second Edition. Philadelphia: Current Medicine, 1995:312, $149.95.

15. Lutz J, editor. *Complications of Interventional Procedures.* New York: Igaku-Shoin, 1995:248, $73.95.

16. Freed M, Grines C, Safian R, editors. *Manual of Interventional Cardiology.* Birmingham, Michigan: Physicians' Press, 1996:750, $75.00.

HEART FAILURE

17. McCall D, Rahimtoola SH, editors. *Heart Failure.* New York: Chapman & Hall, 1995:436, $79.95.

18. Dhalla NS, Beamish RE, Takeda N, Nagano M, editors. *The Failing Heart.* Philadelphia: Lippincott-Raven Publishers, 1995:524, $99.00.

SYSTEMIC HYPERTENSION

19. Messerli FH, Aepfelbacher FC, editors. *Hypertension in Postmenopausal Women.* New York: Marcel Dekker, Inc., 1996:298, $79.80.

20. O'Brien E, Beevers DG, Marshall HJ. *ABC of Hypertension.* Third Edition. London: BMJ Publishing Group, 1995:79, $22.00.

A gem.

ELECTROCARDIOGRAPHY

21. Levine GN, Podrid PJ. *The ECG Workbook. A Review and Discussion of ECG Findings and Abnormalities.* Armonk, New York: Futura Publishing Company, Inc., 1995:550, $74.00.

ARRHYTHMIAS AND CONDUCTION DEFECTS

22. Mandel WJ, editor. *Cardiac Arrhythmias. Their Mechanisms, Diagnosis, and Management.* Third Edition. Philadelphia: JB Lippincott Company, 1995:1266, $165.00.

23. Saksena S, Lüderitz B, editors. *Interventional Electrophysiology. A Textbook.* Second Edition. Armonk, New York: Futura Publishing Company, Inc., 1996:634, $160.00.

24. Vlay SC, editor. *A Practical Approach to Cardiac Arrhythmias.* Second Edition. Boston: Little, Brown and Company, 1996:479, $49.95.

25. Fogoros RN. *Electrophysiologic Testing.* Second Edition. Cambridge, Massachusetts: Blackwell Science, 1995:270, $32.95.

26. DiMarco JP, Prystowsky EN, editors. *Atrial Arrhythmias. State of the Art.* Armonk, New York: Futura Publishing Company, Inc., 1995:432, $70.00.

27. Lüderitz B. *History of the Disorders of Cardiac Rhythm.* Armonk, New York: Futura Publishing Company, 1995:167, $75.00.

A splendid little book.

ECHOCARDIOGRAPHY

28. D'Cruz IA. *Echocardiographic Anatomy. Understanding Normal and Abnormal Echocardiograms.* Stamford, Connecticut: Appleton & Lange, 1996:563, $95.00.

29. Chambers JB. *Clinical Echocardiography.* London: BMJ Publishing Group, 1995:260, $98.00.

30. Roelandt JRTC, Pandian NG, editors. *Multiplane Transesophageal Echocardiography.* New York: Churchill Livingstone, 1996:257, $99.00.

31. Rafferty TD. *Basics of Transesophageal Echocardiography.* New York: Churchill Livingstone, 1995: 190, $85.00.

STRESS TESTING

32. Ellestad MH (main author), Selvester RHS, Mishkin FS, James FW, Mazumi K (contributors). *Stress Testing. Principles and Practice.* Edition 4. Philadelphia: F.A. Davis Company, 1996:593, $69.95.

This is it in stress testing.

NUCLEAR CARDIOLOGY

33. Iskandrian AS, Verani MS. *Nuclear Cardiac Imaging: Principles and Applications.* Second Edition. Philadelphia: F.A. Davis Company, 1996:451, $160.00.

34. Beller GA. *Clinical Nuclear Cardiology.* Philadelphia: W.B. Saunders Company, 1995:387, $95.00.

Both of these books are excellent. Neither is an edited book; one is double authored, the other single authored, both unusual these days. The Beller book is the better buy.

OTHER IMAGING

35. Adachi H, Nagai J. *Three-Dimensional CT Angiography.* Boston: Little, Brown and Company, 1995: 232, $149.95.

Beautiful.

36. Van Der Wall EE, Blanksma PK, Niemeyer MG, Paans AMJ, editors. *Positron Emission Tomography. Viability, Perfusion, Receptors and Cardiomyopathy.* Dordrecht: Kluwer Academic Publishers, 1995:253, $120.00.

37. DePuey EG, Berman DS, Garcia EV, editors. *Cardiac SPECT Imaging.* New York: Raven Press, 1995: 290, $130.00.

Beautiful but expensive. Each page costs 45¢.

CARDIAC CATHETERIZATION

38. Baim DS, Grossman W, editors. *Cardiac Catheterization, Angiography, and Intervention.* Fifth Edition. Baltimore: Williams & Wilkins, 1996:879, $85.00.

This classic is now an edited book.

HEART RATE VARIABILITY

39. Malik M, Camm AJ, editors. *Heart Rate Variability.* Armonk, New York: Futura Publishing Company, Inc., 1995:543, $98.00.

A needed reference.

PHARMACOLOGY AND DRUG THERAPY

40. Opie LH. *Drugs for the Heart.* Fourth Edition. Philadelphia: W.B. Saunders Company, 1995:377, $29.95.

A jewel for the price.

41. Khan MG. *Cardiac Drug Therapy.* Fourth Edition. London: W.B. Saunders Company Ltd., 1995:426, $39.00.

RESUSCITATION

42. Paradis NA, Halperin HR, Nowak RM, editors. *Cardiac Arrest. The Science and Practice of Resuscitation Medicine.* Baltimore: Williams & Wilkins, 1996:981, $139.00.

CARDIOVASCULAR REHABILITATION

43. Fardy PS, Yanowitz FG, with assistance from Wilson PK. *Cardiac Rehabilitation, Adult Fitness, and Exercise Testing.* Third Edition. Baltimore: Williams & Wilkins, 1995:459, $62.50.

PEDIATRIC CARDIOLOGY

44. Nichols DG, Cameron DE, Greeley WJ, Lappe DG, Ungerleider RM, Wetzel RC, editors. *Critical Heart Disease in Infants and Children.* St. Louis: Mosby, 1995:1069, $175.00.

A major text.

45. Gewitz MH, editor. *Primary Pediatric Cardiology.* Armonk, New York: Futura Publishing Company, Inc., 1995:482, $85.00.

46. Gillette PC, Zeigler VL, editors. *Pediatric Cardiac Pacing.* Armonk, New York: Futura Publishing Company, Inc., 1995:254, $45.00.

47. Guntheroth WG. *Crib Death. The Sudden Infant Death Syndrome.* Armonk, New York: Futura Publishing Company, Inc., 1995:439, $72.00.

MOLECULAR CARDIOLOGY

48. Haber E, editor. *Scientific American Molecular Cardiovascular Medicine.* New York: Scientific American, Inc., 1995:338, $49.00.

CARDIOVASCULAR SURGERY

49. Sabiston DC Jr, Spencer FC, editors. *Surgery of the Chest.* Sixth Edition. Volumes I and II. Philadelphia: W.B. Saunders Company, 1995:2174, $295.00.

Beautiful books. Packed full of the latest information.

50. Sabiston DC Jr, editor. *Atlas of Cardiothoracic Surgery.* Philadelphia: W.B. Saunders Company, 1995: 598, $165.00.

51. Waldhausen JA, Pierce WS, Campbell DB, editors. *Surgery of the Chest.* Sixth Edition. St. Louis: Mosby, 1996:656, $125.00.

684 illustrations but lots of wasted space.

52. Harlan BJ, Starr A, Harwin FM. *Manual of Cardiac Surgery.* Second Edition. New York: Springer-Verlag, 1995:378, $185.00.

363 colored drawings.

53. Litwin SB. *Color Atlas of Congenital Heart Surgery.* St. Louis: Mosby, 1996:240, $225.00.

627 four-color intraoperative photographs. Some of the anomalies are difficult to discern.

54. Salerno TA, editor. *Warm Heart Surgery.* London: Arnold, 1995:230, $99.95.

55. Dean RH, Yao JST, Brewster DC, editors. *Diagnosis & Treatment in Vascular Surgery.* Norwalk, Connecticut: Appleton & Lange, 1995:461, $41.95.

CARDIAC TRANSPLANTATION

56. Frazier OH (editor), Macris MP and Radovančević (associate editors). *Support and Replacement of the Failing Heart.* Philadelphia: Lippincott-Raven Publishers, 1996:363, $149.95.

57. Helderman JH, Frist WH, editors. *Grand Rounds in Transplantation.* New York: Chapman & Hall, 1995:233, $69.95.

BASIC CARDIOVASCULAR PATHOPHYSIOLOGY AND ELECTROPHYSIOLOGY

58. Sperelakis N, editor. *Physiology and Pathophysiology of the Heart.* Third Edition. Boston: Kluwer Academic Publishers, 1995:1173, $395.00.

This is a major reference work of basic cardiology focusing primarily on cardiac ultrastructure, electrophysiology, cardiac contractility, ion exchange, and coronary circulation. Each page costs 34¢.

59. Sperelakis N. *Electrogenesis of Biopotentials in the Cardiovascular System.* Boston: Kluwer Academic Publishers, 1995:364, $105.00.

CARDIOVASCULAR PATHOLOGY

60. Stehbens WE, Lie JT, editors. *Vascular Pathology.* London: Chapman & Hall Medical, 1995:797, $169.00.

61. Ho SY, Baker EJ, Rigby ML, Anderson RH. *Color Atlas of Congenital Heart Disease. Morphologic and Clinical Correlations.* London: Mosby-Wolfe, 1995:192, $115.00.

CARDIAC ECONOMICS

62. Ott R, Tanner T, Henderson B, editors. *Managed Care and the Cardiac Patient.* Philadelphia: Hanley & Belfus, Inc., 1995:334, $45.00.

MISCELLANEOUS

63. Daniel WG, Kronzon I, Mügge A, editors. *Cardiogenic Embolism.* Baltimore: Williams & Wilkins, 1996:380, $75.00.

64. Hurst JW. *Cardiac Puzzles.* London: Mosby-Wolfe Medical Communications, 1995:210, $32.95.

Part I of this neat book includes a discussion of the clues the physician must be able to collect from the patient, and Part II includes the presentation of 50 puzzles. The goal of the book appears simple—if one can solve the carefully selected puzzles, he/she will understand most of the principles of cardiovascular medicine. Each puzzle is shown on the right hand page and the discussion is on the back of the page.

65. Weber KT, editor. *Wound Healing in Cardiovascular Disease.* Armonk, New York: Futura Publishing Company, Inc., 1995:320, $88.00.

66. Boudoulas H, Toutouzas PK, Wooley CF, editors. *Functional Abnormalities of the Aorta.* Armonk, New York: Futura Publishing Company, Inc., 1996:384, $85.00.

67. National Diabetes Data Group. *Diabetes in America.* Second Edition. Bethesda, Maryland: National Institutes of Health (NIH Publication No 95-1468), 1995:782, $20.00.

This is a splendid reference volume. Because patients with diabetes mellitus tend to die from complications of atherosclerosis, this book will be of value to cardiovascular specialists. (This book can be obtained from The National Diabetes Information Clearinghouse, National Institute of Diabetes and Digestive and Kidney Diseases, 1 Information Way, Bethesda, Maryland 20892-3560, telephone 301-654-3327.)

68. DeJong JW, Ferrari R, editors. *The Carnitine System. A New Therapeutical Approach to Cardiovascular Diseases.* Dordrecht: Kluwer Academic Publishers, 1995: 393, $250.00.

CARDIOLOGIC HISTORY

69. Neill C, Clark EB. *The Developing Heart: A "History" of Pediatric Cardiology.* Dordrecht: Kluwer Academic Publishers, 1995:169, $62.00.

A needed book.

70. Blackburn H. *On the Trail of Heart Attacks in Seven Countries.* Minneapolis: University of Minnesota, 1995:148, $20.00.

The Seven Countries study was the first to examine systematically the relation among lifestyle, diet, and the roles of heart attack and stroke in contrasting populations. It is the seminal study of cardiovascular disease epidemiology. Dr. Blackburn brings to life the adventures experienced while accumulating the data—both joys and tribulations—in these rural areas around the world.

71. Snellen HA. *Willhem Einthoven (1860–1927). Father of Electrocardiography. Life and Work, Ances-*

tors and Contemporaries. Dordrecht, Kluwer Academic Publishers, 1995:140, $40.00.

A splendid little book.

ANNUAL LITERATURE REVIEWS

72. Schlant RC (editor in chief), Collins JJ Jr, Engle MA, Gersh BJ, Kaplan NM, Waldo AL (editors). *The 1995 Year Book of CARDIOLOGY.* St. Louis: Mosby, 1995 (October):525, $74.95.

73. Roberts WC, Rackley CE, Willerson JT, Mason DT, Parmley WW, Graham TP, Jr. *CARDIOLOGY 1995.* Armonk, New York: Futura Publishing Company, Inc., 1995 (June):499, $69.00.

The Schlant book summarizes 304 articles each appearing in either 1993 or 1994. Comments on each article are provided by the various editors. The Roberts book includes summaries of 723 articles, all published in 1994. Its advantage is the larger number of articles discussed and all articles on the same subject are grouped together to read as a chapter; its disadvantage is the opinions of each author are not always discernible. The higher price of the Schlant book and the fewer numbers of articles summarized translates into 25¢ per article; the Roberts book translates into 10¢ per article. I obviously prefer the Roberts book.

COMMENTS

Of the 73 books mentioned herein, 20 (27%) have a 1996 publication date, which means that this piece, appearing January 1, 1996, is the first medical journal to mention the availability of these 20 books. The pages in the 73 books totalled 38,412, ranging from 79 (*ABC of Hypertension*) to 2,174 (Sabiston and Spencer, *Surgery of the Chest*) (mean 526 pages). The 73 books cost a total of $7,544.50, ranging from $20.00 to $395.00 (mean $103.00); 24 books (33%) cost more than $100.00. The 38,412 pages in the 73 books cost an average of 20¢ each. Of the 73 books, 47 (64%) were edited; 16 (22%) had a single author; 5 (7%) had 2 authors, and the remaining 5 books (7%) had 3 to 6 authors. Only 22 (30%) of the 73 books were published on acid-free (permanent) paper, the same percent as were published on acid-free paper last year. Authors need to stipulate acid-free paper in their contracts with publishers!

William C. Roberts

William Clifford Roberts, MD
Editor in Chief
Baylor University Medical Center
Dallas, Texas 75246

Good Books on Cardiovascular Disease Appearing in 1996

MAJOR GENERAL TEXTBOOKS

1. Braunwald E, editor. *Heart Disease. A Textbook of Cardiovascular Medicine.* Fifth Edition. Philadelphia: WB Saunders, 1997:2052, $125.00 (single volume), $140.00 (2-volume set).

This is the most comprehensive clinical book on cardiovascular disease that has ever appeared. The book has 63 chapters prepared by 81 authors and Braunwald is the author or coauthor of 15 (24%) of them. His editorial pen is clearly evident also in the other 48 chapters. The amount of information per page is incredible. The type size is small but necessary to get this much information in the 1996 pages of text. Additionally, the index has even smaller type and it is 53 pages long. The book has 2551 illustrations, 30 in full color, and 1257 in 2 color. There are 21 new chapters in this new edition. The references are extensive and right up to date. This masterpiece is "a must own" by anyone who even pretends to be a cardiovascular specialist. This book also is the best buy compared to the information included ever published in cardiovascular disease!

2. Giuliani ER, Gersh BJ, McGoon MD, Hayes DL, Schaff HV, editors. *Mayo Clinic Practice of Cardiology.* Third Edition. St. Louis: Mosby, 1996:2007, $129.95.

Fully packed, but I prefer the Braunwald book.

ATLASES

3. Schlant RC, Alexander RW, Lipton MJ, editors. *Diagnostic Atlas* of the *Heart.* New York: McGraw-Hill, 1996:398, $79.00.

4. Crawford MH, editor. *Atlas of Heart Diseases. Heart Disease in the Presence of Disorders of Other Organ Systems.* Volume VI. St. Louis: Mosby, 1996:191, $99.95.

5. Belch JJF, McCollum PT, Stonebridge PA, Walker WF. *Color Atlas of Peripheral Vascular Diseases.* Second Edition. London: Mosby-Wolfe, 1996:138, $69.95.

ARRHYTHMIAS AND CONDUCTION DISTURBANCES

6. Paradis NA, Halperin HR, Nowak RM, editors. *Cardiac Arrest. The Science and Practice of Resuscitation Medicine.* Baltimore: Williams & Wilkins, 1996:981, $99.00.

This book constitutes the first comprehensive treatise dealing exclusively with research and clinical issues in resuscitation medicine. The 53 chapters are produced by 96 contributors.

7. Podrid PJ, Kowey PR, editors. *Handbook of Cardiac Arrhythmia.* Baltimore: Williams & Wilkins, 1996:459, $39.00.

This is considerably more than a "handbook." A very good buy.

8. Waldo AL, Touboul P, editors. *Atrial Flutter. Advances in Mechanisms and Management.* Armonk, New York: Futura, 1996:480, $109.00.

Although there are a number of books on atrial fibrillation, atrial flutter has received far less attention. This book attempts to fill that void.

9. Atlee JL. *Arrhythmias and Pacemakers. Practical Management for Anesthesia and Critical Care Medicine.* Philadelphia: WB Saunders, 1996:465, $60.00.

This book provides in one volume the essential information pertaining to diagnosis and management of cardiac arrhythmias or pacemakers in perioperative and critical care settings.

10. Singer I, editor. *Interventional Electrophysiology.* Baltimore: Williams & Wilkins, 1997:1133, $115.00.

11. Saksena S, Lüderitz B, editors. *Interventional Electrophysiology. A Textbook.* Second Edition. Armonk, New York: Futura, 1996:659, $160.00.

12. Kroll MW, Lehmann MH, editors. *Implantable Cardioverter Defibrillator Therapy: The Engineering-Clinical Interface.* Dordrecht, The Netherlands: Kluwer Academic, 1996:585, $115.00.

13. Deedwania PC, editor. *Circadian Rhythms of Cardiovascular Disorders.* Armonk, New York: Futura, 1997:221, $55.00.

14. Blanc J-J, Benditt D, Sutton R, editors. *Neurally Mediated Syncope: Pathophysiology, Investigations, and Treatment. The Bakken Research Center Series Volume 10.* Armonk, New York: Futura, 1996:171, $55.00.

This book summarizes presentations at a symposium in June 1995 on Neurally Mediated Syncope.

ELECTROCARDIOLOGY AND AMBULATORY MONITORING

15. Chou T-C, Knilans TK. *Electrocardiography in Clinical Practice. Adult and Pediatric.* Fourth Edition. Philadelphia: WB Saunders, 1996:717, $95.00.

Of the 717 pages, 93% were written by Chou and 7% were written by Knilans. Each page is fully packed.

16. Moss AJ, Stern S, editors. *Noninvasive Electrocardiology. Clinical Aspects of Holter Monitoring.* London: WB Saunders, 1996:529, $59.00.

A collection of the newest information derived from the surface electrocardiogram.

ECHOCARDIOGRAPHY

17. St. John Sutton MG, Oldershaw PJ, Kotler MN, editors. *Textbook of Echocardiography and Doppler in Adults and Children.* Second Edition. Cambridge, Massachusetts: Blackwell Science, 1996:1047, $225.00.

A comprehensive book on this subject. In addition to the numerous black and white illustrations, it contains 64 pages of full color illustrations, with at least 4 per page.

18. Otto CM, editor. *The Practice of Clinical Echocardiography.* Philadelphia: WB Saunders, 1997:861, $165.00.

A beautiful book by 62 contributors. Each of the 861 pages is fully packed with information. It contains 1336 illustrations, 162 in full color.

19. Jawad IA. *A Practical Guide to Echocardiography and Cardiac Doppler Ultrasound.* Second Edition. Boston: Little, Brown, 1996:405, $39.95.

20. Kerut EK, McIlwain EF, Plotnick GD. *Handbook of Echo-Doppler Interpretation.* Armonk, New York: Futura, 1996:274, $39.00.

Both the Jaward and the Kerut et al books are very practical and easy-to-read instruction books of echocardiography.

CORONARY ARTERY DISEASE

21. Miller M, Vogel RA. *The Practice of Coronary Disease Prevention.* Baltimore: Williams & Wilkins, 1996:294, $24.95.

A terrific little book. I was asked by the authors to write the foreword and I did. Preventive cardiology is here.

22. Wainwright CL, Parratt JR, editors. *Myocardial Preconditioning.* Austin, Texas: R. G. Landes, 1996:281, $89.95.

23. Fuster V, editor; Stary HC, Chandler AB, Glagov S, Insull W Jr, Rosenfeld ME, Schwartz CJ, Wagner WD, Wissler RD, coeditors. *Syndromes of Atherosclerosis. Correlations of Clinical Imaging and Pathology.* Armonk, New York: Futura, 1996:558, $85.00.

This book contains lots of information on atherosclerotic plaques in the coronary, carotid, and ileofemoral arteries, aorta, and aortosaphenous venous grafts.

24. Willich SN, Muller JE, editors. *Triggering of Acute Coronary Syndromes. Implications For Prevention.* Dordrecht, The Netherlands: Kluwer Academic, 1996:491, $290.00.

A good book but hardly worth $0.59 a page. It's better to buy 2 Braunwald textbooks and give one away.

25. Thompson PL, editor. *Coronary Care Manual.* New York: Churchill Livingstone, 1997:693, $35.00.

A very good book for the money.

26. Gersh BJ, Rahimtoola SH, editors. *Acute Myocardial Infarction.* Second Edition. New York: Chapman & Hall, 1997:848, $99.95.

27. Califf RM, editor. *Atlas of Heart Diseases. Acute Myocardial Infarction and Other Acute Ischemic Syndromes.* Volume VIII. St. Louis: Mosby, 1996:250, $99.95.

A beautiful book under the series editorship of Eugene Braunwald. Book #4 is of the same series.

HEART FAILURE

28. Poole-Wilson PA, Colucci WS, Massie BM, Chatterjee K, Coats AJS, editors. *Heart Failure. Scientific Principles and Clinical Practice.* New York: Churchill Livingstone, 1997:929, $135.00.

A major reference book of 55 chapters by 93 contributors. Maybe the best thus far on this subject.

29. Dhalla NS, Singal PK, Takeda N, Beamish RE, editors. *Pathophysiology of Heart Failure.* Boston: Kluwer, 1996:578, $225.00.

This is a book primarily by basic scientists focusing on fundamental cardiomyopathic processes and ischemic perfusion injury.

30. Spinale GF, editor. *Pathophysiology of Tachycardia-Induced Heart Failure.* Armonk, New York: Futura, 1996:235, $48.00.

A lot on a limited subject.

THROMBOEMBOLISM

31. Pineo GF, Hull R, editors. *Disorders of Thrombosis.* Philadelphia: WB Saunders, 1996:447, $130.00.

32. Hull RD, Raskob GE, Pineo GF, editors. *Venous Thromboembolism: An Evidence-Based Atlas.* Armonk, New York: Futura, 1996:449, $149.00.

A multiauthored fine book.

33. Stein PD. *Pulmonary Embolism.* Baltimore: Williams & Wilkins, 1996:330, $37.95.

This is the best book I've seen on this topic. Much of the data were derived by continuing analysis of the database of the Prospective Investigation of Pulmonary Embolism Diagnosis (PIOPED). Most data presented has been published previously in peer review journals. The book is dedicated to the late Dr. Lewis Dexter, the first to position a catheter in a pulmonary artery, who contributed much to our knowledge on acute pulmonary embolism.

IMAGING

34. Skorton DJ, editor in chief; Schelbert HR, Wolf GL, Brundage BH, associate editors. *Marcus*

Cardiac Imaging, Second Edition, *A Companion to Braunwald's Heart Disease,* Volumes 1 and 2. Philadelphia: WB Saunders, 1996:1218, $195.00.

These 2 volumes with 116 contributors are major works on this subject. Over 1315 illustrations, 72 in color, are included.

35. Gerson MC, editor. *Cardiac Nuclear Medicine.* Third Edition. New York: McGraw-Hill, 1997:830, $120.00.

36. Marwick TH, editor. *Cardiac Stress Testing & Imaging. A Clinician's Guide.* New York: Churchill Livingstone, 1996:638, $75.00.

37. Nienaber CA, Sechtem U, editors. *Imaging and Intervention in Cardiology.* Dordrecht, The Netherlands: Kluwer Academic, 1996:547, $295.00.

A good book but is it worth $0.54 per page? No.

38. Schwaiger M, editor. *Cardiac Positron Emission Tomography.* Boston: Kluwer Academic, 1996:366, $250.00.

This book is for the imaging specialist only.

INTERVENTIONAL CARDIOLOGY

39. Peterson KL, Nicod P, editors. *Cardiac Catheterization. Methods, Diagnosis, and Therapy.* Philadelphia: WB Saunders, 1997:643, $95.00.

This first edition book by 40 contributors will give the Grossman book and the Pepine book a run for their money. It is very well done. Each page is fully packed.

40. Sigwart U, editor. *Endoluminal Stenting.* London: WB Saunders, 1996:601, $79.00.

Eighty chapters by 166 contributors. The major stentors are all here. A very useful book for stentors.

41. Kern MJ, Deligonul U, editors. *The Interventional Cardiac Catheterization Handbook.* St. Louis: Mosby, 1996:556, $44.00.

A nice book by 24 authors. It includes 211 illustrations.

MISCELLANEOUS

42. Smith TW, editor; Antman EM, Bittl JA, Colucci WS, Gotto AM Jr, Loscalzo J, Williams GH, Zipes DP, section editors. *Cardiovascular Therapeutics. A Companion to Braunwald's Heart Disease.* Philadelphia: WB Saunders, 1996:770, $95.00.

In the foreword Eugene Braunwald describes this book as ". . . the most comprehensive, modern text of cardiovascular therapeutics . . . scholarly . . . authoritative . . . landmark text." The intent is to provide the clinician with a practical, evidence-based approach to the optimal management of specific clinical problems. That goal was accomplished.

43. Kupersmith J, Deedwania PC, editors. *The Pharmacologic Management of Heart Disease.* Baltimore: Williams & Wilkins, 1997:581, $39.95.

A superb buy!

44. Khan MG. *Heart Disease Diagnosis and Therapy. A Practical Approach.* Baltimore: Williams & Wilkins, 1996:651, $49.00.

This is a user-friendly text that focuses only on common cardiologic conditions.

45. Sobel BE, editor; Cain ME, Eisenberg PR, associate editors. *Medical Management of Heart Disease.* New York: Marcel Dekker, 1996:566, $99.75.

46. Alpert JS, editor. *Cardiology for the Primary Care Physician.* St. Louis: Mosby, 1996:376, $125.00.

A heavily illustrated book of 43 brief chapters by 65 contributors.

47. Miller SW, editor. *Cardiac Radiology. The Requisites.* St. Louis: Mosby, 1996:447, $75.00.

A very nice book of 820 figures, almost all radiographs. Seven of the 10 chapters were contributed by Dr. Miller. Coronary angiography may be a bit short changed.

48. Mockrin SC, editor. *Molecular Genetics and Gene Therapy of Cardiovascular Disease.* New York: Marcel Dekker, 1996:591, $195.00.

49. Spodick DH. *The Pericardium. A Comprehensive Textbook.* New York: Marcel Dekker, 1997:464, $165.00.

David Spodick is the king of diseases involving the pericardium. He introduced the work "pericardiology" to describe the comprehensive scope of this book. This book is Dr. Spodick's fourth on the subject, but the most comprehensive one. Its drawback is the large price.

50. Boudoulas H, Toutouzas PK, Wooley CF, editors. *Functional Abnormalities of the Aorta.* Armonk, New York: Futura, 1996:398, $85.00.

51. Lanzer P, Lipton M, editors. *Diagnostics of Vascular Diseases. Principles and Technology.* Berlin: Springer, 1997:362, $159.00.

52. Rowlands DJ, editor. *Recent Advances in Cardiology.* New York: Churchill Livingstone, 1996:242, $69.95.

This book has 13 chapters, each covering a different topic. An interesting book.

53. Maccioli GA, editor. *Intra-aortic Balloon Pump Therapy.* Baltimore: Williams & Wilkins, 1997:206, $39.95.

All one needs to know on this subject is in one little book.

CARDIOVASCULAR SURGERY

54. Baue AE, editor; Geha AS, Laks H, Hammond GL, Naunheim KS, coeditors. *Glenn's Thoracic and Cardiovascular Surgery.* Sixth Edition. Volumes I and II. Stamford, Connecticut: Appleton & Lange, 1996:2428, $325.00.

55. Edmunds LH Jr, editor. *Cardiac Surgery in the Adult.* New York: McGraw-Hill, 1997:1632, $195.00.

Contains over 1200 illustrations.

56. Waldhausen JA, Pierce WS, Campbell DB, editors. *Surgery of the Chest.* Sixth Edition. St. Louis: Mosby, 1996:656, $129.00.

57. Doty DB. *Cardiac Surgery. Operative Technique.* St. Louis: Mosby, 1997:431, $179.00.

58. Khonsari S. *Cardiac Surgery. Safeguards and Pitfalls in Operative Technique.* Second Edition. Philadelphia: Lippincott-Raven, 1997:341, $195.00.

59. Harlan BJ, Starr A, Harwin FM. *Illustrated Handbook of Cardiac Surgery.* New York: Springer, 1996:321, $49.00.

Books 57-60 are how to-do-it books.

60. Litwin SB. *Color Atlas of Congenital Heart Surgery.* St. Louis: Mosby, 1996:240, $250.00.

A 4-color atlas of 627 photographs of the heart at operations for congenital heart disease.

61. Svensson LG, Crawford ES. *Cardiovascular and Vascular Disease of the Aorta.* Philadelphia: WB Saunders, 1997:472, $140.00.

This is a beautiful book by 2 masters of surgery of the aorta and its branches. It contains 889 illustrations and extensive text. This book is "a must own" for surgeons dealing with the aorta.

62. Williams GM, Schlossberg L. *Atlas of Aortic Surgery.* Baltimore: Williams & Wilkins, 1997:176, $175.00.

This book, written by the lead author and illustrated by the second author, demonstrates the retroperitoneal approach to the descending thoracic and abdominal aorta. The 99 illustrations alone make this book a collector's item.

63. Borst HG, Heinemann MK, Stone CD. *Surgical Treatment of Aortic Dissection.* New York: Churchill Livingstone, 1996:357. $119.95.

64. Williams JP, editor. *Postoperative Management* of the *Cardiac Surgical Patient.* New York: Churchill Livingstone, 1996:435, $80.00.

BIOLOGICAL AND MECHANICAL REPLACEMENT

65. Smith JA, McCarthy PM, Sarris GE, Stinson EB, Reitz BA, editors. *The Stanford Manual of Cardiopulmonary Transplantation.* Armonk, New York: Futura, 1996:306, $65.00.

66. Akutsu T, Koyanagi H, editors. *Heart Replacement. Artificial Heart 5. The 5th International Symposium on Artificial Heart and Assist Devices, January 26-27, 1995, Tokyo, Japan.* Tokyo: Springer, 1996:424, $289.00.

67. Frazier OH, editor; Macris MP, Radóvančević B, associate editor. *Support and Replacement of the Failing Heart.* Philadelphia: Lippincott-Raven, 1996:363, $149.95.

68. Cooper DKC, Novitsky D, Patterson GA, editors. *The Transplantation and Replacement of Thoracic Organs. The Present Status of Biological and Mechanical Replacement of the Heart and Lungs.* Second Edition. Dordrecht, The Netherlands: Kluwer Academic, 1997:820, $350.00.

CARDIOVASCULAR PATHOLOGY

69. Bharati S, Lev M. *The Pathology of Congenital Heart Disease. A Personal Experience With More Than 6,300 Congenitally Malformed Hearts.* Volumes 1 and 2. Armonk, New York: Futura, 1996:1579, $395.00.

This work is mainly an atlas. It contains hundreds of photographs of hearts and a rare diagram.

70. Manabe H, Yutani C, editors. *Atlas of Ischemic Heart Disease, Clinical and Pathologic Aspects.* New York: Churchill Livingstone, 1997:185, $140.00.

A color atlas focusing exclusively on coronary artery disease. The authors are good illustrators.

71. Virmani R, Farb A, Burke A. *Atlas of Cardiovascular Pathology.* Philadelphia: WB Saunders, 1996:224, $169.00.

This color atlas contains 484 illustrations, most of which are photomicrographs. The emphasis is on tissues excised at operation rather than those retrieved at necropsy. The text consists primarily of facts presented in bullet fashion about the various conditions. Most illustrations are excellent.

CARDIAC PSYCHOLOGY

72. Allan R, Scheidt S, editors. *Heart & Mind. The Practice of Cardiac Psychology.* Washington, DC: American Psychological Association, 1996:510, $49.95.

"Cardiac psychology" is a new phrase. This helps in my view in determining when atherosclerotic events occur, not why they occur. This volume increases awareness of the relation between psychological and physiological factors as they both influence cardiovascular health.

73. Orth-Gomér K, Schneiderman N, editors. *Behavioral Medicine Approaches to Cardiovascular Disease Prevention.* Mahwah, New Jersey: Lawrence Erlbaum Associates, 1996:324, $69.95.

The Allan-Scheidt book is a much better buy.

HEALTHY EATING

74. Page HC, Schroeder JS, Dickson TC. *The Stanford Life Plan for a Healthy Heart.* San Francisco: Chronicle Books, 1996:595, $29.95.

Intended for the lay public.

75. *Texas Heart Institute Heart Owner's Handbook.* New York: John Wiley & Sons, 1996:396, $16.95.

Intended for the lay public.

EXERCISE PROGRAMS

76. Paffenbarger RS Jr, Olsen E. *Lifefit. An Effective Exercise Program for Optimal Health and a Longer Life.* Leeds, United Kingdom: Human Kinetics, 1996:426.

77. Thomas RJ, editor. *The Heart and Exercise: A Practical Guide for the Clinician.* New York: Igaku-Shoin, 1996:140, $29.95.

ANNUAL REVIEWS

78. Roberts WC, Willerson JT, Graham TP Jr, Parmley WW, Rackley CE, Mason DT. *Cardiology 1996.* Armonk, New York: Futura, 1996:513, $75.00.

79. Schlant RC, editor in chief; Collins JJ Jr, Engle MA, Gersh BJ, Kaplan NM, Waldo AL, editors. St. Louis: Mosby, 1996:642, $76.95.

The Roberts book summarizes 784 articles on 515 pages. The Schlant book summarizes roughly half that number on 642 pages.

CARDIOLOGICAL HISTORY

80. Hollman A. *Sir Thomas Lewis. Pioneer Cardiologist and Clinical Scientist.* London: Springer, 1997:300, $75.00.

A splendid book. It also contains 145 figures, a very large number for a biography. Although he was the first to characterize nearly every arrhythmia and conduction disturbance by electrocardiography, Lewis spent only 15 years of his life actively working in cardiology. He founded the journal *Heart* which later became the *British Heart Journal* and has only recently reverted back to the original journal title, *Heart.*

COMMENTS

Of the 80 books mentioned herein, 21 (26%) have a 1997 publication date. The costs of the 78 books intended for physicians (excludes #74 and #75) ranged from $24.95 (#21) to $395.00 (#69) (mean $123.45). Ten books (13%) cost >$200.00 and 14 books (18%) cost <$50.00. The best buys by far were the large general textbooks. The Braunwald cardiology book costs only 6.1 cents/page, and the Giuliani et al cardiology book, 6.5 cents/page. The 2 large cardiovascular surgery textbooks (Baue et al [#54] and Edmunds [#55]) cost 13.4 and 11.9 cents/page, respectively. The 2 major surgery textbooks cost twice as much as the 2 major cardiology textbooks. From the standpoint of cost/page, only 1 book (#25) cost less than the Braunwald book (#1) and it was a manual with far less content per page. The average cost/page for the 78 medical books was 21 cents a page. Eleven books (#4, 5, 24, 37, 38, 58, 60, 62, 66, 70, and 71) each cost >50 cents/page, including 1 (#60) which cost $1.04/page and another (#62) which cost $0.99/page; 9 books (#1, 2, 19, 21, 25, 41, 43, 44 and 72) each cost <10 cents/page.

Some publishers clearly charge more for their books than do others and the quality differential appears to be nonexistent. Of 9 books published by Williams & Wilkins the cost/book ranged from $24.95 to $175.00 (mean $69.00) and the cost per page averaged 13 cents. In contrast, of 6 books published by Kluwer Academic the cost per book ranged from $115.00 to $350.00 (mean $254.00) and the cost per page averaged 45 cents!

Most medical books published in the USA continue to be published on acid paper including those published by WB Saunders, Mosby, Williams & Wilkins, Little-Brown, Churchill Livingstone, McGraw-Hill, and Lippincott-Raven. Only Futura, among the USA publishers, consistently uses acid-free paper. In contrast, most of the European publishers consistently use acid-free paper, including Kluwer Academic and Marcel Dekker. The acid-free books last many lifetimes and the figure reproductions are good; the acid books last a single lifetime and the figures and text are less crisp. The cost of acid paper and acid-free paper of similar weight is similar!

Happy book reading.

William Clifford Roberts, MD
Editor in Chief
Baylor Cardiovascular Institute
Baylor University Medical Center
Dallas, Texas 75246

Good Books on Cardiovascular Disease Appearing in 1997

MAJOR GENERAL TEXTBOOKS

1. Alexander RW, Schlant RC, Fuster V, editors: O'Rourke RA, Roberts R, Sonnenblick EH, associate editors. *Hurst's The Heart, Arteries and Veins,* Ninth Edition. New York: McGraw-Hill 1998:2,722, $130.00 (1 volume), $145.00 (2 volumes).*

2. Topol EJ, editor; Califf RM, Isner JM, Prystowsky EN, Serruys PW, Swain JL, Thomas JD, Thompson PD, Young JB, associate editors. *Textbook of Cardiovascular Medicine,* Philadelphia: Lippincott-Raven 1998:2,732, $99.95.

The latest edition (6th) of the Braunwald book appeared in November 1996 (1997 copyright) and the 9th edition of the original Hurst book—now edited by Alexander, Schlant and Fuster—appeared in November 1997 (1998 copyright). These 2 classics are now joined by Topol's first edition and it certainly will give the other 2 a run for their money. Both the Alexander-Schlant-Fuster book and the Topol book are similar in size (2,722 and 2,732 pages), numbers of chapters (105 and 98), and numbers of contributors (181 and 154). Both weigh the same (approximately 8.5 pounds). The Topol book has smaller type and less space between lines and therefore more content per page. Both are loaded with information. My recommendation is the same as for dictionaries. I have 3 of them that I use regularly. It's good to have all 3 of these major cardiovascular textbooks. Alternating the new one purchased with each new addition is reasonable. These major textbooks are the most cost beneficial books available in cardiovascular disease.

CARDIOVASCULAR PHARMACOTHERAPEUTICS

3. Frishman WH, Sonnenblick EH, editors. *Cardiovascular Pharmacotherapeutics.* New York: McGraw-Hill 1997:1,722, $85.00.

This book contains 74 chapters and 3 appendices and 52 (88%) of the 77 were authored in whole or in part by Bill Frishman. This superb comprehensive text addresses virtually every possible pharmacologic issue that a clinician might face in managing patients with both intrinsic cardiac and noncardiac vascular disease and patients having iotrogenic cardiac and systemic disorders from adverse drug reactions and drug-drug interactions.

GENERAL ANGIOGRAPHY

4. Baum S (vols I and II), Pentecost MJ (vol III), editors. *Abrams' Angiography. Vascular and Interventional Radiology,* Boston: Little, Brown 1997: 2,025 (vols I and II), 1,095 (vol III), $495.00.

Edition 3 appeared in 1983 so the present fourth edition 14 years later contains much new information. Volume III is dedicated entirely to interventional radiology. This is the bible on the entire field of angiography.

CONGENITAL HEART DISEASE

5. Freedom RM, Mawson JB, Yoo S-J, Benson LN. *Congenital heart disease. Textbook of Angiocardiography.* Armonk, NY: Futura 1997: 1,464 (vols I & II), $275.00 (both volumes).*

This is a beautiful book containing over 2,700 figures, most, but not all, are reproductions of 35-mm cineangiocardiograms. Although the focus is mainly angiography, there is much discussion in the text on prevalence, classification, morphologic features, associated malformations, prognosis, and a bit on therapy. The angiograms are accompanied by many diagrams and photographs of heart specimens. This is a *must* book for a pediatric cardiac library.

6. Freedom RM, volume editor; Braunwald E, series editor. *Atlas of Heart Diseases. Congenital Heart Disease, Volume XII.* St. Louis: Mosby 1997:274, $130.00.

A beautiful book consisting essentially of illustrations and legends for them. A big year for Robert Freedom!

7. Perloff JK, Child JS, editors. *Congenital Heart Disease in Adults, 2nd edition.* Philadelphia: W.B. Saunders 1998:393, $110.00.

The first edition of this book appeared in 1991. This 1998 edition represents a considerable expansion, larger page size, smaller type, and more illustrations. It's a must for a well-diversified cardiovascular library of any cardiologist.

8. Moller JH, editor. *Perspectives in Pediatric Cardiology,* Anderson RN, series editor. Volume 6. *Surgery of Congenital Heart Disease. Pediatric Cardiac Care Consortium* 1984–1995. Armonk, NY: Futura 1998:391, $97.00.*

This is a very useful book. It describes results of operations on congenital cardiac malformations pooled from a number of USA medical centers included in the Pediatric Cardiac Care Consortium (PCCC). With 11 years of data, the results of operations allow centers not in the database to compare their results to those included. From 1984 through 1994, data were gathered in 36,855 cardiac operations for a cardiac malformation. Of these, 5,447 were performed on neonates (<29 days), 9,566 on infants (29–365 days), 20,260 on children (1–21 years), and 1,582 on adults (>21 years).

9. Franco KL, editor. *Pediatric Cardiopulmonary Transplantation.* Armonk, NY: Futura 1997:397, $89.00.*

A good book on transplantation of the heart or lung(s) or both in the pediatric age group.

10. Ferencz C, Correa-Villaseñor A, Loffredo CA, Wilson PD. *Perspectives in Pediatric Cardiology. Volume 5. Genetic and Environmental Risk Factors of Major Cardiovascular Malformation: The Baltimore-Washington Infant Study:* 1981–1989, Armonk, NY: Futura 1997:463, $95.00.

This book describes findings in the Baltimore-Washington Infant Study of 4,390 cases of congenital heart disease and 3,572 controls from 6 pediatric cardiology centers involving 53 area hospitals and 800 physicians. Familial and infant characteristics were compiled on all cardiovascular malformations in the defined geographic area of about 100,000 annual births. This is a useful book for cardiovascular pediatricians.

LARGE GENERAL BOOK BUT NOT MAJOR TEXTBOOK

11. Murphy JG, editor. *Mayo Clinic Cardiology Review.* Armonk, NY: Futura 1997:724, $89.00.

This book by 56 contributors is aimed at cardiology fellows preparing for the board examination. Whenever a course or book emphasizes that it would be useful to those preparing for an examination, the number of enrollees and book buyers increases. That will probably be the case with this one. Its cost however is nearly that of the Alexander-Schlant-Fuster or Braunwald or Topol books and there is far more information in the major textbooks.

CORONARY ARTERY DISEASE

12. Yellon DM, Rahimtoola SH, Opie LH, editors. *New Ischemic Syndromes. Beyond Angina and Infarction.* Philadelphia: Lippincott-Raven 1997:237, $49.95.

These "new ischemic syndromes" include silent myocardial ischemia, myocardial stunning and hibernation, and preconditioning. As such it is useful.

13. Geschwind HJ, Kern MJ, editors. *Guidebook to Endovascular Coronary Diagnostic Techniques.* Armonk, NY: Futura 1997:552, $125.00.*

14. Grech ED, Ramsdale DR, editors. *Practical Interventional Cardiology.* St. Louis: Mosby 1997: 413, $99.95.

15. King SB III, Douglas JS Jr, editors. *Atlas of Heart Diseases. Interventional Cardiology. Volume XIII.* St. Louis: Mosby 1997:199, $125.38.*

16. Leon MB, Saftian RD, Freed M. *Interventional Cardiology. Self-Assessment & Review.* Birmingham, Michigan: Physicians' Press 1998:380, $45.00.

The first question-answer book on this topic. Quite useful.

17. Reisman M. *Guide to Rotational Atherectomy.* Birmingham, Michigan: Physicians' Press 1997:317, $59.95.

18. Phillips PS, Kern MJ, Serruys PW. *The Stenter's Notebook.* Birmingham, Michigan: Physicians' Press 1998:211, $49.95.

Also includes 27 color slides of 27 stent designs.

19. Rotterdam Thoraxcentre Group (Serruys PW, editor in chief). *Handbook of Coronary Stents.* St. Louis: Mosby 1997:163, $69.95.

All of the above 7 interventional books (numbers 13–19) are useful to those in this field. The illustrations in the King-Douglas book are wonderful.

20. Talley JD, Mauldin PD, Becker ER, editors. *Cost Effective Diagnosis and Treatment of Coronary Artery Disease.* Baltimore: Williams & Wilkins 1997: 227, $49.95.

It's good, of course, to know the price of cardiovascular medicine. This book is useful in that regard.

21. Klein LW, editor. *Coronary Stenosis Morphology: Analysis and Implication.* Boston: Kluwer Academic 1997:392, $187.00.*

This book contains some useful information, but it is poorly produced by the publisher who nevertheless prices it unrealistically ($187.00).

SYSTEMIC HYPERTENSION

22. Kaplan NM. *Clinical Hypertension, Seventh Edition.* Baltimore: Williams & Wilkins 1998:444, $79.00.

The first edition of this classic appeared in 1973 and subsequent ones have appeared usually every 4 years since. If you buy only 1 book on systemic hypertension, this is the one to have. It's a pleasure to have such a good book authored by a single person (except for 1 chapter).

23. Opie LH, Messerli FH, editors. *Combination Drug Therapy for Hypertension.* New York, NY: Author's Publishing House Lippincott-Raven 1997:178, $49.95.

This is a small and useful book. It is the first to address exclusively the issue of combination drug therapy in systemic hypertension. The book addresses the advantages of combining different antihypertensive drugs (greater potency, fewer side effects, beneficial hemodynamic and neurohumoral interactions). The book covers virtually all possible combinations of 2 drugs among the major classes (diuretics, beta blockers, ACE inhibitors, calcium antagonists, alpha blockers, and angiotensin-receptor inhibitors). Despite the emphasis on combination therapy, whether combination drug therapy reduces cardiovascular morbidity and mortality better than monotherapy, is not answered because it remains unknown.

24. Zanchetti A, Mancia G, editors. Volume 17. *Pathophysiology of Hypertension.* (In: *Handbook of Hypertension.* series editors Birkenhäger WH and Reid JL). Amsterdam: Elsevier 1997:1,102, $465.75.*

25. Hansson L, Birkenhäger WH, editors. Volume 18. *Assessment of Hypertensive Organ Damage.* (In: *Handbook of Hypertension,* series editors Birkenhäger WH and Reid JL). Amsterdam: Elsevier 1997:402, $309.50.*

The latter 2 books contain a lot of information. The 2 together cost $775.25.

ELECTROCARDIOGRAPHY

26. O'Keefe JH Jr, Hammill SC, Freed M. *The Complete Guide to ECGs—1997.* Birmingham, Michigan: Physicians' Press 1997:593, $69.95.

ECHOCARDIOGRAPHY

27. Snider AR, Serwer GA, Ritter SB. *Echocardiography in Pediatric Heart Disease. Second Edition.* St. Louis: Mosby 1997:598, $175.00.

Splendid book.

28. Abuhamad A. *A Practical Guide to Fetal Echocardiography.* Philadelphia: Lippincott-Raven 1997: 127, $80.00.

This book costs nearly 50 cents per page. This topic is also well covered in the Snider-Serwer-Ritter book.

29. Nanda NC, Schlief R, Goldberg BB, editors. *Advances in Echo Imaging Using Contrast Enhancement. Second Edition.* Dordrecht: Kluwer Academic 1997:698, $155.00.*

The first edition of this book appeared in 1993. This new edition, the only book available dealing with contrast echocardiography, has been expanded by 20 chapters and 300 pages. It may be a "must book" for echocardiographers.

30. Siegel RJ, editor. *Intravascular Ultrasound Imaging in Coronary Artery Disease.* New York, NY: Marcel Decker 1998:367, $155.00.

An excellent book.

GENERAL CARDIAC IMAGING

31. Chen JTT, editor. *Essentials of Cardiac Imaging. 2nd edition.* Philadelphia: Lippincott-Raven, 1997:378, $132.50.

Nice general book on a wide range of imaging techniques.

ARRHYTHMIAS, CONDUCTION DISTURBANCES, AND ELECTROPHYSIOLOGY

32. Murgatroyd FD, Camm AJ, editors. *Nonpharmacological Management of Atrial Fibrillation.* Armonk, NY: Futura 1997:536, $120.00.*

Because atrial fibrillation is so common (3 million in the USA, 0.4% of the entire population, 4% of the hospital population, and 40% of patients with congestive heart failure), books on this topic are welcomed. This one contains 34 chapters by 81 contributors and it contains essentially all information available on this topic.

33. El-Sherif N, Lekieffre J, editors. *Practical Management of Cardiac Arrhythmias.* Armonk, NY: Futura 1997:348, $95.00.*

The first part of this book deals with pharmacological treatment of supraventricular and ventricular arrhythmias, and the second part focuses on radiofrequency catheter ablation.

34. Singer I, editor. *Interventional Electrophysiology.* Baltimore: Williams & Wilkins 1997:1,133, $117.00.

This is a major multiauthored textbook on electrophysiology discussing in detail 1) the interventional laboratory itself, 2) radiofrequency ablation, 3) surgical ablation techniques, 4) implantable cardioverter defibrillators, and 5) pacemakers. It also is an attractive book.

35. Daubert JC, Prystowsky EN, Ripart A, editors. *Prevention of Tachyarrhythmias and Cardiac Pacing.* Armonk, NY: Futura 1997:203, $39.50.

36. Barold SS, Mugica J, editors. *Recent Advances in Cardiac Pacing. Goals for the 21st Century.* Armonk, NY: Futura 1998:454, $98.00.*

37. Spooner PM, Joyner RW, Jalife J, editors. *Discontinuous Conduction of the Heart.* Armonk, NY: Futura 1997:569, $95.00.*

This book is "too heavy" for most clinical electrophysiologists. It focuses on "discontinuity in cardiac conduction," which is multidimensional divergence and anisotropy in intertissue and intercellular communication between cardiocytes.

38. Morillo CA, Klein GJ, Yee R, Guiraudon GM. *The Wolff-Parkinson-White Syndrome.* (A part of Clinical Approaches to Tachyarrhythmias edited by Camm AJ, volume 6). Armonk, NY: Futura 1997:143, $24.00.*

39. Schwartz PJ, Matteo PS. *The Long QT Syndrome.* (A part of Clinical Approaches to Tachyarrhythmias edited by Camm AJ, volume 7), Armonk, NY: Futura 1997:108, $24.00.*

40. Schurig L, Gura M, Taibi B, editors. *Educational Guidelines Pacing and Electrophysiology, Second Edition,* Armonk, NY: Futura 1997:621, $45.00.*

This book is directed to the registered nurse, physician assistant, and cardiovascular technician working in the electrophysiology laboratory.

41. Hayes DL, Wang PJ, editors. *Cardiac Pacemakers and Implantable Defibrillators: A Workbook in 3 Volumes.*

Volume 1. Hayes DL, Wang PJ, Irwin ME, Camm AJ. *Cardiac Pacing: A Case Approach.* 1998:102, $25.00.

Volume 2. Wang PJ, Estes NAM, Camm AJ. *Implantable Defibrillators: A Case Approach.* 1998:72, $25.00.

Volume 3. Christiansen JR, Hayes DL. *Transtelephonic Electrocardiography and Troubleshooting: A Case Approach.* 1998:82, $25.00.

In each of the above volumes, a question is posed with an electrocardiographic tracing or radiograph and the answer follows. Each of these books could be smaller because there is much wasted space in each.

SUDDEN CARDIAC DEATH

42. Dunbar SB, Ellenbogen KA, Epstein AE, editors. *Sudden Cardiac Death. Past, Present, and Future.* Armonk, NY: Futura 1997:417, $78.00.*

This book contains 23 chapters contributed by 48 authors, many of whom are recognized leading investigators. A fine book.

43. Skinner DV, Vincent R. *Cardiopulmonary Resuscitation, Second Edition.* Oxford: Oxford University Press 1997:222, $44.00.

This book provides all the theoretical knowledge required to manage a patient having cardiac arrest successfully.

VALVULAR HEART DISEASE

44. Rahimtoola SH, volume editor (Braunwald E, series editor). *Atlas of Heart Diseases. Valvular Heart Disease,* volume XI. St. Louis: Mosby 1997:321, $130.00.

Beautiful book.

CARDIOVASCULAR DISEASE IN WOMEN

45. Julian DG, Wenger NK, editors. *Women and Heart Disease.* St. Louis: Mosby 1997:454, $124.00.

Several books have appeared in recent years on this subject. This one may be the best yet.

46. Forte TM, editor. *Hormonal, Metabolic, and Cellular Influences on Cardiovascular Disease in Women.* Armonk, NY: Futura 1997:365, $85.00.*

This text reviews the information available on the use of estrogen replacement therapy.

EXERCISE TESTING AND EXERCISE TRAINING

47. Jones NL. *Clinical Exercise Testing. Fourth edition.* Philadelphia: WB Saunders 1997:259, $49.95.

The first edition appeared in 1975 and the last one in 1988. The extensively revised present edition represents a considerable expansion. Each page is fully packed.

48. Balady GJ, Piña IL, editors. *Exercise and Heart Failure.* Armonk, NY: Futura 1997:354, $75.00.*

This book focuses on exercise training as a therapeutic intervention in patients with heart failure and in patients who have had cardiac transplantation. It is quite useful and it is edited by 2 recognized experts in this area.

49. Fardy PS, Franklin BA, Porcari JP, Verrill DE, editors. *Training Techniques in Cardiac Rehabilitation.* (Monograph number 3 of Current Issues in Cardiac Rehabilitation edited by Fardy PS), Champaign, Illinois; Human Kinetics 1998:144, $24.00.

This nice little book provides in-depth information about the broad range of exercise based cardiac rehabilitation programs presently available. The first chapter covers exercise activities available for coronary patients and subsequent chapters focus on swimming training, resistance exercise, and innovative calisthenics.

MISCELLANEOUS

50. Sasahara AA, Loscalzo J, editors. *New Therapeutic Agents in Thrombosis and Thrombolysis.* New York: Marcel Dekker 1997:681, $195.00.*

This is a major textbook focusing on hemostasis, thrombosis, and thrombolysis. A splendid book.

51. Mohsenifar Z, Shah PK, editors. *Practical Critical Care in Cardiology.* New York: Marcel Dekker 1998:449, $165.00.*

This fine book provides 16 chapters dealing with the highly complex management of the critically ill cardiac patient.

52. Jackson G, editor. *Difficult Cardiology III.* St. Louis: Mosby 1997:419, $99.50.

This book takes 19 subjects "where opinion is divided," reviews the evidence, and then tries to be as practical as possible. It seems that there are very few topics in cardiology or in any other field for that matter where opinion is not divided, assuming that if it is not 100% it is divided.

53. Elliott HL, editor. *Current Issues in Cardiovascular Therapy.* St. Louis: Mosby 1997:221, $75.00.

This book is similar to the book edited by Jackson (number 52). Fourteen different topics are discussed.

54. Hultgren H. *High Altitude Medicine.* Stanford, California: Hultgren Publications 1997:550, $59.95.

Herb Hultgran is gone and it's a tribute to him that he left this fine book in his final year. The first 11 chapters deal with physiologic effects of high altitude on numerous organ systems. High-altitude diseases—pulmonary edema, acute and chronic mountain sickness, sleep disorders, syncope, retinal hemorrhage, headache, etc.—are discussed in chapters 12–22. Then, sea-level medical conditions—chronic obstructive pulmonary disease, coronary artery disease, and systemic and pulmonary hypertension—that are adversely affected by altitude are discussed. The appendix contains medicolegal aspects of wilderness travel and a list of 74 high-altitude monographs with a succinct summary of each. This book, written by an avid mountain man, will be the ultimate reference source on this subject for a long time to come.

55. Pitt B, Julian D, Pocock S, editors. *Clinical Trials in Cardiology.* London: W.B. Saunders 1997:386, $90.00.*

This fine book reviews critically a number of published major randomized clinical cardiovascular trials, and it considers the standards by which such trials should be evaluated. The authors of the 19 chapters were asked by the editors to give their opinions as to what was learned from each trial, to point out deficiencies in the accumulated data, and to suggest areas for further clinical investigation.

56. Lilly LS, editor. *Pathophysiology of Heart Disease. A Collaborative Project of Medical Students and Faculty.* Second Edition. Baltimore: Williams & Wilkins 1998:401, $29.00.

The first edition of this unique book appeared in 1993 and the present one is an expanded and updated version of the first edition. The book represents a collaborative project of Harvard Medical Students and Faculty. Lilly brought together a group of talented students and faculty to produce a book specifically designed to meet the needs of medical students during their initial encounters with patients with cardiac disease.

57. Grubb BP, Olshansky B, editors. *Syncope: Mechanisms and Management.* Armonk, NY: Futura 1998:416, $89.00.*

This useful book may be the first one to deal comprehensively with syncope and provide useful guidelines for its management.

58. Aronow WS, Stemmer EA, Wilson SE, editors. *Vascular Disease in the Elderly.* Armonk, NY: Futura 1997:574, $120.00.*

A fine book dealing with multiple arterial vascular systems in the elderly and how to manage these problems.

59. Rubanyi GM, Dzau VJ, editors. *The Endothelium in Clinical Practice. Source and Target of Novel Therapies.* New York: Marcel Dekker 1997:551, $195.00.*

The first part of this fine book describes existing and emerging therapies based on endothelial factors and molecules. The second part describes novel therapeutic approaches targeting pathophysiologic processes associated with the vascular endothelium. The last part focuses on the role of endothelium in gene therapy.

60. March KL, editor. *Gene Transfer in the Cardiovascular System. Experimental Approaches and Therapeutic Implications. Boston: Kluwer Academic 1997:516, $119.50.**

This book puts in one place a vast amount of information on gene transfer potentials in the cardiovascular system.

CARDIOVASCULAR SURGERY

61. Sidawy AN, Sumpio BE, DePalma RG, editors. *The Basic Science of Vascular Disease.* Armonk, NY: Futura 1997:904, $175.00.*

This is a major textbook of basic aspects of vascular disease wherever it might occur in the body.

62. Carpentier AF, Chachques JC, Grandjean PA, editors. *Cardiac Bioassist.* Armonk, NY: Futura 1997: 632, $125.00.*

This book provides an up-to-date state of the arteries in ventricular assistance by biological means, i.e., cardiomyoplasty and aortomyoplasty, muscle-powered artificial ventricles and cellular and molecular cardiomyoplasty.

63. Li CM, Chiu R C-J. *Dynamic Cardiomyoplasty. The Mechanisms and Optimization of Programming (volume I).* Armonk, NY: Futura 1997:55, $15.00.*

This small book describes what is currently known about the mechanisms of action of cardiomyoplasty and methods to optimally program the cardiomyostimulator.

SMALL HANDY COAT-POCKET BOOKS

64. Feher MD, Richmond W. *Lipids and Lipid Disorders. Second Edition.* Chicago: Mosby-Wolfe 1997:106, $15.00.

This is mainly a picture book but the pictures are beautiful. It's a good one to have in the pocket at the Lipid Clinic.

65. Froelicher VF, Quaglieti S. *Handbook of Ambulatory Cardiology.* Philadelphia: Lippincott-Raven 1997:397, $24.95.

This is a nice book featuring the ADVIsE approach to patients. The key features of this approach are: 1) myocardial *dysfunction* or damage; 2) myocardial *is*chemia; 3) *valvular* dysfunction; 4) *exercise* capacity (the amount that can be performed), and 5) *arrhythmias* and conduction disturbances.

66. Khan MG, *On Call Cardiology.* Philadelphia: W. B. Saunders 1997:343, $19.50.

The common "on-call" cardiologic problems are discussed here: chest pain, tamponade, aortic dissection, hypotension and shock, acute dyspnea, peripheral and pulmonary edema, bothersome cough, heart failure, tachy- and bradyarrhythmias, severe hypertension, syncope, cardiac arrest, and deep venous thrombosis. Numerous electrocardiograms are illustrated.

67. Patterson DLH. *Clinical Cardiology. Self-Assessment Picture Tests. Second Edition.* London: Mosby-Wolfe 1997:140, $19.95.

Mainly a picture book.

68. Timmis A, Brecker S. *Cardiology. Diagnosis in Color.* London: Mosby-Wolfe 1997:275, $30.00.

A picture book.

69. Sharkey SW. *A Guide to Interpretation of HEMODYNAMIC DATA in the Coronary Care Unit.* Philadelphia: Lippincott-Raven 1997:214, $36.00.

This book describes what can be learned from the Swan Ganz catheter (bedside hemodynamic monitoring).

ANNUAL CARDIOLOGY REVIEW

70. Willerson JT, Roberts WC, Rackley CE, Graham TP Jr., Mason DT, Parmley WW. *Cardiology 1997.* Armonk, NY: Futura 1997:622, $98.00.*

This book summarizes 738 articles published in medical journals in 1996. No other cardiologic annual book contains as much information as does this one.

Jim Willerson did a superb job in putting all this information together under 1 cover. The amount of space between topics has been increased in the 1997 edition compared with the 1996 book and therefore the size of the book has increased without an increase in the number of articles summarized.

CARDIOVASCULAR BOOK WRITTEN PRIMARILY FOR THE LAY PUBLIC

71. DeBakey ME, Gotto AM Jr. *The New Living Heart.* Holbrook, Massachusetts: Adams Media Corporation 1997:495, $17.95.

In 1977 Doctors DeBakey and Gotto published *The Living Heart* which was written to provide the layman with a better understanding of the many different forms of disease of the heart and blood vessels, to indicate what could be done about it, and to suggest what a person could do to help prevent its development. The present book is an expansion and update of the one appearing 20 years ago.

COMMENTS

Each of the 71 books mentioned herein were sent to me by the publisher. Therefore, the books mentioned herein are only those sent to me by the publishers. Of the 71 books, 14 (20%) have a 1998 publication date and 57 (80%) have a 1997 date. The costs of the 70 books intended for physicians or allied health-care givers (excludes #71) ranged from $15.00 to $495.00 (mean $104.95). Twelve books (17%) cost >$150.00 and 20 books (29%) cost <$50.00. The 2 large general cardiovascular texts (#1 and #2) were good buys: the Alexander-Schlant-Fuster book (#1) cost 4.8 cents/page, and the Topol book (#2), 3.7 cents/page.

Most medical books published in the USA continue to be published on acid paper including those published by W. B. Saunders, Mosby, Williams & Wilkins, Little-Brown, and Lippincott-Raven. Only Futura, among the US publishers, consistently uses acid-free paper. In contrast, most of the European publishers consistently use acid-free paper, including Kluwer Academic, Marcel Dekker, and Elsevier. The 30 books (43%) published on acid-free paper herein are marked with an asterisk. The acid free books last many lifetimes; the acid books, a single lifetime. The cost of acid and acid-free paper from most printers is similar!

Happy book reading!

William C. Roberts

William Clifford Roberts, MD
Editor in Chief
Baylor Cardiovascular Institute
Baylor University Medical Center
Dallas, Texas 75246

Good Books on Cardiovascular Disease Appearing in 1998

MAJOR TEXTBOOKS

1. Garson A Jr, Bricker JT, Fisher DJ, Neish SR, editors. *The Science and Practice of Pediatric Cardiology. Second Edition.* Baltimore: Williams & Wilkins, 1998:3072, $395.00.

The first edition of this 2 volume text first appeared in 1990. The second edition clearly establishes this textbook as the best in pediatric cardiology. Each page is fully packed.

2. Topol EJ, editor. *Comprehensive Cardiovascular Medicine.* Philadelphia: Lippincott-Raven 1998: 3311 (2 volumes), $275.00.

This "magnum opus" contains 121 chapters and 3,153 fully packed pages divided into 2 volumes. The entire text and graphics are captured in CD-ROM, enriched with >1,000 images. The book in actuality is an extension of *Textbook of Cardiovascular Medicine,* a single volume of "only" 98 chapters and 2,732 pages, 421 less than the present version. Just like the *Textbook* the *Comprehensive* one is superb, but buy one or the other, not both.

3. Yusuf S, Cairns JA, Camm AJ, Fallen EL, Gersh BJ. *Evidence Based Cardiology.* London: BMJ Books 1998:1123, $225.00.

This is an interesting book. It does not contain as much information as other major textbooks—Braunwald; Alexander-Schlant-Fuster, Willerson, or Topol—but it contains a lot and the recommendations are graded as to the levels of evidence used.

4. Kaiser LR, Kron IL, Spray TL, editors. *Mastery of Cardiothoracic Surgery.* Philadelphia: Lippincott-Raven 1998:976, $175.00.

Although the editors consider it somewhere between a textbook and an atlas, this book is a textbook in my view and a very good one. Each of the 92 chapters is followed by an *Editor's Comments*, including those of another editor when the chapter is written by one of the editors. I particularly liked these commentaries.

CORONARY ARTERY DISEASE

5. Gould KL. *Coronary Artery Stenosis and Reversing Atherosclerosis. Second Edition.* London: Arnold 1999:689, $129.00.

This single-author book is superb and it is nicely priced.

6. Topol EJ, editor. *Textbook of INTERVENTIONAL CARDIOLOGY. Third Edition.* Philadelphia: W.B. Saunders Company 1999:967, $155.00.

This outstanding book of 51 chapters by 82 contributors is packed full of information on this topic.

***7.** Topol EJ, editor. *ACUTE CORONARY SYNDROMES.* New York: Marcel Dekker 1998:628, $99.75.

Once Topol got into books he has gone gangbusters. He and Braunwald are now the dominant cardiologic book editors. This one of 21 chapters by 36 contributors is very good.

8. Brown DL, editor. *Cardiac Intensive Care.* Philadelphia: W.B. Saunders Company 1998:836, $125.00.

This comprehensive book contains 63 chapters by 121 contributors and each page is fully packed.

***9.** Cannon CP, editor. *Management of Acute Coronary Syndromes.* Totowa NJ: Humana Press 1999: 659, $125.00.

This book of 26 chapters by 47 contributors is excellent.

***10.** Wu AHB, editor. *Cardiac Markers.* Totowa, NJ: Humana Press 1998;300, $99.50.

This useful book of 17 chapters by 15 contributors describes the current and future markers for atherosclerotic coronary artery disease and how they are used in clinical practice.

***11.** Clements IP, editor. *The Electrocardiogram in Acute Myocardial Infarction.* Armonk, NY: Futura Publishing Company 1998:260, $65.00.

This useful book of 16 chapters by 18 contributors provides an up-to-date review of the electrocardiogram in acute myocardial infarction.

12. Davies MJ. *Atlas of Coronary Artery Disease.* Philadelphia: Lippincott-Raven 1998:161, $125.00.

This book includes 4 chapters: anatomy of the coronary arteries (contributed by Siew Yen Ho); atherosclerosis; acute ischemic syndromes and coronary progression, and stable angina. The book contains many fine pictures but no numbers.

***13.** Bates ER, Holmes DR, Jr., editors. *Saphenous Vein Bypass Graft Disease.* New York: Marcel Dekker 1998:329, $150.00.

This book is a good one on this topic but it is very expensive.

***14.** Oz MC, Goldstein DJ, editors. *Minimally Invasive Cardiac Surgery.* Iotowa, NJ: Humana Press 1999:237, $125.00.

A wonderful book on this topic.

***15.** Krieger KH, Isom OW, editors. *Blood Conservation in Cardiac Surgery.* New York: Springer-Verlag 1998:683, $89.00.

This book of 27 chapters by 30 contributors is needed. The editors using their algorithm recently completed 100 consecutive coronary bypass operations without a single donor exposure (no red blood cells, no blood factors).

THROMBOSIS

16. Loscalzo J, Schafer AI, editors. *Thrombosis and Hemorrhage, Second Edition.* Baltimore: Williams & Wilkins 1998:1449, $275.00.

The first edition of this book is only 4 years old. This new one in such a short time shows how fast this increasingly complex field of hemostasis is expanding. This book provides a comprehensive review of the pathobiology and clinical disorders of the hemostatic system in 52 chapters by 111 contributors.

17. Verstraete M, Fuster V, Topol EJ, editors. *CARDIOVASCULAR THROMBOSIS. Thrombocardiology and Thromboneurology. Second Edition.* Philadelphia: Lippincott-Raven 1998:871, $129.00.

The first edition *(Thrombosis in Cardiovascular Disorders)* appeared in 1992, and this second edition is large (51 chapters) and better. Its contributors numbered 106 authors. The word *thrombocardiology* was first used by Eugene Braunwald when writing the foreword to the first edition. *Thromboneurology* was added by the editors. This book is useful to cardiologists, neurologists and hematologists, and right up to date.

PREVENTION

***18.** Gotto AM Jr, Lenfant C, Paoletti R, Catapano AL, Jackson AS, editors. *Multiple Risk Factors in Cardiovascular Disease. Strategies of Prevention of Coronary Heart Disease, Cardiac Failure, and Stroke. Dordrecht:* Kluwer Academic Publishers 1998:370, $119.00.

This book of 40 chapters by 81 contributors summarizes proceedings of a meeting held in April 1997.

***19.** LaRosa JC, editor. *Medical Management of Atherosclerosis.* New York: Marcel Dekker 1998:326, $135.00.

This good book of 12 chapters by 21 contributors focuses on therapies to prevent and arrest atherosclerosis.

20. Stone NJ, Blum CB, Winslow E. *Management of Lipids in Clinical Practice. Second Edition.* Caddo, OK: Professional Communications 1998:316, $17.95.

A useful little book which fits nicely into the pocket of the white coat.

ARRHYTHMIAS, CONDUCTION DISORDERS, AND SUDDEN DEATH

***21.** Singer I, Barold SS, Camm AJ, editors. *Nonpharmacological Therapy of Arrhythmias for the 21st Century. The State of the Art.* Armonk, NY: Futura Publishing Company 1998:908, $125.00.

This fine book with 82 contributors discusses in detail catheter ablation techniques, implantable defibrillation therapy, arrhythmia surgery and mapping technologies, and pacing. The book of course is particularly useful to the interventional electrophysiologist.

***22.** Jalife J, Delmar M, Davidenko JM, Anumonwo JMB. *Basic Cardiac Electrophysiology For the Clinician.* Armonk, NY: Futura Publishing Company 1999:306, $55.00.

This book of 8 chapters focuses on basic cardiac electrophysiology but tries to make it understandable for the clinician. I believe they succeed.

***23.** Deal BJ, Wolff GS, Gelband H, editors. *Current Concepts in Diagnosis and Management of Arrhythmias in Infants and Children.* Armonk, NY: Futura Publishing Company 1998:438, $95.00.

This fine book of 14 chapters by 17 contributors actually began in 1977 in a book entitled *Cardiac Arrhythmias in the Neonate, Infant and Child* and in its revision in 1983. The present newly titled book is a comprehensive text intended for physicians who care for neonates, infants, and children with cardiac arrhythmias.

24. Williams EMV, Somberg JC. *Control of Cardiac Rhythm.* Philadelphia: Lippincott-Raven 1998: 186, $93.00.

This fine book provides a thorough historical review and an up-to-date account of the development and current usage of antiarrhythmic therapy.

***25.** Farré J, Moro C, editors. *Ten Years of Radiofrequency Catheter Ablation.* Armonk, New York: Futura Publishing 1998:373, $145.00.

This book of 26 chapters by 71 contributors (only 3 from the USA) is a fine book on this topic.

***26.** Saoudi N, Schoels W, El-Sherif N, editors. *Atrial flutter and fibrillation. From Basic to Clinical Applications.* Armonk, NY: Futura Publishing Company 1998:372, $85.00.

This book of 21 chapters by 66 contributors covers this topic thoroughly.

***27.** Fischer W, Ritter P. *Cardiac Pacing in Clinical Practice.* Berlin: Springer-Verlag 1998:457, $65.00.

A comprehensive text on cardiac pacing by 2 authors.

***28.** Estes NAM III, Salem DN, Wang PJ, editors. *Sudden Cardiac Death in the Athlete.* Armonk, New York: Futura Publishing 1998:600, $89.00.

This book, which contains 34 chapters by 47 contributors, discusses the various causes of sudden death in athletes and how to prevent it.

***29.** Bossaert L, editor. European *Resuscitation Council Guidelines for Resuscitation.* Amsterdam: Elsevier 1998:217, $72.00.

This 1998 edition of the European Resuscitation Council brings together all new and revised Guidelines for Resuscitation that were produced earlier (1992) by the International Liaison Committee on Resuscitation.

30. Weil MH, Tang W, editors. *CPR. Resuscitation of the Arrested Heart.* Philadelphia: W. B. Saunders Company 1999:318, $45.00.

This book of 21 chapters by 37 contributors covers this topic thoroughly.

SYSTEMIC HYPERTENSION

31. Frohlich ED. *Hypertension: Evaluation and Treatment.* Baltimore: William & Wilkins 1998:212, $45.00.

A single-authored book is unusual these days but Frohlich has produced a good one designed specifically for the primary care physician.

32. Hollenberg NK, Volume editor; Braunwald E, Series editor. *Atlas of Heart Diseases. Hypertension: Mechanisms and Therapy. Second Edition.* Philadelphia: Blackwell Science 1998:224, $99.00.

This book of 13 chapters by 19 contributors is beautiful.

HEART FAILURE

33. Rose EA, Stevenson LW, editors. *Management of End-Stage Heart Disease.* Philadelphia: Lippincott-Raven 1998:271, $125.00.

This book contains 21 chapters by 40 contributors. Heart failure patients admitted to the hospital in the USA yearly is approaching 1,000,000 and 100,000 to 200,000 of them have end-stage heart failure. This excellent book discusses the latter group of patients.

34. Colucci WS, editor. Braunwald E, Series Editor. *Atlas of Heart Failure. Cardiac Function and Dysfunction. Second Edition.* Philadelphia: Blackwell Science 1999:208, $99.00.

This book of 12 chapters by 17 contributors is beautiful.

35. Mills RM Jr, Young JB, editors. *Practical Approaches to the Treatment of Heart Failure.* Baltimore: Williams & Wilkins 1998:278, $45.00.

This fine little book of 18 chapters by 13 contributors is a practical guide for diagnosis and treatment of heart failure, a condition affecting nearly 4 million in the USA.

VALVULAR HEART DISEASE

36. Willerson JT, Cohn JN, McAllister HA Jr, Guest editors; Manabe H, Yutani C, editors. *Atlas of VALVULAR HEART DISEASE. Clinical and Pathologic Aspects.* New York: Churchill Livingstone 1998: 166, $145.00.

Pretty pictures, mainly gross specimens, some echocardiograms, no references. This book is a compilation of 130 examples of valvular heart disease contributed by 7 Japanese investigators from primarily the National Cardiovascular Center of Japan. The book apparently was first published in Japan in 1988 and translated into English for the current edition. I can't tell who wrote what.

PEDIATRIC CARDIOLOGY

37. Emmanouilides GC, Allen HD, Riemenschneider TA, Gutgesell HP, editors. *Clinical Synopsis of Moss and Adams' Heart Disease in Infants, Children, and Adolescents, Including the Fetus and Young Adult.* Baltimore: Williams & Wilkins 1998: 911, $49.00.

This very useful book of 35 chapters is a condensed version of the 1824-page fifth edition of "Moss and Adams."

38. Chang AC, Hanley FL, Wernovsky G, Wessel DL, editors. *Pediatric Cardiac Intensive Care.* Baltimore: Williams & Wilkins 1998:574, $89.00.

This book of 34 chapters by 56 multidisciplinary contributors is focused on care of critically ill neonates and children with heart disease both before and after cardiovascular operations.

39. Phoon CKL. *A Guide to Pediatric Cardiovascular Physician Examination. Or How to Survive an Outreach Clinic.* Philadelphia: Lippincott-Raven 1998:142, $34.95.

The first part of this little pocket book is a description of precordial observation, palpation, and auscultation in children. The second part features 100 case descriptions with emphasis on the value of various clinical signs useful in diagnosing specific cardiac anomalies and in assessing their severity.

ELECTROCARDIOGRAPHY AND MONITORING

***40.** Bayés de Luna A. *Clinical Electrocardiography: A Textbook. 2nd Updated Edition.* Armonk, New York: Futura Publishing Company 1998:398, $125.00.

Professor Bayés de Luna is one of the world's best interpreters of electrocardiograms. He has produced a single-authored authoritative book.

41. Marriott HJL. *Pearls & Pitfalls in Electrocardiography. Pithy, Practical Pointers. Second Edition.* Baltimore: Williams & Wilkins 1998:167, $33.00.

This single-authored book presents one beautifully-cropped electrocardiogram after another. The tracings were selected by the author because the subject was either not known or misunderstood or because it has practical value in diagnosis.

42. Mark JB. *Atlas of Cardiovascular Monitoring.* New York: Churchill Livingstone 1998:362, $75.00.

This single-authored book provides considerable information obtained from standard cardiovascular monitoring modalities. There is a good bit of wasted space on many pages.

ECHOCARDIOGRAPHY

43. Valdes-Cruz LM, Cayre RO, editors. *Echocardiographic Diagnosis of Congenital Heart Disease.*

An Embryologic and Anatomic Approach. Philadelphia: Lippincott-Raven 1999:572, $205.00.

This superb book of 35 chapters by 8 contributors is a comprehensive textbook on echocardiographic diagnosis of congenital heart disease.

44. Nanda NC, Domanski MJ. *Atlas of Transesophageal Echocardiography.* Baltimore: Williams & Wilkins 1998:521, $165.00.

Beautiful illustrations but much wasted space. When opening the book, the first few pages separated from the spine. This separation would not have occurred had the book been string bound.

45. Oh JK, Seward JB, Tajik AJ. *The Echo Manual. Second Edition.* Philadelphia: Lippincott-Raven 1999:278, $129.00.

This book of 21 chapters is tightly packed and excellent.

46. Drose JA, editor. *Fetal Echocardiography.* Philadelphia: W. B. Saunders Company 1998:300, $65.00.

This book, which contains 21 chapters by 15 contributors, provides descriptions of sonographic technique and diagnosis and insights into management both before and after birth. The reproductions are excellent and each one is well labeled.

CARDIAC CATHETERIZATION

47. Pepine CJ, Hill JA, Lambert CR, editors. *Diagnostic and Therapeutic Cardiac Catheterization. Third Edition.* Baltimore: Williams & Wilkins 1998: 1066, $99.00.

This book, which contains 44 chapters by 66 contributors, is a complete text on all aspects of cardiac catheterization. My copy of the book "cracked" near its center when I first opened it. The book is not string bound, for if it was, that would not have happened.

IMAGING (PET, SPECT, MRI, IVUS, EBCT)

***48.** Higgins CB, Ingwall JS, Pohost GM, editors. *Current and Future Applications of Magnetic Resonance in Cardiovascular Disease.* Armonk, New York: Futura Publishing Company 1998:560, $130.00.

This book contains 30 chapters by 78 contributors and provides an enormous amount of information on magnetic resonance imaging and magnetic resonance spectroscopy regarding their usefulness in clinical diagnosis and as investigative tools in cardiovascular disease.

***49.** Van Der Wall EE, Blanksma PK, Niemeyer MG, Vaalburg W, Crijns HJGM, editors. *Advanced Imaging in Coronary Artery Disease. PET, SPECT, MRI, IVUS, EBCT.* Dordrecht: Kluwer Academic Publishers 1998:348, $130.00.

This book of 20 chapters by 54 contributors is an outgrowth of the second European Conference on Cardiac PET Research held in May 1998. The usefulness of the various cardiac imaging modalities are well presented.

***50.** Iskandrian AE, Verani MS, editors. *New Developments in Cardiac Nuclear Imaging.* Armonk, New York: Futura Publishing Company 1998:288, $85.00.

This fine book of 13 chapters by 22 authors discusses primarily the newer technologies and radiopharmaceuticals in cardiac nuclear imaging.

***51.** Bogaert J, Duerinckx AJ, Rademakers FE, editors. *Magnetic Resonance of the Heart and Great Vessels. Clinical Applications.* Berlin: Springer-Verlag 1999:284, $189.00.

This book of 15 chapters by 21 contributors describes essential features of cardiovascular magnetic resonance imaging in a clear didactic fashion.

MISCELLANEOUS

52. Goldman L, Braunwald E, editors. *Primary Cardiology.* Philadelphia: W. B. Saunders Company 1998:526, $60.00.

This user-friendly superb book of 31 chapters by 29 contributors is intended primarily for primary care physicians and general internists. The book is loaded with algorithms, flow diagrams, and practice guidelines, all in color: diagnostic approaches in blue, therapeutic recommendations in green.

53. Opie LH. The Heart. *Physiology, from Cell to Circulation. Third Edition.* Philadelphia: Lippincott-Raven 1998:637, $68.00.

This splendid single-authored book of 20 chapters comprehensively presents basic cardiovascular science and integrates it into clinical cardiology.

54. Pashkow FJ, Dafoe WA, editors. *Clinical Cardiac Rehabilitation: A Cardiologist's Guide. Second Edition.* Baltimore: Williams & Wilkins 1999:565, $89.50.

This book of 26 chapters by 50 contributors is superb. This second edition appears 7 years after the first and contains 6 new chapters. Preventive cardiology is well covered.

***55.** Elkayam U, Gleicher N, editors. *CARDIAC PROBLEMS IN PREGNANCY. Diagnosis and Management of Maternal and Fetal Heart Disease. Third Edition.* New York: Wiley-Liss 1998:773, $199.00.

This comprehensive book by 81 contributors contains 54 chapters, quite a few more than in the second edition 7 years ago. I suspect that this is the best book on this topic.

56. Wenger NK, editor. *Cardiovascular Disease in the Octogenarian and Beyond.* London: Martin Dunitz 1999:439, $150.00.

Even though I authored 1 of the 30 chapters, this book is a splendid one.

***57.** Alpert MA, Alexander JK, editors. *THE HEART AND LUNG IN OBESITY.* Armonk, New York: Futura Publishing Company 1998:253, $81.00.

This book of 12 chapters by 9 contributors concerns primarily the cardiovascular and pulmonary effects of severe or morbid obesity. These authors have done an excellent job on a very important topic, one effecting thousands of Americans.

58. Chien KR, chief editor; Breslow JL, Leiden

JM, Rosenberg RD, Seidman CE, section editors. *Molecular Basis of Cardiovascular Disease. A Companion to BRAUNWALD'S HEART DISEASE.* Philadelphia: W. B. Saunders Company, 1999:637, $135.00.

This beautiful book of 25 chapters by 55 contributors is filled with important concepts and explanations in this exploding field.

***59.** Borer JS, Somberg JC, editors. *Cardiovascular Drug Development. Protocol Design and Methodology.* New York: Marcel Dekker 1999:232, $130.00.

This book of 19 chapters and 4 panel discussions by 7 contributors focuses on 5 areas: heart failure, systemic hypertension, arrhythmias, hyperlipidemia and myocardial ischemia. The didactic expositions are followed by panel discussions. I have not seen a book quite like this one. It is very readable and useful.

60. Lipshultz SE, editor. *Cardiology in AIDS.* New York: Chapman & Hall 1998:513, $59.95.

This book of 30 chapters by 49 contributors is the first to focus on vascular and cardiac complications of HIV infection and AIDS. It is a good reference work.

***61.** De Mello WC, Janse MJ, editors. *Heart Cell Communication in Health and Disease.* Boston: Kluwer Academic Publishers 1998:295, $139.00.

This book of 10 chapters by 12 contributors is an extensive review of different aspects of heart-cell communication including the role of gap junction in heart development, the molecular biology of gap junctions, the biophysics of intercellular channels, the control of junctional conductance, and the influence of gap junctions on impulse propagation.

***62.** Reeves JT, Weir EK, editors. *Pulmonary Edema.* Armonk, New York: Futura Publishing Company 1998:411, $98.00.

This book of 26 chapters by 51 contributors describes basic research investigations on an important topic.

CARDIOLOGY ANNUALS

***63.** Willerson JT, Roberts WC, Rackley CE, Graham TP Jr, Mason DT, Parmley WW. *Cardiology 1998.* Armonk, New York: Futura Publishing Company 1998:611, $98.00.

Willerson has done a magnificent job in pulling together the best articles on cardiovascular disease the previous year. He has added interviews of prominent cardiovascular leaders at the end—Eric J. Topol, Michael E. DeBakey, Denton A. Cooley, James T. Willerson, and Joseph S. Alpert.

64. Schlant RC, editor in chief; Collins JJ Jr; Gersh BJ, Graham TP, Kaplan NM, Waldo AL, editors. *1998 The Year Book of Cardiology.* St. Louis: Mosby 1998:552, $79.00.

This book is the 38th in the series. Of course, I prefer book #63.

HISTORY

***65.** Roberts CS. *Stoking the Fire. A Surgical Memoir of London.* Armonk, New York: Futura Publishing Company 1999:184, $40.00.

This is my physician son's second book. Of course I think it is wonderful.

COMMENTS

Of the 65 books mentioned herein, 8 (12%) were single-authored; 4 (6%) had 2 authors; 2 (3%), three authors; 1 (2%), four authors; 1 (1%), five authors; 1 (2%), six authors, and 47 (72%) were edited books with usually numerous contributors. The publication date in 15 books (23%) was 1999, and in the other 50 books (77%), 1998. Acid-free, i.e., permanent paper was used in 29 books (45%) (Each is designated by an asterisk.), and acid paper in the other 36 books (55%). The publishers using acid-free paper were Elsevier, Futura, Humana, Kluwer Academic, Marcel Dekker, and Springer-Verlag. The graphics also are better on acid-free paper than on acid paper. Too many books? Probably so, but not too many *good* books.

William C. Roberts

William Clifford Roberts, MD
Baylor University Medical Center
Dallas, Texas 75246

Good Books in Cardiovascular Disease Appearing in 1999

GENERAL TEXTBOOKS

1. Murphy JG, editor in chief, *Mayo Clinic Cardiology Review, Second Edition*, Philadelphia: Lippincott Williams & Wilkins, 2000:1381, $99.95.

This is an interesting and useful book. It is an outgrowth of the syllabus for the Mayo Cardiovascular Review Course. The first chapter is entitled "The Cardiology Boards" and it describes how they are presented annually. The subsequent 85 chapters succinctly present essential information on each topic. Many chapters are followed by multiple choice questions (>600 in all). The type is large, making for easy reading. The 76 contributors provide descriptions in italics of each reference at the end of each chapter. Placing the word "Review" in the book's title will increase sales.

2. Dalla Volta S, editor in chief; Bayés de Luna A, Jezek V, Brochier ML, Mortensen SA, Dienstl F, Poole-Wilson PA, editors. *Cardiology.* London: McGraw-Hill International 1999:880, $75.00.

This large book by 126 contributors is practical and user friendly and nicely priced. The numbers of references after each of the 81 chapters are relatively few.

3. Grenvik A, Senior Editor; Ayres SM, Holbrook PR, Shoemaker WC, editors. *Textbook of Critical Care, Fourth Edition.* Philadelphia: W.B. Saunders 2000:2227, $165.00.

This book, the bible of critical care, contains 202 chapters by 342 authors. The latter include pulmonologists, cardiologists, traumatologists, neurologists, neurosurgeons, cardiothoracic surgeons, and transplant surgeons. The book is divided into 15 sections, only 1 of which focuses on cardiovascular problems.

4. Taylor GJ, editor. *Primary Care Management of Heart Disease.* St. Louis: Mosby 2000:658, $69.00.

This book by 61 contributors is of course directed to the primary care physician. Although not encyclopedic, most cardiac subjects are at least touched on. The chapter on cardiomyopathies is 8 pages with 6 references. It contains 53 useful tables and 51 figures. The last 82 pages provide detailed information on 128 drugs used by cardiologists. Each chapter is authored by a primary care physician and a cardiologist.

***5.** Chesler E, editor. *Clinical Cardiology in the Elderly. Second Edition.* Armonk, New York: Futura Publishing 1999:837, $165.00.

Herein are 32 chapters by 43 contributors. Cardiology is rapidly becoming a condition of the "elderly" (undefined). This book covers most cardiovascular conditions seen in older folks and it covers them well.

***6.** Tresch DD, Aronow WS, editors. *Cardiovascular Disease in the Elderly Patient. Second Edition*, Revised and Expanded. New York: Marcel Dekker 1999:807, $150.00.

This second edition is comprehensive and well done. I like this book better than the Chesler one, but maybe it is because I authored a chapter.

7. Constant J. *Bedside Cardiology, Fifth Edition*, Philadelphia: Lippincott Williams & Wilkins 1999: 342, $49.95.

This single authored book focuses primarily on physical signs in the cardiac patient and what causes them. The author uses the question–answer approach to discuss each topic. The book contains many excellent figures including numerous phonocardiograms. This fine book describes diagnosis, with emphasis on auscultation, and avoids therapy.

CORONARY ARTERY DISEASE

***8.** Nash IS, Fuster V, editors. *Efficacy of Myocardial Infarction Therapy. An Evaluation of Clinical Trials Evidence.* New York: Marcel Dekker 1999:493, $195.00.

This book by 39 contributors is a real contribution. It is divided into 3 parts: therapies with established efficacy, therapies without established efficacy, and alternative strategies. Each of the 41 chapters focuses on a major trial. This is "a must-have book."

***9.** Lincoff AM, Topol EJ, editors. *Platelet Glycoprotein IIb/IIIa Inhibitors in Cardiovascular Disease.* Totowa, New Jersey: Humana Press 1999:369, $125.00.

This book by 28 contributors is a comprehensive overview of the preclinical and clinical development and uses of the glycoprotein II/b/IIIa receptor antagonists.

***10.** Timmis GC, editor. *Thrombolytic Therapy.* Armonk, New York: Futura Publishing 1999:357, $98.00.

This splendid book by 47 contributors brings together essentially all the important information showing the effectiveness of thrombolytic therapy for patients with acute myocardial infarction.

11. Sclarovsky S, editor. *Electrocardiography of Acute Myocardial Ischaemic Syndromes*. London: Martin Dunitz 1999:226, $120.00

When I opened this attractive book it separated from the spine. Thus, the printer and binder did not do their jobs properly. Nevertheless, the book is a bit unusual for an electrocardiographic one in that it provides extensive and illuminating explanations for each of the many electrocardiograms.

12. Isner JM, Kearney M. *Atherosclerosis: Pathology of the Vasculature in Live Patients*. London: W.B. Saunders 1999:112, $99.00.

This atlas provides in color mainly photomicrographs of portions of atherectomy specimens retrieved during life from many patients. It certainly is the best and indeed the only book on this subject in existence.

***13.** Grines CL, Savu MA, Tejada LA. *Interventional Cardiology. The Essentials for the Boards. Questions and Answers, Clinical Cases and Pearls*. Armonk, New York: Futura Publishing 1999:291, $39.00.

For those about to take the new interventional cardiology boards, I suspect that this book will be extremely useful.

14. Kutryk MJB, Serruys PW. *Coronary Stenting: Current Perspectives. A Companion to the* Handbook of Coronary Stents. London: Martin Dunitz 1999:318, $65.00.

These 2 authors review what is known about coronary stenting, its indications, and the use of adjunctive therapies. This book needs to be purchased and read quickly because the field changes so rapidly.

***15.** Panza JA, Cannon RO III, editors. *Endothelium, Nitric Oxide, and Atherosclerosis: From Basic Mechanisms to Clinical Implications*. Armonk, New York: Futura Publishing 1999:320, $75.00.

This valuable book by 36 contributors is divided into 4 sections that include in-depth discussions of the discovery, biological roles, and regulation of endothelial nitric oxide; the basic mechanisms that lead to endothelial dysfunction in cardiovascular disease; clinical studies of impaired endothelial dysfunction, and therapeutic strategies that might ameliorate endothelial dysfunction.

ATHEROSCLEROTIC PREVENTION

***16.** Grundy SM, editor. *Cholesterol-Lowering Therapy. Evaluation of Clinical Trial Evidence*. New York: Marcel Dekker 2000:329, $150.00.

This fine book by 28 contributors brings together all the recent clinical trials of cholesterol-lowering therapy. It is nice to have all this information in the same place.

17. Gotto AM Jr, Pownall HJ. *Manual of Lipid Disorders. Reducing the Risk of Coronary Heart Disease. Second Edition*. Baltimore: Williams & Wilkins 1999:402, $24.95.

This is an excellent book. I use it frequently. It contains an amazing number of references for such a small volume.

***18.** Wong ND, editor in chief; Black HR, Gardin JM, associate editors. *Preventive Cardiology*. New York: McGraw-Hill 2000;630, $65.00.

This book by 42 contributors is a comprehensive and large book on this subject.

HEART FAILURE

19. Hosenpud JD, Greenberg BH, editors. *Congestive Heart Failure. Pathophysiology, Diagnosis, and Comprehensive Approach to Management. Second Edition*. Philadelphia: Lippincott Williams & Wilkins 2000:858, $140.00.

A large comprehensive book on this topic by 75 contributors.

20. Colucci WS, editor. *Atlas of Heart Failure. Cardiac Function and Dysfunction. Second Edition*. Philadelphia: Blackwell Science:1999:approximately 300 (pages not numbered continuously), $125.00.

A beautiful book by 17 contributors. There is essentially no text. The text consists of the legends for the figures.

21. Katz AM. *Heart Failure. Pathophysiology, Molecular Biology and Clinical Management*. Philadelphia: Lippincott Williams & Wilkins 2000:381, $65.00.

A single-authored scholarly book that focuses on basic underlying mechanisms.

SYSTEMIC HYPERTENSION

22. Oparil S, Weber MA, editors. *Hypertension: A Companion to Brenner and Rector's* The Kidney. Philadelphia: W.B. Saunders 2000:757, $95.00.

This book by 138 contributors is packed full of information on this subject.

23. Beevers DG, MacGregor GA. *Hypertension in Practice. Third Edition*. London: Martin Dunitz 1999: 286, $89.95.

An excellent, practical, and easily readable book.

***24.** McCarty R, Blizard DA, Chevalier RL, editors. *Development of the Hypertensive Phenotype: Basic and Clinical Studies*. Amsterdam: Elsevier 1999: 693, $370.50.

This book is the 19th in the *Handbook of Hypertension* series. The 62 contributors focus on the endogenous (genetic) and exogenous (environmental) components contributing to the pathogenesis of essential hypertension. The price ($370.50) will probably limit it to libraries.

ARRHYTHMIAS AND CONDUCTION DISTURBANCES, ELECTROPHYSIOLOGY

25. Zipes DP, Jalife J, editors. *Cardiac Electrophysiology. From Cell to Bedside. Third Edition*. Philadelphia: W.B. Saunders 2000:1111, $230.00.

This book by 233 contributors is the bible on this subject.

26. Kastor JA. *Arrhythmias. Second Edition.* Philadelphia: W.B. Saunders 2000:603, $125.00.

This single authored very readable book, appearing 6 years after the first edition, is divided into 4 sections: history, supraventricular tachyarrhythmias, ventricular arrhythmias, and bradyarrhythmias. The clinical effects of these arrhythmias as well as illustrative electrocardiograms and electrophysiologic studies are presented. The numbers of references are enormous– "... all relevant publications for the 30 years proceeding the summer of 1998. . .."

27. Gillette PC, Garson A, Jr, editors. *Clinical Pediatric Arrhythmias, Second Edition.* Philadelphia: W.B. Saunders 1999:339, $125.00.

The information in this edition is more succinct and understandable than in the first edition. The 24 contributors have produced a fine book.

28. Sutton R, Rydén L, Bourgeois I, editors. *The Foundations of Cardiac Pacing. Part II. An Illustrated Guide to Rate Variable Pacing.* Armonk, New York: Futura Publishing 1999:540, $98.00.

VALVULAR HEART DISEASE

29. Alpert JS, Dalen JE, Rahimtoola SH, editors. *Valvular Heart Disease. Third Edition.* Philadelphia: Lippincott Williams & Wilkins 2000:478, $65.00.

This book by 29 contributors is well done.

30. Otto CM. *Valvular Heart Disease.* Philadelphia: W.B. Saunders 1999:468, $115.00.

Of the 18 chapters in this book, all but 2 were written by Otto. It is a superb, highly recommended book.

***31.** Vlessis AA, Bolling SF, editors. *Endocarditis. A Multidisciplinary Approach to Modern Treatment.* Armonk, New York: Futura Publishing 1999:425, $98.00.

There has not been a book on this subject in a while. The 28 contributors provide one.

CONGENITAL HEART DISEASE

***32.** Lock JE, Keane JF, Perry SB, editors. *Diagnostic and Interventional Catheterization in Congenital Heart Disease. Second Edition.* Boston: Kluwer Academic Publishers 2000:377, $125.00.

This book by 18 contributors is probably the first on this topic for pediatric interventionalists. The 3 editors have gathered together the leaders in this field and produced a fine book.

33. Angelini P, editor. *Coronary Artery Anomalies. A Comprehensive Approach.* Philadelphia: Lippincott Williams & Wilkins 1999:200, $149.00.

This fine book focuses on coronary anomalies in patients both with and without other congenital cardiac anomalies. The book is packed with coronary angiograms illustrating the various abnormal origins and courses of these anomalies. This book is particularly useful for those working in cardiac catheterization laboratories.

PERIPHERAL ARTERIAL DISEASE

34. Calligaro KD, Dougherty MJ, Hollier LH, editors. *Diagnosis and Treatment of Aortic and Peripheral Arterial Aneurysms.* Philadelphia: W.B. Saunders 1999:365, $98.00.

This book by 69 contributors, 64 of whom are surgeons, provides a fine update on this important topic.

***35.** Nienaber CA, Fattori R, editors. *Diagnosis and Treatment of Aortic Diseases.* Dordrecht: Kluwer Academic 1999:278, $127.00.

This book by 8 authors focuses on aortic dissection, aneurysm, trauma, inflammation (aortitis), inherited disorders, and aortic arch malformations. Each page costs 46 cents.

36. Heuser RR, editor. *Peripheral Vascular Stenting For Cardiologists.* London: Martin Duntiz 1999: 174, $99.95.

This book by 18 contributors describes interventions for the carotid, renal, abdominal aorta, iliac, femoral and popliteal arteries. For interventionalists involved in these areas, the book should be useful.

ELECTROCARDIOGRAPHY

37. Stein E. *Rapid Analysis of Electrocardiograms. A Self-Study Program. Third Edition.* Philadelphia: Lippincott Williams & Wilkins 2000:390, $32.95.

This simply written, amply illustrated book is a good one on this topic. My only criticisms are the presence of blank space on many pages and the use of xerographic copies periodically of electrocardiograms.

ECHOCARDIOGRAPHY

38. Otto CM. *Textbook of Clinical Echocardiography. Second Edition.* Philadelphia: W.B. Saunders 2000:443, $105.00.

This single-authored book is superb. It is intended for those new to echocardiography. The illustrations are clear and cropped. A list of annotated references are included at the end of each chapter.

39. Oh JK, Seward JB, Tajik AJ. *The Echo Manual. Second Edition.* Philadelphia: Lippincott Williams & Wilkins 1999:278, $129.00.

Nice book. Excellent illustrations. It appears only 4 years after the first edition.

CARDIAC FUNCTION TESTING

40. Froelicher VF, Myers JN. *Exercise and the Heart. Fourth Edition.* Philadelphia: W.B. Saunders 2000:456, $65.00.

Fine book. Fully packed. The type is light which makes reading a bit more difficult than it should be.

41. Wasserman K, Hansen JE, Sue DY, Casaburi R, Whipp BJ. *Principles of Exercise Testing & Interpretation Including Pathophysiology and Clinical Applications. Third Edition.* Philadelphia: Lippincott Williams & Wilkins 1999:556, $65.00.

This book describes how to evaluate patients with

exercise intolerance using the pathophysiology of exercise gas exchange as the frame of reference. Electrocardiograms during exercise are not presented. This book probably will be more useful to the pulmonologist than the cardiologist.

*42. Dilsizian V, editor. *Myocardial Viability: A Clinical and Scientific Treatise.* Armonk, New York: Futura Publishing 2000:448, $125.00.

This fine book by 27 contributors bridges together basic cellular physiology and clinical decision making as it relates to myocardial viability.

*43. Germano G, Berman DS, editors. *Clinical Gated Cardiac SPECT.* Armonk, New York: Futura Publishing 1999:387, $125.00.

This book of 12 chapters by 13 contributors appears to be the first monograph dedicated to the performance, interpretation, and applications of gated single-photon emission computed tomography (SPECT). Because SPECT has emerged as the most common approach to myocardial perfusion imaging, this book is particularly useful.

CARDIAC SURGERY

44. Guo-Wei HE, editor. *Arterial Grafts for Coronary Artery Bypass Surgery. A Textbook for Cardiovascular Clinicians and Researchers.* Singapore: Springer 1999:449, $64.00.

This book by 50 contributors consists of 37 chapters. My son, who is a cardiovascular surgeon and favors all-arterial grafts, bought this book, read it, and told me it was useful.

45. Cohen RG, Mack MJ, Fonger JD, Landreneau RJ, editors. *Minimally Invasive Cardiac Surgery.* St. Louis: Quality Medical Publishing 1999:359, $245.00.

This is a superb book of 38 chapters by 82 authors in a rapidly developing field. Most illustrations are in color.

46. Ennker J, editor. *Cardiac Surgery and Concomitant Disease.* New York: Springer 1999:324, $59.00.

The contributions in this book were originally presented at a symposium in Baden-Baden, Germany, October 1997. The symposium focused on problems of concomitant diseases in patients referred for cardiac surgery, mainly coronary bypass, including diseases of the liver, lungs, kidneys, skeletal muscle, endocrine organs, connective tissue and hematologic tissues, and increased body weight.

*47. Attar S, editor. *Hemostasis in Cardiac Surgery.* Armonk, New York: Futura Publishing 1999: 262, $74.00.

This book by 17 contributors is divided into 4 sections: basic hemostatic alterations produced by cardiopulmonary bypass; blood transfusions and blood conservation; diagnosing coagulopathy and their therapy.

*48. Whittaker P, Abela GS, editors. *Direct Myocardial Revascularization: History, Methodology, Technology.* Boston: Kluwer Academic 1999:202, $162.00.

49. Yao JST, Pearce WH, editors. *Practical Vascular Surgery.* Stamford, Connecticut: Appleton & Lange 1999:542, $155.00.

This book by 68 contributors focuses on standard vascular surgical procedures rather than newer endovascular techniques. It is more comprehensive than the Calligaro-Dougherty-Hollier book.

50. Shumacker HB Jr. A Dream of the Heart. *The Life of John H. Gibbon, Jr. Father of the Heart-Lung Machine.* Santa Barbara, California: Fithian Press 1999:297, $24.95.

The heart-lung machine was one of the most important advances of the twentieth century. Dr. Shumacker provides a splendid story of its developer.

MISCELLANEOUS

51. Hennekens CH, chief editor. Buring JE, Manson JE, Ridker PM, section editors. *Clinical Trials in Cardiovascular Disease. A Companion to Braunwald's Heart Disease.* Philadelphia: W.B. Saunders 1999:472, $130.00.

This excellent book by 58 contributors is divided into 3 parts: methodology of doing randomized clinical trials; treatment trials including interventions for acute myocardial ischemia and secondary prevention, and primary presentation trials. This book puts in one place comprehensive discussions of the major clinical trials in cardiovascular disease.

52. Chien KR, editor. Breslow JL, Leiden JM, Rosenberg RD, Seidman CE, section editors. *Molecular Basics of Cardiovascular Disease. A Companion to BRAUNWALD'S HEART DISEASE.* Philadelphia: W.B. Saunders 1999:637, $140.00.

This is a splendid book. It should be part of every young cardiologist's library. This book is modern academic cardiology at its best.

53. Kaplan JA, editor; Reich DL and Konstadt SN, associate editors. *Cardiac Anesthesia, Fourth Edition.* Philadelphia: W.B. Saunders 1999:1411, $279.00.

This is the classic on this topic since its first edition in 1979. Each new edition has been larger than the preceding one. Each of the 1411 pages is fully packed.

*54. Kern MJ, editor. *Hemodynamic Rounds, Second Edition.* New York: Wiley-Liss 1999:329, $64.95.

Of the 42 chapters in this book, Mort Kern is the author or coauthor in all 42 (100%). He is joined by 21 coauthors. The focus is on interpretation of pressure tracings which are plentiful and well reproduced. It is a good book for those in the cardiac catheterization laboratory.

*55. Rubanyi GM, editor. *Angiogenesis in Health and Disease. Basic mechanisms and Clinical Applications.* New York: Marcel Dekker 2000:552, $195.00.

This book by 96 contributors provides an in-depth review of the basic sciences and therapeutic application of angiogenesis research.

*56. Share L, editor. *Hormones and the Heart in Health and Disease.* Totowa, New Jersey: Humana Press 1999:258, $99.50.

This useful book by 29 contributors focuses on

hormones and autocoids that are secreted by the heart or that act on it, including natriuretic peptides, adrenomedullin, urocortin, adrenocortical hormones, renin and angiotensin, catecholamines, vasopressin, insulin, kinins, endothelin, nitric oxide, eicosanoids, estrogen and androgen.

*__57.__ Caplan LR, Hurst JW, Chimowitz MI. *Clinical Neurocardiology*. New York: Marcel Dekker 1999:498,$195.00.

*__58.__ Sarret M, Kher A, Toulemonde F, editors. *Low Molecular Weight Heparin Therapy. An Evaluation of Clinical Trials Evidence.* New York: Marcel Dekker 1999:474, $165.00.

This book by 27 contributors is it on this subject.

59. Williams RA, editor. *The Athlete and Heart Disease. Diagnosis Evaluation & Management.* Philadelphia: Lippincott Williams & Wilkins 1999:333, $89.95.

This book is the best one so far on this topic.

60. Fletcher GF, Grundy SM, Hayman LL, editors. *Obesity: Impact on Cardiovascular Disease.* Armonk, New York: Futura Publishing 1999:377, $69.00.

Because of the growing problem of obesity, the American Heart Association in 1998 sponsored a conference on the impact of obesity on cardiovascular disease. This book by 29 contributors is an outgrowth of that conference. This is a superb and needed book.

61. Goldstein DJ, Stunkard AJ, editors. *The Management of Eating Disorders and Obesity.* Totowa, New Jersey: Humana Press 1999:367, $99.50.

Obesity is a topic that cardiovascular specialists need to focus on. Few patients with coronary artery disease are at ideal body weight. This book by 37 contributors is by leaders in this field and a good place to begin.

62. Reaven GM, Laws A, editors. *Insulin Resistance. The Metabolic Syndrome X.* Totowa, New Jersey: Humana Press 1999:374, $145.00.

This is a hot topic and done by the leaders in this field. Insulin resistance is too important to be left entirely to the endocrinologists. Cardiologists see this syndrome daily. It is all in this book.

*__63.__ Bogaert J, Duerinckx AJ, Rademakers FE, editors. *Magnetic Resonance of the Heart and Great Vessels. Clinical Applications.* Berlin: Springer 1999: 284, $161.00.

This book by 18 contributors provides a description of the essential features of cardiovascular magnetic resonance imaging.

*__64.__ Willerson JT, Roberts WC, Rackley CE, Graham TP Jr, Mason DT, Parmley WW. *Cardiology 1999*, Armonk, New York: Futura Publishing 1999: 774, $125.00.

This is the 19th volume in this series. Dr. Willerson did a masterful job in putting together the information published in 1998.

COMMENTS

The 64 books mentioned herein, 7 (11%) had a single author, 5 (8%) had 2 authors, 2 (3%) had 3 authors, and 1 each had 5 and 6 authors; the remaining 46 (72%) were edited books with multiple contributors. The 64 books ranged in cost from $24.95 to $370.50 (mean $118.00). Twenty-four books (38%) were published on acid-free (permanent) paper, and 40 (62%) were published on acid paper. Unfortunately, the 2 largest US publishers (Lippincott Williams & Wilkins and W.B. Saunders) use only acid paper. 1999 was a good year for books on cardiovascular disease.

William C. Roberts

William Clifford Roberts, MD
Baylor Cardiovascular Institute
Baylor University Medical Center
Dallas, Texas 75246

Good Books in Cardiovascular Disease Appearing in 2000

MAJOR CARDIOVASCULAR TEXTS

***1.** Fuster V, Alexander RW, O'Rourke RA, editors. *Hurst's The Heart. Tenth Edition.* New York: McGraw-Hill Medical Publishing Division 2001: 2660, $150.00 (single), 2-volume set $165.00.

This is the first major textbook published on acid-free paper! It contains 98 chapters by 190 contributors. Each page is fully packed. It is loaded with unusually fine illustrations and tables. A superb book.

2. Willerson JT, Cohn JN, editors. *Cardiovascular Medicine, Second Edition.* New York: Churchill Livingston 2000:2344, $165.00.

This book of 127 chapters by 194 contributors represents a second edition of the book which appeared initially in 1995. It will compete effectively with the Braunwald, Hurst, and Parmerly texts. These texts are too big to carry around or place on one's lap. I was surprised to find that the sources of some illustrations were not indicated.

3. Crawford MH, DiMarco JP, editors. *Cardiology.* London: Mosby 2001:1600, $165.00.

This huge book by 280 contributors is divided into 8 major sections, each of which is color-coded with a different color. The text is comprehensive and the figures, many in color, are excellent. The 2 editors write (preface) that the book "Although comprehensive . . . is not intended to be encyclopedic." It looks comprehensive to me. A nice additional major text book.

4. Allen HD, Gutgesell HP, Clark EB, Driscoll DJ, editors. *Moss and Adams' Heart Disease in Infants, Children, and Adolescents, Including the Fetus and Young Adult.* Philadelphia: Lippincott Williams & Wilkins 2001:1614, $259.00.

This book of 75 chapters by 112 contributors is of course a major text in this field. Being in 2 volumes requires the repeating of the table of contents and index and of a small introductory chapter (I prefer single volume books). The book is very well done.

5. Moller JH, Hoffman JIE, editors, *Pediatric Cardiovascular Medicine*, New York: Churchill Livingston 2000:1004, $225.00.

This book of 64 chapters by 100 contributors is a major textbook of pediatric cardiology. Although not as large or as heavy as some textbooks on this subject, I found it surprisingly thorough. Each page is fully packed.

CARDIOLOGY IN PRIMARY CARE

***6.** Branch WT, Jr., Alexander RW, Schlant RC, Hurst JW, editors. *Cardiology in Primary Care.* New York: McGraw-Hill Medical Publishing Division 2000:940, $75.00.

This book by 71 contributors is larger than previous books on this topic. It contains no photographs but many useful tables and diagrams.

7. Alpert JS, editor. *Cardiology for the Primary Care Physician, 3rd edition.* Philadelphia: Current Medicine 2001:456, $125.00.

The 75 contributors have produced 46 beautifully illustrated chapters, This book is not a substitute for an excellent text on this subject but the illustrations and diagrams are highly useful.

CORONARY ARTERY DISEASE

***8.** Topol EJ, editor. *Acute Coronary Syndromes. Second Edition Revised and Expanded.* New York: Marcel Dekker 2001:862, $99.95.

The first edition of the book appeared in 1998 so this one is a 2-year update. The 45 contributors produce 28 excellent chapters.

***9.** Aliot E, Clémanty J, Prystowsky EN, editors. *Fighting Sudden Cardiac Death. A Worldwide Challenge.* Armonk, New York: Futura Publishing Company 2000:724, $225.00.

This book by 125 contributors is very comprehensive, more so than other books I have seen on this subject.

***10.** Cohn PE. *Silent Myocardial Ischemia and Infarction. Fourth Edition.* New York: Marcel Dekker 2000:327, $125.00.

A single-authored book, something rare today, but how refreshing. The last edition was published in 1993 so this edition is a large update on a subject that receives less addition than the past.

11. Alpert JS, Francis GS. *Handbook of Coronary*

*Published on acid-free (permanent) paper.

Care, Sixth Edition. Philadelphia: Lippincott Williams & Wilkins 2000:222, $35.95.

A very useful book which fits into a coat pocket.

ATHEROSCLEROTIC PREVENTION

***12.** Foody JM, editor. *Preventive Cardiology. Strategies for the Prevention and Treatment of Coronary Artery Disease*. Totowa, New Jersey: Humana Press 2001:366, $99.50.

Eighteen good chapters by 27 contributors.

13. Betteridge DJ, editor. *Lipids and Vascular Disease. Current Issues*. London: Martin Dunitz 2000: 262, $95.00.

This book of 18 chapters by 27 contributors is not comprehensive but it is nicely done.

14. Wilson PWF, editor. *Atlas of Atherosclerosis. Risk Factors and Treatment. Second Edition*. Philadelphia: Current Medicine 2000:269, $135.

The 22 contributors produce 13 beautifully illustrated chapters.

SYSTEMIC HYPERTENSION

***15.** Weber MA, editor. *Hypertension Medicine*. Totowa, New Jersey: Humana Press 2001:462, $89.50.

The 49 contributors produce 41 chapters, nearly all of which are useful to the practicing physician.

16. Messerli FH, editor. *The ABCs of Antihypertensive Therapy. Second Edition*. Philadelphia: Lippincott Williams & Wilkins 2000:325, $49.00.

This book of 25 chapters by 39 contributors provides a practical and authoritative guide to the drug treatment of systemic hypertension. This book is fully packed and highly useful.

17. Hollenberg NK, volume editor; Braunwald E, series editor. *Atlas of Heart Diseases Hypertension Volume I. Hypertension: Mechanisms and Therapy. Third Edition*. Philadelphia: Current Medicine 2001: 327, $125.00.

The 22 contributors produced 15 beautiful chapters.

***18.** White W.B., editor. *Blood Pressure Monitoring in Cardiovascular Medicine and Therapeutics*. Totowa, New Jersey: Humana Press 2001:309, $99.00.

For those interested in home and ambulatory blood pressure monitoring, this is it. Twenty-one contributors produce 13 chapters.

***19.** Bulpitt CJ, editor. *Epidemiology of Hypertension Volume 20 in Series Handbook of Hypertension* edited by Birkenäger WH and Reid JL. Amsterdam: Elsevier 2000:706, $275.00.

Forty chapters by 66 contributors. This book represents an update on volume 6 in the series having to do with epidemiology of systemic hypertension. The book, although fully packed, is expensive (39 cents/page).

***20.** Rubin PC, editor. *Hypertension in Pregnancy. Volume 21 in the Series Handbook of Hypertension* edited by Birkenhäger WH and Reid JL. Amsterdam: Elsevier 2000:374, $275.00.

This book of 17 chapters by 22 contributors is an update of volume 10 in this series. The cause of preeclampsia remains unclear and therapy has not changed in any major degree in a number of years. This book provides a great deal of information but it is expensive information (74 cents/page).

HEART FAILURE

21. Katz AM. *Heart Failure. Pathophysiology, Molecular Biology and Clinical Management*. Philadelphia: Lippincott Williams & Williams 2000:381, $69.00.

As Eugene Braunwald stated in the foreword, "Single-authored, comprehensive medical texts on complex subjects are now a great rarity . . ." but such is the case with this book.

22. McMurray JJV, Cleland JGF, editors. *Heart Failure in Clinical Practice. Second Edition*. London: Martin Dunitz 2000:343, $95.00.

This book of 20 chapters by 42 contributors reviews in easy fashion this important field.

23. Gibbs CR, Davies MK, and Lip GYH, editors. *ABC of Heart Failure*. London: BMJ Books 2000:46, $30.50.

This book of 10 chapters by 9 contributors represents previously published articles in the *British Medical Journal* in a short but useful presentation of a condition which if untreated has a prognosis worse than many forms of cancer. The illustrations, diagrams, and tables are excellent.

ARRHYTHMIAS AND CONDUCTION DISTURBANCES, ELECTROPHYSIOLOGY

***24.** Spooner PM, Rosen MR, editor. *Foundations of Cardiac Arrhythmias. Basic Concepts and Clinical Approaches*. New York: Marcel Dekker 2001:820, $165.00.

For the electrophysiologists, this book by 58 contributors looks useful.

***25.** Ovsyshcher IE, editor. *Cardiac Arrhythmias and Device Therapy: Results and Prospectives for the New Century*. Armonk, New York: Futura Publishing Company 2000:423, $115.00.

This book of 50 chapters by 65 contributors covers basic electrophysiology, including genetics and the molecular base of arrhythmias; invasive and noninvasive clinical electrophysiology; and cardiac pacing and defibrillation.

***26.** Woosley RL, Singh SN, editors. *Arrhythmia Treatment and Therapy. Evaluation of Clinical Trial Evidence*. New York: Marcel Dekker 2000:373, $175.00.

This book of 18 chapters by 41 contributors brings together in 1 volume the results of the most influential clinical trials of antiarrhythmias in the last 20 years. The final chapter summarizes the trials that are currently underway and provides a glimpse of the future.

27. Lip GYH. *Atrial Fibrillation in Clinical Practice*. London: Martin Dunitz 2001:234, $70.00.

A single-authored good book.

***28.** Quan L, Franklin WH, editors. *Ventricular*

Fibrillation. A Pediatric Problem. Armonk, New York: Futura Publishing Company 2000:302, $95.00.

This topic has received little attention in the pediatric age group. It represents a full exploration of a fortunately very uncommon problem.

***29.** Mazgalev TN, Tchou PJ, editors. *Atrial-AV Nodal Electrophysiology: A View from the Millennium.* Armonk, New York: Futura Publishing Company 2000:501, $130.00.

This book of 29 chapters by 74 contributors focuses on the atrioventricular node, both its anatomy and electrophysiology. It provides an enormous amount of information on this topic.

30. Hayes DL, Lloyd MA, Friedman PA. *Cardiac Pacing and Defibrillation: A Clinical Approach.* Armonk, New York: Futura Publishing Company 2000: 600, $89.00.

This book by 3 authors from the Mayo Clinic provides very practical clinical information on cardiac pacing and defibrillation. For those involved in pacing and defibrillation this is a very useful book.

31. Moses HW, Moulton KP, Miller BD, Schneider JA. *A Practical Guide to Cardiac Pacing. Fifth Edition.* Philadelphia: Lippincott Williams & Wilkins 2000:206, $39.95.

This book of 10 chapters by the 4 authors acquaints the reader with basic principles and terminology of cardiac pacing.

***32.** Hayes DL, Wang PJ. *Cardiac Pacemakers and Implantable Defibrillators: A Multi-Volume Workbook. Volume 4. ICDs and Pacemakers.* Armonk, New York: Futura Publishing Company 2000: 120, $29.00.

These 2 authors present 25 cases with various pacemaker problems, and 30 cases with various problems involving implantable defibrillators. For those interested in or involved with this area this workbook is useful.

***33.** Huang SKS, Wilber DJ, editors. *Radiofrequency Catheter Ablation of Cardiac Arrhythmias. Basic Concepts and Clinical Applications. Second Edition.* Armonk, New York: Futura Publishing Company 2000:884, $135.00.

This book by 81 contributors brings up to date the techniques and tools of radiofrequency ablation. Since the first reported use of radiofrequency energy for ablative procedures in 1987 the numbers of these procedures performed annually in the USA has risen to >100,000. This excellent book is divided into 7 parts: fundamental aspects of radiofrequency energy application; ablation of atrial tachycardia and flutter; its use in atrial fibrillation; its use in atrioventricular nodal reentrant tachycardia; in accessory pathways; in ventricular tachycardia; and miscellaneous topics.

***34.** Tentori MC, Segura EL, Hayes DL, editors. *Arrhythmia Management in Chagas' Disease.* Armonk, New York: Futura Publishing Company 2000: 156, $65.00.

This book by 24 contributors concerns the most common cause of atrioventricular block in South America, namely Chagaś disease. However, an estimated 500,000 persons residing in the USA are infected with *Trypanosoma cruzi.* Some of these cases in the USA are misdiagnosed as idiopathic dilated cardiomyopathy or ischemic cardiomyopathy. This book, although on a limited subject in the USA, is quite useful.

***35.** Franz MR, editor. *Monophasic Action Potentials. Bridging Cell and Bedside.* Armonk, New York: Futura Publishing Company 2000:884, $159.00.

This book of 50 chapters by 114 contributors is a magnum opus on monophasic action potential recordings. It is the first comprehensive account of the nature and use of MAPs and how they can help in the understanding of repolarization-related electrophysiology and its abnormalities that lead to arrhythmias.

***36.** Olsson SB, Amlie JP, Yuan S, editors. *Dispersion of Ventricular Repolarization: State of the Art.* Armonk, New York: Futura Publishing Company 2000:330, $125.00.

This book of 20 chapters by 56 contributors focuses on the role of dispersion of ventricular repolarization (DVR) in the pathophysiology of malignant ventricular arrhythmias and its prognostic role in several patient groups.

VALVULAR HEART DISEASES

***37.** Boudoulas H, Wooley CF, editors. *Mitral Valve: Floppy Mitral Valve, Mitral Valve Prolapse, Mitral Valve Regurgitation. Second Revised Edition.* Armonk, New York: Futura Publishing Company 2000:753, $145.00.

This book by 35 contributors consists of 27 chapters, 11 (41%) of which were written by the editors, who in addition, authored an "introduction" to each of the 18 different sections. This is a long book on a single subject, but it is a good one.

CONGENITAL HEART DISEASE

38. Allan L, Hornberger LK, Sharland G, editors. *Textbook of Fetal Cardiology.* London: Greenwich Medical Media Limited 2000:596, $199.00.

This book by 29 contributors (60% by the 3 editors) provides relatively short descriptions and beautiful illustrations of most of the congenital anomalies that can be diagnosed by echocardiography of the fetus. I highly recommend this book to anyone doing this procedure in the fetus.

***39.** Edwards BS, Edwards JE. *Jesse E. Edwards' Synopsis of Congenital Heart Disease.* Armonk, New York: Futura Publishing Company 2000:136, $72.00.

What a pleasure to see this highly illustrated book (57 figures, 246 individual drawings, 19 gross photographs) by the king of cardiovascular pathology and his devoted physician son. The relatively brief text represents a few notes to the beautiful music.

ELECTROCARDIOGRAPHY

***40.** Fisch C, Knoebel SB. *Electrocardiography of Clinical Arrhythmias.* Armonk, New York: Futura Publishing Company 2000:407, $49.00.

This richly illustrated practical book shows how to

diagnose the various arrhythmias from the surface electrocardiogram. The first part of the book focuses primarily on the electrocardiography of the arrhythmias most commonly encountered, and the second part focuses on the mechanisms of arrhythmogenesis and the deductive processes used to reach the diagnoses of complex arrhythmias. Every cardiologist could benefit from this book.

41. Fowler NO. *Clinical Electrocardiographic Diagnosis. A Problem-Based Approach.* Philadelphia: Lippincott Williams & Wilkins 2000:244, $49.95.

Another book on electrocardiograms. Yes. But this one is by Noble Fowler and therefore it is worth taking a look at. Each page presents 1 or 2 twelve-lead electrocardiograms and a caption providing a brief clinical history. The accompanying text is exceedingly short but good.

***42.** Osterhues H-H, Hombach V, Moss AJ, editors. *Advances in Noninvasive Electrocardiographic Monitoring Techniques*. Dordrecht: Kluwer Academic Publishers 2000:493, $175.00.

This book by 45 contributors focuses on the various forms of electrocardiography such as the standard 12-lead electrocardiogram; high resolution, ambulatory and exercise electrocardiography; and related domains such as magnetocardiography, newer signal detection and analysis techniques, and ambulatory blood pressure monitoring. The price, however, is too much.

EXERCISE TESTING

43. Franklin BA (Senior Editor); Whaley MH and Howley ET (Associate Editors). *American College of Sport Medicine's Guidelines For Exercise Testing and Prescription. Sixth Edition.* Philadelphia: Lippincott Williams & Wilkins 2000:368, $29.95.

This is the sixth edition of this book, the first appearing in 1975 and the fifth one in 1995. The fifth edition sold about 100,000 copies, making it one of the largest medical publications. This is a superb book on this subject.

ECHOCARDIOGRAPHY

44. Wiegers SE, Plappert T, St. John Sutton M, editors. *Echocardiography in Practice. A Case-Oriented Approach.* London: Martin Dunitz 2001:536, $149.00.

This beautifully prepared book contains 150 chapters by 21 contributors, all but 3 of whom are located at the University of Pennsylvania Medical Center. Each chapter is a case presentation with all images from the single patient.

CARDIOVASCULAR IMAGING

45. Pohost GM, O'Rourke RA, Berman DS, Shah PM, editors. *Imaging in Cardiovascular Disease.* Philadelphia: Lippincott Williams & Wilkins 2000: 976, $149.00.

This superb book of 66 chapters by 101 contributors provides a comprehensive and up-to-date reviews of each of the cardiovascular imaging techniques presently available including ultrasound-based methods, myocardial perfusion techniques, radionuclide methods for evaluating cardiac ventricular function and metabolism, computed tomography and electron-beam computed tomography, and magnetic resonance imaging including spectroscopy. Following the discussion of each imaging technique, there is a section on clinical applications.

***46.** Iskandrian AE, Van Der Wall EE, editors. *Myocardial Viability. 2nd Completely Revised Edition.* Dordrecht: Kluwer Academic Publishers 2000: 240, $118.00.

This book of 11 chapters by 19 contributors updates the first edition published in 1994. The techniques include positron emission tomography, thallium-201, technetium-99m-labeled perfusion tracers, fatty acid SPECT imaging, FDG SPECT, angiography, echocardiography, and magnetic resonance imaging.

CARDIAC CATHETERIZATION AND INTERVENTION

47. Baim DS, Grossman W, editors. *Grossman's Cardiac Catheterization, Angiography, and Intervention, Sixth Edition.* Philadelphia: Lippincott Williams & Wilkins 2000:943, $125.00.

This book of 35 chapters by 32 contributors is called by the editors ". . . the leading text of invasive cardiology." They are probably correct, but the Pepine book on this subject is giving them some competition. For those in the cardiac catheterization laboratory this book is highly useful.

48. Ellis SG, Holmes DR Jr, editors. *Strategic Approaches in Coronary Intervention. Second Edition.* Philadelphia: Lippincott Williams & Wilkins 2000:622, $99.00.

This book by 103 contributors comes just 4 years after the first edition and it provides a comprehensive review of interventional cardiology in its 36 chapters. It's well done.

49. Colombo A, Tobis J, editors. *Techniques in Coronary Artery Stenting.* London: Martin Dunitz 2000:422, $108.00.

The 11 contributors produce 24 chapters, most of which are beautifully illustrated.

50. Waksman R, Serruys PW, editors. *Handbook of Vascular Brachytherapy. Second Edition.* London: Martin Dunitz 2000:238, $50.00.

Whether radiation will prove useful is unclear (at least to me). I am doubtful. This small book of 26 chapters by 61 contributors updates this field. The first edition appeared only 2 years earlier.

CARDIOVASCULAR SURGERY

51. Gewertz BL, Schwartz LB, editors. *Surgery of the Aorta and Its Branches.* Philadelphia: W.B. Saunders Company 2000:479, $165.00.

This book by 2 editors, 11 associate editors, and 71 contributors is authored by vascular surgeons and of course intended for them. Both text and illustrations are excellent.

52. Baumgartner WA, Stuart RS, Gott VL,

Schlossberg L, editors. *Atlas of Cardiac Surgery*. Philadelphia: Hanley & Belfus 2000:264, $195.00.

This book authored by the 4 editors plus 5 contributors is essentially a collection of 193 drawings by the finest medical illustrator of the last half of the 20th century, namely Leon Schlossberg, a talented and splendid man who died on December 19, 1999. I also had the privilege of working with Leon Schlossberg when I was at the NIH. Mr. Schlossberg prepared >500 illustrations for me during the many years I worked with him.

***53.** Steinberg JS, editor. *Atrial Fibrillation After Cardiac Surgery*. Boston: Kluwer Academic Publishers 2000:169, $125.00.

This book of 10 chapters by 16 contributors focuses on the most common arrhythmic complication of cardiac surgery. It brings a lot of information on this topic to a single location.

***54.** Goldstein DJ, Oz MC, editors. *Cardiac Assist Devices*. Armonk, New York: Futura Publishing Company 2000:444, $115.00.

This book by 70 contributors brings up to date in one place the field of mechanical circulatory support. Because only an estimated 1 in 25 who could greatly benefit from a heart transplant actually receives a donor organ, cardiac mechanical assist devices are needed. The book of 30 chapters by leaders in this field is divided into 3 sections: general aspects of mechanical support; extracorporeal and intracorporeal devices; and future devices.

MISCELLANEOUS

55. Marso SP, Griffin BP, Topol EJ, editors. *Manual of Cardiovascular Medicine*. Philadelphia: Lippincott Williams & Wilkins 2000:878, $39.95.

This book of 58 chapters by 44 contributors, most of whom are or were cardiology fellows at the Cleveland Clinic Foundation, provides a huge amount of cardiologic information that fits into a pocket of the white coat. The price is also reasonable (4.5 cents/page).

56. Sharis PJ, Cannon CP. *Evidence-Based Cardiology*. Philadelphia: Lippincott Williams & Wilkins 2000:368, $39.95.

This double-authored book is filled with cardiologic information and it readily fits into the coat pocket.

57. Opie LH, editor; Gersh BJ, co-editor. *Drugs for the Heart*. Fifth Edition. Philadelphia: W.B. Saunders Company 2001:426, $39.95.

This book of 11 chapters by 10 contributors represents a concise yet complete presentation of cardiac pharmacology and therapeutics. The diagrams and tables are superb and the references are up to date.

58. Mancia G, editor. *Angiotensin II Receptor Antagonists in Perspective*. London: Martin Dunitz 2000:175, $65.00.

This small book of 9 chapters by 14 contributors provides much information on the angiotensin II blockers.

***59.** Thompson PD, editor. *Exercise and Sports Cardiology*. New York: McGraw-Hill Medical Publishing Division 2001:504, $75.00.

The 21 chapters by 30 contributors embodies virtually all aspects of exercise and sports in cardiovascular medicine. It fits, as Eric Topol emphasizes in his foreword, an unmet need in cardiovascular medicine.

60. McManus BM (volume editor); Eugene Braunwald (series editor). *Atlas of Cardiovascular Pathology for the Clinician*. Philadelphia: Current Medicine 2001:290, $125.00.

The 30 contributors present 17 beautifully illustrated chapters.

61. Perloff JK. *Physical Examination of the Heart and Circulation. Third Edition*. Philadelphia: W.B. Saunders Company 2000:340, $34.95.

This is it on this subject by the master of the physical examination of the heart and circulation!

***62.** Schnall PL, Belkić K, Landsbergis P, Baker D, editors. *Occupational Medicine. The Workplace and Cardiovascular Disease*. Philadelphia: Hanley & Belfus 2000:334, $39.00.

The 14 chapters by 38 contributors discusses specific features of the work environment, the locus in which adults spend most of their awake hours, which contribute to cardiovascular disease including systemic hypertension. The authors introduce the word "econeurocardiology" to describe the theoretical constructs of work stress as it relates to cardiovascular disease.

***63.** Roberts WC. *Facts and Ideas From Anywhere*. Armonk, New York: Futura Publishing Company 2000:172, $39.00.

This single-authored book includes the from-the-editor columns entitled "Facts and Ideas From Anywhere" appearing in the *Baylor University Medical Center Proceedings* from April 1994 through April 2000. A total of 560 topics, many of which concern cardiovascular disease, are commented upon. Of course, I think this is a fine book.

COMMENTS

Of the 63 books mentioned herein, 50 (79%) were edited and therefore multiauthored; 6 (10%) were single authored; 5 (8%) were by 2 authors; and 1 each by either 3 or 4 authors. Of the 63 books, 15 (24%) contained a 2001 publication date, and the remaining 48 (76%), a 2000 date. Thirty (48%) were published on acid-free (permanent) paper and 33 (52%) on acid paper. Unfortunately, the 2 largest US publishers (Lippincott Williams & Wilkins and W.B. Saunders) use only acid paper. The 63 books ranged in cost from $29.00 to $275.00 (mean $113.00). The year 2000 was a good year for new cardiovascular books!

William C. Roberts

William Clifford Roberts, MD
Baylor Heart and Vascular Center
Baylor University Medical Center
Dallas, Texas 75246

Good Books in Cardiovascular Disease Appearing in 2001

MAJOR CARDIOVASCULAR TEXTBOOKS

1. Braunwald E, Zipes DP, Libby P, editors. *Heart Disease. A Textbook of Cardiovascular Medicine. Sixth Edition.* Philadelphia: WB Saunders Company 2001:2385, $145.00 (single volume), and $165.00 (2 volumes).

This is the sixth edition in 21 years of this classic, and the first in which Braunwald was not the sole editor. The 72 chapters were written by 103 contributors. Each page is maximally packed with information. I suspect that there is more information in this cardiovascular textbook than in any text on this topic ever published. If one can have only one book in cardiovascular medicine, this is the one to have.

2. Lilly LS. *Heart Disease Review and Assessment to accompany Braunwald/Zipes/Libby: Heart Disease, Sixth Edition.* Philadelphia: WB Saunders Company 2001:268, $59.00.

This book provides >700 questions and answers related to the sixth edition of Braunwald's *Heart Disease*. All information is cross-referenced to pertinent sections of the Braunwald text, including the CD-ROM version of the text. Questions with answers are the easiest way for me to learn. Highly recommended.

3. Becker RC, Alpert JS, editors. *Cardiovascular Medicine. Practice and Management.* London: Arnold 2001:825, $98.50.

This textbook of 41 chapters by 62 contributors provides clear, concise, practical, and science-oriented guidelines that have direct applicability to routine practice in both ambulatory and hospital-based settings. Patient management is the book's theme.

4. Rosendorff C, editor. *Essential Cardiology Principles and Practice.* Philadelphia: WB Saunders 2001: 895, $65.00.

This book of 43 chapters by 73 contributors is not an all-inclusive textbook of cardiology but it does contain the information cardiologists need to practice well. The type is relatively small so that the amount of information per page is impressive.

5. Allen HD, Clark EB, Gutgesell HP, Driscoll DJ, editors. *Moss and Adams' Heart Disease in Infants, Children, and Adolescents Including the Fetus and Young Adult. Sixth Edition.* Volumes I and II. Philadelphia: Lippincott Williams & Wilkins 2001:1564, $269.00.

Beautiful book in 2 volumes by 113 contributors.

*__6.__ Rudolph AM. *Congenital Diseases of the Heart: Clinical-Physiological Considerations. Fully Revised and Updated Second Edition.* Armonk, New York: Futura Publishing 2001:808, $98.00.

The first edition of this book appeared in 1974 and the new one 25 years later is similar in that it is single authored and contains few figures, virtually all of which are diagrams. Nevertheless, wisdom exudes from the pages and every pediatric cardiologist could learn from this wise author.

CORONARY ARTERY DISEASE

*__7.__ Hurst JW, Morris DC, editors. "*Chest Pain→*" Armonk, New York: Futura Publishing 2001:514, $79.00.

This book of 52 chapters by 30 contributors is worth owning. It is not going out of date next year! It discusses "chest pain" in patients with herpes zoster, costochondritis, thoracic outlet syndromes, chest wall syndromes, shoulder-hand syndromes, bursitis and arthritis of the shoulder, joint disease of the cervical or thoracic spine, Mondor's syndrome, cervical disc syndrome, brachial plexus neuropathy, mediastinal emphysema, pleuritis, pneumothorax, pulmonary embolism, "café" coronary, esophageal mobility disorders, gastroesophageal reflex, esophageal rupture, esophageal stenosis, esophagitis, etc.

*__8.__ Adams JE III, Apple FS, Jaffe AS, Wu AHB, editors. *Markers in Cardiology: Current and Future Clinical Applications.* Armonk, New York: Futura 2001:272, $79.00.

A timely and needed book of 20 chapters by 46 contributors.

9. de Bono D, Sobel BE, editors. *Acute Coronary*

*Published on acid-free (permanent) paper.

Syndromes. Oxford: Blackwell Science 2001:308, $99.00.

This is an excellent book of 17 chapters by 32 contributors. Bert Sobel in the preface pays a beautiful tribute to the late David de Bono.

10. Stansfeld S, Marmot M, editors. *Stress and the Heart. Psychosocial Pathways to Coronary Heart Disease*. London, UK: BMJ Books 2002:304, $49.95.

This fine book of 16 chapters by 22 contributors discusses various "risk factors" to coronary disease, including hostility, social isolation, job strain, depression, and socioeconomic inequality among others. Every cardiologist could learn a lot from this book.

CORONARY INTERVENTION

11. Stack RS, Roubin GS, O'Neill WW, editors. *Interventional Cardiovascular Medicine. Principles and Practice*. New York: Churchill Livingstone 2002: 976, $189.00.

This book of 50 chapters by 93 investigators is the bible on this topic. It needs to be in the library of all interventional cardiologists.

12. Norell MS, Perrins EJ, editors. *Essential Interventional Cardiology*. Philadelphia: WB Saunders 2001:420, $55.00.

This book of 29 chapters by 34 contributors, nearly all of whom are from the United Kingdom, describe current practices of percutaneous coronary intervention.

***13.** Abela GS, editor. *Myocardial Revascularization. Novel Percutaneous Approaches*. New York: Wiley-Liss 2002:278, $119.00.

This is an intriguing, highly recommended book of 19 chapters by 53 contributors.

***14.** Nguyen TN, Saito S, Hu D, Dave V, Grines CL, editors. *Practical Handbook of Advanced Interventional Cardiology*. Armonk, New York: Futura 2001:586, $49.00.

This handbook of 28 chapters by 58 contributors provides much practical information for the interventional cardiologist.

***15.** Uchida Y. *Coronary Angioscopy*. Armonk, New York: Futura Publishing 2001:274, $80.00.

This is the first book on this topic and it is by a pioneer in coronary angioscopy. For those interested in this topic, this is it.

***16.** Salerno TA, Ricci M, Karamanoukian HL, D'Ancona G, Bergsland J, editors. *Beating Heart Coronary Artery Surgery*. Armonk, New York: Futura Publishing 2001:278, $75.00.

This book of 22 chapters by 36 contributors puts in one place a great deal of information about this important development in coronary bypass surgery.

***17.** D'Ancona G, Karamanoukian HL, Ricci M, Salerno TA, Bergsland J. *Intraoperative Graft Patency Verification in Cardiac and Vascular Surgery*. Armonk, New York: Futura Publishing 2001:248, $80.00.

This book describes various methods to confirm that grafts, both coronary and noncoronary ones, are patent and that they provide adequate flow to tissues at rest and during exercise.

SYSTEMIC HYPERTENSION

18. MacGregor GA, Kaplan NM. *Hypertension. Second Edition*. Oxford: Health Press 2001:72, $19.95.

A neat little book on an extremely important subject. About 50% of persons in the Western World have systolic blood pressures >140 mm Hg or diastolic pressures >90 mm Hg, or both, and yet <20% of them have their elevated pressures controlled. The way to prevent stroke, aortic dissection, abdominal aortic aneurysm, and heart failure is to prevent systemic hypertension and this book helps in that regard.

19. Sibai BM, editor. *Hypertensive Disorders in Women*. Philadelphia: WB Saunders 2001:262, $89.00.

This book by 19 contributors focuses on recent developments in the prevention and management of systemic hypertension in women, mainly young women, and includes those in nonpregnant and pregnant women, and preconception counseling of women with hypertension.

HEART FAILURE

20. Young JB, Mills RM. *Clinical Management of Heart Failure. First Edition*. Caddo, Oklahoma: Professional Communications 2001:320, $24.95.

This little pocket book focuses primarily on the treatment of heart failure.

CONGENITAL HEART DISEASE

21. Johnson WH Jr, Moller JH. *Pediatric Cardiology*. Philadelphia: Lippincott Williams & Wilkins 2001:326, $29.95.

A nice handbook.

***22.** Gatzoulis MA, Murphy DJ Jr, editors. *The Adult with Tetralogy of Fallot. The ISACCD Monograph Series*. Armonk, New York: Futura Publishing Company 2001:95, $29.50.

This monograph of 6 chapters by 22 contributors is the first of a series on common topics in adult congenital heart disease co-sponsored by the International Society of Adult Congenital Cardiac Disease (ISACCD) and Futura Media Services.

ELECTROCARDIOLOGY AND ELECTROPHYSIOLOGY

23. Surawicz B, Knilans TK. *Chou's Electrocardiography in Clinical Practice. Adult and Pediatric.*

Fifth Edition. Philadelphia: WB Saunders 2001:709, $99.00.

This is a splendid book. Dr. Te-Chuan Chou, the author of the first 4 editions, died on November 30, 1995. Borys Surawicz revised and updated the first 27 chapters (629 pages) on adult electrocardiography and Timothy K. Knilans contributed the 4 chapters (56 pages) on pediatric electrocardiography. This is a book worth owning.

24. Wagner GS. *Marriott's Practical Electrocardiography. Tenth Edition.* Philadelphia: Lippincott Williams & Wilkins 2001:475, $49.95.

Books do not go through 10 editions unless they are excellent and certainly this one is. The Marriott-Wagner electrocardiograms are well trimmed and the waves very clear. There is more clear or empty space than is necessary.

*__25.__ Ganz LI, editor. *Management of Cardiac Arrhythmias.* Totowa, New Jersey: Humana Press 2002: 527, $125.00.

This book by 42 contributors shows the tremendous development in this field in the treatment of arrhythmias. It shows how cardiac electrophysiology has evolved from a purely diagnostic to an interventional field. Radiofrequency catheter ablation and implantable cardioverter-defibrillators are now standard, even in outpatient procedures.

26. Rimmerman CM, Jain AK. *Interactive Electrocardiography. CD-ROM with Workbook.* Philadelphia: Lippincott Williams & Wilkins 2001:654, $99.95.

This book and CD-ROM contain 631 digital high-quality electrocardiograms, essentially 1 per page, with 3 blank lines for written interpretation beneath each electrocardiogram. Eric Topol in his foreword calls it "an unparalleled work . . . destined to become a classic [which] . . . takes the field of electrocardiography to a new height . . ."

27. Chung EK. *Pocket Guide to ECG Diagnosis. Second Edition.* Malden, Massachusetts: Blackwell Science 2001:508, $45.00.

This little book describes the common electrocardiographic abnormalities including arrhythmias. On the left page is information on the electrocardiographic abnormality, which is on the right page.

*__28.__ Hurst JW. *Interpreting Electrocardiograms Using Basic Principles and Vector Concepts.* New York: Marcel Dekker 2001:317, $165.00.

Willis Hurst has taught electrocardiography by the vector approach for 50 years. As a medical student Dr. Hurst introduced me to Robert P. Grant's splendid book (*Clinical Electrocardiography. The Spatial Vector Approach.* New York: McGraw-Hill 1957:225) and it is one of the prize possessions in my cardiovascular library. In 1991, Hurst published *Ventricular Electrocardiography*, a beautiful book, which also stressed the vector approach and which was dedicated to Robert Grant (1915–1966). Hurst's newest book, a splendid one, is about the same size as Grant's 1957 book, and it deals with the basic principles used to determine the direction and size of the electrical forces that produce the P, QRS, S-T, and T waves.

29. Tighe DA, Cook JR, Schweiger MJ, Chung EK. *Pocket Guide to ECG Diagnosis. Second Edition.* Malden, Massachusetts: Blackwell Science 2001:239, $29.95.

This pocket book or manual describes the drugs used in patients with cardiovascular disease.

30. Garratt C. *Mechanisms and Management of Cardiac Arrhythmias.* London, UK: BMJ Books 2001: 176, $49.95.

A single-authored neat little book that fits into a white-coat pocket.

31. Ellenbogen KA, Wood MA, editors. *Cardiac Pacing and ICDs. Third Edition.* Malden, Massachusetts 2002:530, $49.95.

This book of 10 chapters by 12 contributors focuses on pacemakers and implantable cardioverter-defibrillators.

32. Kusumoto FM, Goldschlager NF, editors. *Cardiac Pacing For the Clinician.* Philadelphia: Lippincott Williams & Wilkins 2001:404, $99.00.

This good book of 17 chapters by 25 contributors provides current information on pacemakers and defibrillators for the non-electrophysiologist.

*__33.__ Israel CW, Barold SS, editors. *Advances in the Treatment of Atrial Tachyarrhythmias: Pacing, Cardioversion, and Defibrillation.* Armonk, New York: Futura 2002:446, $127.00.

This is the first book devoted solely to the rapidly expanding options to prevent and terminate atrial tachyarrhythmias electrically. Forty investigators contributed the 20 chapters.

34. Singer I, editor. *Interventional Electrophysiology. Second Edition.* Philadelphia: Lippincott Williams & Wilkins 2001:858, $175.00.

A major electrophysiology book by 74 contributors.

35. Walsh EP, Saul JP, Triedman JK, editors. *Cardiac Arrhythmias in Children and Young Adults With Congenital Heart Disease.* Philadelphia: Lippincott Williams & Wilkins 2001:516, $150.00.

This is a major text on this topic. It consists of 25 chapters by 21 contributors.

36. Balaji S, Gillette PC, Case CL, editors. *Cardiac Arrhythmias after Surgery for Congenital Heart Disease.* London, UK: Arnold 2001:360, $98.50.

This book of 18 chapters by 23 contributors attempts to describe what is known about arrhythmias developing after cardiac surgery for congenital heart disease.

*__37.__ Zeighler VL, Gillette PC, editors. *Practical Management of Pediatric Cardiac Arrhythmias.* Armonk, New York: Futura 2001:422, $69.00.

This book of 8 chapters by 13 contributors describes various arrhythmias and their management in children.

*38. Oto A, Breithardt G, editors. *Myocardial Repolarization. From Gene to Bedside.* Armonk, New York: Futura 2001:402, $105.00.

This book of 25 chapters by 56 contributors focuses on the electrical behavior of myocardial cells in health and disease, on the use of the electrocardiogram for the evaluation of repolarization of the ventricular myocardium, and on drugs used to treat arrhythmias and how to avoid serious drug-induced arrhythmias.

39. Zareba W, Maison-Blanche P, Locati EH, editors. *Noninvasive Electrocardiology in Clinical Practice.* Armonk, New York: Futura 2001:489, $98.00.

This book of 25 chapters by 54 contributors, mainly European, describes noninvasive electrophysiology that attempts to reconcile comprehensive invasive electrophysiology with conventional surface electrocardiography by extracting from the latter more extensive information.

*40. Rosenbaum DS, Jalife J, editors. *Optical Mapping of Cardiac Excitation and Arrhythmias.* Armonk, New York: Futura 2001:458, $99.00.

This unique book of 23 chapters by 36 contributors bridges the gap between basic science and clinical electrophysiology.

ECHOCARDIOGRAPHY

41. Wiegers SE, Plappert T, St John Sutton M, editors. *Echocardiography in Practice. A Case-Oriented Approach.* London: Martin Dunitz 2001:536, $175.00.

A major book by 21 contributors. This book presents one case after another. The illustrations are magnificent. My only criticism is that there is too much blank space on too many pages, and that increases the book's cost.

42. Linker DT. *Practical Echocardiography of Congenital Heart Disease. From Fetus to Adult.* New York: Churchill Livingstone 2001:203, $105.00.

Nice book.

CARDIAC IMAGING

43. DePuey EG, Garcia EV, Berman DS, editors. *Cardiac SPECT Imaging. Second Edition.* Philadelphia: Lippincott Williams & Wilkins 2001:349, $149.95.

This book of 16 chapters by 26 contributors focuses on myocardial perfusion single-photon emission computed tomography (SPECT), the most widely used noninvasive imaging modality for the diagnosis and management of patients with coronary artery disease. If this is your interest, this is your book.

44. Manning WJ, Pennell DJ, editors. *Cardiovascular Magnetic Resonance.* New York: Churchill Livingstone 2002:472, $120.00.

This fine book of 35 chapters by 65 contributors, as stated by Eugene Braunwald in the foreword, is "detailed, authoritative, yet eminently readable." Cardiovascular magnetic resonance combines unsurpassed image quality of the heart with blood flow, myocardial perfusion, angiography, oxygen saturation, temperature, and chemical composition. Cardiovascular magnetic resonance is rapidly becoming the preferred method for determining cardiac anatomy and function.

CARDIOVASCULAR PATHOLOGY

45. Silver MD, Gotlieb AI, Schoen FJ, editors. *Cardiovascular Pathology. Third Edition.* New York: Churchill Livingstone 2001:808, $295.00.

46. Virmani R, Farb A, Burke A, Atkinson JB. *Cardiovascular Pathology. Second Edition.* (Volume 40 in the Series MAJOR PROBLEMS IN PATHOLOGY). Philadelphia: WB Saunders 2001:541, $99.00.

MISCELLANEOUS

*47. Johnstone MT, Veves A, editors. *Diabetes and Cardiovascular Disease.* Totowa, New Jersey: Humana Press 2001:458, $125.00.

This book of 24 chapters by 51 contributors covers this topic admirably.

48. Alpert JS, editor; Aurigemma GP, Balady GJ, Chaitman BR, Crawford MH, Epstein AE, Francis GS, Gersony WM, Harrington RA, Wenger NK, associate editors. *The AHA Clinical Cardiac Consult.* Philadelphia: Lippincott Williams & Wilkins 2001: 311, $59.95.

This book by 85 contributors covers 150 topics discussed under 6 headings: basics, diagnosis, treatment, medications, follow-up, and miscellaneous. Three of these headings are briefly discussed on each page. I guess that this format would be appealing to some physicians. Some columns are mainly blank space. I prefer a cardiologic textbook but that is only 1 view.

49. Cannon CP, O'Gara PT, editors. *Critical Pathways in Cardiology.* Philadelphia: Lippincott Williams & Wilkins 2001:260, $59.95.

This book of 24 chapters by 33 contributors presents critical pathways (standardized documents or computer order sets incorporating new cost-effective therapies) or "best practices" as developed by leaders in their areas. This is an interesting and useful book.

50. Katz AM. *Physiology of the Heart. Third Edition.* Philadelphia: Lippincott Williams & Wilkins 2001:718, $99.00.

This book, which is reaching "classic" status, describes the biophysical basis of cardiac function. Katz emphasizes that "virtually every important physiological, pharmacological, or pathological change in cardiac function arises from alterations in the physical and chemical processes that are responsible for the heart beat."

***51.** Bers DM. *Excitation—Contraction Coupling and Cardiac Contractile Force. Second Edition.* Dordrecht: Kluwer Academic 2001:427, $147.00.

This single-authored book is similar to Arnold Katz's book. It provides an overview of calcium regulation in cardiac muscle cells, particularly with respect to excitation-contraction coupling and the control of cardiac contractile force.

***52.** Goldhaber SZ, Ridker PM, editors. *Thrombosis and Thromboembolism.* New York: Marcel Dekker 2002:365, $165.00.

This book of 20 chapters by 28 contributors (19 from Boston) focuses on hypercoagulability, acute coronary syndromes, venous thromboembolism, and diagnostic laboratory and catheter interventions for both arterial and venous thromboembolism.

53. Sutherland J. *Blackwell's Primary Care Essentials: Cardiology.* Malden, Massachusetts: Blackwell Science 2001:304, $38.95.

This handbook is intended for the primary care physician as a guide to cardiology. The book contains 200 abbreviations, not including those in the references. That's too many!

54. Hoekstra JW, editor. *Handbook of Cardiovascular Emergencies. Second Edition.* Philadelphia: Lippincott Williams & Wilkins 2001:494, $39.95.

This pocket book of 45 chapters by 51 contributors is fully packed and quite useful.

***55.** Nguyen TN, Hu D, Saito S, Dave V, Rocha-Singh K, Grines CL, editors. *Management of Complex Cardiovascular Problems. The Consultant's Approach.* Armonk, New York: Futura 2002:409, $54.00.

This book of 18 chapters by 64 contributors describes some of the most difficult problems faced by cardiovascular specialists.

***56.** Young DB. *Role of Potassium in Preventive Cardiovascular Medicine.* Boston: Kluwer Academic Publishers 2001:219, $165.00.

There are about 3,500 mmol of potassium in the body, only 65 mmol of which is present in the blood and extracellular fluids. Potassium plays a major role in nerve conduction and for enabling skeletal and cardiac muscle contraction. Dr. Young has investigated potassium for >25 years. As Dr. John Laragh states in his foreword "David's book is a must for me and for all other Kalomaniacs."

57. Franklin BA, Noakes T, Brusis OA. *Active Cardiac Rehabilitation.* Kempele, Finland: Polar Electro 2001:82, $1.75.

This booklet is an outgrowth of Dr. Barry Franklin's 1999 booklet entitled "Post Cardiac: Physical Activity & Healthy Lifestyle" published by the same publisher. Both of these booklets are very useful for cardiac patients undergoing rehabilitation. The earlier edition (1999) costs only $1.00.

58. Khan MG. *On Call Cardiology. Second Edition.* Philadelphia: WB Saunders 2001:486, $28.00.

A nice fully packed pocket book of cardiology.

59. Estafanous FG, Barash PG, Reves JG, editors. *Cardiac Anesthesia. Principles and Clinical Practice. Second Edition.* Philadelphia: Lippincott Williams & Wilkins 2001:1035, $199.00.

This book of 33 chapters by 60 contributors must be the most comprehensive on this topic.

60. Liu MB, Davis K. *Lessons From a Horse Named Jim.* A Clinical Trials Manual From The Duke Clinical Research Institute. Durham, North Carolina: Duke Clinical Research Institute 2001:279, $69.95.

In 1901, a horse named Jim was used to prepare an antitoxin for diphtheria. After the death of 13 children who received the antitoxin, investigators discovered that the horse had developed tetanus and therefore had contaminated the antitoxin. As a result, Congress passed the Biologic Control Act of 1902, giving the government regulatory power over antitoxin and vaccine development. This book describes the process of conducting clinical trials, both its theory and its practice. A very useful book for those involved in clinical trials.

GOOD READS

***61.** Kastor JA. *Mergers of Teaching Hospitals in Boston, New York, and Northern California.* Ann Arbor, Michigan: The University of Michigan Press 2001:487, $59.50.

This beautifully researched and written book describes the conditions that led to mergers of some of the USA's top teaching hospitals: The Massachusetts General and Brigham and Women's hospitals in Boston; the Presbyterian and New York hospitals in New York City; and the teaching hospitals of the University of California, San Francisco, and Stanford University.

62. Blackburn H. *PK. Irreverent Memoirs of a Preacher's Kid.* Published by Henry Blackburn 1999: 152, $15.00.

63. Blackburn H. *If It Isn't Fun . . . A Memoir from a Different Sort of Medical Life. Volume 1. The First 30 Years, 1942–72.* Published by Henry Blackburn 2001:443, $15.00.

I have not laughed in years as much as I did while reading these 2 memoirs by Henry Blackburn, who is a splendid writer and wonderful storyteller. Henry was also one of the very best epidemiologists—preventive cardiologists of the 20th century! I highly recommend these 2 books to anyone who enjoys a good laugh. The pages are filled with them.

COMMENTS

Of the 63 books mentioned herein, 37 (59%) were edited and multiauthored; 14 (22%) were single authored, and the remainder had from 2 to 5 authors. Of the 63 books, 9 (14%) had a 2002 publication date; 53 (84%) a 2001 date, and 1, a 1999 date. Twenty (32%) were published on acid-free (permanent) paper, and 43 (68%) on acid paper. Only books sent to me were included in this review. Thus, I suspect that some good books appearing in 2001 were omitted from this list. For any omissions, I apologize.

William C. Roberts

William Clifford Roberts, MD
Baylor Heart and Vascular Institute
Baylor University Medical Center
Dallas, Texas 75246

Good Books in Cardiovascular Disease Appearing in 2002

MAJOR CARDIOVASCULAR TEXTBOOKS

1. Topol EJ, editor; Califf RM, Prystowsky EN, Thompson PD, Isner JM, Swain JL, Thomas JD, Young JB, associate editors. *Textbook of Cardiovascular Medicine.* Second Edition. Philadelphia: Lippincott Williams & Wilkins 2002:2210, $234.75.

This edited book of 112 chapters by 182 contributors is superb. It comes only 4 years after the first edition appeared. This book has to be compared with other textbooks on cardiovascular disease. The latest (2001) Braunwald-Zipes-Libby textbook contains 2,362 pages and more content per page. The Willerson-Cohn textbook (2000) contains 2,344 pages and also is more densely packed than the Topol book. The Fuster-Alexander-O'Rourke textbook (2001) contains 2,660 pages. All 4 are good. Does one buy the latest or the one most densely packed with information?

2. Anderson RH, Baker EJ, Macartney RFJ, Rigby ML, Shinebourne EA, Tynan M, editors. *Paediatric Cardiology.* 2nd Edition. London: Churchill Livingstone 2002:2059, $399.00 (2 volumes).

The first edition of this edited book appeared 15 years ago in 1987. The present edition contains 75 chapters by 74 contributors. The 6 editors are from London, UK, and more of the contributors are from UK than from any other country. The book (2 volumes) is very comprehensive. The illustrations for the most part are excellent but diagrams are relatively few in number.

*3. Lanzer P, Topol EJ, editors. *Pan Vascular Medicine. Integrated Clinical Management.* Berlin: Springer 2002:1941, $199.00.

This book of 133 chapters by 300 contributors is a comprehensive state-of-the-art review of current vascular medicine.

*4. Frishman WH, Sonnenblick EH, Sica DA, editors. *Cardiovascular Pharmacotherapeutics.* Second Edition. New York: McGraw-Hill 2003:1072, $159.00.

This book of 51 chapters and 8 appendixes by 115 contributors appears 6 years after the first edition. It provides updated information on drugs used in patients with cardiovascular disease. The sections of the book include clinical pharmacology, patient compliance issues, new drug development, the placebo effect, pharmacoeconomics, and a chapter on history of cardiac drug development.

5. Antman EM, editor; Colucci WS, Gotto AM Jr, Josephson ME, Loscalzo J, Oparil S, Popma JJ, section editors. *CARDIOVASCULAR THERAPEUTICS. A Companion to Braunwald's Heart Disease.* Second Edition. Philadelphia: WB Saunders Company, 2002:1213, $149.00.

This edited book of 55 chapters and 3 appendixes by 112 contributors discusses cardiovascular therapeutics, which includes drugs, catheter-based interventions, and surgical procedures. This is a good book but most of the information in it appears also in Braunwald-Zipes-Libby's *Heart Disease.*

6. Yusuf S, Cairns JA, Camm AJ, Fallen EL, Gersh BJ, editors. *Evidence-based Cardiology.* Second Edition. London, UK: BMJ Books, 2003:968, $165.00.

This book of 74 chapters by 132 contributors is intriguing and very readable. Within the text or tables of each chapter the therapeutic recommendations are graded according to the level of evidence (Grade A [level 1a, 1b, 1c, 1d], B [level 2, 3, 4], and C [level 5]), supporting the recommendation. This book is not as comprehensive as the Braunwald, Fuster, Topol, or Willerson textbooks, but not nearly as heavy.

SYSTEMIC HYPERTENSION

7. Mancia G, Chalmers J, Julius S, Saruta T, Weber MA, Ferrari AU, Wilkinson IB, editors. *Manual of Hypertension.* London: Churchill Livingstone, 2002: 706, $89.00.

This book of 45 chapters by 74 contributors (59 [80%] from non-USA countries) is soft-covered and called a "manual." It contains a lot of information on hypertension but a lot of space on each page is blank. If the space on each page had been better utilized, the book would have been much smaller, weighed less, and cost less.

8. Moser M. *The Treatment of Hypertension. A Story of Myths, Misconceptions, Controversies, and Heroics.* Second Edition. New York: Le Jacq Communications, 2002:94, $17.00.

A neat little book.

CORONARY HEART DISEASE

*9. Hasdai D, Berger PB, Battler A, Holmes DR Jr, editors. *Cardiogenic Shock. Diagnosis and Treatment.*

Totowa, New Jersey: Humana Press, 2002:381, $135.00.

This book of 21 chapters by 41 contributors focuses mainly on shock caused by coronary artery disease but it also discusses shock associated with valvular, primary myocardial, pericardial, and congenital cardiac diseases. It describes well various percutaneous and thoracotomy-inserted left ventricular assist devices. This is a good book, but a full cardiology textbook can be purchased for the same price.

*10. Ellestad MH, Amsterdam EA, editors. *Exercise Testing: New Concepts for the New Century*. Boston: Kluwer Academic Publishers, 2002:183, $135.00.

This book of 17 chapters by 29 contributors describes present-day modes of exercise testing as a measure of cardiac function. The basic modalities of exercise electrocardiography by treadmill and bicycle have been extended, of course, by noninvasive cardiac imaging techniques, including scintigraphy and echocardiography during exertion and pharmacologic stress, and all these methods and their sensitivities and specificities are discussed in this little but fine book.

*11. Cannon CP, editor. *Management of Acute Coronary Syndromes*. Second Edition. Totowa, New Jersey: Humana Press, 2003:781, $135.00 (soft cover $99.50).

This book of 27 chapters by 54 contributors is superb.

12. Stansfeld S, Marmot M, editors. *Stress and the Heart. Psychosocial Pathways to Coronary Heart Disease*. London: BMJ Books, 2002:304, $49.95.

This book of 16 chapters by 22 contributors brings much information on this topic together under 1 cover.

*13. Sobel BE, Schneider DJ, editors. *Medical Management of Diabetes and Heart Disease*. New York: Marcel Dekker, 2002:292, $125.00.

This book of 16 chapters by 22 contributors is a good one on this topic.

*14. Brown DL, editor. *Cardiovascular Plaque Rupture*. New York: Marcel Dekker, 2002:519, $195.00.

This book of 23 chapters by 58 contributors is a good book for those who put their faith in plaque rupture as the cause of coronary events. I am not in that camp. I believe that plaque rupture is important in acute myocardial infarction, but not in angina pectoris or in sudden coronary death.

*15. Fuster V, editor. *Assessing and Modifying the Vulnerable Atherosclerotic Plaque*. Armond, New York: Futura, 2002:379.

This book of 19 chapters by 45 contributors is similar to the Brown book (14). I believe that plaque quantity is far more important than plaque vulnerability. Nevertheless, this is a good book.

*16. Kromhout D, Menotti A, Blackburn H, editors. *Prevention of Coronary Heart Disease. Diet, Lifestyle and Risk Factors in the Seven Countries Study*. Norwell, Massachusetts: Kluwer Academic Publishers, 2002:267, $135.00.

This book of 18 chapters by 7 contributors—mainly the 3 editors—is superb. It is my kind of book.

THROMBOSIS, THROMBOEMBOLISM, THROMBOLYSIS, BLEEDING

17. Loscalzo J, Schafer AI, editors. *Thrombosis and Hemorrhage*. Third Edition. Philadelphia: Lippincott Williams & Wilkins, 2003:1142, $225.00.

This is a major textbook of 57 chapters by 99 contributors. The first edition appeared in 1994, the second in 1998, and the third in 2002 (although the copyright is 2003). This book is now approaching classic status. It contains most of what is known about bleeding and thrombotic disorders. Each page is fully packed and the illustrations are excellent. Highly recommended!

*18. Sasahara AA, Loscalzo J, editors. *New Therapeutic Agents in Thrombosis and Thrombolysis*. Second Edition, Revised and Expanded. New York: Marcel Dekker, 2003:707, $195.00.

This book of 42 chapters by 91 contributors focuses on therapy of bleeding and clotting disorders. It compliments rather than duplicates the Loscalzo and Schafer book.

*19. Goldhaber SZ, Ridker PM, editors. *Thrombosis and Thromboembolism*. New York: Marcel Dekker, 2002:365, $195.00.

This book of 20 chapters by 28 contributors, 19 of whom are in Boston, provides up-to-date information on a fast-moving field.

PERCUTANEOUS CORONARY INTERVENTION

20. Topol EJ, editor. *Textbook of Interventional Cardiology*. 4th Edition. Philadelphia: WB Saunders, 2003:1123, $169.00.

This book of 53 chapters by 88 contributors is superb and comprehensive. The first edition appeared in 1994, the third in 1999, and now the fourth just 3 years later (it was published in late 2002.). This field is changing so fast that 3 years is plenty of time between editions.

21. Stack RS, Roubin GS, O'Neill WW, editors. *Interventional Cardiovascular Medicine. Principles and Practice*. 2nd Edition. New York: Churchill Livingstone, 2002:976, $194.00.

This book of 50 chapters by 93 authors is comprehensive. The Topol book on this topic is a bit more up to date, more compact, and less expensive.

22. Morrison DA, Serruys PW, editors. *High-Risk Cardiac Revascularization and Clinical Trials*. London: Martin Dunitz, 2002:580, $99.00.

This book of 37 chapters by 49 contributors is very good.

23. Grech ED, Ramsdale DR, editors. *Practical Interventional Cardiology*. Second Edition. London: Martin Dunitz 2002:486, $150.00.

A book of 36 chapters by 65 contributors is good but not nearly as comprehensive as either the Topol or Stack books.

24. Serruys PW, Rensing B, editors. *Handbook of Coronary Stents*. Fourth Edition. London: Martin Dunitz, 2002:366, $75.00.

This book of 43 chapters by 67 contributors provides much information on each of the various stents used in coronary arteries. The book could have been more compact.

25. Serruys PW, Colombo A, Leon MB, Kutryk MJB, editors. *Coronary Lesions. A Pragmatic Approach.* London: Martin Dunitz, 2002:364, $115.00.

This book of 21 chapters by 49 contributors is good.

26. Colombo A, Stankovic G. *Colombo's Tips and Tricks in Interventional Cardiology.* London: Martin Dunitz, 2002:63, $115.00.

This "book" consists primarily of 4 CD-ROMS concerning (1) general approach, (2) value of intravascular ultrasonic imaging, (3) direct coronary atherectomy, and (4) cutting balloon angioplasty. Each CD contains several case discussions. This looks to be useful to the interventionist.

*27. Tcheng JE, editor. *Primary Angioplasty in Acute Myocardial Infarction.* Totowa, New Jersey: Humana Press, 2002:182, $99.50.

This book of 10 chapters by 17 contributors provides superb data about direct percutaneous coronary intervention as primary therapy for patients with acute myocardial infarction. The book's editor is not the author of any chapter.

ECHOCARDIOGRAPHY

28. Otto CM, editor. *The Practice of Clinical Echocardiography.* Second Edition. Philadelphia: W.B. Saunders Company, 2002:977, $195.00.

The second edition of this book, which first appeared in 1997, has 44 chapters by 73 contributors. I find little wrong with this book. It is fully packed with information and the illustrations are well cropped and clear.

*29. Nanda NC, Sorrell VL, editors. *Atlas of Three-Dimensional Echocardiography.* Armonk, New York: Futura Publishing Company, 2002:272, $199.00.

This book of 13 chapters by 13 contributors (9 of the 13 chapters are by both editors only) is probably the best on this topic. The illustrations are excellent and color is used in many. The cost is steep ($1.37 a page) and there is a good bit of wasted space on many pages.

ARRHYTHMIAS

30. Podrid PJ, Kowey PR, editors. *Cardiac Arrhythmia: Mechanisms, Diagnosis & Management.* Second Edition. Philadelphia: Lippincott Williams & Wilkins, 2002:992, $159.00.

Superb!

31. Murgatroyd FD, Krahn AD, Klein GJ, Yee RK, Skanes AC. *Handbook of Cardiac Electrophysiology. A Practical Guide to Invasive EP Studies and Catheter Ablation.* London, UK: REMEDICA Publishing, 2002:248, $120.00.

This beautiful book is filled with one electrophysiologic tracing after another illustrating the various atrial and ventricular arrhythmias. This is a nice book to get a feel of day-to-day electrophysiology.

32. Macle L. *Pulmonary Vein Recordings. A Practical Guide to the Mapping and Ablation of Atrial Fibrillation.* London, UK: REMEDICA Publishing, 2002:125.

A single-authored book showing one electrophysiologic tracing after another of pulmonary venous circumferential mapping and ablation for atrial fibrillation.

*33. Zipes DP, Haïssaguerre M, editors. *Catheter Ablation of Arrhythmias.* Second Edition. Armonk, New York: Futura Publishing Company, 2002:448, $98.00.

This book of 19 chapters by 66 contributors (45 [68%] from non-USA nations) brings together presentations at the Bordeaux symposium in May 2001. The field of electrophysiology, of course, has exploded since the first catheter ablation procedure was performed in March 1982. Publications of symposia presentations infrequently produce chapters of uniform excellence. I think money is better spent buying the best electrophysiology textbook.

CARDIOVASCULAR DISEASE IN WOMEN

34. RETAC. *Radiofrequency Catheter Ablation for the Treatment of Cardiac ARRHYTHMIAS. A Practical Atlas with Illustrative Cases.* Armonk, New York: Futura, 2002:377.

An atlas of 38 cases contributed by 30 physicians in Europe.

35. Douglas PS, editor. *Cardiovascular Health and Disease in Women.* Second Edition. Philadelphia: WB Saunders Company, 2002:545, $125.00.

This book of 29 chapters by 53 contributors, 29 (55%) of whom are women, is excellent. The first edition appeared in 1993 and much has happened in these last 9 years. I like this book very much. Each page is fully packed.

36. Wilansky S, Willerson JT, editors. *Heart Disease in Women.* New York: Churchill Livingstone, 2002:672, $129.95.

This book of 41 chapters by 95 contributors, 58 (61%) of whom reside in Houston, is well done. Not all of the chapters, however, focus exclusively on women. Although the book is useful, a major cardiovascular text of >2,000 pages can be purchased for almost the same price.

MISCELLANEOUS

*37. Page E, Fozzard HA, Solaro RJ, editors. *HANDBOOK OF PHYSIOLOGY. A Critical, Comprehensive Presentation of Physiological Knowledge and Concepts. Section 2: The Cardiovascular System. VOLUME 1: The Heart.* Oxford: Oxford University Press, 2002:822, $198.95.

This edited book of 21 chapters by 41 contributors contains essays on mechanisms underlying normal and abnormal physiology of the heart. This book is not for the practicing cardiologist but it will be useful to many cardiovascular researchers.

38. Crawford MH, editor. *Current Diagnosis &*

Treatment in Cardiology. Second Edition. New York: Lange Medical Books/McGraw-Hill, 2003:627, $59.95.

A book of 37 chapters by 52 contributors is very good for the price.

39. Kirklin JK, Young JB, McGiffin DC, editors. *Heart Transplantation*. New York: Churchill Livingstone, 2002:883, $229.00.

This book by 17 contributors is superb, unquestionably the best so far on this topic.

*40. Cooper LT Jr., editor. *Myocarditis. From Bench to Bedside*. Totowa, New Jersey: Humana Press, 2003:621, $175.00.

This book of 24 chapters by 60 contributors is comprehensive and beautifully presented. If the amount of space between lines was reduced, the size of the book would be reduced considerably.

41. Alpert JS, Ewy GA. *Manual of Cardiovascular Diagnosis and Therapy*. Fifth Edition. Philadelphia: Lippincott Williams & Wilkins, 2002:424, $39.95.

This 30-chapter book has just 2 authors. It is packed full of useful cardiologic information and it can fit into the pocket of the white coat.

42. Park MK. *The Pediatric Cardiology Handbook*. Third Edition. St. Louis: Mosby 2003:311, $34.95.

The first edition of this little pocket book appeared in 1991, the second in 1997. It would be particularly useful for the fellow in training in pediatric cardiology.

*43. Edwards NM, Maurer MS, Wellner RB, editors. *Aging, Heart Disease and its Management. Facts and Controversies*. Totowa, New Jersey: Humana Press, 2003:389, $125.00.

An excellent book of 20 chapters by 35 contributors.

*44. Coffman JD, Eberhardt RT, editors. *Peripheral Arterial Disease. Diagnosis and Treatment*. Totowa, New Jersey: Humana Press, 2003:356, $129.50.

This book of 19 chapters by 27 contributors is useful and needed. I have a major beef with this book, however, when it comes to risk factors for peripheral arterial disease. In chapter 1, dyslipidemia is listed as third from the top in the list of risk factors and it consists of 3 sentences. The insulin resistance syndrome, listed as one of the "new potential risk factors," consists of a full page, and endothelial problems goes on for just over 8 pages. In chapter 3, hyperlipidemia is listed in the discussion of atherosclerotic risk factors as number 3 and in only a single paragraph. In chapter 9, under "traditional risk factors" dyslipidemia is listed as factor number 4. Peripheral arterial atherosclerosis does not occur in patients who for decades have serum total cholesterol levels <150 mg/dl, low-density lipoprotein cholesterol levels <100 mg/dl, and high-density lipoprotein cholesterol levels >20 mg/dl, irrespective of how many cigarettes are smoked or how high the systemic arterial blood pressure resides chronically. The prevention of atherosclerosis systemically requires serum cholesterol levels that occur naturally in vegetarians.

*45. Constant J. *Essentials of Bedside Cardiology with a Complete Course in Heart Sounds and Murmurs on CD*. Second Edition. Totowa, New Jersey: Humana Press, 2003:298, $89.50.

A wonderful book by a single author.

46. Gray HH, Dawkins KD, Simpson IA, Morgan JM. *Lecture Notes on Cardiology*. Fourth Edition. London: Blackwell Science, 2002:274, $39.95.

This is a short, nonedited book on the essentials of cardiology for the general practitioner or general internist. It is quite readable and the illustrations and boxes of summarizing points are helpful.

47. Kloner RA, Birnbaum Y. *Cardiovascular Trials Review*. 7th Edition. Darien, CT: LeJacq Communications, 2002:1532, $89.00.

A total of 698 of cardiovascular trials are summarized.

48. Weisse AB. *Heart to Heart. The Twentieth-Century Battle Against Cardiac Disease*. New Brunswick, New Jersey: Rutgers University Press, 2002: 415, $30.00.

This book reproduces conversations between Weisse and 16 leaders in cardiovascular disease including 8 cardiologists, 6 surgeons, and 2 basic scientists. It is good reading. There is much space between the lines so the book could have been much more compact.

49. Borer JS, Isom OW, editors. *Pathophysiology, Evaluation and Management of Valvular Heart Diseases*. Framington, CT: S. Karger Publishers, 2002: 218, $156.50.

Good but expensive ($0.72 per page).

*50. Wadden TA, Stunkard AJ, editors. *Handbook of Obesity Treatment*. New York: The Guiford Press, 2002:624, $65.00.

This book of 27 chapters by 47 contributors is not a "handbook." It is heavy, fully packed, and highly useful. Most cardiologic patients are overweight and cardiologists need to know more about this topic. Body mass index needs to be elevated to a "vital sign." Lowering body weight even as little as 5% lowers blood lipid levels, blood pressure, and blood glucose levels. Not many drugs do all 3.

51. Piscatella JC, Franklin BA. *Take a Load Off Your Heart. 109 Things You Can Actually Do to Prevent, Halt or Reverse Heart Disease*. New York: Workman Publishing, 2003:379, $14.95.

I am a major fan of both of these authors. This book is terrific! The first chapter asks 67 practical questions about cardiovascular disease and then answers them. Other sections demonstrate how to assess risk, to manage daily stress, to manage diet, and to make exercise a habit! The book is extremely readable, practical, and both physician and nonphysician can learn much from it. I particularly recommend it to individuals who would like to prevent atherosclerotic disease and to patients with overt atherosclerotic disease.

52. Silverman ME, Murray TJ, Bryan CS, editors. *The Quotable OSLER*. Philadelphia: American College of Physicians, 2003:283, $30.00.

It is difficult to get too much of Sir William Osler! The editors sifted through the 1,500 publications of

Osler to pick up some wise, inspiring, educational, and amusing observations or some of historic interest. A total of 812 quotes are reproduced, each with its source. Highly recommended!

COMMENTS

Some good books appeared in 2002! Of the 52 mentioned herein, 14 (27%) have a 2003 publication date, and 21 (40%) were published on acid-free paper. (They are marked with an asterisk.)

William C. Roberts

William Clifford Roberts, MD,
Editor in Chief
Baylor Heart & Vascular Institute
Baylor University Medical Center
Dallas, Texas

Good Books in Cardiology Appearing in 2003

This is my 20th column on "Good Books in Cardiology . . ." since the first one in 1984. The present column is based only on the books sent to me by publishers in 2003, so surely some "good books" will be missing from this piece.

MAJOR CARDIOVASCULAR TEXTBOOKS

1. Kouchoukos NT, Blackstone EH, Doty DB, Hanley FL, Karp RB. *Kirklin/Barratt-Boyes Cardiac Surgery. Morphology, Diagnostic Criteria, Natural History, Techniques, Results, and Indications.* Third Edition. Philadelphia: Churchill Livingstone, 2003:1–1073 (volume 1), 1075–1938, (volume 2); Index 1–83, $349.00.

This is a great book! The 1986 and 1993 editions of the book were written almost entirely by John Kirklin and Sir Brian Barratt-Boyes. Of the 5 authors of the present edition, 4 trained under Dr. Kirklin at the University of Alabama Medical Center in Birmingham. All chapters presented in the second edition have been substantially revised. Each chapter was rewritten with input from at least 2 of the 5 authors. After review of each edited chapter by the primary author, the chapter was forwarded to Dr. Blackstone, who served as the final arbiter of each chapter.

As in the 2 previous editions, Part I discusses basic concepts of cardiac surgery and Parts II to VI discuss specific acquired and congenital diseases of the heart and great vessels. Of the 55 chapters in the 2 volumes, 29 (53%) concern various congenital malformations.

Each chapter begins with a detailed outline of its content. The chapters having to do with specific disease entities, stenotic atherosclerotic coronary artery disease, for example, follow the format of *definition, historical note, morphology, clinical features, and diagnostic criteria, natural history, technique of operation, special features of postoperative care, results,* and *indications for operation.*

The references in each chapter are extensive and done interestingly as in the 2 previous editions. They are arranged in alphabetical order by first author and numbered consecutively under each letter. Reference A8 for example indicates the eighth reference under the letter A; reference W4 represents the fourth reference under the letter W. This innovation was originated by Kirklin in the first edition of this classic. This method allows for easy retrieval by the reader and easy organization by the author. Each reference includes as many as 6 authors, and if there are more, "et al" is used I prefer the listing of all authors because the last one may be the most important or the most recognized author).

Before anyone concludes that this book is useful only to cardiovascular surgeons, a look at chapter 6 (surely by Dr. Blackstone) would be in order. This 97-page chapter entitled "Generating knowledge from information, data, and analyses" is a scholarly masterpiece and applies to all disciplines of medicine.

There is little to criticize in this book. Kirklin should be most proud of his trainees.

2. Mavroudis C, editor, Backer CL, associate editor. *Pediatric Cardiac Surgery.* Third Edition. Philadelphia: Mosby, 2003:875; $239.00.

This book of 48 chapters by 52 contributors is very useful for surgeons dealing with patients with malformations of the heart and great vessels. The illustrations throughout were predominantly prepared by a single illustrator (Rachid F. Idriss), and they provide a nice uniformity throughout the book. Highly recommended.

ELECTROCARDIOGRAPHY

*3. Wellens HJJ, Gorgels APM, Doevendans PA. *The ECG in Acute Myocardial Infarction and Unstable Angina. Diagnosis and Risk Stratification.* Boston: Kluwer Academic Publishers, 2003:132; $116.00.

4. Khan MG. *Rapid ECG Interpretation.* Second Edition. Philadelphia: Saunders, 2003:338; $34.95.

5. Hampton JR. *The ECG in Practice.* Fourth Edition. Edinburgh: Churchill Livingstone, 2003:420; $24.95.

6. Hampton JR. *The ECG Made Easy.* Sixth Edition. Edinburgh: Churchill Livingstone, 2003:150; $24.95.

7. Hampton JR. *150 ECG Problems.* Second Edition. Edinburgh: Churchill Livingstone, 2003:309; $24.95.

Each year several books on interpretation of electrocardiograms appear. This year is no exception. I recommend the Khan book, and 1 of the 3 Hampton books, namely *The ECG in Practice.* The Wellens book is interesting because of the reputation of the investigators, but the reproductions of the electrocardiograms leave something to be desired and there is wasted space on numerous pages. It bothers me to see abbreviations in titles of books or articles.

*Asterisks indicate that the book was published on acid-free (permanent) paper.

STRESS TESTING

*8. Ellestad MH. *Stress Testing. Principles and Practice*. Fifth Edition. Oxford: Oxford University Press, 2003:546; $79.95.

This book—now in its 5th edition—is the bible of exercise stress testing. The 1st edition appeared in 1975 and the 5th edition, 28 years later. Each chapter in this new edition has been much revised. *Take home* messages are now sprinkled throughout most chapters. Two new chapters provide information on exercise echocardiography and exercise testing in heart failure. Ellestad writes so that the reading is easy. This is a very important book in cardiology.

*9. Marwick TH. *Stress Echocardiography. Its Role in the Diagnosis and Evaluation of Coronary Artery Disease*. 2nd Edition. Boston: Kluwer Academic Publishers, 2003:255; $95.00.

This single-authored book of 8 chapters focuses on echocardiographic detection of ischemic myocardium by direct visualization of regional left ventricular dysfunction. Marwick makes the case that exercise echocardiography enhances the accuracy of exercise electrocardiography in diagnosing myocardial ischemia, primarily by providing greater sensitivity for its detection. A nice but expensive book (37¢ per page).

CARDIAC IMAGING

10. Konstadt SN, Shernan SK, Oka Y, editors. *Clinical Transesophageal Echocardiography. A Problem-Oriented Approach.* Second Edition. Philadelphia: Lippincott Williams & Wilkins, 2003:452; $199.00.

This book of 28 chapters is beautifully prepared, full of illustrations, and enjoyable to read.

*11. Iskandrian AE, Verani MS, editors. *Nuclear Cardiac Imaging. Principles and Applications*. Third Edition. Oxford: Oxford University Press, 2003:511; $179.00.

This edition, consisting of 26 chapters by 40 contributors, appears barely 5 years after edition 2, an indication of the rapid pace of scientific advancement in nuclear cardiology. The book focuses primarily on myocardial perfusion imaging (perhaps 90% of all nuclear cardiologic imaging procedures), but it also comprehensively discusses radionuclide angiography, metabolic and receptor imaging, and positron emission tomography. This book appears to be a superb one on this subject.

*12. Wackers FJ Th, Bruni W, Zaret BL. *Nuclear Cardiology: The Basics. How to Set Up and Maintain a Laboratory*. Totowa, New Jersey: Humana Press, 2004:300; $99.50.

This book appears to be the first to provide information on how to establish and run a state-of-the art nuclear cardiology laboratory, an important topic since nearly 8 million are now performed annually in the USA. The book accomplishes its purpose.

13. Weissman NJ, Adelmann GA, editors. *Cardiac Imaging Secrets*. Philadelphia: Hanley & Belfus, 2004:395; $34.95.

This book of 63 chapters by 25 contributors provides a fairly in-depth review of current methods of evaluating various functional and structural cardiac changes in cardiac disease. Echocardiographic, hemodynamic, radiographic, nuclear, computer tomographic imaging, magnetic resonance imaging, and intravascular ultrasonic imaging of the heart in various cardiovascular conditions are discussed. The price is also right.

SYSTEMIC HYPERTENSION

14. Egan BM, Basile JN, Lackland DT, editors. *Hypertension*. Philadelphia: Hanley & Belfus, 2004: 487; $29.95.

This is a book of 42 chapters by 67 contributors, many of whom are leaders in this field. By age 50, nearly 50% of Americans have systemic systolic arterial pressures >140 mm Hg or diastolic pressures >90 mm Hg, or both; by age 60 that percent approaches 60%; by age 70, 70%; by age 80, 80%, and by age 90, 90%. Only about 30% of patients with hypertension are having their pressures controlled. That percentage would improve if this book was read and information brought to patients. A good book.

CORONARY ARTERY DISEASE

15. Théroux P, editor. *Acute Coronary Syndromes. A Companion to Braunwald's Heart Disease.* Philadelphia: Saunders, 2003:752; $149.00.

This book of 50 chapters by 95 contributors is superb. The content of Braunwald's HEART DISEASE "Companion" books needs to be compared with the same subject matter in HEART DISEASE to determine the additional value of these "companion" books.

16. Califf RM. *Acute Coronary Syndromes. ACS Essentials*. Royal Oak, Michigan: Physicians' Press, 2003:193; $16.95.

This little inexpensive book is a concise, practical, and authoritative guide for the management of patients with unstable angina pectoris and acute myocardial infarction. It readily fits into the white-coat pocket. This book integrates the latest clinical guidelines and the results of trials into therapy. Highly recommended.

*17. Dhalla NS, Chockalingam A, Berkowitz HI, Singal PK, editors. *Frontiers in Cardiovascular Health*. Boston: Kluwer Academic Press, 2003:595; $189.00.

This book of 41 chapters by many contributors (no list provided) covers a broad range of cardiovascular topics.

18. de Marchena E, Ferreira AC, editors. *Interventional Cardiology Secrets*. Philadelphia: Hanley & Belfus, 2003:385; $39.95.

This book of 61 chapters by 81 contributors asks questions and then answers them. Each chapter provides a set of questions which are answered. I like the format. The book is well done.

*19. Faergeman O. *Coronary Artery Disease. Genes, Drugs and the Agricultural Connection*. Amsterdam: Elsevier Science, 2003:182; $35.00.

This is a terrific book. It focuses exclusively on

coronary artery disease and what produces it. Faergeman writes well: "...Each of us can choose to eat less meat and drink less milk, but as long as we, as nations, continue to produce ever increasing amounts of meat and milk, some of us will consume them... and ... atherosclerotic disease will continue to rise... The food we choose to produce determines the need for cardiologists and heart surgeons... the choices ... for ... health are therefore not only on the level of health care policy [but] ... also on the level of food policy and agricultural policy." Highly recommended.

HEART FAILURE

20. Mann DL, editor. *Heart Failure. A Companion to Braunwald's Heart Disease*. Philadelphia: Saunders. 2004:812; $145.00.

This book of 47 chapters by 85 contributors is expensive, but the best of the 4 books on heart failure listed here. It is beautifully prepared and in depth. Highly recommended.

21. Jessup M, McCauley KM, editors. *Heart Failure: Providing Optimal Care*. Elmsford, New York: Blackwell Publishing/Futura Division, 2003:264; $69.95.

This book of 14 chapters by 18 contributors provides practical information on diagnosis and management of patients with heart failure.

*22. Jessup ML, Loh E, editors. *Heart Failure. A Clinician's Guide to Ambulatory Diagnosis and Treatment*. Totowa, New Jersey: Humana Press, 2003: 360; $99.50.

This book of 21 chapters by 28 contributors focuses on outpatient management of heart failure.

*23. Matsumori A, editor. *Cardiomyopathies and Heart Failure: Biomolecular, Infectious and Immune Mechanisms*. Boston: Kluwer Academic Publishers, 2003:531; $182.00.

This book of 38 chapters by 138 contributors (average 3.6 per chapter) focuses on basic and clinical aspects of many nonischemic cardiomyopathies. This book will be of limited interest to the heart failure clinician.

ARRHYTHMIAS, CONDUCTION DISTURBANCES, SYNCOPE, AND DEVICES

24. Lip GYH, Godtfredsen J, editors. *Cardiac Arrhythmias*. Edinburgh: Mosby, 2003:399; $129.00.

This book of 21 chapters by 14 contributors is a very useful book on arrhythmias. The format is pleasing and the graphics are excellent.

*25. Gussak I, Antzelevitch C, editors: Hammill SC, Shen W-K, Bjerregaard P, coeditors. *Cardiac Repolarization. Bridging Basic and Clinical Science*. Totowa, New Jersey: Humana Press, 2003:548; $175.00.

This book of 23 chapters by 47 contributors focuses on ventricular repolarization and the latest developments in cardiac electrophysiology. The book appears comprehensive and surely will be useful to electrophysiologists. The price is steep (32¢/page).

*26. Shenasa M, Borggrefe M, Breithardt G, editors. *Cardiac Mapping*. Second Edition. Elmsford, New York: Blackwell Publishing/Futura Division, 2003: 816; $174.95.

This book of 40 chapters by 105 contributors focuses on cardiac mapping of the various arrhythmias. It should be a useful reference for the interventional electrophysiologist.

27. Benditt D, Blanc J-J, Brignole M, Sutton R, editors. *The Evaluation and Treatment of Syncope. A Handbook for Clinical Practice*. Elsmsford, New York: Blackwell Publishers/Futura Division, 2003: 231; $65.00.

This book of 18 chapters consists of guidelines on the diagnosis and treatment of syncope formulated by the European Society of Cardiology. The book attempts to answer 5 questions: What are the diagnostic criteria for causes of syncope? What is the preferred approach to the diagnostic workup in various subgroups of patients with syncope? How should patients with syncope be risk stratified? When should patients with syncope be hospitalized? Which treatments are likely to be effective in preventing syncope recurrences?

VALVULAR HEART DISEASE

28. Otto CM, editor. *Valvular Heart Disease*. Second Edition. Philadelphia: Saunders, 2004:598; $159.00.

This is an excellent book of 20 chapters, 16 of which were written entirely by Dr. Otto; in 2 others she was a coauthor, and 2 were written by other contributors. This is far more than an echocardiographic book. All aspects of valvular disease are discussed. Each page is fully packed.

29. Borer JS. *Contemporary Diagnosis and Management of Valvular Heart Disease*. Newtown, Pennsylvania: Handbooks in Health Care Co., 2003:277; $19.95.

Jeff Borer in recent years has focused particularly on valvular heart disease and he has written extensively on this topic. This little book, which readily fits into a white-coat pocket, provides easily readable information on this topic.

CONGENITAL HEART DISEASE

30. Perloff JK. *The Clinical Recognition of Congenital Heart Disease,* 5th Edition. Philadelphia: Saunders, 2003:614; $149.00.

The first edition of this classic appeared in 1970 and the last edition in 1994. As Dr. Perloff states in the preface "...the clinical recognition of congenital heart disease remains an exciting discipline in logical thinking, a stimulating challenge, and a gratifying source of self-education. Therein lies the essence of my book." The phrase "logical thinking" is the essence of Joe Perloff, a dear friend, who has taught me much. This is a must book for those dealing with patients with congenital malformations of the heart and great vessels.

31. Gatzoulis MA, Webb GD, Daubeney PEF, editors. *Diagnosis and Management of Adult Congenital Heart Disease*. Edinburgh: Churchill Livingstone, 2003:517; $129.00.

This book of 56 chapters by 81 contributors, including a foreword by Dr. Joseph K. Perloff, focuses on those patients with congenital heart disease who survive into adulthood. As one who, years ago, also edited a book on congenital heart disease in adults, I find this one to be of excellent quality. Most of the illustrations are superb. Color is frequent in tables and figures.

MISCELLANEOUS

32. Braunwald E, Goldman L, editors. *Primary Cardiology*. Second Edition. Philadelphia: Saunders, 2003:721; $89.95.

This book of 38 chapters by 45 contributors is intended to be an authoritative, yet user-friendly, text for primary care physicians, general internists, and any physician not specializing in cardiovascular diseases. The book has beautifully achieved that purpose. Putting color on many of the figures and photographs enhances the reading.

33. Rutherford JD, editor. *Cardiology Core Curriculum. A Problem-Based Approach*. London: BMJ Books, 2003:623; $69.95.

This edited book of 18 chapters by 24 contributors, about half of whom are or were at the University of Texas Southwestern Medical Center in Dallas, provides information on major topics in heart disease. The amount of information is less, of course, than in the major cardiovascular texts. The book is more for the noncardiologist interested in heart disease than for the cardiologist.

34. Khan MG. *Cardiac Drug Therapy*. Sixth Edition. Philadelphia: Saunders, 2003:542; $44.95.

This single-authored book is amazingly detailed and informative. It can fit into the pocket of the white coat.

*35. Lincoff AM, editor. *Platelet Glycoprotein IIB/IIIA Inhibitors in Cardiovascular Disease*. Second Edition. Totowa, New Jersey: Humana Press, 2003: 476; $149.50.

This book of 21 chapters by 33 contributors provides extensive information on this topic.

*36. Weintraub WS, editor. *Cardiovascular Health Care Economics*. Totowa, New Jersey: Humana Press 2003:436; $135.00.

This book of 22 chapters by 38 contributors puts in one place a huge amount of information on cardiovascular health-care economics. Its purpose is to show how cardiovascular services can be rationally valued, that is, how outcomes can be assessed, how cost can be derived, and how choices can be rationally made. This book was needed. All of us need to think more in terms of value for cardiovascular services rendered.

*37. Bales CW, Ritchie CS, editors. *Handbook of Clinical Nutrition and Aging*. Totowa, New Jersey: Humana Press, 2004:698; $145.00.

This book of 31 chapters by 63 contributors is not necessarily cardiology, but it focuses on nutrition in older adults. Cardiology now mainly focuses on patients >65 years of age, and cardiologists in general are not experts on nutrition. This book helps to fill that nutritional void. I like it.

*38. Fraser GE. *Diet, Life Expectancy, and Chronic Disease. Studies of Seventh-Day Adventists and Other Vegetarians*. Oxford: Oxford University Press, 2003:371; $59.95.

This excellent book summarizes studies—particularly in Seventh-day Adventists—which support the benefits of a vegetarian diet in decreasing the frequency of atherosclerotic disease and certain cancers and increasing life expectancy.

39. Randall OS, Randall D. *Menu for Life. African Americans Get Healthy, Eat Well, Lose Weight, and Live Beautifully*. New York: Broadway Books, 2003: 305; $22.95.

Black health, on average, in the USA is not good. Obesity, diabetes mellitus, and systemic hypertension are more prevalent in the black community in the USA than in the white community. These 2 investigators provide a spark to reverse this trend.

40. Chung EK. *100 Questions & Answers About Heart Attack and Related Cardiac Problems*. Boston: Jones and Bartlett Publishers, 2004:164; $16.95.

This book is Dr. Chung's 100th. It is one of several "100 Questions & Answers" books published by Jones and Bartlett. Others are about prostate gland, breast, lung, colorectal, pancreatic, dermal, and brain cancers, and leukemia, erectile dysfunction, Parkinson's disease, and bone marrow and stem-cell transplantation. The book is intended mainly for the lay public.

41. Halle AA III. *Heart Healthy. How to Prevent a Heart Attack*. St. Louis: A. Arthur Halle, 2003:139; $19.95.

This book is intended mainly for the lay public. It was privately printed.

42. Nasser WK. *Near to My Heart. An American Dream*. Indianapolis: Nasco Publishing Company, 2003:105; $18.95.

Bill Nasser, a cardiologist who built the largest private-practice cardiology group in the world, has had 4 aortic valve replacements and 1 liver transplantation. This book summarizes the trials and tribulations of his life. For each book sold—and 12,000 have been sold—$100.00 was given to St. Vincent's Childrens Hospital in Indianapolis. As a result, over $200,000 was donated to that hospital. The donors included industry and wealthy supporters. Bill Nasser made no money from his book.

William C. Roberts

William Clifford Roberts, MD
Editor in Chief
Baylor Heart & Vascular Institute
Baylor University Medical Center
Dallas, Texas

Good Books in Cardiovascular Disease Appearing in 2004

This is my 21st column on "Good Books in Cardiovascular Disease." The present column is based only on the books sent to me by publishers in 2004, so surely some "good books" will be missing from this piece.

MAJOR CARDIOVASCULAR TEXTBOOKS

1. Zipes DP, Libby P, Bonow RO, Braunwald E, editors. *Braunwald's Heart Disease. A Textbook of Cardiovascular Medicine.* Seventh edition. Philadelphia: Saunders (Elsevier), 2005: 2256, $269.00 (single volume); 2400, $289.00 (2 volumes).

A 12-pound book of 87 chapters by 122 contributors. The preface of this great book by the authors describes its contents beautifully and how this 7th edition differs from the previous one. The book's appearance has changed considerably: the cover now shows a holographic magnetic resonance image of a heart alternating between ventricular systole and diastole. Most of the 569 tables and 1,503 figures are now in color. Each page is packed full: the print size is relatively small but adequate, the space between lines small but adequate, and figures, tables, and print extend to near the pages' edges. Indeed, I have never seen a medical book with such maximal use of each page. Also, now an e-edition is available and it provides electronic access to the entire book and enables the reader to download any figure or table to his or her own computer and to use them in a Power Point format for lectures. In addition to the figures and tables in the book, the accompanying CD contains additional images and video clips. Important articles appearing between editions 7 and 8 (the one due out in 2009) will be scanned and summarized and posted on the e-edition site and updated *weekly*. The index—73 pages of it— also includes, for the first time potential conflicts of interest for all contributors. The 51 chapters in the 6th edition have been retained, but all are upgraded and thoroughly revised. In addition, 36 new chapters have been included. The 10 general topics—preventive cardiology, atherosclerotic cardiovascular disease, arrhythmias, sudden death, syncope, and so forth—are color-coded in the side margins for easy access. References included in each chapter have generally been limited to sources published in 1998 or later. If you buy 1 cardiology book, this is the one to get.

2. Crawford MH, DiMarco JP, Paulus WJ. *Cardiology.* Second Edition. Edinburgh: Mosby (Elsevier), 2004: 1702, $159.00.

A 10-pound book of 212 chapters by 275 contributors. The book is divided into 8 major sections and each section is color-coded for easy searching: Atherosclerosis is green, Ischemic Heart Disease, brown; Hypertensive Heart Disease, purple; and so forth This is a good and comprehensive textbook—as good as the Braunwald one, no. All figures are collected together in an attached CD-ROM.

CARDIOVASCULAR SURGERY

***3.** Little AG, editor. *Complications in Cardiothoracic Surgery. Avoidance and Treatment.* Elmsford, New York: Futura (Blackwell), 2004: 454, $99.00.

A book of 21 chapters by 35 contributors. A useful book but the major cardiovascular surgery textbooks are more cost-effective.

4. Hallett JW Jr, Mills JL, Earnshaw JJ, Reekers JA, editors. *Comprehensive Vascular and Endovascular Surgery.* Edinburgh: Mosby (Elsevier), 2004: 712, $199.00.

A book of 46 chapters by 83 contributors. This is a timely book combining input from vascular surgeons, interventional radiologists, and vascular medicine specialists sometimes presenting opposing views regarding therapy for disorders involving arteries, veins, and lymphatics. Most diagrams are in color. A superb book.

5. Yang SC, Cameron DE, editors. *Current Therapy in Thoracic and Cardiovascular Surgery.* Philadelphia: Mosby (Elsevier), 2004: 833, $159.00.

A book of 222 short concise chapters by 334 contributors! The first edition of this book appeared in 1986, eighteen years before the present one. The 2 new editors plan on subsequent books appearing every 3 years. Cardiac surgery involves about half of the book and thoracic surgery, the other half. The book is packed full, the illustrations are good, and the chapters "run on" to each other saving space. An interesting book.

6. Leung JM, editor. *Cardiac and Vascular Anesthesia. The Requisites in Anesthesiology.* St. Louis: Mosby (Elsevier), 2004: 216, $79.95.

A book of 13 chapters by 15 contributors. This is a relatively succinct coverage of cardiac and vascular anesthesia.

***7.** Edwards NM, Chen JM, Mazzeo PA, editors. *Cardiac Transplantation.* The Columbia University

*Asterisks indicate that the book was published on acid-free (permanent) paper.

Medical Center/New York–Presbyterian Hospital Manual. Totowa, New Jersey: Humana Press, 2004: 283, $125.00.

A book of 12 chapters by 20 contributors describing cardiac transplantation in about 1,600 patients at these 2 major university hospitals. I like this kind of book, which I believe will be useful to those in this arena.

ARRHYTHMIAS AND CONDUCTION DISTURBANCES

8. Zipes DP, Jalife J, editors. *Cardiac Electrophysiology. From Cell to Bedside.* Fourth Edition. Philadelphia: Saunders (Elsevier), 2004: 1144, $259.00.

A book of 120 chapters by 245 contributors. Its all here—both the basic and the clinical.

9. Malik M, Camm AJ, editors. *Dynamic Electrocardiography.* Elmsford, New York: Futura (Blackwell), 2004: 637, $140.00

This book of 64 chapters by 112 contributors takes electrocardiography to another level. The advanced signal analyses and processing techniques applied to the electrocardiographic signal allow extraction of additional clinically important information, and they are discussed in this book.

*__10.__ Chen S-A, Haïssaguerre M, Zipes DP, editors. *Thoracic Vein Arrhythmias.* Malden, Massachusetts: Futura (Blackwell), 2004: 352, $135.95.

This book of 28 chapters by 74 contributors focuses on the importance of the pulmonary veins in the genesis of atrial arrhythmias. It is very well done.

11. Kowey P, Naccarelli GV, editors. *Atrial Fibrillation.* New York: Marcel Dekker, 2005: 365, $ 99.95.

A book of 14 chapters by 25 contributors. It is nice to have all this information on this common arrhythmia in one place.

12. Hayes DL, Wang PJ, Sackner-Bernstein J, Asirvatham SJ. *Resynchronization and Defibrillation for Heart Failure. A Practical Approach.* Oxford, UK: Futura (Blackwell), 2004: 228, $60.00.

A timely book.

CARDIAC IMAGING

13. Otto CM. *Textbook of Clinical Echocardiography.* Third Edition. Philadelphia: Saunders (Elsevier), 2004: 541, $129.00.

This single-authored book is beautifully done.

14. Heller GV, Hendel RC, editors. *Nuclear Cardiology. Practical Applications.* New York: McGraw-Hill, 2004: 369, $79.95.

A useful book of 24 chapters by 29 contributors.

*__15.__ Schoepf UJ, editor. *CT of the Heart. Principles and Applications.* Totowa, New Jersey: Humana Press, 2005: 407, $195.00.

This book of 38 chapters by 63 authors is timely and beautifully done.

MISCELLANEOUS

16. Mehta JL, editor. *Statins: Understanding Clinical Use.* Philadelphia: Saunders (Elsevier), 2004: 334, $39.95.

This soft-back book of 16 chapters by 30 contributors concerns statins, the best drug available for preventing and arresting atherosclerosis. This is a superb little book!

*__17.__ Aronow WS, Fleg JL, editors. *Cardiovascular Disease in the Elderly.*Third Edition. Revised and Expanded. New York: Marcel Dekker, 2004: 847, $195.00.

This book of 32 chapters by 52 contributors is surely the best one available on this topic. Cardiac patients are getting older and adult cardiology now is mainly geriatric medicine, depending on how "elderly" is defined.

18. Manson JE, Buring JE, Ridker PM, Gaziano JM, editors. *Clinical Trials in Heart Disease. A Companion to Braunwald's Heart Disease.* Second Edition. Philadelphia: Saunders (Elsevier), 2004: 434, $129.00.

This book of 32 chapters by 62 contributors focuses on results of clinical trials involving treatment of acute coronary ischemia, arrhythmias, heart failure, and primary and secondary prevention. Clinical trials, of course, have become the principal method of judging the efficacy and safety of interventions. This book gathers many of them together in one location.

19. St. John Sutton M, Rutherford JD, editors. *Clinical Cardiovascular Imaging. A Companion to Braunwald's Heart Disease.* Philadelphia: Saunders (Elsevier), 2004: 486, $129.00.

This book of 16 chapters by 63 contributors compares the varying imaging techniques for quantitating cardiac ventricular function and myocardial perfusion and assessing cardiac metabolism.

20. Chien KR. *Molecular Basis of Cardiovascular Disease. A Companion to Braunwald's Heart Disease.* Second Edition. Philadelphia: Saunders (Elsevier), 2004: 713, $145.00.

This book of 33 chapters by 69 contributors does what the title says. I suspect that it is a bit "heavy" for most cardiovascular specialists.

*__21.__ Topol EJ, editor. *Acute Coronary Syndromes.* Third Edition. Revised and Expanded. New York: Marcel Dekker, 2005: 763, $99.75.

This book of 32 chapters by 46 contributors focuses, of course, on acute coronary syndromes. Overall, it is well done and heavily referenced.

22. Runge MS, Ohman EM, editors, with illustrations by Netter FH. *Netter's Cardiology.* Teterboro, New Jersey: Icon Learning Systems, 2004: 664, $79.95.

This book of 65 chapters by 86 contributors is a mini-cardiology textbook with generous sprinklings of Dr. Netter's illustrations throughout. Separately, the Netter Cardiology Collection can be purchased on CD-ROM.

23. Spittell JA Jr. *Peripheral Vascular Disease for Cardiologists. A Clinical Approach.* Elmsford, New York: Futura (Blackwell), 2004: 134, $54.95.

This single-authored little book is useful.

24. Portman RJ, Sorof JM, Ingelfinger JR. *Pediatric Hypertension.* Totowa, New Jersey: Humana Press, 2004: 492, $145.00.

A book of 27 chapters by 40 contributors. Although there are numerous books on hypertension, few have focused on hypertension in infants, children, and adolescents. This is a very useful and well-done book.

*__25.__ Kloner RA, editor. *Heart Disease and Erectile Dysfunction.* Totowa, New Jersey: Humana Press, 2004: 300, $99.50.

A useful book of 18 chapters by 24 contributors, including cardiologists, urologists, physiologists, and a psychologist.

26. Jackson G. *Sex, the Heart and Erectile Dysfunction.* London, UK: Taylor & Francis, 2004: 70, $17.95.

A single-authored useful pocketbook on an important topic.

*__27.__ Stein RA, Oz MC, editors. *Complementary and Alternative Cardiovascular Medicine.* Totowa, New Jersey: Humana Press, 2004: 286, $99.50.

A book of 16 chapters by 26 contributors concerning complementary and alternative medical therapies for patients with cardiovascular disease. These therapies include herbs and supplements, various botanical medicines, vitamins, oils and fats, nutrachemicals, meditation, prayer, massage, acupuncture, chelation, energy, and homeopathy. It is useful having this information in one volume.

*__28.__ Mansoor GA, editor. *Secondary Hypertension. Clinical Presentation, Diagnosis, and Treatment.* Totowa, New Jersey: Humana Press, 2004: 352, $99.50.

A book of 17 chapters by 26 contributors. All of the secondary causes are here.

*__29.__ Morganroth J, Gussak I. *Cardiac Safety of Noncardiac Drugs. Practical Guidelines for Clinical Research and Drug Development.* Totowa, New Jersey: Humana Press, 2005: 361, $165.00.

This book of 18 chapters by 27 contributors provides expert practical advice to researchers in industry and academics on establishing new product safety, predicting regulatory actions, and getting the drug to market. The most common cause of new drug discontinuations, cause of disapproval from marketing, and removal from the market after approval is a drug's effect on cardiac repolarization, which is identified by increasing duration of the QTc interval on the electrocardiogram. For those in this arena, I am sure that this book will be useful.

30. Blackburn H. *It Isn't Always Fun. A Memoir from a Different Sort of Medical Life. Volume II. The Second 30 Years: 1972 to 2002.* Privately published 2004: 415, $15.00.

Volume I appeared in 2001. Dr. Blackburn, a renowned cardiovascular epidemiologist, knows how to write and his memory is incredible. If you want some good reading loaded with humor, get both volumes. To get his books, email him at: blackburn@epi.umn.edu.

OVERLOOKED 2003 BOOK

*__31.__ Cohn LH, Edmunds LH Jr, editors. *Cardiac Surgery in the Adult.* Second Edition. New York: McGraw-Hill, 2003: 1573, $250.00.

This superb 9-pound book was received after last year's book column had gone to press. It contains 65 chapters contributed by 48 contributors, 19 new chapters since the first edition. This is the first major textbook I have seen in years printed on acid-free paper.

William C. Roberts

William Clifford Roberts, MD
Editor in Chief
Baylor Heart and Vascular Institute
Baylor University Medical Center
Dallas, Texas

Good Books in Cardiology Appearing in 2005

This is my 22nd column on "Good Books in Cardiology . . ." since the first one in 1984. The present column is based only on the books sent to me by publishers in 2005, so surely some "good books" will be missing from this piece.

General Cardiology Texts

*__1.__ Rosendorff C, editor. *Essential Cardiology Principles and Practice*. Second Edition. Totowa, New Jersey: Humana Press 2005: 865, $135.00.

This book of 44 chapters by 81 contributors is well done and useful. The problem lies in the fact that the major comprehensive cardiology texts (Braunwald, Hurst, Willerson, etc) can be purchased for almost the same price.

*__2.__ Khan MG. *Encyclopedia of Heart Diseases*. Amsterdam: Elsevier 2006: 653, $129.95.

This book actually does fulfill a definition of encyclopedia ("A comprehensive reference work containing articles on a wide range of subjects on numerous aspects of a particular field, usually arranged alphabetically." [*The American Heritage Dictionary*, Second College Edition, 1982]). It contains 91 short chapters all written by the same author, and they are arranged in alphabetical order—aging and the heart, alcohol and the heart, altitude and pulmonary edema, anatomy of the heart and circulation, etc. I like it.

*__3.__ Runge MS, Patterson C, editors. *Principles of Molecular Cardiology*. Totowa, New Jersey: Humana Press 2005: 617, $175.00.

This book of 32 chapters by 74 contributors provides a broad and up-to-date treatment of molecular biology of cardiovascular diseases. Certainly this book shows quite thoroughly the direction in which cardiology is moving.

*__4.__ Gerstenblith G, editor. *Cardiovascular Disease in the Elderly*. Totowa, New Jersey: Humana Press 2005: 418, $135.00.

This book of 15 chapters by 25 contributors is an excellent one on this topic.

5. Wenger NK, Collins P, editors. *Women & Heart Disease*. Second Edition. London: Taylor & Francis 2005: 640, $149.00.

This book of 43 chapters by 81 contributors is well done. As Dr. Wenger said in an editorial in 2004, "You've come a long way, baby." I guess that we also need a book "Men & Heart Disease." The female heart, a tender one, is highly susceptible to heart disease, and those susceptibilities are fully discussed in this fine book.

* Asterisks indicate that the book was published on acid-free (permanent) paper.

Coronary Artery Disease

6. Fuster V, Topol EJ, Nabel EG, editors. *Atherothrombosis and Coronary Artery Disease*. Second Edition. Philadelphia: Lippincott Williams & Wilkins 2005: 1636, $149.00.

A superb book 105 chapters by 187 contributors. This must be the largest book so far focusing entirely on atherosclerosis and coronary artery disease. The leaders in the various areas are contributors to this splendid book. Surprisingly, 1 editor contributed to 4 chapters, and each of the other 2 contributed to 1 chapter each. This is a book I will retain.

7. Becker RC, Harrington RA, editors. *Clinical, Interventional, and Investigational Thrombo-Cardiology*. Boca Raton, Florida: Taylor & Francis 2005: 731, $199.95.

This book of 20 chapters, each with many subdivisions, by 65 contributors carefully details the connection between thrombosis and cardiovascular disease. It is well done.

*__8.__ Dauerman H, Sobel BE, editors. *Pharmacoinvasive Therapy in Acute Myocardial Infarction*. Boca Raton, Florida: Taylor & Francis 2005: 246, $149.95.

This little book of 10 chapters by 19 contributors summarizes well the modern therapy for patients with acute myocardial infarction.

9. Camenzind E, de Scheerder IK, editors. *Local Drug Delivery for Coronary Artery Disease*. London: Taylor & Francis 2005; 594, $85.00.

This book of 64 chapters by 91 contributors focuses well on an important area in heart disease.

10. Ellis SG, Holmes DR Jr, editors. *Strategic Approaches in Coronary Intervention*. Third Edition. Philadelphia: Lippincott Williams & Wilkins 2006: 546, $139.00.

This book of 51 chapters by 95 contributors is a must for the interventional cardiologist. It's all here.

11. Serruys PW, Gershlick AH, editors. *Handbook of Drug-Eluting Stents*. London: Taylor & Francis 2005: 369, $65.00.

This book of 40 chapters by 99 contributors summarizes work of the pioneers, basic researchers, and clinical trialists involved in the development of drug-eluting stents. The result, hardly a handbook, is a well done compendium on this topic.

12. White CJ, editor. *Drug-Eluting Stents*. London: Taylor & Francis 2005: 154, $49.95.

This book of 14 chapters by 14 contributors, all from the Ochsner Clinic Foundation in New Orleans, is not as comprehensive as the Serruys and Gershlick book.

13. Colombo A, Stankovic G, editors. *Colombo's Tips &*

Tricks with Drug-Eluting Stents. London: Taylor & Francis 2005: 252, $169.95.

This book of 10 major chapters with numerous case presentations by 18 contributors, including 2 CD-ROM attachments, surely must be useful to interventional cardiologists.

***14.** Laham RJ, Baim DS, editors. *Angiogenesis and Direct Myocardial Revascularization*. Totowa, New Jersey: Humana Press 2005: 357, $145.00.

This book of 13 chapters by 31 contributors summarizes this topic very well.

Hypertension

15. Oparil S, Weber MA, editors. *Hypertension. A Companion to Brenner and Rector's The Kidney*. Philadelphia: Elsevier Saunders 2005: 872, $99.00.

A book of 79 chapters by 153 contributors. There are many books on hypertension, something present in about 65 million Americans, and this one is clearly one of the better ones. Most are smaller and less comprehensive than this 5-pound book.

16. Kaplan NM. Kaplan's *Clinical Hypertension*. Ninth Edition. Philadelphia: Lippincott Williams & Wilkins 2006: 518, $99.00.

Except for the single chapter on hypertension in childhood and adolescence, all other 15 chapters and 446 pages were written by Kaplan, who is a masterful synthesizer of information on this topic. For those who treat patients with hypertension, this is a book to have.

***17.** Prisant LM, editor. *Hypertension in the Elderly*. Totowa, New Jersey: Humana Press 2005: 531, $135.00.

This book of 24 chapters by 29 contributors focuses on the huge body of patients "with the largest body of outcomes, trial data, but the poorest blood pressure control." It is a fine book. I prefer, however, to avoid the use of the word "elderly" which is not used uniformly in all the chapters.

***18.** Fennell JP, Baker AH, editors. *Hypertension. Methods and Protocols*. Totowa, New Jersey 2005: 501, $135.00.

This book of 29 chapters by 73 contributors is exclusively for researchers in hypertension.

Heart Failure

***19.** Dec GW, editor; DiSalvo T, Hajjar RJ, Semigram MJ, associate editors. *Heart Failure. A Comprehensive Guide to Diagnosis and Treatment*. New York: Marcel Dekker 2005: 582, $179.95.

This book of 25 chapters by 45 contributors focuses on a very major problem in cardiology, namely heart failure. It is well done.

20. Shaddy RE, Wernovsky G, editors. *Pediatric Heart Failure*. Boca Raton, Florida: Taylor & Francis 2005: 897, $199.95.

This book of 23 chapters by 42 contributors covers causes and management of heart failure in the fetus, neonate, and children.

Exercise Testing

21. Wasserman K, Hansen JE, Sue DY, Stringer WW, Whipp BJ. *Principles of Exercise Testing and Interpretation Including Pathophysiology and Clinical Applications*. Fourth Edition. Philadelphia: Lippincott Williams & Wilkins 2005: 585, $89.95.

A book of 85 chapters by the 5 authors. It appears to be a scholarly book.

22. Williams MA, editor in chief. *AACVRR [American Association of Cardiovascular and Pulmonary Rehabilitation] Cardiac Rehabilitation Resource Manual. Promoting Health and Preventing Disease*. Fifth Edition. Champaign, Illinois: Human Kinetics 2006: 214, $45.00.

This book of 13 chapters by 23 contributors provides reviews of topics critical to the understanding of the basis for cardiac rehabilitation and secondary prevention. It forms the basis of the *AACVPR's Guidelines for Cardiac Rehabilitation and Secondary Prevention.*

Echocardiography

23. Feigenbaum H, Armstrong WF, Ryan T. *Feigenbaum's Echocardiography*. Sixth Edition. Philadelphia: Lippincott Williams & Wilkins 2005: 709, $149.00.

The first edition appeared in 1972, and now the sixth in 2005. This edition is the first where Feigenbaum was not the sole author. The illustrations are far superior to those in earlier editions. This book is now a classic.

24. Roldan CA, editor. *The Ultimate Echo Guide*. Philadelphia: Lippincott Williams & Wilkins 2005: 254, $95.00.

Nice book of 16 chapters by 12 contributors.

25. St. John Sutton MG, Maniet A. *Mitral Valve Transesophageal Echocardiography*. London: Taylor & Francis 2006: 318, $85.00.

A well-done book by just 2 authors. The anatomic and echocardiographic illustrations are superb.

26. Savage RM, Aronson S, editors; Thomas JD, Slernan SK, Smedira NG, Shanewise JS, Wallace L, associate editors. *Comprehensive Textbook of Intraoperative Transesophageal Echocardiography*. Philadelphia: Lippincott Williams & Wilkins 2005: 745, $199.00.

A splendid book of 38 chapters by 73 contributors. For cardiologists called into the operating room to interpret these echocardiograms, this book appears to be essential. Many of the figures could have been cropped and then they could have been reproduced larger.

27. Mintz GS. *Intracoronary Ultrasound.* London: Taylor & Francis 2005: 408, $75.00.

This single-authored book is loaded with illustrations, and would be useful to anyone involved in intravascular ultrasonic imaging.

28. Schoenhagen P, DeFranco A, Nissen SE, Tuzcu EM, editors. *IVUS Made Easy.* London: Taylor & Francis 2006: 114, $34.95.

This book of 6 chapters by the 4 authors plus 2 contributing authors is loaded with beautiful illustrations. For those interested in this topic, this book is a bargain.

29. Kronzon I, Tunick PA. *Challenging Cases in Echocardiography.* Philadelphia: Lippincott Williams & Wilkins 2005: 219, $120.00.

It's just what it says it is. There is almost as much blank (white) space on each page as that for illustrations and brief text. In other words, there is a lot of wasted space. The illustrations need to be trimmed (cropped) and blown up. Too expensive.

Computed Tomography

*__30.__ Schoepf UJ, editor. *CT of the Heart. Principles and Applications.* Totowa, New Jersey: Humana Press 2005: 407, $195.00.

This book on a hot topic contains 38 chapters by 62 contributors. The illustrations are superb. The book will be very useful for those in this field.

Nuclear Cardiology

31. Zaret BL, Beller GA, editors. *Clinical Nuclear Cardiology. State of the Art and Future Directions.* Third Edition. Philadelphia: Elsevier Mosby 2005: 749, $165.00.

The first edition appeared in 1993 and the second in 1999. The book consists of 43 chapters by 81 contributors. If nuclear cardiology is your thing, it would be wise to have this book.

Electrophysiology

32. Saksena S, Camm AJ, senior editors; Boyden PA, Dorian P, Goldschlager N, associate editors. *Electrophysiological Disorders of the Heart.* Philadelphia: Elsevier Churchill Livingstone 2005: 1035, $219.00.

A book of 49 chapters by 116 contributors providing an excellent overview of current knowledge on mechanisms and management of cardiac arrhythmias.

33. Kohl P, Sachs F, Franz MR, editors. *Cardiac Mechano-Electric Feedback and Arrhythmias. From Pipette to Patient.* Philadelphia: Elsevier Saunders 2005: 423, $149.00.

This book of 42 chapters by 72 contributors focuses on various facets of the mechano-sensitive heart. It is not meant for the day-to-day practicing cardiologist.

Peripheral Vascular Disease

34. Mansour MA, Labropoulos N, editors. *Vascular Diagnosis.* Philadelphia: Elsevier Saunders 2005: 573, $139.00.

This book of 54 chapters by 100 contributors concerns the detection and management of peripheral vascular disease. It is a beautifully produced book.

35. Zwiebel WJ, Pellerito JS, editors. *Introduction to Vascular Ultrasonography.* Fifth Edition. Philadelphia: Elsevier Saunders 2005: 723, $99.00.

This book of 35 chapters by 30 contributors is intended for non-cardiac peripheral vascular specialists. For those in this arena, I am sure the book will be useful.

36. Heuser RR, Biamino G, editors. *Peripheral Vascular Stenting.* Second Edition. London: Taylor & Francis 2005: 204, $89.95.

This book of 17 chapters by 24 contributors will be useful for the peripheral vascular interventionalists.

Cardiovascular Surgery

37. Sellke FW, editor in chief; del Nido PJ, Swanson SJ, editors. *Sabiston & Spencer Surgery of Chest.* Seventh Edition, Volumes I and II. Philadelphia: Elsevier Saunders 2005: 2351, $299.00.

A book of 129 chapters by 252 contributors. There is little to criticize in these 2 volumes, which together weigh 16 pounds. Just don't let either volume fall on your toes. The new editors have maintained the excellence initiated by Sabiston and Spencer.

38. Rutherford RB, editor in chief. *Vascular Surgery.* Sixth Edition. Volumes I and II. Philadelphia: Elsevier Saunders 2005: 2576, $299.00.

This book has 1 editor in chief, 3 associate editors, 12 assistant editors, and 242 contributors for its 176 chapters. This is a "must-have" book for vascular surgeons. Its 17+ pounds requires that it either be at the office or at home. Transportation back and forth would be difficult.

39. Rutherford RB, editor in chief; Cronenwett JL, Krupski WC, Gloviczki P, Ouriel K, Johnston KW, Sidawy AN, associate editors. *Review of Vascular Surgery. Companion to Vascular Surgery, 6th edition.* Second Edition. Philadelphia: Elsevier Saunders 2005: 217, $59.95.

A question-and-answer companion book. A great way to learn.

*__40.__ Iaizzo PA, editor. *Handbook of Cardiac Anatomy, Physiology, and Devices.* Totowa, New Jersey: Humana Press 2005: 469, $175.00.

This book of 33 chapters by 44 contributors is far from a "handbook." It is divided into 3 areas: anatomy, physiology and assessment, and devices and therapies. I'm not certain which group or groups would find this book most useful. For those involved with cardiovascular devices, there is good information here.

41. Baim DS, editor. *Grossman's Cardiac Catheterization, Angiography and Intervention*. Seventh Edition. Philadelphia: Lippincott Williams & Wilkins 2006: 807, $135.00.

This book of 34 chapters by 34 contributors has become a classic! This new edition also provides a DVD-ROM that contains >150 cases covering a broad range of classic findings, specific procedures, anomalies, and complications.

Miscellaneous

42. Walsh RA editor; Schneider M, Vatner S, Marban E, Seidman J, Seidman C, associate editors. *Molecular Mechanisms of Cardiac Hypertrophy and Failure*. London: Taylor & Francis 2005: 736, $165.00.

This book of 41 chapters by 78 contributors is for the research cardiologist and focuses on the mechanisms of abnormal cardiac function in heart failure, the molecular mechanisms responsible for arrhythmogenesis, and the molecular genetic basis of cardiomyopathy.

*__43.__ Codario RA. *Type 2 Diabetes, Pre-Diabetes, and the Metabolic Syndrome. The Primary Care Guide to Diagnosis and Management*. Totowa, New Jersey 2005: 247, $89.50.

This single-authored book focuses, of course, on diabetes mellitus and the metabolic syndrome, probably simply stages of the same disease process which has devastating effects on the heart.

44. Nichols WW, O'Rourke MF. *McDonald's Blood Flow in Arteries. Theoretical, Experimental and Clinical Principles*. Fifth Edition. London: Hodder Arnold 2005: 607, $225.00.

The first edition of this book appeared in 1960 and now, 45 years later, the fifth. For students of pulsatile blood flow,this is it.

45. Frishman WH, Weintraub MI, Micozzi MS, editors. *Complementary and Integrative Therapies For Cardiovascular Disease*. St. Louis: Elsevier Mosby 2005: 429, $51.95.

This book of 27 chapters by 40 contributors focuses on non-conventional medicine. The editors indicate that in the USA more visits are made to nonconventional "healers" than to physicians at an annual cost of $30 billion. This is a thorough and scholarly book on this topic.

*__46.__ Roberts WC. *Facts and Ideas from Anywhere 2000 to 2005*. Dallas: Baylor Health Care System 2006: 180 (privately published).

This book is a compilation of from-the-editor columns by WCR appearing in the *Baylor University Medical Center Proceedings* from 2000 to 2005. A total of 431 subject items are covered in the 22 columns and many of the items concern cardiovascular disease and its prevention.

William Clifford Roberts, MD
Editor in Chief
Baylor Heart & Vascular Institute
Baylor University Medical Center
Dallas, Texas

Good Books in Cardiovascular Disease Appearing in 2006

Major Textbooks

1. Topol EJ, editor, Calif RM, Prystowsky EN, Thomas JD, Thompson PD, associate editors. *Textbook of Cardiovascular Medicine.* Third Edition. Philadelphia: Lippincott Williams & Wilkins 2007:1,628, $229.00.

A book of 110 chapters by 197 contributors. It is certainly an authoritative reference textbook in cardiovascular medicine. It is accompanied by a DVD with >1,000 digital images and multimedia video clips that bring the text alive. Each page is fully packed. Excellent illustrations. Highly recommended. A beautiful book.

2. Creager MA, Dzau VJ, Loscalzo J. *Vascular Medicine. A Companion to Braunwald's Heart Disease.* Philadelphia: Saunders Elsevier 2006:1,000, $149.00.

This comprehensive book of 66 chapters by 110 contributors concerns non-coronary vascular disease. It is probably the bible on this topic. It involves many varieties of specialists including internists, cardiologists, vascular surgeons, and interventional cardiologists.

3. Griffin BP, Rimmerman CM, Topol EJ, editors. *The Cleveland Clinic Cardiology Board Review.* Philadelphia: Lippincott Williams & Wilkins 2007:809, $129.00.

A book of 60 chapters by 87 contributors. The phrase "board review" attracts buyers to books and enrollees to meetings. I prefer Topol's *Textbook of Cardiovascular Medicine.*

General Cardiology but Not in Depth

4. Nixon JV (Ian), editor. Aurigemma GP, Bolger AF, Chaitman BR, Crawford MH, Fletcher GF, Francis GS, Gersony WM, Harrington RA, Ott P, Wenger NK, Alpert JS (co-editor). *The AHA Clinical Cardiac Consult.* Second Edition. Philadelphia: Lippincott Williams & Wilkins 2007: 400, $69.95.

This book of 354 topics by 135 contributors is owned by the Council on Clinical Cardiology of the American Heart Association. Each topic is no more than 2 pages in length and divided into 5 major subheadings: basic, diagnosis, treatment, medication (drugs), and follow-up. The topics are listed alphabetically as in an encyclopedia. I guess the book is useful. Much space is blank on many pages.

*5. Crawford MH, Srivathson K, McGlothlin DP, editors. *Current Consult Cardiology.* New York: Lange Medical Books/McGraw-Hill 2006:350, $64.95.

This book is similar to the Nixon one. A total of 356 topics are covered, each in alphabetical order, and each no more than 2 pages and 6 columns in length. Each topic is divided into "differential diagnosis" and "key diagnostic and treatment points for all major disorders in cardiology." The 6-column format leads to much wasted space in the lower portions of most pages. The bit-sized bits of information may be good in the computer age, but it is not my preference.

Preventive Cardiology

6. Gotto AM Jr, Toth PP, editors. *Comprehensive Management of High Risk Cardiovascular Patients.* New York: Informa Healthcare 2007:770, $199.95.

An authoritative and lucid book of 21 chapters by 44 contributors. Superb.

7. Foody JM, editor. *Preventive Cardiology. Insight into the Prevention and Treatment of Cardiovascular Disease.* Totawa, New Jersey: Humana Press 2006:346, $99.50.

This book of 17 chapters by 27 contributors is well done and useful for both general internists and cardiologists.

8. Lauer RM, Burns TL, Daniels SR, editors. *Pediatric Prevention of Atherosclerotic Cardiovascular Disease.* Oxford: Oxford University Press 2006:378, $69.95.

A good book of 18 chapters by 34 contributors.

9. Ridker PM, Rifai N, editors. *C-Reactive Protein and Cardiovascular Disease.* Montreal, Canada: Medi Edition 2006:393, $68.99.

This book of 24 chapters by 37 contributors is a comprehensive focus on the biology, clinical importance, and laboratory evaluation of high-sensitivity C-reactive protein. This topic is obviously a hot one, and this book puts together in one place a huge amount of information on this important protein.

Heart Failure

10. Hosenpud JD, Greenberg BH, editors. *Congestive Heart Failure.* Third Edition. Philadelphia: Lippincott Williams & Wilkins 2007:845, $169.00.

A book of 49 chapters by 92 contributors. Since the first edition in 1994, many changes and innovations have occurred in the diagnosis and management of patients with heart failure. This book is comprehensive and very well done.

Hemostasis and Thrombosis

11. Colman RW, Marder VJ, Clowes AW, George JN, Goldhaber SZ, editors. *Hemostatis and Thrombosis. Basic Principles and Clinical Practice.* Fifth Edition. Philadelphia: Lippincott Williams & Wilkins (A Wolters Kluwer Company) 2006:1,827, $299.00.

A comprehensive book of 123 chapters by 190 contributors is the classic in this important field. Each page is fully packed and each chapter is fully referenced. This book covers the entire broad field of thrombotic and bleeding disorders.

Cardiovascular Disease in Women

12. Winn HN, Dellsperger KC, editors. *Cardiovascular Disease in Women.* Abingdon, Oxon: Informa Healthcare 2006:178, $159.66.

This book of 12 chapters by 26 contributors is one of several on this topic and is useful but not exceptional.

Cardiomyopathy

*13. Maron BJ, Salberg L. *Hypertrophic Cardiomyopathy. For Patients, Their Families and Interested Physicians.* Second Edition. Malden, Massachusetts: Blackwell Publishing 2006:113, $26.95.

This little book by today's leader in hypertrophic cardiomyopathy describes the nature of the disease, its genetics, and methods for screening, diagnosis, and estimating prognosis. Additionally, it provides recommendations on lifestyle for both physicians and patients.

Arrhythmias and Conduction Defects

14. Huang SKS, Wood MA, editors. *Catheter Ablation of Cardiac Arrhythmias.* Philadelphia: Saunders Elsevier 2006: 691, $149.00.

This comprehensive beautifully prepared book of 34 chapters by 82 contributors looks to be the best on catheter ablation for cardiac arrhythmias.

15. Bennett DH. *Cardiac Arrhythmias. Practical Notes on Interpretation and Treatment.* Seventh Edition. New York: Oxford University Press 2006:384, $57.50.

This single-authored book of 27 chapters provides a non-comprehensive but practical guide to diagnosis and management of the more frequent cardiac arrhythmias.

*16. Sternick EB, Wellens HJJ. *Variants of Ventricular Preexcitation. Recognition and Treatment.* Malden, Massachusetts: Blackwell Futura 2006:152, $84.95.

This double-authored book of 9 chapters offers insight into the many variant forms of preexcitation that are not well recognized. As such, it is useful.

Valvular Heart Disease

17. Hijazi ZM, Bonhoeffer P, Feldman T, Ruiz CE, editors. *Transcatheter Valve Repair.* London: Taylor & Francis 2006:382, $95.00.

A hot topic and already a book on it! This one has 34 chapters by 70 contributors and will be of interest to cardiac interventionalists doing or planning to do these procedures.

18. Butchart EG, Gohlke-Bärwolf C, Antunes MJ, Hall RJC, editors. *Heart Valve Disease. A Guide to Patient Management after Surgery.* Milton Park, Abingdon, Oxon: Informa Healthcare 2006:199, $131.37.

This book of 19 chapters by 29 contributors is interesting and new, and will be useful to both adult cardiologists and cardiac surgeons.

Pediatric Cardiology

19. Mullins CE, editor. *Cardiac Catheterization in Congenital Heart Disease: Pediatric and Adult.* Malden, Massachusetts: Blackwell Futura 2006:932, $225.00.

This single-authored book of 31 chapters occupying 932 pages is a tour-de-force. It represents the largest single-authored medical text I have seen since Dr. Arthur Guyton's 11 editions of *Textbook of Physiology*, every page of which was written by him. Mullins' book is a must for those dealing with patients with congenital heart disease.

20. Kearns-Jonker M, editor. *Congenital Heart Disease. Molecular Diagnostics.* Totowa, New Jersey: Human Press 2006:278, $99.50.

This book of 15 chapters by 31 contributors describes a series of techniques currently used to identify the molecular basis for cardiovascular disease. For those involved in this area, surely this book will be useful.

21. Driscoll DJ. *Fundamentals of Pediatric Cardiology.* Philadelphia: Lippincott Williams & Wilkins (a Wolters Kluwer company) 2006:176, $69.95.

This single-authored book of 14 chapters is directed to primary care physicians who care for infants and children with congenital heart disease. Driscoll emphasizes that it is not necessary for non-pediatric cardiologists to know about each of the congenital cardiac malformations, but that it is important to be able to determine that the patient has: congenital heart disease; cyanotic or non-cyanotic variety; heart failure or excessive pulmonary blood flow; or requires urgent detailed evaluation and treatment. A useful little book by a very experienced pediatric cardiologist.

Electrocardiography

22. Ferry DR. *ECG in 10 Days.* Second Edition. New York: McGraw-Hill Medical 2007:320, $39.95.

This single-authored book has 10 chapters—one for each of 10 days. There have been literally 100s of books published on electrocardiography and each tends to possess some special feature. If one studied thoroughly each of these chapters for 10 days, the likelihood is that one could be a fairly decent electrocardiographer, a fairly unusual creation in modern-day cardiology.

23. Bayés de Luna A, Fiol-Sala M, Antman EM. *The 12-Lead ECG in ST Elevation Myocardial Infarction. A Practical Approach For Clinicians.* Malden, Massachusetts: Blackwell Futura 2007:112, $59.95.

A little book of 6 chapters focuses exclusively on ST-elevation acute myocardial infarction.

24. Hung-Chi Lue with the collaboration of Yung-Chang Lai, Mei-Hwan Wu, Jou-Kou Wang, Ming-Lon Young, Yung-Ching Chang, Shu-Jen Yeh, and Jiuana-Huey Lin. *ECG in the Child and Adolescent. Normal Standards and Percentile Charts.* Malden, Massachusetts: Blackwell Publishing 2006:86, $89.95.

This book will be useful to the field. These authors have gathered electrocardiographic data in over 1,800 normal infants, children, and adolescents. They have produced a unique monograph displaying numerous normal standards and percentile charts.

Echocardiography

25. Oh JK, Seward JB, Tajik AJ. *The Echo Manual.* Third Edition. Philadelphia: Lippincott Williams & Wilkins 2006: 431, $159.00.

Although 18 of the 23 chapters are entirely by the book's 3 authors, 11 others contribute to the other 5 chapters. This book comes from the Mayo Clinic, where there are 45 echocardiography physicians and more than 90 sonographers. The book is beautifully done. Although a few of the illustrations could be cropped, virtually all are excellent. This book is one of the very best on this topic.

*26. Solomon SD, editor, with Bulwer B. *Essential Echocardiography. A Practical Handbook with DVD.* Totowa, New Jersey: Humana Press 2007:458, $150.00.

This book of 23 chapters by 23 contributors provides a practical and scholarly overview of echocardiography today. The illustrations are extensive and well selected. The superb paper quality brings them out fully.

27. Plappert T, St John Sutton MG. *The Echocardiographers' Guide.* Milton Park, Abingdon, Oxon: Informa Healthcare 2006:186, $55.00.

This double-authored book of 12 chapters contains echocardiographic images on most major cardiovascular diseases. The pictures are well-cropped and superb. This is a nice echo book to own.

28. Natale A, editor. Wilber DJ, Rhodes JF Jr, Reddy V, Raviele A, Jordaens L, Kalman JM, co-editors. *Intracardiac Echocardiography in Interventional Electrophysiology.* Abingdon, Oxon: Informa Healthcare 2006:156, $100.00.

This book of 13 chapters by 40 contributors in beautifully prepared and focuses on a highly specialized area.

Exercise Testing

29. Froelicher VF, Myers J. *Exercise and the Heart.* Fifth Edition. Philadelphia: Saunders Elsevier 2006:524, $89.00.

This double-authored splendid book has become a classic. Each page of the 14 chapters is fully packed.

Cardiac Imaging

30. Lee VS. *Cardiovascular MRI. Physical Principles to Practical Protocols.* Philadelphia: Lippincott Williams & Wilkins (a Wolters Kluwer Company) 2006:402, $89.95.

This single-authored book of 22 chapters is well done. Abbreviations in titles of books are to be avoided.

31. Higgins CB, de Roos A, editors. *MRI and CT of the Cardiovascular System.* Second Edition. Philadelphia: Lippincott Williams & Wilkins (a Wolters Kluwer Company) 2006:656, $159.00.

This book of 38 chapters by 80 contributors is almost certainly the best on this topic. It includes both the heart and the peripheral vascular system. Again, abbreviations in titles of books are to be avoided.

*32. Dilsizian V, Pohost GM, editors. *Cardiac CT, PET and MR.* Malden, Massachusetts: Blackwell Futura 2006: 262, $125.00.

This book of 11 chapters by 22 contributors focuses on positron emission tomography, cardiovascular magnetic resonance, and cardiac computed tomography, techniques that provide non-invasive coronary angiograms, delineation of the arterial wall, and corresponding functional data on myocardial perfusion, metabolism, and viability. Same criticism as in #30 and #31.

*33. Germano G, Berman DS, editors. *Clinical Gated Cardiac SPECT.* Second Edition. New York: Blackwell Futura 2006:367, $150.00.

This book of 14 chapters by 17 contributors is well done. For those in this field, it will be very useful.

Cardiac Catheterization and Vascular Angiography

34. Baim DS, editor. *Grossman's Cardiac Catheterization, Angiography, and Intervention.* Seventh Edition. Philadelphia: Lippincott Williams & Wilkins (A Wolters Kluwer Company) 2006:807, $135.00.

This comprehensive book of 34 chapters by 34 contributors has changed with time and remains the first and classic in this field. The accompanying DVD-CDROM contains >150 cases covering a broad range of classic findings. The case examples can be transferred into one's own computer for educational purposes.

35. Uflacker R, editor. *Atlas of Vascular Anatomy. An Angiographic Approach.* Second Edition. Philadelphia: Lippincott Williams & Wilkins 2007:905, $229.00.

This book covers the entire vascular system, and therefore, would be more useful to the non-cardiac interventionalist than the cardiac one. Although there are 5 contributors in addition to the editor, their names are not listed on the title page of each of the 24 chapters. That should be corrected in future editions. Most illustrations, and particularly, the drawings by Josè Falcetti are superb.

Percutaneous Intervention

*36. King SB III, Yeung AC, editors. *Interventional Cardiology.* New York: McGraw-Hill Medical 2007:600, $135.00.

This book of 71 chapters by 117 contributors is beautifully prepared and intended, of course, for the interventional cardiologist. For this subspecialty group, this book appears to be a "must have."

37. Seung-Jung P, Mintz GS, editors. *Handbook of Left Main Stem Disease.* Abingdon, Oxon: Informa Healthcare 2006:178, $150.26.

This good book of 7 chapters by 17 contributors may be the first on this topic.

38. Kern MJ, editor. Berger PB, Block PC, Klein LW, Luskey WK, Uretsky BF, associate editors. *SCAI Interventional Cardiology Board Review Book.* Philadelphia: Lippincott Williams & Wilkins 2007:301, $129.00.

A book of 29 chapters by 42 contributors. I like this book. Again, playing on the phrase "board review book."

39. Mukherjee D, Cho L, Moliterno DJ, Gilbreath DA, editors. *900 Questions: An Interventional Cardiology Board Review.* Philadelphia: Wolters Kluwer 2007:368, $89.95.

These questions and answers were contributed by 62 contributors and concern 40 topics (chapters). If I were soon to take the cardiology boards, I would purchase this book and study it.

*40. Bridges CR, Horvath KA, Chiu R C-J, editors. *Myocardial Laser Revascularization.* Malden, Massachusetts: Blackwell Futura 2006:174: $95.00.

This book of 13 chapters by 19 contributors will surely be useful to those involved in this very specialized area.

41. Lanzer P, editor. *Mastering Endovascular Techniques. A Guide to Excellence.* Philadelphia: Lippincott Williams & Wilkins 2007:460, $149.00.

A book of 15 chapters by 42 contributors. Includes both coronary and non-coronary interventions.

*42. Saw J, Exaire JE, Lee DS, Yadav JS, editors. *Handbook of Complex Percutaneous Carotid Intervention.* Totowa, New Jersey: Humana Press 2007:334, $185.00.

This book of 24 chapters by 17 contributors focuses, of course, on the percutaneous intravascular approach to carotid arterial narrowing. Whether this intravascular approach (angioplasty ± stenting) will win out over the extravascular approach (endarterectomy) remains to be seen. At any rate, the intravascular approach is gaining in popularity.

Cardiac Physical Examination

43. Ranganathan N, Sivaciyan V, Saksena FB. *The Art and Science of Cardiac Physical Examination with Heart Sounds and Pulse Wave Forms on CD.* Totowa, New Jersey: Humana Press 2006:411, $99.50.

A book of 11 chapters by the 3 authors. Obviously, this area of cardiology is presently being neglected. Most of this information, however, is also present in the major cardiac textbooks (Braunwald, Hurst, Topol, Willerson).

Cardiac Physiology

44. Katz AM. *Physiology of the Heart.* Fourth Edition. Philadelphia: Lippincott Williams & Wilkins (A Wolters Kluwer Company) 2006:644, $99.00.

This single-authored comprehensive book of 16 chapters has become a classic. It focuses on both the normal and abnormal heart on many levels—cellular, subcellular, molecular, genetic—and how they effect cardiac function.

Cardiac Pharmacology

45. Mancia G, editor. *Angiotensin II Receptor Antagonists. Current Perspectives.* Second Edition. Milton Park, Abingdon, Oxon: Informa Healthcare 2006:218, $206.61.

This book of 11 chapters by 23 contributors describes the use of angiotensin II antagonists in several conditions—myocardial infarction, systemic hypertension, renal failure, diabetes mellitus, heart failure, metabolic syndrome and preventing stroke. It also compares the various AT1 inhibitors. Its price is inappropriate!

Miscellaneous

*46. Morrow DA, editor. *Cardiovascular Biomarkers. Pathophysiology and Disease Management.* Totowa, New Jersey: Humana Press 2006:620, $175.00.

This book of 34 chapters by 52 contributors is superb and fills a major void among books on cardiovascular disease. Highly recommended.

*47. Clark LT, editor; McFarlane SI, associate editor. *Cardiovascular Disease and Diabetes.* New York: McGraw Hill Medical 2007:635, $75.00.

This book of 22 chapters by 40 contributors, all but one of whom have professional addresses in New York City, puts in one publication a great deal of information on cardiovascular problems in patients with diabetes mellitus.

48. McAllister HA, Jr, Willerson JT, editors. *Ten Years of Images from CIRCULATION, Journal of the American Heart Association.* Dallas: American Heart Association 2007:231, $59.95.

This book includes 148 separate case images. I enjoy single case studies and splendid images, so I applaud the editors and the American Heart Association for publishing this monograph.

Non-Human Cardiology

49. Xu Q, editor. *A Handbook of Mouse Models of Cardiovascular Disease.* West Sussex, UK: John Wiley & Sons 2006:387, $200.00.

This "handbook" of 29 chapters occupying 387 pages by 68 contributors puts together in one place a large amount of information on experimentally-produced heart disease in mice. For those working in this area, this book will be useful.

Comments

Of the 49 books commented on in this piece, 16 (33%) have a 2007 publishing date and the others a 2006 publishing date. Only 14 (29%) were published on acid-free (permanent) paper. (They are indicated by an asterisk.) The prices of the books keep rising. These 49 ranged from $26.95 to $299.00 (mean $125.03).

William Clifford Roberts, MD
Editor in Chief
Baylor Heart & Vascular Institute
Baylor University Medical Center
Dallas, Texas

Good Books in Cardiovascular Diseases Appearing in 2007 and in Early 2008

Major Textbooks

1. Libby P, Bonow RO, Mann DL, Zipes DP, editors; Braunwald E, Founding editor and E-dition editor. Braunwald's Heart Disease. A Textbook of Cardiovascular Medicine. Eighth Edition. Philadelphia: Saunders Elsevier 2008: 2273, $189.00 (single volume), $199.00 (2-volume set).

2. *Fuster V, O'Rourke RA, Walsh RA, Poole-Wilson P, editors; King SB III, Roberts R, Nash IS, Prystowsky EN, associate editors. Hurst's The Heart. Twelfth Edition. New York: McGraw Hill Medical 2008:2540, $179.00 (single volume), $199.00 (2-volume set).

3. *Willerson JT, Cohn JN, Wellens HJJ, Holmes DR Jr, editors. Cardiovascular Medicine, Third Edition. London: Springer-Verlag 2008:2926, $199.00.

Miscellaneous

4. Waksman R, Serruys PW, Schaar J, editors. *The Vulnerable Plaque*. Second Edition. London: informa healthcare, 2007:490, $129.95.

5. *Vogel JHK, Krucoff MW, editors. *Integrative Cardiology: Complementary and Alternative Medicine for the Heart*. New York: McGraw-Hill Medical, 2007:595, $69.95.

6. *De Caterina R, Libby P, editors. *Endothelial Dysfunctions and Vascular Disease*. Malden, Massachusetts: Blackwell Futura, 2007:416, $134.95.

7. Dzau VJ, Liew C-C, editors. *Cardiovascular Genetics and Genomics for the Cardiologist*. Malden, Massachusetts: Blackwell Futura, 2007:308, $144.95.

8. *Nguyen TN, Hu D, Kim M-H, Grines CL, editors. *Management of Complex Cardiovascular Problems: The Evidence-Based Medicine Approach*. Malden, Massachusetts: Blackwell Futura, 2007:451, $69.95.

9. *Leri A, Anversa P, Frishman WH, editors. *Cardiovascular Regeneration and Stem Cell Therapy*. Malden, Massachusetts: Blackwell Futura, 2007:229, $134.95.

10. *Kraus WE, Keteyian SJ, editors. *Cardiac Rehabilitation*. Totowa, New Jersey: Humana Press, 2007:307, $99.00.

11. *Oakley C, Warnes CA, editors. *Heart Disease in Pregnancy*. Second Edition. Malden, Massachusetts: Blackwell (BMJ Books), 2007:354, $114.95.

12. Phibbs B. *The Human Heart: A Basic Guide to Heart Disease*. Second Edition. Philadelphia: Wolters Kluwer/ Lippincott Williams & Wilkins, 2007:229, $59.95.

13. Watson RR, Larson DF, editors. *Immune Dysfunction and Immunotherapy in Heart Disease*. Malden, Massachusetts: Blackwell Futura, 2007:308, $150.00

14. Sutherland JA. *The Little Black Book of Cardiology*. Second Edition. Sudbury, Massachusetts: Jones & Bartlett, 2007:385, $45.95.

15. Wollert KC, Field LJ, editors. *Rebuilding the Infarcted Heart*. London: informa healthcare, 2007:200, $159.95.

16. Aggarwal R, Ferenczi E, Muirhead N, Francis D. *One Stop Doc: Cardiology*. London: Hodder Arnold, 2007:136, $21.99.

17. Shishehbor MH, Wang T, Askari AT, Penn MS, Topol EJ, editors. *Management of the Patient in the Coronary Care Unit*. Philadelphia: Lippincott Williams & Wilkins, 2008:338, $69.95.

18. *Wackers FJTh, Bruni W, Zaret BL. *Nuclear Cardiology, the Basics: How to Set Up and Maintain a Laboratory*. Second Edition. Totowa, New Jersey: Humana Press, 2008:433, $99.50.

19. Abedin Z, Conner R. *ECG Interpretation: The Self-Assessment Approach*. Second Edition. Malden, Massachusetts: Blackwell Futura, 2008:233, $59.95.

20. *Stouffer GA, editor. *Cardiovascular Hemodynamics for the Clinician*. Malden, Massachusetts: Blackwell Futura, 2008:302, $65.00.

Mainly for the Lay Public

21. Elefteriades JA, Cohen LS. *Your Heart: An Owner's Guide*. Amherst, New York: Prometheus, 2007:415, $20.00.

22. Flanigan RJ, Sawyer KF. *Longevity Made Simple: How to Add 20 Good Years to Your Life: Lessons from Decades of Research*. Denver, Colorado: Williams Clark, 2007:195, $12.95.

23. Cooper KH, Cooper TC, with Proctor W. *Start Strong, Finish Strong*. New York: Avery, 2007:408, $24.95.

24. Agatston A. *The South Beach Heart Program: The 4-Step Plan That Can Save Your Life*. New York: Rodale, 2007:291, $25.95.

25. Graboys TB, with Zheutlin P. *Life in the Balance: A Physician's Memoir of Life, Love, and Loss With Parkinson's Disease and Dementia*. New York: Sterling, 2007: 196, $19.95.

Systemic Hypertension

26. Korner P. *Essential Hypertension and Its Causes: Neural and Non-Neural Mechanisms*. Oxford, United Kingdom: Oxford University Press, 2007:690, $120.25.

Heart Failure

27. St. John Sutton M, Box JJ, Jessup M, Brugada J, Schalij MJ, editors. *Cardiac Resynchronization Therapy*. London: informa healthcare, 2007:324, $254.95.

28. *Abraham WT, Krum H, editors. *Heart Failure: A Practical Approach to Treatment*. New York: McGraw-Hill Medical, 2007:322, $85.95.

29. *Kenny T. *The Nuts and Bolts of Cardiac Resyn-*

* Printed on acid-free paper.

chronization Therapy. Malden, Massachusetts: Blackwell Futura, 2007:218, $54.95.

30. *McCarthy PM, Young JB, editors. *Heart Failure: A Combined Medical and Surgical Approach*. Malden, Massachusetts: Blackwell Futura, 2007:314, $99.95.

31. *McIvor M. *Establishing a Heart Failure Program: The Essential Guide*. Third Edition. Malden, Massachusetts: Blackwell Futura, 2007:161, $145.00.

Arrhythmias, Conduction Disturbances, Electrocardiography, and Electrophysiology

32. *Khan MG. *Rapid ECG Interpretation*. Third Edition. Totowa, New Jersey: Humana Press, 2008:416, $79.50.

33. Hayes DL, Asirvatham SJ. *Dictionary of Cardiac Pacing, Defibrillation, Resynchronization, and Arrhythmias*. Second Edition. Minneapolis, Minnesota: Cardiotext, 2007:302, $98.50.

34. Natale A, Wazni O, editors. *Handbook of Cardiac Electrophysiology*. London: informa healthcare, 2007:383, $90.00.

35. *Abedin Z, Conner R. *Essential Cardiac Electrophysiology With Self Assessment*. Malden, Massachusetts: Blackwell Futura, 2007:295, $44.95.

36. *Grubb BP. *The Fainting Phenomenon: Understanding Why People Faint and What to Do About It*. Second Edition. Malden, Massachusetts: Blackwell Futura, 2007:135, $24.95.

Congenital Heart Disease

37. Kirby ML. *Cardiac Development*. Oxford, United Kingdom: Oxford University Press, 2007:273, $164.33.

38. Sievert H, Qureshi SA, Wilson N, Hijazi ZM, editors. *Percutaneous Interventions for Congenital Heart Disease*. London: informa healthcare, 2007:606, $279.95.

39. *Mond HG, Karpawich PP. *Pacing Options in the Adult Patient With Congenital Heart Disease*. Malden, Massachusetts, 2007:136, $65.00.

Imaging

40. Rimington H, Chambers JB, editors. *Echocardiography: A Practical Guide to Reporting*. Second Edition. London: informa healthcare, 2007:148, $50.00.

41. Shiota T, editor. *3D Echocardiography*. London: informa healthcare, 2007:166, $84.00.

42. Nanda NC, Domanski MJ, editors. *Atlas of Transesophageal Echocardiography*. Second Edition. Philadelphia: Lippincott Williams & Wilkins, 2007:641, $199.00.

43. Regar E, van Leeuwen TG, Serruys PW, editors. *Optical Coherence Tomography in Cardiovascular Research*. London: informa healthcare, 2007:338, $165.00.

44. *Marwick TH, Yu C-M, Sun JP, editors. *Myocardial Imaging: Tissue Doppler and Speckle Tracking*. Malden, Massachusetts: Blackwell Futura, 2007:321, $150.00.

45. Bury B, Dickinson C, Sheard K, Thorley P. *Myocardial Perfusion Scintigraphy: From Request to Report*. London: informa healthcare, 2007:160, $129.95.

46. Gerber TC, Kantor B, Williamson EE, editors. *Computed Tomography of the Cardiovascular System*. London: informa healthcare, 2007:518, $284.95.

Cardiovascular Interventions

47. Kipshidze NN, Moses JW, Fareed J, Serruys PW, editors. *Textbook of Interventional Cardiovascular Pharmacology*. London: informa healthcare, 2007:646, $199.00.

48. Rooke TW, Sullivan TM, Jaff MR, editors. *Vascular Medicine and Endovascular Interventions*. Columbia, Maryland: Blackwell Futura, 2007:331, $99.95.

49. Raman SV, Grodecki PV, Cook SC, Garcia MJ. *Cardiovascular Multidetector CT Angiography*. London: informa healthcare, 2007:181, $174.95.

50. Eeckhout E, Lerman A, Carlier S, Kern M, editors. *Handbook of Complications During Percutaneous Cardiovascular Interventions*. London: informa healthcare, 2007:319, $179.95.

51. *Duckers HJ, Nabel EG, Serruys PW, editors. *Essentials of Restenosis for the Interventional Cardiologist*. Totowa, New Jersey: Humana Press, 2007:458, $134.95.

52. Dangas GD, Mehran R, Moses JW, editors. *Handbook of Chronic Total Occlusions*. London: informa healthcare, 2007:237, $90.00.

53. Columbo A, Stankovic G, editors. *Problem Oriented Approaches in Interventional Cardiology*. London: informa healthcare, 2007:286, $199.95.

54. *Nguyen TN, Colombo A, Hu D, Grines CL, Saito S, editors. *Practical Handbook of Advanced Interventional Cardiology: Tips and Tricks*. Third Edition. Malden, Massachusetts: Blackwell, 2008:616, $103.95.

Cardiac Surgery

55. *Cohn LH, editor. *Cardiac Surgery in the Adult*. Third Edition. New York: McGraw-Hill Medical, 2008:1704, $265.00.

56. *Yuh DD, Vricella LA, Baumgartner WA, editors. *The Johns Hopkins Manual of Cardiothoracic Surgery*. New York: McGraw-Hill Medical, 2007:1464, $159.00.

57. Slaughter MS, editor. *Cardiac Surgery in Chronic Renal Failure*. Malden, Massachusetts: Blackwell Futura, 2007:98, $74.95.

Noncoronary Vascular Disease

58. *Stein PD. *Pulmonary Embolism*. Second Edition. Malden, Massachusetts: Blackwell Futura, 2007:476, $124.95.

59. Schillinger M, Minar E, editors. *Complications in Peripheral Vascular Interventions*. London: informa healthcare, 2007:239, $95.00.

60. Moussa I, Rundek T, Mohr JP, editors. *Asymptomatic Carotid Artery Stenosis Risk Stratification and Management*. London: informa healthcare, 2007:210, $75.00.

Preventive Cardiology

61. Steinberg D. *The Cholesterol Wars: The Skeptics vs. the Preponderance of Evidence*. Amsterdam, The Netherlands: Elsevier (Academic Press), 2007:227, $69.95.

William Clifford Roberts, MD
Editor in Chief
Baylor University Medical Center
Dallas, Texas

Good Books in Cardiovascular Disease Appearing in 2008

General Cardiology

1. Griffin BP, Topol EJ, editors. *Manual of Cardiovascular Medicine*. Third Edition. Philadelphia: Wolters Kluwer/Lippincott Williams & Wilkins, 2009:1015, $79.95.
2. Aronow WS, Fleg JL, Rich MW, editors. *Cardiovascular Disease in the Elderly*. Fourth Edition. New York: Informa Healthcare, 2008:865, $299.95.
3. Baliga RR, Eagle KA, editors. *Practical Cardiology: Evaluation and Treatment of Common Cardiovascular Disorders*. Second Edition. Philadelphia: Wolters Kluwer/Lippincott Williams & Wilkins, 2008:770, $69.95.
4. *Swanton RH, Banerjee S. *Swanton's Cardiology: A Concise Guide to Clinical Practice*. Sixth Edition. Malden, Massachusetts: Blackwell Futura, 2008: 686, $100.00.
5. Cuculich PS, Kates AM, editors. *The Washington Manual, Cardiology, Subspecialty Consult*. Second Edition. Philadelphia: Wolters Kluwer/Lippincott Williams & Wilkins, 2009:458, $39.95.
6. Daniels DV, Rockson SG, Vagelos R, editors. *Concise Cardiology. An Evidence-Based Handbook*. Philadelphia: Lippincott Williams & Wilkins, 2008:271, $42.95.

Coronary Artery Disease

7. Durstine JL, Moore GE, LaMonte MJ, Franklin BA, editors. *Pollock's Textbook of Cardiovascular Disease and Rehabilitation*. Champaign, Illinois: Human Kinetics, 2008:411, $89.00.
8. Angiolillo DJ, Kastrati A, Simon DI, editors. *Clinical Guide to the Use of Antithrombotic Drugs in Coronary Artery Disease*. London, United Kingdom: Informa Healthcare, 2008:276, $189.95.
9. *Mitchell ARJ, West NEJ, Leeson P, Banning AP, editors. *Cardiac Catheterization and Coronary Intervention*. Oxford, United Kingdom: Oxford University Press, 2008:282, $69.50.
10. *de Lemos JA, editor. *Biomarkers in Heart Disease*. Malden, Massachusetts: Blackwell Futura, 2008: 238, $125.00.
11. Bhatt DL, editor. *Platelets in Cardiovascular Disease*. London, United Kingdom: Imperial College Press, 2008:218, $98.00.
12. Feinstein SB, editor. *Non-Invasive Surrogate Markers of Atherosclerosis*. London, United Kingdom: Informa Healthcare, 2008:125, $119.95.

Arrhythmia and/or Conduction Defect

13. Josephson ME. *Clinical Cardiac Electrophysiology: Techniques and Interpretations*. Fourth Edition. Philadelphia: Wolters Kluwer/Lippincott Williams & Wilkins, 2008:922, $210.00.
14. *Natale A, Jalife J, editors. *Atrial Fibrillation: From Bench to Bedside*. Totowa, New Jersey: Humana Press, 2008:453, $99.50.
15. Calkins H, Jai P, Steinberg JS, editors. *A Practical Approach to Catheter Ablation of Atrial Fibrillation*. Philadelphia: Wolters Kluwer/Lippincott Williams & Wilkins, 2008:371, $110.00.
16. Zimetbaum PJ, Josephson ME, editors. *Practical Clinical Electrophysiology*. Philadelphia: Wolters Kluwer/Lippincott Williams & Wilkins, 2009:304, $110.00.
17. *Al-Ahmad A, Callans D, Hsia H, Natala A, editors. *Electroanatomical Mapping: An Atlas for Clinicians*. Malden, Massachusetts: Blackwell Futura, 2008:268, $120.00.
18. Kenny T. *The Nuts and Bolts of Cardiac Pacing*. Chichester, United Kingdom: Wiley-Blackwell, 2008: 171, $60.00.

Electrocardiography

19. Wagner GS. *Marriott's Practical Electrocardiography*. Eleventh Edition. Philadelphia: Wolters Kluwer/ Lippincott Williams & Wilkins, 2008:468, $75.00.
20. *Wang PJ, Al-Ahmad A, Hsia HH, Zei PC, editors. *Ventricular Arrhythmias and Sudden Cardiac Death*. Malden, Massachusetts: Blackwell Futura, 2008:345, $150.00.
21. *Bayés de Luna A, Fiol-Sala M. *Electrocardiography in Ischemia Heart Disease: Clinical and Imaging Correlations and Prognostic Implications*. Malden, Massachusetts: Blackwell Futura, 2008:332, $125.00.
22. Houghton AR, Gray D. *Making Sense of the ECG: A Hands-On Guide*. Third Edition. London, United Kingdom: Hodder Arnold, 2008:292, $25.92.
23. *Mattu A, Brady W. *ECGs for the Emergency Physician 2*. Malden, Massachusetts: Blackwell Futura, 2008:211, $55.00.

Imaging

24. Rubin GD, Rofsky NM, editors. *CT and MR Angiography: Comprehensive Vascular Assessment*. Phila-

* Printed on acid-free paper.

delphia: Wolters Kluwer/Lippincott Williams & Wilkins, 2009:1316, $269.00.

25. *Kwong RY, editor. *Cardiovascular Magnetic Resonance Imaging*. Totowa, New Jersey: Humana Press, 2008:749, $179.00.
26. *Iskandrian AE, Garcia EV, editors. *Nuclear Cardiac Imaging: Principles and Applications*. Fourth Edition. Oxford, United Kingdom: Oxford University Press, 2008:732, $195.50.
27. Biederman RWW, Doyle M, Yamrozik J. *The Cardiovascular MRI Tutorial: Lectures and Learning*. Philadelphia: Wolters Kluwer/Lippincott Williams & Wilkins, 2008:378, $185.00.
28. *Heller GV, Mann A, Handel RC, editors. *Nuclear Cardiology: Technical Applications*. New York: McGraw Hill Medical, 2009:336, $75.00.
29. *Sabharwal N, Leong CY, Kelion A. *Nuclear Cardiology*. Oxford, United Kingdom: Oxford University Press, 2008:231, $69.50.
30. Faletra FF, Pandian NG, Ho SY. *Anatomy of the Heart by Multislice Computed Tomography*. Oxford, United Kingdom: Wiley-Blackwell, 2008:125, $99.95.

Heart Failure

31. *Cheuk-Man Y, Hayes DL, Auricchio A, editors. *Cardiac Resynchronization Therapy*. Second Edition. Malden, Massachusetts: Blackwell Futura, 2008: 444, $100.00.
32. *Kearney M, editor. *Chronic Heart Failure*. Oxford, United Kingdom: Oxford University Press, 2008: 130, $24.95.

Peripheral Vascular Disease

33. Heuser RR, Henry M, editors. *Textbook of Peripheral Vascular Interventions*. Second Edition. London, United Kingdom: Informa Healthcare, 2008: 908, $299.95.
34. Kandarpa K, editor. *Peripheral Vascular Interventions*. Philadelphia: Wolters Kluwer/Lippincott Williams & Wilkins, 2008:577, $184.00.
35. Sangiorgi G, Holmes DR Jr, Rosenfield K, Hopkins LN, Spagnolia LG, editors. *Carotid Atherosclerotic Disease: Pathologic Basis for Treatment*. London, United Kingdom: Informa Healthcare, 2008:362, $179.95.

Metabolic Cardiology

36. *Hansen BC, Bray GA, editors. *The Metabolic Syndrome: Epidemiology, Clinical Treatment, and Underlying Mechanisms*. Totowa, New Jersey: Humana Press, 2008:401, $149.00.
37. *Fisman EZ, Tenenbaum A, editors. *Cardiovascular Diabetology: Clinical, Metabolic and Inflammatory Facets*. Basel, Switzerland: Karger, 2008:174, $180.00.
38. *Feinglos MN, Bethel MA, editors. *Type 2 Diabetes Mellitus: An Evidence-Based Approach to Practical Management*. Totowa, New Jersey: Humana Press, 2008:474, $139.00.

Pulmonary Hypertension

39. *Hill NS, Farber HW, editors. *Pulmonary Hypertension*. Totowa, New Jersey: Humana Press, 2008:444, $145.00.
40. Barst RJ, editor. *Pulmonary Arterial Hypertension: Diagnosis and Evidence Based Treatment*. Chichester, United Kingdom: John Wiley & Sons, Ltd., 2008:256, $100.00.

Miscellaneous

41. Yagel S, Silverman NH, Gembruch U, editors; Cohen SM, associate editor. *Fetal Cardiology: Embryology, Genetics, Physiology, Echocardiographic Evaluation, Diagnosis and Perinatal Management of Cardiac Disease*. Second Edition. New York: Informa Healthcare, 2009:780, $499.95.
42. Field JM, editor in chief. *The Textbook of Emergency Cardiovascular Care and CPR*. Philadelphia: Wolters Kluwer/Lippincott Williams & Wilkins, 2009:610, $129.00.
43. Perloff JK, Child JS, Aboulhosn J. *Congenital Heart Disease in Adults*. Third Edition. Philadelphia: Saunders Elsevier, 2008:504, $165.00.
44. Opie LH, editor; Gersh BJ, co-editor. *Drugs for the Heart*. Seventh Edition. Philadelphia: Saunders Elsevier, 2009:502, $64.95.
45. *Mongero LB, Beck JR, editors. *On Bypass: Advanced Perfusion Techniques*. Totowa, New Jersey: Humana Press, 2008:576, $129.00.
46. Yim PJ, editor. *Vascular Hemodynamics: Bioengineering and Clinical Perspectives*. Hoboken, New Jersey: Wiley-Blackwell, 2008:346, $125.00.
47. Cho L, Griffin BP, Topol EJ, editors. *The Cardiology Intensive Board Review Question Book*. Philadelphia: Wolters Kluwer/Lippincott Williams & Wilkins, 2009:385, $89.00.
48. Diethrich EB, Ramaiah VG, Kpodonu J, Rodriquez-Lopez JA. *Endovascular and Hybrid Management of Thoracic Aorta: A Case-Based Approach*. Chichester, United Kingdom: Wiley-Blackwell, 2008:308, $160.00.
49. *Burgess JH. *Doctor to the North: Thirty Years Treating Heart Disease Among the Inuit*. Montreal, Canada: McGill-Queen's University Press, 2008:168, $34.95.

William Clifford Roberts, MD
Editor in Chief
Baylor Heart and Vascular Institute
Baylor University Medical Center
Dallas, Texas 75246

Good Books in Cardiovascular Disease Appearing in 2009

General Textbooks

1. Camm AJ, Lüscher TF, Serruys PW, editors. *The ESC Textbook of Cardiovascular Medicine*. Second Edition. Oxford, United Kingdom: Oxford University Press, 2009:1398, $395.00.
2. Yusuf S, Cairns JA, Camm AJ, Fallen EL, Gersh BJ, editors. *Evidence-Based Cardiology*. Third Edition. Oxford, United Kingdom: Wiley-Blackwell, 2010: 218, $299.95.
3. O'Rourke RA, Walsh RA, Fuster V, editors. *Hurst's the Heart Manual of Cardiology*. Twelfth Edition. New York: McGraw-Hill Medical, 2009:750, $59.95.
4. Ferdinand KC, editor. *Educational Review Manual in Cardiovascular Disease*. New York: Castle Connolly Graduate Medical Publishing, 2009:642, $99.95.
5. *Crawford MH, editor. *Current Diagnosis & Treatment Cardiology*. Third Edition. New York: McGraw-Hill Medical, 2009:574, $71.95.

Coronary Artery Disease

6. Hutchison SJ. *Complications of Myocardial Infarction: Clinical Diagnostic Imaging Atlas*. Philadelphia: Saunders Elsevier 2009:280, $169.00.
7. Antoniucci D, editor. *Primary Angioplasty: Mechanical Interventions for Acute Myocardial Infarction*. Second Edition. New York: Informa Healthcare, 2009:246, $299.95.
8. Waksman R, Ajani AE, editors. *Pharmacology in the Catheterization Laboratory*. Hoboken, New Jersey: Wiley-Blackwell, 2010:379, $149.95.
9. Wiviott SD, editor. *Antiplatelet Therapy in Ischemic Heart Disease*. Dallas, Texas: American Heart Association, 2009:289, $125.00.
10. Januzzi JL Jr, editor. *Cardiac Biomarkers in Clinical Practice*. Sudbury, Massachusetts: Jones & Bartlett, 2011:892, $69.95.
11. *Peacock WF, Cannon CP, editors. *Short Stay Management of Chest Pain*. New York: Humana Press, 2009:271, $189.00.
12. Waksman R, Saito S, editors. *Chronic Total Occlusions: A Guide to Recanalization*. Chichester, United Kingdom: Wiley-Blackwell, 2009:198, $125.00.
13. Pundziūte G, editor. *Imaging of Coronary Atherosclerosis With Multi-Slice Computed Tomography*. Leiden, The Netherlands: Leiden, 2009.
14. Califf RM, Roe MT. *ACS Essentials*. Third Edition. Sudbury, Massachusetts: Physicians' Press, 2010:228, $24.95.

Preventive Cardiology

15. Ballantyne CM, editor. *Clinical Lipidology: A Companion to Braunwald's Heart Disease*. Philadelphia: Saunders Elsevier, 2009:608, $169.00.
16. Kwiterovich PO Jr, editor. *The Johns Hopkins Textbook of Dyslipidemia*. Philadelphia: Wolters Kluwer/Lippincott Williams & Wilkins, 2010:303, $89.95.
17. Kokkinos P. *Physical Activity and Cardiovascular Disease Prevention*. Sudbury, Massachusetts: Jones & Bartlett, 2010:418, $78.95.
18. *Bendich A, Deckelbaum RJ, editors. *Preventive Nutrition: The Comprehensive Guide for Health Professionals*. Fourth Edition. New York: Humana Press, 2010:862, $169.00.
19. Hobbs FDR, Arroll B, editors. *Cardiovascular Risk Management*. Chichester, United Kingdom: John Wiley & Sons, 2009:90, $45.00.

Systemic Hypertension

20. Kaplan NM, Victor RG. *Kaplan's Clinical Hypertension*. Tenth Edition. Philadelphia: Wolters Kluwer/Lippincott Williams & Wilkins, 2010:469, $99.00.
21. Frohlich ED, Ventura HO. *Hypertension: An Atlas of Investigation and Management*. Oxford, United Kingdom: Clinical Publishing, 2009:144, $99.95.
22. Kaplan NM, Weber MA. *Hypertension Essentials 2010*. Second Edition. Sudbury, Massachusetts: Physicians' Press, 2010:102, $24.95.

Arrhythmias and Conduction Disturbances and Electrocardiography

23. Zipes DP, Jalife J, editors. *Cardiac Electrophysiology: From Cell to Bedside*. Fifth Edition. Philadelphia: Saunders Elsevier, 2009:1155, $299.00.
24. Issa ZF, Miller JM, Zipes DP. *Clinical Arrhythmology and Electrophysiology: A Companion to Braunwald's Heart Disease*. Philadelphia: Saunders Elsevier, 2009:520, $199.00.
25. Baltazar RF. *Basic and Bedside Electrocardiography*. Philadelphia: Wolters Kluwer/Lippincott Williams & Wilkins, 2009:464, $79.95.
26. Stroobandt RX, Barold SS, Sinnaeve AF. *Implantable Cardioverter-Defibrillators: Step by Step: An Illustrated Guide*. Chichester, UK: Wiley-Blackwell, 2009:427, $69.95.
27. Ho RT. *Electrophysiology of Arrhythmias: Practical Images for Diagnosis and Ablation*. Philadelphia: Wolters Kluwer/Lippincott Williams & Wilkins, 2010:388, $99.00.
28. Kenny T. *The Nuts and Bolts of Paced ECG Interpretation*. Chichester, United Kingdom: Wiley-Blackwell, 2009:480, $75.00.
29. Macle L, Weerasooriya R, Scavee C, Jaïs P. *Pulmonary Vein Recordings: A Practical Guide to the Mapping and Ablation of Atrial Fibrillation*. Minneapolis, Minnesota: Cardiotext, 2009:163, $79.00.
30. Thaler MS. *The Only EKG Book You'll Ever Need*. Sixth Edition. Philadelphia: Wolters Kluwer/Lippincott Williams & Wilkins, 2010:336, $59.95.
31. O'Keefe JH Jr, Hammil SC, Freed MS, Pogwizd SM. *The ECG Criteria Book*. Second Edition. Sudbury, Massachusetts: Physicians' Press, 2010:184, $24.95.

32. Houghton AR, Gray D. *Making Sense of the ECG Cases for Self-Assessment*. London, United Kingdom: Hodder Arnold, 2009:290, $31.00.

Heart Failure

33. Abraham WT, Baliga RR, editors. *Cardiac Resynchronization Therapy in Heart Failure*. Philadelphia: Wolters Kluwer/Lippincott Williams & Wilkins 2010: 182, $129. 00.

Valvular Heart Disease

34. Otto CM, Bonow RD, editors. *Valvular Heart Disease: A Companion to Braunwald's Heart Disease*. Third Edition. Philadelphia: Sanders Elsevier, 2009: 468, $179.00.
35. *Wang A, Bashore TM, editors. *Valvular Heart Disease*. New York: Humana Press, 2009:536, $269.00.

Congenital Heart Disease

36. *Wyszynski DF, Correa-Villasenor A, Graham TP, editors. *Congenital Heart Defects: From Origin to Treatment*. Oxford, United Kingdom: Oxford University Press, 2009:560, $129.95.
37. Eidem BW, Cetta F, O'Leary PW, editors. *Echocardiography in Pediatric and Adult Congenital Heart Disease*. Philadelphia: Wolters Kluwer/Lippincott Williams & Wilkins, 2010:500, $229.00.
38. Hijazi ZM, Feldman T, Chetham JP, Sievert H, editors. *Complication During Percutaneous Interventions for Congenital and Structural Heart Disease*. London, United Kingdom: Informa Healthcare, 2009:360, $349.95.
39. Warnes CA, editor. *Adult Congenital Heart Disease*. Dallas, Texas: American Heart Association, 2009: 271, $125.00.

Peripheral Arterial Disease

40. *Dieter RS, Dieter RA Jr, Dieter RA II, editors. *Peripheral Arterial Disease*. New York: McGraw-Hill Medical, 2009:1104, $129.00.
41. *Saw J, editor. *Carotid Artery Stenting: The Basics*. New York: Humana Press, 2009:276, $189.00.
42. Hutchison SJ. *Aortic Diseases: Clinical Diagnostic Imaging Atlas*. Philadelphia: Saunders Elsevier, 2009: 374, $169.00.
43. Donnelly R, London NJM, editors. *ABC of Arterial and Venous Disease*. Second Edition. Chichester, United Kingdom: Wiley-Blackwell, 2009:104, $47.00.

Cardiovascular Imaging

44. Garcia MJ, editor. *Noninvasive Cardiovascular Imaging: A Multi-Modality Approach*. Philadelphia: Wolters Kluwer/Lippincott Williams & Wilkins, 2010:744, $199.00.
45. Hutchison SJ. *Pericardial Diseases: Clinical Diagnostic Imaging Atlas*. Philadelphia: Saunders Elsevier, 2009:288, $169.00.

Miscellaneous

46. Freedman JE, Loscalzo J, editors. *New Therapeutic Agents in Thrombosis and Thrombolysis*. Third Edition. New York: Informa Healthcare, 2009:700, $299.95.
47. Opie LH, Gersh BJ, editors. *Drugs for the Heart*. Seventh Edition. Philadelphia: Sanders Elsevier, 2009:512, $69.95.
48. Fuster V, editor. *The AHA Guidelines and Scientific Statements Handbook*. Dallas, Texas: American Heart Association (Wiley-Blackwell), 2009:376, $100.00.
49. Roden D, editor. *Cardiovascular Genetics and Genomics*. Dallas, Texas: American Heart Association (Wiley-Blackwell), 2009:265, $125.00.
50. Perloff JK. *Physical Examination of the Heart and Circulation*. Fourth Edition. Shelton, Connecticut: People's Medical, 2009:274, $49.95.
51. Ballastas HC, Durston S, Kelly MM, Ramirez MN, Roberson AR, Trujillo LA. Auscultation Skills. *Breath & Heart Sounds*. Fourth Edition. Philadelphia: Wolters Kluwer/Lippincott Williams & Wilkins, 2010:240, $54.95.
52. Regensteiner JG, Reusch JEB, Stewart KJ, Veves A, editors. *Diabetes and Exercise*. New York: Humana Press, 2009:317, $179.00.
53. Ferdinand KC, Armani A, editors. *Cardiovascular Disease in Racial and Ethnic Minorities*. Totowa, New Jersey: Humana Press, 2009:331, $129.00.
54. Piscatella JC. *Positive Mind, Healthy Heart: Take Charge of Your Cardiac Health, One Day at a Time*. New York: Workman, 2010:314, $10.95.
55. *Doroghazi RM. *The Physician's Guide to Investing: A Practical Approach to Building Wealth*. Second Edition. New York: Humana Press, 2009:425, $29.95.

The books included herein were selected from books sent to me for review in 2009 and in January 2010. Noninclusion indicates that the book was not sent to me. Of the 55 books included herein, 34 were organized by 1 to 5 editors, and the other 21 were written by 1 to 6 authors. Only 9 were printed on acid-free paper (denoted by asterisks).

William Clifford Roberts, MD
Editor in Chief
Baylor Heart & Vascular Institute
Dallas, Texas

Good Books in Cardiovascular Disease Appearing in 2010

Major Textbooks

1. Crawford MH, DiMarco JP, Paulus WJ, editors. *Cardiology*. 3rd ed. Philadelphia, Pennsylvania: Mosby Elsevier, 2010:1984, $264.00.

2. Anderson RH, Baker EJ, Penny DJ, Redington AN, Rigby ML, Wernovsky G, editors. *Pediatric Cardiology*. 3rd ed. Philadelphia, Pennsylvania: Churchill Livingston/ Elsevier, 2010:1344, $299.00.

Physiology

3. Katz AM. *Physiology of the Heart*. 5th ed. Philadelphia, Pennsylvania: Lippincott Williams & Wilkins 2010: 576, $99.00.

4. Levick JR. *An Introduction to Cardiovascular Physiology*. 5th ed. London, United Kingdom: Hodder Arnold, 2010:430, $49.95.

5. Levick JR. *Cardiovascular Physiology: Questions for Self Assessment With Illustrated Answers*. London, United Kingdom: Hodder Arnold, 2010:266, $34.95.

Prevention

6. Vissers MN, Kastelein JJP, Stroes ES, editors. *Evidence-Based Management of Lipid Disorders*. Harley, United Kingdom: TFM, 2010:313, $99.00.

*7. Das UN. *Metabolic Syndrome Pathophysiology: The Role of Essential Fatty Acids*. Ames, Iowa: John Wiley, 2010:284, $179.99.

*8. Sniderman A, Durrington P. *Fast Facts: Hyperlipidemia*. 5th ed. Oxford, United Kingdom: Health Press, 2010: 142, $15.50.

9. Bell DSH, O'Keefe JH. *Metabolic Syndrome Essentials*. Sudbury, Massachusetts: Jones & Bartlett Learning, 2010:90, $24.95.

10. Piscatella JC, Franklin BA. *Take a Load Off Your Heart! 109 Things You Can Actually Do to Prevent, Halt and Reverse Heart Disease*. New York, New York: Workman, 2011:365, $14.95.

Imaging

11. Zaret BL, Beller GA, editors. *Clinical Nuclear Cardiology: State of the Art and Future Directions*. 4th ed. Philadelphia, Pennsylvania: Mosby Elsevier, 2010:896, $189.00.

12. Lang RM, Goldstein SA, Kronzon I, Khandheria BK, editors. *Dynamic Echocardiography*. St. Louis, Missouri: Saunders Elsevier, 2011:496, $229.00.

*13. Fogel MA, editor. *Principles and Practice of Cardiac Magnetic Resonance in Congenital Heart Disease: Form, Function, and Flow*. Chichester, United Kingdom: John Wiley, 2010:480, $174.95.

14. Bulwer BE, Rivero JM. *Echocardiography Pocket Guide: The Transthoracic Examination*. Sudbury, Massachusetts: Jones & Bartlett, 2010:336, $59.00.

15. Gray AT. *Atlas of Ultrasound-Guided Regional Anesthesia*. Philadelphia, Pennsylvania: Saunders Elsevier, 2010:365, $165.00.

16. Taylor AJ, editor. *Atlas of Cardiovascular Computed Tomography: An Imaging Companion to Braunwald's Heart Disease*. Philadelphia, Pennsylvania: Saunders Elsevier, 2010:304, $179.00.

17. Kramer CM, Hundley WG, editors. *Atlas of Cardiovascular Magnetic Resonance Imaging: An Imaging Companion to Braunwald's Heart Disease*. Philadelphia, Pennsylvania: Saunders Elsevier, 2010:376, $179.00.

18. Nanda NC, Hsiung MC, Miller AP, Hage FG. *Live/ Real Time 3D Echocardiography*. Chichester, United Kingdom: John Wiley, 2010:312, $269.95.

19. Nicholls SJ, Worthley SG, editors. *Cardiovascular Imaging for Clinical Practice*. Sudbury, Massachusetts: Jones & Bartlett, 2010:386, $95.95.

20. Sun JP, Felner JM, Merlino JD, editors. *Practical Handbook of Echocardiography: 101 Cases*. Chichester, United Kingdom: John Wiley, 2010:368, $124.95.

21. Sridharan S, Price G, Tann O, Hughes M, Muthurangu V, Taylor AM. *Cardiovascular MRI in Congenital Heart Disease: An Imaging Atlas*. New York, New York: Springer, 2010:164, $139.00.

22. Russo RJ. *Intravascular Ultrasound Pocket Guide*. 7th ed. Sudbury, Massachusetts: Jones & Bartlett, 2010:108, $21.95.

Arrhythmias

23. Yan G-X, Kowey PR, editors. *Management of Cardiac Arrhythmias*. 2nd ed. New York, New York: Humana, 2010:485, $239.00.

24. Al-Ahmad A, Ellenbogen KA, Natale A, Wang PJ, editors. *Pacemakers and Implantable Cardioverter Defibrillators. An Expert's Manual*. Minneapolis, Minnesota: Cardiotext, 2010:480, $149.00.

25. Steinberg JS, Mittal S, editors. *Electrophysiology: The Basics: A Companion Guide for the Cardiology Fellow During the EP Rotation*. Philadelphia, Pennsylvania: Lippincott Williams & Wilkins, 2009:240, $72.95.

26. Kotar SL, Gessler JE. *The Complete Guide to Ambulatory Cardiac Monitoring and Full Disclosure Telemetry*. Sudbury, Massachusetts: Jones & Bartlett Learning, 2010:236, $69.95.

Heart Failure

27. Barold SS, Stroobandt RX, Sinnaeve AF. *Cardiac Pacemakers and Resynchronization: Step-by-Step: An Illustrated Guide*. 2nd ed. Chichester, United Kingdom: John Wiley, 2010:480, $69.95.

* Printed on acid-free paper.

*28. Marin-Garcia J. *Heart Failure: Bench to Bedside*. New York, New York: Humana, 2010:470, $269.00.

*29. Maisel WH, editor. *Device Therapy in Heart Failure*. New York, New York: Humana, 2010:400, $239.00.

Percutaneous Interventions

30. Haase J, Schäfers H-J, Sievert H, Waksman R, editors. *Cardiovascular Interventions in Clinical Practice*. Chichester, United Kingdom: John Wiley, 2010:744, $299.95.

31. Watson S, Gorski KA, editors. *Invasive Cardiology: A Manual for Cath Lab Personnel*. 3rd ed. Sudbury, Massachusetts: Jones & Bartlett Learning, 2010:646, $80.95.

*32. Hijazi ZM, Feldman T, Abdullah Al-Qbandi MH, Sievert H, editors. *Transcatheter Closure of ASDs and PFOs: A Comprehensive Assessment*. Minneapolis, Minnesota: Cardiotext, 2010:459, $169.00.

33. Thakur R, Natale A, editors. *Transseptal Catheterization and Interventions*. Minneapolis, Minnesota: Cardiotext, 2010:256, $99.00.

34. Meier B, editor. *Current Best Practice in Interventional Cardiology*. Chichester, United Kingdom: John Wiley, 2010:232, $149.95.

35. Ragosta M. *Cardiac Catheterization: An Atlas and DVD*. Philadelphia, Pennsylvania: Saunders Elsevier, 2009:208, $165.00.

36. Grech ED, editor. *ABC of Interventional Cardiology*. 2nd ed. Chichester, United Kingdom: John Wiley, 2011:120, $38.00.

Miscellaneous

*37. Naghavi M, editor. *Asymptomatic Atherosclerosis: Pathophysiology, Detection and Treatment*. New York, New York: Humana, 2010:624, $239.00.

*38. Kumar D, Elliott P, editors. *Principles and Practice of Clinical Cardiovascular Genetics*. Oxford, United Kingdom: Oxford University Press, 2010:624, $155.00.

39. Tighe DA, Tran MT, Donovan JL, Cook JR. *Cardiology Drug Guide, 2010*. Sudbury, Massachusetts: Jones & Bartlett Learning, 2010:558, $55.95.

*40. Freemark M, editor. *Pediatric Obesity: Etiology, Pathogenesis and Treatment*. New York, New York: Humana, 2010:516, $239.00.

41. Griffiths MJD, Cordingley JJ, Price S, editors. *Cardiovascular Critical Care*. Chichester, United Kingdom: John Wiley, 2010:504, $129.95.

42. Nixon JV, editor. *The AHA Clinical Cardiac Consult*. 3rd ed. Philadelphia, Pennsylvania: Lippincott Williams & Wilkins, 2010:400, $84.95.

43. Gatzoulis MA, Webb GD, Broberg CS, Uemura H, editors. *Cases in Adult Congenital Heart Disease*. Philadelphia, Pennsylvania: Elsevier Health Science Division, 2010:560, $169.00.

44. Weir MR, editor. *Evidence-Based Management of Hypertension*. Harley, United Kingdom: TFM, 2010:300, $99.00.

*45. Askari AT, Lincoff AM, editors. *Antithrombotic Drug Therapy in Cardiovascular Disease*. New York, New York: Humana, 2010:475, $269.00.

46. Committee on Public Health Priorities to Reduce and Control Hypertension, Institute of Medicine. *A Population-Based Policy and Systems Change Approach to Prevent and Control Hypertension*. Washington, DC: National Academies Press, 2010:236, $49.00.

*47. Mousa SA, editor. *Anti-Coagulants, Antiplatelets, and Thrombolytics: Methods in Molecular Biology*. 2nd ed. New York, New York: Humana, 2010:316, $139.00.

48. Brusch JL, editor. *Endocarditis Essentials*. Sudbury, Massachusetts: Jones & Bartlett Learning, 2010:264, $24.95.

49. Betts T, Bull S, Dwight J. *Cardiology: Clinical Cases Uncovered*. Chichester, United Kingdom: John Wiley, 2010:256, $42.95.

50. Alonso A, McManus DD, Fisher DZ. *Dx/Rx—Peripheral Vascular Disease*. Sudbury, Massachusetts: Jones & Bartlett Learning, 2010:204, $34.95.

51. Kowey P, with Fox ML. *Lethal Rhythm*. Philadelphia, Pennsylvania: Pavilion, 2010:234, $17.90.

52. Cannon CP, Steinberg BA. *Evidence-Based Cardiology*. 3rd ed. Philadelphia, Pennsylvania: Lippincott, Williams & Wilkins, 2010:480, $59.95.

53. Sauer H, Shah AM, Laurindo FRM, editors. *Studies on Cardiovascular Disorders*. New York, New York: Humana, 2010:400, $204.00.

54. Toth PP, Cannon CP, editors. *Comprehensive Cardiovascular Medicine in the Primary Care Setting*. New York, New York: Humana, 2010:603, $199.43.

55. Bojar RM. *Manual of Perioperative Care in Adult Cardiac Surgery*. 5th ed. Chichester, United Kingdom: John Wiley, 2011:832, $64.95.

56. Martin VB. *The Celestial Society: A Life in Medicine*. Bloomington, Indiana: Xlibris, 2010:743, $23.99. (This book is about Dr. George Burch, the author's father.)

*57. Cooper DKC. *Open Heart: The Radical Surgeons Who Revolutionized Medicine*. New York, New York: Kaplan, 2010:448, $26.99.

58. Weisse AB. *Notes of a Medical Maverick*. New York, New York: iUniverse, 2010:220, $14.00.

*59. Roberts WC. *Facts and Ideas from Anywhere, 2006-2010*. Dallas, Texas: Baylor Health Care System, 2011:212. ("From the Editor" columns published in the *Baylor University Medical Center Proceedings* in a 5-year period.)

William Clifford Roberts, MD
Editor in Chief
Baylor Heart and Vascular Institute
Dallas, Texas

Good Books in Cardiovascular Disease Appearing in 2011

Major Textbooks in Cardiovascular Surgery

*1. Cohn LH, editor. Cardiac Surgery in the Adult. Fourth Edition. New York: McGraw Hill 2012:1448, $299.00.

2. Franco KL, Thourani VH, editors. Cardiothoracic Surgery Review. Philadelphia: Wolters Kluwer|Wolters Kluwer|Lippincott Williams & Wilkins 2012:1770, $279.00.

Cardiac Imaging

3. Ho VB, Reddy GP, editors. Cardiovascular Imaging, Volumes I and II. Philadelphia: Elsevier Saunders 2011: 1729, $329.00.

4. Pahlm O, Wagner GS, editors. Multimodal Cardiovascular Imaging. Principles and Clinical Applications. New York: McGraw Hill Medical 2011:444, $149.00.

5. Koster NK, editor. Cardiovascular Imaging Review. Philadelphia: Elsevier Saunders 2011:171, $99.00.

6. Otto CM, Schwaegler RG, Freeman RV. Echocardiography Review Guide. Companion to the Textbook of Clinical Echocardiography. Second Edition. Philadelphia: Elsevier Saunders 2011:426, $109.00.

7. Silverman DI, Manning WJ. The Complete Guide to Echocardiography. Sudbury, Massachusetts: Jones & Bartlett Learning 2012:346, $94.95.

*8. Vegas A. Perioperative Two-Dimensional Transesophageal Echocardiography. A Practical Handbook. New York: Springer 2012:235, $59.95.

9. Perrino AC Jr, Reeves ST, Glas K, editors. Practice of Perioperatve Transesophageal Echocardiography: Essential Cases. Philadelphia: Wolters Kluwer|Lippincott Williams & Wilkins 2011:384, $132.95.

10. Halpern EJ, editor. Clinical Cardiac CT: Anatomy and Function. Second Edition. New York: Thieme 2011: 425, $149.95.

11. Iskandrian AE, Garcia EV, editors. Atlas of Nuclear Cardiology: Imaging Companion to Braunwald's Heart Disease. Philadelphia: Elsevier Saunders 2012:453, $179.00.

12. Rychik J, Tian Z, editors. Fetal Cardiovascular Imaging: A Disease-Based Approach. Philadelphia: Elsevier Saunders 2012:511, $149.00.

Arrhythmias and Conduction Disturbances

13. Ellenbogen KA, Kay GN, Lau CP, Wilkoff BL, editors. Clinical Cardiac Pacing, Defibrillation and Resynchronization Therapy. Fourth Edition. Philadelphia: Elsevier Saunders 2011:1085, $299.00.

*14. Friedman PA, Rott MA, Wokhlu A, Asirvatham SJ, Hayes DL. A Case-Based Approach to Pacemakers, ICDs, and Cardiac Resynchronization. Questions for Examination Review and Clinical Practice, Volumes I and II. Minneapolis: cardiotext 2011:442, $99.00.

15. Huang SKS, Wood MA, editors. Catheter Ablation of Cardiac Arrhythmias. Second Edition. Philadelphia: Elsevier Saunders 2011:650, $195.00.

16. Bredikis AJ, Wilber DJ, editors. Cryoblation of Cardiac Arrhythmias. Philadelphia: Elsevier Saunders 2011: 241, $149.00.

17. Wren C. Concise Guide to Pediatric Arrhythmias. Oxford: Wiley-Blackwell 2011:189, $64.95.

*18. Kowey PR, Mohmand-Borkowski A, Burke JF. Clinical Management of Atrial Fibrillation. West Islip, New York: Professional Communications 2011:400, $24.95.

19. Garcia MAB, Khairy P, Macle L, Nattel S, editors. Electrophysiology for Clinicians. Minneapolis: cardiotext 2011:254, $69.00.

20. Purves PD, Klein GJ, Leong-Sit P, Yee R, Skanes AC, Gula LJ, Krahn AD. Cardiac Electrophysiology: A Visual Guide for Nurses, Techs, and Fellows. Minneapolis: cardiotext 2011:139, $89.00.

21. Olshansky B, Chung MK, Pogwizd SM, Goldschlager N. Arrhythmia Essentials. Sudbury, Massachusetts: Jones & Bartlett Learning 2012:343, $34.95.

Miscellaneous

*22. Frishman WH, Sica DA, editors. Cardiovascular Pharmacotherapeutics. Third Edition. Minneapolis: cardiotext 2011:775, $199.00.

23. Nicols WW, O'Rourke MF, Vlachopoulos C, with a contribution from Hoeks AP, Reneman RS. McDonald's Blood Flow in Arteries: Theoretical, Experimental and Clinical Principles. Sixth Edition. London: Hodder Arnold 2011:755, $245.00.

*24. Tse HF, Lip GYH, Coats AJS, editors. Oxford Desk Reference: Cardiology. New York: Oxford University Press 2011:448, $149.50.

25. Ardehali R, Perez M, Wang P, editors. A Practical Approach to Cardiovascular Medicine. Chichester, UK: Wiley-Blackwell 2011:302, $69.95.

26. Ragosta M, editor. Cases in Interventional Cardiology. St. Louis: Elsevier Saunders 2011:335, $99.95.

27. Gatzoulis MA, Webb GD, Daubeney PEF, editors. Diagnosis and Management of Adult Congenital Heart Disease. Second Edition. Philadelphia: Elsevier Saunders 2011: 508, $195.00.

28. Mann DL, editor. Heart Failure. A Companion to Braunwald's Heart Disease. Second Edition. Philadelphia: Elsevier Saunders 2011:902, $174.00.

*29. Flynn JT, Ingelfinger JR, Portman RJ, editors. Pediatric Hypertension. Second Edition. New York: Humana Press (Springer Science) 2011:618, $239.00.

30. Davies MG, Lumsden AB, editors, Vykoukal D, assistant editor. Venous Thromboembolic Disease: Contem-

* Acid-free Paper.

porary Endovascular Management. Minneapolis: cardiotext 2011:242, $99.00.

31. Heywood JT, Burnett JC Jr, editors. The Cardiorenal Syndrome: A Clinician's Guide to Pathophysiology and Management. Minneapolis: cardiotext 2012:235, $89.00.

***32.** Jaff MR, White CJ, editors. Vascular Disease: Diagnostic and Therapeutic Approaches. Minneapolis: cardiotext 2011:582, $99.00.

33. Rajagopalan S, Dean SM, Mohler ER III, Mukherjee D, editors. Manual of Vascular Diseases. Second Edition. Philadelphia: Wolters Kluwer|Lippincott Williams & Wilkins 2012:626, $79.95.

34. Casserly IP, Sachar R, Yadav JS, editors. Practical Peripheral Vascular Intervention. Second Edition. Philadelphia: Wolters Kluwer|Lippincott Williams & Wilkins 2011: 466, $134.95.

35. Allan R, Fisher J, editors. Heart and Mind. The Practice of Cardiac Psychology. Second Edition. Washington, DC: American Psychological Association 2012:524, $39.95.

36. Byrne CD, Wild SH, editors. The Metabolic Syndrome. Second Edition. Chichester, UK: Wiley-Blackwell 2011:366, $116.95.

***37.** Codario RA. Type 2 Diabetes, Pre-Diabetes, and the Metabolic Syndrome. Second Edition. New York: Humana Press (Springer) 2011:367, $99.00.

38. Mancini M, Ordovas JM, Riccardi G, Rubba P, Strazzullo P, editors. Nutritional and Metabolic Bases of Cardiovascular Disease. Chichester, UK: Wiley-Blackwell 2011:463, $159.95.

***39.** Cohen IS, Gaudette GR, editor. Regenerating the Heart: Stem Cells and the Cardiovascular System. New York: Humana Press (Springer) 2011:556, $239.00.

40. Moorjani N, Viola N, Ohri SK, editors. Key Questions in Cardiac Surgery. Harley, UK: tfm Publishing 2011: 502, $99.00.

Cardiovascular History

***41.** Cooley DA. 100,000 Hearts: A Surgeon's Memoir. Austin: Dolph Briscoe Center for American History, The University of Texas at Austin 2012:267, $29.95.

42. Edwards BS, Moller JH, editors. Jesse E. Edwards: His Legacy to Cardiovascular Medicine. Stamford, CT: Science International Corp 2011:389, $85.00.

William Clifford Roberts, MD
Baylor Heart and Vascular Institute of
Baylor University Medical Center
Dallas, Texas

Good Books in Cardiovascular Disease Appearing in 2012 and Early 2013

Major Textbooks

1. Allen HD, Driscoll DJ, Shaddy RE, Feltes TF. *Moss and Adams' Heart Disease in Infants, Children, and Adolescents: Including the Fetus and Young Adults*. 8th ed. Volumes I & II. Philadelphia, Pennsylvania: Lippincott Williams & Wilkins, 2013:1683, $369.99.

*2. Murphy JG, Lloyd MA, editors-in-chief; Brady PA, Olson LJ, Shields RC, assoc eds. *Mayo Clinic Cardiology: Concise Textbook*. 4th ed. New York, New York: Oxford University Press, 2013:1091, $175.00.

Preventive Cardiology

3. Erdman JW Jr, Macdonald IA, Zeisel SH, eds. *Present Knowledge in Nutrition*. 10th ed. Ames, Iowa: Wiley-Blackwell, 2012:1305, $169.99.
4. Kontush A, Chapman MJ. *High-Density Lipoproteins: Structure, Metabolism, Function, and Therapeutics*. Hoboken, New Jersey: John Wiley & Sons, 2012:605, $141.00.
5. Pearson D, Grace C. *Weight Management: A Practitioner's Guide*. Chichester, United Kingdom: Wiley-Blackwell, 2012:278, $63.99.

*6. DeBakey ME, Gotto AM Jr. *The Living Heart in the 21st Century*. Amherst, New York: Prometheus Books, 2012:317, $20.00.

7. Piscatella JC, Piscatella B. *The Healthy Heart Cookbook: Over 650 Recipes for Every Day and Every Occasion*. New York, New York: Black Dog & Leventhal Publishers, 2013:448, $19.95.
8. Franklin B, Sweetgall R. *One Heart, Two Feet. Enhancing Heart Health, One Step at a Time*. Clayton, Missouri: Creative Walking, 2013:157, $13.00.

Electrocardiography and Electrophysiology

9. Das MK, Zipes DP. *Electrocardiography of Arrhythmias: A Comprehensive Review. A Companion to Cardiac Electrophysiology: From Cell to Bedside*. Philadelphia, Pennsylvania: Saunders, 2012:496, $84.95.
10. Podrid P, Malhotra R, Kakkar R, Noseworthy PA. *Podrid's Real-World ECGs: A Master's Approach to the Art and Practice of Clinical ECG Interpretation, Volume 1, The Basics*. Minneapolis, Minnesota: Cardiotext Publishing, 2013:402, $69.00.
11. Rimmerman CM. *Electrocardiography Review: A Case-Based Approach*. Philadelphia, Pennsylvania: Lippincott Williams & Wilkins, 2012:350, $81.99.
12. Ho SY, Ernst S. *Anatomy for Cardiac Electrophysiologists: A Practical Handbook*. Minneapolis, Minnesota: Cardiotext, 2012:264, $139.00.
13. Al-Ahmad A, Callans DJ, Hsia HH, Natale A, Oseroff O, Wang PJ, eds. *Hands-On Ablation: The Expert's Approach*. Minneapolis, Minnesota: Cardiotext, 2013:496, $229.00.

Echocardiography

14. Roldan CA, ed. *The Ultimate Echo Guide*. 2nd ed. Philadelphia, Pennsylvania: Lippincott Williams & Wilkins, 2012:368, $146.99.
15. Pai RG, Varadarajan P, Chandraratna PAN, Malik S, eds. *Echocardiography: A Case Studies Based Approach*. Burlington, Maine: Jones & Bartlett Learning, 2013:574, $179.00.
16. Kane GC, Oh JK. *Echocardiography: A Case-Based Review*. Philadelphia, Pennsylvania: Lippincott Williams & Wilkins, 2013:346, $164.99.
17. Rasalingam R, ed., MaKan M, Pérez JE, assoc. eds. *The Washington Manual of Echocardiography*. Philadelphia, Pennsylvania: Lippincott Williams & Wilkins, 2013:303, $76.99.
18. Lang RM, Shernan SK, Shirali GS, Mor-Avi V, eds. *Comprehensive Atlas of 3D Echocardiography*. Philadelphia, Pennsylvania: Lippincott Williams & Wilkins, 2013:382, $225.99.
19. Savage RM, Aronson S, eds. *Basic Perioperative Transesophageal Echocardiography: A Multimedia Review*. Philadelphia, Pennsylvania: Lippincott Williams & Wilkins, 2013:231, $125.99.

Nuclear Cardiology

20. Jaber WA, Cerqueira MD, eds. *Nuclear Cardiology Review: A Self-Assessment Tool*. Philadelphia, Pennsylvania: Lippincott Williams & Wilkins, 2013:183, $79.95.

Interventional Diagnosis and Percutaneous Cardiac Interventions

21. Carroll JD, Webb JG, eds. *Structured Heart Disease Interventions*. Philadelphia, Pennsylvania: Lippincott Williams & Wilkins, 2012:416, $183.99.
22. Moussa ID, Bailey SR, Colombo A, eds. *Complications of Interventional Cardiovascular Procedures. A Case-Based Atlas*. New York, New York: Demos Medical, 2012:344, $175.00.
23. Hanna EB, Glancy DL. *Practical Cardiovascular Hemodynamics. With Self-Assessment Problems*. New York, New York: Demos Medical, 2013:402, $85.00.

Manuscript received April 9, 2013; revised manuscript received and accepted April 9, 2013.

*24. Anwaruddin S, Martin JM, Stephen JC, Askari AT, eds. *Cardiovascular Hemodynamics: An Introductory Guide*. New York, New York: Humana Press, 2013:340, $159.00.
25. Nguyen T, Hu D, Chen SL, Kim M-H, Saito S, Grines C, Gibson CM, Bailey SR, eds. *Practical Handbook of Advanced Interventional Cardiology. Tips and Tricks*. 4th ed. Chichester, United Kingdom: Wiley-Blackwell, 2013:686, $99.95.
26. Cohen HA, ed. *Transradial Access. Techniques for Diagnostic Angiography and Percutaneous Intervention*. Minneapolis, Minnesota: Cardiotext, 2013:209, $89.00.

Cardiac Biomarkers

27. Maisel AS, ed. *Cardiac Biomarkers: Expert Advice for Clinicians*. New Delhi, India: Jaypee Brothers Medical Publishers, 2012:238, $40.00.

Systemic Hypertension

28. McFarlane SI, Bakris GL. *Diabetes and Hypertension: Evaluation and Management*. New York, New York: Humana Press, 2012:190, $149.00.
*29. Koch CA, Chrousos GP, eds. *Endocrine Hypertension. Underlying Mechanisms and Therapy*. New York, New York: Humana Press, 2013:317, $159.00.

Heart Failure

*30. Bakris GL, ed. *The Kidney in Heart Failure*. New York, New York: Springer, 2012:248, $159.00.
*31. Peacock WF, ed. *Short Stay Management of Acute Heart Failure*. 2nd ed. New York, New York: Humana Press, 2012:347, $189.00.
32. Piña IL, Madigan EA, eds. *Heart Failure: Strategies to Improve Outcomes*. Minneapolis, Minnesota: Cardiotext, 2013:144, $39.00.

Coronary Artery Disease

*33. Tomanek RJ. *Coronary Vasculature. Development, Structure-Function, and Adaptations*. New York, New York: Springer, 2013:276, $189.00.

Cardiomyopathy

34. Picken MM, Dogan A, Herrera GA, eds. *Amyloid and Related Disorders: Surgical Pathology and Clinical Correlations*. New York, New York: Humana Press, 2012:425, $219.00.

Congenital Heart Disease

35. Perloff JK, Marelli AJ. *Perloff's Clinical Recognition of Congenital Heart Disease*. 6th ed. Philadelphia, Pennsylvania: Saunders, 2012:559, $189.00.

Peripheral Vascular Disease

36. Mohler ER III, Litt HI, eds. *Atlas of Vascular Medicine: A Case-Based Approach to Current Management*. New York, New York: Demos Medical, 2012:216, $125.00.

Miscellaneous

*37. Patterson C, Willis MS, eds. *Translational Cardiology: Molecular Basis of Cardiac Metabolism, Cardiac Remodeling, Translational Therapies and Imaging Techniques*. New York, New York: Humana Press, 2012:543, $189.00.
*38. Homeister JW, Willis MS, eds. *Molecular and Translational Vascular Medicine*. New York, New York: Humana Press, 2012:335, $159.00.
39. Slovut DP, Dean SM, Jaff MR, Schneider PA, eds. *Comprehensive Review in Vascular and Endovascular Medicine*. Minneapolis, Minnesota: Cardiotext, 2012:355, $109.00.
40. Kumar D, ed. *Genomics and Health in the Developing World*. New York, New York: Oxford University Press, 2012:1501, $250.00.
41. Hollenberg S, Heitner S. *Cardiology in Family Practice: A Practical Guide*. 2nd ed. New York, New York: Humana Press, 2012:159, $49.95.
42. Elefteriades JA, Tribble C, Geha AS, Siegel MD, Cohen LS. *The House Officer's Guide to ICU Care. Fundamentals of Management of the Heart and Lungs*. 3rd ed. Minneapolis, Minnesota: Cardiotext, 2013:512, $49.95.
*43. Wong CJ, Hamlin NP, eds. *The Perioperative Medicine Consult Handbook*. New York, New York: Springer, 2013:283, $39.95.
44. Basso C, Valente M, Thiene G, eds. *Cardiac Tumor Pathology*. New York, New York: Humana Press, 2013:197, $149.00.
45. Griffin PB, ed., Callahan TD, Manon V, assoc. ed. *Manual of Cardiovascular Medicine*. 4th ed. Philadelphia, Pennsylvania: Lippincott Williams & Wilkins, 2013:1171, $99.99.
46. Eidem BW, Cannon BC, Chang AC, Cetta F. *Pediatric Cardiology Board Review*. Philadelphia, Pennsylvania: Lippincott Williams & Wilkins, 2013:251, $144.99.
*47. Supino PG, Borer JS, eds. *Principles of Research Methodology: A Guide for Clinical Investigators*. New York, New York: Springer, 2012:276, $149.00.

*Acid-free paper.

William Clifford Roberts, MD
Editor in Chief
Baylor Heart & Vascular Institute
Dallas, Texas

Good Books in Cardiovascular Disease Appearing in 2013 and Early 2014

Cardiology Textbooks

1. Chatterjee K, Anderson M, Heistad D, Kerber RE, editors. Cardiology: An Illustrated Textbook. New Delhi: Jaypee Brothers Medical Publishers 2013:2099 (Volumes 1 & 2), $231.00.
*2. Rosendorff C, editor. Essential Cardiology: Principles and Practice. Third Edition. New York: Springer 2013:823, $205.48.
3. Katritsis DG, Gersh BJ, Camm AJ. Clinical Cardiology: Current Practice Guidelines. Oxford: Oxford University Press 2013:737, $115.00.

The Chatterjee 2-volume book is the first major cardiologic textbook to appear in some time. It is fully packed (maximal content per page) and well illustrated. I see no need for the subtitle ("An Illustrated Textbook"). The Rosendorff book is in its third edition, less than half the length of the Chatterjee volumes, contains far fewer color illustrations, but nevertheless is "reasonably comprehensive." The Katritsis soft-cover book is a rather concise guide to most cardiovascular conditions with the most recent guidelines in a summarized tabulated format.

Heart Failure

4. Semigran MJ, Shin JT, editors. Heart Failure. Second Edition. Boca Raton: CRC Press 2013:487, $205.48.
*5. Morgan JA, Naka Y, editors. Surgical Treatment for Advanced Heart Failure. New York: Springer 2013:199, $189.00.

The Semigran-Shin book, a second edition of the one which appeared 5 years earlier, is comprehensive except for discussions of left and right ventricular assist devices and cardiac transplantation. The Morgan-Naka book fills in that void.

Congenital Heart Disease

6. Moodie DS, editor. Clinical Management of Congenital Heart Disease from Infancy to Adulthood. Minneapolis: cardiotext 2014:378, $129.00.
7. Richardson RR, editor. Atlas of Pediatric Cardiac CTA. Congenital Heart Disease. New York: Springer 2013:128, $139.00.

The Moodie, although shorter than many of the older textbooks on congenital heart disease, is well done and easily readable. The small (128 pages) Richardson book focuses entirely on cardiac computed tomographic angiography in congenital heart disease. The images are beautiful—many in color—but much space is wasted.

Electrocardiography and Electrophysiology

8. Wagner GS, Strauss DG. Marriott's Practical Electrocardiography. Twelfth Edition. Philadelphia: Wolters Kluwer|Lippincott Williams & Wilkins 2014:532, $99.99.
9. Podrid P, Malhotra R, Kakkar R, Noseworthy PA. Podrid's Real-World ECGs. Volume 3, Conduction Abnormalities 3: a Master's Approach to the Art and Practice of Clinical ECG Interpretation. Minneapolis: cardiotext 2013:481, $89.00.
10. Levine GN. Arrhythmias 101. The Ultimate Easy-to-Read Introductory Book to Arrhythmias. New Delhi: Jaypee Brothers Medical Publishers 2013:98, $36.00.
11. Abedin Z. Essential Cardiac Electrophysiology. The Self-Assessment Approach. Second Edition. Chichester, West Sussex, UK: Wiley-Blackwell 2013:511, $69.95.

The Wagner-Strauss book is the 12th edition started years ago by Henry J.L. Marriott. If one buys a single book on electrocardiography this is the one to purchase. The electrocardiograms are displayed as Marriott did originally—no wasted space—with the various complexes in black on pink-blocked paper. The Podrid book focuses entirely on conduction abnormalities. The 104-page Levine book displays the electrocardiograms in easy-to-read fashion but despite its attractive format much space is wasted. The Abedin second edition is a single-authored book which provides the basics of electrophysiology.

Echocardiography

12. Otto CM. Textbook of Clinical Echocardiography. Fifth Edition. Philadelphia: Elsevier Saunders 2013:552, $179.00.
13. Siegel RJ (Editor in Chief); Beigel R (Assistant Editor); Gurudevan SV, Shiota T, Tolstrup K, Wunderlich N, (Editors). Complex Cases in Echocardiography. Philadelphia: Wolters Kluwer|Lippincott Williams & Wilkins 2014:175, $149.99.
*14. Houghton AR. Making Sense of Echocardiography. A Hands-On Guide. Second Edition. Boca Raton: CRC Press 2013:328, $55.95.

The Otto book, now in its fifth edition, has become a classic. It is beautifully done. The Siegel book is new and contains 120 "complex" cases with more than 400 supplementary videos online and 295 questions and answers. The 10 cases in the latter portion provide numerous echocardiograms in pull-out format

*Printed on acid-free paper.

for each case. The Houghton book is primarily a primer for those learning echocardiography for the first time. Many of the images are a bit small.

Cardiac Catheterization

15. Moscucci M, editor. Grossman & Baim's Cardiac Catheterization, Angiography, and Intervention. Eighth Edition. Philadelphia: Wolters Kluwer|Lippincott Williams & Wilkins 2014:1141, $229.99.
16. Hanna EB, Glancy DL. Practical Cardiovascular Hemodynamics With Self-Assessment Problems. New York: demos Medical 2013:402, $85.00.

The classic Grossman & Baim's book, now edited by Moscucci, is now in its eighth edition and it remains the bible in this arena. It is a fully packed beautifully done book. The Hanna-Glancy book is a new one in this area. It provides in-depth understanding of hemodynamic wave forms and tracings in various cardiovascular conditions. The unique features are the individual case tracings in the latter half of the book and the detailed explanations provided for each tracing. This portion of the book is particularly instructive.

Miscellaneous

*17. Zygmunt J Jr, Pichot O, Dauplaise T. Practical Phlebology: Venous Ultrasound. Boca Raton: CRC Press 2013:170, $139.95.
*18. Comerota AJ. Practical Phlebology: Deep Vein Thrombosis. Boca Raton: CRC Press 2014:131, $95.95.
*19. Aronow WS, Fleg JL, Rich MW, editors. Tresch and Aronow's Cardiovascular Disease in the Elderly. Fifth Edition. Boca Raton: CRC Press 2014:786, $219.95.
*20. Luks AM, Glenny RW, Robertson HT. Introduction to Cardiopulmonary Exercise Testing. New York: Springer 2013:145, $49.95.
21. Jackson E. An Ageless Woman's Guide to Heart Health. Your Path to Lifelong Wellness. Ann Arbor, Michigan: Spry Publishing 2013:272, $15.95.
22. Brill JB. Blood Pressure Down. The 10-Step Plan to Lower Your Blood Pressure in 4 Weeks—Without Prescription Drugs. New York: Three Rivers Press 2013:338, $15.00.
*23. Silverman B, Adler S. Your Doctors' Manners Matter: Better Health Through Civility in the Doctor's Office and in the Hospital. Alpharetta, Georgia: Booklogix 2014:185, $10.95.
*24. Roberts CS. Selected Roberts Papers: Seven Generations of a Southern Lineage. Bloomington, Indiana: iUniverse 2013:542, $42.95.

The Tresch and Aronow's book is now in its fifth edition. The only thing I do not like about this book is the word "elderly" because some people reach that stage at age 50 and others at 80 have not reached that stage. Cardiology has become a specialty of the "elderly." Most heart attacks now are in this age group. The average age of aortic valve replacement at my institution, for example, for aortic stenosis is now 72 years. Thus, this book is a useful one. The Luks book is a pocket-sized one on cardiopulmonary exercise testing. The 2 phlebology books are small but instructive. The Jackson book is intended primarily for the non-physician but certainly physicians can learn from it. The pocket-sized Silverman-Adler is full of insightful observations and thoughtful suggestions by 2 physicians who have devoted their careers to patient care and promoting professionalism. Highly recommend. The Roberts (Charles Stewart) book provides biographical notes and reproductions of some publications and private papers of men in 7 generations in their paternal Roberts lineage. Three of the 7 were physicians or surgeons specializing in cardiovascular disease. Of course I like this book.

William Clifford Roberts, MD
Baylor Heart and Vascular Institute
Baylor University Medical Center
Dallas, Texas

Good Books in Cardiovascular Disease Received in 2014 and in Early 2015

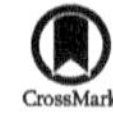

Major Textbooks

1. Mann DL, Zipes DP, Libby P, Bonow RO, editors. *Braunwald's HEART DISEASE: A Textbook of Cardiovascular Medicine*, Volumes 1 and 2, 10th edition. Philadelphia, Pennsylvania: Elsevier Saunders 2015:1943, $211.91.

This book of about 2,000 pages probably contains more information than any cardiovascular book ever published! Each page is fully packed, the illustrations are superb, the references are numerous but of small font such that they do not occupy a great deal of space. The 139 contributors of the 71 chapters are representative of the best of the cardiologic profession. It also includes a disclosure index and 54 pages for chapter listings. If there is one book to purchase in cardiology, this is the one. And it is kept up to date online by Eugene Braunwald himself. It may be more worthwhile each month to read this book than all the cardiologic journals put together. And the most recent guidelines follow each appropriate chapter.

Lipids

2. Ballantyne CM, editor. *Clinical Lipidology: A Companion to Braunwald's HEART DISEASE*, 2nd edition. Philadelphia, Pennsylvania: Elsevier Saunders 2015:550, $143.07.

This 550-page book with 99 contributors is an offshoot of Braunwald's Heart Disease. It too is packed full as is Braunwald's HEART DISEASE. Lipid therapy (statins, ezetimibe, etc.) is changing the face of atherosclerosis. Coronary events are decreasing and cardiac mortality is decreasing despite waist circumferences' increasing. Highly recommended.

Diabetes Mellitus

3. McGuire DK, Marx N, editors. *Diabetes in CARDIOVASCULAR DISEASE: A Companion to Braunwald's HEART DISEASE.* Philadelphia, Pennsylvania: Elsevier Saunders 2015:398, $179.55.

These editors have put together another of the Braunwald textbook offshoots with an up-to-date by 65 contributors. With caloric intake increasing and physical activity decreasing around the world, obesity has reached pandemic proportions and diabetes mellitus is one of the major consequences. These editors gather the best to produce 31 chapters connecting diabetes mellitus to cardiovascular disease.

Arrhythmias and Conduction Disturbances

4. *Asirvatham SJ, editor in chief; Cha Y-M, Friedman PA, associate editors. *Mayo Clinic Electrophysiology Manual.* New York, New York: Oxford University Press 2014:711, $175.28.
5. Huang SKS, Miller JM, editors. *Catheter Ablation of Cardiac Arrhythmias*, 3rd edition. Philadelphia, Pennsylvania: Elsevier Saunders 2015:775, $353.63.

The Huang-Miller book has the format of one of the Braunwald offshoot books but is not part of that series. The book is a third edition, the first one appearing in 2006. I suspect that this book represents the best in this arena and it is provided by 95 contributors. The Asirvatham book is of similar size but is not as eloquently prepared.

Systemic Hypertension

6. Kaplan NM, Victor RG. *Kaplan's Clinical Hypertension*, 11th edition. Philadelphia, Pennsylvania: Wolters Kluwer 2015:461, $94.99.
7. *Ram CVS. *Hypertension: A Clinical Guide.* Boca Raton, Florida: CRC Press 2014:136, $51.03.

The Kaplan book is the classic in this area. Not many books survive through 11 editions! Kaplan is one of the world's very best teachers on the topic of hypertension. The Ram book comes from the same institution, is much smaller, and far less complete.

Peripheral Vascular Disease

8. Zeller T, Cissarek T, Gray WA, Kröger K, editors; Wojciuk J, Assistant editor. *Vascular Medicine: Therapy and Practice*, 2nd edition. Stuttgart, Germany: Thieme 2014:520, $209.49.

This is a full textbook on peripheral vascular disease with 72 contributors. Which authors provided which chapters are difficult to determine.

Echocardiography

9. Eidem BW, O'Leary PW, Cetta F, editors. *Echocardiography in Pediatric and Adult Congenital Heart Disease*, 2nd edition. Philadelphia, Pennsylvania: Wolters Kluwer 2015:720, $261.24.

Manuscript received March 18, 2015; revised manuscript received and accepted March 18, 2015.

* Printed on acid-free paper.

10. Sorrell VL, Jayasuriya S, editors. *Questions Tricks and Tips for the ECHOCARDIOGRAHY BOARDS.* Philadelphia, Pennsylvania: Wolters Kluwer 2015:483, $94.99.

The Eidem-O'Leary-Cetta book represents a second edition, a statement that the first edition did very well. Echocardiography is so important for evaluation of patients with congenital heart disease it is now hard to consider what this specialty was like without this "instrument of precision." This book appears to be essential for those in this area.

The Sorrell-Jayasuriya book provides >700 questions and >350 videos. An interesting book. Some of the echocardiograms could have been cropped.

Cardiovascular Computed Tomography

11. Hutchison SJ, Merchant N. *Principles of Cardiac and Vascular Computed Tomography.* Philadelphia, Pennsylvania: Elsevier Saunders 2015:572, $79.55.

This book is loaded with nice illustrations and most chapters have videos available. There may be as many illustrations as words. Nice book!

Invasive Cardiology

12. Bertrand OF, Rao SY, editors. *Best Practices for Transradial Approach in Diagnostic Angiography and Intervention.* Philadelphia, Pennsylvania: Wolters Kluwer 2015:359, $132.99.

The transradial approach is becoming more and more popular. This detailed book shows how to do it well. The transradial approach to percutaneous coronary intervention varies a great deal worldwide, about 20% in the USA and 80% in China. Nice book!

Miscellanous

13. Maron BJ, Salbert L. *A Guide to Hypertrophic Cardiomyopathy for Patients, Their Families, and Interested Physicians*, 3rd edition. Oxford, UK: Wiley Blackwell 2014:140, $34.15.
14. Cuculich PS, Kates AM, editors. DeFer TM, series editor. *Cardiology Subspecialty Consult.* The Washington Manual Subspecialty Consult Series. 3rd edition. Philadelphia, Pennsylvania: Wolters Kluwer 2014:513, $74.50.
15. Rubboli A, Eeckhout E, Lip GYH, editors. *Percutaneous Coronary Intervention in the Patient on Oral Anticoagulation.* Oxford, UK: Oxford University Press 2014:75, $35.00.

The Maron-Salbert book is primarily for families with one or more members with hypertrophic cardiomyopathy (HC), a condition occurring in 1 in 500 people, a percent identical to that of homozygous familial hypercholesterolemia. Barry Maron is now the king of this condition, having devoted most of his professional life studying patients with HC. Lisa Salberg is one of several family members with HC so she is a magnificent voice for this condition from the patient standpoint. She founded the Hypertrophic Cardiomyopathy Association (HCMA), a patient advocacy organization devoted to this disease. This little book is filled with useful information on HC for both families and physicians.

The Rubboli-Eeckhout-Lip book is another white-coat pocket-sized reference on this topic.

Cardiovascular History

16. *Fye WB. *Caring for the Heart: Mayo Clinic and the Rise of Specialization.* Oxford, UK: Oxford University Press 2015:704, $37.95.
17. Winters WL Jr, with Parish B. *Houston Hearts: A History of Cardiovascular Surgery and Medicine and The Methodist DeBakey Heart and Vascular Center of Houston Methodist Hospital.* Houston, Texas: Elisha Freeman Publishing 2014:549, $27.97.

The Fye book records major developments in the diagnosis and treatment of heart disease in the 20th century, explains how the Mayo Clinic evolved from a family practice in Minnesota into one of the world's leading medical centers, and shows how the invention of new technologies and procedures promoted specialization among physicians and surgeons. Dr. Fye is the planets foremost medical historian and his scholarship shows through on every page. This book is far more than a Mayo Clinic history. It probably should be required reading for any cardiologist or cardiovascular surgeon.

The Winters-Parish book is also masterly done and describes how Houston and especially the Methodist Hospital and Dr. Michael E. DeBakey changed Houston from a family-practice center to one of the world's finest medical centers. It also shows the importance of physicians working smoothly with hospital administrators to produce an outstanding medical center.

Novels Written by Cardiologists

18. Kowey PR. *THE EMPTY NET: A Philip Sarkis Mystery.* Philadelphia, Pennsylvania: Pavilion Press 2014:351, $27.90.
19. Doroghazi RM. *The Alien's Secret.* Columbia, Missouri: Compass Flower Press 2014:454, $22.84.

The first cardiologist—electrophysiologist—to produce a couple of mystery novels was Dr. Douglas P. Zipes. Dr. Peter R. Kowey, another electrophysiologist, published *Deadly Rhythm* in 2012 and now just 2 years later comes *The Empty Net.* These are spellbinders. He is a superb storyteller.

Robert M. Doroghazi practiced cardiology for 25 years in Springfield, Missouri, and then became a financial advisor and author of a popular financial letter which I have subscribed to from its beginning. I was recently surprised to receive *The Alien's Secret*, his first novel. Doroghazi is a talented guy and has produced a suspenseful novel.

Comments

The first "Good Books in Cardiovascular Disease" was produced in 1983 and briefly discussed 80 books. Each year subsequently this column has appeared. The number of books received each year seems to be falling such that this column commented on only 19 books. Possibly, publishers are sending me fewer books. Writing provides a good record of our profession and specialty so I hope that authors will continue to write them and publishers will continue to publish them.

William C. Roberts, MD
Baylor Heart and Vascular Institute
Baylor University Medical Center
Dallas, Texas

Editorial Board Meetings

The AJC Editorial Board Meeting—1984

The Editorial Board of The American Journal of Cardiology meets once a year at the Annual Scientific Sessions of The American College of Cardiology. In addition to the gathering of about 75 of the 118 Editorial Board members, 25 manuscript reviewers who are not Board members also attended the March 1984 meeting. After introducing the publishing staff, the Editor discussed the following items:

1. *The number of manuscripts reviewed in 1983 by the 118 AJC Editorial Board members.* Ten members (9%) reviewed more than 10 manuscripts, 58 (48%) reviewed 6 to 10 manuscripts, and 50 (42%), 1 to 5 manuscripts. The editor, of course, is indebted to all manuscript reviewers, but special thanks were extended to the 10 persons who reviewed more than 10 manuscripts during the single year. The 10 were: C. Richard Conti, Michael M. Crawford, Jeffrey M. Isner, Barry J. Maron, Joel Morganroth, Carl J. Pepine, Joseph K. Perloff, Robert Roberts, Grace S. Wolff and Barry Zaret.

2. *Stylistic changes made in the Journal since the 1983 Board meeting.* These changes included centering of the article's title and authors on the title page (previously, each was "flush left"), and the insertion of the Journal's name, volume number, page numbers and year of publication as the final item in the article's abstract.

3. *Numbers of pages and articles, types of articles, numbers and titles of symposia, figures and tables published in the AJC in 1983 and comparison to those published in the 3 other major USA cardiologic journals and to those of 3 English-language foreign cardiologic journals.* These comparisons were published in the March 1, 1984, issue of the AJC and a reprint of that article was provided to those in attendance.[1]

4. *Awards for the 3 best Brief Reports in the AJC in 1983.* In January 1984 the editor asked Dr. Howard B. Burchell, former Editor of *Circulation*, if he would be willing to review the 81 Brief Reports published in the AJC in 1983 and pick, in his view, the 3 best ones. Dr. Burchell kindly agreed, and elsewhere in this issue his selections are described.[2] We will provide a certificate recognizing this award to each of the 7 authors of the 3 Brief Reports selected by Dr. Burchell. The publisher is providing a modest honorarium to Dr. Burchell for his considerable efforts.

5. *Relocating the editorial office to a new address in Bethesda.* The new office, which opened in March 1984, is nicer and more conveniently located than the previous office.

6. *Recent acquisition of a computer for the editorial office.* It is expected that the efficiency of manuscript processing will be improved by computerization.

7. *Revised "Instructions to Authors" page.* The revised Instructions, published in January 1984, are the second revision issued during the present editorship.

8. *Improved quality of paper for reprints of articles published in the AJC.* The quality of the paper for reprints was upgraded in July 1983.

9. *Best utilization of the space occasionally available on the last page of original articles.* About a year ago, quotations were occasionally inserted into that space. The editor is now considering its utilization for book reviews, and brief vignettes on cardiologic topics.

10. *A suggested new logo for the AJC.* Few physicians currently recognize the present AJC logo and a more simple one was suggested by the editor.

11. *Reduced subscription rate to AJC to medical students, house officers and cardiology and cardiovascular surgery fellows.* The wording on the subscription card implies that the rate for medical students, house officers and fellows is for 1 year only, when in fact that reduced rate is effective for the entire time the subscriber is in one of these positions. In mid-1984, the subscription card will be rephrased to clarify the ambiguous wording.

12. *Questions and comments.* The meeting was then opened for discussion of any item concerning the AJC by any board or non–Board member in attendance. The following questions were asked from the floor:

How does the editor handle manuscripts with split rec-

ommendations, one advising acceptance and the second advising rejection? About 85% of manuscripts submitted to the AJC are sent to 2 reviewers. Often, 1 reviewer recommends acceptance and the second, rejection. The split decision is the most frequent occurrence, considerably more common than either 2 recommendations of acceptance or 2 of rejection. After thorough personal study of the manuscript and of each review, with consideration of the relative expertise and stature of each of the 2 reviewers, the editor usually "bites the bullet" and makes a decision on the manuscript of tentative acceptance (with revision) or rejection. The editor tries not to resort to a third reviewer when the first 2 reviewers had opposing recommendations. To seek a third reviewer starts the review process all over again and delays the final decision on the manuscript by several weeks. When, however, the editor feels uncomfortable with the subject matter of the manuscript, finds neither reviewers' comments convincing, or is unable to arrive at an independent decision that he feels comfortable with, a third review is sought.

On the review form there are 2 categories of acceptance and 2 of rejection: "definitely accept" and "probably accept" and "definitely reject" and "probably reject." When a "definitely reject" is counterbalanced by a "definitely accept," the decision may be particularly difficult. The most common circumstance is a "probably accept" recommendation from 1 reviewer and a "probably reject" recommendation from the other. Only a rare manuscript gets 2 "definitely accept" recommendations. Its occurrence is so unusual that the editor usually indicates its occurrence to the submitting author. Few manuscripts receive 2 recommendations of "definitely reject," probably because about 15% of submitted manuscripts are rejected outright by the editor. Even more helpful to the editor than an "acceptance" or "rejection" recommendation are the reviewers' comments about the manuscript. The editor is surprised periodically by seeing extremely negative reviewers' comments with an "acceptance" recommendation, or the reverse, positive comments with a "rejection" recommendation.

Why do some manuscripts appear to receive only 1 review? A single review of a manuscript is unusual. Occasionally, only 1 review is sought with a Brief Report but 2 reviews are sought for all original investigations. The major reason a manuscript appears to receive only 1 review is that the editor generally makes a decision on a manuscript after 6 weeks even if only 1 of the 2 reviews has been received. When the late review is received it is then forwarded to the author. The editor believes it is unfair to authors to retain their manuscripts for 6 to 8 weeks or longer. The editor has been pleased that the decisions on manuscripts made on the basis of only 1 review—and this is an unusual circumstance—generally is in agreement with the recommendation or comments of the tardy reviewer.

This question allowed the editor to emphasize the importance of prompt reviewing. The period allowed for review of a manuscript is 3 weeks. However, the number "3" needs explanation. It is the total period from the day the manuscript leaves the editorial office to the day it arrives back. The mails being what they are, this generally means a week for transport of the manuscript to the reviewer and another week for transport from the reviewer back to the editorial office. Thus, the reviewer really has only about 1 week in which to review the manuscript. The editor suggests that the manuscript be briefly examined by the reviewer the day it is received. This brief initial examination might allow the reviewer to have a few days to contemplate the manuscript's subject before actually preparing the review. Also, if a colleague happens to be an expert on the subject of the manuscript, the colleague's opinion can be sought early rather than late.

The most annoying feature of 1 late review is that it is generally translated into 2 late reviews. If 1 review is returned in 3 weeks, and the second in 6 weeks, the promptness of the prompt reviewer is neutralized by the lateness of the late reviewer. Thus, any 1 late review means, for practical purposes, 2 late reviews.

How much editing is expected by a reviewer when reviewing a manuscript written by one whose native language is not English? Very little is expected. The opinion sought of the reviewer is primarily that of scientific merit. Of course, any suggestions to shorten the manuscript or means to present data in a more understandable way is much appreciated.

Why was the percent of experimental articles, i.e., those concerning nonhuman subjects, published in the AJC in 1983 relatively small? In 1983, 8% of the articles published in the AJC were of experimental studies. In contrast, this percent in *Circulation* was 24, in the *Journal of the American College of Cardiology* (JACC) 14, and in the *American Heart Journal* (AHJ), 12. These percentages, however, provide an incomplete picture of the data. The absolute number of actual experimental articles published is more meaningful. Although only 8% of the articles published in the AJC in 1983 were experimental, because the total number of articles published was large—643—the number of experimental articles also was relatively large—52, more than the 48 in JACC and the 47 in AHJ because the total number of articles published in those 2 journals was much smaller than in the AJC.

Although publication of experimental studies has a place in a clinical cardiology journal, I do not want them to represent more than 10% of the total. Furthermore, the experimental articles in general are the longest ones submitted, probably because the review process for the experimental articles is more strenuous than that for the clinical articles. The authors of the experimental articles are often "covering their flanks" for any possible criticism from reviewers. The editor is eager to decrease the length of most experimental studies, either before or after the reviewing process.

Why the 3 half-size extra regular issues (January 15, March 15 and May 15) rather than making the first issue of each of these 3 months much larger? The editor asked the publisher to respond to this question. Robert Brawn responded that there is a publishing principle that an issue that is too large produces reader fatigue and the increased content is lost. At some point, increased content requires the publication of 1 or more additional issues. Although not discussed, the additional issues provide increased exposure of the *Journal*, which may translate into increased subscribers and advertisers.

Does the editor plan on selecting 1 or more Associate or Assistant Editors? The editor responded by stating that he is fearful of diffusing the responsibility of his position, at least in the relatively early stages of his editorship. Some editors have selected 4 associate editors and then apportioned responsibility for the manuscript processing and selection relatively equally among the 5 of them. Personally, I have never been particularly pleased as an author when having to deal on a particular manuscript with an associate editor rather than the editor himself/herself. When the editor's responsibility is spread out among a group, no 1 person then has complete familiarity with all the manuscripts. I like communicating with all the authors. I personally take responsibility for the care of their manuscript. In 1 cardiology journal, an assistant editor selects reviewers for all the manuscripts—sometimes by phone with the managing editor—and the editor does not see a manuscript until it is back from reviewers. This procedure also prevents any immediate rejection or acceptance decision on a manuscript. The selection of reviewers is a major decision on any manuscript because that selection may well determine a manuscript's fate. This selection therefore should be the responsibility of the editor.

I would like to have an assistant or associate editor for the purpose of running the entire operation when I am away for 1 or 2 weeks. At the moment, it is virtually impossible to be gone for more than 2 or 3 days at any time. Thus, eventually, an associate editor will be selected. This selection also will comfort the publisher in case of an unexpected absence on the editor's part. With such a short lag time (average 3.5 months from acceptance to publication) in the AJC, any relatively short absence in the editor's office could disrupt the publishing process.

What percent of articles received had already been submitted to another journal or subsequently published elsewhere? Of course, the editor has no way of knowing the answer to the first part of this question. The editor has seen a number of articles rejected in the AJC appear in other prominent journals.

This question raises another issue, namely that of an author's attempting to hide the fact that his/her manuscript has been rejected by another journal. This fact does not bother me. Actually, I would welcome receiving the reviews from the Jounal that previously had rejected the manuscript now being submitted to the AJC. In this way, a rereview process might not be necessary, depending on the extent that the authors revised their manuscript or rebutted the criticisms of the previous reviewers. I am certain that some manuscripts receive numerous reviews and that this excessive reviewing simply saturates the system and may decrease time available for reviewing of previously unreviewed manuscripts.

Thus, it is the poorer manuscripts that receive the most reviews, a situation that diminishes the time available for reviewers to provide suggestions to improve the manuscripts of initial high quality.

When further questions were not forthcoming, the meeting was adjourned to a reception provided by the publisher.

William C. Roberts, MD
Editor-in-Chief

References

1. **Roberts WC.** Comparison of 7 English-language cardiology journals for 1983. Am J Cardiol 1984;53:862–869.
2. **Burchell HB.** The "best" (?) three brief reports in *The American Journal of Cardiology*—1983. Am J Cardiol 1984;53: 1453–1454.

The AJC Editorial Board Meeting—1985

The Editorial Board of *The American Journal of Cardiology* meets once a year, at the Annual Scientific Sessions of the American College of Cardiology. In addition to the gathering of about 75 of the 127 board members, about 25 non-Board members but frequent manuscript reviewers also attended the March 12, 1985, meeting. After introducing the publishing staff and the 2 Associate Editors, the following items were discussed:

1. *Names of board members reviewing the most manuscripts in 1984.* The top AJC manuscript reviewer in 1984 was Joel Morganroth, who reviewed 12 manuscripts, all within the allotted time period (3 weeks from the time the manuscript leaves the editorial office until it is returned). Barry J. Maron and David J. Sahn each reviewed 11 manuscripts. Each of 6 board members reviewed 9 manuscripts: Jon Abrams, C. Richard Conti, Robert DeBusk, Robert J. Myerburg, Nathaniel Reichek and David H. Spodick. Each of 8 board members reviewed 8 manuscripts: Michael H. Crawford, Stephen E. Epstein, William Ganz, Fredrick A. Heupler, Jr, L. David Hillis, Robert A. O'Rourke, Joseph K. Perloff, and Melvin M. Scheinman. Seven manuscripts were reviewed by each of 19 board members and of the 19, seven reviewed each manuscript within the allotted time period: Agustin Castellanos, George A. Diamond, Robert L. Feldman, Abdulmassih S. Iskandrian, Navin Nanda, Norman Silverman and Andrew G. Wallace. The remaining 91 Board members (72% of the board) reviewed 6 or fewer manuscripts for the AJC in 1984. The Editor is enormously appreciative of the unselfish efforts extended by the manuscript reviewers on behalf of the AJC. The Editor also is aware that the AJC is not the only journal for which board members review manuscripts.

2. *Names of non-Board members reviewing the most manuscripts for the AJC in 1984.* Although the AJC editorial board numbers 127 members, an additional nearly 1,110 scientists reviewed manuscripts for the AJC in 1984. The non-Board physician reviewing the most manuscripts for the AJC in 1984 was Lowell W. Perry, with 8 manuscripts. Tied for second were Joseph Alpert and Alfred E. Buxton, each with 7. Ten non-Board members each reviewed 6 manuscripts: Bruce S. Alpert, James E. Lock, G. B. John Mancini, Richard S. Meltzer, Eric L. Michelson, Philip J. Podrid, Philip R. Reid, Robert Slutsky, Bruce F. Waller and Hein J. Wellens. Five manuscripts were reviewed by Ernest Craige, Richard S. Crampton, Antonio DeLeon, Nicholas L. DePace, James E. Doherty, Arthur Garson, Adolph M. Hutter, George J. Klein, Martin J. Lipton, Fred Morady, Philip Samet, and Harvey L. Waxman. The Editor extends his sincere thanks to these non-Board reviewers who, at least to this point, have received no recognition for their efforts in behalf of the AJC.

3. *Analysis of the numbers of editorial (non-advertising) pages and of types of articles published in the AJC in 1984.* In the 15 regular issues in 1984, a total of 3,403 editorial pages were published, and 3,077 were used for the 747 articles. An average of 256 article pages and 62 articles were published each month in the AJC in 1984.

4. *Analysis of the numbers of Brief Reports published in the AJC in 1984.* This item was summarized in the March 1, 1985, From-the-Editor column in the AJC. Two hundred four Brief Reports were published in 1984. These constituted 27% of the 747 articles and 10% (308 pages) of the 3,077 pages used for articles.

5. *Comparison of numbers of articles and pages published in the AJC in 1958, its first year of publication; in 1982, the last year of the previous editorship; and in 1983 and 1984, the first 2 years in which all articles were se-*

TABLE I ***American Journal of Cardiology***

Year	No. of Articles	No. of Pages	Average Pages/ Article	Subscription Cost
1958	117	778	6.6	$12.00
1982	389	3,332	7.6	$50.00
1983	643	3,471	4.9	$52.00
1984	747	3,403	4.1	$55.00

TABLE II **Changes in the 4 Major USA Cardiologic Journals, 1983 Compared with 1984**

	1983	1984	Change
AJC			
Pages for articles	3,130	3,077	−2%
No. of articles	643	747	+14%
AHJ			
Pages for articles	2,096	2,392	+12%
No. of articles	392	466	+16%
Circulation			
Pages for articles	2,793	2,252	−19%
No. of articles	362	294	−19%
JACC			
Pages for articles	2,569	2,682	+4%
No. of articles	337	371	+9%

TABLE III Symposia Published in *The American Journal of Cardiology* in 1984

No.	Date	Subject of Symposium	Guest Editor(s)	No. of Articles	No. of Pages (Articles)	Industry Sponsor
1	January 27	Systemic hypertension	Norman M. Kaplan	14	64 (58)	Pfizer
2	February 27	Flecainide acetate	J. Thomas Bigger	24		
3	June 15	Percutaneous transluminal coronary angioplasty	Kenneth M. Kent Suzanne M. Mullin Eugene R. Passamani	35	167 (146)	0
4	June 25	Metoprolol for AMI	Ake Hjalmarson	9	56 (50)	AB Hasle
5	July 30	Bretylium	Lon Castle	6	40 (46)	Am Critical Care
6	August 13	Lorcainide	John C. Somberg	9	64 (54)	Janssen
7	August 27	Cholestyramine	Robert I. Levy	8	56 (41)	Mead Johnson
8	November 14	Propafenone	Douglas P. Zipes	12	80 (73)	Knoll
9	December 21	Early intervention in AMI	Charles E. Rackley	9	40 (31)	CIBA-GEIGY

lected by the present editor. These items are summarized in Table I.

6. *Analysis of the numbers of pages and types of articles* published in the *American Heart Journal* (AHJ), *Circulation* and the *Journal of the American College of Cardiology* (JACC) *in 1984 in comparison to the AJC.*

7. *Changes in the numbers of editorial pages and numbers of articles published* in the AJC, the AHJ, *Circulation* and the JACC *in 1984 compared to 1983.* These items are summarized in Table II.

8. *Symposia published in the AJC in 1984.* The subject matter, names of guest editors, numbers of editorial pages, and numbers of articles in each of the 9 symposia are summarized in Table II. Eight symposia were underwritten by industry.

9. *Review of stylistic changes having occurred in the AJC in the past 34 months and review of new stylistic changes proposed by the publisher for the AJC.* This item occupied about 1 hour of discussion, and centered on whether or not additional stylistic changes were useful and, if so, what form they should take. The answers have not been fully resolved. The lengthy discussion on this item prevented the free-for-all question and answer period that has generally characterized the AJC Editorial Board meetings in the past.

After nearly 90 minutes of discussion, the meeting was adjourned to a reception provided by the publisher.

William C. Roberts

William C. Roberts, MD
Editor in Chief

AJC Editorial Board Meeting—1986

Most medical journals have an editorial board meeting each year. The AJC is no exception. Its meeting is held each year at the time of the Annual Scientific Sessions of the American College of Cardiology. The editorial board meeting has 4 purposes: (1) to say "thanks" to the board members for their contributions to the *Journal*, primarily their reviews of manuscripts; (2) to inform the board members on happenings with the *Journal* the previous year; (3) to inform board members of plans for the *Journal* for the present year; and (4) to seek advice from and answer questions raised by board members.

The first half of the 1986 meeting was used by the editor to summarize happenings in the *Journal* in 1985 and to outline projected happenings in 1986. The second half of the meeting was a question-and-answer session between the editor and board members. The following items were discussed:

(1) *Numbers of manuscripts received:* In 1985, 1,735 manuscripts were received. Of this number, 1,000 were received by 22 July 1985. From 18 July 1985 until 1 October 1985 all submitted manuscripts were returned to authors because of a reduction in number of editorial pages from 1 August 1985 until 31 December 1985.

(2) *Numbers of manuscripts reviewed by all AJC board members in 1985:* Of the 1,732 manuscripts received, 587 (34%) were sent to 1 or more AJC board members for review and the other manuscripts were reviewed by non-board members. Of these 587 manuscripts, 499 (85%) were full-length reports and 88 (15%) were brief reports. Of the 587 manuscripts sent to board members, the reviews were returned to the editorial office within the allotted time (≤3 weeks) for 385 manuscripts (66%) and outside the allotted time for 173 manuscripts (29%); 29 manuscripts (5%) were returned not reviewed (out of town, etc.).

(3) *Numbers of manuscripts received for review by each AJC board member in 1985:* The numbers of manuscripts sent to board members are summarized in Figure 1 and ranged from no manuscripts (3 members) to 11 manuscripts (1 member). The average number of manuscripts received for review by the 131 AJC board members in 1985 was 4.5.

(4) *AJC board members receiving the most manuscripts in 1985 for review: Barry J. Maron* received 11 manuscripts (7). (The number in parentheses represents the number of full-length reports and the difference between the number in parentheses and the first number mentioned represents the number of brief reports received.) Ten manuscripts were received for review by *Agustin Castellanos* (7), *Lowell W. Perry* (4) and *Melvin M. Scheinman* (8). Of these 41 manuscripts received by these 4 super reviewers, the reviews in 37 (90%) were returned to the editor within the allotted time, and only 2 (5%) were returned non-reviewed. Each of 5 board members reviewed 9 manuscripts: *Robert L. Feldman* (8), *Frank I. Marcus* (6), *Carl J. Pepine* (7), *Nathaniel Reichek* (7) and *Allan M. Ross* (5). Each of 8 board members received 8 manuscripts and only 1 of the 64 was returned non-reviewed: *D. Woodrow Benson, Jr.* (5), *Robert O. Bonow* (8), *Alfred E. Buxton* (7), *Brian G. Firth* (7), *L. David Hillis* (8), *Leonard N. Horowitz* (8), *Navin C. Nanda* (5), and *David H. Spodick* (8). Each of 10 board members received 7 manuscripts and only 1 of the 70 manuscripts was returned non-reviewed: *Joseph A. Franciosa* (7), *Lawrence D. German* (7), *Jeffrey M. Isner* (4), *Mark E. Josephson* (7), *John A. Kastor* (7), *Kenneth M. Kent* (6), *Joel Morganroth* (7), *Randolph Patterson* (7), *Phillip J. Podrid* (6) and *Ralph Shabetai* (7).

(5) *Top reviewers among non-board members:* Over two-thirds of manuscripts received in 1985 were sent to 1 or

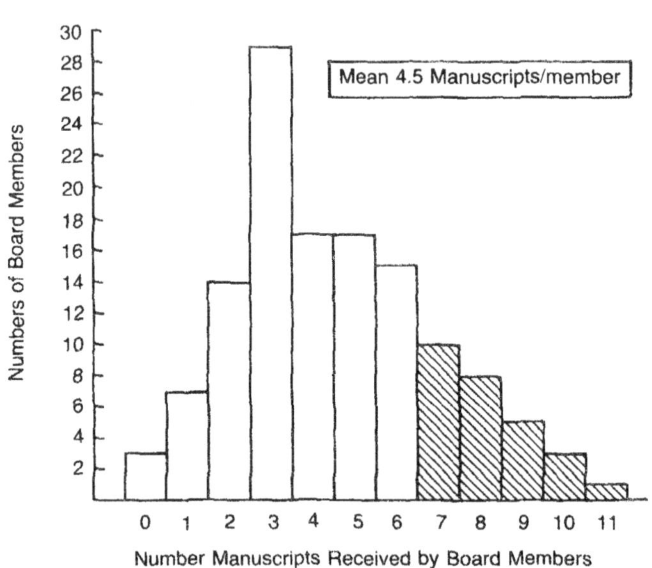

more of 1,200 investigators who are not AJC board members but who serve as manuscript reviewers for the AJC. The top non-board reviewers in 1985 were: *Jai Agarwal* (3), *Wilbert S. Aronow* (7) and *Pamela S. Douglas* (2). Each of these 3 physicians reviewed 7 manuscripts, each of the 21 manuscripts was reviewed within the allotted time, and none was returned non-reviewed. Each of 10 non-board members reviewed 6 manuscripts, none was returned non-reviewed, and only 6 (10%) of the 60 manuscripts were returned outside the allotted time: *William F. Armstrong* (3), *Robert A. Bauernfeind* (4), *Ernest Craige* (6), *Gregory J. Dehmer* (5), *Nicholas L. DePace* (3), *Ha Dinh* (4), *Toby R. Engel* (5), *William H. Gaasch* (5), *Arthur Labovitz* (5) and *David C. Levin* (2).

(6) *Number and types of manuscripts published:* In 1985, 645 articles, an average of 54 each month, were published in the 16 regular issues of the AJC. Of this number, 432 (67%) were full-length reports, 172 (27%) were brief reports, 16 (2%) were editorials, and 25 (4%) were From-the-Editor and The-AJC-25-Years Ago columns.

(7) *Letters to the editor:* Forty Letters to the Editor, 16 with replies, occupying 21 pages, were published in 1985. In contrast, 80 letters, 38 with replies, occupying 36 pages, were published in 1984. Whenever a letter is accepted it is sent immediately to the managing editor in the publisher's office. The understanding is that letters are prepared for printing and set in galley form quickly so that when pages are available they can be filled in their entirety with already prepared letters. It is the editor's desire to shorten the lag time for letters to the same as that for manuscripts, which for presently submitted manuscripts averages 4.5 months. Lag time is the interval between acceptance of a manuscript or letter and its publication.

(8) *Budgeted and used pages for articles:* In 1985, 3,172 editorial (non-advertising) pages for articles were budgeted. During the first 6 months, 1,636 editorial pages were published, 50 pages (3%) over budget. During the last 6 months, 987 editorial pages were published, or 778 pages (38%) below budget. For all of 1985, 2,623 editorial pages were published in the 16 regular issues of the *Journal*.

(9) *Budgeted pages for articles for 1986:* For the 16 regular issues in 1986, 2,694 pages are budgeted: 1,350 pages for the first half of the year and 1,344 pages for the second half. It is likely, however, that the actual number of pages published in 1986 will exceed the budgeted number.

(10) *Symposia published in 1985:* Fifteen symposia, all sponsored by pharmaceutical companies, were published in 1985. These are listed in the March 1, 1986, From-the-Editor column. Including the June 1, 1985, index issue which included abstracts of all full-length articles in the January-June 1985 AJC, 31 separate issues of the AJC appeared in 1985. Readership surveys have indicated that the symposium issues are popular with the readers. In contrast to the 15 symposia published in 1985, 9 symposia were published in 1984 and 5 in 1983.

(11) *Format changes in 1985:* The editorial-board page and contents-in-brief pages were changed to a 3-column format and contents-with-abstracts pages to a 1-column format. Additionally, the type style used throughout all editorial pages was changed in 1985. The type used for references is now smaller than that used previously. The type changes were necessitated by a change in the printing process.

(12) *Format changes in 1986:* Change to a 3-column format for all full-length and brief articles is still under consideration. The 3-column format allows greater flexibility with figures and tables, although it does not increase the numbers of words per page compared to the present 2-column format. The *Journal* cover likely will undergo change also.

(13) *Desire to simplify the AJC logo:* The possibility of designing a new, understandable logo was raised again.

After the above items were discussed by the editor, the floor was opened to questions and comments. The following issues were raised:

(1) *Copy editing:* One board member believed that manuscripts accepted for publication in the *Journal* received too much copy editing. The editor does not see manuscripts (except his own) after they have been copy edited. Thus, it is necessary for an author to call the editor's attention to changes considered inappropriate by authors. The editor often makes editorial changes in manuscripts, but these changes are made before the manuscript is returned to an author for revision. In this way the author has the option to disagree with the editor and disallow the editor's change. Any changes made in a revised manuscript by the editor are so described in the editor's acceptance letter to the author. Copy editing of medical manuscripts will be the subject of a separate piece in the future.

(2) *Guidelines for guest editors of supplements:* This idea was proposed by Dr. Donald C. Harrison and was well received by board members and the editor. This proposal is particularly timely because of the large number of symposia being published yearly. These guidelines will be developed and shared with the readership.

(3) *Second monthly regular issues of the AJC:* Beginning in 1983, in addition to the large regular issues dated the first day of each month, smaller regular issues dated the 15th of the month began appearing. Three such issues appeared in 1983 and in 1984, and in 1985 four such issues appeared (February 15, April 15, September 15 and November 15). These smaller regular issues have averaged about 100 editorial pages and the larger regular issues, about 210 editorial pages. A board member questioned the usefulness of the smaller regular issues and expressed the view that he wished his own manuscripts be published in the first-of-the-month

large regular issue and not the smaller ones. I did not get the feeling that this viewpoint was unanimous with the board. These smaller issues help to keep the lag time relatively short. The alternative, of course, is to make each of the first of the month regular issues larger. This decision is the publisher's.

(4) *Brief reports:* Several board members apparently believe that too many brief reports are published in the *Journal* and other board members have directly opposing viewpoints. I like the brief reports and hear many favorable comments on them. As outlined in the February 1, 1986, From-the-Editor column, only 54% of the brief reports in 1985 were single case studies and I suspect that the percent that will be single case studies in 1986 will be even smaller.

(5) *Experimental type manuscripts:* Several months ago the editor began declining all full-length experimental-type manuscripts, i.e., those dealing with nonhuman subjects, in order to reduce the lag time from the present average of 4.5 to 3.5 months, and to better manage the huge increase in number of manuscripts submitted in view of the decrease in numbers of editorial pages available. This decision was not an easy one, but since the experimental-type manuscripts tend to be the longest and probably the least read, this decision appeared appropriate. This decision will be reevaluated in several months.

Views of readers on items discussed in this piece or other matters are welcomed by the editor.

William C. Roberts

William C. Roberts, MD
Editor in Chief

Annual AJC Editorial Board Meeting—March 1987

This year's AJC board meeting was held March 10, 1987, in New Orleans, Louisiana, at the time of the Annual Scientific Sessions of the American College of Cardiology. The meeting began by introducing Paul J. Carnese, Publisher of the Yorke Medical Group, who announced that Cahners Publishing Company was now the owner of Technical Publishing Company. The purchase was made in late 1986. Cahners Publishing Company publishes over 50 magazines now, including the Yorke Medical Group, comprising *The American Journal of Cardiology*, *The American Journal of Medicine*, *The American Journal of Surgery* and *Cutis*. Its other medical publication is *Emergency Medicine*. Paul introduced Carroll V. Dowden, Group Vice President of Cahners Publishing Company, and he emphasized how pleased Cahners was in having acquired the Yorke Medical Group and that Cahners would strongly support its editorial endeavors. I had spent several hours with Carroll Dowden, Paul Carnese and Kenton T. Finch, publisher of the Yorke Symposia, earlier in the day, and I came away from the discussions enormously pleased with the new owner and convinced that Cahners has every intent to support strongly the editorial endeavors of the AJC.

The remainder of the first half of the 1-hour meeting was used by the editor to summarize happenings in the *Journal* in 1986, and the second half was a question-and-answer session between editor and board members. The following items were discussed:

(1) *Number of manuscripts reviewed by all AJC board members in 1986:* Of the 1,598 manuscripts received in 1986, 664 (42%) were sent to 1 or more board members for review and the other manuscripts were reviewed by non-board members. Of these 664 manuscripts, 591 (89%) were full-length reports and 73 (11%) were brief reports. Of the 664 manuscripts sent to board members, the reviews were returned to the editorial office within the allotted time (≤3 weeks) for 521 manuscripts (78%) and outside the allotted time for 143 manuscripts (22%); 39 manuscripts (6%) were returned not reviewed (out of town, etc.)

(2) *Numbers of manuscripts received for review by each AJC board member in 1986:* The numbers of manuscripts sent to board members are summarized in Figure 1 and ranged from no manuscripts (3 members) to 11 manuscripts (3 members). The average number of manuscripts received for review by the 130 AJC board members in 1986 was 5.1.

(3) *AJC board members reviewing the most manuscripts in 1986: Carl J. Pepine* (11) and *Lowell W. Perry* (8) each reviewed 11 manuscripts. (The number in parentheses represents the number of full-length reports and the difference between the number in parentheses and the first number mentioned represents the number of brief reports reviewed). Ten manuscripts were reviewed by *Joseph Alpert* (10) and *Robert L. Feldman* (6). Of the 42 manuscripts reviewed by these 4 superb reviewers, only 1 was returned late (>3 weeks). Each of 5 board members reviewed 9 manuscripts: *Robert Bonow (8), Leonard N. Horowitz (9), Jeffrey M. Isner (7), Kenneth M. Kent (4) and Navin C. Nanda (6)*. Each of 10 board members reviewed 8 manuscripts: *George A. Beller* (8), *Alfred E. Buxton* (8), *Agustin Castellanos* (7), *C. Richard Conti* (8), *Michael H. Crawford* (8), *Edward D. Freis* (7), *L. David Hillis* (7), *Joel Morganroth* (8), *David H. Spodick* (6), and *James T. Willerson* (8). Of the 80 manuscripts reviewed by these last 10 board members, 75 were full-length reports and 77 (96%) of the 80 were returned within the allotted time period. Each of 10 board members reviewed 7 manuscripts: *Brian G. Firth* (7), *Bernard J. Gersh* (7), *John A Kastor* (7), *Joseph Lindsay, Jr.* (5), *Jawahar Mehta* (6), *Robert J. Myerburg* (7), *Philip J. Podrid* (7), *Nathaniel Reichek* (7), *Allan M. Ross* (7) and *Melvin M. Scheinman* (7). Of the 70 manuscripts reviewed by these 10 board members, 67 were full-length reports and 63 (90%) of the 70 were reviewed within the allotted time period.

(4) *Top reviewers among non-board members:* Over two-thirds of manuscripts received in 1986 were sent to 1 or more of nearly 1,300 investigators who are not AJC board members but who serve as manuscript reviewers for the AJC. Each of 5 non-board members reviewed 8 manuscripts for the AJC in 1986: *Abdul S. Abbasi* (5), *Jeffrey Anderson* (8), *Pamela S. Douglas* (7), *Julius M. Gardin* (6) and *Morris N. Kotler* (7). Of the 40 manuscripts reviewed by these superb reviewers, 36 (90%) reviews were returned within the allotted time period. Each of 3 non-board members reviewed 7 manuscripts for the AJC in 1986: *Anthony N. DeMaria* (7), *George J. Klein* (7) and *Hugh D. Allen* (4). Each of 6 non-board members reviewed 6 manuscripts for the AJC in 1986: *Masood Akhtar* (4), *William F. Armstrong* (3), *Richard W. Asinger* (3), *Thomas M. Bashore* (6), *Andrew J. Buda* (3), *Premindra A.N. Chandraratna* (4), *Nicholas L. DePace* (5), *James C. Dillon* (4), *Fetnat M. Fouad* (6), *Jay Hollman* (4), *J. O'Neal Humphries* (4), *William B. Kannel* (4), *Richard S. Meltzer* (5), *Florence H. Sheehan* (5), *Robert J. Siegel* (3) and *David D. Waters* (5).

(5) *Top 15 reviewers for the AJC during past 4 years, 1983–1986:* Table I lists the names and numbers of manuscripts

TABLE I Top 15 Reviewers for the AJC 1983–1986 Listed According to Number of Manuscripts (MS) Reviewed

Name	No. MS Reviewed	No. LR	No. BR	No. On Time
1. Barry J. Maron	46	39	7	36
2. Jeffrey M. Isner	38	31	7	31
2. Carl J. Pepine	38	35	3	31
4. Joel Morganroth	36	35	1	35
5. L. David Hillis	34	33	1	33
6. Nathaniel Reichek	33	31	2	23
6. Melvin M. Scheinman	33	31	2	33
8. Agustin Castellanos	32	27	5	30
8. C. Richard Conti	32	32	0	31
10. David H. Spodick	31	28	3	31
10. Brian G. Firth	31	29	2	31
10. Allan M. Ross	31	27	4	25
10. Navin C. Nanda	31	25	6	22
14. Leonard N. Horowitz	28	28	0	24
14. Barry L. Zaret	28	28	0	14
Totals	502	459 (91%)	43 (9%)	430 (86%)

BR = brief reports; LR = long reports.

reviewed by the top 15 reviewers for the AJC during the present editorship. The editor is enormously indebted to these persons for their enormous contribution to the success of this *Journal.*

(6) *Number and types of manuscripts published:* In 1986, 616 articles, an average of 51 each month, were published in the 16 regular issues of the AJC. Of this number, 412 (67%) were full-length reports, 160 (26%) were brief reports, 21 (3%) were editorials, and 23 (4%) were From-the-Editor and The-AJC-25-Years-Ago columns.

(7) *Letters to the editor:* Forty letters, 8 with replies, occupying 17 pages, were published in 1986. The lag time between acceptance of a letter for publication is several months longer than the lag time between acceptance of a manuscript and its publication. It is the editor's desire to shorten the lag time for letters to the same as that for manuscripts, which at present is 4 months. The lag time is the interval between acceptance of a manuscript or a letter and its publication.

(8) *Budgeted and used pages for articles and letters to the editor:* In late 1985, a total of 2,694 pages for articles and letters to the editor were budgeted for 1986 for the regular issues (excludes supplements). During the first 6 months of 1986, 1,389 pages for articles and letters were published or 39 (3%) over budget. During the last 6 months of 1986, 1,344 pages were budgeted for articles and letters and 1,255 pages or 89 (7%) below budget were published. Thus, for the year 50 pages (2%) below budget were published. Considerable variability occurred in the number of editorial pages published in the 12 first-of-the-month regular issues. The March 1, 1986, issue, for example, contained 207 editorial pages and the December 1, 1986, issue, only 121 editorial pages.

(9) *Budgeted pages for articles and letters for 1987.* For the 16 regular issues in 1987, 2,672 pages are budgeted and the number is equally divided in the 2 halves of the year. Relatively similar numbers of pages must be published each month to maintain a relatively similar accept-and-reject policy each month, to control and maintain a short lag time, and to inform authors at the time of acceptance of their manuscripts precisely which month they can expect their article to appear. I have been assured that there will be more flexibility in numbers of editorial pages available for 1987 compared to the 2 previous years.

TABLE II Statements of Ownership, Management and Circulation of the Four USA Cardiology Journals in 1986

Journal	Issue	No. Copies Printed of Each Issue	No. Copies Distributed	Paid Circulation
AJC	11/86	31,000	30,000	22,500
Circulation	11/86	28,500	22,000	21,000
AHJ	11/86	13,500	12,500	12,000
JACC	12/86	24,000	20,000	19,000

(10) *Symposia published in 1986.* Thirteen symposia including 143 articles and 823 pages were published in the AJC in 1986. The 16 regular issues plus the 13 symposia indicate that 29 separate issues of the AJC were published in 1987.

(11) *Evaluation of the usefulness of the AJC compared to that of other major USA cardiology journals.* Determining the usefulness of a publication is far more difficult than counting the numbers of pages or types of articles published in it. One method of evaluation is the number of subscribers. Table II shows the numbers of subscribers and the numbers of copies distributed from the AJC, *Circulation, American Heart Journal* and the *Journal of the American College of Cardiology* as recorded to the nearest 500 in the "statement of ownership, management and circulation" for these 4 journals as of November or December 1986. The AJC has the largest paid circulation and the largest number of copies distributed.

Another possible means of evaluating the usefulness of a journal is to determine the number of its articles reviewed in annual or monthly review books or journals. The annual yearbook of cardiology titled *CARDIOLOGY 1986* summarized more articles published in 1985 from the AJC than from any other journal, but that fact may be biased because WCR is the editor

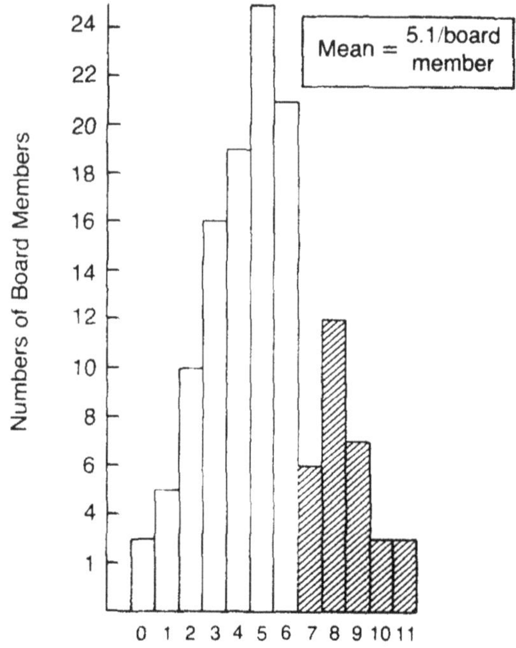

FIGURE 1. Bar graph showing the numbers of manuscripts received by the 130 AJC board members in 1986.

TABLE III Sources of Articles Summarized in 1986 YEAR BOOK OF CARDIOLOGY*

Journal	No. (%)
1. *Amercian Journal of Cardiology*	60 (19%)
2. *Journal of American College of Cardiology*	31 (10%)
3. *Circulation*	25† (8%)
4. *Journal of Thoracic & Cardiovascular Surgery*	25 (8%)
5. *American Heart Journal*	21 (7%)
6. *New England Journal of Medicine*	17 (6%)
7. *British Heart Journal*	16 (5%)
8. *Hypertension*	10 (3%)
9. Others	104 (34%)
Totals	309 (100%)

*Harvey WP, Kirkendall WM, Laks H, Resnekov L, Rosenthal A, Sonnenblick EH, editors. 1986 Yearbook of Cardiology, Chicago:Year Book Medical Publishers, 1986:364.

†Ten of the 25 were in the surgical supplement.

and major contributor of that book.[1] The 1986 YEARBOOK OF CARDIOLOGY, in contrast, is published by the Year Book Publishers and none of the 6 editors of that publication are involved with the AJC. As shown in Table III, the AJC was the source of the largest number of articles summarized in that publication, namely 60, and the journal next most frequently referenced was the *Journal of the American College of Cardiology*, with 31 articles cited.

A monthly controlled circulation journal called *Cardiology Board Review* and edited by Dr. Peter F. Cohn contains 8 or 9 articles monthly and each is a condensed version of an original article published in a peer-review journal. Table IV summarizes the journals containing the original articles from which the condensed articles were derived in a recent 12-month period. The AJC was the source of the most articles and the *Journal of the American College of Cardiology* was next.

(12) *Areas for improvement in the AJC.* Like any publication there are areas for improvement. Most important is the stabilization of the number of pages published in each of the 12 first-

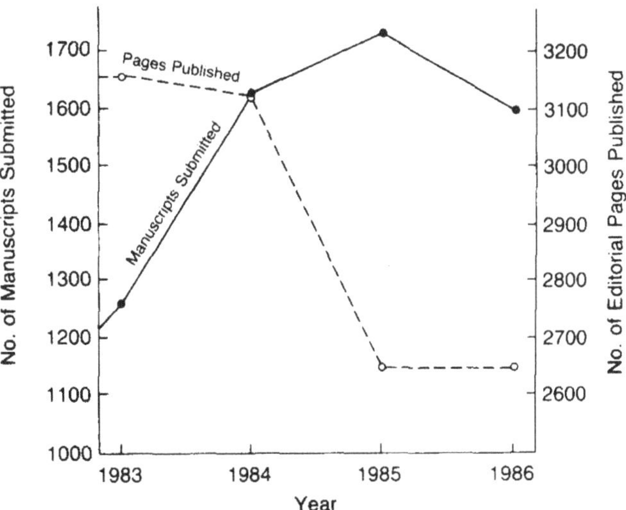

FIGURE 2. Graph showing the numbers of manuscripts submitted and numbers of editorial pages (for articles and letters to the editor) published in the past 4 years (1983, 1984, 1985, 1986). In 1982, 1,100 manuscripts were submitted and about 3,200 editorial pages were published.

TABLE IV Sources of Articles in *Cardiology Board Review*—February 1986-January 1987

Journal	Number (%)
American Journal of Cardiology	28 (25%)
Journal of American College of Cardiology	27 (25%)
Circulation	15 (14%)
American Heart Journal	15 (14%)
New England Journal of Medicine	6 (5%)
British Heart Journal	5 (5%)
Annals of Internal Medicine	3 (3%)
Other	11 (10%)
Totals	110 (100%)

of-the-month regular issues and in the 4 extra regular issues. For each of the 12 first-of-the-month regular issues, 192 editorial pages (for articles and letters to the editor) are budgeted for 1987, and 92 pages for each of the 4 regular extra issues (scheduled for February 15, April 15, September 15 and November 15). It is also the publisher's intent that these regular numbers be maintained throughout 1987.

An increase in the number of editorial pages available in 1987 compared to the 2 previous years would be welcomed by the editor. As shown in Figure 2, the numbers of manuscripts submitted continues to be high and the numbers of editorial pages available less than ideal. The last year of the previous editorship was 1982 and in that year 1,100 manuscripts were received and 3,200 editorial pages (for articles and letters to the editor) were published, By 1984 the numbers of manuscripts submitted had increased to 1,628, and about 3,100 editorial pages were published. During 1985 and 1986, the numbers of manuscripts submitted continued to be high (1,727 in 1985 and 1,598 in 1986) but the number of editorial pages published was about 450 less than in 1983 and 1984. (Each published page is roughly equivalent to 4.5 manuscript pages.) Because of the large number of manuscripts submitted in light of the reduction during the past 2 years of numbers of editorial pages available, publication of experimental-type manuscripts (those involving non-human subjects) in the AJC was discontinued and this policy will continue unless the numbers of editorial pages available increase. In 1986 the AJC published in its regular issues an average of 220 editorial pages (those for articles and letters to the editor) each month (total 2,647); the *American Heart Journal*, an average of 204 each month (total 2,450) (excludes symposia underwritten by pharmaceutical companies); *Circulation*, an average of 234 (total 2,808); and the *Journal of the American College of Cardiology*, an average of 242 pages monthly (total 2,908).

Another area for improvement is quicker mailing of each of the regular issues of the AJC. During a 9-month period (June 1986–February 1987) I received the first-of-the-month regular issue of the AJC at my NIH office on day 15 of the month on the cover of the Journal. In contrast, I received at my NIH office the regular issue of the *American Heart Journal* on day 11, *Circulation* on day 8, and the *Journal of the American College of Cardiology* on day 4. I am anxious that that AJC arrive in the subscriber's mailbox on day 1 of each month.

After the above items were discussed by the editor, the floor was opened to questions and comments. The following issues were raised:

(1) *Value of symposia*: One question concerned the value of symposia sponsored by pharmaceutical companies and pub-

lished in the AJC. During the past 5 years in the USA, there has been a striking increase in the number of industry-sponsored symposia in certain peer-review journals. In 1983, the AJC published 3 industry-sponsored symposia; in 1984, nine; in 1985, fifteen, and in 1986, thirteen. The symposia have the same format as the regular journal issues except that they are devoid of advertisements.

I support publication, within certain guidelines, of the symposia in otherwise peer-review journals for several reasons, and I believe most (>90%) board members have a similar view:

(a) The symposia place in a single issue a great deal of information on a single subject. Thus, they provide considerable amounts of information on a single product, drug or medical device. Usually in each industry-sponsored symposium several of the published articles provide background information on the topic, which only indirectly relates to the drug or medical device produced by the sponsor of the symposium.

(b) The symposia are provided as a "bonus" to the journal subscriber. The publisher bills the symposium sponsor on a per page basis. The symposia published in the AJC contain no advertisements, and thus the articles in the symposia are actually easier to read than are the peer-reviewed articles in the regular issues of the journal, in which ads are interspersed between articles or groups of articles.

(c) Publication of industry-sponsored symposia provides profit to the publisher, and some of the profit can be used to provide additional editorial pages in the regular issues of the journal.

An obvious real or potential disadvantage of publishing industry-sponsored symposia is that the articles about the drug or device produced by the sponsor of the symposium may be biased toward their drug or device compared with those produced by their competitors. There are some safeguards, however, against excessive bias.

(a) A strong guest editor of the symposium can guard against excesses because his/her reputation is "on the line." Whenever I am approached about interest in publishing a symposium in the AJC, the questions I ask are first, "Who is the guest editor? Who are the physician and/or scientists participating in the symposium? What is the subject matter of the symposium"? A quality guest editor generally assures a quality symposium.

(b) Another safeguard is review of symposium manuscripts by participants in the symposium. It is impossible to have the symposium manuscripts reviewed in the same manner as the manuscripts submitted for publication to the regular issues of the journal. Symposia manuscripts, however, can be improved by review by other symposia contributors, not for accept-or-reject recommendations but for suggestions for improvement only. Because symposia manuscripts are not reviewed in the same manner as manuscripts submitted to the regular issues of the journal and because the content of the symposia manuscripts may be have been published in part or in total previously, it is essential that each symposium be published under separate cover from the regular issues and also that the symposia be bound in a volume of their own at the end of each year, separate from that of the regular issues.

(c) Another check on quality of symposia is the editor of the peer review journal in which the symposium is to be published. In the AJC, the final decision regarding publication of an industry-sponsored symposium or any part of it is that of the editor in chief. There is, however, some pressure on the editor from medical participants in the symposium, from the pharmaceutical or medical device company, and from the publisher to accept symposia because of the benefit to sponsor, publisher and the physician participants. The guest editor and symposium contributors benefit because they are paid a fee by the symposium sponsor. The journal editor is not rewarded financially by acceptance of an industry-sponsored symposium for publication.

In the final analysis, the proceedings of a symposium sponsored by a pharmaceutical or medical device company will be published if both sponsor and medical contributors are desirous of publication. The symposium may be published privately by the sponsor or the symposium may be published by a recognized medical journal. I favor the latter path because it has far more checks on biases and overstatements than the former path. Additionally, I suspect that authors put more effort into their contributions when they realize that the proceedings will be published in a well-recognized medical journal than when a symposium is to be published privately by the sponsor.

(2) *Smaller extra regular issues appearing on day 15 of February, April, September and November.* At the 1986 board meeting, Dr. Bernard Gersh expressed the view that authors do not like their articles to appear in the 4 smaller regular issues, much preferring the larger first of the month regular issues. During recent months Dr. Gersh polled his cardiologic colleagues at the Mayo Clinic and he found that >90% of his colleagues also preferred that their articles appear in the larger 12 regular issues rather than in the smaller 4 issues. Most board members, I suspect, prefer 12 larger regular issues with elimination of the 4 smaller regular issues. This subject will be discussed further with the new owner of the AJC during this year. The possibility of having more regular issues each of the same size and at regular intervals also will be discussed.

(3) *Interval between publication of an article in the AJC and receipt of reprints of that article from the publisher:* This complaint is heard periodically and it was noted by the publisher.

(4) *The necessity of miniabstracts for the "contents with abstracts" was raised:* Both the AJC and *Journal of the American College of Cardiology* publish abstracts of articles in the elongated table of contents. The reason is that advertisements in apposition to the "contents with abstracts" provide a premium to the publisher. Additionally, some readers cut the abstracts with the title and authors for filing and retrieval purposes.

(5) *Status of experimental studies:* Experimental-type manuscripts, those involving nonhuman subjects, are not being accepted by the AJC and this policy will continue until the numbers of editorial pages are substantially increased.

The meeting was adjourned to a reception provided by the publisher.

Views of readers on items discussed in this piece or other matters are welcomed by the editor.

William C. Roberts

William C. Roberts, MD
Editor in Chief

1. Roberts WC (ed.), Rackley CE, Willerson JT, Graham TP Jr, Pacifico AD, Karp RB. *Cardiology 1986. New York: Yorke Medical Books, 1986:1–444.*

AJC Editorial Board Meeting—March 1988

The annual editorial board meeting of *The American Journal of Cardiology* this year was held in Atlanta, Georgia, on March 29, 1988, at the time of the Annual Scientific Sessions of the American College of Cardiology. It was my pleasure to introduce the new Publishing Director of the Yorke Medical Group, Martin W. Morgan. He briefly described Yorke's parent company, Cahners Publishing Company, emphasizing that quality of editorial is of primary importance both to him and to his company. He pointed out that advertising and subscription support follow quality editorial and that Cahners had done several readership surveys and 1 focus group study since he became publisher in July 1987, and that more readership surveys will be done. Mr. Morgan then announced that the graphic design of the Journal was changing as of July 1, 1988, and examples of the new design and layout of the table of contents, title pages of the various sections and cover were shown. The table of contents with abstracts may be discontinued in 1989. A public relations program for the Journal has been initiated; press releases and occasionally copies of the best AJC manuscripts are being sent to a number of scientific and news reporters for release at the time of the article's publication in the AJC. The publisher further announced that the mailing date of the Journal was being reset so that subscribers will soon receive their issues on or very near the day of the month printed on the Journal's cover. Short-term free subscriptions of the AJC to cardiologists are being discontinued. Despite a relatively large investment in recent months by Cahners in the Journal, the subscription cost in 1988 is the same as in 1987.

After returning to the podium, I emphasized to the board the importance of having the publisher's support and stated how much I had enjoyed working with this vigorous new publisher.

The following items were then discussed:

(1) *Number of manuscripts reviewed by AJC board members in 1987:* Of the 1,525 manuscripts received in 1987, 662 were sent to board members for review and the other 863 manuscripts were reviewed by non-board members. Of the 662 manuscripts, 554 (84%) were long reports and 108 (16%) were brief reports or case reports. Of the 662 manuscripts sent to board members, the reviews of 555 (84%) were returned to the editorial office within the allotted time (≤3 weeks); 26 manuscripts (4%) were returned not reviewed (out of town, etc.).

(2) *Numbers of manuscripts received for review by each AJC board member in 1987:* The number of manuscripts sent to board members is summarized in Figure 1 and ranged from none (5 members) to 12 manuscripts (1 member). The average number of manuscripts received for review by the 141 board members in 1987 was 4.7. As shown in Table I, the 106 adult cardiologists on the board reviewed the most manuscripts (mean 5.2), the 13 cardiac surgeons the least (mean 1.8) and the pediatric cardiologists (mean 3.7) and related specialists (mean 4.2) were intermediate.

(3) *AJC board members reviewing the most manuscripts in 1987:* Joel Morganroth (11) and David H. Spodick (9) each reviewed 11 manuscripts. (The number in parentheses represents the number of full-length reports and the difference between the number in parentheses and the first number mentioned represents the number of brief reports or case reports reviewed.) Ten manuscripts were reviewed by Richard B. Devereux (8), Frank I. Marcus (9) and Barry J. Maron (7). Each of 7 board members reviewed 9 manuscripts: Joseph S. Alpert (9), Robert L. Feldman (8), Frank A. Finnerty (9), Fred Morady (6), Navin C. Nanda (6), Melvin M. Scheinman (7) and James T. Willerson (9). Each of 11 board members reviewed 8 manuscripts: George A. Beller (7), Robert Bonow (8), Agustin Castellanos (7), Michael H. Crawford (6), Harvey Feigenbaum (6), Arthur Garson, Jr. (4), Spencer B. King, III, (8), Robert A. Kloner

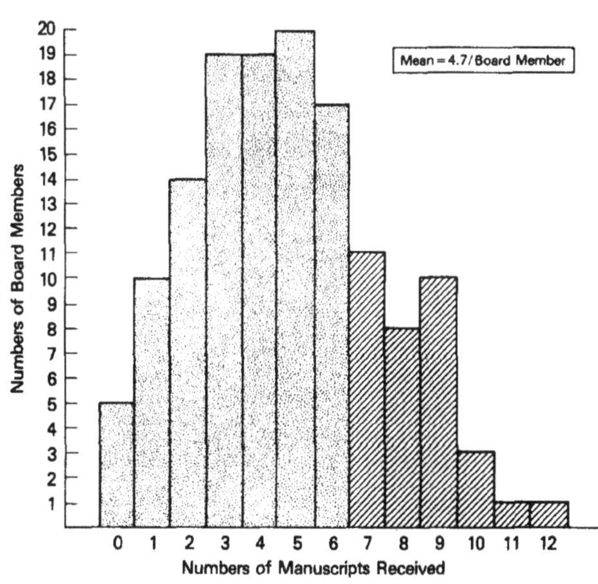

FIGURE 1. Diagram showing numbers of manuscripts sent to AJC board members in 1987.

TABLE I Numbers and Types of Manuscripts Sent to AJC Board Members in 1987 According to Board Specialty

	No. on Editorial Board	No. MS Sent (No. per Reviewer)	No. LR	No. BR	No. Returned on Time	No. Returned without Review
Adult cardiologists	106	554 (5.2)	480	74	458 (83%)	19 (3%)
Pediatric cardiologists	16	59 (3.7)	41	18	54 (92%)	0
Cardiac surgeons	13	24 (1.8)	20	4	23 (96%)	0
Related specialists*	6	25 (4.2)	13	12	20 (80%)	7 (28%)
Total	141	662 (4.7)	554 (84%)	108 (16%)	555 (84%)	26 (4%)

* Four pathologists and 2 radiologists.
BR = brief report; LR = long reports; MS = manuscript.

TABLE II Top 25 Reviewers and Numbers of Manuscripts Reviewed for the AJC from 1983 to 1987

	No. Manuscripts Reviewed	No. on Time	No. LR	No. BR
1. Barry J. Maron*	56	46	46	10
2. Joel Morganroth	47	46	46	1
3. Carl J. Pepine*	46	37	42	4
4. Jeffrey M. Isner	44	38	36	8
5. Robert Bonow	43	23	42	1
6. David H. Spodick	42	42	38	4
6. Melvin M. Scheinman	42	42	38	4
8. Nathaniel Reilchek	41	32	39	2
9. Augustin Castellanos	40	40	33	7
9. Navin C. Nanda*	40	30	31	9
11. Michael H. Crawford	39	33	36	3
12. C. Richard Conti	38	37	37	1
12. Frank I. Marcus*	38	26	32	6
12. Allan M. Ross	38	33	34	4
15. George A. Beller	36	27	34	2
15. Robert L. Feldman*	36	35	30	6
15. L. David Hillis*	36	35	35	1
15. James T. Willerson*	36	36	36	0
19. Brian G. Firth	35	35	33	2
19. Robert A. Kloner	35	29	30	5
21. Barry L. Zaret	34	21	33	1
22. Joseph S. Alpert*	33	32	33	0
23. Robert A. O'Rourke	31	29	30	1
24. Richard B. Devereux	30	16	28	2
24. Leonard N. Horowitz	30	28	30	0

* These 8 board members never returned a manuscript without its being reviewed. Of the other 17 top reviewers, 37 manuscripts (an average of 2.2 per board member) were returned without being reviewed.
Abbreviations as in Table I.

(4), Robert Myerburg (7), Carl J. Pepine (7) and Nathaniel Reichek (8). Each of 8 board members reviewed 7 manuscripts: Peter F. Cohn (6), Donald C. Harrison (7), Carl V. Leier (7), Joseph Lindsay, Jr, (7), Michael Mock (7), Lowell W. Perry (2), Robert Roberts (7) and Allan M. Ross (7). Of the 259 manuscripts reviewed by the 31 aforementioned board members, 228 (88%) were reviewed within the allotted time period (≤3 weeks).

(4) *Top reviewers among non-board members:* Over two-thirds of the manuscripts received in 1987 were sent to 1 or more of nearly 1,300 investigators who are not board members but who serve as manuscript reviewers for the AJC. The top non-board reviewer for the AJC in 1987 was David R. Holmes, Jr., (8) who reviewed 8 manuscripts. Abdul S. Abbasi (7), Marc Cantin (6), George J. Klein (4), Miguel S. Quinones (6), Andrew Selwyn (7), Eric Topol (6) and Ron Vlietstra (7) each reviewed 7 manuscripts. Each of 10 non-board members reviewed 6 manuscripts: Harisios Boudoulas (6), Kanu Chatterjee (6), Jay N. Cohn (4), Gregory Dehmer (6), Anthony N. DeMaria (4), Lawrence D. German (3), K. Lance Gould (5), James C. Huhta (6), Jay W. Mason (5) and Leonard Scherlis (6). Each of 7 non-board members reviewed 5 manuscripts: Lewis C. Becker (5), Nora F. Goldschlager (5), William B. Kannel (4), Zuhdi Labadidi (4), Randolph P. Martin (5), Denis Roy (4) and George A. Williams (5).

(5) *Top 25 reviewers for the AJC in the last 5 years:* The names of the board members who reviewed the most manuscripts for the AJC from 1983 through 1987 are listed in Table II. Of the 966 manuscripts reviewed by these 25 board members, 828 (86%) were returned to the editorial office in the allotted time period and several reviewers were never late with a single manuscript during the 5-year period. The quality of the reviews by these 25 board members is predictably outstandings. I am enormously indebted to these 25 board members for their extraordinary contribution to the success of the Journal.

(6) *Number and types of manuscripts published in the AJC in 1987 and comparison to* Circulation *and to the* Journal of the American College of Cardiology (JACC)*:* As shown in Table III, 695 articles (an average of 58 each month) occupying 2,810 pages were published in the regular issues of the AJC in 1987. Circulation published 331 articles (average 28 a month) occupying 2,772 pages, and JACC published 382 articles (average 32 a month) occupying 2,729. The average length of an article in the AJC in 1987 was 4.04 pages; in Circulation, 8.37 pages and in JACC, 7.14 pages.

The numbers of pages for articles and letters to the editor published in the AJC in each of the past 5 years and the number of manuscripts received during each of these years is displayed in Figure 2. The number of pages for articles and letters budgeted in 1988 in the AJC is about 125 less than in 1987, but the new graphic design is expected to increase content per page by at least 5%.

(7) *Symposia published in 1987:* Nineteen symposia including 279 articles occupying 1,576 pages were published in the AJC in 1987, a larger number than in any of the preceding 4 years (Table IV).

(8) *Evaluation of the usefulness of the AJC compared to that of other major USA cardiology journals:* Determining the useful-

TABLE III Numbers of Pages and Numbers and Percents of Articles Published in Three Major USA Cardiology Journals in 1987

	American Journal of Cardiology	Circulation	Journal of the American College of Cardiology
Number of pages	3,228	2,856	2,999
For articles (pages/article) (% of pages)	2,810 (4.04) (87%)	2,772 (8.37) (97%)	2,729 (7.14) (91%)
For letters (number) [no. with replies]	23 (45) [18]	0	23 (28) [15]
For staff and editorial board	16	12	24
For contents in brief	50	26	24
For contents with abstracts	202	0	93
For information for authors	16	4	24
For volume indexes	101	37	53
For other	10	5	29
Number of articles (mean/month)	695 (58)	331 (28)	382 (32)
Coronary artery disease	180 (27%)	57 (17%)	82 (22%)
Arrhythmias and conduction disturbances	83 (12%)	25 (8%)	55 (14%)
Systemic hypertension	28 (4%)	8 (2%)	3 (1%)
Congestive heart failure	25 (3%)	8 (2%)	16 (4%)
Valvular heart failure	30 (4%)	16 (5%)	22 (6%)
Cardiomyopathy	14 (2%)	6 (2%)	12 (3%)
Congenital heart disease	31 (4%)	22 (7%)	21 (6%)
Miscellaneous	26 (4%)	31 (9%)	29 (8%)
Methods	24 (3%)	3 (1%)	9 (2%)
Experimental studies	0	111 (34%)	55 (14%)
Historical studies	7 (1%)	1 (0.3%)	2 (0.5%)
Brief reports	117 (17%)	0	0
Case reports	86 (12%)	0	23 (6%)
Editorials	38* (6%)	43 (13%)	53 (14%)

* Includes 12 From-the-Editor columns.

ness of a publication is far more difficult than counting the numbers of pages or types of articles published. One method of evaluation is the number of subscribers. Table V shows the numbers of subscribers and numbers of copies distributed from the *AJC*, *Circulation*, *JACC* and the *American Heart Journal* (*AHJ*) as recorded to the nearest 500 in the "statement of ownership, management and circulation" for these 4 journals as of November or December 1987. The AJC has the largest paid circulation and it, of course, is not associated with a professional society.

Another possible means of evaluating the usefulness of a journal is to examine the number of its articles reviewed in annual or monthly review books or journals. A monthly controlled circulation journal called *Cardiology Board Review* and edited by Dr. Peter F. Cohn contains 8 or 9 articles monthly and each is a condensed version of an original article published in a peer-review journal. Table VI summarizes the journals containing the original articles from which the condensed articles were derived in 1987. As in 1986, the AJC was the source of the most articles.

(9) *Request for more high-quality editorials:* I would like to increase the number of editorials published annually in the AJC from 38 to perhaps 50. The editorial's length should be determined by the message delivered. One-point editorials can be short. Multiple-point editorials might best be characterized as editorial reviews.

(10) *Faster publishing of letters to the editor:* For the past 2 years, the lag time (period from acceptance to publication) for letters has been excessive. By July 1988, however, the significant lag time for letters will have vanished. It would be ideal to have a shorter lag time for letters than for regular manuscripts because most letters are comments on or criticisms of recently published articles or editorials. The present interval from acceptance of a manuscript to its publication in the AJC averages 4 months.

TABLE IV Symposia in the AJC, 1983 to 1987

Year	No. of Symposia	No. of Articles	No. of Pages
1983	5	60 (12)	326 (62)
1984	9	126 (14)	703 (78)
1985	15	192 (13)	1161 (77)
1986	13	143 (11)	823 (63)
1987	19	279 (15)	1576 (83)

TABLE V Statement of Ownership, Management and Circulation of the Four Major USA Cardiology Journals in 1987

Journal	Issue	Mean No. Copies Printed/mo*	Mean No. Copies Distributed/mo*	Mean Paid Circulation/mo*
AJC	11/87	31,350	29,100	22,000
Circulation	11/87	26,050	21,700	20,850
JACC	12/87	25,100	21,500	20,800
AHJ	11/87	13,700	12,900	12,100

* For each of the preceding 12 months.

(11) *Reminder to authors to supply several names of nonlocal, nonbiased reviewers for their manuscripts:* Editors have no monopoly on choosing the best reviewers of manuscripts. No one should be more knowledgeable of experts in the subject of a manuscript than the authors of the manuscript. Thus, I urge authors to supply names—preferably 5 and when they are non-

TABLE VI Sources of Articles in Cardiology Board Review in 1987

Journal	No. (%)
American Journal of Cardiology	33 (30.6%)
Journal of the American College of Cardiology	27 (25.0%)
Circulation	14 (13.0%)
American Heart Journal	13 (12.0%)
Annals of Internal Medicine	6 (5.6%)
American Journal of Medicine	5 (4.6%)
New England Journal of Medicine	5 (4.6%)
British Heart Journal	5 (4.6%)
Total	108 (100%)

board members also their addresses—of nonbiased, nonlocal potential reviewers of their manuscripts. For my own manuscripts, careful consideration of ideal reviewers is begun long before the particular research project is finished. I urge other investigators to consider this avenue more often. It is necessary for an author to supply several names because almost certainly some of the potential reviewers will already have a manuscript for review and a second manuscript is not sent to a reviewer who already possesses one, unless the second manuscript is a brief report or case report.

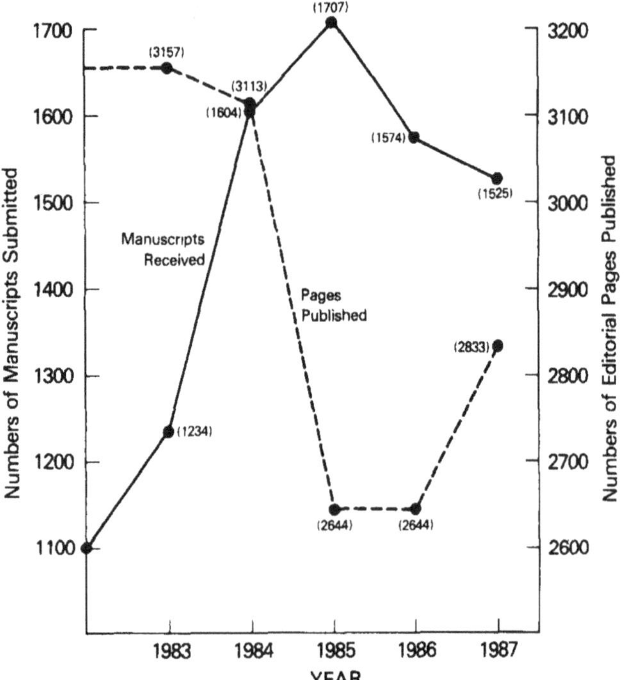

FIGURE 2. Manuscripts received and editorial pages (for articles and letters) published in the AJC 1983 through 1987.

The floor was then opened for questions and comments. The issue raised was the *uneven quality of symposia*. Some symposia are excellent and some are not. There is no way that manuscripts for symposia can be reviewed on a peer-review basis similar to that of the nonsymposia manuscripts. I urge guest editors of symposia to have symposia contributors review each other's manuscripts. One guest editor had the sponsoring pharmaceutical company provide a large honorarium to each of 2 investigators who reviewed all 15 or so manuscripts of that symposium. I found the reviews, however, in this one instance not very helpful. The manuscripts in that symposium already were excellent.

When someone contacts me about the possibility of publishing a symposium in the AJC, I first want to know who the guest editor will be and then the names of the participants. Many leaders in cardiology have served as guest editors of symposia in the AJC. In 1987 alone, guest editors included *Eugene Braunwald, Edward D. Frohlich, Spencer B. King III, Desmond Julian, Aram V. Chobanian, Leonard Horowitz, Attilio Maseri, Joel Morganroth, Bernard Lown* and *Jonathan Abrams*. The guest editors must accept the major quality-control role with their symposia. I spend one night reviewing each symposium—not much maybe, but that was 19 nights in 1987.

When pharmaceutical companies pay nice honoraria for presentations and expenses for participation in lovely resort settings, they are in a position to expect and require high quality presentations and manuscripts from their invitees. Presenters at symposia must be informed long in advance of their presentation that the symposium will be published and that a manuscript is expected at the time of the symposium. If honoraria and expenses are withheld until the manuscript is delivered, manuscripts are more likely to be delivered in timely fashion and publication of the symposium proceedings then is not unduly delayed.

One of the bonuses of symposia is that they generally contain 1 or more review articles. Although the information in symposia is not always new, publication of the symposium proceedings provides a great deal of information in 1 place on a single subject. The question-and-answer sessions also are often published and they are appealing in my view.

The symposia in the AJC should be bound at the end of the year in a single volume separate from that of the regular issues. To emphasize that symposia are clearly different from the regular issues of the AJC, the publisher soon will alter the cover of the symposia issues so that they have a different appearance from the regular issues.

I welcome suggestions to improve symposia and other portions of the Journal. The meeting was adjourned to a fine reception.

William C. Roberts

William C. Roberts, MD
Editor-in-Chief

Editorial Board Meeting of The American Journal of Cardiology—March 1989

The annual editorial board meeting of *The American Journal of Cardiology* (AJC) this year was held in Anaheim, California, March 21, at the time of the Annual Scientific Sessions of the American College of Cardiology. The major purposes of the editorial board meeting were to say "thanks" to the 138 board members for their enormous help during the previous year, to pay particular tribute to those board members reviewing the most manuscripts during 1988, to summarize AJC publication figures in 1988, to summarize new developments affecting the AJC since the last board meeting and to receive input from board members through their comments and questions.

The meeting began by introducing Joe Navitsky, the new publisher of the AJC, with whom I am enormously pleased to be working. I am confident that he will provide significantly more editorial pages for the *Journal* than have been provided in the past 3 years, and, therefore, this leadership change is a boost to both readers and authors. Not only was there a change in publisher in 1988, but the director of Cahners' 16 publications in New York changed in 1988. The new director is Robert Brawn, who had initially chosen me to be the *Journal*'s second editor in 1982, and who obviously is enormously familiar with the *Journal*. After introducing other publishing staff in attendance, the following items were discussed:

(1) *Introduction of new board members:* Twenty physicians (Table I) were added to the board in 1989, and they were introduced. New board members are selected entirely on their record as nonboard reviewers for the AJC. It is easy to select the new board members. The card files of the 1,200 or so nonboard AJC reviewers are reviewed and the 15 or 20 with the best reviewing records are selected. I had not met before this meeting several board members selected this year. Many other nonboard reviewers are deserving of board status, but all obviously cannot be chosen. It is hoped that the most deserving, however, will eventually become board members.

The task of eliminating about 10% of the board members each year is getting progressively more difficult. The reason is because most board members do a superb job. The elimination process is also done by the numbers. The card file of each board member is reviewed near the end of the calendar year; those members with the largest numbers of reviews returned late or manuscripts returned without review are deleted. Thus, each AJC board member determines his or her longevity on the AJC editorial board. Although it makes the editor's task a bit easier politically, set terms for board members is not a policy of the AJC.

(2) *Numbers of manuscripts received for review by each AJC board member in 1988:* The numbers of manuscripts sent to each board members in 1988 are summarized in Figure 1, and they ranged from none (8 members) to 12 manuscripts (1 member) (mean 4.6). The numbers and types of manuscripts sent (95% actually reviewed) to the 4 types of specialists on the board are summarized in Table II. The 103 adult cardiologists on the board were sent 533 manuscripts (mean 5.2/member); the 17 pediatric cardiologists were sent 59 manuscripts (mean 3.5); the 14 cardiac surgeons were sent 27 manuscripts (mean 1.9); and the 4 cardiac radiologists or pathologists were sent 15 manuscripts (mean 3.7). Of the 634 manuscripts sent to board members, only 30 (5%) were returned without review (out of town, etc.), and 56 manuscripts (9%) were returned late.

(3) *AJC board members reviewing the most manuscripts in 1988:* The 15 top AJC reviewers in 1988 are listed in Table III. Dr. Jeffrey M. Isner was number 1, and Joel Morganroth was number 2. Table IV lists the 19 board reviewers who each reviewed 7 manuscripts in 1988.

(4) *Numbers of pages and articles published in the regular issues of the AJC in 1988 and in the previous five years:* These are summarized in Table V. Of the 3,043 editorial pages (nonrevenue earning) published in the AJC in 1988, 2,680 pages were for articles (2,642 pages), letters (26 pages) and abstracts (12 pages) (from the cardiology section of a pediatric meeting). The remaining 363 pages (12%) were for table of contents, indexes, etc. A total of 636 articles, an average of 53 a month, were published in the regular issues in 1988.

(5) *Number and types of articles published in the AJC in 1988 and comparison to* Circulation *and* The Journal of The American College of Cardiology (*JACC*)*:* As shown in Table VI, fewer pages but more articles were published in the AJC in 1988 than in either Circulation or JACC. The shorter average length of articles in the AJC (4.15 pages) than in Circulation (8.80 pages) or JACC (6.56 pages) and the slightly greater content per page of articles in the AJC makes this possible. Table VI also displays other differences in 1988 among these 3 USA cardiology journals. No experimental articles (those involving nonhuman animals) were published in the AJC (except for a few in the Brief Reports sec-

tion) whereas 53 (12% of articles) were published in JACC and 104 (31% of articles) in Circulation. A unique feature of the AJC is the large number of Brief Reports published (152 [24% of articles]) whereas neither of the other 2 journals publish brief reports. Over a third of the Brief Reports published had been submitted initially as full-length manuscripts. The Brief Report section is not a Case Report section. The Case Report section numbered 53 articles in 1988; all had 1 to 3 case descriptions. The percentages of the full-length articles involving coronary artery disease, arrhythmias and conduction disturbances, congestive heart failure, valvular heart disease, cardiomyopathy, congenital heart disease, miscellaneous conditions and methods were similar among the 3 journals.

(6) *Numbers of symposia published in the AJC in 1988 and in the previous five years:* These are summarized in Table VII.

(7) *Specific symposia in the AJC in 1988, their guest editors and sponsors:* These are listed in Table VIII. A total of 252 articles occupying 1,393 pages were published in those symposia in 1988. Adding the 636 articles occupying 2,642 pages published in AJC's regular issues in 1988, a total of 888 articles occupying 4,035 pages were published in the AJC in 1988.

(8) *Developments affecting the AJC since the last editorial board meeting (March 1988):* In April 1988 the Brief Report section was divided into 2 sections; one called Brief Reports and reserved for manuscripts describing clinical investigations but providing only 1 or 2 major findings, and one called Case Reports and reserved for manuscripts containing actual case descriptions. Both reports are limited in numbers of manuscript pages and references.

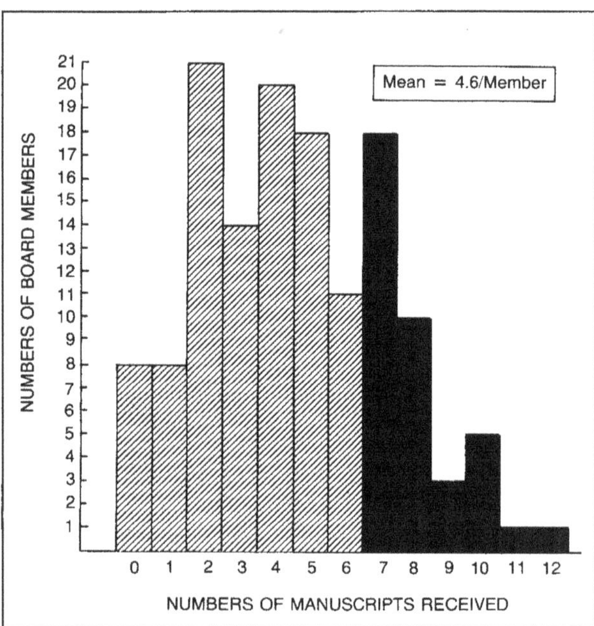

FIGURE 1. Numbers of manuscripts sent to AJC Board Members in 1988.

TABLE I New AJC Board Members—1989

1. Masood Akhtar
2. Hugh D. Allen
3. Jack Ferlinz
4. Jeffrey M. Hoeg
5. Kenneth Hossack
6. Adolph M. Hutter, Jr.
7. William B. Kannel
8. George J. Klein
9. Lloyd W. Klein
10. John Kostis
11. Melvin L. Marcus
12. Randolph P. Martin
13. Franz H. Messerli
14. Eugene R. Passamani
15. James L. Ritchie
16. Jeffrey Saffitz
17. A. Rebecca Snider
18. Eric Topol
19. Robert Vogel
20. David D. Waters

In July 1988, graphic and redesign changes, which took nearly a year to formulate, were introduced. These changes, I believe, have been well received.

In October 1988, the new publisher of the AJC and the new director of Cahners' publications in New York came on board.

In January 1989 the bimonthly publishing schedule for the regular issues of the AJC began. The regular issues now are published on the first and fifteenth of 10 months of the year; only the first of the month issue will appear in August and December. In 1990 the publisher has indicated that he will likely introduce 2 regular issues in both August and December as well so relatively soon the bimonthly distribution of the regular issues will include all 12 months. The bimonthly schedule is flowing smoothly.

In late 1988 the regular issues began appearing earlier each month. The first of the month regular issues now are published the last day or so of the preceding month and now the first of the month issue should be in the subscribers' hands during the first week of each month.

The long lag time for letters has now been shortened to that of manuscripts, namely slightly less than 3 months from acceptance date to publication date. We, therefore, publish manuscripts after their acceptance faster than either the American Heart Association or the American College of Cardiology publishes their annual meeting abstracts after they are accepted.

(9) *Evaluation of the usefulness of the AJC compared to that of other major USA cardiology journals:* Determining the usefulness of a publication is more difficult than counting the numbers of pages or types of articles published. One method of evaluation is the number of subscribers. Table IX shows the numbers of subscribers and numbers of copies distributed from the AJC, Circulation and JACC as recorded to the nearest 50 in the "statement of ownership, management and circulation" as appeared in the November 1988 issue of each journal. The paid circulation of each of the 3 journals is similar.

TABLE II Numbers and Types of Manuscripts Sent to AJC Board Members in 1988 According to Specialty of Board Member

Specialty	No. on Editorial Board	No. MS Sent (No./ Reviewer)	No. LR	No. BR	No. CR	No. (%) MSS Returned on Time	No. (%) MSS Returned Late	No. (%) MSS Returned Without Review
Adult cardiologist	103	533 (5.2)	491	20	22	461 (87)	45 (8)	27 (5)
Pediatric cardiologist	17	59 (3.5)	47	3	9	53 (90)	5 (8)	1 (2)
Cardiac surgeon	14	27 (1.9)	22	0	5	25 (93)	2 (7)	0
Radiologist or pathologist	4	15 (3.7)	9	2	4	9 (60)	4 (27)	2 (13)
Total	138	634 (4.6)	569 (90%)	25 (4%)	40 (6%)	548 (86)	56 (9)	30 (5)

BR = brief report; CR = case report; LR = long report; MS = manuscript.

TABLE III Top 15 AJC Reviewers in 1988 and Numbers of Manuscripts Reviewed for the AJC in 1988

Name	No. MSS Reviewed	LR	BR	CR	No. MSS Reviewed on Time
1. Jeffrey M. Isner	12	10	1	1	12
2. Joel Morganroth	11	11	0	0	11
3. Michael H. Crawford	10	10	0	0	9
4. Pamela S. Douglas	10	10	0	0	10
5. Fred Morady	10	8	0	2	10
6. Leonard N. Horowitz	9	9	0	0	9
7. Barry J. Maron	9	6	0	3	8
8. Arthur J. Moss	9	9	0	0	8
9. Melvin M. Scheinman	9	9	0	0	9
10. Jeffrey Anderson	8	7	1	0	7
11. Peter F. Cohn	8	8	0	0	7
12. Pablo Denes	8	8	0	0	7
13. James E. Lock	8	4	1	3	7
14. Bramah N. Singh	8	7	0	1	5
15. David H. Spodick	8	5	0	3	8

Abbreviations as in Table II.

TABLE IV Reviewers of Seven Manuscripts for the AJC in 1988

Name	No. MSS Reviewed	LR	BR	CR	No. MSS Reviewed on Time
1. Lionel M. Bargeron	7	6	0	1	7
2. George A. Beller	7	7	0	0	7
3. Richard O. Cannon, III	7	6	1	0	7
4. C. Richard Conti	7	7	0	0	7
5. Robert F. DeBusk	7	7	0	0	7
6. Myrvin H. Ellestad	7	5	2	0	7
7. Julius M. Gardin	7	7	0	0	5
8. Harold L. Kennedy	7	7	0	0	4
9. Kenneth M. Kent	7	5	1	1	4
10. Frank I. Marcus	7	7	0	0	7
11. Jawahar Mehta	7	6	1	0	7
12. Robert J. Myerburg	7	7	0	0	7
13. Navin C. Nanda	7	7	0	0	7
14. Carl J. Pepine	7	6	1	0	6
15. Philip J. Podrid	7	6	0	1	6
16. Charles E. Rackley	7	7	0	0	6
17. Allan M. Ross	7	7	0	0	5
18. Ralph Shabetai	7	5	1	1	6
19. Douglas P. Zipes	7	7	0	0	7

Abbreviations as in Table II.

Beginning in January 1989, Merck Sharp & Dohme contracted with the publisher to distribute the AJC free of charge to cardiology fellows in the USA during 1989 and 1990. With these additional subscribers the AJC has the largest paid circulation of the 3 journals listed in Table IX.

Another possible means of evaluating the usefulness of a journal is to examine the number of its articles reviewed in annual or monthly review books or journals. A monthly controlled circulation journal called *Cardiology Board Review* and edited by Dr. Peter F. Cohn contains 5 to 12 articles monthly and each is a condensed version of an original article published in a peer-reviewed journal. Table X summarizes the journals containing the original articles from which the condensed articles were derived in 1988. As in both 1986 and 1987, the AJC was the source of the most articles.

(10) *Request for more high quality editorials:* I would like to increase the number of editorials and editorial reviews in the AJC. The editorial's length should be determined by the message delivered. One-point editorials should be short. Multiple-point editorials might best be characterized as editorial reviews.

(11) *Reminder to authors to supply several names of nonlocal, nonbiased reviewers for their manuscripts:* Editors have no monopoly on choosing the best reviewers of manuscripts. No one should be more knowledgeable of experts in the subjects of a manuscript than the authors of the manuscript. Thus, I urge authors to supply names—preferably 5 and when they are nonboard members also their addresses—of nonbiased, nonlocal potential reviewers of their manuscripts. It is necessary for an author to supply several names because almost certainly some of the potential reviewers will already have a manuscript for review and a second manuscript is not sent to a reviewer who already possesses one, unless the second manuscript is a brief report or a case report. Presently, in only about 20% of manuscripts submitted have authors provided names of potential reviewers. After studying for several years reviews by reviewers suggested by authors, I am impressed that in general they are of higher quality than those selected by the AJC's editor or associate editors, and that the author-chosen reviewers are not more favor-

TABLE V Number of Pages and Articles Published in the Regular Issues of *The American Journal of Cardiology* from 1983 to 1988

	1983	1984	1985	1986	1987	1988
No. of pages	3,435	3,403	3,014	3,004	3,228	3,043
For articles	3,130	3,077	2,623	2,627	2,810	2,642
For letters (no.)	27 (53)	36 (80)	21 (40)	17 (40)	23 (45)	26 (60)
For abstracts	0	0	0	10	10	12
For staff and board	15	15	17	17	16	16
For contents in brief	28	31	44	44	50	51
For contents with abstracts	142	145	207	179	202	194
For information for authors	12	15	17	15	16	17
For indexes	79	69	70	86	101	85
For other	2	15	15	10	0	0
No. of articles	643	747	645	616	695	636
Mean/month	54	62	54	51	58	53
Pages/article	4.87	4.12	4.07	4.26	4.04	4.15

TABLE VI Number of Pages and Types of Articles Published in the Regular Issues of *The American Journal of Cardiology, Journal of the American College of Cardiology* and *Circulation* in 1988

	American Journal of Cardiology	Journal of the American College of Cardiology	Circulation
No. of pages (mean/month)	3,043 (254)	3,224 (269)	3,268 (272)
For articles (pages/article)	2,642 (4.15)	2,921 (6.56)	2.973 (8.80)
For letters (no.) [no. with replies]	26 (60) [18]	24 (30) [20]	5 (4) [0]
For abstracts	12	0	16
For staff and editorial board	16	36	18
For contents in brief	51	25	31
For contents with abstracts	194	101	29
For information for authors	17	36	12
For volume indexes	85	54	42
For miscellaneous	0	27	142
No. of articles (mean/month)	636 (53)	445* (37)	338* (28)
Coronary artery disease	158 (24.8%)	104 (23.4%)	77 (22.8%)
Arrhythmias and conduction defects	77 (12.1%)	58 (13.0%)	37 (11.0%)
Systemic hypertension	25 (3.9%)	6 (1.3%)	11 (3.2%)
Congestive heart failure	10 (1.6%)	9 (2.0%)	7 (2.1%)
Valvular heart disease	32 (5.0%)	24 (5.4%)	25 (7.4%)
Cardiomyopathy	13 (2.0%)	10 (2.3%)	6 (1.8%)
Congenital heart disease	29 (4.6%)	31 (7.0%)	20 (5.9%)
Miscellaneous	31 (4.9%)	38 (8.5%)	20 (5.9%)
Methods	9 (1.4%)	9 (2.0%)	2 (0.6%)
Experimental studies	0 (0)	53 (11.9%)	104 (30.8%)
Historical studies	5 (0.8%)	1 (0.002%)	0 (0)
Brief reports	152 (23.9%)	0 (0)	0 (0)
Case reports	53 (8.3%)	5 (1.1%)	0 (0)
AJC 25 years ago	7 (1.1%)	—	—
Editorials and editorial reviews	24 (3.8%)	97 (21.8%)	28 (8.3%)
From the editor	11 (1.7%)	0	1 (0.3%)

* These articles were categorized as if they had been submitted to The American Journal of Cardiology.

TABLE VII Symposia in the AJC From 1983 to 1988

Year	No. of Symposia	No. of Articles	No. of Pages
1983	5	60 (12)	326 (62)
1984	9	126 (14)	703 (78)
1985	15	192 (13)	1,161 (77)
1986	13	143 (11)	823 (63)
1987	19	279 (15)	1,576 (83)
1988	19	252 (13)	1,393 (73)

Numbers in parentheses equal mean number per issue.

able to a manuscript than are editor-selected reviewers. Indeed, many manuscripts have been reviewed by 1 author-selected reviewer and by 1 editor-selected reviewer and the author-selected reviewer recommended rejection and the editor-selected reviewer recommended acceptance of the manuscript.

The floor was then opened to questions and comments from board members:

(1) *What was the manuscript acceptance rate in 1988?* In 1988, 1,496 manuscripts were submitted and 636 manuscripts were published. Some manuscripts sub-

TABLE VIII Symposia in *The American Journal of Cardiology* in 1988

Number	Month, Day	Symposium Title	Guest Editor(s)	Articles	Pages	Sponsor	Date of Symposium	Interval (months) Symposium to Publication
A	January 15	Arrhythmia Therapy (Disopyramide)	Eric N. Prystowsky	13	116	G. D. Searle	February 27–March 1, 1987	10
B	January 29	Silent Myocardial Ischemia	James J. Morris, Jr.	7	31	CIBA-GEIGY	March 7, 1987	11
C	February 10	Systemic Hypertension (Celiprolol)	Giuseppe Mancia John L. Reid	14	59	Rorer International Pharmaceuticals	September 6, 1986	16
D	February 24	Rilmenidine	Colin T. Dollery Michel E. Safar	20	103	Institute de Recherches Internationales Servier and Laboratoires Biopharma	September 7, 1986	17
E	March 25	Nitrates	Adam Schneeweiss Marija Weiss	19	83	Schwarz Pharma	March 31, 1987	12
F	April 21	Silent Myocardial Ischemia	David P. Lauler	9	49	Marion Laboratories	September 10–12, 1987	7
G	May 9	Angioplasty, Valvuloplasty and Atherectomy	Donald S. Baim	19	117	Advanced Cardiovascular Systems (Eli Lilly)	June 8–9, 1987	12
A	July 11	Congestive Heart Failure	Jay N. Cohn Karl Swedberg John Kjekshus	15	83	Merck Sharp & Dohme	March 27–28, 1987	15
B	July 25	Hypercholesterolemia (Probucol)	John T. Gwynne Colin J. Schwartz	15	81	Merrell Dow	November 13–14, 1987	8
C	August 11	Dopexamine HCl	Paul G. Hugenholtz	16	88	Fisons plc	September 12–13, 1987	11
D	August 25	Flecainide	Jeffery L. Anderson Edward L. C. Pritchett	12	67	3M Riker	October 23–26, 1987	10
E	September 9	Congestive Heart Failure	Hanjörg Just Helmut Drexler Robert Zelis	23	114	F. Hoffman-LaRoche	December 4–5, 1987	9
F	October 1	Cardiovascular Equipment	Joseph C. Greenfield, Jr.	8	44	0	—	—
G	October 5	Systemic Hypertension, Kidney and Calcium	Edward D. Frolich	21	120	Marion Laboratories	April 7–9, 1988	6
H	October 19	Arrhythmias	Raymond L. Woosley	7	49	Bristol Laboratories	March 26, 1988	7
I	November 3	Arrhythmias	Ezra A. Amsterdam Thomas B. Graboys	7	27	A. H. Robins	November 13–14, 1987	12
J	November 11	Lovastatin	David W. Bilheimer	6	49	Merck Sharp & Dohme	March 26, 1988	8
K	December 6	Interventional Cardiology	Robert A. Vogel	7	29	Mallinckrodt	March 26, 1988	9
L	December 20	Encainide	Gerald V. Naccarelli Hein J. J. Wellens	14	84	Bristol Laboratories	June 3–4, 1988	6

TABLE IX Statement of Ownership, Management and Circulation of the 3 Major USA Cardiology Journals in 1988

Journal	Issue	Mean No. Copies Printed/mo*	Mean No. Copies Distributed/mo*	Mean Paid Circulation/mo*
AJC	11/88	29,100	27,950	21,500
Circulation	11/88	27,150	21,700	20,850
JACC	11/88	26,600	22,600	21,700

* For each of the preceding 12 months to the nearest 50.

TABLE X Sources of Articles in *Cardiology Board Review* in 1988

Journal	No.
American Journal of Cardiology	33
Journal of the American College of Cardiology	23
Circulation	13
American Heart Journal	9
British Heart Journal	6
Annals of Internal Medicine	6
New England Journal of Medicine	6
American Journal of Medicine	4
Catheterization and Cardiovascular Diagnosis	1
Total	101

mitted in 1988 were not published until 1989 and some manuscripts published in 1988 had been submitted in 1987. The acceptance rate therefore is roughly 40%. Many manuscripts declined in 1988 were good ones and I am sure that many accepted ones could have been better. I am not of the school that a low acceptance rate necessarily indicates a high quality rate. Many articles appearing in the AJC are quite different from the manuscripts as they appeared when initially submitted to the AJC. Some manuscripts when initially submitted were as long as 14 text pages (those before the references) and these have been reduced to 4-text page brief reports. These manuscripts are accepted but actually they have little resemblance to the manuscripts as they appeared when initially submitted. If the AJC published only long reports, i.e., no Brief Reports or Case Reports, the acceptance rate would be about 25% and as a consequence the amount of information provided to readers by the AJC would be reduced substantially. Thus, in my view, the quality of a journal publication is not determined by the percent of submitted manuscripts declined but the quality of those published and the one is not necessarily indicative of the other.

(2) *What percent of manuscripts published in the AJC come from the USA and what percent from non-USA countries?* This percent has not been determined in recent years. In 1984, 70% of the articles published in the AJC came from the USA and 30% from non-USA countries.[1] I think the percent of manuscripts submitted from non-USA nations has increased in recent years, and, therefore, the percent published probably has also.

(3) *What is the average time interval from manuscript submission to notification of authors of the accept or reject decision, and is the mail service slowing this process significantly?* This interval has not been calculated for any year during my 7-year editorship. I suspect that the interval averages about 30 days. A few manuscripts require 3 months because of late return of reviews or because one or both of the reviewers initially selected returned the manuscript nonreviewed and then it had to be sent to 1 or 2 new reviewers. Occasionally a reviewer returns a manuscript nonreviewed after having retained the manuscript for 30 days or so. The latter circumstance is "no-no" number 1 for reviewers. Many decisions on Case Reports are made the day the manuscripts arrive in the editorial office. Most of the immediate decisions are "rejects." Occasionally an immediate decision is made on editorials. These immediate manuscript decisions counterbalance the few manuscripts in which the review process is excessively delayed. I suspect that the manuscript review process in the AJC is shorter than most journals. Manuscript reviewers are assigned to nearly all submitted manuscripts on the day of their arrival in the editorial office, and the manuscripts are mailed to reviewers the next office working day. By Sunday night of every week the editor's and associate editors' desks are always clean: all manuscripts have been assigned, all revised manuscripts have been accepted or returned to authors for further change and decisions have been made on all manuscripts in which both reviews have been received.

Reviewers for long (full-length) reports are chosen mainly by the associate editors and those for Brief Reports, Case Reports and Editorials are chosen by me. All reviewed manuscripts and all revised manuscripts are placed on my desk for review and decision.

Whether the mail service is adversely affecting the manuscript-processing time is uncertain. Reviewers of manuscripts for the AJC are allotted 3 weeks, and that interval is from the time the manuscript leaves the editorial office until it is due back in that office. Because many manuscripts in the USA require 1 week to arrive at the reviewer's office and another week to be returned by mail, the actual time to review the manuscript and get the review back to the editorial office within the allotted interval is only 7 to 10 days. Thus, it is recommended that reviewers at least quickly examine the manuscript for review the day it arrives so that the review will have some time to be thoughtfully considered.

(4) *Could reviews be returned to the editorial office by FAX?* Yes. Dr. Larry Cohn asked this question. The suggestion in the question is a superb one and we will put our FAX number on the reviewer form. Even if the review is returned by FAX, however, the authors' manuscript with figures and tables and the prepaid return envelope still need to be returned to the editorial office.

(5) *If an author has been accused or proven to have produced fraudulent published data in the past, does the AJC have a policy on subsequent manuscripts submitted by that author?* No. The editor requested suggestions on this matter. I tend to believe that each manuscript should be considered on the basis of its own merits without consideration of past author performance. In my view, incorrect data in manuscripts are infrequently on the

basis of fraudulence; they are far more likely the result of careless collection of data. Whether incorrect published data are intentional, i.e., fradulent, or nonintentional, i.e., careless, however, errors are errors and wrong results may be the consequence.

(6) *What is the AJC policy regarding manuscripts resulting from industry-supported research and are authors advised to submit statements regarding their association with the supporting industry?* Manuscripts based on research supported by industry are processed in the same manner as other manuscripts considered for the regular issues of the *Journal.* I agree with the policy of *The New England Journal of Medicine* that authors presenting results of industry-sponsored research should indicate in the manuscript their financial involvement with the company supporting the research. In general, I believe it unwise for physicians involved in industry-supported research to own stocks or have stock options in the company supporting their research. Incidently, I also believe it unwise for editors of medical journals to own stocks in pharmaceutical or medical equipment companies. For the record, I do not own stock in any pharmaceutical or medical equipment company.

(7) *Does the AJC keep records on the manuscript recommendations of the reviewers?* No. Some reviewers, however, appear to be excessively critical and others, excessively noncritical. I have learned that it is possible to reliably predict the manuscript recommendations of some reviewers. We could gather data on this question, but I would not be certain what to do with it. This type of data might produce bias in the selectors of reviewers of manuscripts.

The meeting was adjourned to a reception provided by the publisher. Comments from readers on any of the above items are welcomed.

William C. Roberts

William C. Roberts, MD
Editor in Chief

1. Roberts WC. Country of origin of articles in the AJC in 1984. *Am J Cardiol 1985;56:380.*

Editorial Board Meeting of The American Journal of Cardiology—March 1990

The annual editorial board meeting of The American Journal of Cardiology (AJC) this year was held in New Orleans, Louisiana, on March 20 at the time of the Annual Scientific Sessions of the American College of Cardiology. The major purposes of the meeting were to say "thanks" to the 148 board members for their enormous help during the previous year, to pay particular tribute to those board members reviewing the most manuscripts during 1989, to summarize AJC publication figures during 1989, and to receive input from board members through their questions and comments.

(1) *Introduction of new board members:* Fifteen physicians (Table I) were added to the board beginning January 1990, and they were introduced. New board members are selected entirely on their record as nonboard reviewers for the AJC. It is easy to select the new members. The card files of the 1,300 or so nonboard AJC reviewers are reviewed and the 15 or 20 with the best reviewing records are selected. Many other nonboard reviewers are deserving of board status, but all obviously cannot be chosen. It is hoped that the most deserving, however, will eventually become board members.

The task of eliminating about 10% of the board members each year is getting progressively more difficult because most board members do a superb job. The card file of each board member is reviewed after the end of the calendar year; those members with the largest numbers of reviews returned late or manuscripts returned without review are deleted. Thus, each AJC board member determines his or her longevity on the AJC editorial board.

TABLE I New AJC Board Members Beginning in January 1990

1. David G. Benditt
2. William E. Boden
3. Kanu Chatterjee
4. Gregory J. Dehmer
5. James S. Forrester
6. Gary S. Francis
7. Jerome L. Fleg
8. W. Bruce Fye
9. Sidney Goldstein
10. David R. Holmes, Jr.
11. Richard E. Kerber
12. Eric L. Michelson
13. Natesa Pandian
14. Nanette K. Wenger
15. Salim Yusuf

(2) *Numbers of manuscripts received for review by each AJC board member in 1989:* A total of 1,740 manuscripts were submitted to the AJC in 1989, a 13% increase compared to the 1,525 submitted in 1988. The numbers and types of manuscripts sent (95% actually reviewed) to the 4 types of specialists on the board are summarized in Table II. The 148 board members were sent 812 manuscripts to review, an average of 5.5 per member: 751 (95%) were reviewed on time (3 weeks from the mailing date to receiving date from the Bethesda, Maryland, editorial office); 22 manuscripts (3%) were not reviewed within this time period, and 39 manuscripts (5%) were returned without review. As shown in Table II, the 112 adult cardiologists reviewed the most manuscripts (a mean of 6.0), and the 13 cardiac surgeons reviewed the least (a mean of 2.1). The numbers of manuscripts actually reviewed by the board members are summarized in Figure 1.

(3) *AJC board members reviewing the most manuscripts in 1989:* The 14 top reviewers in 1989 are listed in Table III. Drs. Joel Morganroth and David Spodick were tops. Tables IV to VI list board members reviewing 9, 8 and 7 manuscripts, respectively, during 1989.

(4) *Numbers of pages and articles and types of articles published in the AJC in 1989 and comparison to* Circulation *and* The Journal of the American College of Cardiology (JACC)*:* These numbers are summarized in Table VII. The AJC published 2,922 pages in 1988. Fewer pages but more articles were published in the AJC in 1989 than in either Circulation or JACC. The AJC published 699 articles in 1989, a 9% increase compared to the 636 published in 1988. The shorter average length of articles in the AJC (4.15 pages) than in Circulation (8.55 pages) or JACC (6.60 pages) and the slightly greater

TABLE II Numbers and Types of Manuscripts Sent to AJC Board Members in 1989 According to Specialty of Board Member

Specialty	No. on Board	No. MSS Sent (No./Reviewer)	No. LR	No. BR	No. CR	No. (%) Reviews on Time	No. (%) Reviews Late	No. (%) MSS Returned Without Review
Adult cardiologist	112	676 (6.0)	650	23	3	624 (92%)	20 (3%)	32 (5%)
Pediatric cardiologist	19	93 (4.9)	86	6	1	89 (96%)	1 (1%)	3 (3%)
Cardiac surgeon	13	27 (2.1)	23	1	1	24 (89%)	1 (4%)	2 (7%)
Radiologist or pathologist	4	16 (4.0)	16	0	0	14 (88%)	0	2 (12%)
Total	148	812 (5.5)	775 (95%)	30	5	751 (92%)	22 (3%)	39 (5%)

BR = brief report; CR = case report; LR = long report; MSS = manuscripts.

content per page of articles in the AJC made this possible. Table VII also displays other differences among these 3 USA cardiology journals. No experimental articles (those involving nonhuman animals) were published in the AJC (except for a few in the Brief Reports section) whereas 59 (11% of articles) were published in JACC and 98 (26% of articles) in Circulation. A unique feature of the AJC is the large number of Brief Reports published (187 [27% of articles]) whereas neither of the other 2 journals publish brief reports. Over a third of the Brief Reports published were originally submitted as full-length manuscripts. The AJC published 68 Case Reports (10% of articles) in 1989; all had 1 to 3 case descriptions. Relatively few editorials were published in the AJC in 1989 (32 [4.5% of articles]) compared to Circulation (61 [16% of articles]) and JACC (163 [31% of articles]). The percentages of full-length articles on the various types of heart diseases varied slightly among the 3 journals. The AJC published more on systemic hypertension than did the other 2 journals combined (26 [4%] vs 6 [1%] vs 8 [2%]), and fewer articles on congenital heart disease than JACC (22 vs 38) but more than Circulation (6 articles). All articles published in either JACC or Circulation were categorized as if they had been submitted to the AJC.

(5) *Symposia published in the AJC in 1989:* The AJC published 20 symposia in 1989, one more than in 1988, and they are listed in Table VIII along with their guest editors and sponsors. A total of 232 articles occupying 1,240 pages were published in the 20 symposia.

(6) *Developments affecting the AJC since the last editorial board meeting (March 1989):* In 1989, the regular issues of the AJC appeared every 2 weeks except during the months of August and December when they appeared only once. In 1990, the regular issues will appear twice a month for all 12 months, rather than for just 10 months.

The section of the journal previously called *Letters* was changed in January 1990 to *Readers' Comments*. Nearly all published "letters" are responses to articles published in the AJC and the name change is intended to reflect this fact. Additionally, letters (to the editor) are actually intended to be comments to the readers so that "letters" is not an accurate description. Finally, authors of "letters" to be published tend to write them on their own stationery, single spaced and without titles, and the name change may help in having *Readers' Comments* prepared in a form similar to that of other manuscripts. It is nearly impossible to edit a single spaced "letter" or any other single-spaced manuscript.

(7) *Evaluation of the usefulness of the AJC:* Determining the usefulness of a publication is more difficult than counting the numbers of pages or types of articles published. Of course, the numbers of paid subscribers is an important index. The number of paid subscribers of the AJC is approximately 22,000. In addition to this number the publisher sends out several thousand copies on a rotational basis to potential new subscribers.

Another possible means of evaluating the usefulness of a journal is to examine the number of its articles reviewed in annual or monthly review books or journals. A monthly controlled circulation journal called Cardiolo-

TABLE III Top 14 AJC Reviewers in 1989 and Numbers of Manuscripts Reviewed

Name	No. MSS Reviewed	LR	BR	CR	No. Reviewed on Time
1. Joel Morganroth	13	13	0	0	13
1. David H. Spodick	13	12	1	0	13
3. Abdulmassih S. Iskandrian	12	11	0	1	12
4. Richard O. Cannon, III	11	11	0	0	11
4. Robert L. Feldman	11	11	0	0	10
4. Lowell W. Perry	11	11	0	0	11
4. Eric J. Topol	11	11	0	0	10
8. Bernard R. Chaitman	10	10	0	0	10
8. Pamela S. Douglas	10	9	1	0	10
8. Julius M. Gardin	10	9	1	0	10
8. Leonard N. Horowitz	10	10	0	0	10
8. Jeffrey M. Isner	10	9	1	0	10
8. Spencer B. King, III	10	10	0	0	10
8. Robert A. Kloner	10	9	1	0	10

Abbreviations as in Table II.

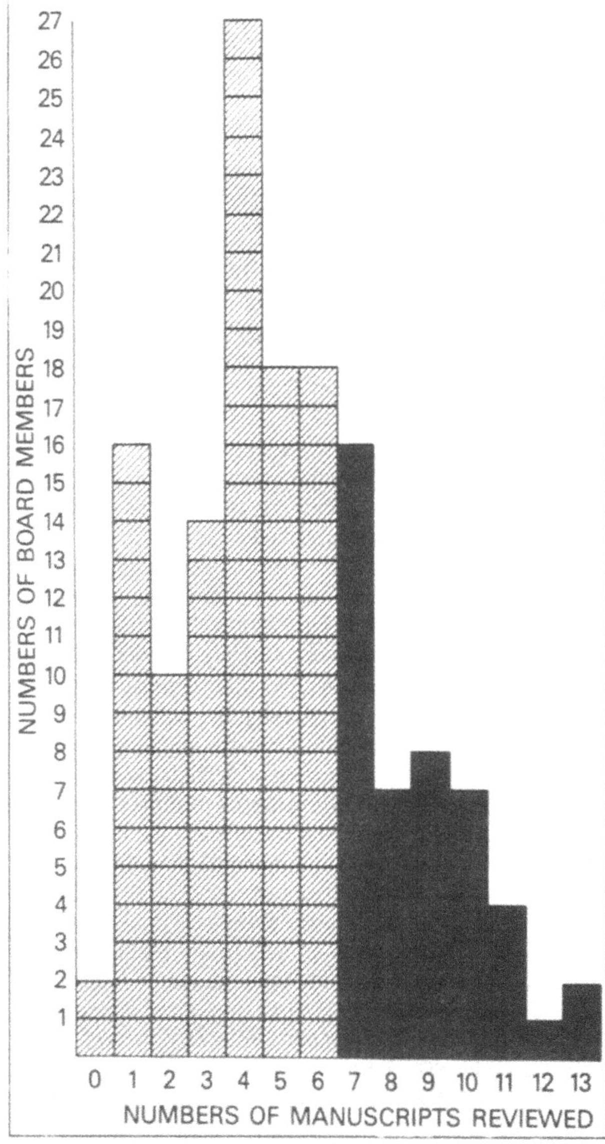

FIGURE 1. Number of manuscripts reviewed by AJC board members in 1989.

TABLE IV Reviewers of Nine Manuscripts for the AJC in 1989

Name	No. MSS Reviewed	LR	BR	CR	No. Reviewed on Time
1. Peter F. Cohn	9	9	0	0	9
2. Robert F. DeBusk	9	9	0	0	8
3. Frank A. Finnerty, Jr.	9	8	1	0	9
4. Kenneth M. Kent	9	9	0	0	8
5. Arthur J. Moss	9	8	1	0	9
6. Carl J. Pepine	9	9	0	0	9
7. Nathaniel Reichek	9	9	0	0	9

Abbreviations as in Table II.

TABLE V Reviewers of Eight Manuscripts for the AJC in 1989

Name	No. MSS Reviewed	LR	BR	CR	No. Reviewed on Time
1. Jeffrey Anderson	8	7	1	0	7
2. George A. Beller	8	8	0	0	8
3. Michael H. Crawford	8	8	0	0	7
4. Pablo Denes	8	8	0	0	7
5. William H. Gaasch	8	8	0	0	8
6. Eugene R. Passamani	8	8	0	0	8
7. Nelson B. Schiller	8	6	2	0	8

Abbreviations as in Table II.

TABLE VI Reviewers of Seven Manuscripts for the AJC in 1989

Name	No. MSS Reviewed	LR	BR	CR	No. Reviewed on Time
1. Robert O. Bonow	7	7	0	0	6
2. George A. Diamond	7	7	0	0	7
3. Myrvin H. Ellestad	7	6	1	0	7
4. Carl V. Leier	7	7	0	0	7
5. Joseph Lindsay, Jr.	7	6	0	1	7
6. Fred Morady	7	7	0	0	7
7. Robert J. Myerburg	7	7	0	0	7
8. Bertram Pitt	7	7	0	0	7
9. Philip J. Podrid	7	6	1	0	7
10. Melvin M. Scheinman	7	7	0	0	7
11. Barry L. Zaret	7	7	0	0	7
12. Warren G. Guntheroth	7	7	0	0	7
13. Howard P. Gutgesell	7	6	1	0	7
14. Grace S. Wolff	7	6	1	0	7

Abbreviations as in Table II.

gy Board Review and edited by Dr. Peter F. Cohn contains 5 to 12 articles monthly and each is a condensed version of an article originally published in a peer-reviewed journal. Table IX summarizes the journals containing the original articles from which the condensed articles were derived in 1989. As in 1986, 1987 and 1988, the AJC was the source of the most articles.

(8) *Request for more high quality editorials:* I think that it would be useful to increase the number of editorials and editorial reviews published in the AJC. The editorial's length should be determined by the complexity of the message delivered. One-point editorials should be short, and multiple-point ones longer.

(9) *Reminder to authors to supply several names of nonlocal, nonbiased reviewers for their manuscripts:* Editors have no monopoly on choosing the best reviewers of manuscripts. No one should be more knowledgeable of experts in the subject of a manuscript than the authors of the manuscript. Thus, I urge authors to supply names—preferably 5 and when they are nonboard members their addresses also—of nonbiased, nonlocal potential reviewers of their manuscripts. It is necessary for an author to supply several names because almost certainly some of the potential reviewers will already have a manuscript for review and a second manuscript is not sent to a reviewer who already possesses one, unless the second manuscript is a brief report or a case report. Presently, in only about 20% of manuscripts submitted have authors provided names of potential reviewers. After studying for several years reviews by reviewers suggested by authors, I am impressed that in general they are of higher quality than those selected by the AJC's editor or associate editors, and that the author-chosen reviewers are not more favorable to a manuscript than are editor-selected reviewers. Indeed, many manuscripts have been reviewed by 1 author-selected reviewer and by 1 editor-selected reviewer and the author-selected reviewer recommended rejection and the editor-selected reviewer recommended acceptance of the manuscript.

(10) *Effectiveness of the policy of blind reviews of all manuscripts:* During the past 8 years authors requesting a blind review of their manuscripts have had their wishes honored. The blind review has been accomplished by the authors providing a separate title page containing the manuscript's title without the names of authors or their institution. The title page containing the authors' and institution's names of course was not submitted to the reviewer. During these past 7 years this author-requested optional blind review process has been used relatively infrequently (probably about 10% of submitted manuscripts) and then almost entirely by authors from less well-known medical centers. On September 1, 1989, a new policy was instituted, and that was to send all manuscripts for blind review, and that policy has been in effect to the present. I have received only 1 letter from a board member commenting on the blind review policy for all manuscripts and 2 paragraphs from that letter are the following:

> "This is the first manuscript that I have received where I was asked to do a blinded review. I would like to express my personal objection at being asked to do this. On the one hand a blinded review could be construed to insure fairness in the review process. On the other hand, a number of groups do poor quality work which is written up quite nicely and which time after time fails to stand the test of time and is refuted by most other reputable groups. If I receive a manuscript with an enthusiastic endorsement of some new antiarrhythmic drug or device, I would place much more emphasis on that report if it came from a laboratory which had over

TABLE VII Number of Pages and Types of Articles Published in the Regular Issues of *The American Journal of Cardiology, Journal of the American College of Cardiology* and *Circulation* in 1989

	American Journal of Cardiology	Journal of the American College of Cardiology	Circulation
No. of pages	3,356	3,818	3,824
For articles (mean/month) [pages/article]	2,903 (242) [4.15]	3,471 (289) [6.60]	3,274 (273) [8.55]
For letters (number) [number with replies]	19 (36) [7]	25 (25) [15]	18 (16) [8]
For staff, editorial board	22	28	24
For contents in brief	77	28	39
For contents with abstracts	230	122	96
For boxed abstracts (for card files)	0	0	117
For information for authors	24	28	24
For volume indexes	75	63	51
For miscellaneous	11*	53†	181‡
No. of articles (mean/month)	699 (58)	526 (44)	383 (32)
Coronary artery disease	172 (24.6%)	100 (19.0%)	76 (19.8%)
Arrhythmias and conduction defects	70 (10.0%)	52 (9.9%)	25 (6.5%)
Systemic hypertension	26 (3.7%)	6 (1.1%)	8 (2.1%)
Congestive heart failure	19 (2.7%)	11 (2.1%)	15 (3.9%)
Valvular heart disease	22 (3.1%)	32 (6.1%)	17 (4.4%)
Cardiomyopathy	9 (1.3%)	22 (4.2%)	11 (2.9%)
Congenital heart disease	22 (3.1%)	38 (7.2%)	6 (1.6%)
Methods	14 (2.0%)	14 (2.7%)	6 (1.6%)
Experimental studies	0	59 (11.2%)	98 (25.6%)
Historical studies	3 (0.4%)	4 (0.8%)	0
Miscellaneous	55 (7.9%)	15 (2.9%)	59 (15.4%)
Brief reports	187 (26.8%)	0	0
Case reports	68 (9.7%)	9 (1.7%)	0
Editorials and editorial reviews	22 (3.1%)	163 (31.0%)	61 (15.9%)
From the editor	10 (1.4%)	0	1 (0.3%)

* Includes 42 abstracts of the cardiology section of a pediatric society.
† Includes items related to The American College of Cardiology.
‡ For American Heart Association News, Meetings Calendar, list of names of nonboard reviewers of manuscripts submitted to Circulation and table of contents of Circulation Research, Hypertension, Arteriosclerosis and Japan Heart Journal.

the years presented well-balanced pictures in all of their publications. On the other hand, my review would be influenced somewhat if it came from a laboratory that was always enthusiastic about every single compound or device to come along and which had close relationships with industry that might result in this ongoing string of glowing reports of new therapies.

"While there may be certain inherent biases in my review in this regard, I try to be as objective as possible about each individual review and the above factors only play a minor role in my final decision. In general, I think each manuscript should stand on its own merit. However, if I am on the fence about whether or not a manuscript should be accepted or rejected, knowledge of the quality of work from the laboratory from which it is submitted would definitely influence my decision one way or the other. Finally, in these days where there is so much potential for conflict of interest due to various financial and other relationships between authors and the subjects about which they are publishing, knowledge of the individual investigators is extremely important. Not that this should in any way influence whether the manuscript is published, but it would permit the reviewer to point out potential conflicts of interest to the editor and be certain that the authors have disclosed them to the editor."

The concept of reviewing all submitted manuscripts blindly was discussed by several board members. Several board members commented that they were able to identify the authors and their institutions readily from the authors' references to their own institutions in the manuscripts, or from the mention of the name of their institution in the text of the manuscript. Authors' names frequently are left on the backs of figures and tables. Thus, although the manuscript-review process is intended to be blinded, authors of the manuscripts actually often prevent a blind review process. After considerable discussion a vote was taken. It appeared that about one-half of the editorial board members present favored the blind review policy for all manuscripts, and that the other one-half were against it.

Discussed briefly were mechanisms by which data could be obtained comparing reviewer comments and recommendations of the same manuscript reviewed blindly by one reviewer and in a nonblinded fashion by the other reviewer. The problem here, of course, is that the same reviewer cannot review the same manuscript in both a blinded and in a nonblinded fashion. It would be easy, however, to send the same manuscript for a blinded review to one reviewer and for a nonblinded review to the other reviewer and simply add up the recommendations (definitely accept, probably accept, definitely reject, probably reject) for a large number of manuscripts of those reviewed blindly compared to those reviewed nonblindly. This policy will be instituted on April 1, 1990, for at least several months.

Questions on other subjects from board members followed:

TABLE VIII Symposia Published in the AJC in 1989

	1989 Date of Publication	Subject of Symposium	Guest Editor(s)	Sponsor	Number Articles	Number Pages for Articles	Interval (months) Symposium to Publication
A	January 3	Phosphodiesterase inhibitors	Edmund H. Sonnenblick	Winthrop	11	53	8
B	January 17	Systemic hypertension (triamterene/hydrochlorothiazide)	Norman K. Hollenberg	Lederle	8	41	9
C	February 2	Acute hypertension (urapidil)	Antoon Amery Hugo Van Aken	ByK Gulden	13	50	10
D	February 21	Congestive heart failure (enalapril)	William W. Parmley	Merck, Sharp & Dohme	8	37	16
E	March 7	Myocardial ischemia	Chuichi Kawai Dirk L. Brutsaert John Ross, Jr.	Otsuka	22	120	20
F	October 1	Technologic equipment	Joseph C. Greenfield Jr.	—	4	42	—
G	April 18	Magnesium deficiency (MgCl)	David P. Lauler	GD Searle	8	46	7
H	May 2	Cardiovascular disease in the elderly	Thomas C. Cesario	Warner-Lambert	13	59	14
I	June 5	Systemic hypertension (labetalol)	William H. Frishman J. David Wallin Alberto Zanchetti	Key	16	78	11
J	June 20	Angina pectoris and congestive heart failure (nicorandil)	Stanley H. Taylor Kazuzo Kato	Rhône Poulenc Sante and Chugai	15	85	8
A	July 5	Thrombolysis in myocardial infarction (Eminase) [APSAC]	Jeffrey L. Anderson	Beecham	8	42	6
B	July 18	Myocardial infarction	William C. Roberts	DuPont	9	43	7
C	August 2	George E. Burch Festschrift	Thomas D. Giles Gary E. Sander	Musser-Burch Society, Department of Medicine Tulane University	11	60	—
D	August 15	Urapidil	Pieter A. van Zwieten	ByK Gulden Lomberg GmbH	8	39	9
E	September 5	Cardiovascular imaging	Carl L. Tommaso Gerald L. Wolf	Winthrop	11	63	6
F	September 19	Nifedipine	William H. Frishman	Pfizer	12	69	?
G	October 3	Lipids	John T. Gwynne	Merrell Dow	6	38	6
H	October 17	Nicardipine	William W. Parmley	Syntex	8	41	26
I	November 7	Amiodipine	Arnold Schwartz Pieter A. van Zwieten	Pfizer	17	137	24
J	December 5	Arrhythmia treatment	A. John Camm Yoshio Watanabe Kazuo Yamada	Roussel and Chugai	24	97	10
20					232	1,240	Mean 12

(1) *How often is a third review requested on a manuscript that has received 1 accept recommendation and 1 reject recommendation?* Probably 20% of the time. If I feel comfortable with the subject of the manuscript, I make a decision after 2 reviews despite the opposite recommendations by the 2 reviewers. Often also a reviewer might recommend rejection of a manuscript but the reviewers' comments and criticisms are such that the recommendation could just as easily have been accept. Also, when 1 reviewer is extremely favorable toward a manuscript, the extremely positive review often neutralizes the negative review. The status of the 2 reviewers also is helpful. When 1 reviewer is a senior well-respected investigator and the other reviewer is a young beginning investigator, these factors are taken into consideration. Younger reviewers in general tend to be more critical I believe than the older reviewers. The 2 views often provide a nice balance. Thus, in general, I try not to seek a third review, because it means that the review process starts all over again and the decision on disposition of the manuscript is delayed. When a third review is requested I send the reviews of the first 2 reviewers to the third reviewer so that he or she better understands the issue of the particular manuscript at hand. Numerical data on the frequency of a third review will be recorded beginning April 1, 1990.

Recently, in a few manuscripts receiving strongly opposing recommendations (definitely accept from 1 reviewer and definitely reject from the other reviewer), I have returned the manuscript immediately to the reviewer (before returning it to the authors) who recommended definitely reject with the review of the reviewer who had recommended definitely accept requesting that the reviewer point out to me the incorrect judgments of the favorable reviewer. This process has not been carried out yet in sufficient numbers of manuscripts to form a judgment on this process.

(2) *Should one reviewer of a manuscript be provided with the name of the other reviewer of the same manuscript?* At present, each reviewer of a manuscript sent to the AJC is provided the review of the other reviewer. The other reviewer's name, however, is camouflaged so that it is rarely discernible. The consensus was that the names of the 2 reviewers should not be revealed to each other. Thus, the present system of name concealment will re-

main. The exception, as mentioned earlier, is when a third review is sought and then the names of the first 2 reviewers are disclosed to the third reviewer.

(3) *Are any manuscripts accepted without review?* The answer depends on whether or not the editor is considered a reviewer. If the editor is considered a reviewer, the answer is no. If the editor is not considered a reviewer, the answer is yes. Although most are sent for outside review, some editorials that are accepted are not sent out for review. An occasional case report or brief report is accepted after review by the editor only. Many case reports are declined without outside review. Nearly all Brief Reports and all long reports are sent to 2 reviewers. An occasional manuscript is returned from 1 reviewer without review, and if the review by the other reviewer appears to be a particularly good one, a decision on that manuscript is made without seeking a second review.

(4) *If a manuscript is declined by another journal, can the reviews provided by that journal be submitted with the manuscript if it is then submitted to the AJC?* Yes. This policy was instituted in January 1985 and 3 paragraphs from that piece were as follows[1]:

> "An unfortunate principle of the peer-review process is that the best manuscripts receive the fewest reviews and the worst manuscripts receive the most reviews. The best manuscripts are usually accepted by the first journal to which they are sent. Therefore, they receive 1 to 3 reviews, depending on the policy of the particular journal; the manuscript usually is revised to varying degrees, and then accepted. The process for the less-than-superb or the inferior manuscript is not so rapid. The first journal to which the manuscript is sent may acquire 2 reviews for it, and when neither reviewer recommends acceptance and the editor agrees, the manuscript with the reviews is returned to the submitting author. Then the latter usually submits the manuscript to another journal, ideally after having revised the manuscript as suggested by the reviewers from the first submission. The editor of the journal receiving the previously rejected manuscript then sends it to 2 more reviewers—on occasion, to one who happened to have reviewed the manuscript for the first journal. These reviewers in turn often also provide unfavorable recommendations for the manuscript for the first journal. The editor then returns the rejected manuscript to the authors, who in turn send it to another journal with or without additional revisions. The duplication process continues.
>
> "To prevent this depletion of reviewers' energies and also to prevent further publication delay, I suggest to authors who submit a manuscript rejected by another journal to the AJC that the authors enclose copies of all reviews from the previous journal, a copy of the original manuscript, 3 copies of the revised manuscript, and a response to all items raised by all reviewers from the previous journal. In other words, the response to the reviews from the previous journal should be identical to the response given reviews had they been sent from the AJC. This procedure might allow the AJC editor to make a rapid accept or reject decision on the manuscript, or it might allow him to send the manuscript for reexamination to only 1 reviewer rather than 2. . . .
>
> "I would welcome a thorough evaluation of this time-saving process and I will do my best not to be offended because the manuscript had not been sent initially to the AJC. I also urge other editors of cardiovascular journals to adopt the same procedure, because all 4 major USA cardiovascular journals essentially use the same pool of reviewers. The concept needs full testing so that the energies for reviewing will be conserved and those energies expended will be utilized more effectively and efficiently."

TABLE IX Sources of Articles in *Cardiology Board Review* in 1989

Journal	No. (%)
American Journal of Cardiology	23 (27.1)
Journal of the American College of Cardiology	18 (21.1)
American Heart Journal	13 (15.3)
Circulation	13 (15.3)
American Journal of Medicine	6 (7.1)
Archives of Internal Medicine	5 (5.9)
Annals of Internal Medicine	3 (3.5)
New England Journal of Medicine	3 (3.5)
British Heart Journal	1 (1.2)
Total	85 (100)

This process has been in effect now for 5 years, and I believe that it has been useful. Occasionally, authors who submit their manuscript with previous reviews do not send the manuscript as it appeared when it had been initially submitted. We then call the authors and request that they send the "unrevised" manuscript, and we learn that the authors made no revisions of their manuscript before it was sent to the AJC despite 2 or more reviews from the journal to which it had been submitted earlier. When I learn that authors made no effort to revise or respond to the reviews received from the journal to which it had been submitted previously, I usually return the manuscript to the authors. Nearly all of our manuscripts can be improved when we take into consideration the views of reviewers, and not to do so is an insult to the review process and a sign of a lack of desire for excellence on the part of authors. I believe that we have received some first-class manuscripts by this procedure.

(5) *How often do authors provide suggestions for reviewers of their submitted manuscripts?* Although we have not kept records, I estimate that about 20% of authors provide names of potential reviewers. I would like to see this percent over 75%. I am convinced that scholarly authors can identify reviewers of their manuscripts better than can editors. I do not know how to substantiate this view.

(6) *Dr. William Ganz questioned the policy of the lack of experimental (nonhuman) type articles in the AJC, suggesting that this policy might diminish the prestige of the AJC, particularly in the eyes of young investigators.* This issue is an important one. The decision

to eliminate publication of experimental studies (except in the Brief Report section of the journal) was made in 1986, at the time when the number of pages published in the journal was dramatically reduced. The reduction actually was short-lived (1 year) due to a change in ownership, but subsequently the numbers of manuscripts received has increased far in excess of the numbers of pages available. (In 1989 we received 1,740 manuscripts; in 1982 the number was 1,100, and in 1982 we published 300 more pages than in 1989.) Because experimental manuscripts are usually the longest of any submitted, it is simply not possible to keep the lag time (interval from acceptance of a manuscript to its publication) short, and accept experimental manuscripts. I am convinced that our having the shortest lag time of any peer-reviewed cardiology journal in the world (4 months) encourages authors to send us manuscripts that might otherwise be sent to another journal. We publish manuscripts in a shorter time period than are abstracts published at the annual scientific sessions of either The American Heart Association or The College of Cardiology. Additionally, several readership surveys have indicated that the experimental articles are usually the least read portions of the journal. And our subscribers are paid ones independent of any society. Until the number of pages published in the AJC increases substantially I believe it best for the journal to remain a purely clinical one.

(9) *How many paid subscribers to the AJC are in non-USA countries?* The publisher indicated that this number was approximately 4,000. The non-USA pool of potential subscribers, of course, is a large one, and mechanisms to increase this number are presently being discussed.

The board members were thanked for coming and the meeting was adjourned to a reception provided by the publisher. The editor welcomes comments from readers on any item(s) (or others) discussed herein.

William C. Roberts

William Clifford Roberts, MD
Editor in Chief

1. Roberts WC. A suggestion to lighten the load of manuscript reviewing. *Am J Cardiol 1985;55:247.*

Editorial Board Meeting of The American Journal of Cardiology — 5 March 1991

The annual editorial board meeting of *The American Journal of Cardiology* (AJC) this year was held in Atlanta, Georgia, on March 5 at the time of the Annual Scientific sessions of *The American College of Cardiology*. The major purposes of the meeting were to say "thanks" to the 160 board members for their enormous help during the previous year, to pay particular tribute to those board members reviewing the most manuscripts in 1990, and to receive input from board members through the questions and comments.

(1) *Introduction of new board members:* Ten physicians (Table I) were added to the board beginning January 1991, and they were introduced. New board members are selected entirely on their record as non–board reviewers for the AJC. It is easy to select the new members. The card files of the 1,400 or so non–board AJC reviewers are reviewed and the 10 or so with the best reviewing records are selected. The task of eliminating 10 or so board members each year is getting to be extraordinarily difficult because nearly all board members do a superb job. The card file of each board member is reviewed near the end of the calendar year and those members with the largest numbers of reviews returned late or manuscripts returned without review are deleted. Thus, each board member determines his/her longevity on the AJC board.

(2) *Numbers of manuscripts received for review by each AJC board member in 1990:* A total of 1,725 manuscripts were received in 1990, a 5% increase over 1989, a 20% increase over 1988, and a 60% increase over 1982, the first year of the present editorship. The numbers and types of manuscripts sent (96% actually reviewed) to the 4 types of specialists on the board are summarized in Table II. The 160 board members were sent 844 manuscripts to review, an average of 5.2 per member: 788 (93%) were reviewed on time (3 weeks from the mailing date to receiving date from the Bethesda, Maryland, editorial office); only 20 manuscripts (3%) were not reviewed within this time period; and 36 manuscripts (4%) were returned without review.

(3) *AJC board members reviewing the most manuscripts in 1990:* The top 13 reviewers (the "double-digit guys") in 1990 are listed in Table III. An attempt was made in 1990 to send no more than 10 manuscripts to any AJC board member. (I am certainly aware that AJC board members also review many manuscripts for

TABLE I New Editorial Board Members for 1991

1. J. Thomas Bigger, Jr.
2. Peter C. Block
3. Kenneth M. Borow
4. Richard B. Devereux
5. William D. Edwards
6. Sidney O. Gottlieb
7. Geoffrey O. Hartzler
8. Raymond G. McKay
9. Catherine M. Otto
10. Augusto D. Pichard

TABLE II Numbers and Types of Manuscripts Sent to AJC Board Members in 1990 According to Speciality of Board Member

Speciality	No. on Board	No. MSS Sent (No./Reviewer)	No. LR	No. BR	No. CR	No. (%) Reviews on Time	No. (%) Reviews Late	No. (%) MSS Returned Without Review
Adult cardiologist	124	720 (5.8)	679	38	3	683 (95%)	15 (2%)	22 (3%)
Pediatric cardiologist	18	78 (4.3)	65	11	2	66 (85%)	2 (2%)	10 (13%)
Cardiac surgeon	14	28 (2.0)	28	0	0	26 (93%)	1 (3.5%)	1 (3.5%)
Radiologist or pathologist	4	18 (4.5)	17	1	0	13 (72%)	2 (11%)	3 (17%)
Totals	160	844 (5.2)	789 (93%)	50	5	788 (93%)	20 (3%)	36 (4%)

BR = brief reports; CR = case reports; LR = long reports; MSS = manuscripts.

other medical journals.) Tables IV to VII list board members reviewing 9, 8, 7 and 6 manuscripts, respectively, in 1990.

(4) *Numbers of pages and articles and types of articles published in the AJC in 1990:* These data are presented in Table VIII. A total of 662 articles were published in 3,001 pages in 1990, an average of 55 articles a month with each having an average length of 4.53 pages. Among the 448 long reports, 205 (46%) concerned coronary artery disease; 66 (15%), arrhythmias and conduction disturbances; 33 (7%), congestive heart failure; 27 (6%), congenital heart disease; 24 (5%), valvular heart disease; and 20 (4%), systemic hypertension. Miscellaneous conditions (43 [10%]), cardiomyopathy (14 [3%]), methods (14 [3%]) and historical studies (2 [<1%]) comprised small percentages of the 448 long reports. Additionally, 158 brief reports, 23 case reports, and 33 editorials were published. I would like to increase the numbers of articles on systemic hypertension. The percentage of brief reports—the unique feature of the AJC—concerning coronary artery disease is much less than that comprising the long reports.

(5) *Symposia published in the AJC in 1990:* Twenty symposia were published in 1990, the same number as in 1989. Each is published under separate white cover from the regular issues under blue cover.

(6) *Country of origin of articles in the AJC in 1990:* The country of origin of articles in the AJC was last tabulated for 1984 and for that year 70% of the articles published were from the USA and 30% were from non-USA countries.[1] Of the 662 articles published in the

TABLE III Top AJC Board Reviewers in 1990 and Numbers of Manuscripts Reviewed

Name	No. MSS Reviewed	LR	BR	CR	No. Reviewed on Time
1. Jawahar Mehta	12	12	0	0	12
2. Robert L. Feldman	11	11	0	0	11
2. William B. Kannel	11	11	0	0	11
4. Michael H. Crawford	10	9	1	0	10
4. Pablo Denes	10	9	1	0	10
4. Julius M. Gardin	10	9	1	0	10
4. David R. Holmes, Jr.	10	9	1	0	10
4. Abdulmassih S. Iskandrian	10	8	1	1	10
4. Carl V. Leier	10	9	1	0	10
4. Fred Morady	10	9	1	0	10
4. Melvin M. Scheinman	10	10	0	0	10
4. David H. Spodick	10	7	3	0	10
4. Salim Yusuf	10	10	0	0	10
Totals	134	123 (92%)	10	1	134 (100%)

Abbreviations as in Table II.

TABLE IV Reviewers of Nine Manuscripts for the AJC in 1990

Name	No. MSS Reviewed	LR	BR	CR	No. Reviewed on Time
1. Robert O. Bonow	9	8	1	0	7
2. Pamela S. Douglas	9	9	0	0	9
3. Joseph A. Franciosa	9	8	1	0	9
4. Leonard N. Horowitz	9	9	0	0	9
5. Jeffrey M. Isner	9	9	0	0	9
6. Joel Morganroth	9	9	0	0	9
7. Eugene R. Passamani	9	8	1	0	9
8. Joseph K. Perloff	9	7	2	0	9
9. Philip J. Podrid	9	9	0	0	9
10. Nathaniel Reichek	9	9	0	0	9
11. Eric J. Topol	9	8	1	0	9
Totals	99	93 (94%)	6	0	97 (98%)

Abbreviations as in Table II.

TABLE V Reviewers of Eight Manuscripts for the AJC in 1990

Name	No. MSS Reviewed	LR	BR	CR	No. Reviewed on Time
1. George A. Beller	8	8	0	0	8
2. Richard O. Cannon, III	8	8	0	0	8
3. Frank A. Finnerty, Jr.	8	8	0	0	8
4. William H. Gaasch	8	8	0	0	8
5. L. David Hillis	8	7	1	0	8
6. Spencer B. King, III	8	8	0	0	8
7. Frank I. Marcus	8	8	0	0	7
8. Franz H. Messerli	8	8	0	0	7
9. Robert J. Myerburg	8	8	0	0	8
10. Natesa Pandian	8	7	1	0	8
11. Bramah N. Singh	8	8	0	0	8
12. James T. Willerson	8	8	0	0	8
Totals	96	94 (98%)	2	0	94 (98%)

Abbreviations as in Table II.

TABLE VI Reviewers of Seven Manuscripts for the AJC in 1990

Name	No. MSS Reviewed	LR	BR	CR	No. Reviewed on Time
1. Peter F. Cohn	7	7	0	0	7
2. Gregory J. Dehmer	7	7	0	0	7
3. Jack Ferlinz	7	7	0	0	7
4. Bernard Gersh	7	7	0	0	7
5. Richard E. Kerber	7	7	0	0	7
6. Robert A. Kloner	7	7	0	0	7
7. Joseph Lindsay, Jr.	7	6	1	0	7
8. Bertram Pitt	7	7	0	0	7
9. Robert Roberts	7	7	0	0	7
10. Nelson B. Schiller	7	5	2	0	7
11. Ralph Shabetai	7	6	1	0	7
12. Pravin M. Shah	7	7	0	0	6
13. Nanette K. Wenger	7	5	2	0	7
14. Howard P. Gutgesel	7	6	1	0	7
15. Lowell W. Perry	7	2	3	2	7
Totals	105	93 (89%)	10	2	104 (99%)

Abbreviations as in Table II.

AJC in 1990, 65% were from the USA and 35% were from non–USA countries (Table IX).

(7) *Sources of articles in Cardiology Board Review in 1990:* A possible means of evaluating the usefulness of a journal is to examine the number of its articles reviewed in annual or monthly review books or journals. A monthly controlled circulation journal called *Cardiology Board Review* and edited by Dr. Peter F. Cohn contains 5 to 12 articles monthly and each is a condensed version of an article originally published in a peer-reviewed journal. Table X summarizes the journals containing the original articles from which the condensed articles were derived in 1990. As in 1986, 1987, 1988, and 1989, the AJC was the source of the most articles.

(8) *Reminder to authors to supply several names of nonlocal nonbiased reviewers for their manuscripts:* Editors have no monopoly on choosing the best reviewers of manuscripts. No one should be more knowledgeable of experts in the subject of a manuscript than the authors of the manuscript. Thus, I urge authors to supply names—preferably 5 and when they are non–board members their addresses also—of nonbiased, nonlocal potential reviewers of their manuscripts. It is necessary for an author to supply several names because almost certainly some of the potential reviewers will already have a manuscript for review and a second manuscript is not sent to a reviewer who already possesses one, unless the second manuscript is a brief report or a case report. Currently, in only about 20% of manuscripts submitted have authors provided names of potential reviewers. After studying for several years reviews by reviewers suggested by authors, I am impressed that the author-chosen reviewers are of

TABLE VII Reviewers of Six Manuscripts for the AJC in 1990

Name	No. MSS Reviewed	LR	BR	CR	No. Reviewed on Time
1. Joseph S. Alpert	6	4	2	0	6
2. George A. Diamond	6	6	0	0	6
3. Jeffrey M. Hoeg	6	6	0	0	6
4. G. B. John Mancini	6	6	0	0	6
5. Francis E. Marchlinski	6	6	0	0	6
6. Arthur J. Moss	6	6	0	0	6
7. Robert A. O'Rourke	6	6	0	0	6
8. Carl J. Pepine	6	5	1	0	4
9. Allan M. Ross	6	6	0	0	6
10. Douglas P. Zipes	6	6	0	0	6
11. James E. Lock	6	5	1	0	6
Totals	66	62 (94%)	4	0	64 (97%)

Abbreviations as in Table II.

TABLE VIII Numbers of Pages and Numbers and Types of Articles Published in the American Journal of Cardiology in 1990

Number of Pages	3498
For Articles (Average 4.53 Pages/Article)	3,001 (85.79%)
For Readers' Comments (Number) [Number with Replies]	20(40) (11)
For Staff, Editorial Board	24
For Contents in Brief	83 (2.37%) } (9.03%)
For Contents with Abstracts	233 (6.66%) } (9.03%)
For Boxed Abstracts in Advertising Pages	0
For Information for Authors	24
For Abstracts Within Editorial Pages	10
For Volume Indexes	103 (2.94%)
Number of Articles (Mean/Month)	662 (55/Month)
Coronary Artery Disease	205 (30.97%)
Arrhythmias and Conduction Disturbances	66 (9.97%)
Systemic Hypertension	20 (3.02%)
Congestive Heart Failure	33 (4.98%)
Valvular Heart Disease	24 (3.63%)
Cardiomyopathy	14 (2.11%)
Congenital Heart Disease	27 (4.08%)
Methods	14 (2.11%)
Experimental Studies	0 (0)
Historical Studies	2 (0.30%)
Miscellaneous	43 (6.50%)
Brief Reports	158 (23.87%)
Case Reports	23 (3.47%)
Editorials and Editorial Reviews	25 (3.78%)
From the Editor Columns	8 (1.21%)

TABLE IX Country of Origin of Articles in the AJC in 1990

Country	Number (%) of Articles
1. USA	432 (65%)
2. Italy	34 (5%)
3. Canada	33 (5%)
4. Germany	25 (4%)
5. Japan	22 (3%)
6. United Kingdom	20 (3%)
7. Scandinavia	17 (3%)
8. Israel	14 (2%)
9. France	12 (2%)
10. The Netherlands	12 (2%)
11. Australia	6 (1%)
12. Belgium	5 (1%)
13. Others	30 (4%)
Total	662 (100%)

TABLE X Sources of Articles Published in Cardiology Board Review in 1990

Journal	No. (%) of Articles
1. American Journal of Cardiology	22 (29.3%)
2. Journal of the American College of Cardiology	19 (25.3%)
3. New England Journal of Medicine	12 (16.0%)
4. Circulation	7 (9.3%)
5. American Journal of Medicine	5 (6.7%)
6. American Heart Journal	3 (4.0%)
7. Annals of Internal Medicine	3 (4.0%)
8. Archives of Internal Medicine	3 (4.0%)
9. British Heart Journal	1 (1.3%)
Total	75 (100%)

high quality and that the author-chosen reviewers are not more favorable to a manuscript than are editor-selected reviewers. Indeed, many manuscripts have been reviewed by 1 author-selected reviewer and by 1 editor-selected reviewer and the author-selected reviewer recommended rejection and the editor-selected reviewer recommended acceptance of the manuscript.

Questions and comments on other subjects from board members follow:

(1) *What was the acceptance rate in the AJC in 1990?* Approximately 38%. A total of 1,725 manuscripts were submitted to the AJC in 1990, and 662 manuscripts were published in the AJC in 1990. Some manuscripts published in 1990, however, had been submitted in 1989, and some manuscripts submitted in 1990 were not published until 1991. Thus, I do not know the precise percentage of the 1,725 manuscripts submitted in 1990 which will be published. The acceptance rate, however, is approximately 38%. The acceptance rate is a bit deceptive because many manuscripts initially submitted as long reports are published as brief reports. If it were not for the brief report section, the acceptance rate would be much lower.

(2) *Has there been a readership survey on the desirability of 2 regular issues of the AJC each month versus only 1 regular issue each month?* No. Last year was the first year of having 2 regular issues of the AJC each month or a total of 24 regular issues in the year. (In 1989, 22 regular issues were published.) A vote was held among board members present and *all* favored a single regular monthly issue over 2 regular issues each month. With 24 regular issues each year plus approximately 20 symposium issues each year, some AJC publication is received by a subscriber nearly every week.

(3) *Does it cost more to publish 2 regular issues a month compared to publishing only 1 regular issue monthly?* Yes. The mailing costs, paper costs (covers, table of contents, instructions to authors, etc.) are greater, but advertising revenue is greater—not great enough, however, to counterbalance the increased publishing expenses.

(4) *Editorial board members were asked if they like the Brief Reports section of the Journal.* The response was strongly yes. One board member suggested having a final summary sentence for each report and this suggestion will be acted on.

(5) *What is the lag time currently between acceptance of a manuscript and its publication?* At present, the period is between 3.5 and 4.0 months. During most of 1990 it was 4 months. This short lag time, in my view, is one of the most attractive features of the AJC to authors.

(6) *Why not publish the Instructions to Authors only once in each volume (twice a year)?* Currently the Instructions are published in each of the 24 regular issues. The Instructions occupy a single page and the managing editor likes to use this page anywhere in the journal as "a filler." Thus, the present policy will stay.

(7) *Add a statement in the Instructions to Authors about the policy of submission of manuscripts, declined by another journal, with the reviews from the other journal and the authors responses to them:* This suggestion is a good one and it will be carried out. I am pleased with the policy of making rapid decisions on manuscripts declined by other journals. It is incumbent upon authors submitting each manuscript, however, to respond in detail to each suggestion by the previous reviewers and to submit to the AJC the manuscript initially submitted to the previous journal, as well as the revised manuscript. Too often, the previous reviews are submitted to the AJC and only a single manuscript. The authors are then asked to submit to the AJC a copy of the manuscript initially submitted to the other journal, and when it is sent to the AJC it is no different than the manuscript initially submitted to the AJC. In other words, the authors have totally ignored the suggestions of the reviewers and have made no changes in their manuscript. This conduct is disrespectful of the review process. Virtually all of our manuscripts can be improved by responding to reviewers' suggestions.

(8) *The desirability of reinstituting the policy of publishing experimental studies* (those involving nonhuman animals) *was raised by a board member:* Some background. From its beginning in 1958 most issues of the AJC have contained 1 or more experimental-type articles. In 1983, fifty-two (10%) of the 529 long reports (excludes brief reports, case reports and editorials) in the AJC were experimental studies.[2] Experimental studies comprised 64 (13%) of the 500 long reports in the AJC in 1984,[3] and 49 (11%) of the 432 long reports in 1985.[4] In 1986 only 4 experimental studies were published as long reports,[5] and since that time none has been published. An occasional experimental study, however, continues to be published in the brief report section of the journal. Although approximately 10% of the long reports in the journal until 1986 were experimental studies, these studies occupied a higher percentage of the editorial pages because experimental studies tend to be longer than the clinical studies.

In 1982, the first year of the present editorship, approximately 1,100 manuscripts were submitted and over 3,300 pages of articles were published. By 1986, the number of manuscripts submitted had risen to approximately 1,600 (a 31% increase) and the numbers of editorial pages available for articles had fallen to approximately 2,650 (a 20% decrease). In 1990, the numbers of manuscripts submitted had further risen to 1,725, but the number of pages for articles had increased to 3,001.[6] The decision to eliminate the publication of experimental studies in 1986 was made because of the increased volume of manuscripts submitted along with the decreased numbers of editorial pages available, and the knowledge that the experimental studies were in general the longest manuscripts and the ones least read according to readership surveys. Thus, the AJC since 1986 has been a purely clinical journal.

The other 3 major USA paid-subscription cardiology journals publish many experimental-type manuscripts.[6] Of the 419 long reports (excludes 109 editorials) published in *Circulation* in 1990, one hundred and thirty-two (32%) were experimental studies; of the 393 long reports (excludes 141 editorials and 6 case reports) published in the *Journal of the American College of Cardiology* in 1990, fifty (13%) were experimental studies; and of the 300 long reports (excludes 168 case reports, 12 brief reports, and 9 editorials) published in the *American Heart Journal* in 1990, 29 (10%) were experimental studies.[6] The percentage of pages occupied by the experimental studies in these 3 cardiology journals was greater than the percentage of articles composed of these studies. In contrast to *The American Journal of Cardiology* (and also the *American Heart Journal*), both *Circulation* and the *Journal of the American College of Cardiology* have a substantial automatic readership base (I believe about 18,000) because these 2 journals are received by members of their respective societies (American Heart Association and American College of Cardiology) as part of the membership dues. The readers of the AJC, in contrast, subscribe to the journal because they like what they find in it, and it is difficult, in my view, to keep a substantial readership base (22,000—approximately the same as *Circulation* and the *Journal of the American College of Cardiology*) by publishing experimental studies.

Suggestions by board members included limiting the number of experimental studies published in the AJC to 2 per month, limiting of the length of experimental-type manuscripts, and processing for review only those experimental-type manuscripts that had clearly clinically applicable implications, and returning without review the other experimental-type manuscripts submitted.

A show of hands indicated that approximately 60% of board members present favored the reinstitution of publication of experimental studies as long reports and that approximately 40% favored the present policy of not publishing experimental studies (except in the brief report section of the journal). At the reception following the meeting, many board members encouraged me to continue the present policy: "Do not meddle with success"; "keep it a purely clinical journal"; "if a written ballot had been taken at the meeting, the present policy would have won." After considerable thought, I plan to continue with the present policy because the editorial pages allocated for 1991 will not be quite as large as 1990; the content per page will decrease beginning April 1991 for the publisher has decided to increase the size of the type which will decrease the number of columns and words per column; the number of manuscripts submitted probably will continue to rise, and maintaining an extremely short lag time between manuscript acceptance and publication will be far more difficult if the door is opened to experimental-type manuscripts which are usually long. I would welcome comments from readers on this or other topics.

The meeting was adjourned to a reception provided by the publisher.

William C. Roberts

William Clifford Roberts, MD
Editor in Chief

1. Roberts WC. Country of origin of articles in the AJC in 1984. *Am J Cardiol* 1985;56:380.

2. Roberts WC. Comparison of 7 English-language cardiology journals for 1983. *Am J Cardiol* 1984;53:862–869.

3. Roberts WC. Analysis of page utilization and types of articles published in four major American cardiology journals in 1984. *International J Cardiol* 1985;8:353–360.

4. Roberts WC. The AJC in 1986. *Am J Cardiol* 1987;59:391–392.

5. Roberts WC. The AJC in 1987. *Am J Cardiol* 1988;61:672–674.

6. Roberts WC. Comparison of the four major USA cardiology journals in 1990: a look at 51 kilograms (112 pounds) of journals and over 15,000 editorial pages. *Am J Cardiol* 1991;67:551–554.

Editorial Board Meeting of *The American Journal of Cardiology* on 14 April 1992

The annual editorial board meeting of *The American Journal of Cardiology* (AJC) in 1992 was held in Dallas, Texas, on April 14 at the time of the Annual Scientific Sessions of *The American College of Cardiology*. The major purposes of the meeting were to say "thanks" to the 164 board members for their enormous help during the previous year, to pay particular tribute to the board members reviewing the most manuscripts in 1991, and to receive input from board members through questions and comments.

1. Introduction of new board members: Fifteen physicians (Table I) were added to the board beginning January 1992, and they were introduced. New board members are selected entirely on their record as non-board reviewers for the AJC. It is relatively easy to select the new board members. The card files of the 1,400 or so non-board AJC reviewers are reviewed and the 15 or so with the best reviewing records are selected. Usually about a similar number of members are eliminated from the board. In 1991, however, all board members did such a superb job that none could be readily removed. In the future some infrequently- or inadequately-used board members will have to be eliminated to make room for the many non-board reviewers deserving of board status.

2. Number of manuscripts sent for review to board members in 1991: A total of 1,615 manuscripts were received in the Bethesda, Maryland, editorial office in 1992 (This number does not include the manuscripts for the supplement issues.), and 984 of them were sent to the 4 types of specialists on the board (Table II). Of the 984 manuscripts, an average of 6.0 per board member, 938 (95%) were reviewed on time (3 weeks from the mailing date to the receiving date), only 18 (2%) were not reviewed within the 3-week period, and 45 manuscripts (4%) were returned without review.

3. AJC board members reviewing the most manuscripts in 1991: The top 16 reviewers in 1991 are listed in Table III; of the 235 manuscripts reviewed by these 16 members, the reviews in 228 (97%) were returned on time. Table IV lists the 19 board members reviewing 9 or 8 manuscripts in 1991; of the 159 manuscripts reviewed by them, all reviews were received within the 3-week time period. Table V lists the 22 members who each reviewed 7 manuscripts in 1991; of the 154 manuscripts reviewed, 150 (97%) were reviewed on time. The reviewing records of these 62 board members (representing 38% of the board members) is truly remarkable!

4. Numbers of pages and articles and types of articles published in the AJC in 1991: These data are presented in Table VI. A total of 680 articles were published on 3,165 pages in 1991, an average of 57 articles a month, with each having an average length of 4.65 pages. These numbers represent a 5% increase (3,001 to 3,165) in the numbers of pages for articles and a 3% increase (662 to 680) in the numbers of articles published in 1991 compared to 1990. The reasons for the increase in articles published in 1991 was a 13% increase in the number of brief reports (158 to 182) published, a 6% decrease in the numbers of long reports (448 to 421) published, and a 5% increase in the numbers of pages published. An editorial stylistic change was made in the *Journal* beginning April 15, 1991, and this change resulted in an approximately 15% decrease in the content per page on the pages without tables or figures. The size type used and the space between lines were

TABLE I New Editorial Board Members Beginning January 1992

1. Daniel S. Berman
2. Robert M. Califf
3. S. Ward Casscells, III
4. John Douglas
5. David Faxon
6. Nancy C. Flowers
7. Victor F. Froelicher, Jr.
8. Stephen P. Glasser
9. Joseph Loscalzo
10. Richard C. Pasternak
11. John S. Schroeder
12. Prediman K. Shah
13. Burton Sobel
14. George W. Vetrovec
15. William B. White

TABLE II Numbers and Types of Manuscripts Sent to AJC Board Members According to Specialty of Board Member

Specialty	Number on Board	No. MSs Sent (No./Reviewer)	No. LR	No. BR	No. CR	No. (%) Reviews on Time	No. (%) Reviews Late	No. (%) MSs Returned Without Review
Adult cardiologist	131	836 (6.4)	805	24	7	785 (94%)	16 (2%)	35 (4%)
Pediatric cardiologist	15	91 (6.1)	80	11	0	85 (93%)	1 (1%)	5 (6%)
Cardiac surgeon	13	37 (2.8)	33	2	2	34 (92%)	0	3 (8%)
Radiologist or pathologist	5	20 (4.0)	20	0	0	17 (85%)	1 (5%)	2 (10%)
TOTALS	164	984 (6.0)	938 (95%)	37 (4%)	9 (1%)	921 (94%)	18 (2%)	45 (4%)

BR = brief report; CR = case report; LR = long report; MSs = manuscripts.

returned to the pre-April 15, 1991, format in January 1992. Thus, 1992 should show an increase in number of articles published if the number of pages published remains at the same level as in 1991. The types of long reports published in 1991 are shown in Table II.

5. Symposia published in the AJC in 1991: Nine symposia were published in 1991, a 45% decrease (20 to 9) from 1990 (Table VII). Each symposium is published under separate white cover from the regular issues which are published under blue cover.

6. Numbers of manuscripts submitted in 1991 and the acceptance rate: Table VIII summarizes the numbers of manuscripts submitted to the AJC in each of the last 5

TABLE III Top AJC Board Reviewers in 1991 and Number of Manuscripts Reviewed

Name	No. MSs Reviewed	LR	BR	CR	No. Reviewed on Time
1. Joseph S. Alpert	14	14	0	0	14
2. Eric J. Topol	13	12	1	0	13
3. Peter C. Block	12	12	0	0	12
3. Richard O. Cannon, III	12	12	0	0	12
3. Pamela S. Douglas	12	10	2	0	12
3. L. David Hills	12	12	0	0	12
3. Joel Morganroth	12	10	2	0	12
8. J. Thomas Bigger, Jr.	11	9	2	0	9
8. Michael H. Crawford	11	11	0	0	11
8. David R. Holmes, Jr.	11	10	1	0	11
8. Fred Morady	11	10	1	0	11
8. Arthur J. Moss	11	11	0	0	10
8. Bramah N. Singh	11	10	1	0	11
8. James E. Lock	11	8	3	0	8
8. Lowell W. Perry	11	8	3	0	11
16. George A. Beller	10	10	0	0	10
16. Robert O. Bonow	10	10	0	0	9
16. Gregory J. Dehmer	10	10	0	0	10
16. Richard B. Devereux	10	9	0	1	10
16. George A. Diamond	10	10	0	0	10
16. Nanette K. Wenger	10	9	1	0	10
TOTALS (21)	235	217 (92%)	17 (7%)	1 (<1%)	228 (97%)

Abbreviations as in Table II.

TABLE IV Reviewers of 9 and 8 Manuscripts for the AJC in 1991

Name	No. MSs Reviewed	LR	BR	CR	No. Reviewed on Time
22. Pablo Denes	9	9	0	0	9
22. Robert L. Feldman	9	9	0	0	9
22. Gary S. Francis	9	9	0	0	9
22. Leonard N. Horowitz	9	9	0	0	9
22. Jeffrey M. Isner	9	8	1	0	9
22. Natesa Pandian	9	7	1	1	9
22. David H. Spodick	9	9	0	0	9
29. Bernard R. Chaitman	8	8	0	0	8
29. Kanu Chatterjee	8	8	0	0	8
29. John P. DiMarco	8	7	1	0	8
29. Joseph A. Franciosa	8	8	0	0	8
29. Bernard Gersh	8	7	1	0	8
29. Abdulmassih S. Iskandrian	8	8	0	0	8
29. Carl V. Leier	8	8	0	0	8
29. Jawahar Mehta	8	7	0	1	8
29. Eugene R. Passamani	8	8	0	0	8
29. Florence H. Sheehan	8	8	0	0	8
29. James T. Willerson	8	8	0	0	8
29. A. Rebecca Snider	8	8	0	0	8
TOTALS (19)	159	153 (96%)	4 (3%)	2 (1%)	159 (100%)

Abbreviations as in Table II.

TABLE V Reviewers of 7 Manuscripts for the AJC in 1991

Name	No. MSs Reviewed	LR	BR	CR	No. Reviewed on Time
41. William E. Boden	7	7	0	0	7
41. Agustin Castellanos	7	7	0	0	7
41. William H. Gaasch	7	7	0	0	7
41. Julius M. Gardin	7	7	0	0	7
41. Robert E. Goldstein	7	7	0	0	7
41. Sidney O. Gottlieb	7	7	0	0	7
41. William B. Kannel	7	7	0	0	7
41. Kenneth M. Kent	7	7	0	0	6
41. George J. Klein	7	7	0	0	7
41. Frank I. Marcus	7	7	0	0	7
41. Richard S. Meltzer	7	7	0	0	7
41. Franz H. Messerli	7	6	1	0	7
41. Robert J. Myerburg	7	7	0	0	7
41. Robert A. O'Rourke	7	7	0	0	7
41. Carl J. Pepine	7	6	1	0	6
41. Augusto D. Pichard	7	6	1	0	7
41. Bertram Pitt	7	7	0	0	6
41. Philip J. Podrid	7	7	0	0	7
41. Melvin M. Scheinman	7	7	0	0	7
41. David D. Waters	7	7	0	0	7
41. Arthur Garson, Jr.	7	7	0	0	7
41. Barry J. Maron	7	6	1	0	6
TOTALS (22)	154	150 (97%)	4 (3%)	0	150 (97%)

Abbreviations as in Table II.

TABLE VI Numbers of Pages and Articles Published in *The American Journal of Cardiology* in 1991

Number of Pages	3,672		
For Articles		3,165	(86%)
For Readers' Comments		38 (59)*[22]†	(1%)
For Staff, Editorial Board		24	(<1%)
For Contents in Brief		74	(2%)
For Contents with Abstracts		234	(6%)
For Information for Authors		23	(<1%)
For Meeting Abstracts		10	(<1%)
For Volume Indexes		104	(3%)
Number of Articles	680		
Long Reports		421	(62%)
Coronary Artery Disease		203 (48%)	
Arrhythmias and Conduction Disturbances		66 (16%)	
Systemic Hypertension		21 (5%)	
Congestive Heart Failure		16 (4%)	
Valvular Heart Disease		31 (7%)	
Cardiomyopathy		15 (4%)	
Congenital Heart Disease		18 (4%)	
Cardiovascular Pharmacology		2 (<1%)	
Miscellaneous		42 (10%)	
Methods		7 (2%)	
Historical Studies		0	
Brief Reports		182	(27%)
Case Reports		41	(6%)
Editorials		25	(4%)
From-the-Editor columns		11	(1%)

*Numbers of Readers' Comments (formerly Letters to the Editor) published.
†Numbers of replies published.

TABLE VII Symposia Published in *The American Journal of Cardiology* in 1991

	1991 Date of Publication	Subject of Symposium	Guest Editor(s)	Sponsor	No. of Articles	No. of Discussions	No. of Pages	Interval (mos) Symposium to Publication
A	January 25	Adjunctive therapies in thrombolysis	Robert Roberts	Genentech	6	0	32	—
B	April 22	Beta blockers in hypertension	Kikou Arakawa Pieter A. van Zwieten	Sandoz	9	0	50	10
C	May 6	Congestive heart failure	William W. Parmley	ICI Pharmaceuticals	11	3	54	23
D	May 21	Nuclear cardiovascular imaging	Mario S. Verani	Fujisawa Pharmaceutical Company	7	0	56	11
A	July 24	Hypertriglyceridemia	Gerd Assmann Antonio M. Gotto, Jr. Rodolfo Paoletti	Parke-Davis	12	0	42	—
B	September 3	Unstable angina pectoris	Giuseppe Speccia Diego Ardissino William C. Roberts	Boehringer Ingelheim	15	0	141	11
C	November 4	Unstable angina pectoris	James S. Forrester	Marion Merrell Dow	14	0	77	11
D	November 18	Ventricular remodeling and unloading after myocardial infarction	Marc A. Pfeffer Eugene Braunwald	Bristol-Myers Squibb	16	0	131	7
E	December 5	Thrombolytic therapy	Joseph S. Alpert Harvey D. White	Smith Klein Beecham	9	1	48	8

years, and the acceptance rates. In 1991, a total of 1,615 manuscripts were submitted, a 6% decrease compared to the number submitted in 1990, and 680 (42%) were accepted for publication. The acceptance rate averaged 40% for the past 5 years. The only reason this percent is this high is because many of the submitted *long reports* are converted into *brief reports* for publication. Approximately 50% of the brief reports published were originally submitted as long reports. If the AJC did not publish brief reports — and I consider them to be a major feature of the AJC — the acceptance rate in 1991 would have been 31% rather than 42%.

TABLE VIII Numbers of Manuscripts Submitted to AJC in Last Five Years (Excludes Symposia)

Year	Number Manuscripts Submitted	Number Manuscripts Published	Percent Published
1987	1,525	695	46%
1988	1,479	636	43%
1989	1,651	526	32%
1990	1,717	662	38%
1991	1,615	680	42%
TOTALS	7,987	3,199	40%

7. Reminder to authors to supply several names with addresses of nonlocal nonbiased reviewers for their manuscripts: Editors have no monopoly on choosing the best reviewers of manuscripts. No one should be more knowledgeable of experts in the subject of a manuscript than the authors of the manuscript. Thus, I urge authors to supply names — preferably 5, and when they are nonboard members their addresses also — of nonbiased, nonlocal potential reviewers for their manuscripts. It is necessary for an author to supply several names because almost certainly some of the potential reviewers will already have a manuscript for review and a second manuscript is not sent to a reviewer who also possesses one, unless the second manuscript is a brief report or a case report. Currently, in only about 20% of manuscripts submitted have authors provided names of potential reviewers. After studying for nearly 10 years reviews by reviewers suggested by authors, I am impressed that the author-suggested reviewers are of high quality and that the author-suggested reviewers are not more biased to a manuscript than are editor-selected reviewers. Indeed, many manuscripts have been reviewed by 1 author-suggested reviewer and by 1 editor-selected reviewer and the author-selected reviewer recommended rejection and the editor-selected reviewer recommended acceptance of the manuscript.

The meeting was then opened to comments and questions from board members:

1. What is the number of paid subscribers to the AJC? These data are published each year in the *Journal* — indeed in all medical journals — in the *Statement of Ownership, Management and Circulation.* This "statement" was published in the November 1, 1991, issue of the AJC. The average numbers of copies of each issue during the preceding 12 months were the following: total copies printed = 32,500 (rounded off to nearest 100); total paid and/or requested circulation = 22,100; free distribution by mail, carrier or other means = 8,600; total distribution = 30,700; copies not distributed = 1,800.

2. How have the Federal Drug Administration guidelines impacted on the AJC? The only effect has been on the number of symposia published, which fell nearly 50% in 1991 compared to 1990. The decrease in numbers of symposia published, however, appears to be a transient one. In 1992, for example, the number of symposia scheduled to be published is similar to the number published yearly before the FDA guidelines were released, namely about 20/year.

3. Why not publish a brief abstract at the beginning of each brief report as is done at the beginning of each long report? The reason this has not been done is to save space. The last paragraph of each brief report, however, should summarize the major message of the report. The brief reports are published in back-to-back format and therefore the insertion of a summary statement at the beginning of each brief report is a bit more cumbersome than is the case with the long reports.

4. Does the AJC use acid-free paper for its editorial pages? Unfortunately, the answer is no. But other major journals including *The New England Journal of Medicine, The Journal of the American Medical Association, Circulation,* and *The American Heart Journal* are published on acid paper (non-permanent paper). *The Annals of Internal Medicine* switched to acid-free (permanent) paper in November 1991. The consequences of the use of acid paper for editorial pages (defined by many publishers as non-income producing pages) were discussed in a recent editorial in the *Journal.*[1] In my view, it is a disgrace to use acid paper for editorial pages of peer-reviewed medical journals, but I am convinced that alkaline paper will become standard for all peer-reviewed medical publications in the USA by the year 2000 and probably sooner. In January 1987, for example, only 4% of the 3,050 titles of *Index Medicus* were published on acid-free paper. By October 1991, 48% of the titles of *Index Medicus* were known to be published on acid-free paper. In 1987 acid-free paper was in short supply in the USA and 2 manufacturers had a virtual monopoly on it in North America. Today an estimated 35 paper manufacturers provide acid-free paper, such that today it is probably easier to purchase acid-free paper than acid paper. Once paper producers convert from acid to acid-free paper making, it is cheaper, less corrosive to machinery, requires less water, and is less polluting to produce the alkaline paper than the acid paper and for comparable weight paper, the alkaline paper is no more expensive than is the acid paper. Another factor pushing conversion toward alkaline paper is the increased sensitivity or awareness of the problem by paper producers, publishers, authors, and purchasers of print publications. A major impetus toward conversion to acid-free paper has come from the federal government of the USA. In October 1990 Congress passed Public Law 101-423 which requires the use of acid-free paper for publications of enduring value produced by the Government Printing Office, the largest printer in the world. In 1991, 77% of the paper used by the Government Printing Office was alkaline, and by 1996, 100% will be alkaline. Medical publications also should benefit by this law in due course. Many ads in our medical publications are on acid-free paper. Surely our manuscripts deserve to be published on alkaline paper, even if it is of lower weight than that used for the ads. The most productive period of human beings has been the last 140 years and most publications during this period have been on acid paper and therefore they have or soon will vanish into dust. A good quality of toilet paper and paper towels now consists of acid-free paper. Surely if some of our toilet paper can be alkaline, most of our medical publications, including all our peer-reviewed journals, can use a paper of at least similar quality.

5. Is it necessary to publish the Instructions to Authors in each of the 24 issues of the Journal? No. But the 1-page "Instructions" is often used as a filler. I would prefer to shorten the *Contents in Brief,* which occupied 74 pages in 1991, to no more than 1 or 2 pages per issue, as a better page-saving device. Even better would be to drastically reduce or eliminate the *Contents with Abstracts* which occupied 234 pages in 1991.

6. Is the quality of scientific writing getting better? I believe that the quality of the writing by authors from English-speaking countries continues to improve. The problem is that the number of manuscripts being submitted to USA medical journals, including the AJC, by authors residing in countries where the native language is not English is increasing. The latter manuscripts require much editorial effort.

7. Should the abstract format be changed to a structured format which has recently been adapted by The American Journal of Medicine, The Annals of Internal Medicine, Circulation, Journal of the American Medical Association, and The New England Journal of Medicine, among others? These structured formats include separate paragraphs for each of the separate categories, which generally include such items as *background, methods, results,* and *conclusions* (*New England Journal of Medicine* and *Circulation*), or *objective, design, setting, patients, primary outcome measure, results,* and *conclusion* (*Annals of Internal Medicine, Journal of the American Medical Association*). The addition of the subheadings, and the separation of each subheading into separate paragraphs adds to the length of the abstract. Additionally, there is usually some redundancy in the structured abstracts because each subheading requires at least some statement. Most abstracts in the AJC presently are single paragraphs. I prefer, at least for now, the present AJC abstract format rather than the structured one.

8. Would it be better to have an even right margin for the AJC abstracts or an uneven right margin as it is presently? The uneven right margin was one recommended by a design consultant when the AJC style was changed several years ago. The bold type of the abstract might make the even right margin more cumbersome to achieve than if the type was not of the bold variety. Board members appeared to prefer an even right border for the abstract, and that view appears reasonable to me. An effort will be made to make this change.

9. Should the AJC reestablish the policy of publishing experimental-type studies (those involving non-human animals)? This item was discussed at length at the 1991 board meeting,[2] and this item continues to be a concern of editorial board members. About one half of those members present favored the publication of experimental studies and the other half favored a continuation of the current policy, i.e., the publication of experimental studies only if they are short enough to fit into the brief report section of the *Journal.* The problem is simply that experimental-type manuscripts are usually the longest ones submitted, the numbers of editorial pages available do not predictably increase, and the number of clinical studies submitted remains large. During the first 3 months of 1992 the numbers of manuscripts submitted rose substantially compared to the first 3 months of 1991. If the current numbers continue for all 12 months of 1992, a total of 1,920 manuscripts will be submitted in 1992 and the number of editorial pages available in 1992 is approximately the same as in 1991. If experimental-type manuscripts were accepted, the numbers of clinical studies accepted would decrease, and probably the interval between the acceptance of a manuscript and its publication would increase. Currently, this interval ("lag time") is 3.5 months, and I am convinced that this short interval is a major factor in attracting superb clinical manuscripts into the AJC. Another factor to consider is that the largest numbers of AJC subscribers are private practitioners who probably would find the experimental-type articles of considerably less use to them than the clinical articles. If the publisher were able to provide let's say an additional 200 pages per year on top of the currently budgeted editorial pages, then the publication of the experimental studies would be more reasonable. But the 200-page commitment from the publisher would have to be a long-term commitment and not simply a single year commitment. An important feature of the AJC at the moment I believe is that it is a purely clinical journal. It is one where every attempt is made to treat both readers and authors respectfully and to publish good clinical manuscripts as rapidly as possible. The large number of paid subscribers suggests that the present policy is working satisfactorily. Thus, for the moment the present policy will remain unless additional pages set aside for experimental studies are provided by the publisher.

The meeting was adjourned to a reception provided by the publisher.

William C. Roberts

William Clifford Roberts, MD
Editor in Chief

1. Roberts WC. Alkaline paper and preserving the record. *Am J Cardiol* 1991;68:1729–1732.
2. Roberts WC. Editorial board meeting of The American Journal of Cardiology — 5 March 1991. *Am J Cardiol* 1991;67:1033–1037.

Editorial Board Meeting of *The American Journal of Cardiology* in March 1993

The annual meeting of *The American Journal of Cardiology* (AJC) in 1993 was held in Anaheim, California, on March 16 at the time of the Annual Scientific Sessions of *The American College of Cardiology*. The meeting's purpose was to thank the 178 board members for their enormous help during the previous year, to pay particular tribute to those reviewing the most manuscripts in 1992, and to receive input from board members through questions and comments. The meeting went as follows:

1. *Introduction of new board members:* Eight physicians (Table I) were added to the board beginning January 1993 and they were introduced. New board members are selected entirely on their record as non-board reviewers for the AJC. Their selection is based on review of the card files of the approximately 1,400 non-board AJC reviewers and those with the best reviewing records are selected. No board members were eliminated in 1992 because of superior performance of nearly all members, but in the near future some infrequently- or inadequately-used board members will have to be eliminated to provide places for many non-board reviewers deserving of board status.

2. *Numbers of manuscripts sent for review to board members in 1992:* A total of 1,873 manuscripts were received in the editorial office in 1992 (This number does not include the manuscripts for the supplement issues.), and 1,107 of them were sent to at least 1 board member (Table II). Of the 1,107 manuscripts, an average of 6.2 per board member, 1,025 (93%) were reviewed on time (3 weeks from the day the manuscript was sent from and returned to the editorial office), 60 (5%) were not reviewed within the 3-week period, and 22 manuscripts (2%) were returned without review (Table II).

3. *AJC board members reviewing the most manuscripts in 1992:* The top 18 reviewers are listed in Table III. Each reviewed 10 manuscripts in 1992 and all were reviewed on time. Table IV lists the 9 board members who each reviewed 9 manuscripts during the year; Table V lists the 15 board members who each reviewed 8 manuscripts, and Table VI lists the 21 board members who each reviewed 7 manuscripts in 1992. The reviewing records of the 63 board members listed in Tables III to VI are truly remarkable, and these board members represent 35% of the total board. The editor also is fully aware that the AJC is not the only medical journal for which these board members review manuscripts.

4. *Numbers of pages and articles and types of articles published in the AJC in 1992:* These data are listed in Table VII. A total of 711 articles (an average of 59 per month) were published on 3,211 pages (an average of 268 per month) in 1992. The average length of each article was 4.52 pages. These numbers represent a 1% increase (3,165 to 3,211) in the numbers of pages for articles and a 4% increase (680 to 711) in the number of articles published in 1992 compared to 1991 (Table VIII). Although 3,211 pages were used for articles, an additional 540 editorial pages (i.e., a non-revenue producing page [a non-ad page]) (13%) were used for publishing Readers' Comments (46 pages), abstracts of a pediatric cardiology meeting, for staff and editorial board members, for contents in brief, for contents with extended abstracts (256 pages), for *Information for Authors,* and for volume indexes (108 pages). Of the 711 articles published, 487 (68.5%) were long reports, 166 (23.3%) were brief reports, 31 were case reports (4.4%), and 27 (3.9%) were editorials.

5. *Numbers of manuscripts submitted in 1992 and acceptance rate:* Table VIII summarizes the numbers of

TABLE I New AJC Board Members Beginning January 1993

1. Jeffrey A. Brinker
2. Robert J. Cody
3. Jean S. Kan
4. Michael McGoon
5. Jeffrey J. Popma
6. James B. Seward
7. Galen S. Wagner
8. Redford B. Williams

TABLE II Numbers and Types of Manuscripts Sent to AJC Board Members in 1992 According to Specialty of Board Member

Specialty	Number on Board	Number MSS Sent (No./Reviewer)	No. LR	No. BR	No. CR	Number (%) Reviews on Time	Number (%) Reviews Late	No. (%) MSS Returned Without Review
Adult cardiologist	145	961 (6.6)	929	28	4	888 (92%)	54 (6%)	19 (2%)
Pediatric cardiologist	15	83 (5.5)	74	4	5	79 (95%)	3 (4%)	1 (1%)
Cardiac surgeon	13	38 (2.9)	36	2	0	34 (89%)	3 (8%)	1 (3%)
Related specialist	5	25 (5.0)	23	0	2	24 (96%)	0	1 (4%)
Totals	178	1107 (6.2)	1062	34	11	1025 (93%)	60 (5%)	22 (2%)

BR = brief report; CR = case report; LR = long report; MSS = manuscripts.

TABLE III Reviewers of 10 Manuscripts for the AJC in 1992

Name	Number Manuscripts Reviewed	LR	BR	CR	Number Reviewed on Time
1. George A. Beller	10	10	0	0	10
2. Bernard R. Chaitman	10	10	0	0	10
3. Michael H. Crawford	10	10	0	0	10
4. Robert L. Feldman	10	10	0	0	10
5. Frank A. Finnerty, Jr.	10	10	0	0	10
6. Gary S. Francis	10	10	0	0	10
7. William H. Gaasch	10	10	0	0	10
8. L. David Hillis	10	10	0	0	10
9. Abdulmassih S. Iskandrian	10	10	0	0	10
10. Jeffrey M. Isner	10	10	0	0	10
11. William B. Kannel	10	10	0	0	10
12. Harold L. Kennedy	10	9	1	0	10
13. Arthur J. Moss	10	10	0	0	10
14. Joseph K. Perloff	10	10	0	0	10
15. Philip J. Podrid	10	10	0	0	10
16. Nathaniel Reichek	10	10	0	0	10
17. David O. Spodick	10	10	0	0	10
18. James T. Willerson	10	10	0	0	10

Abbreviations as in Table II.

TABLE IV Reviewers of 9 Manuscripts for the AJC in 1992

Name	Number Manuscripts Reviewed	LR	BR	CR	Number Reviewed on Time
1. William E. Boden	9	8	1	0	9
2. Robert M. Califf	9	9	0	0	7
3. Richard O. Cannon, III	9	9	0	0	9
4. David R. Holmes, Jr.	9	9	0	0	9
5. George J. Klein	9	8	1	0	9
6. Carl V. Leier	9	9	0	0	9
7. Fred Morady	9	9	0	0	9
8. Joel Morganroth	9	8	1	0	9
9. Eric J. Topol	9	8	1	0	9

Abbreviations as in Table II.

manuscripts submitted in the last 5 years, and the acceptance rate for articles in which a final decision was made during that particular year. The 1,873 manuscripts submitted in 1992 represent a submission rate of 5.8 manuscripts for every day of the year, or 8.1 manuscripts submitted for each of the 5 official work days each week, or 40.5 manuscripts submitted per week. Some manuscripts accepted in 1992, for example, had been submitted in 1991 and some manuscripts submitted in 1992 were not accepted until 1993. Of the 1,873 manuscripts submitted in 1992, 664 (35%) were eventually accepted. The 4% increase in the numbers of manuscripts published in 1992 compared to 1991 resulted primarily from a reduction (3%) in the average length of each article (4.65 to 4.52 pages) and only a slight (1%) increase in the numbers of editorial pages published. If the AJC did not publish brief reports — and I consider them to be the unique feature of the AJC — the acceptance rate in 1992 would have been approximately 30% rather than 38% or 35%.

The numbers of manuscripts submitted have continued to increase in 1993. In January and February alone 341 manuscripts were submitted in 1993, 303 in 1992, and 257 in 1991. The numbers of editorial pages, however, are not increasing, and in 1993 there probably will

TABLE V Reviewers of 8 Manuscripts for the AJC in 1992

Name	Number Manuscripts Reviewed	LR	BR	CR	Number Reviewed on Time
1. Jeffrey Anderson	8	8	0	0	8
2. Barry J. Maron	8	7	1	0	8
3. Peter C. Block	8	8	0	0	8
4. Robert O. Bonow	8	8	0	0	7
5. Pablo Denes	8	8	0	0	8
6. Pamela S. Douglas	8	8	0	0	8
7. Kenneth M. Kent	8	8	0	0	5
8. Lloyd W. Klein	8	8	0	0	8
9. Francis E. Marchlinski	8	7	1	0	8
10. Frank I. Marcus	8	8	0	0	8
11. Jawahar Mehta	8	8	0	0	8
12. Robert J. Myerburg	8	8	0	0	8
13. Navin C. Nanda	8	7	1	0	7
14. Charles E. Rackley	8	8	0	0	7
15. Douglas P. Zipes	8	8	0	0	8

Abbreviations as in Table II.

TABLE VI Reviewers of 7 Manuscripts for the AJC in 1992

Name	Number Manuscripts Reviewed	LR	BR	CR	Number Reviewed on Time
1. Masood Akhtar	7	7	0	0	6
2. Joseph S. Alpert	7	7	0	0	7
3. Michael E. Cain	7	6	1	0	7
4. Gregory J. Dehmer	7	7	0	0	7
5. George A. Diamond	7	6	1	0	7
6. John Douglas	7	7	0	0	4
7. Jack Ferlinz	7	7	0	0	7
8. John A. Kastor	7	7	0	0	7
9. Spencer B. King, III	7	7	0	0	5
10. Robert A. Kloner	7	7	0	0	7
11. Arthur J. Labovitz	7	7	0	0	7
12. Raymond G. McKay	7	7	0	0	6
13. Franz H. Messerli	7	7	0	0	6
14. Carl J. Pepine	7	7	0	0	4
15. Bertram Pitt	7	7	0	0	5
16. Melvin M. Scheinman	7	7	0	0	7
17. John S. Schroeder	7	6	1	0	7
18. Bramah N. Singh	7	7	0	0	5
19. Hugh D. Allen	7	7	0	0	7
20. James E. Lock	7	7	0	0	7
21. Lowell W. Perry	7	6	1	0	7

Abbreviations as Table II.

be fewer editorial pages than in 1992 because of a reduction in anticipated advertising revenue. Thus, the acceptance rate in 1993 almost certainly will be less than in 1992.

6. *Symposia published in the AJC in 1992:* Fifteen symposia were published in 1992, a 40% increase over the number published in 1991 (Table IX). These 15 symposia included 165 articles and 4 discussion sections occupying 979 editorial pages. No advertisements appear in the symposia issues which are published under separate and different-colored cover from that of the regular issues. Most symposia were guest edited by one or more major leaders in cardiology.

7. *Sources of articles published in* Cardiology Board Review *in 1992:* The controlled journal *Cardiology Board Review,* edited by Dr. Peter F. Cohn, publishes shortened versions of articles previously published in peer-reviewed journals. Of the 82 articles published in

TABLE VII Numbers of Pages and Types of Articles Published in the Regular Issues of *The American Journal of Cardiology* in 1992 (volumes 69 and 70)

Number of pages	3,751			
For articles (mean/month) [pages/article]	3,211	(268)	[4.52]	87%
For *Readers' Comments* (number) [number replies]	46	(53)	[14]	
For abstracts (cardiologic section of a pediatric society)	11			
For staff, editorial board	24	(<1%)		
For contents in brief	73	(2%)		
For contents with abstracts	256	(7%)		
For *Information for Authors*	22	(<1%)		
For volume indexes	108	(3%)		
Number of articles (mean/month)	711	(59)		
Long reports	487	→	68.5%	
Coronary artery disease		201	(43.1%)	
Preventive cardiology		9	(1.8%)	
Arrhythmias and conduction defects		73	(15.0%)	
Systemic hypertension		22	(4.5%)	
Congestive heart failure		31	(6.4%)	
Valvular heart disease		36	(7.4%)	
Cardiomyopathy		23	(4.7%)	
Congenital heart disease		20	(4.1%)	
Miscellaneous		54	(11.1%)	
Methods		14	(2.9%)	
Cardiovascular pharmacology		4	(0.5%)	
Historic studies		0		
Brief reports	166	→	23.3%	
Case reports	31	→	4.4%	
Editorials	23	→	3.2%	
From-the-editor columns	4	→	0.6%	

TABLE VIII Numbers of Manuscripts Submitted, Articles and Editorial Pages Published, Percent Published, and Average Length of Each Article in the AJC in the Last 5 Years

Year	Number Manuscripts Submitted	Number Manuscripts Published	Percent Published	Number Editorial Pages For Articles	Average Pages Per Article
1988	1,479	636	43%	2642	4.15
1989	1,651	699	32%	2903	4.15
1990	1,717	662	32%	3001	4.53
1991	1,615 } 14% ↑	680 } 4% ↑	42%	3165 } 1%↑	4.65
1992	1,873	711	38%	3211	4.51

1992, 23 (28%) came from the AJC, 17 from *Circulation,* and 15 from *The Journal of the American College of Cardiology* (Table X).

8. *Removal of mailing wrappers covering the AJC:* About mid-1992 the cellophane mailing wrappers were removed from the journal. The lack of these wrappers caused damage to some issues during the mailing, and as a consequence the mailing wrappers were restored in early 1993.

9. *Merger of company which publishes the AJC with another major publishing company:* It was announced in September 1992 that Reed International PLC, which is the parent of Cahners Publishing Company, the publisher of the AJC, will merge with Elsevier N.V., the publisher of *The Journal of the American College of Cardiology,* in January 1993. Reed, of Britain, specializes in trade, consumer and travel publications. Netherlands-based Elsevier is the world's leading publisher of scientific journals with approximately 1,000 scientific titles. The combined stock valuations give the merger a value of just under 10 billion dollars.

10. *Reminder to authors to supply several names with addresses of non-local, non-biased reviewers for their manuscripts:* Editors have no monopoly on choosing the best reviewers of manuscripts. No one should be more knowledgeable of experts in the subject of a manuscript than the authors of the manuscript. Thus, I urge authors to supply names — preferably 5, and when the names are non-board members also the addresses — of non-biased, non-local potential reviewers for their manuscripts. It is necessary for an author to supply several names because almost certainly some of the potential reviewers will already have a manuscript for review and a second manuscript is not sent to a reviewer who also possesses one, unless the second manuscript is a brief report or a case report. Currently, in only about 20% of manuscripts submitted have authors provided names of potential reviewers. After studying for over 10 years reviews by author-suggested reviewers, I am impressed that the author-suggested reviewers are of high quality and that the author-suggested reviewers are not more biased to a manuscript than are editor-selected reviewers. Indeed, many manuscripts have been reviewed by 1 author-suggested reviewer and by 1 editor-selected reviewer and the author-selected reviewer recommended rejection and the editor-selected reviewer recommended acceptance of the manuscript.

The meeting was then opened to comments and questions from board members:

1. *Has any progress been made toward using acid-free paper in the AJC?* No. Acid-free paper *is used* in the AJC. Many of the advertisements are published on

No.	1992 Date of Publication	Subject of Symposium	Guest Editor(s)	Sponsor(s)	Number of Articles	Discussions Included	Number of Pages	Interval (months) Symposium to Publication
A	January 3	Thrombolytic agents	Richard C. Becker Joel M. Gore	Genentech	9	0	82	—
B	March 6	Myocardial ischemia and diltiazem	Peter F. Cohn Robert S. Gibson	Marion Merrell Dow	9	+	46	15
C	April 2	Hypertension and quinapril	James A. Schoenberger	Park-Davis	10	0	64	9
D	April 9	Angina pectoris and bepridil	Richard Gorlin	McNeil Pharmaceutical and Wallace Laboratories	15	0	88	8
E	April 30	Hypertension and nifedipine-SR (sustained release)	Aram V. Chobanian	Miles	8	0	42	6
F	May 7	Complex angioplasty	Robert A. Vogel	Mallinckrodt	6	0	32	13
A	August 20	Supraventricular arrhythmias and flecainide	Robert J. Myerburg Pedro Brugada	3M Pharmaceuticals	12	+	74	12
B	September 24	Nitroglycerin	Jonathan Abrams	CIBA-GEIGY	15	0	104	16
C	October 8	Congesive heart failure and lisinopril	Lars Ryden	ICI Pharmaceuticals	28	0	153	11
D	October 29	Systemic hypertension and trandolapril	John H. Laragh Giuseppe Mancia	Roussel Uclaf Cardiovascular	10	0	66	4
E	November 5	Cardiac imaging and thallium-201	Mario S. Verani	Mallinckrodt Medical	6	0	34	12
F	November 16	Myocardial ischemia	Peter F. Cohn	Marion Merrell Dow	10	+	48	11
G	November 27	Antianginal therapy, particularly nitrates	William H. Frishman	Wyeth-Ayerst Boehringer Mannheim	14	+	76	9
H	December 14	Triglycerides	Yechezkiel Stein Antonio M. Gotto, Jr.	Parke-Davis	6	0	31	14
I	December 21	Cardioprotection	William H. Frishman	Astra Pharmaceuticals	7	0	39	13
15	Totals				165	4	979	(mean = 11)

TABLE IX Symposia Published in *The American Journal of Cardiology* in 1992

acid-free paper! The paper used for the editorial pages, however, is not acid-free. As discussed in a previous piece in this column,[1] more and more peer-reviewed scientific journals are being published on alkaline, i.e., permanent paper. Plenty of alkaline paper is now available in the USA such that all peer-reviewed medical journals could be published on this type paper. Eventually, in my view, permanent paper will be required for all medical journals listed in the Index Medicus. It is my understanding that Elsevier uses acid-free paper for all of their scientific publications. This fact also with the fact that the publisher of the AJC has now merged with Elsevier makes me hopeful that the AJC will be published on acid-free paper in the foreseeable future.

2. *What are the numbers of subscribers to the AJC?* The statement of ownership, management and circulation published in the November 1, 1992, issue of the AJC indicates that the AJC has nearly 22,000 paid and/or requested mail subscriptions as of October 1992. Another 7,350 copies are mailed of each issue on a complimentary basis. These free copies are sent out on a rotating basis seeking paid subscriptions.

3. *What percentage of subscribers to the AJC are in the USA and what percentage are outside the USA?* The publisher indicated that there are about 16,000 domestic and 6,000 foreign paid subscribers.

4. *What happens to manuscripts submitted to the AJC and declined?* I do not know. Frequently, I see an article in another journal which I know had earlier been declined by the AJC. The percentage of articles declined by one journal and eventually published in another journal is unknown as far as I know.

TABLE X Sources of Articles in *Cardiology Board Review* in 1992

Journal	Number of Articles
1. American Journal of Cardiology	23 (28%)
2. Circulation	17 (21%)
3. Journal of the American College of Cardiology	15 (18%)
4. Annals of Internal Medicine	6 (7%)
5. Archives of Internal Medicine	5 (6%)
6. New England Journal of Medicine	5 (6%)
7. American Heart Journal	4 (5%)
8. American Journal of Medicine	4 (5%)
9. British Heart Journal	3 (4%)
	82 (100%)

5. *Why not have an abstract for the brief reports?* Currently, there are no subheadings in the brief report and case report sections of the journal. Subheadings are not used in these sections simply to save space. An attempt has been made to encourage authors to provide a summary statement at the end of each brief or case report but that desire has not been enforced and it should be. A suggestion was made by a board member to put this final summarizing statement in bold type. That suggestion would highlight the message without taking up more space. Thanks.

6. *Should the abstract format be changed to a structured one, something adapted by several prominent*

journals in recent years? This question also was posed at the 1991 editorial board meeting. The structured formats include separate paragraphs for each of the separate categories, which generally include such items as *background, methods, results,* and *conclusions (New England Journal of Medicine)* or *objective, design, setting, patients, primary outcome measure, results, and conclusions (Annals of Internal Medicine, Journal of the American Medical Association).* The addition of subheadings, and the separation of each subheading into separate paragraphs adds to the length of the abstract. Additionally, there is usually some redundancy in the structured abstracts because each subheading requires at least some statement. Most abstracts in the AJC currently are single paragraphs. I still prefer the present AJC abstract format rather than the structured one.

7. *Could the quality of the paper used for the editorial pages be improved?* Yes it could. Will it? This decision of course is that of the publisher. The cost of paper continues to increase faster than the inflation rate. Possibly the merger with Elsevier will lead to a change in the quality of paper used in the AJC.

8. *Why not accept fewer manuscripts, only those that are outstanding, and maybe even expand some of them?* This question concerns editorial philosophy. Cardiology is an extremely broad area. Some readers are pediatric cardiologists and they of course focus only on articles applicable to them. The echocardiographers probably focus mainly on articles affecting them. The same can be said of the electrophysiologists, nuclear cardiologists, interventionalists, cardiovascular radiologists, and pathologists. Cardiovascular surgeons need their share of articles in the AJC. Thus, if the numbers of articles are diminished some of the cardiovascular subspecialists will not get their share of appropriate articles. The AJC publishes far more articles than any cardiovascular journal in the world. The only reason we are able to do so is because we publish many brief reports and our long reports are shorter on the average than those of other peer-reviewed cardiology journals. From the standpoint of the editor, brief reports demand considerable editorial time since about half of them were initially submitted as long reports. And finally, there is no such thing as universal agreement as to which are the excellent articles. An article may be excellent in the mind of one reader (or reviewer) and poor in the mind of another reader (or reviewer). Walt Whitman and Herman Melville were considered poor writers in their lifetimes![2] Some medical articles also are not considered outstanding until years after their publication.

The publisher presented the editor with a beautiful pen and pencil set in appreciation of 10 years of editorship, and the editor was grateful. The meeting was adjourned to a reception provided by the publisher.

William C. Roberts

William Clifford Roberts, MD
Editor in Chief

1. Roberts WC. Alkaline paper and preserving the record. *Am J Cardiol* 1991;68:1729–1732.
2. Roberts WC. Reviews of classic books and ineptness of reviewers: lessons for judges of medical manuscripts. *Am J Cardiol* 1987;59:922–923.

Proceedings of the Editorial Board Meeting of *The American Journal of Cardiology* on March 14, 1994

The 1994 meeting of the editorial board of *The American Journal of Cardiology* (AJC) was held on March 14 in Atlanta, Georgia, at the time of the Annual Scientific Sessions of The American College of Cardiology. The meeting's purpose was to review AJC publication results in 1993, to recognize particularly those AJC board members reviewing the most manuscripts in 1993, and to receive through questions and comments input from the board members present. The meeting went as follows:

1. *Introduction of Mr. Ken Senerth, the new Publishing Director:* Mr. Senerth reviewed briefly the results of the Reed-Elsevier merger in 1993 and how that merger affects the AJC. The AJC now is part of Excerpta Medica, formerly a part of Elsevier, and the publishing office has moved from New York City to Belle Mead, New Jersey. I met with Mr. Senerth recently and came away convinced that the AJC will continue to reside in good hands. One immediate result of the merger is that the AJC soon (by July 1994 anyway) will be printed for the first time on neutral pH paper rather than on acid paper, the non-permanent variety! In contrast, *The New England Journal of Medicine, The Journal of the American Medical Association, Circulation,* and *The American Heart Journal* all will continue to be printed on acid paper, which will vanish into ashes in 50 years.[1]

The number of paid subscribers to the AJC in 1993 was approximately 21,500. Additionally, another 7,500 receive the journal free on a rotational (3 month) basis in an attempt to attract new subscribers. The total recipients of each issue, therefore, are about 29,000, the largest of any peer-reviewed cardiology journal in the world.

2. *Introduction of the new Associate and Assistant Editors (Table I):* The editorial office of the AJC was moved from Bethesda, Maryland, to Dallas, Texas, in April 1993. This move necessitated the replacement of Doctors William P. Baker and Paul A. Tibbits who had served the journal from 1985 to 1993 with distinction and unselfishness. I will miss them. The new team is as follows:

John D. Rutherford, MD, Associate Editor. John, who was born in Wanganui, New Zealand, and trained in internal medicine and cardiology in Auckland, New Zealand, currently is Professor of Medicine, University of Texas Southwestern Medical Center in Dallas, and holds the Gail Griffiths Chair in Cardiology at that institution. John came to Dallas from the Brigham and Women's Hospital in Boston, Massachusetts, where he was co-director of the clinical cardiology service. As Associate Editor, John will serve as editor in chief for 12 weeks a year, at which time I will take a vacation from the editor's chair. After 12 years without a substitute, I welcome John with open arms.

Doctors **Azam Anwar, Samuel J. DeMaio, Michael N. Sills, Rolando M. Solis, and Peter John Wells** will

TABLE I New Associate and Assistant Editors

Associate Editor
John D. Rutherford
Assistant Editors
Azam Anwar
Samuel J. DeMaio
Michael N. Sills
Rolando M. Solis
Peter J. Wells

TABLE II New Editorial Board Members Beginning January 1994

1. Martin A. Alpert
2. Donald S. Baim
3. Elias H. Botvinick
4. Gerald Dorros
5. Stephen Ellis
6. Toby R. Engel
7. Barry A. Franklin
8. Paul C. Gillette
9. Thomas P. Graham, Jr.
10. Gary V. Heller
11. Charles B. Higgins
12. Sanjiv Kaul
13. Morton J. Kern
14. John D. Kugler
15. Leslie W. Miller
16. Douglass A. Morrison
17. Gerald V. Naccarelli
18. J. V. Nixon
19. Maria-Teresa Olivari
20. Robert J. Siegel
21. Steven N. Singh
22. Carole A. Warnes
23. Donald A. Weiner
24. Paul G. Yock

TABLE III Numbers and Types of Manuscripts Sent to AJC Board Members in 1993 According to Specialty of Board Member

Specialty	Number on Board	Number of MSS Sent (no./reviewer)	No. LR	No. BR	No. CR	Number (%) Reviewed on Time	Number (%) Reviewed Late	No. (%) Returned Without Review
Adult cardiologist	151	700	675	24	1	579 (83%)	67 (9%)	54 (8%)
Pediatric cardiologist	15	56	52	3	1	49 (87%)	2 (4%)	5 (9%)
Cardiac surgeon	12	27	26	1	0	19 (70%)	6 (22%)	2 (8%)
Related specialist	6	22	20	2	0	16 (73%)	2 (9%)	4 (18%)
Totals	184	805 (4.38)	773 (96%)	30 (4%)	2 (<1%)	663 (82%)	77 (10%)	65 (8%)

BR = brief report; CR = case report; LR = long reports; MSS = manuscripts.

TABLE IV Reviewers of 9 and 8 Manuscripts for the AJC in 1993

Name	Number of Manuscripts Reviewed	LR	BR	CR	Number Reviewed on Time
David H. Spodick	9	9	0	0	9
Richard O. Cannon, III	8	8	0	0	8
Gegory J. Dehmer	8	7	1	0	8
Richard B. Devereux	8	8	0	0	7
L. David Hillis	8	8	0	0	8
Abdulmassih S. Iskandrian	8	8	0	0	8
Arthur Labovitz	8	8	0	0	8
Fred Morady	8	7	1	0	8
Nelson B. Schiller	8	7	1	0	7
Arthur Garson, Jr.	8	8	0	0	8

Abbreviations as in Table III.

TABLE V Reviewers of 7 Manuscripts for the AJC in 1993

Name	Number of Manuscripts Reviewed	LR	BR	CR	Number Reviewed on Time
Robert O. Bonow	7	7	0	0	4
Bernard Chaitman	7	7	0	0	7
Michael H. Crawford	7	7	0	0	7
Gary S. Francis	7	7	0	0	7
Victor F. Froelicher, Jr.	7	7	0	0	7
Carl V. Leier	7	6	1	0	6
Barry J. Maron	7	6	1	0	4
Jawahar Mehta	7	6	1	0	6
Franz H. Messerli	7	7	0	0	5
Catherine M. Otto	7	7	0	0	7
Jeffrey J. Popma	7	7	0	0	6
Melvin M. Scheinman	7	7	0	0	7
Eric J. Topol	7	7	0	0	7
Nanette K. Wenger	7	7	0	0	7

Abbreviations as in Table III.

serve as Assistant Editors. Each comes into the editorial office 1 day a week, and assigns reviewers for each of the long reports and brief reports. The case reports, editorials and manuscripts with reviews by other journals which declined them go directly to my desk. The assistant editors also pick out manuscripts that are not deemed worthy of review, and these manuscripts undergo further in-house scrutiny before a final decision. I am pleased to have these 5 Assistant Editors, each of whom is a part of the Baylor faculty in Dallas. Doctors Anwar, DeMaio, and Solis are invasive therapeutic cardiologists, Dr. Wells focuses on electrophysiology, and Dr. Sills' special interest is echocardiography.

3. *Introduction of new AJC board members:* Twenty-four new members were added to the board beginning January 1994 (Table II) and they were introduced. New board members are selected entirely on their record as non-board reviewers for the AJC. Selection is based on review of card files of approximately 1,400 non-board AJC reviewers and those with the best reviewing records are selected. Board members determine their longevity on the AJC board by the quality and promptness of their reviews. Each year it gets more and more difficult to eliminate board members because nearly all have outstanding reviewing records.

4. *Numbers of manuscripts sent for review to board members in 1993:* A total of 1,997 manuscripts were received in the editorial office in 1993 (this number does not include the manuscripts for the supplement issues), and 805 of them were sent to at least 1 of the 184 AJC board members, an average of 4.38 manuscripts sent to each board member in 1993: 663 (82%) were reviewed on time, 77 (10%) were returned to the office late (>3 weeks from date of mailing from the AJC office), and 65 (8%) were returned without review (Table III). The percentage reviewed late or returned without review is higher than any previous year of my editorship.

5. *AJC board members reviewing the most manuscripts in 1993:* The top AJC reviewer in 1993 was **Dr. David H. Spodick** who reviewed 9 manuscripts, all within the allotted 3-week time period (Table IV). Nine reviewers reviewed 8 manuscripts (Table IV), 14 reviewers reviewed 7 manuscripts (Table V), and 20 AJC board members reviewed 6 manuscripts in 1993 (Table VI). The reviewing record of the 44 board members who reviewed either 9, 8, 7 or 6 manuscripts during the year is truly remarkable, and these board members represent 24% of the total board. The editor also is fully aware that the AJC is not the only medical journal for which the board members review manuscripts. Indeed, David H. Spodick, our top reviewer, is himself an editor of a cardiologic journal.

TABLE VI Reviewers of 6 Manuscripts for the AJC in 1993

Name	Number of Manuscripts Reviewed	LR	BR	CR	Number Reviewed on Time
Hugh D. Allen	6	6	0	0	6
Jeffrey Anderson	6	6	0	0	6
J. Thomas Bigger, Jr.	6	6	0	0	3
Robert J. Cody	6	6	0	0	4
Peter F. Cohn	6	6	0	0	6
John P. DiMarco	6	6	0	0	6
Robert L. Feldman	6	6	0	0	6
Jerome L. Fleg	6	6	0	0	6
Joseph A. Franciosa	6	6	0	0	5
William H. Gaasch	6	6	0	0	6
Jeffrey M. Isner	6	5	0	1	6
Spencer B. King, III	6	6	0	0	6
George J. Klein	6	6	0	0	6
G. B. John Mancini	6	5	1	0	4
Richard S. Meltzer	6	6	0	0	6
Navin Nanda	6	5	1	0	6
Philip J. Podrid	6	6	0	0	5
Nathaniel Reichek	6	5	1	0	6
John R. Wilson	6	6	0	0	4
Barry L. Zaret	6	6	0	0	6

Abbreviations as in Table III.

6. *Numbers of pages and articles and types of articles published in the AJC in 1993:* These data are listed in Table VII. A total of 650 articles (an average of 54 per month) were published on 2,890 pages (an average of 241 per month) in 1993. The average length of each article was 4.45 pages, a 1% decrease compared with 1992 (Table VIII). In 1993 a total of 1,997 manuscripts were submitted (a 6% increase from 1992 when 1,873 manuscripts were submitted) and 619 (31%) were accepted, a 7% decrease from 1992 when 664 manuscripts were accepted. In 1993, 650 manuscripts were published, a 9% decrease from the 711 published in 1992. The number of editorial pages used for articles in 1993 was 2,890, a 10% decrease from the 3,211 published in 1992. Thus, 1993 was a difficult year, a year in which the most manuscripts were received and the number of editorial pages published was less than that in any of the past 12 years of my editorship. The reason for the fewer number of editorial pages is due to the fewer number of advertising pages, a situation that affected nearly all large clinical medical journals in 1993. Nevertheless, of the 4 major cardiologic journals published in the USA *(American Heart Journal, AJC, Circulation,* and *Journal of the American College of Cardiology),* the AJC received the second largest number of advertisements. The only reason the AJC publishes as many articles as it does is because the journal publishes many brief reports, 209 or 32% of the articles in 1993. Only 19 case reports were published in 1993.

7. *Numbers of editorial pages published in 1993 in the 4 major USA cardiologic journals:* These data are listed in Table IX. The AJC published the fewest number of editorial pages of the 4 in 1993. Table X lists the number of editorial pages published in these 4 journals during the first 3 months of 1994.

8. *Symposia published in the AJC in 1993:* Thirteen symposia were published in the AJC in 1993 (Table XI).

TABLE VII Numbers of Pages and Articles and Types of Articles Published in the Regular Issues of the AJC in 1993 (volumes 71 and 72)

Number of pages	3,395			
For articles (mean/month) [pages/article]	2,890	(241)	[4.45]	85.12%
For *Readers' Comments* (number) [number replies]	37	(64)	[12]	1.09%
For abstracts*	10			0.29%
For staff, editorial board	24			0.71%
For contents in brief	73			2.15%
For contents with abstracts	235			6.92%
For *Information for Authors*	24			0.71%
For volume indexes	102			3.00%
Number of articles (mean/month)	650	(54)		
Long reports	397			61.08%
Coronary artery disease		173	43.58%	
Preventive cardiology		9	2.27%	
Arrhythmias and conduction defects		60	15.11%	
Systemic hypertension		17	4.28%	
Congestive heart failure		11	2.77%	
Valvular heart disease		32	8.06%	
Cardiomyopathy		19	4.79%	
Congenital heart disease		23	5.79%	
Miscellaneous		36	9.07%	
Methods		11	2.77%	
Cardiovascular pharmacology		3	0.75%	
Historic studies		3	0.75%	
Brief reports	209			32.15%
Case reports	19			2.92%
Editorials	20			3.08%
From-the-Editor columns	5			0.77%

*From Section of Cardiology, American Academy of Pediatrics.

The 13 symposia, 2 less than in 1992, included 167 articles occupying 1,076 pages. No advertisements appear in the symposia issues, which are published under separate cover (and a different-colored cover) from that of the regular issues. Most symposia were guest edited by 1 or more major leaders in cardiology.

9. *Sources of articles published in* Cardiology Board Review *in 1993:* The controlled journal *Cardiology Board Review,* edited by Dr. Peter F. Cohn, publishes shortened versions of articles previously published in peer-reviewed journals. Of the 71 articles published in 1993, 33 (46%) came from the AJC, 11 (15%) from the *Journal of the American College of Cardiology,* and 6 (8%) from *Circulation* (Table XII).

10. *Reminder to authors to supply several names with addresses of nonlocal, nonbiased reviewers for their manuscripts:* Editors have no monopoly on choosing the best reviewers of manuscripts. No one should be more knowledgeable of experts in the subject of a manuscript than the authors of the manuscript. Thus, I urge authors to supply names—preferably 5, and when the names are non-board members also the addresses—of nonbiased, nonlocal potential reviewers for their manuscripts. It is necessary for an author to supply several names because almost certainly some of the potential reviewers will already have a manuscript for review and a second manuscript is not sent to a reviewer who also possesses one, unless the second manuscript is a brief report or a case report. Currently, in only about 20% of manuscripts

TABLE VIII Numbers of Manuscripts Submitted and Accepted, Numbers of Editorial Pages Published, and Average Length of Each Article in the AJC in 1992 and 1993

Year	Number of Manuscripts Submitted	Number (%) Manuscripts Accepted	Number of Manuscripts Published	Number of Editorial Pages for Articles Published	Average Length Per Article
1992	1873	664 (35%)	711	3211	4.51
1993	1997	619 (31%)	650	2890	4.45
	(6% ↑)	(7% ↓)	(9% ↓)	(10% ↓)	(1% ↓)

TABLE IX Numbers of Editorial Pages Published in 1993 in *The American Journal of Cardiology* (AJC), *American Heart Journal* (AHJ), *Circulation,* and *The Journal of the American College of Cardiology* (JACC)

Journal	For Articles, Editorials, and Letters	For Indexes
AJC	2,927	102
AHJ	3,336 (12%>)	90
Circulation	5,100 (43%>)	68
JACC	3,818 (23%>)	65

TABLE X Numbers of Editorial Pages Published in the January, February, and March 1994 Issues of *The American Journal of Cardiology, American Heart Journal, Circulation,* and *The Journal of the American College of Cardiology*

Journal	For Articles, Editorials, and Letters
American Journal of Cardiology	626
American Heart Journal	726 (14%>)
Circulation	1,494 (139%>)
Journal of the American College of Cardiology	989 (37%>)

submitted have authors provided names of potential reviewers. After studying reviews by author-suggested reviewers for nearly 12 years, I am impressed that the author-suggested reviewers are of high quality and that the author-suggested reviewers are not more biased toward a manuscript than are editor-selected reviewers. Indeed, many manuscripts have been reviewed by 1 author-suggested reviewer and by 1 editor-selected reviewer and the author-selected reviewer recommended rejection while the editor-selected reviewer recommended acceptance of the manuscript.

The meeting was then opened to comments and questions from board members:

1. *How has the process of rapid decision for manuscripts declined by other journals and accompanied by their previous reviews and responses worked at the AJC?* I think well. This process was initiated several years ago in an attempt to preserve the energies of reviewers. In general, the worst manuscripts get the most reviews and the best manuscripts get the fewest reviews. When a manuscript is declined by another journal, the author may submit the manuscript to the AJC with the reviews from the other journal and with responses to each of the comments or suggestions in the previous reviews. Both the manuscript initially submitted to the other journal and the revised manuscript should be sent to the AJC. In other words, the process should be looked at as if the manuscript had initially been submitted to the AJC and the reviewers had been picked by the AJC. These manuscripts go immediately to my desk and usually an immediate decision is made—either decline, accept with further revision, or accept as is.

This process has allowed the AJC to pick up some excellent manuscripts declined after long review processes by *The New England Journal of Medicine* or other journals. Some authors request the expeditious review process but fail to submit the manuscript originally submitted to the other journal or the previous reviews or the responses to the reviews. The AJC editorial office then must call the corresponding author and request a copy of the manuscript previously submitted to the other journal, the reviews, or the authors' responses to the reviewers' comments. Too often in these circumstances it becomes apparent that the manuscript submitted to the AJC is identical to the manuscript previously submitted to the other journal. In other words, despite good reviews, the authors elected not to change their manuscript one iota or to respond in any way to the comments of the reviewers. To disregard the efforts of reviewers is disrespectful and detrimental to the quality of manuscripts and to the review process itself. Authors who ignore reviewers' comments without altering their manuscript, or at least rebutting appropriately, in general are not viewed favorably.

2. *Would it be better to publish the AJC once a month rather than twice a month?* The publisher went to biweekly publication of the journal several years ago as a means of increasing advertising revenue and it worked. At the time of the change the AJC editorial board voted unanimously against the move to biweekly publication and urged continuation of the monthly publication schedule. Another vote was held at the present meeting and now the board unanimously voted in favor of the twice-a-month over the once-a-month publication. There are differing viewpoints on whether or not the publication costs increase when the journal is published twice a month rather than once a month. Certainly, the biweekly is not less expensive. *Circulation,* incidentally, will soon go to the twice-a-month schedule.

3. *Why not eliminate the contents-with-abstracts section in each issue of the journal?* This section, which also is carried by *Circulation* and *The Journal of the*

TABLE XI Symposia Published in *The American Journal of Cardiology* in 1993

No.	1993 Pub. Date	Subject of Symposium	Guest Editor(s)	Sponsors	Articles	Discussions Included	Pages	Time (mos): Symposium to Publication
A	Jan 21	Aldosterone and antialdosterone therapy	David P. Lauler	Searle	9	0	54	17
B	Feb 25	Antioxidants and lipids	Antonio M. Gotto, Jr.	Marion Merrell Dow	7	+	42	10
C	Mar 25	Carvedilol or bucindolol for heart failure	Michael B. Fowler	SmithKline Beecham & Boehringer Mannheim GmbH	10	0	70	—
D	May 20	Intracoronary Doppler guidewire flow velocity	Morton J.Kern H. Vernon Anderson	Cardiometrics	10	0	86	14
E	June 24	Perindopril for hypertension and heart failure	Giuseppe Mancia	Institut de Recherces Internationales Servier	12	0	68	10
A	Aug 12	Sotalol for ventricular arrhythmias	Jeffrey L. Anderson	Bristol-Myers Squibb & Berlex Laboratories	12	0	85	24
B	Aug 26	QTc interval prolongation	Joel Morganroth	Marion Merrell Dow	12	+	59	10
C	Sept 9	Endothelial and vascular smooth muscle and their secretions	John O. Parker Thomas W. Smith	Schwarz-Pharma	12	0	68	11
D	Sept 30	Familial hypercholesterolemia	Diane E. Bild Roger R. Williams	Merck Sharpe & Dohme & the publisher of AJC	15	0	84	14
E	Oct 18	Directional atherectomy	Donald S. Bain Patrick L. Whitlow	Devices for Vascular Intervention	16	0	108	20
F	Nov 26	Amiodarone and arrhythmias	Bramah N. Singh Steven N. Singh	Wyeth-Ayerst Laboratories	18	0	124	12
G	Dec 16	Thrombolysis	John Ambrose Diego Ardissino Giuseppe Specchia	Boehringer Ingelheim Italia, SpA & Policlinico San Matteo, IRCCS	26	0	180	7
H	Dec 30	Fosinopril	Michael A. Weber	Bristol-Myers Squibb	8	0	48	8
13					167 (13)	2	1,076 (83)	7–24 (13)

TABLE XII Sources of Articles in *Cardiology Board Review* in 1993

Journal	Number of Articles
1. *American Journal of Cardiology*	33 (46%)
2. *Journal of the American College of Cardiology*	11 (15%)
3. *American Heart Journal*	8 (11%)
4. *Circulation*	6 (8%)
5. *Archives of Internal Medicine*	5 (7%)
6. *Annals of Internal Medicine*	4 (6%)
7. *British Heart Journal*	3 (4%)
8. *New England Journal of Medicine*	1 (1%)
	71 (100%)

American College of Cardiology, allows the publisher to charge a premium for advertisements appearing in apposition to the abstracts. A vote was held and only 1 board member favored the retention of the contents-with-abstracts section. The elimination of this section would save over 200 editorial pages a year, and if the saved pages were used for articles, over 50 additional articles could be published in the AJC each year. In the days of reduced advertising pages, the elimination of the contents-with-abstracts section would appear to be a cost-effective move. The cost of each editorial page for 29,000 copies printed 24 times a year was estimated several years ago to be about $300. Today it must be much more.

4. *Is an attempt made to choose at least 1 editorial board member as a reviewer for each manuscript?* It depends on the type of manuscript submitted. Case reports, for example, are virtually never sent to board members. All case reports go directly to my desk and most are declined immediately. Long reports authored by board members historically have gone to 1 or more other board member for review. I would say that an attempt is made to send most long reports to at least 1 board member but we follow no standard procedure in this matter. Board members usually are not sent brief reports for review. When editorials are sent for review, nearly always 1 and usually 2 board members are selected.

5. *Is it necessary to place portions of the brief reports in italics?* No. The methods and result sections—although not labeled as such—of the brief reports have been in italics since this section was initiated 12 years ago. The purpose was to separate the original portion of the report from the introduction and discussion portions —again not labeled as such—of the report. We can look into using a different type of Roman type. I too agree that italics are more difficult to read than Roman type. David Spodick has been urging this change, also, for some time.

6. *Will conversion to submission of a disk with the revised manuscript speed up the editorial processing time?* We think so. Submission of a disk saves us 2 steps—retyping an edited manuscript and proofreading the retyped manuscript.

7. *What about developing a glossary in the Instruction to Authors of most commonly used abbreviations?* This topic was the subject of a from-the-editor column in this journal in April 1983 (AJC 51:A9–A10). It is time to address this subject again and a separate column of this subject will appear soon.

8. *What about providing a summary in bold type for each brief report?* This was started about a year ago but it has been done only sporadically. I think it is a good idea and we will be more consistent in the future.

9. *Will free subscriptions for the cardiology fellows in the USA be continued?* Yes. We are continuing this program, and are currently seeking a sponsor.

The meeting was adjourned to a wonderful reception provided by the publisher. Comments on any item discussed in this piece are welcomed.

William Clifford Roberts, MD
Editor in Chief
Baylor University Medical Center
Dallas, Texas

1. Roberts WC. Alkaline paper and preserving the record. *Am J Cardiol* 1991;68: 1729–1732.

Proceedings of the Editorial Board Meeting of *The American Journal of Cardiology* on March 21, 1995

The 1995 meeting of the editorial board of *The American Journal of Cardiology* (AJC) was held on March 21 in New Orleans, Louisiana, at the time of the Annual Scientific Sessions of The American College of Cardiology. The meeting's purpose was to review AJC publication results for 1994, to recognize particularly those AJC board members reviewing the most manuscripts in 1994, to present a few of my own views on manuscripts, to receive input through questions and comments from the board members present, and to recognize the top 14 reviewers on the editorial board of the AJC during the past 13 years. The meeting went as follows:

1. *Introduction of Mr. Robert Weidner, the Publisher of the AJC:* Mr. Weidner welcomed the board members and thanked them for coming. Bob indicated that the journal was healthy despite some fall off, as in virtually all medical journals, in the number of advertisements appearing in the journal. He warned that a reduction, compared with previous years, in advertisements will probably continue for some time.

2. *Introduction of new AJC board members:* Thirteen new members were added to the board beginning in January 1995 (Table I) and they were introduced. New board members are selected entirely on their record as non-board reviewers of the AJC. Selection is based on review of card files of nearly 2,000 non-board AJC reviewers and those with the best reviewing records are selected. Board members determine their longevity on the AJC board by the quality and promptness of their reviews. Each year it gets more and more difficult to eliminate board members because nearly all have good reviewing records.

3. *Numbers of manuscripts sent for review to board members in 1994:* A total of 1,783 manuscripts were received in the editorial office in 1994 (this number does not include the manuscripts for the supplement issues),[1] and 849 of them were sent to at least 1 of the 198 AJC board members. An average of 4.29 manuscripts were sent to each board member in 1994: 682 (80%) were reviewed on time, 65 (8%) were returned to the office late (>3 weeks from date of mailing from the AJC office), and 102 (12%) were returned without review (Table II). The percent of manuscripts returned without review by board members was the highest during any of the nearly 13 years of my editorship. This larger number may reflect inappropriate choices of reviewers by the editors as well as insufficient time to provide reviews by the potential reviewers.

4. *AJC board members reviewing the most manuscripts in 1994:* The top AJC reviewers in 1994 were Doctors Fred Morady and L. David Hillis, both of whom reviewed 11 manuscripts, all within the 3-week time period (Table III). Dr. Navin C. Nanda reviewed 10 manuscripts (Table III); Doctors Peter C. Block and Peter F. Cohn reviewed 9 manuscripts and 6 board members reviewed 8 manuscripts (Table III). Ten board members reviewed 7 manuscripts, all within the allotted time (Table IV), and 21 board members reviewed 6 manuscripts (Table V). The reviewing records of the 42 board

TABLE I New AJC Board Members Beginning January 1995

Rodney H. Falk
Ted Feldman
Stanley J. Goldberg
Samuel Z. Goldhaber
K. Lance Gould
Paul A. Grayburn
Robert E. Kleiger
Paul Kligfield
James E. Muller
Marc A. Silver
Mark E. Silverman
Thomas Spray
Frans Wackers

TABLE II Numbers and Types of Manuscripts Sent to AJC Board Members in 1994 According to Board Member Specialty

Specialty	Number on Board	Number MSs sent (No./reviewer)	No. LR	No. BR	No. CR	No. E	No. (%) reviewed on time	No. (%) reviewed late	No. (%) MSs returned without review
Adult cardiology	163	735 (4.51)	632 (86%)	95 (13%)	3 (<1%)	5 (<1%)	590 (80%)	57 (8%)	88 (12%)
Pediatric cardiology	17	59 (3.47)	46 (78%)	12 (20%)	1 (2%)	0 —	49 (83%)	4 (7%)	6 (10%)
Cardiac surgery	10	29 (2.90)	25 (86%)	2 (7%)	2 (7%)	0 —	22 (76%)	2 (7%)	5 (17%)
Related specialty	8	26 (3.25)	21 (81%)	4 (15%)	0 —	1 (4%)	21 (81%)	2 (8%)	3 (11%)
TOTALS	198	849 (4.29)	724 (85%)	113 (13%)	6 (<1%)	6 (<1%)	682 (80%)	65 (8%)	102 (12%)

BR = brief report; CR = case report; E = editorial; LR = long report; MSs = manuscripts; No. = number.

TABLE III Top Reviewers of Manuscripts for the AJC in 1994						
Name	Number of manuscripts reviewed	LR	BR	CR	E	Number reviewed on time
Fred Morady	11	10	0	1	0	11
L. David Hillis	11	10	1	0	0	11
Navin C. Nanda	10	7	3	0	0	10
Peter C. Block	9	8	1	0	0	9
Peter F. Cohn	9	8	1	0	0	9
Gregory J. Dehmer	8	6	2	0	0	8
Gerald Fletcher	8	6	2	0	0	8
Nancy C. Flowers	8	7	1	0	0	8
Abdulmassih S. Iskandrian	8	7	1	0	0	8
Jeffrey J. Popma	8	6	2	0	0	2
David H. Spodick	8	8	0	0	0	8

Abbreviations as in Table II.

members who reviewed 11, 10, 9, 8, 7, or 6 manuscripts during 1994 are truly remarkable, and these board members represent 21% of the total board. The editor also is fully aware that the AJC is not the only medical journal for which the board members review manuscripts.

5. *Numbers of pages and articles and types of articles published in the AJC in 1994:* These data are listed in Table VI. A total of 604 articles (an average of 50 per month) were published on 2,493 pages (an average of 208 per month) in 1994. The average length of each article was 4.13 pages, a 7% decrease compared with 1993 (Table VII). In 1994, a total of 1,783 manuscripts were submitted, an 11% reduction from 1993, and 509 manuscripts (29%) were accepted, an 18% decrease from 1993. Although 604 manuscripts (Table VI) were published in 1994 in the AJC, some of those manuscripts had been submitted in 1993 and some of the manuscripts submitted in 1994 will not be published until 1995. The number of editorial pages for articles in the AJC in 1994 was 2,493, a 14% decrease compared with 1993. Of the 604 articles actually published in 1994, 341 (56%) were long reports, and 221 (37%) were brief reports. Many articles submitted as long reports eventually are published as brief reports. The brief reports section of the AJC is the unique portion of the AJC in my view.

6. *Symposia published in the AJC in 1994:* Five symposia were published in the AJC in 1994 (Table VIII) compared to 13 published in 1993. Already in 1995, 16 symposia are scheduled for publication. No advertisements, of course, appear in the symposia issues, which are published under separate cover and a different colored cover from that of the regular issues. The guest editors of most symposia are major leaders in cardiology around the world.

7. *Reminder to authors to supply several names with addresses of non-local, non-biased reviewers for their manuscripts:* Editors have no monopoly on choosing the best reviewers of manuscripts. No one should be more knowledgeable of experts in the subject of the manuscript than the author of the manuscript. Thus, I urge authors to supply names—preferably 5, and when the names are non-board members, also their addresses—of non-local, non-biased, potential reviewers of their manuscripts. It is necessary for an author to submit several names because almost certainly some of the potential reviewers will already have a manuscript for review and a second manuscript is not sent to a reviewer already having one unless 1 of the 2 manuscripts is a brief report or case report. Currently, about 20% of the authors supply names of potential reviewers for their manuscripts. After studying the reviews of authors' suggested reviewers for nearly 13 years, I am impressed that the authors' suggested reviewers are of high quality and that the authors' suggested reviewers are no more biased toward their manuscripts than are editor-selected reviewers. Indeed, many manuscripts have been reviewed by 1 author-suggested reviewer and 1 editor-suggested reviewer, and the author-suggested reviewer recommended rejection while the editor-suggested reviewer recommended acceptance of the manuscript.

8. *Changes in the AJC in 1994:* The cover, table of contents, and article title pages were altered and the changes appeared with the January 1, 1995 issue. The

TABLE IV Reviewers of 7 Manuscripts for the AJC in 1994					
Name	LR	BR	CR	E	Number reviewed on time
Jeffrey Anderson	6	1	0	0	7
George A. Beller	7	0	0	0	7
William E. Boden	4	1	0	2	7
Robert M. Califf	7	0	0	0	7
Sanjiv Kaul	7	0	0	0	7
Morton J. Kern	6	1	0	0	7
Carl V. Leier	7	0	0	0	7
Barry J. Maron	7	0	0	0	7
Raymond G. McKay	6	1	0	0	7
D. Woodrow Benson Jr.	5	2	0	0	7

Abbreviations as in Table II.

TABLE V Reviewers of 6 Manuscripts for the AJC in 1994					
Name	LR	BR	CR	E	Number reviewed on time
Joseph S. Alpert	4	2	0	0	6
Thomas M. Bashore	5	1	0	0	6
Robert O. Bonow	5	1	0	0	1
Michael E. Cain	5	1	0	0	6
Richard O. Cannon III	6	0	0	0	6
Michael H. Crawford	6	0	0	0	6
Myrvin H. Ellestad	5	1	0	0	6
Robert L. Feldman	5	1	0	0	6
Joseph A. Franciosa	5	1	0	0	6
William H. Gaasch	4	2	0	0	6
Julius M. Gardin	6	0	0	0	4
Donald C. Harrison	4	2	0	0	6
Geoffrey O. Hartzler	6	0	0	0	6
David R. Holmes Jr.	5	1	0	0	5
Joseph Lindsay Jr.	5	1	0	0	6
Richard S. Meltzer	6	0	0	0	6
Maria-Teresa Olivari	6	0	0	0	6
Joseph K. Perloff	5	1	0	0	6
Nelson B. Schiller	6	0	0	0	6
Eric J. Topol	5	1	0	0	6
Nanette K. Wenger	5	1	0	0	6

Abbreviations as in Table II.

new publication process allows text to be included more closely around figures and tables than in the past. These stylistic changes yield an increased content per page. Beginning July 1995 the "contents with abstracts" will be eliminated and then the number of editorial pages available for articles will increase by approximately 150 yearly.

9. *Review of technical features required of manuscripts submitted to the AJC:* With the industry-wide reduction in advertising revenue, the number of editorial pages available in scientific journals has diminished in recent years. As a consequence, pressure for the editorial pages has never been greater. When I became editor of the AJC in 1982, about 3,300 editorial pages were published yearly, and approximately 1,100 manuscripts were received yearly. Today, we have about 2,500 editorial pages for articles and we now receive about 1,800 manuscripts yearly. The publication of numerous brief reports allows the number of total articles published in the AJC each year to remain high. But longer articles are becoming shorter. We no longer have unlimited space for long discussions, long introductions, or long abstracts. The methods and results sections are the heart of any manuscript and they need to be in exquisite detail, but the other portions must now be limited. I agree with Doctor John Shaw Billings'[1] comment on manuscripts submitted to medical journals: "the author must have something to say, say it, stop as soon as it is said, and give the article a proper title." Clear, precise writing has never been more in demand than at present. The introduction ideally should be a single paragraph filling no more than one-half page typed double-spaced. The abstract should occupy no more than a single page typed double-spaced.[2] The discussion section must be limited, usually to no more than 3 double-spaced typed pages. If manuscripts concern 30 patients or less, a table showing the findings in each of those 30 patients with no more than 1 line across is usually preferred over a table showing only pooled data.[3,4] More focus needs to be on tables and figures.[5] When the message of the manuscript can be shown graphically, the manuscript is usually a good one. The AJC usually limits its references to no more than 30 in a long report and to 20 in a brief report. Preparing references tells much about the scholarship of the authors.[6] Examples of good and not so good titles were shown.[7] Subtitles are usually avoided in the AJC.[7] Abbreviations should be kept to a minimum, no more than 3 per manuscript and usually limited to phrases in the article's title.[8] And finally, it is wise to read the Instructions to Authors before submitting a manuscript to a journal.[9,10] Clues to the editor's pleasures and displeasures can often be detected from the Instructions to Authors.

TABLE VI Numbers of Pages and Articles and Types of Articles Published in the Regular Issues of the AJC in 1994

Number of pages	2,921			
For articles (mean/month) [pages/article]	2,493	(208)	[4.13]	85%
For *Readers' Comments* (number) [number replies]	31	(46)	[11]	1%
For staff, editorial board	34			1%
For contents in brief	70			2%
For contents with abstracts	187			6%
For *Information for Authors*	24			1%
For volume indexes	82			3%
Number of articles (mean/month)	604	(50)		
Long reports	341			56%
Coronary artery disease		154	45%	
Preventive cardiology		12	4%	
Arrhythmias and conduction defects		55	16%	
Systemic hypertension		16	5%	
Congestive heart failure		8	2%	
Valvular heart disease		21	6%	
Cardiomyopathy		14	4%	
Congenital heart disease		22	6%	
Miscellaneous		25	7%	
Methods		10	3%	
Cardiovascular pharmacology		1	<1%	
Historical studies		3	<1%	
Brief reports	221			37%
Case reports	23			4%
Editorials	12			2%
From-the-Editor columns	7			1%

TABLE VII Numbers of Manuscripts Submitted, Articles and Editorial Pages Published, Percent Published, and Average Length of Each Article in the AJC in the Past 5 Years

Year	Number of manuscripts submitted	Number of manuscripts published	Percent accepted	Number of editorial pages for articles	Average pages per article
1990	1,717	662	39%	3,001	4.53
1991	1,615	680	42%	3,165	4.65
1992	1,873	664	35%	3,211	4.51
1993	1,997	619	31%	2,890	4.45
1994	1,783* (11%↓)†	509 (18%↓)†	29% (2%↓)†	2,493 (14%↓)†	4.13 (7%↓)†

*Of these 1,783 manuscripts, 860 (48%) came from medical centers in the USA, and 332 (39%) were accepted; 923 manuscripts (52%) came from non-USA medical centers, and 177 (19%) were accepted.
†Comparison of 1994 to 1993.

The meeting was opened to comments and questions from board members:

1. *How many subscribers does the AJC presently have?* The publisher indicated that the AJC has approximately 19,000 paid subscribers, and that 9,000 to 11,000 journals of each issue also are sent to non-paid subscribers, mainly to general internists, in an attempt to acquire new paid subscribers.

2. *Why not publish only 1 regular issue each month, rather than 2?* This issue arose at the editorial board meeting in 1994 and the board voted overwhelmingly in favor of only 1 regular issue per month. As I recall, only 1 board member preferred 2 issues per month. The mailing expenses and costs of covers, etc., would of course be less if the journal was published only once a month instead of twice per month. At the moment, each subscriber receives 24 issues of the regular blue-covered issues per year, and in 1995 we expect from 15 to 20 symposia to be published, which means that the subscriber in 1995 will receive just over 40 issues.

Editorial Board Meeting of *The American Journal of Cardiology*, March 21, 1995, New Orleans, Louisiana

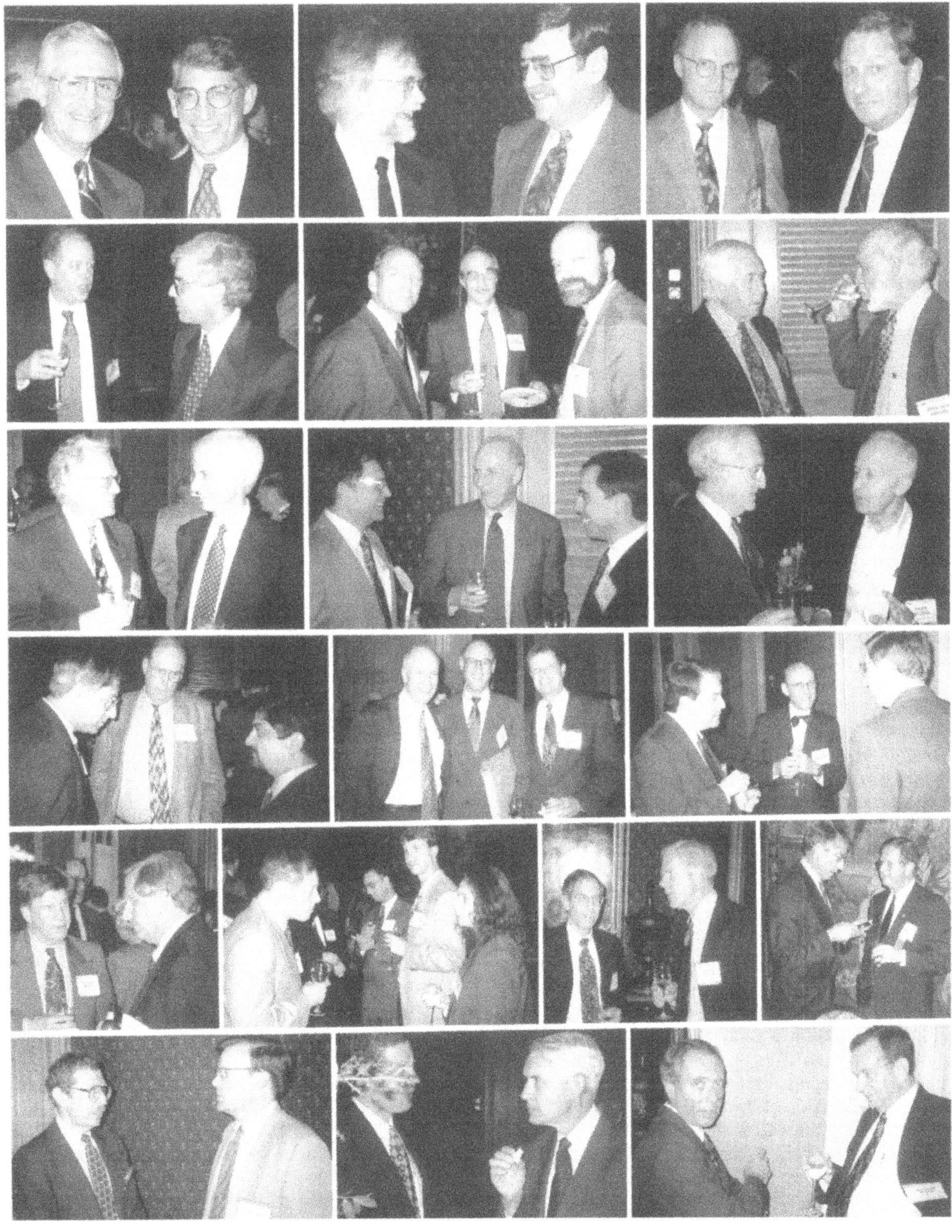

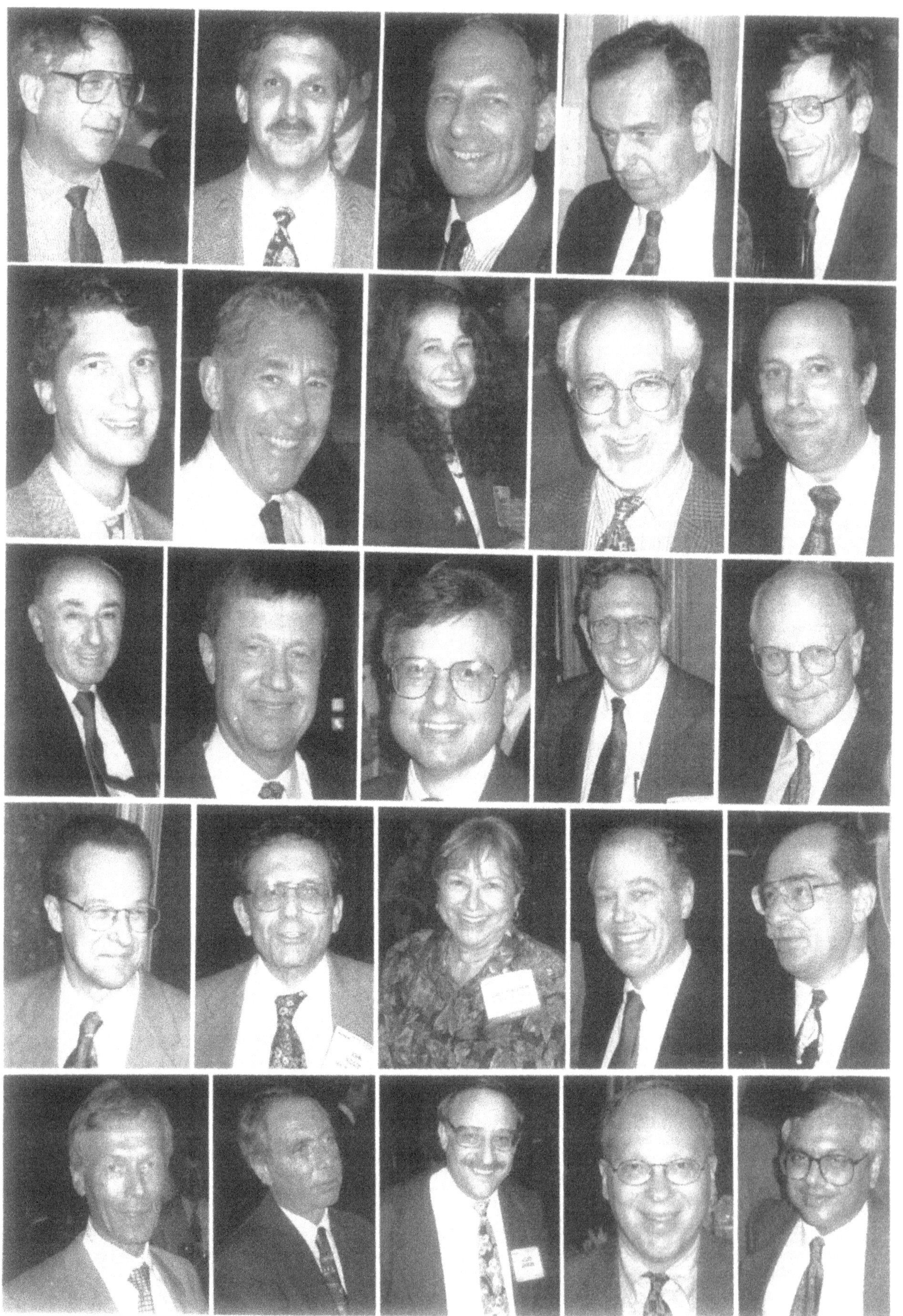

TABLE VIII Symposia Published in the AJC in 1994

Supplement	1994 Publication date	Subject of symposium	Guest editor(s)	Sponsors	Articles	Pages	Time (mos.) symposium to publication
A	Jan 27	Amlodipine	William H. Frishman	Pfizer Labs	10	58	—
B	Mar 10	Diltiazem	Peter F. Cohn	Marion Merrell Dow	10	44	15
C	April 7	Trandolapril	Bernard Swynghedauw A. John Camm	Roussel UCLAF Cardiovascular	8	50	19
D	May 26	Fluvastatin	W. Virgil Brown	Sandoz Pharmaceuticals	9	61	19
A	Dec 22	Rilmenidine	John H. Laragh	Servier	10	65	30
TOTALS					47	278	mean: 21

3. *How does the new editorial director impact on the editor in chief?* The new editorial director, Kathleen Dallessio, is responsible for the editorial quality of the journals in her group. She is Excerpta Medica's in-house voice for the editorial content and the editorial board. The position, in my view, is a statement that Excerpta Medica is quite serious about editorial content. The company believes that *editorial value* is the primary reason for success of any medical journal.

4. *Does Excerpta Medica plan on reviewing its policy regarding requests for permission to reproduce figures and tables previously published in the AJC?* Excerpta Medica is currently reviewing its permissions guidelines in order to ensure that its policy protects copyrighted material and is equitable to all parties.

Awards to the 14 most outstanding reviewers for the AJC during the last 13 years: The publisher prepared a nice plaque for each of the 14 most outstanding AJC reviewers during my nearly 13 years of editorship (Figure 1). The names of the 14 awardees are listed in Table IX. These men all deserve our heartiest thanks for taking the most time to make all of our manuscripts better.

The meeting was adjourned to a splendid reception provided by the publisher.

William C. Roberts

William Clifford Roberts, MD
Editor in Chief
Baylor University Medical Center
Dallas, Texas 75246

TABLE IX The 14 Most Outstanding Reviewers for AJC During the Last 13 Years

Michael H. Crawford
Jeffrey M. Isner
Barry J. Maron
Joel Morganroth
Carl J. Pepine
David H. Spodick
L. David Hillis
Robert O. Bonow
Joseph S. Alpert
George A. Beller
James T. Willerson
C. Richard Conti
Melvin M. Scheinman
Frank I. Marcus

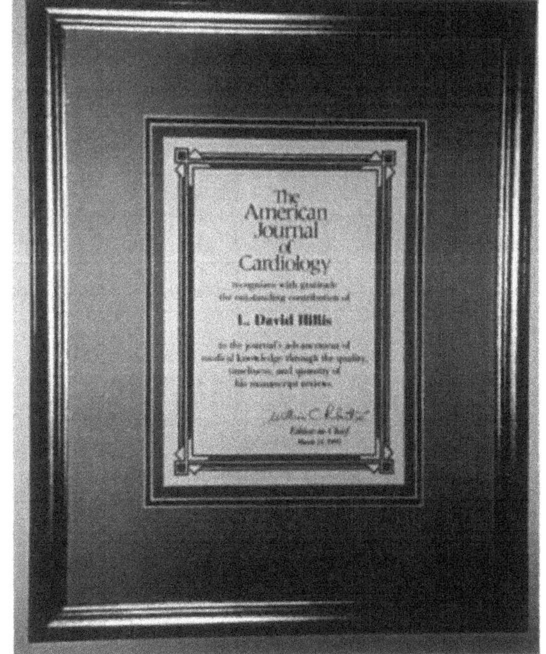

FIGURE 1. One of the plaques awarded to the 14 most outstanding reviewers of the AJC during the last 13 years.

1. Chapman CB. Order Out of Chaos: John Shaw Billings and America's Coming of Age. Canton, Massachusetts: Watson Publishing International, 1994:420.
2. Roberts WC. The summary: the manuscript's bottom line. *Am J Cardiol* 1983;52:A3.
3. Roberts WC. Making clinical studies involving many patients useful to the single patient. *Am J Cardiol* 1990;65:1408.
4. Roberts WC. Oft-repeated requests to authors from an editor of a cardiology journal. *Am J Cardiol* 1991;68:1121–1122.
5. Roberts WC. The search for the masterful figure. *Am J Cardiol* 1987;60:633–634.
6. Roberts WC. References: a clue to scholarship. *Am J Cardiol* 1983;51:A9–A10.
7. Roberts WC. The article's title. *Am J Cardiol* 1985;56:210–212.
8. Roberts WC. Abbreviations in the AJC. *Am J Cardiol* 1983;51:A9–A10.
9. Roberts WC. Studying the "Instructions to Authors" before final typing of a manuscript for submission to a medical journal. *Am J Cardiol* 1984;52:398.
10. Roberts WC. Further comments on the "Instructions to Authors." *Am J Cardiol* 1984;54:470.

I would like to thank all those who took the time to write me concerning my piece about my mother—"Ruby Viola Holbrook Roberts (1903–1994)" (*Am J Cardiol* 1994;74:1078). Your thoughtful and touching comments are greatly appreciated.

William C. Roberts

Proceedings of the Editorial Board Meeting of *The American Journal of Cardiology* on March 26, 1996

The 1996 meeting of the editorial board of *The American Journal of Cardiology* (AJC) was held on March 26 in Orlando, Florida, at the time of the Annual Scientific Sessions of the American College of Cardiology. The meeting went as follows:

1. *Numbers of manuscripts sent for review to board members in 1995:* A total of 1,844 manuscripts were received in the editorial office in 1995 (This number does not include the manuscripts for the supplement issues.), and 877 (48%) of them were sent to at least 1 of the 205 AJC board members (Table I). An average of 4.28 manuscripts were sent to each board member in 1995: 714 (81%) of the 877 manuscripts were reviewed in a timely fashion (<3 weeks from the date of mailing from the AJC office), and 94 (11%) were returned without review.

2. *Numbers and types of manuscripts sent to AJC*

TABLE I Numbers and Types of Manuscripts Sent to *AJC* Board Members in 1995 According to Board-Member Specialty

Specialty	Number on Board	Number MSs Sent (no./reviewer)	No. LR	No. BR	No. CR	No. E	No. (%) Reviewed on Time	No. (%) Reviewed Late	No. (%) MSs Returned Without Review
Adult cardiology	169	733 (4.34)	620 (85%)	98 (13%)	11 (1.5%)	4 (<1%)	599 (82%)	54 (7%)	80 (11%)
Pediatric cardiology	18	82 (4.56)	59 (72%)	20 (24%)	3 (4%)	0 —	68 (83%)	7 (8.5%)	7 (8.5%)
Cardiac surgery	10	27 (2.70)	17 (63%)	7 (26%)	3 (11%)	0 —	22 (82%)	3 (11%)	2 (7%)
Related specialty	8	35 (4.34)	25 (71%)	10 (29%)	0 —	0 —	25 (72%)	5 (14%)	5 (14%)
TOTALS	205	877 (4.28)	721 (82%)	135 (15%)	17 (2%)	4 (<1%)	714 (81%)	69 (8%)	94 (11%)

BR = brief report; CR = case report; E = editorial; LR = long report; MSs = manuscripts; No. = number.

TABLE II Numbers and Types of Manuscripts Sent to *AJC* Board Members in Each of the Last 9 Years

Year	Number on Board	Number of MSs Sent (no./reviewer)	No. LR	No. BR	No. CR	No. (%) Reviewed on Time	No. (%) Reviewed Late	No. (%) MSs Returned Without Review
1995	205	877 (4.3)	721 (82%)	135 —	17 —	714 (81%)	69 (8%)	94 (11%)
1994	198	849 (4.3)	724 (85%)	113 —	6 —	682 (80%)	65 (8%)	102 (12%)
1993	184	805 (4.4)	773 (96%)	30 —	2 —	663 (82%)	77 (10%)	65 (8%)
1992	178	1,107 (6.2)	1,062 (96%)	34 —	11 —	1,025 (93%)	60 (5%)	22 (2%)
1991	164	984 (6.0)	938 (95%)	37 —	9 —	921 (94%)	18 (2%)	45 (4%)
1990	160	844 (5.2)	789 (93%)	50 —	5 —	788 (93%)	20 (3%)	36 (4%)
1989	148	812 (5.5)	775 (95%)	30 —	5 —	751 (92%)	22 (3%)	39 (5%)
1988	138	634 (4.6)	569 (90%)	25 —	40 —	548 (86%)	56 (9%)	30 (5%)
1987	141	662 (4.7)	554 (84%)	108 —	— —	554 (84%)	82 (12%)	26 (4%)
TOTALS = 9		7,574 (5.0)	6,905 (91%)	562 (8%)	95 (1%)	6,646 (88%)	469 (6%)	459 (6%)

Abbreviations as in Table I.

TABLE III Board Members Reviewing the Most Manuscripts for the *AJC* in 1995

Name	Number of Manuscripts Reviewed	Long Reports	Brief Reports	Case Reports	Number Reviewed on Time
Paul A. Grayburn	9	9	0	0	9
Robert A. Kloner	9	7	2	0	9
David J. Sahn	9	7	2	0	6
Hugh D. Allen	8	4	3	1	7
Joseph S. Alpert	8	8	0	0	8
Agustin Castellanos	8	8	0	0	7
Pablo Denes	8	7	1	0	7
William H. Gaasch	8	6	1	1	8
Abdulmassih S. Iskandrian	8	7	1	0	8
Jeffrey M. Isner	8	7	1	0	8
Fred Morady	8	7	1	0	8
Robert J. Myerburg	8	8	0	0	5
Nathaniel Reichek	8	7	1	0	8
John R. Wilson	8	7	1	0	8
TOTALS 14	115	99 (86%)	14 (12%)	2 (2%)	106 (92%)

TABLE IV Board Members Reviewing 7 Manuscripts for the *AJC* in 1995

Name	Number of Manuscripts Reviewed	Long Reports	Brief Reports	Case Reports	Number Reviewed on Time
Bruce S. Alpert	7	6	1	0	7
Robert O. Bonow	7	7	0	0	2
Richard O. Cannon III	7	6	1	0	7
Bernard R. Chaitman	7	7	0	0	7
Robert J. Cody	7	7	0	0	7
Gregory J. Dehmer	7	7	0	0	7
Eric Eichhorn	7	7	0	0	7
Gary S. Francis	7	5	2	0	7
Spencer B. King III	7	7	0	0	6
James E. Lock	7	4	2	1	5
Barry J. Maron	7	4	2	1	7
Franz H. Messerli	7	6	1	0	3
Gerald B. Naccarelli	7	7	0	0	7
Navin C. Nanda	7	7	0	0	7
Lowell W. Perry	7	4	3	0	7
David H. Spodick	7	4	3	0	7
TOTALS 16	112	95 (85%)	15 (13%)	2 (2%)	100 (89%)

TABLE V Board Members Reviewing 6 Manuscripts for the *AJC* in 1995

Name	Number of Manuscripts Reviewed	Long Reports	Brief Reports	Case Reports	Number Reviewed on Time
Donald S. Baim	6	6	0	0	6
Thomas M. Bashore	6	6	0	0	5
George A. Beller	6	5	1	0	6
J. Thomas Bigger, Jr.	6	5	1	0	3
William E. Boden	6	6	0	0	6
Alfred E. Buxton	6	5	1	0	4
John S. Child	6	4	2	0	6
Michael H. Crawford	6	5	1	0	5
Pamela S. Douglas	6	5	1	0	6
Stephen Ellis	6	5	1	0	6
Joseph A. Franciosa	6	3	1	2	4
Victor F. Froelicher, Jr.	6	6	0	0	6
W. Bruce Fye	6	4	2	0	4
L. David Hillis	6	4	2	0	6
Robert E. Kleiger	6	5	1	0	5
Joseph Lindsay, Jr.	6	6	0	0	6
Douglas P. Zipes	6	5	1	0	6
TOTALS 17	102	85 (83%)	15 (15%)	2 (2%)	90 (88%)

TABLE VI Numbers of Pages, Articles, and Types of Articles Published in the Regular Issues of the *AJC* in 1995

Number of pages	2,869			
For articles (mean/month) [pages/article]	2,570	(214)	[3.85]	
For *Readers' Comments* (number) [replies]	34	(52)	[4]	
For staff, editorial board	48			
For contents in brief	79			
For contents with abstracts	49			
For *Instructions to Authors*	14			
For volume indexes	75			
Number of articles (mean/month)	668	(56)		
Long reports	354			53%
Coronary artery disease		171		
Preventive cardiology		17		
Arrhythmias and conduction defects		49		
Systemic hypertension		9		
Congestive heart failure		20		
Valvular heart disease		19		
Cardiomyopathy		8		
Congenital heart disease		19		
Miscellaneous		26		
Methods		12		
Cardiovascular pharmacology		2		
Historical studies		2		
Brief reports	268			40%
Case reports	18			3%
Editorials	24			4%
From-the-Editor columns	4			<1%

board members in each of the last 9 years: These data are summarized in Table II. The percentage of manuscripts returned without review is higher in the last 2 years than in any of the previous 7 years.

3. *AJC board members reviewing the most manuscripts in 1995:* The top AJC reviewers in 1995 were Doctors Paul A. Grayburn, Robert A. Kloner, and David J. Sahn, each of whom reviewed 9 manuscripts (Table III). The names of the 11 reviewers of 8 manuscripts also are listed in Table III. Sixteen board members reviewed 7 manuscripts (Table IV), and 17 board members reviewed 6 manuscripts (Table V). The reviewing records of the 47 board members reviewing 9, 8, 7, and 6 manuscripts is truly remarkable, and these board members represent 23% of the total board. The editor is also aware that the AJC is not the only medical journal for which the board members review manuscripts.

4. *Numbers of pages and articles and types of articles published in the AJC in 1995:* These data are listed in Table VI. A total of 668 articles, an average of 56 a month, were published on 2,570 pages, an average of 214 a month, in 1995. The average length of each article was 3.85 pages.

TABLE VII Numbers of Manuscripts Submitted and Published and Numbers of Editorial Pages Published in the *AJC* 1983–1995

Year	Number of Manuscripts Submitted	Number of Manuscripts Published	Percent Accepted	Number of Editorial Pages for Articles	Average Pages Per Article
1995	1,844*	668*	36%	2,570	3.85
1994	1,783	604	34%	2,493	4.13
1993	1,997	619	31%	2,890	4.45
1992	1,873	664	35%	3,211	4.51
1991	1,615	680	42%	3,165	4.65
1990	1,717	662	38%	3,001	4.53
1989	1,740	699	40%	2,903	4.15
1988	1,496	636	42%	2,642	4.15
1987	1,525	695	46%	2,810	4.04
1986	1,574	616	39%	2,627	4.26
1985	1,707	645	38%	2,623	4.07
1984	1,604	747	46%	3,077	4.12
1983	1,234	643	52%	3,130	4.87

* Of the 1,844 manuscripts submitted in 1995, 603 have been published or accepted and 80 have been tentatively accepted pending review. Thus, the acceptance rate for manuscripts actually submitted in 1995 was 37%.

Editorial Board Meeting of *The American Journal of Cardiology*, March 26, 1996, Orlando, Florida

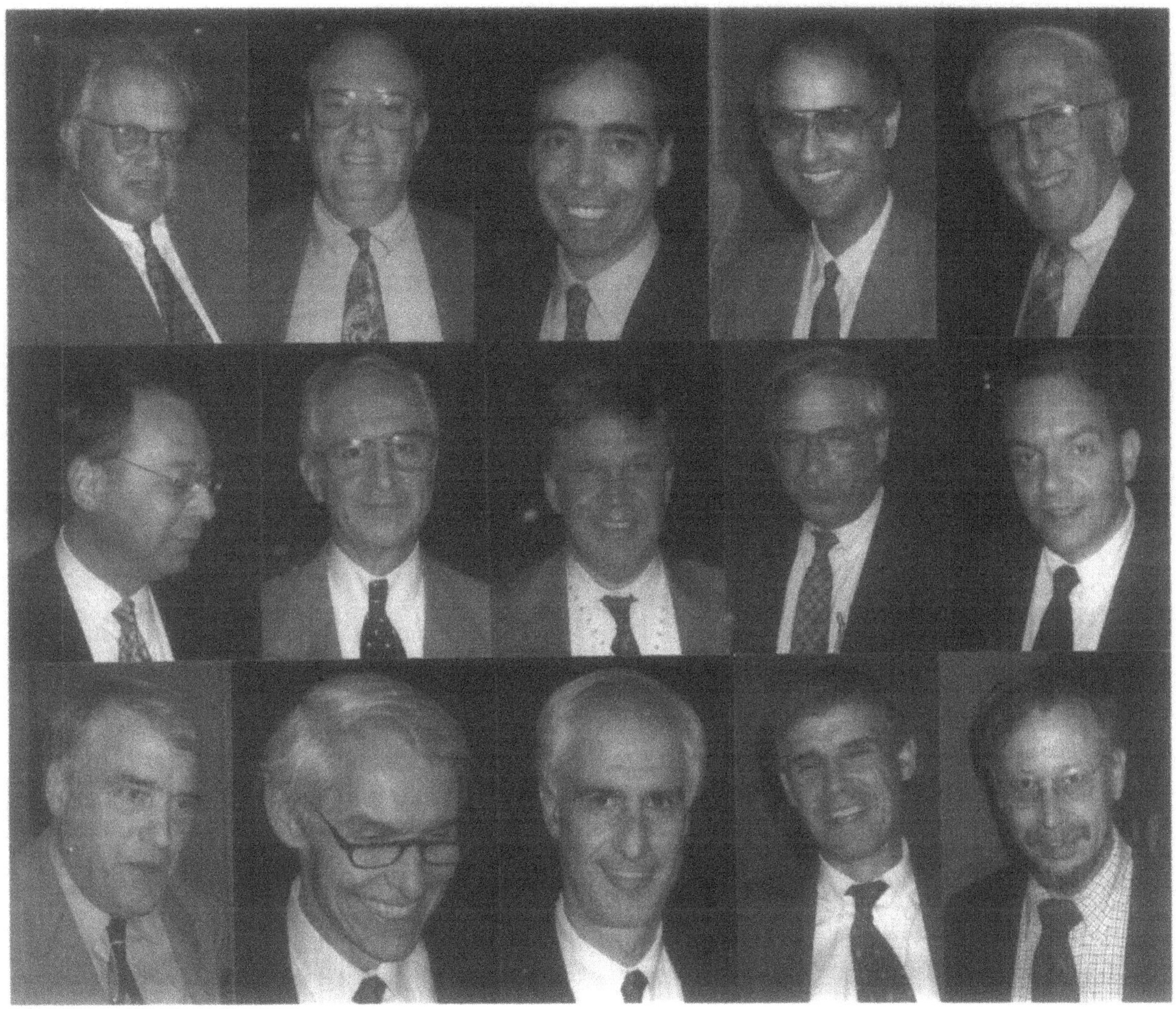

5. *Numbers of manuscripts submitted, number published, percent accepted, numbers of editorial pages used for articles, and average pages per article in each year 1983 through 1995:* These are listed in Table VII. The first full year of editorship for the present editor was 1983. Although the percentage of submitted manuscripts accepted is about one third in recent years, virtually all originally submitted manuscripts are revised considerably before they are accepted. Many manuscripts submitted as long reports, for example, are eventually published as brief reports. The brief report section of the AJC is the unique feature of the journal.

6. *Countries of origin and acceptance rates of manuscripts submitted in 1995:* These data are presented in Table VIII.

7. *Numbers of pages for articles and letters published in the regular issues of the 4 major USA cardiologic journals in 1995:* These data are summarized in Table IX.

8. *Symposia published in the AJC in 1995:* The 11 symposia are listed in Table X.

9. *Numbers of symposia and numbers of articles and pages in each of the 13 years of the present editorship:* These are listed in Table XI. A total of 173 symposia including 2,144 articles and 12,236

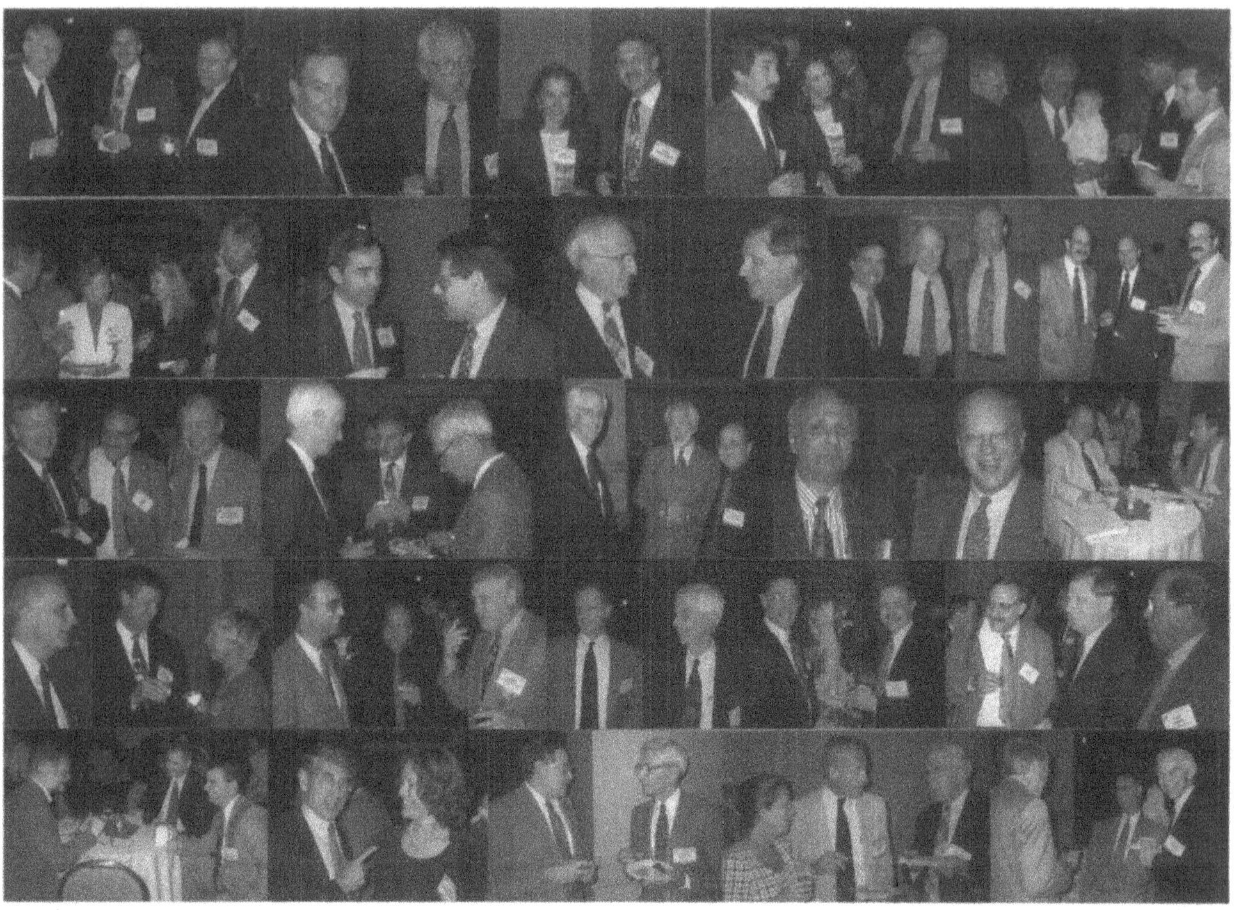

editorial pages were published in the AJC from 1983 through 1995.

10. *Articles originally published in the AJC and summarized in another journal:* Dr. Peter Cohn edits *Cardiology Board Review* which summarizes articles previously published in peer-reviewed journals. Of the 50 articles published in *Cardiology Board Review* in 1995, the AJC was the source of 16 (32%) of them (Table XII). Thank you Dr. Cohn!

TABLE VIII Origin of Manuscripts Submitted to the *AJC* in 1995 and the Number and Percent Accepted

	Number Submitted	Number (%) Accepted
USA	911 (49%)	380 (42%)
Non–USA	931 (51%)	303 (33%)
Japan	170	43 (25%)
Italy	120	36 (30%)
France	82	17 (21%)
Germany	81	29 (36%)
United Kingdom	59	24 (41%)
Netherlands	56	24 (43%)
China	42	12 (29%)
Israel	41	17 (41%)
Spain	31	6 (19%)
Canada	25	16 (64%)
Australia	24	14 (58%)
Switzerland	20	4 (20%)
Turkey	20	3 (15%)
Finland	17	7 (41%)
Greece	17	6 (35%)
India	17	4 (23%)
Sweden	15	6 (40%)
Austria	14	5 (36%)
Hong Kong	12	2 (17%)
Denmark	10	6 (60%)
Others	58	22 (38%)

The meeting was then opened to comments and questions from board members:

1. *Why not publish the AJC once a month rather than twice a month?* A vote was held. Of the estimated 115 board members in attendance, all but 2 favored the once/month schedule, rather than the twice/month schedule.

2. *Does Excerpta Medica, the publisher of the AJC, plan to review its policy regarding requests for*

TABLE IX Numbers of Pages for Articles and Letters Published in the 4 Major USA Cardiologic Journals in 1995

Journal	Pages for Articles & Letters	Percent Difference from AJC	Pages for Index
AJC	2,604	—	75
AHJ	2,564	−2%	63
Circ.	6,639	+61%	88
JACC	3,502	+26%	66

AHJ = American Heart Journal; *AJC* = American Journal of Cardiology; *Circ.* = Circulation; *JACC* = Journal of the American College of Cardiology.

TABLE X Symposia Published in the *AJC* in 1995

Supplement	1995 Publication Date	Subject of Symposium	Guest Editor(s)	Sponsor(s)	Articles	Pages	Interval (mo) Symposium to Publication
A	January 19	Prostacyclin	Robert O. Bonow Nazzareno Galiè Mihai Gheorghiade Bruno Magnani		12	73	14
B	February 23	Atherothrombosis	William C. Roberts Jack Hirsh H. Bryan Brewer, Jr. R. Wayne Alexander	Dupont Pharma	20	97	13
C	March 23	Bari and EAST Trials (PTCA-vs-CABG)	Robert L. Frye Spencer B. King III George Sopko Katherine M. Detre	NIH & AJC	7	59	—
D	April 13	Cardiac imaging	Timothy Bateman	Mallinckrodt Medical, Inc.	11	78	14
E	April 27	Nisoldipine	Shahbudin H. Rahimtoola Willem J. Remme	Bayer AG	13	76	10
F	June 16	Delapril	Sergio Dalla-Volta	Chiesi Farmaceutici SpA	10	55	—
A	July 13	Fluvastatin	Gustav Schonfeld James Shephard	Sandoz Pharma Ltd.	30	142	11
B	August 24	Trimetazidine	Attilio Maseri	Groupe de Recherche Servier–Les Laboratoires Biopharmaceutiques de France	10	49	11
C	September 28	Pravastatin	Frank M. Sacks Marc A. Pfeffer Eugene Braunwald	Bristol-Myers Squibb	20	126	8
D	November 2	Enalapril	Miguel M. Iriarte Antonio Bayés de Luna Bernard Swynghedauw	Merck, Sharpe & Dohme	12	63	8
E	November 24	Perindopril	Jay N. Cohn	Groupe de Recherche Servier, France	11	54	14
TOTALS 11		—	—	—	156	872	11 (mean)

permission to reproduce figures and tables previously published in the AJC? The restriction policy put into place in 1994 has been rescinded. Authors no longer will have to pay a fee to Excerpta Medica to reproduce their tables and figures previously published in the AJC.

3. *At what stage of a multicenter trial might the AJC be willing to publish the trial's protocol?* This

TABLE XI Symposia Published in the *AJC* 1983–1995

Year	Number of Symposia	Number of Articles	Number of Pages
1995	11	156	872
1994	5	47	278
1993	13	167	1,076
1992	15	165	979
1991	9	99	631
1990	20	226	1,169
1989	20	232	1,240
1988	19	252	1,393
1987	19	279	1,576
1986	13	143	832
1985	15	192	1,161
1984	9	126	703
1983	5	60	326
13	173 (n = 13)	2,144 (mean/issue = 12)	12,236 (mean/issue = 71)

TABLE XII Sources of Articles in *Cardiology Board Review* in 1995

Journal	Number of Articles
1. *American Journal of Cardiology*	16 (32%)
2. *Journal of the American College of Cardiology*	12 (24%)
3. *Circulation*	6 (12%)
4. *American Heart Journal*	5 (10%)
5. *New England Journal of Medicine*	4 (8%)
6. *Archives of Internal Medicine*	3 (6%)
7. *Annals of Internal Medicine*	3 (6%)
8. *British Heart Journal*	1 (2%)
	50 (100%)

question was raised by the associate editor, Dr. John Rutherford, who led the discussion on this item. Protocols to be considered for publication must be short and not submitted until all patients have been entered into the study. Lengthy discussions justifying the trial will not be published. The AJC is willing to publish some study protocols with the understanding that the AJC will be strongly considered as the publication site of the major results manuscript.

The meeting was adjourned to a splendid reception provided by the publishers.

William C. Roberts

William Clifford Roberts, MD
Editor in Chief
Baylor University Medical Center
Dallas, Texas 75246

Proceedings of the Editorial Board Meeting of *The American Journal of Cardiology* on 17 March 1997

The 1997 meeting of the editorial board of *The American Journal of Cardiology* (AJC) was held on March 17 in Anaheim, California, at the time of the Annual Scientific Sessions of The American College of Cardiology. The meeting's purpose was to review AJC publication results for 1996, to recognize particularly those AJC board members reviewing the most manuscripts in 1996, and to receive input from the board members. The meeting went as follows:

1. *Introduction of Mr. David Dionne, the Associate Publisher of the York Medical Group, which includes the AJC:* Mr. Dionne indicated that the journal was healthy, and that he was glad to be a part of it.

2. *Introduction of new AJC board members:* Twenty-three new members were added to the board beginning in January 1997 (Table I), and they were introduced. New members are selected entirely on their record as non-board reviewers of the AJC. Selection is based on review of card files of nearly 2,000 non-board AJC reviewers and those with the best reviewing records are selected. Board members determine their longevity on the AJC board by the quality and promptness of their reviews. Each year it gets more and more difficult to eliminate board members because nearly all have good reviewing records.

TABLE I New Board Members Beginning 1997

William F. Armstrong	Allan S. Jaffe
Richard W. Asinger	Richard Lange
Gary John Balady	Robert Meidell
Eric Bates	John W. Moore
Monty M. Bodenheimer	E. Magnus Ohman
Jeffrey S. Borer	Milton Packer
Harisios Boudoulas	Carl J. Pepine
Anthony N. DeMaria	Ronald M. Peshock
Nicholas L. DePace	Barry D. Rutherford
Kenneth A. Ellenbogen	Byron F. Vandenberg
Julius Gardin	Mario Verani
Nora F. Goldschlager	

3. *Numbers of manuscripts sent for review to board members in 1996:* A total of 1,930 manuscripts were received in the editorial office in 1996 (This number does not include the manuscripts for the supplement issues.), and 818 of them were sent to at least 1 of the 205 AJC board members. An average of 3.99 manuscripts were sent to each board member in 1996: 669 (82%) were reviewed on time, 78 (10%) were returned to the office late (>3 weeks from date of mailing from the AJC office), and 71 (8%) were returned without review (Table II).

4. *AJC board members reviewing the most manuscripts in 1996:* The top AJC reviewer in 1996 was Dr. Paul A. Grayburn who reviewed 12 manuscripts and returned each of them during the allotted 3-week period. Dr. Pablo Denes reviewed 11 manuscripts and returned each one within the allotted time period. Dr. Fred Morady reviewed 10 manuscripts and returned each within the allotted time period. Drs. Joseph Alpert, Donald S. Bain,

TABLE II Numbers and Types of Manuscripts Sent to *AJC* Board Members in 1996 According to Board-Member Specialty

Specialty	Numbers on Board	Number MSs sent (no./reviewer)	No. LR	No. BR	No. CR	No. E	No. (%) Reviewed on Time	No. (%) Reviewed Late	No. (%) MSs Returned Without Review
Adult cardiology	169	730 (4.32)	627 (86%)	89 (12%)	4 (<1%)	10 (1%)	599 (82%)	71 (10%)	60 (8%)
Pediatric cardiology	18	47 (2.61)	39 (83%)	6 (13%)	1 (2%)	1 (2%)	42 (90%)	3 (6%)	2 (4%)
Cardiovascular surgery	10	17 (1.70)	13 (76%)	2 (12%)	2 (12%)	0	11 (65%)	2 (12%)	4 (23%)
Related specialties	8	24 (3.00)	16 (67%)	7 (29%)	1 (4%)	0	17 (71%)	2 (8)	5 (21%)
Totals	205	818 (3.99)	695 (85%)	104 (13%)	8 (1%)	11 (1%)	669 (82%)	78 (10%)	71 (8%)

BR = brief report; CR = case report; E = Editorial; LR = long report; MSs = manuscripts; No. = numbers.

TABLE III Top Reviewers of Manuscripts for the *AJC* in 1996

Name	Numbers of Manuscripts Reviewed	LR	BR	CR	E	Number Reviewed On Time
1. Paul A. Grayburn	12	10	2	0	0	12
2. Pablo Denes	11	9	2	0	0	11
3. Fred Morady	10	9	1	0	0	10
4. Joseph Alpert	9	8	0	0	1	9
4. Donald S. Baim	9	8	1	0	0	5
4. Robert L. Feldman	9	9	0	0	0	9
4. Navin C. Nanda	9	9	0	0	0	9
8. Richard O. Cannon III	8	5	3	0	0	8
8. Bernard O. Chaitman	8	5	2	0	1	8
8. Stephen Ellis	8	8	0	0	0	8
8. L. David Hillis	8	8	0	0	0	8
8. Robert E. Kleiger	8	7	1	0	0	8
8. Joseph Lindsay, Jr.	8	6	1	1	0	8
8. Arthur J. Moss	8	6	2	0	0	5
8. David H. Spodick	8	4	4	0	0	8
Totals	133	111 (83%)	19 (14%)	1 (1%)	2 (2%)	126 (95%)

Abbreviations as in Table II.

TABLE IV Reviewers of 7 Manuscripts for the *AJC* in 1996

Name	Numbers of Manuscripts Reviewed	LR	BR	CR	E	Number Reviewed On Time
16. Michael E. Cain	7	6	1	0	0	6
16. Robert M. Califf	7	5	2	0	0	6
16. Pamela S. Douglas	7	7	0	0	0	7
16. W. Bruce Fye	7	6	1	0	0	7
16. William H. Gaasch	7	7	0	0	0	7
16. David R. Holmes, Jr.	7	7	0	0	0	7
16. John A. Kastor	7	6	1	0	0	6
16. Kenneth M. Kent	7	6	1	0	0	6
16. Robert A. Kloner	7	7	0	0	0	7
16. Barry J. Maron	7	5	2	0	0	5
16. Richard S. Meltzer	7	6	1	0	0	7
16. Robert A. O'Rourke	7	5	2	0	0	6
Totals	84	73	11	0	0	77 (92%)

Abbreviations as in Table II.

TABLE V Reviewers of 6 Manuscripts for the *AJC* in 1996

Name	Numbers of Manuscripts Reviewed	LR	BR	CR	E	Number Reviewed On Time
28. Robert O. Bonow	6	6	0	0	0	4
28. Peter F. Cohn	6	6	0	0	0	6
28. Michael H. Crawford	6	5	1	0	0	6
28. John Douglas	6	6	0	0	0	2
28. Eric Eichhorn	6	6	0	0	0	6
28. Gerald Fletcher	6	4	1	0	1	6
28. Gary S. Francis	6	5	1	0	0	6
28. Victor F. Froelicher, Jr.	6	6	0	0	0	6
28. K. Lance Gould	6	4	2	0	0	4
28. Abdulmassih S. Iskandrian	6	6	0	0	0	6
28. Jeffrey M. Isner	6	6	0	0	0	4
28. Francis E. Marchlinski	6	6	0	0	0	6
28. Melvin M. Scheinman	6	6	0	0	0	6
28. Prediman K. Shah	6	5	1	0	0	3
28. Nanette K. Wenger	6	4	0	0	2	6
28. Hugh D. Allen	6	4	1	1	0	6
28. Charles B. Higgins	6	4	2	0	0	5
Totals	102	89	9	1	3	88 (86%)

Abbreviations as in Table II.

TABLE VI Numbers of Manuscripts Submitted and Published and Numbers of Editorial Pages Published in the *AJC* 1983–1996					
Year	Number of Manuscripts Submitted	Number of Manuscripts Published	Percent Accepted	Number of Editorial Pages for Articles	Average Pages Per Article
1996	1,930*	701*	36%	2,775	3.96
1995	1,844	668	36%	2,570	3.85
1994	1,783	604	34%	2,493	4.13
1993	1,997	619	31%	2,890	4.45
1992	1,873	664	35%	3,211	4.51
1991	1,615	680	42%	3,165	4.65
1990	1,717	662	38%	3,001	4.53
1989	1,740	699	40%	2,903	4.15
1988	1,496	636	42%	2,642	4.15
1987	1,525	695	46%	2,810	4.04
1986	1,574	616	39%	2,627	4.26
1985	1,707	645	38%	2,623	4.07
1984	1,605	747	46%	3,077	4.12
1983	1,234	643	52%	3,130	4.87

*Of the 1,930 manuscripts submitted in 1996, 701 have been published, accepted, or tentatively accepted pending revision.

TABLE VII Numbers of Pages, Articles, and Types of Articles Published in the Regular Issues of the *AJC* in 1996	
Number of pages	3,053
For articles (mean/month) [pages/article]	2,775 (231) [4.22] (91%)
For Readers' Comments (number) [replies]	29 (52) [4] (1%)
For staff, editorial board	48 (2%)
For contents	98 (3%)
For Instructions to Authors	20 (<1%)
For volume indexes	79 (3%)
For contents with abstracts	4 (<1%)
Number of articles (mean/month)	658 (55)
Long reports	333 (51%)
Coronary Artery Disease	163
Preventive Cardiology	11
Arrhythmias & Conduction Disturbances	40
Systemic Hypertension	13
Congestive Heart Failure	22
Valvular Heart Disease	18
Cardiomyopathy	7
Congenital Heart Disease	16
Miscellaneous	25
Methods	13
Cardiovascular Pharmacology	4
Historical Studies	1
Interviews	2 (<1%)
Brief Reports	273 (41%)
Case Reports	20 (3%)
Editorials	25 (4%)
From-the-Editor columns	5 (1%)

Robert L. Feldman, and Navin C. Nanda, each reviewed 9 manuscripts in 1996, and 8 board members reviewed 8 manuscripts in 1996 (Table III). Twelve board members reviewed 7 manuscripts in 1996, and of the 84 manuscripts reviewed by them 77 (92%) were reviewed within the allotted 3-week time period (Table IV). Seventeen board members each reviewed 6 manuscripts in 1996. The reviewing records of the 44 board members who reviewed 6 or more manuscripts during 1996 are truly remarkable, and these board members represent 21% of the total board. The editor also is fully aware that the AJC is not the only journal for which AJC board members review manuscripts.

5. *Numbers of manuscripts submitted and published and numbers of editorial pages published in the AJC in 1983–1996:* In 1996, a total of 1,930 manuscripts were received: 611 have been accepted or published and 90 others are tentatively accepted pending revision. Thus, potentially 701 of these 1,930 manuscripts probably will be published in the AJC. Table VI lists the numbers of manuscripts submitted and published, and the numbers of editorial pages published in the AJC in 1983 through 1996.

6. *Numbers of pages, articles, and types of articles published in the regular issues of the AJC in 1996:* These data are listed in Table VII. A total of 658 articles, an average of 55 per month, were published on 2,775 pages, an average of 231 per month, in 1996. The average length of each article was 4.22 pages; 29 additional editorial pages were used for 52 Readers' Comments (letters to the editor) with 4 replies. Of the 658 articles published in 1996, 333 (51%) were long reports, 273 (41%) were brief reports, 20 (3%) were case reports, 30 (5%) were editorials, and 2 were interviews (Eric J. Topol and W. Bruce Fye). The most unique feature of the AJC is the brief reports and probably over half of those eventually published as brief reports were originally submitted as long reports. Interviews of prominent figures in cardiovascular medicine and surgery were initiated in 1996 and they will continue.

7. *Symposia published in the AJC in 1996:* A total of 11 supplements were published in the AJC in 1996 (Table VIII). No advertisements, of course, appear in the supplement issues, which are published under separate cover with a different color from that of the regular issues. The guest editors of most of

TABLE VIII Supplements(s) Published in the *AJC* in 1996

S	1996 Date of Publication	Subject of Symposium	Guest Editor(s)	Sponsor	Article	Pages	Interval (months) Symposium to Publication
A	January 25	Supraventricular arrhythmias	Douglas P. Zipes	3M Pharmaceuticals	12	95	20
B	February 22	Indapamide	Norman M. Kaplan	Groupe de Recherche Servier	8	30	20
C	May 30	Nitrates in heart failure	Uri Elkayam	G. Phol-Boskamp GmbH	8	51	24
D	June 20	Verapamil	Louis Guize Nina Rehnqvist	Knoll AG	7	36	22
3A	August 14	Transcatheter cardiovascular therapeutics	Martin B. Leon Gary S. Mintz	Cordis	10	52	6
4A	August 29	Sotalol	Bramah N. Singh Ralph Lazzara	Berlex	10	72	35
5A	September 12	Implantable cardioverter defibrillators	Richard N. Fogoros Antonio Raviele	CPI/Guidant	24	141	18
6A	September 26	Fluvastatin	Jerome D. Cohen	Sandoz	6	41	—
8A	October 17	Ibutilide	Albert L. Waldo Craig M. Pratt	Pharmacia & Upjohn	9	52	9
9A	November	Mibefradil	Craig M. Pratt	F. Hoffman-La Roche AG	5	23	7
12A	December 19	Reteplase	Richard W. Smalling	Boehringer Mannheim	6	27	9
11	Totals				105 (m10)	620 (m56)	(m15)

the supplement issues are major leaders in cardiology around the world.

8. *Reminder to authors to supply several names with addresses of non-biased reviewers for their manuscripts:* Editors have no monopoly on choosing the best reviewers of manuscripts. No one should be more knowledgeable of experts in the subject of the manuscript than the author of the manuscript. Thus, I urge authors to supply names—preferably 5, and their addresses—of non-local, non-biased potential reviewers of their manuscripts. It is necessary for an author to submit several names because almost certainly some of the potential reviewers will already have a manuscript for review and a second manuscript is not sent to a reviewer already having 1, unless 1 of the 2 manuscripts is a Brief Report or Case Report. Currently, about 20% of the authors supply names of potential reviewers for their manuscripts. After studying the reviews of author-suggested reviewers for 15 years, I am impressed that the author-suggested reviewers are of high quality, and that the author-suggested reviewers are no more biased toward their manuscripts than are editor-selected reviewers. Indeed, many manuscripts have been reviewed by 1 author-suggested reviewer and 1 editor-suggested reviewer, and the author-suggested reviewer recommended rejection while the editor-suggested reviewer recommended acceptance of the manuscript.

9. *A plea for publication of the AJC on acid-free paper:* Nearly every year at the editorial board meeting I bring up the topic of publication of the AJC on acid paper. Only 1 cardiology journal published in the USA is published on acid-free paper. Acid-free paper, of course, is permanent paper and will not vanish into dust in 40 to 50 years as will the acid paper. Furthermore, acid-free paper allows the figures to be have a sharper and crisper appearance, compared to when they are published on acid paper. It is my understanding that acid-free paper is no longer more expensive than acid paper.

10. *Review of technical features for manuscripts submitted to the AJC:* Because the AJC receives nearly 2,000 manuscripts annually and because the number of editorial pages published is limited, it is essential that each manuscript be of appropriate length so that we can nevertheless publish well over 600 manuscripts yearly. The publication of numerous Brief Reports allows the number of total articles published in the AJC each year to remain high. But longer articles are becoming shorter. We no longer have unlimited space for long discussions, long introductions, or long abstracts. The methods and results sections are the heart of any manuscript and they need to be in exquisite detail, but the other portions must now be limited. I agree with Dr. John Shaw Billings' comment on manuscripts submitted to medical journals: ''The author must have something to say, say it, stop as soon as it is said, and give the article a proper title.'' Clear, precise writing has never been more in demand than at the present. The introduction ideally should be a single paragraph filling no more than one-half page typed double spaced. The abstract should occupy no more than a single page typed double spaced. The discussion section must be limited, usually to no more than 3 double-spaced typed pages. If manuscripts concern 30 patients or less, a table showing the findings in each of those 30 patients with no more than 1 line across is usually preferred over a table showing only pool data. More focus, in my view, needs to be on tables and figures. When the message of the manuscript can

be shown graphically, the manuscript is usually a good one. The AJC usually limits references to no more than 30 in a long report and to 20 in a brief report. Preparing references tells much about the scholarship of the authors. Examples of good and not so good titles have been discussed previously in this column. Subtitles are usually avoided in the AJC. Abbreviations should be kept to a minimum, no more than 3 per manuscript, and usually limited to phrases in the articles' title. Acronyms are not considered abbreviations. Finally, it is wise to read the Instructions to Authors before submitting a manuscript to this journal. Clues to the editor's pleasures and displeasures can often be detected from the Instructions to Authors.

11. *Discussion regarding electronic publishing:* Ms. Belinda Kerkhof, who recently moved from the Elsevier office in Amsterdam to New York, is working on getting several Elsevier cardiovascular journals available electronically. A product is not presently available, but by this time next year, almost certainly one will be. Electronic publishing is here to stay, and we all must get more familiar with it.

No time was left for questions and comments from board members this year which is the first editorial board meeting in 15 years where this was the case. Comments from readers are always welcomed.

William C. Roberts

William Clifford Roberts, MD
Editor in Chief
Baylor University Medical Center
Dallas, Texas 75246

Proceedings of the Editorial Board of *The American Journal of Cardiology* on 30 March 1998

The 1998 meeting of the editorial board of *The American Journal of Cardiology* (AJC) was held on March 30, 1998, at the time of The Annual Scientific Sessions of the American College of Cardiology. The meeting's purpose was to review AJC publication results for 1997, to recognize particularly those AJC board members reviewing the most manuscripts in 1997, and to receive input from the board members. The meeting went as follows:

1. *Introduction of Mr. David Dionne, the Associate Publisher at Elsevier Science, Inc., New York, which includes the AJC:* Mr. Dionne, who introduced the publishing staff, indicated that the journal was healthy.

2. *Numbers of manuscripts sent for review to board members in 1997:* A total of 1,898 manuscripts were received in the editorial office in 1997 (This number does not include the manuscripts for the supplement issues.): 763 of them were sent to at least 1 of the 220 AJC board members (Table I). An average of 3.47 manuscripts was sent to each board member in 1997: 620 (81%) were reviewed on time, 68 (9%) were returned to the office late (>3 weeks from date of mailing from the AJC editorial office), and 75 (10%) were returned without review.

3. *AJC board members reviewing the most manuscripts in 1997:* The top 28 reviewers (13%) for the AJC in 1997 are listed in Table II. Dr. Joseph S. Alpert was the top reviewer for 1997. He reviewed 10 manuscripts and all 10 were returned within the allotted time.

4. *Numbers of manuscripts submitted and published and numbers of editorial pages published in the AJC in 1983–1997:* In 1997, a total of 1,898 manuscripts were received: 693 have been accepted or published and 90 others are tentatively accepted pending revision. Thus, potentially 768 of these 1,898 manuscripts probably will be published in the AJC. Table III lists the numbers of manuscripts submitted and published and the numbers of editorial pages published in the AJC in 1983 through 1997.

5. *Numbers of pages, articles, and types of articles published in the regular issues of the AJC in 1997:* These data are listed in Table IV. A total of 826 articles were published on 3,328 pages, an average of 69 per month, in 1997. The average length of each article was 4.03 pages; 32 additional editorial pages were used for publication of 45 Readers' Comments (Letters to the Editor) and 6 replies. Of the 826 articles published in 1997, 357 (43%) were long reports, 409 (50%) were brief reports, 23 (3%) were case reports, 24 (3%) were editorials, and 9 (1%) were From-the-Editor columns. Four interviews were published in the AJC in 1997. The unique feature of the AJC is the Brief Reports and probably about 75% of them were initially submitted as Long Reports. The brief-report section allows the number of manuscripts to be published in the AJC to be quite large.

6. *Interviews in the AJC:* A total of 16 interviews have now been done and these are listed in Table V. Interviews numbers 7–16 will be published in 1998.

7. *Symposia published in the AJC in 1997:* A total of 17 supplements were published in the AJC in 1997 and these are listed in Table VI. No advertisements, of course, appear in the supplement issues, which are published under separate cover with a different color from that of the regular issues. The guest editors of most of the supplement issues are major leaders in cardiology around the world.

8. *Reminder to authors to supply several names with addresses of potential nonbiased reviewers for their manuscripts:* Editors have no monopoly on choosing the best reviewers of manuscripts. No one should be more knowledgeable of experts in the subject of the manuscript than the author of the manuscript. Thus, I urge authors to supply names—preferably 5, and their addresses—of nonlocal, nonbiased potential reviewers of their manuscripts. It is necessary for an author to submit several names because almost certainly some of the potential reviewers will already have a manuscript for review and a second manuscript is not sent to a reviewer already having 1, unless 1 of the 2 manuscripts is a Brief Report or Case Report. Currently, about <20% of the authors supply names of potential reviewers of their manuscripts. After studying the reviews of author-suggested reviewers for 15 years, I am impressed that the author-suggested reviewers are of high quality, and that the author-suggested reviewers are no more biased toward the manuscripts than are editor-selected reviewers. Indeed, many manuscripts have been reviewed by 1 author-suggested reviewer and 1 editor-suggested re-

TABLE I Numbers and Types of Manuscripts Sent to *AJC* Board Members 1997										
Specialty	Number On Board	Number Manuscripts Sent (No./Reviewer)	No. LR	No. BR	No. CR	No. E	No. (%) Reviewed on Time	No. (%) Reviewed Late	No. (%) Returned Without Review
Adult Cardiology	186	663 (3.56)	574 (87%)	75 (11%)	11 (2%)	3 (<1%)	540 (81%)	60 (9%)	63 (10%)
Pediatric Cardiology	18	60 (3.33)	51 (85%)	7 (12%)	1 (1.5%)	1 (1.5%)	47 (78%)	7 (12%)	6 (10%)
Cardiovascular Surgery	9	18 (2.00)	13 (72%)	1 (6%)	4 (22%)	0	16 (89%)	0	2 (11%)
Related specialties	7	22 (3.14)	18 (82%)	3 (14%)	1 (4%)	0	17 (77%)	1 (5%)	4 (18%)
TOTALS	220	763 (3.47)	656 (86%)	86 (11%)	17 (2%)	4 (1%)	620 (81%)	68 (9%)	75 (10%)

BR = brief report; CR = case report; E = editorial; LR = long report.

TABLE II Top 28 Reviewers (Top 13%) of Manuscripts for the AJC in 1997						
Name	Numbers of Manuscripts Reviewed	LR	BR	CR	E	Number Reviewed on Time
1. Joseph S. Alpert	10	9	0	1	0	10
2. Eric Eichhorn	9	9	0	0	0	9
2. William H. Gaasch	9	9	0	0	0	9
2. Morton Kern	9	8	1	0	0	9
2. Navin C. Nanda	9	8	1	0	0	9
6. Agustin Castellanos	8	5	3	0	0	8
6. Abdulmassih S. Iskandrian	8	6	1	0	1	7
6. Kenneth M. Kent	8	8	0	0	0	7
6. Robert Roberts	8	8	0	0	0	8
10. George Beller	7	7	0	0	0	7
10. Michael E. Cain	7	6	0	1	0	7
10. Pamela S. Douglas	7	7	0	0	0	7
10. L. David Hillis	7	7	0	0	0	7
10. Barry J. Maron	7	4	1	2	0	5
10. Warren G. Guntheroth	7	5	1	1	0	7
10. Charles B. Higgins	7	7	0	0	0	6
17. Richard O. Cannon III	6	5	1	0	0	6
17. Michael H. Crawford	6	5	0	1	0	6
17. Victor F. Froelicher, Jr.	6	5	1	0	0	6
17. Norman M. Kaplan	6	5	0	1	0	4
17. Sanjiv Kaul	6	3	3	0	0	6
17. Robert A. Kloner	6	4	2	0	0	6
17. Fred Morady	6	5	1	0	0	6
17. Carl J. Pepine	6	6	0	0	0	4
17. Augusto D. Pichard	6	4	2	0	0	3
17. Douglas P. Zipes	6	5	1	0	0	5
17. Thomas P. Graham, Jr.	6	5	1	0	0	4
17. John D. Kugler	6	6	0	0	0	5

Abbreviations as in Table I.

viewer, and the author-suggested reviewer recommended rejection while the editor-suggested reviewer recommended acceptance of the manuscript.

9. *A plea for publication of the AJC on acid-free paper:* Nearly every year at the editorial board meeting I bring up the topic of publication of the AJC on acid-free paper. Only 1 cardiology journal published in the USA is published on acid-free paper. Acid-free paper, of course, is permanent paper and will not vanish into dust in 40 to 50 years as will the acid paper. Furthermore, acid-free paper allows the figures to be have a sharper and crisper appearance, compared to when they are published on acid paper.

10. *Review of technical features for manuscripts*

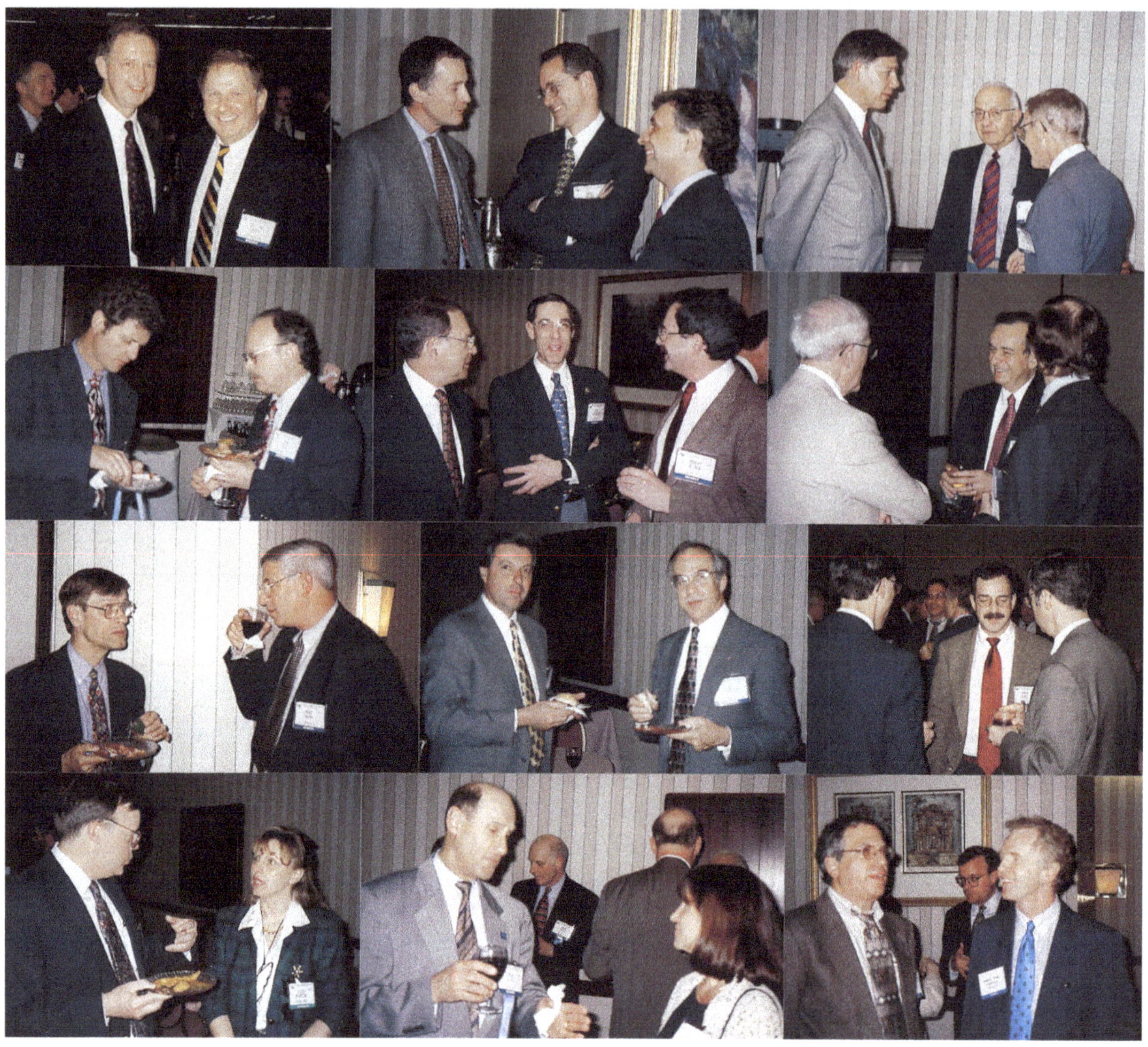

Photographs of Board members taken at the reception (by WCR).

submitted to the AJC: Because the AJC receives nearly 2,000 manuscripts annually and because the number of editorial pages published is limited, it is essential that each manuscript be of appropriate length so that we can nevertheless publish well over 600 manuscripts yearly. The publication of numerous Brief Reports allows the number of total articles published in the AJC each year to remain high. But longer articles are becoming shorter. We no longer have unlimited space for long discussions, long introductions, or long abstracts. The methods and results sections are the heart of any manuscript and they need to be in exquisite detail, but the other portions must now be limited. I agree with Dr. John Shaw Billings' comment on manuscripts submitted to medical journals: "The author must have something to say, say it, stop as soon as it is said, and give the article a proper title." Clear, precise writing has never been more in demand than at present. The introduction ideally should be a single paragraph filling no more than one-half page typed double spaced. The abstract should occupy no more than a single page typed double spaced. The discussion section must be limited, usually to no more than 3 double-spaced typed pages. If manuscripts concern 30 patients or less, a table showing the findings in each of those 30 patients with no more than 1 line across is usually preferred over a table showing only pool data. More focus, in my view, needs to be on tables and figures. When the message of the manuscript can be shown graphically, the manuscript is usually a good one. The AJC usually limits references to no more than 30 in a long report and to 20 in a brief report. Preparing references tells much about the scholarship of the authors. Examples of good and not so good titles have been discussed previously in this column. Subtitles are usually avoided in the AJC. Abbreviations should be kept to a minimum, no more than 3 per manuscript, and usually

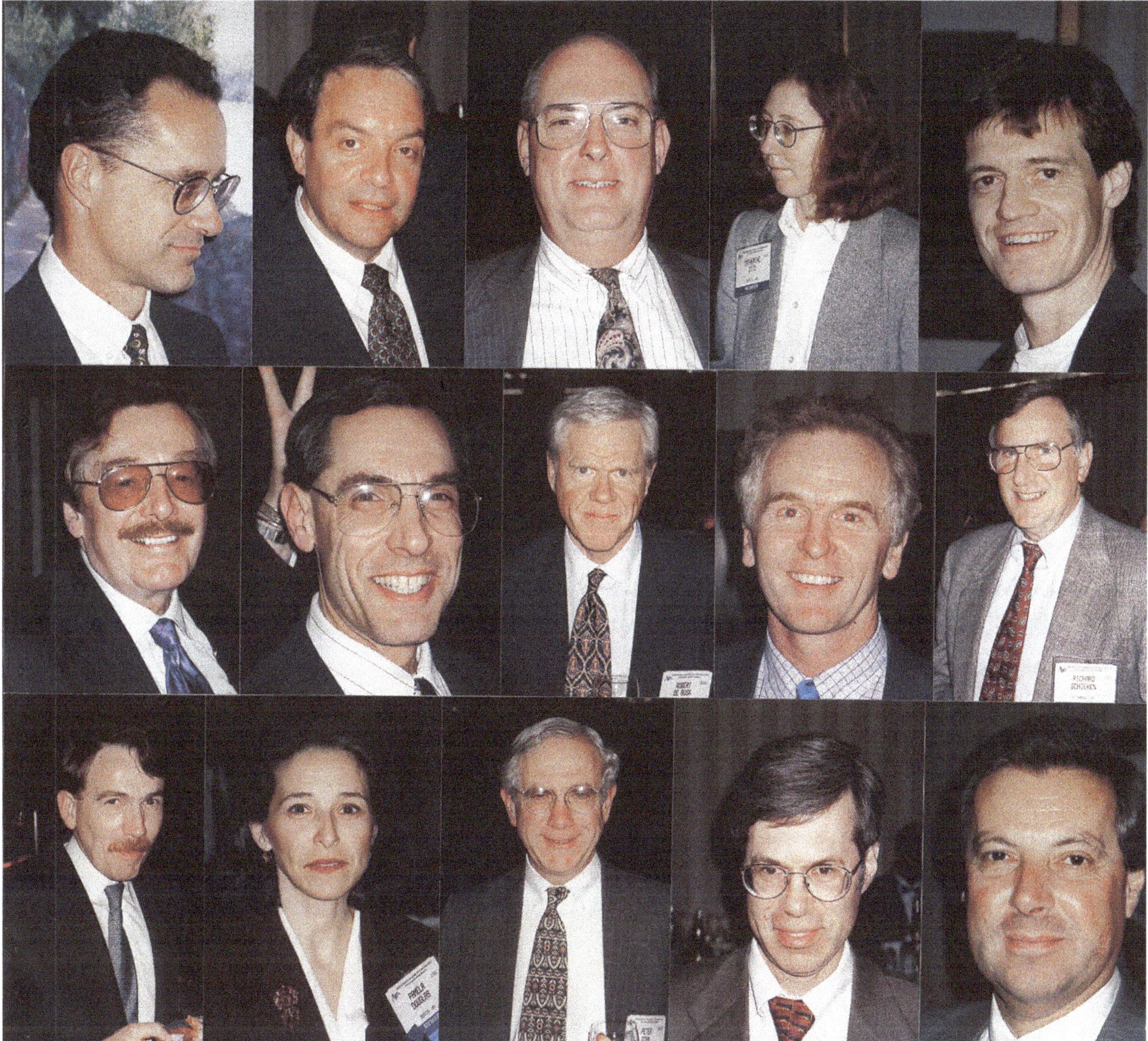

Photographs of Board members taken at the reception (by WCR).

TABLE III Numbers of Manuscripts Submitted and Published and Numbers of Editorial Pages Published in the *AJC* 1983–1997

Year	Number of Manuscripts Submitted	Number of Manuscripts Published or Accepted	Percent Accepted	Number of Editorial Pages for Articles	Average Pages Per Article
1997	1,898*	768	40%	3,328	4.03
1996	1,930	701	36%	2,775	3.96
1995	1,844	668	36%	2,570	3.85
1994	1,783	604	34%	2,493	4.13
1993	1,997	619	31%	2,890	4.45
1992	1,873	664	35%	3,211	4.51
1991	1,615	680	42%	3,165	4.65
1990	1,717	662	38%	3,001	4.53
1989	1,740	699	40%	2,903	4.15
1988	1,496	636	42%	2,642	4.15
1987	1,525	695	46%	2,810	4.04
1986	1,574	616	39%	2,627	4.26
1985	1,707	645	38%	2,623	4.07
1984	1,605	747	46%	3,077	4.12
1983	1,234	643	52%	3,130	4.87

*Of the 1,898 manuscripts submitted in 1997, 768 have been published or definitely or tentatively accepted pending revision.

TABLE IV Numbers of Pages, Articles, and Types of Articles Published in the Regular Issues of *The American Journal of Cardiology* in 1997		
	Volumes 79 & 80 January–December 1997	
Numbers of pages	3,656	
For articles (mean/month) [pages/article]	3,328	(91.03%)
For Readers' Comments (number) [replies]	32(45)[6]	(00.87%)
For staff, editorial board	48	(1.31%)
For contents and abstracts	122	(3.34%)
For Instructions to Authors	27	(0.74%)
For volume indexes	99	(2.71%)
Number of articles (mean/month)	826(69)	
Long reports	357	(43.22%)
Coronary artery disease	183	
Preventive cardiology	9	
Arrhythmias & conduction disturbances	64	
Systemic hypertension	9	
Congestive heart failure	15	
Valvular heart disease	19	
Cardiomyopathy	12	
Congenital heart disease	17	
Miscellaneous	14	
Methods	10	
Cardiovascular pharmacology	4	
Historical studies	1	
Interviews	4	(0.48%)
Brief reports	409	(49.51%)
Case reports	23	(2.78%)
Editorials	24	(2.91%)
From the Editor columns	9	(1.09%)

TABLE V Interviews in the *AJC*

1. Eric Jeffrey Topol (July 1, 1996)
2. W. Bruce Fye (August 1, 1996)
3. James Thornton Willerson (February 15, 1997)
4. Michael Ellis DeBakey (April 1, 1997)
5. Denton Arthur Cooley (April 15, 1997)
6. Joseph Stephan Alpert (May 1, 1997)
7. John Willis Hurst (February 15, 1998)*
8. Jesse Efrem Edwards (April 1, 1998)
9. John Webster Kirklin (April 15, 1998)
10. Howard Bertram Burchell (May 1, 1998)
11. William Howard Frishman (June 1, 1998)
12. Robert Ogden Bonow (June 15, 1998)
13. Eugene Braunwald (July 1, 1998)
14. Joseph Cholmondeley Greenfield (July 15, 1998)
15. David Coston Sabiston, Jr. (August 1, 1998)
16. Norman Meyer Kaplan (August 15, 1998)
17. Robert McKinnon Califf (September 1, 1998)

*Interviewer = Mark Silverman.

limited to phrases in the articles' title. Acronyms are not considered abbreviations. Finally, it is wise to read the Instructions to Authors before submitting a manuscript to this journal. Clues to the editor's pleasures and displeasures can often be detected from the Instructions to Authors.

11. *Publishing the AJC electronically:* Mr. David Dionne discussed what we might expect from this technology in the near future. He stated that the full text and graphics of all 1,200 Elsevier journals were in the process of being posted on the Internet through **Science Direct,** a new on-line host system developed and owned by Elsevier Science. He mentioned that the first group of journals being posted, 350 journals in clinical medicine and the life sciences, would go live in mid–1998 and that the balance of 850 to 900 journals would be accessible by years' end. Eighty (80) to 100 journals are now posted on **Science Direct.** Mr. Dionne encouraged the board members to access the Web site to review the journals' Tables of Contents and other features for free at **http://www.sciencedirect.com.**

Mr. Dionne also remarked that Elsevier has created another on-line service for cardiologists, titled **CardioSource,** which is now in the final phase of beta-testing. **CardioSource** contains the full text of 11 Elsevier journals in the field of cardiology, including *Journal of the American College of Cardiology, The American Journal of Cardiology, Cardiovascular Research, The Lancet,* and 7 other Elsevier journals.

Mr. Dionne explained that while **Science Direct** is

TABLE VI Supplement(s) Published in the *AJC* in 1997							
S	1997 Date of Publication	Subject	Guest Editor(s)	Sponsor	Articles	Pages	Interval (months) Symposium to Publication
6A	March 20	Prevention of sudden cardiac death (Mirowski Symposium)	Morton M. Mower	CPI - Guidant	8	43	11
10A	May 22	Calcium antagonists (Nisoldipine)	Murray Epstein	Zeneca Pharmaceuticals	8	43	6
12A	June 19	Adenosine	Ami E. Iskandrian	Fujisawa USA and MEDCO Research	9	48	8
12B	June 26	Acute coronary syndromes (Nitrates)	Prediman K. Shah Daniel S. Berman	Key Pharmaceuticals	6	35	7
3A (A)	August 4	Autocrine and paracrine signaling in myocardial ischemia	Guenther J. Dietze Heinrich Taegtmeyer	Max Grundig Foundation	24	167	12
4A (B)	August 18	Acute ischemic syndromes (Eptifibatide)	Harvey D. White	COR Therapeutics and Key Pharmaceuticals	8	48	13
4B (C)	August 21	Mibefradil	Thomas D. Giles	F. Hoffman - LaRoche	7	46	—
4C (D)	August 28	Stroke	Elsa-Grace V. Giardina	Janssen Pharmaceutica	5	39	9
5A (E)	September 4	Unstable coronary syndromes (Fragmin)	Alexander G.G. Turpie Lars Wallentine	Pharmacia & Upjohn	15	67	7
5B (F)	September 11	Impact of MADIT	Albert L. Waldo Myron L. Weisfeldt	CPI/Guidant	7	46	10
7A	October	Transcatheter Cardiovascular Therapeutics (Abstracts)	—	Elsevier Science	—	75	—
8A (G)	October 23	Class III antiarrhythmic agents	Braman N. Singh Gunter Breithardt	Bertex Laboratories	12	104	11
8B (H)	October 30	Managing coronary disease and heart failure	Marvin A. Konstam Thomas A. Pearson William C. Roberts Sidney C. Smith, Jr.	Merck	18	90	9
9A (I)	November 6	Mibefradil	Victor J. Dzau	Roche Laboratories	7	42	8
9B (J)	November 13	Metoprolol	Sidney Goldstein Ake Hjalmarson	Astra, Sweden	12	58	12
10A (K)	November 20	New approaches to coronary intervention	Donald S. Baim Katherine M. Detre Robert D. Safian	Cook, Inc Devices for Vascular Intervention Johnson & Johnson SciMed Life Systems	12	105	—
11A (L)	December 4	Carvedilol	Wilson S. Colucci Michael R. Bristow	Smith-Kline Beecham Pharmaceuticals	8	58	21
TOTALS	17	—	—	—	166	1119	Mean 10

directed toward end-users at institutional libraries and cuts across all subject areas of science, engineering, and medicine, **CardioSource** is geared specifically to the practicing cardiologist. The Site has a powerful search engine and includes other important features in addition to the full text of the 11 journals, including a 24-hour Reuters Newsfeed of medical news, a database of major clinical trials in cardiovascular medicine, an updated listing of over 200 professional medical meetings, an on-line cardiology forum, and links to related Web sites. If you wish to participate in the final phase of beta-testing **CardioSource,** Mr. Dionne tells me that you can go to **http://www.cardiosource.com** for registration and testing instructions. You also get free access to all the journals in **CardioSource** through the end of 1998.

The meeting was followed by a fine reception provided by the publisher.

William C. Roberts

William Clifford Roberts, MD
Editor in Chief
Baylor University Medical Center
Dallas, Texas 75246

Proceedings of the Editorial Board Meeting of *The American Journal of Cardiology* on 9 March 1999

The 1999 meeting of the Editorial Board of *The American Journal of Cardiology* (AJC) was held on 9 March 1999 at the time of the Annual Scientific Sessions of The American College of Cardiology. The meeting's purpose was to review *AJC* publication results for 1998, to recognize particularly those *AJC* board members reviewing the most manuscripts in 1998, and to receive input from board members. The meeting went as follows:

1. *Introduction of Mr. David Dionne, the Associate Publisher at Elsevier Science, Inc., New York, which includes the AJC*: Mr. Dionne welcomed the board members and introduced the publishing staff.

2. *Introduction of new AJC board members*: Nineteen new members were added to the board beginning in January 1997 (Table I), and they were introduced. New members are selected entirely on their record as non-board reviewers of the *AJC*. Selection is based on review of card files of nearly 2,000 non-board *AJC* reviewers and those with the best reviewing records are selected. Board members determine their longevity on the *AJC* board by the quality and promptness of their reviews.

3. *Numbers of manuscripts sent for review to board members in 1998*: A total of 1,992 manuscripts were received in the editorial office in 1998. (This number does not include the manuscripts for the supplement issues.): Of these 1,992 manuscripts, 728 were from medical centers in the USA and 318 (44%) were accepted for publication; 1,264 manuscripts submitted were from non-USA countries and 323 (26%) were accepted for publication. The total acceptance rate of manuscripts submitted for the regular issues in 1998 was 32%. A total of 847 of the manuscripts were sent to at least 1 of the 219 *AJC* board members (Table II). An average of 3.9 manuscripts were sent to each board member in 1998: 122 (14%) were returned without review and 725 (86%) were reviewed: 70% on time and 30% >3 weeks after the manuscript was mailed from the editorial offices (late reviews). The percentage of manuscripts returned without review and the percentage late were larger than any of the other 17 years of my editorship.

4. *AJC board members reviewing the most manuscripts in 1998*: The top *AJC* reviewer in 1998 was Dr. Eric Eichhorn who reviewed 11 manuscripts and returned each of them during the allotted 3-week period (Table III). Dr. Navin C. Nanda reviewed 9 manuscripts and also returned each promptly. Dr. Douglas P. Zipes reviewed 8 manuscripts and returned 7 promptly. The names of board members reviewing 7 and 6 manuscripts also are listed in Table III.

5. *Numbers of pages, articles, and types of articles published in the regular issues of the AJC in 1998*: These data are listed in Table IV. A total of 664 articles, an average of 55 per month, were published on 3,048 pages, an average of 254 per month, in 1998. The average length of each article was 4.59 pages. An additional 35 pages were used to publish 37 Readers' Comments (letters to the editor). Of the 664 articles published, 355 (53%) were long reports, 263 (40%) were brief reports, 16 (2%) were case reports, 17 (2%) were editorials, and 13 (4%) were for interviews of prominent cardiovascular specialists. The most unique feature of the *AJC* is the brief reports and well over half of those eventually published as brief reports were originally submitted as long reports. Table V lists the cardiovascular specialists whose interviews have appeared in the *AJC*.

6. *Symposia published in the AJC in 1998*: A total of 22 supplements were published in the *AJC* in 1998 (Table VI). No advertisements, of course, appear in the supplement issues, which are published under separate cover with a different color from that of the regular issues. The guest editors of most of the sup-

TABLE I New Board Members as of January 1999

Ezra A. Amsterdam	Charles Landau
Thomas C. Andrews	Gary S. Mintz
Martial G. Bourassa	David M. Mirvis
L. Maximilian Buja	Gerald V. Naccarelli
Kanu Chatterjee	Erik Magnus Ohman
Prakash C. Deedwania	Antonio Pacifico
Michael J. Domanski	Arshed Quyyumi
Uri Elkayam	Charles S. Roberts
N.A. Mark Estes, III	William M. Rogers
John A. Farmer	Ross J. Simpson, Jr.
David P. Faxon	Sidney C. Smith, Jr.
Mihai Gheorghiade	Peter C. Spittell
Raymond J. Gibbons	Lynne W. Stevenson
Steven A. Goldstein	Jonathan M. Tobis
J. Anthony Gomes	Renu Virmani

TABLE II Numbers of Manuscripts Sent to *AJC* Board Members in 1998

Board members	219
Manuscripts assigned	847 (3.9/member)
Long reports	678
Brief reports	136
Case reports	30
Editorials	3
Manuscripts returned without review	122 (14%)
Manuscripts reviewed	725 (86%)
On time	70%
Late	30%

TABLE III Top Reviewers for the *AJC* in 1998

Board Member	Number Reviewed	On Time	LR	BR	CR	E
Eric Eichhorn	11	11	10	1	0	0
Navin C. Nanda	9	9	8	1	0	0
Douglas P. Zipes	8	7	7	1	0	0
Bernard R. Chaitman	7	6	5	2	0	0
John P. DiMarco	7	1	5	2	0	0
Ted Feldman	7	6	4	3	0	0
Julius M. Gardin	7	3	5	2	0	0
Howard P. Gutsegell	7	6	7	0	0	0
Robert A. Kloner	7	7	7	0	0	0
David H. Spodick	7	7	5	2	0	0
Joseph S. Alpert	6	6	5	1	0	0
Thomas M. Bashore	6	2	6	0	0	0
Eric R. Bates	6	4	6	0	0	0
Harisios Boudoulas	6	5	5	1	0	0
Agustin Castellanos	6	6	6	6	0	0
Gregory J. Dehmer	6	6	6	0	0	0
Myrvin H. Ellestad	6	6	3	3	0	0
Sidney Goldstein	6	4	6	0	0	0
L. David Hillis	6	6	4	2	0	0
Ami E. Iskandrian	6	6	6	0	0	0
Allan S. Jaffe	6	5	5	1	0	0
Morton J. Kern	6	6	4	2	0	0
Richard Lange	6	0	6	0	0	0
Robert J. Myerburg	6	4	6	0	0	0
Robert A. O'Rourke	6	4	5	1	0	0
E. Magnus Ohman	6	6	5	1	0	0
Prediman K. Shah	6	2	4	2	0	0
Marc A. Silver	6	2	5	1	0	0
David D. Waters	6	6	6	0	0	0

BR = Brief Report; CR = Case Report; E = Editorial; LR = Long Report.

plement issues are major leaders in cardiovascular disease around the world.

7. *Reminder to authors to supply several names with addresses of non-biased reviewers for their manuscripts*: Editors have no monopoly on choosing the best reviewers of manuscripts. No one should be more knowledgeable on experts in the subject of the manuscript than the author of the manuscript. Thus, I urge authors to supply names—preferably 5, and their address—of non-local, non-biased potential reviewers of their manuscripts. It is necessary for an author to submit several names because almost certainly some of the potential reviewers will already have a manuscript for review and a second manuscript is not sent to a reviewer already having one. Currently, only about 10% of authors supply names of potential reviewers for their manuscripts. After studying the reviews of author-suggested reviewers for 17 years, I am impressed that the author-suggested reviewers are of high quality, and that the author-suggested reviewers are no more biased toward their manuscripts than the editor-selected reviewers. Indeed, many manuscripts have been reviewed by one author-suggested reviewer and by one editor-suggested reviewer, and the author-suggested reviewer recommended rejection, while the editor-suggested reviewer recommended acceptance of the manuscript.

TABLE IV Number of Pages and Articles Published in the Regular Issues of the *AJC* in 1998

	Volumes 81 & 82 January–December 1998
Number of pages	3,376
For articles	3,048 (90%)
For Readers' comments (number)[replies]	35 (1%)
For staff, editorial board	48 (1%)
For contents with abstracts	107 (3%)
For Instructions to Authors	46 (1%)
For volume indices	92 (3%)
Number of articles	664
Long reports	355 (53%)
Coronary artery disease	183 (52%)
Preventive cardiology	12 (3%)
Arrhythmia & conduction defects	36 (10%)
Systemic hypertension	13 (4%)
Congestive heart failure	25 (7%)
Valvular heart disease	15 (4%)
Cardiomyopathy	10 (3%)
Congenital heart disease	12 (3%)
Miscellaneous	31 (9%)
Methods	16 (5%)
Cardiovascular pharmacology	1 (<1%)
Historical studies	1 (<1%)
Interviews	13 (4%)
Brief reports	263 (40%)
Case reports	16 (2%)
Editorials	14 (2%)
For-the-editor columns	3 (<1%)

TABLE V Interviews Published in the *AJC*

Eric Jeffrey Topol (July 1, 1996)
W. Bruce Fye (August 1, 1996)
James Thornton Willerson (February 15, 1997)
Michael Ellis DeBakey (April 1, 1997)
Denton Arthur Cooley (April 15, 1997)
Joseph Stephan Alpert (May 1, 1997)
Jesse Efrem Edwards (April 1, 1998)
John Webster Kirklin (April 15, 1998)
Howard Bertram Burchell (May 15, 1998)
William Howard Frishman (June 1, 1998)
Robert Ogdon Bonow (June 15, 1998)
Eugene Braunwald (July 1, 1998)
Joseph Cholmondeley Greenfield (July 15, 1998)
David Coston Sabiston, Jr. (August 1, 1998)
Norman Mayer Kaplan (August 15, 1998)
Robert McKinnon Califf (September 1, 1998)
Bernard John Gersh (November 1, 1998)
Dean James Kereiakes (November 15, 1998)
Jeffrey Michael Isner (January 1, 1999)
Scott Montgomery Grundy (January 15, 1999)
Burton Elias Sobel (February 1, 1999)
Robert Anthony O'Rourke (April 1, 1999)
David Kempton Cartwright Cooper (April 15, 1999)
Spencer Bidwell King III (May 1, 1999)
Robert Roberts (May 15, 1999)

TABLE VI Supplement(s) Published in the *AJC* in 1998

Suppl.	1998 Date of Publication	Subject of Symposium	Guest Editor(s)	Sponsor	Articles	Pages	Interval (mo) Symposium to Publication
A	January 8	Nitroglycerin Therapy	Jonathan Abrams Uri Elkayam	Key Pharmaceuticals	11	76	15
B	February 26	Statins in Hyperglyceridemia	Scott M. Grundy	Merck & Co.	13	73	6
C	March 12	Atrial Fibrillation	Craig M. Pratt Albert L. Waldo	3M Pharmaceuticals	7	45	18
D	March 19	Antiarrhythmic Drugs	Craig M. Pratt A. John Camm	Proctor & Gamble Pharmaceuticals	7	46	6
E	April 9	Transcatheter Cardiovascular Therapeutics	Martin B. Leon Gary S. Mintz	Merck US Human Health	11	62	6
F	April 23	Guidelines—Lipid Lowering Agents	Carlos A. Dujovne	Multiple Companies	29	94	19
–	May 22	Nisoldipine in Hypertension	Murray Epstein	Zenec Pharmaceuticals	8	48	17
G	June 18	Echocardiography	Armando Dagianti Harvey Feigenbaum	Pfizer Italiana S.p.A. Merck Sharpe & Dohme Italia S.p.A.	24	121	15
H	August 6	Coronary Artery Disease	Karl B. Swedberg Eugene Braunwald	Knoll AG	6	30	11
I	August 20	Cardiac Arrhythmias	Eric N. Prystowsky	Berlex Laboratories	9	62	–
J	August 27	Cerivastatin	Gilbert R. Thompson	Bayer AG	9	55	18
K	September 3	Trimetazidine	Roberto Ferrari	Servier Research Group	10	67	21
L	September 10	Enoxaparin	Jawed Fareed Alexander G.G. Turpie	Rhône Poulenc Rorer	8	36	14
M	September 24	Fluvastatin	Antonio M. Gotto, Jr.	Novartis Pharmaceutical	7	38	–
–	October	Abstracts-Transcatheter Cardiovascular Therapeutics	–	–	–	151	0
N	October 16	Atrial Fibrillation	James A. Reiffel John Camm	Knoll Pharmaceutical	14	92	5
P	October 22	Anticoagulant Therapy	Eric J. Topol D. W. Harvey	The Medicines Company	10	68	7
Q	November 5	Cholesterol Lowering	Antonio M. Gotto, Jr.	Kos Pharmaceuticals	6	50	–
R	November 12	Hypertension in Diabetes	Murray Epstein	Bayer AG	11	44	3
S	November 19	Endothelial Function	Carl J. Pepine	Parke-Davis	21	64	8
T	November 26	Preventing Coronary Disease	Caldwell B. Esselstyn, Jr.	Parke-Davis & Pfizer	20	94	14
U	December 17	Extended-Release Niacin	John R. Guyton Peter O. Kwiterovich, Jr.	Kos Pharmaceuticals	13	86	9
22					254	1,502	mean=12

8. *Need for publication of the* AJC *on acid-free paper*: Nearly every year at the editorial board meeting I bring up the topic of publication of the *AJC* on acid-free paper. Only 1 cardiology journal published in the USA is now published on acid-free paper. Acid-free paper, of course, is permanent paper and will not vanish into dust in 40 to 50 years as will the acid paper. Furthermore, acid-free paper allows the figures to have a sharper and crisper appearance, compared to when they are published on acid paper. The publisher indicated that the journal in 1999 will not be published on acid-free paper, but that the quality of the paper soon will be changed to a better grade of acid paper.

9. *Review of technical features for manuscripts submitted to the* AJC: Because the *AJC* receives nearly 2,000 manuscripts annually and because the number of editorial pages published is limited, it is essential that each manuscript be of appropriate length so that we can publish well over 600 manuscripts yearly. The publication of numerous brief reports allows the number of total articles published in the *AJC* each year to remain high. But longer articles are becoming shorter. We no longer have unlimited space for long discussions, long introductions, or long abstracts. The methods and results sections are the heart of any manuscript and they need to be in exquisite detail, but the other portions must now be limited. I agree with Dr. John Shaw Billings' comment on manuscripts submitted to medical journals: "The author must have something to say, say it, stop as soon as it is said, and give the article a proper title." Clear, precise writing has never been more in demand than at the present. The introduction ideally should be a single paragraph filling no more than one-half page, typed double spaced. The abstract should occupy no more than a single page typed double spaced. The discussion section usually must be limited to no more than 3 double-spaced typed pages. If manuscripts concern 30 patients or less, a table showing the findings in each of those 30 patients with no more than 1 line

across is usually preferred over a table showing only pooled data. More focus, in my view, needs to be on tables and figures. When the message of the manuscript can be shown graphically, the manuscript is usually a good one. The *AJC* usually limits references to no more than 30 in long reports and to 20 in brief reports. Preparing references tells much about the scholarship of the authors. Examples of good and not so good titles have been discussed previously in this column. Subtitles are usually avoided in the *AJC*. Abbreviations should be kept to a minimum, no more than 3 per manuscript, and usually limited to phrases in the articles' title. Acronyms are not considered abbreviations. Finally, it is wise to read the Instructions to Authors before submitting a manuscript to this journal. Clues to the editor's pleasures and displeasures can often be detected from the Instructions to Authors.

10. *Publishing the AJC electronically*: Mr. David Dionne discussed what we might expect from this technology in the near future. He stated that the full text and graphics of all 1,200 Elsevier journals are now posted on the Internet through **Science Direct**, a new on-line host system developed and owned by Elsevier Science. **Science Direct** is directed toward end-users at institutional libraries and cuts across all subject areas of science, engineering, and medicine. Mr. Dionne encouraged the board members to access the Web site to review the journals' tables of contents and other features for free at http://www.sciencedirect.com.

Mr. Dionne also remarked that Elsevier has available another on-line service for cardiologists, titled **CardioSource**, which contains the full text of 12 Elsevier journals in the field of cardiology, including *Journal of the American College of Cardiology*, *The American Journal of Cardiology*, *Cardiovascular Research*, *The Lancet*, and 7 other Elsevier journals. **CardioSource** is geared specifically to the practicing cardiologist. The site has a powerful search engine and includes other important features in addition to the full text of the 12 journals, including a 24-hour Reuters Newsfeed of medical news, a superb database of over 500 major clinical trials in cardiovascular medicine, an updated listing of over 300 professional medical meetings, an on-line cardiology forum, and links to related Web sites.

The meeting was followed by a fine reception provided by the publisher.

William C. Roberts

William Clifford Roberts, MD
Editor in Chief
Baylor University Medical Center
Dallas, Texas 75246

Proceedings of the Editorial Board Meeting of *The American Journal of Cardiology* on 14 March 2000

The 2000 meeting of the Editorial Board of *The American Journal of Cardiology* (AJC) was held on 14 March at the time of the Annual Scientific Sessions of The American College of Cardiology. The meeting's purpose was to review *AJC* publication results for 1999, to recognize particularly those *AJC* board members reviewing the most manuscripts in 1999, and to receive criticisms and suggestions from board members on how to improve the journal. The meeting went as follows:

1. *Introduction of Mr. David Dionne, the Associate Publisher at Elsevier Science, Inc., New York, which includes the AJC:* Mr. Dionne welcomed the board members, and thanked them for their help.

2. *Numbers of manuscripts submitted and published and numbers of editorial pages published in the AJC 1983–1999 (Table I):* A total of 2,170 manuscripts were received in the editorial office in 1999. (This number does not include the manuscripts for the supplement issues.) This is the largest number ever received in a single year by the *AJC,* and represents an 8% increase over 1998. Of the 2,170 manuscripts, 1,083 were from medical centers in the USA and 1,087 manuscripts were submitted from non-USA countries. The total acceptance rate of manuscripts submitted for the regular issues in 1999 was 32%. (Some of them of course were not published until 2000.) The only reason the acceptance rate is as high as it is is because of the large number of brief reports published. Most of the manuscripts published as brief reports originally were submitted as long reports.

3. *Numbers and types of manuscripts sent to AJC board members in 1999 according to board member specialty (Table II):* The 224 *AJC* board members were sent 992 manuscripts to review in 1999, an average of 4.43 manuscripts/board member; 94 (9%) were returned without review.

4. *AJC board members reviewing the most manuscripts in 1999 (Table III):* The top *AJC* reviewer in 1999 was Dr. John Kostis who reviewed 12 manuscripts and returned each of them during the allotted 3-week period. Drs. Joseph A. Franciosa and Morton J. Kern each reviewed 11 manuscripts and they also returned each promptly. The board members reviewing 10, 9, and 8 manuscripts also are listed in Table III.

5. *Numbers of pages, articles, and types of articles published in the regular issues of the AJC in 1999 (Table IV):* A total of 680 articles were published on 3,015 pages. An additional 38 pages were used to publish 42 Readers' Comments (letters to the editor). Of the 680 articles published, 360 (53%) were long reports, 268 (39%) were brief reports, 21 (3%) were case reports, 21 (3%) were editorials, and 10 (1%) were for interviews of prominent cardiovascular specialists. The unique feature of the *AJC* is the brief report section. Table V lists the cardiovascular specialists whose interviews have appeared in the *AJC.*

6. *Symposia published in the AJC in 1999 (Table VI):* A total of 18 supplements were published in the *AJC* in 1999. No advertisements, of course, appear in the supplement issues, which are published under separate cover with a different color from that of the regular issues. The guest editors of these symposia are for the most part major leaders in cardiovascular disease around the world.

7. *Reminder to authors to supply several names with addresses of nonbiased reviewers for their manuscripts:* Editors have no monopoly on choosing the

TABLE I Numbers of Manuscripts Submitted and Published and Numbers of Editorial Pages Published in the *AJC* 1983–1999

Year	Number of Manuscripts Submitted	Number of Manuscripts Published or Accepted	Percent Accepted	Number of Editorial Pages for Articles
1999	2,170	703	32%	3,015
1998	1,992	631	31%	2,598
1997	1,898	768	40%	3,328
1996	1,930	701	36%	2,775
1995	1,844	668	36%	2,570
1994	1,783	604	34%	2,493
1993	1,997	619	31%	2,890
1992	1,873	664	35%	3,211
1991	1,615	680	42%	3,165
1990	1,717	662	38%	3,001
1989	1,740	699	40%	2,903
1988	1,496	636	42%	2,642
1987	1,525	695	46%	2,810
1986	1,574	616	39%	2,627
1985	1,707	645	38%	2,623
1984	1,605	747	46%	3,077
1983	1,234	643	52%	3,130

TABLE II Numbers and Types of Manuscripts Sent to AJC Board Members in 1999 According to Board Member Specialty

Specialty	Number on Board	Number Manuscripts Sent (no./reviewer)	No. LR	No. BR	No. (%) Returned Without Review
Adult cardiology	196	875 (4.47)	678	197	81
Pediatric cardiology	14	58 (4.14)	36 (62%)	22 (38%)	8 (14%)
Cardiac surgery	6	27 (4.50)	16 (59%)	11 (41%)	3 (11%)
Related specialists	8	32 (4.00)	26 (81%)	6 (19%)	2 (6%)
TOTALS	224	992 (4.43)	756 (76%)	236 (24%)	94 (9%)

BR = brief report; LR = long report.

TABLE III Top 30 (13%) AJC Board Member Reviewers in 1999

Name	Number Manuscripts Reviewed	Long Reports	Brief Reports
John Kostis	12	8	4
Joseph A. Franciosa	11	11	0
Morton J. Kern	11	10	1
Jonathan Abrams	10	9	1
Harisios Boudoulas	10	8	2
Jack Ferlinz	10	7	3
Erik Magnus Ohman	10	9	1
Robert Vogel	10	7	3
Jeffrey Saffitz	10	8	2
Ezra Amsterdam	9	6	3
Stephen P. Glasser	9	8	1
Sanjiv Kaul	9	8	1
Robert A. Kloner	9	7	2
David D. Waters	9	8	1
Eric Bates	8	6	2
Marc Cohen	8	7	1
John Douglas	8	5	3
Myrvin H. Ellestad	8	7	1
David Faxon	8	8	0
Ted Feldman	8	5	3
Gerald Fletcher	8	7	1
Harold L. Kennedy	8	4	4
Gary S. Mintz	8	5	3
Robert J. Myerberg	8	8	0
Navin C. Nanda	8	6	2
James L. Ritchie	8	6	2
John C. Somberg	8	6	2
Jonathan M. Tobis	8	7	1
Lowell W. Perry	8	5	3
Charles S. Roberts	8	6	2

best reviewers of manuscripts. No one should be more knowledgeable on experts in the subject of the manuscript than the authors of the manuscript. Thus, I urge authors to supply names—preferably 5, and their addresses—of nonlocal, nonbiased potential reviewers of their manuscripts. It is necessary for an author to submit several names because almost certainly some of the potential reviewers will already have a manuscript for review and a second manuscript is not sent to a reviewer already having one. Currently, only about 10% of authors supply names of potential reviewers for their manuscripts. After studying the re-

TABLE IV Number of Pages, Articles, and Types of Articles Published in the Regular Issues of *The American Journal of Cardiology* in 1999

	Volumes 83 & 84 January–December 1999
Number of pages	3,361 (100%)
For articles	3,015 (90%)
For Reader's Comments (number)[replies]	38(42)[7] (1%)
For staff, editorial board	48 (1%)
For contents with abstracts	110 (3%)
For Instructions to Authors	48 (1%)
For volume indexes	102 (3%)
Number of articles	680 (4.43 pages/article)
Long reports	360 (53%)
Coronary artery disease	185
Preventive cardiology	14
Arrhythmia & conduction disturbances	29
Systemic hypertension	14
Congestive heart failure	24
Valvular heart disease	19
Cardiomyopathy	14
Congenital heart disease	25
Miscellaneous	21
Methods	11
Cardiovascular pharmacology	3
Historical studies	1
Interviews	10 (1%)
Brief reports	268 (39%)
Case reports	21 (3%)
Editorials	16 (2%)
For-the-editor columns	5 (1%)

TABLE V Interviews Published in the AJC

Eric Jeffrey Topol (July 1, 1996)
W. Bruce Fye (August 1, 1996)
James Thronton Willerson (February 15, 1997)
Michael Ellis DeBakey (April 1, 1997)
Denton Arthur Cooley (April 15, 1997)
Joseph Stephan Alpert (May 1, 1997)
Jesse Efrem Edwards (April 1, 1998)
John Webster Kirklin (April 15, 1998)
Howard Bertram Burchell (May 15, 1998)
William Howard Frishman (June 1, 1998)
Robert Ogdon Bonow (June 15, 1998)
Eugene Braunwald (July 1, 1998)
Joseph Cholmondeley Greenfield (July 15, 1998)
David Coston Sabiston, Jr. (August 1, 1998)
Norman Mayer Kaplan (August 15, 1998)
Robert McKinnon Califf (September 1, 1998)
Bernard John Gersh (November 1, 1998)
Dean James Kereiakes (November 15, 1998)
Jeffrey Michael Isner (January 1, 1999)
Scott Montgomery Grundy (January 15, 1999)
Burton Elias Sobel (February 1, 1999)
Robert Anthony O'Rourke (April 1, 1999)
David Kempton Cartwright Cooper (April 15, 1999)
Spencer Bidwell King III (May 1, 1999)
Robert Roberts (May 15, 1999)
Eugene Auston Stead, Jr (September 15, 1999)
Bertram Pitt (October 1, 1999)
Christopher John Dillon Packard (November 15, 1999)
Terje Rolf Pedersen (November 15, 1999)

TABLE VI Supplements Published in the AJC in 1999

	1999 Date of Symposium to Publication	Subject of Symposium	Guest Editor(s)	Sponsor	Articles	Pages	Interval (mo) Publication
A	January 21	Recommendations for management of heart failure	Milton Packer Jay N. Cohn	Twelve Companies	3	38	—
B	February 18	Hemostasis after cardiac operations	Stephen Scheidt	Bayer	8	52	11
C	March 4	Sildenafil citrate	Randall M. Zusman	Pfizer	6	44	—
D	March 11	Implantable defibrillator	Günter Breithardt Jerónimo Farré David L. Hayes	CPI Guidant	41	245	4
E	May 6	Glycoprotein IIb/IIIa agents	Spencer B. King III	Searle	5	20	6
F	May 13	Hyperglyceridemia	Steven M. Haffner	Abbott	7	35	6
G	May 20	Sodium-hydrogen exchange inhibition	Pierre Théroux	Hoechst Marion Roussel	5	25	9
H	June 17	Mediators and mechanics of cardiac hypertrophy and failure	Heinrich Taegtmeyer Guenther J. Dietze	Max Grundig Foundation	20	98	9
I	June 24	Levosimendan	Julius Gy. Papp	Orion	7	28	14
J	July 8	Insulin resistance	Henry N. Ginsberg	Parke-Davis	9	48	10
K	July 22	Angiotensin II receptor antagonists	Hans R. Brunner	Boehringer Ingelheim Glaxo Wellcome	7	28	4
L	August 19	Amlodipine	Milton Packer Alan B. Miller	Pfizer	5	33	23
M	September 2	Lepirudin	Gianni Tognoni	Hoechst Marion Roussel	6	31	12
N	September 9	Sildenafil citrate	Robert A. Kloner	Pfizer	5	23	10
P	September 22	Transcatheter cardiovascular therapeutics abstracts	—	Elsevier Science	—	125	—
Q	October 21	Vasovagal syncope	Daniel M. Bloomfield	Roberts Pharmaceuticals	6	46	5
R	November 4	Amiodarone	Bramah N. Singh	Wyeth-Ayerst	25	173	12
S	November 18	Angiotensin II blockade	Alan H. Gradman	AstraZeneca	7	41	10
18					172	1,133	mean = 10

views of author-suggested reviewers for 18 years, I am impressed that the author-suggested reviewers are of high quality, and that the author-suggested reviewers are no more biased toward their manuscripts than the editor-selected reviewers. Indeed, many manuscripts have been reviewed by one author-suggested reviewer and by one editor-suggested reviewer, and the author-suggested reviewer recommended rejection, while the editor-suggested reviewer recommended acceptance.

8. *Publishing the AJC electronically:* Mr. David Dionne discussed what we might expect from this technology in the near future. He stated that the full text and graphics of all 1,200 Elsevier journals are now posted on the Internet through **Science Direct,** a new on-line host system developed and owned by Elsevier Science. **Science Direct** is directed toward end-users at institutional libraries and cuts across all subject areas of science, engineering, and medicine. Mr. Dionne encouraged the board members to access the Web site to review the journals' tables of contents and other features for free at *http://www.sciencedirect.com.*

Mr. Dionne also remarked that Elsevier has available another on-line service for cardiologists, titled **CardioSource,** which contains the full text of 12 Elsevier journals in the field of cardiology, including the *Journal of the American College of Cardiology, The American Journal of Cardiology, Cardiovascular Research, The Lancet,* and 7 other Elsevier journals. **CardioSource** is geared specifically to the practicing cardiologist. The site has a powerful search engine and includes other important features in addition to the full text of the 12 journals, including a 24-hour Reuters Newsfeed of medical news, a superb database of over 500 major clinical trials in cardiovascular medicine, an updated listing of over 300 professional medical meetings, an on-line cardiology forum, and links to related Web sites.

The meeting was followed by a fine reception provided by the publisher.

William C. Roberts

William Clifford Roberts, MD
Editor in Chief
Baylor University Medical Center
Dallas, Texas 75246

Proceedings of the Editorial Board Meeting of *The American Journal of Cardiology* on 19 March 2001

The 2001 meeting of the Editorial Board of *The American Journal of Cardiology* (AJC) was held on 19 March at the time of the Annual Scientific Sessions of the American College of Cardiology. The meeting's purpose was to review *AJC* publication results for 2000, to recognize particularly those *AJC* board members reviewing the most manuscripts in 2000, and to receive criticisms and suggestions from board members on how to improve the journal. The meeting went as follows:

1. *Introduction of Mr. Joshua R. Spieler, the Associate Publisher at Elsevier Science, Inc., New York, which includes the AJC:* Mr. Spieler welcomed the board members, and thanked them for their help, and introduced his staff.

2. *Introduction of new AJC board members beginning in 2000:* These were Eugene H. Blackstone, Dean J. Kereiakes, Carl J. Lavie, Richard L. Page, and Miguel Zabalgoitia.

3. *AJC board members reviewing the most manuscripts in 2000 (Table 1):* The top *AJC* reviewer in 2000 was Dr. Harold L. Kennedy who reviewed 8 manuscripts and returned each one of them during the allotted 3-week period.

4. *Numbers of manuscripts submitted and published and numbers of editorial pages published in the AJC 1983–2000 (Table 2):* A total of 2,226 manuscripts were received in the editorial office in 2000. (This number does not include the manuscripts for the supplement issues). This is the largest number ever received in a single year by the *AJC* and represents a 3% increase over 1999. Of the 2,226 manuscripts received, 630 (28%) were either published or accepted for publication and 1,596 (72%) were declined. Of the 2,226 manuscripts received in 2000, 1,078 were from the USA and 329 (33%) of them were accepted; a total of 1,148 manuscripts were submitted from non-USA countries and 271 (24%) of them accepted for publication. Some of the 630 accepted manuscripts of those submitted in 2000 of course will not be published until 2001. The only reason the acceptance rate (presently 28%) is as high as it is, is because of the large number of brief reports published. Over 80% of manuscripts published as brief reports had originally been submitted as long reports.

5. *Numbers of pages, articles, and types of articles published in the regular issues of the AJC in 2000 (Table 3):* A total of 648 articles were published on 2,926 pages in 2000. An additional 38 pages were used to publish 37 Readers' Comments (letters to the editor). Of the 648 articles published, 343 (51%) were long reports, 287 (42%) were brief reports, 8 (1%) were case reports, 22 (3%) were editorials, and 6 were interviews of prominent cardiovascular specialists. The unique feature of the *AJC* is the brief report section. Some of the articles published in 2000 of course had been submitted in 1999.

6. *Interviews published in the AJC:* Table 4 summarizes the interviews published in the *AJC* through year 2000. A number also are planned for 2001.

TABLE 1 *American Journal of Cardiology* Editorial Board Top Reviewers for 2000

Board Member	Number of Manuscripts Reviewed
Harold L. Kennedy	8
Raymond G. McKay	7
Jonathan Abrams	7
Eric Bates	7
Rodney H. Falk	7
Jack Ferlinz	7
Sanjiv Kaul	7
Carl J. Lavie	7
Joseph A. Franciosa	7
Stephen P. Glasser	7
Frank I. Marcus	7
Robert A. O'Rourke	7
James L. Ritchie	7
Jonathan M. Tobis	7
Eric J. Topol	7
Ezra Amsterdam	6
Jeffrey Anderson	6
Harisios Boudoulas	6
Jeffrey A. Brinker	6
Bernard R. Chaitman	6
Marc Cohen	6
Gerald Dorros	6
Myrvin Ellestad	6
Stephen Ellis	6
Ted Feldman	6
Robert E. Goldstein	6
John Kostis	6
Erik Magnus Ohman	6
Hector O. Ventura	6
Robert Vogel	6

TABLE 2 Numbers of Manuscripts Submitted and Published and Numbers of Editorial Pages Published in the *AJC* 1983–2000 (During the Tenure of WCR)

Year	Number of Manuscripts Submitted	Number of Manuscripts Published or Accepted	Percent Accepted	Number of Editorial Pages for Articles	Average Pages Per Article
2000	2,226	630	28%	2,926	4.64
1999	2,170	703	32%	2,745	3.90
1998	1,992	631	31%	2,598	4.11
1997	1,898	768	40%	3,328	4.03
1996	1,930	701	36%	2,775	3.96
1995	1,844	668	36%	2,570	3.85
1994	1,783	604	34%	2,493	4.13
1993	1,997	619	31%	2,890	4.45
1992	1,873	664	35%	3,211	4.51
1991	1,615	680	42%	3,165	4.65
1990	1,717	662	38%	3,001	4.53
1989	1,740	699	40%	2,903	4.15
1988	1,496	636	42%	2,642	4.15
1987	1,525	695	46%	2,810	4.04
1986	1,574	616	39%	2,627	4.26
1985	1,707	645	38%	2,623	4.07
1984	1,605	747	46%	3,077	4.12
1983	1,234	643	52%	3,130	4.87

TABLE 3 Number of Editorial Pages and Numbers and Types of Articles Published in *The American Journal of Cardiology* in 2000 (Volumes 85 + 86)

Number of editorial pages—total	3,292	(100%)
For articles	2,926	(89%)
For Readers' Comments (number) [replies]	38 (37) [4]	(1%)
For staff & editorial board	48	(1%)
For contents with abstracts	116	(4%)
For Instructions to Authors	46	(1%)
For Interactive Grand Rounds	14	(<1%)
For volume indexes	104	(3%)
Number of articles—total	648	(100%)
For Long reports	343	(51%)
Coronary artery disease	170	
Preventive cardiology	19	
Arrhythmia & conduction disturbances	30	
Systemic hypertension	7	
Congestive heart failure	26	
Valvular heart disease	21	
Cardiomyopathy	12	
Congenital heart disease	25	
Miscellaneous	14	
Methods	15	
Cardiovascular pharmacology	3	
Historical studies	1	
For Brief Reports	287	(42%)
For Case Reports	8	(1%)
For Interviews	6	(1%)
For Editorials	20	(3%)
For From-the-Editor column	2	(<1%)
For Interactive Grand Rounds	12	(2%)

7. *Symposia published in the AJC in 2000 (Table 5):* A total of 13 supplements including 132 articles and 888 pages were published in 2000. No advertisements, of course, appear in the supplement issues, which are published under separate cover with a different color from that of the regular issues. The guest editors of these symposia are for the most part major leaders in cardiovascular disease around the world.

TABLE 4 Interviews Published in the AJC

Eric Jeffrey Topol	July 1, 1996
W. Bruce Fye	August 1, 1996
James Thornton Willerson	February 15, 1997
Michael Ellis DeBakey	April 1, 1997
Denton Arthur Cooley	April 15, 1997
Joseph Stephan Alpert	May 1, 1997
Jesse Efrem Edwards	April 1, 1998
John Webster Kirklin	April 15, 1998
Howard Bertram Burchell	May 15, 1998
William Howard Frishman	June 1, 1998
Robert Ogdon Bonow	June 15, 1998
Eugene Braunwald	July 1, 1998
Joseph Cholmondeley Greenfield	July 15, 1998
David Coston Sabiston, Jr.	August 1, 1998
Norman Mayer Kaplan	August 15, 1998
Robert McKinnon Califf	September 1, 1998
Bernard John Gersh	November 1, 1998
Dean James Kereiakes	November 15, 1998
Jeffrey Michael Isner	January 1, 1999
Scott Montgomery Grundy	January 15, 1999
Burton Elias Sobel	February 1, 1999
Robert Anthony O'Rourke	April 1, 1999
David Kempton Cartwright Cooper	April 15, 1999
Spencer Bidwell King III	May 1, 1999
Robert Roberts	May 15, 1999
Eugene Auston Stead, Jr	September 15, 1999
Bertram Pitt	October 1, 1999
Christopher John Dillon Packard	November 15, 1999
Terje Rolf Pedersen	November 15, 1999
Francis Robicsek	June 1, 2000
Richard John Bing	July 1, 2000
Valentin Fuster	July 15, 2000
Henry Arthur Solomon	July 15, 2000
Harvey Stanley Hecht	November 1, 2000
Myrvin Harold Ellestad	December 1, 2000

8. *Reminder to authors to supply several names with addresses of nonbiased reviewers for their manuscripts:* Editors have no monopoly on choosing the best reviewers of manuscripts. No one should be more knowledgeable on experts in the subject of the manuscript than the authors of the manuscript. Thus, I urge authors to supply names—preferably at least 3 or 4, and their addresses—of nonlocal, nonbiased potential reviewers of their manuscripts. It is necessary for an author to submit several names because almost certainly some of the potential reviewers will already have a manuscript for review and a second manuscript is not sent to a reviewer already having one. Currently, about 20% of authors supply names of potential reviewers for their manuscripts. After studying the reviews of author-suggested reviewers for 19 years, I am impressed that the author-suggested reviewers are of high quality, and the author-suggested reviewers are no more biased toward their manuscripts than the editor-selected reviewers. Indeed, many manuscripts have been reviewed by one author-suggested reviewer and by one editor-suggested reviewer, and the author-suggested reviewer recommended rejection, while the editor-suggested reviewer recommended acceptance.

9. *Publishing the* AJC *electronically:* Mr. Spieler discussed what we can expect from this technology now and in the future. He stated that the full text and graphics of all 1,200 Elsevier journals are now posted on the Internet through **ScienceDirect**, an on-line host

TABLE 5 Symposia in *The American Journal of Cardiology* in 2000							
	Date of Publication	Subject of Symposium	Guest Editor(s)	Sponsor of Symposium	Article	Pages	Interval (mo) Symposium and Publications
A	February 10	Improving lipid management	Christie M. Ballantyne	Merck	9	56	4
B	March 9	Acute coronary syndromes	Richard R. Miller	Genentech	9	64	4
C	April 27	Acute coronary syndromes	Howard C. Herrmann	Centocor	8	51	—
D	May 25	Atrial fibrillation	Eric N. Prystowsky	Berlex	7	52	6
E	June 22		Sidney C. Smith, Jr.	Johnson & Johnson Merck Consumer Pharmaceuticals	5	23	7
F	July 20	Sexual activity and cardiac risk	John B. Kostis Harin Padma-Nathan Raymond C. Rosen	Bayer AG, Genupro, Lilly-ICOS, Merck, Pfizer, Pharmacia & Upjohn, Schering-Plough, TAP, and Zonagen	16	68	13
G	August 17	Echocardiography	Armando Dagianti	Merck Sharpe & Dohme Halia S.p.a.	17	60	18
H	August 24	Management after percutaneous coronary intervention	Andrew P. Selwyn	Pfizer	6	32	—
I	October 16	Transcatheter cardiovascular Therapeutics—Program and Abstracts		Elsevier Science	—	145	—
J	October 19	Acute coronary syndromes	David D. Waters Peter Libby		7	52	7
K	November 2	Ablation, pacing, implantable cardioverter-defibrillator	Joseph Brugada Richard G. Charles Eric N. Prystowsky	Guidant Corporation	27	168	7
L	December 21	Raising low high-density lipoprotein levels	Thomas A. Pearson William E. Boden	Kos	13	65	12
M	December 28	Acute coronary syndromes	Robert M. Califf	Aventis	8	52	13
Total: 13					132	888	(mean 9)

system developed and owned by Elsevier Science. **ScienceDirect** is directed toward end-users at institutional libraries and cuts across all subject areas of science, engineering, and medicine. Mr. Spieler encouraged the board members to access the Web site to review the journals' tables of contents and other features for free at http://www.sciencedirect.com.

Mr. Spieler also remarked that Elsevier has available another on-line service for cardiologists, titled **Cardiosource** (http://www.cardiosource.com), which contains the full text of 17 Elsevier journals in the field of cardiology, including *Journal of the American College of Cardiology, The American Journal of Cardiology, Cardiovascular Research, and The Lancet.* **Cardiosource** is geared specifically to the practicing cardiologist. The site has a powerful search engine and includes other important features in addition to the full text of the 17 journals, including a 24-hour Reuters Newsfeed of medical news, a superb database of clinical trials in cardiovascular medicine, personalized alerting features, an updated listing of over 300 professional medical meetings, an on-line cardiology forum, and links to related Web sites.

The meeting was followed by a fine reception provided by the publisher.

William C. Roberts

William Clifford Roberts, MD
Editor in Chief
Baylor University Medical Center
Dallas, Texas 75246

Proceedings of the Editorial Board Meeting of *The American Journal of Cardiology* on 18 March 2002

The 2002 meeting of the Editorial Board of *The American Journal of Cardiology* (*AJC*) was held on 18 March at the time of the Annual Scientific Sessions of the American College of Cardiology. The meeting's purpose was to review *AJC* publication results for 2001, to recognize particularly those *AJC* board members reviewing the most manuscripts in 2001, and to receive criticisms and suggestions from board members on how to improve the journal. The meeting went as follows:

1. *Introduction by Mr. Josh Spieler of Mr. Todd Hummel, the new Associate Publisher at Elsevier Science, Inc., Philadelphia, which includes the* AJC: Mr. Spieler welcomed the board members, thanked them for their help, and described new acquistions and developments at Elsevier, the publisher of the AJC, and of about 2,000 other scientific journals.

2. *Introduction of new* AJC *board members appointed in 2001:* Two new board members were appointed in 2001, Dr. Bruce R. Brodie and Dr. Alan B. Miller.

3. *AJC board members reviewing the most manuscripts in 2001 (Table 1):* The top *AJC* reviewer in 2001 was Dr. David H. Spodick, who reviewed 6 manuscripts and returned each of them during the allotted 3-week period. The AJC has the names of over 1,700 reviewers in its computer system.

TABLE 1 Top *American Journal of Cardiology* Editorial Board Reviewers in 2001

Board Member	Number of Manuscripts
David H. Spodick	6
Jeffrey A. Brinker	5
Bernard R. Chaitman	5
Marc Cohen	5
Stephen G. Ellis	5
Toby R. Engel	5
Stephen P. Glasser	5
David R. Holmes, Jr.	5
Harold L. Kennedy	5
Morton J. Kern	5
Carl J. Lavie	5
G.B. John Mancini	5
Randolph P. Martin	5
Raymond G. McKay	5
Jawahar L. Mehta	5
David M. Mirvis	5
Eugene R. Passamani	5
Mark E. Silverman	5
Robert A. Vogel	5
David D. Waters	5
Miguel A. Zabalgoitia	5

4. *Numbers of editorial pages published and numbers of manuscripts published in the regular issues of the* AJC *in 2001 (Table 2):* A total of 3,230 editorial pages (nonadvertising pages) were published in the regular issues of the *AJC* in 2001. These included 2,862 pages for articles, 37 pages for Readers' Comments, and the remaining 332 pages (10%) for listings of the staff and editorial board, contents with abstracts, instructions to authors, volume indexes, and interactive grand rounds. A total of 701 articles were published in the regular issues of the *AJC* in 2001, including 292 long

TABLE 2 Number of Editorial Pages and Articles Published in *The American Journal of Cardiology* in 2001 (volumes 87 + 88) (nonsymposium issues)

Number of editorial pages—total	3,230 (100%)
Articles	2,862 } (90%)
Reader's Comments (number)[replies]	37 (39) [3] } (90%)
Staff & editorial board	48 (1%)
Contents with abstracts	121 (4%)
Instructions to Authors	48 (1%)
Volume indexes	113 (3%)
Interactive Grand Rounds	1 (<1%)
Number of articles—total	701 (100%)
Long reports	292 (42%)
Brief Reports	370 (53%)
Case Reports	7 (<1%)
Interviews	3 (<1%)
Editorials	26 (4%)
From-the-Editor columns	3 (<1%)

TABLE 3 Types of Articles in the Long Reports Published in *The American Journal of Cardiology* in 2001

Coronary artery disease	156
Preventive cardiology	17
Arrhythmia & conduction disturbances	22
Systemic hypertension	13
Congestive heart failure	18
Valvular heart disease	12
Cardiomyopathy	7
Congenital heart disease	21
Miscellaneous	16
Methods	6
Cardiovascular pharmacology	3
Historical studies	1

TABLE 4 Numbers of Articles and Editorial Pages for Articles and Readers' Comments Published in the Regular Issues of *The American Journal of Cardiology* 1983–2001

	Pages for Articles	Pages for Readers Comments	Total	Number of Articles	Numbers of Readers' Comments	Brief Reports (% of Articles)
1983	3,130	27	3,157	643	53	81 (13%)
1984	3,077	36	3,113	747	80	204 (27%)
1985	2,623	21	2,644	645	40	172 (27%)
1986	2,627	17	2,644	616	40	160 (26%)
1987	2,810	23	2,833	695	45	203 (29%)
1988	2,646	26	2,672	636	60	152 (24%)
1989	2,903	19	2,922	699	36	187 (27%)
1990	3,001	20	3,021	662	40	158 (24%)
1991	3,165	38	3,203	680	59	182 (27%)
1992	3,211	46	3,257	711	53	166 (23%)
1993	2,890	37	2,927	650	64	209 (32%)
1994	2,493	31	2,524	604	46	221 (37%)
1995	2,570	34	2,604	668	52	268 (40%)
1996	2,775	29	2,804	658	52	273 (41%)
1997	3,328	32	3,360	826	45	409 (49%)
1998	3,048	35	3,083	664	37	263 (40%)
1999	3,015	38	3,053	680	42	268 (39%)
2000	2,926	38	2,964	648	37	287 (42%)
2001	2,862	37	2,899	701	39	370 (53%)
19 Years	55,100	584	55,642	12,833	920	4,233 (33%)

TABLE 5 Interviews Published in the *AJC*

Eric Jeffrey Topol	(July 1, 1996)	Francis Robicsek	(June 1, 2000)
W. Bruce Fye	(August 1, 1996)	Richard John Bing	(July 1, 2000)
James Thronton Willerson	(February 15, 1997)	Valentin Fuster	(July 15, 2000)
Michael Ellis DeBakey	(April 1, 1997)	Henry Arthur Solomon	(July 15, 2000)
Denton Arthur Cooley	(April 15, 1997)	Harvey Stanley Hecht	(November 1, 2000)
Joseph Stephan Alpert	(May 1, 1997)	Myrvin Harold Ellestad	(December 1, 2000)
Jesse Efrem Edwards	(April 1, 1998)	Melvin Mayer Scheinman	(March 1, 2001)
John Webster Kirklin	(April 15, 1998)	James Stuart Forrester, III	(December 1, 2001)
Howard Bertram Burchell	(May 15, 1998)	Carl J. Pepine	(December 15, 2001)
William Howard Frishman	(June 1, 1998)	Kenneth Hardy Cooper	(February 1, 2002)
Robert Ogdon Bonow	(June 15, 1998)	Watkins Proctor Harvey	(February 15, 2002)
Eugene Braunwald	(July 1, 1998)	Joseph Kayle Perloff	(March 1, 2002)
Joseph Cholmondeley Greenfield	(July 15, 1998)	Charles Richard Conti	(March 15, 2002)
David Coston Sabiston, Jr.	(August 1, 1998)	William Watts Parmley	(May 1, 2002)
Norman Mayer Kaplan	(August 15, 1998)	Dean Michael Ornish	
Robert McKinnon Califf	(September 1, 1998)	George Allan Beller	
Bernard John Gersh	(November 1, 1998)	Arthur Garson, Jr.	
Dean James Kereiakes	(November 15, 1998)		
Jeffrey Michael Isner	(January 1,1999)		
Scott Montgomery Grundy	(January 15, 1999)		
Burton Elias Sobel	(February 1, 1999)		
Robert Anthony O'Rourke	(April 1, 1999)		
David Kempton Cartwright Cooper	(April 15, 1999)		
Spencer Bidwell King, III	(May 1, 1999)		
Robert Roberts	(May 15, 1999)		
Eugene Auston Stead, Jr.	(September 15, 1999)		
Bertram Pitt	(October 1, 1999)		
Christopher John Dillon Packard	(November 15, 1999)		
Terje Rolf Pedersen	(November 15, 1999)		

reports (42%), 370 brief reports (53%), 26 editorials, and 7 or fewer case reports, interviews, and from-the-editor columns. Of the 370 brief reports published, 278 (75%) had been submitted initially as long reports and 92 (25%) had been submitted initially as brief reports. This means, of course, that many of the submitted long reports were shortened to brief reports. The brief reports, of course, allow the *AJC* to publish many more articles than would be possible if only long reports were published.

5. *Types of articles in the long reports published in the* AJC *in 2001:* These are listed in Table 3.

6. *Numbers of pages for articles and Readers' Comments published and numbers of articles, Readers' Comments, and Brief Reports published in the* AJC *from 1983 to 2001 (during the editor-in-chief*

TABLE 6 Numbers of Manuscripts Submitted and Published in *The American Journal of Cardiology* 1983–2001			
Year	Number of Manuscripts Submitted	Number of Manuscripts Published or Accepted	Percent Accepted
1983	1,234	643	52%
1984	1,605	747	46%
1985	1,707	645	38%
1986	1,574	616	39%
1987	1,525	695	46%
1988	1,496	636	42%
1989	1,740	699	40%
1990	1,717	662	38%
1991	1,615	680	42%
1992	1,873	664	35%
1993	1,997	619	31%
1994	1,783	604	34%
1995	1,844	668	36%
1996	1,930	701	36%
1997	1,898	768	40%
1998	1,992	631	31%
1999	2,170	703	32%
2000	2,226	630	28%
2001	2,068	682	33%

TABLE 7 Sources of Manuscripts Submitted to *The American Journal of Cardiology* in 2001		
Source	Submitted	Accepted
Non-USA	1,065 (51%)	289 (27%)
USA	1,003 (49%)	393 (39%)
Totals	2,068 (100%)	682 (33%)

tenure of WCR): These are tabulated for each of the 19 years in Table 4.

7. *Number of interviews published in the* AJC*:* Table 5 lists the interviews published (and 3 others completed) in the *AJC* and the dates of the issues in which they were published.

8. *Numbers of manuscripts submitted and accepted each year from 1983 to 2001:* These are listed in Table 6.

9. *Sources of manuscripts submitted to the* AJC *in 2001:* In 2001, a total of 2,068 manuscripts were submitted and 682 (33%) were accepted or published (Table 7). Of the 2,068 manuscripts, 1,065 (51%) came from non-USA countries and 289 (27%) were accepted; of the 1,003 (49%) from the USA, 393 (39%) were accepted.

10. *Symposia published in the* AJC *in 2001 (Table 8):* A total of 14 supplements, including 108 articles and 703 pages were published in 2001. No advertisements, of course, appear in the supplement issues, which are published under separate cover with a different color from that of the regular issues. The guest editors of these symposia are for the most part major leaders in cardiovascular disease around the world.

11. *Numbers of symposia and numbers of articles and pages in symposia in the* AJC *1983 to 2001:* These are shown in Table 9.

12. *Comparison of numbers of editorial pages and articles published in the regular (nonsymposium) issues of the* AJC*, Journal of the American College of Cardiology, Circulation, and American Heart Journal in 2001:* These data are shown in Table 10.

13. *Reminder to authors to supply several names with addresses of nonbiased and nonlocal reviewers*

TABLE 8 Symposia in *The American Journal of Cardiology* in 2001							
	Date of Publication	Subject of Symposium	Guest Editor(s)	Sponsor of Symposium	Articles	Pages	Interval (months) Symposium to Publication
A	February 16	Surrogate markers of atherosclerosis and development of drugs	Michael H. Davidson	Astra Zeneca	6	41	8
B	March 8	The ideal lipid-lowering agent	Antonio M. Gotto, Jr. Anders G. Olsson	Astra Zeneca	8	36	8
C	April 19	Pressure, platelets, plaque and angiotensin II	Kikuo Arakawa Michael A. Weber	Sankyo	8	44	8
D	June 28	Claudication and cilostazol	Craig M. Pratt Anthony J. Comerota	Otsuka and Pharmacia	6	48	—
E	July 19	Atherosclerotic imaging	Paolo Raggi	Pfizer	20	87	5
F	August 16	Managing hyperlipidemia	Antonio M. Gotto, Jr.	Pfizer	8	40	—
G	September 11	Transcatheter Cardiovascular Therapeutics abstracts	Martin B. Leon Gregg W. Stone	—	—	147	—
H	September 20	Postprandial state	Harold E. Lebovitz	Bayer	7	36	—
I	October 4	Blood pressure and perindopril	Suzanne Oparil	Solvay	6	40	—
J	October 11	Atorvastatin	Stephen Brunton	Pfizer	10	52	17
K	October 18	Lipids and statins	Andrew P. Selwyn Jeffrey J. Popma	Pfizer	10	43	7
L	November 8	Quinapril	Victor J. Dzau	Pfizer	6	20	28
M	November 21	Amlodipine, quinapril, atorvastatin	Alan B. Miller	Pfizer	4	25	20
N	December 20	Fenofibrate	Neil R. Poulter	Fournier	9	44	—
14					108	703	5–28 (mean 13)

TABLE 9 Numbers of Symposia and the Numbers of Articles and Pages in Symposia in *The American Journal of Cardiology* 1983–2001

Year	Number of Symposia	Number of Articles	Number of Pages
1983	5	60	341
1984	9	126	567
1985	15	192	1,161
1986	13	143	823
1987	19	279	1,576
1988	19	252	1,393
1989	20	232	1,240
1990	20	226	1,169
1991	9	99	631
1992	15	165	979
1993	13	167	1,076
1994	5	47	278
1995	11	156	872
1996	11	105	620
1997	17	166	1,119
1998	22	254	1,502
1999	18	172	1,133
2000	13	132	888
2001	14	108	703
19 Years	268	3,081	18,071

for their manuscripts: Editors have no monopoly on choosing the best reviewers of manuscripts. No one should be more knowledgeable on experts in the subject of the manuscript than the authors of the manuscript. Thus, I urge authors to supply names—preferably at least 3 or 4 and their addresses—of nonlocal, nonbiased potential reviewers of their manuscripts. It is necessary for an author to submit several names because almost certainly some of the potential reviewers will already have a manuscript for review and a second manuscript is not sent to a reviewer already having one. Of the 2,086 manuscripts submitted in 2001, only 244 (12%) of the authors supplied names of potential reviewers for their manuscripts. After studying the reviews of author-suggested reviewers for 20 years, I am impressed that the author-suggested reviewers are of high quality, and the author-suggested reviewers are no more biased towards their manuscripts than the editor-selected reviewers. Indeed, many manuscripts have been reviewed by one author-suggested reviewer and by one editor-suggested reviewer, and the author-suggested reviewer recommended rejection, while the editor-suggested reviewer recommended acceptance.

TABLE 10 Comparison of Numbers of Editorial Pages and Articles published in the Regular (nonsymposium) Issues of the *AJC, JACC, Circulation,* and *AHJ* in 2001

	AJC	*JACC*	*Circulation*	*AHJ*
Number of editorial pages	2,899	4,383	6,332	2,189
Number of articles	701	641	1,105	320
Pages/article	4.13	6.84	5.73	6.84

The meeting produced many comments and suggestions from the editorial board members. The meeting was followed by a fine reception provided by the publisher.

William C. Roberts

William Clifford Roberts, MD
Editor in Chief
Baylor Heart and Vascular Institute
Baylor University Medical Center
Dallas, Texas 75246

Proceedings of the Editorial Board Meeting of *The American Journal of Cardiology* on 31 March 2003

The 2003 meeting of the Editorial Board of *The American Journal of Cardiology* (*AJC*) was held on 31 March at the time of the Annual Scientific Sessions of the American College of Cardiology. The meeting's purpose was to review the *AJC* publication results for 2002, to recognize particularly those *AJC*-board members reviewing the most manuscripts in 2002, and to receive criticisms and suggestions from the board members on how to improve the journal. The meeting went as follows:

1. *Introduction of the new publisher, Ms. Christine B. Rullo, who in turn introduced the Elsevier Science staff:* Ms. Rullo welcomed the board members, thanked them for their help, and described new developments at Elsevier, the publisher of the *AJC* and of about 2,000 other scientific journals.

2. *Introduction of new* AJC *board members appointed in 2002:* These are listed in Table 1.

3. AJC *board members reviewing the most manuscripts in 2002:* These are listed in Table 2.

4. *Numbers of editorial pages published and numbers of manuscripts published in regular issues of the* AJC *in 2002:* A total of 3,201 editorial pages (non-advertising pages) were published in regular issues of the *AJC*in 2002 (Table 3). These included 2,835 pages for articles, 37 pages for Readers' Comments, and the remaining 321 pages (10%) for listings of the staff and editorial board, contents with abstracts, instructions to authors, and volume indexes. A total of 680 articles were published in regular issues of the *AJC* in 2002, including 270 long reports (40%), 363 brief reports (53%), 28 editorials, 7 case reports, 7 interviews, and 4 from-the-editor columns. Of the 363 brief reports published, 268 (74%) had been submitted initially as long reports and 95 (26%) had been submitted initially as brief reports. These numbers and percentages were virtually identical to those published in 2001. The brief reports, of course, allow the *AJC*to publish many more articles than would be possible if only long reports were published.

5. *Types of long report articles published in the* AJC *in 2002:* These are listed in Table 3.

6. *Numbers of pages for articles and Readers' Comments published and numbers of articles, Readers' Comments, and Brief Reports published in the* AJC *from 1983 to 2002 (during the present editor-in-*

TABLE 1 New Board Members Beginning in 2002

Bruce R. Brodie
Lawrence S. Cohen
James A. de Lemos
Michael R. Gold
Jamshid Shirani
Robert L. Wilensky

TABLE 2 Top *American Journal of Cardiology* Editorial Board Reviewers in 2002

Board Member	No. of Manuscripts
Jeffrey Anderson	6
Robert F. DeBusk	6
Gerald F. Fletcher	6
Julius M. Gardin	6
L. David Hillis	6
Morton J. Kern	6
Charles E. Rackley	6
Miguel Zabalgoitia	6

TABLE 3 Number of Editorial Pages and Articles Published in *The American Journal of Cardiology* in 2002 (volumes 89 + 90) (non-symposium issues)

Number of editorial pages—total	3201 (100%)
Articles	2835 (89%)
Readers' Comments (number) [replies]	45 (42) [5] (1%)
Staff & editorial board	48 (1%)
Contents with abstracts	114 (4%)
Instructions to authors	46 (1%)
Volume indexes	113 (4%)
Number of articles—total	680 (100%)
Long reports	270 (40%)
Coronary artery disease	141
Preventive cardiology	22
Arrhythmia & conduction	18
Systemic hypertension	7
Heart failure	20
Valvular heart disease	7
Cardiomyopathy	10
Congenital heart disease	14
Miscellaneous	21
Methods	7
Cardiovascular pharmacology	2
Historical studies	1
Brief Reports	363 (53%)
Case Reports	7 (1%)
Interviews	7 (1%)
Editorials	28 (4%)
From-the-Editor columns	4 (<1%)
Memoriam	1 (<1%)

TABLE 4 Number of Articles and Editorial Pages for Articles and Readers' Comments Published in Regular Issues of *The American Journal of Cardiology* 1983–2002

Year	Pages for Articles	Pages for Readers' Comments	Total	Number of Articles	Numbers of Readers' Comments	Brief Reports (% of articles)
1983	3,130	27	3,157	643	53	81 (13%)
1984	3,077	36	3,113	747	80	204 (27%)
1985	2,623	21	2,644	645	40	172 (27%)
1986	2,627	17	2,644	616	40	160 (26%)
1987	2,810	23	2,833	695	45	203 (29%)
1988	2,646	26	2,672	636	60	152 (24%)
1989	2,903	19	2,922	699	36	187 (27%)
1990	3,001	20	3,021	662	40	158 (24%)
1991	3,165	38	3,203	680	59	182 (27%)
1992	3,211	46	3,257	711	53	166 (23%)
1993	2,890	37	2,927	650	64	209 (32%)
1994	2,493	31	2,524	604	46	221 (32%)
1995	2,570	34	2,604	668	52	268 (40%)
1996	2,775	29	2,804	658	52	273 (41%)
1997	3,328	32	3,360	826	45	409 (49%)
1998	3,048	35	3,083	664	37	263 (40%)
1999	3,015	38	3,053	680	42	268 (39%)
2000	2,926	38	2,964	648	37	287 (42%)
2001	2,862	37	2,899	701	39	370 (53%)
2002	2,835	45	2,880	680	45	363 (53%)
20 Years	57,935	629	58,522	13,513	965	4,596 (34%)

TABLE 5 Interviews Published in *The American Journal of Cardiology*

Eric Jeffrey Topol	(July 1, 1996)	Bertram Pitt	(October 1, 1999)
W. Bruce Fye	(August 1, 1996)	Christopher John Dillon Packard	(November 15, 1999)
James Thornton Willerson	(February 15, 1997)	Terje Rolf Pedersen	(November 15, 1999)
Michael Ellis DeBakey	(April 1, 1997)	Francis Robicsek	(June 1, 2000)
Denton Arthur Cooley	(April 15, 1997)	Richard John Bing	(July 1, 2000)
Joseph Stephan Alpert	(May 1, 1997)	Valentin Fuster	(July 15, 2000)
Jesse Efrem Edwards	(April 1, 1998)	Henry Arthur Solomon	(July 15, 2000)
John Webster Kirklin	(April 15, 1998)	Myrvin Harold Ellestad	(December 1, 2000)
Howard Bertram Burchell	(May 15, 1998)	Melvin Mayer Scheinman	(March 1, 2001)
William Howard Frishman	(June 1, 1998)	James Stuart Forrester, III	(December 1, 2001)
Robert Ogdon Bonow	(June 15, 1998)	Carl J. Pepine	(December 15, 2001)
Eugene Braunwald	(July 1, 1998)	Kenneth Hardy Cooper	(February 1, 2002)
Joseph Cholmondeley Greenfield	(July 15, 1998)	Watkins Proctor Harvey	(February 15, 2002)
David Coston Sabiston, Jr.	(August 1, 1998)	Joseph Kayle Perloff	(March 1, 2002)
Norman Mayer Kaplan	(August 15, 1998)	Charles Richard Conti	(March 15, 2002)
Robert McKinnon Califf	(September 1, 1998)	William Watts Parmley	(May 1, 2002)
Bernard John Gersh	(November 1, 1998)	Dean Michael Ornish	(August 1, 2002)
Dean James Kereiakes	(November 15, 1998)	Dean Towle Mason	(December 15, 2002)
Jeffrey Michael Isner	(January 1, 1999)	George Allan Beller	(January 15, 2003)
Scott Montgomery Grundy	(January 15, 1999)	Leslie David Hillis	(February 1, 2003)
Burton Elias Sobel	(February 1, 1999)	Douglas Peter Zipes	(April 1, 2003)
Robert Anthony O'Rourke	(April 1, 1999)	Nanette Kass Wenger	(May 15, 2003)
David Kempton Cartwright Cooper	(April 15, 1999)	Edward David Frolich	(2003)
Spencer Bidwell King, III	(May 1, 1999)	Arthur Garson, Jr.	(2003)
Robert Roberts	(May 15, 1999)	Andrew Peter Selwyn	(2003)
Eugene Auston Stead, Jr.	(September 15, 1999)	Magdi Habib Yacoub	(2003)

chief's tenure): These are tabulated for each of the 20 years in Table 4.

7. *Interviews published in the* AJC*:* Table 5 lists the interviews published and 6 others scheduled for publication in 2003.

8. *Numbers of manuscripts submitted and accepted each year from 1983 through 2002:* These are listed in Table 6. The manuscripts published or accepted are a bit different from the numbers listed in Table 4 because some of the manuscripts submitted in 2002 were not published until 2003. That holds true for all of the 20 years in which data are shown. Of the 2,171 manuscripts submitted in 2002, 683 (31%) were accepted. This percentage is higher than in some other cardiology journals because so many of the long reports are converted into brief reports. Otherwise, the percent would be much lower. The numbers of editorial pages available for articles in the *AJC* have been relatively constant over the past 20 years. The average pages per article of those published in each of the 20 years are

TABLE 6 Numbers of Manuscripts Submitted and Published and Numbers of Editorial Pages Published in *The American Journal of Cardiology*, 1983–2002

Year	No. of Manuscripts Submitted	No. of Manuscripts Published or Accepted	Percent Accepted	No. of Editorial Pages for Articles	Average Pages Per Article
1983	1,234	643	52%	3,130	4.87
1984	1,605	747	46%	3,077	4.12
1985	1,707	645	38%	2,623	4.07
1986	1,574	616	39%	2,627	4.26
1987	1,525	695	46%	2,810	4.04
1988	1,496	636	42%	2,642	4.15
1989	1,740	699	40%	2,903	4.15
1990	1,717	662	38%	3,001	4.53
1991	1,615	680	42%	3,165	4.65
1992	1,873	664	35%	3,211	4.51
1993	1,997	619	31%	2,890	4.45
1994	1,783	604	34%	2,493	4.13
1995	1,844	668	36%	2,570	3.85
1996	1,930	701	36%	2,775	3.96
1997	1,898	768	40%	3,328	4.33
1998	1,992	631	31%	2,598	4.11
1999	2,170	703	32%	2,745	3.90
2000	2,226	630	28%	2,926	4.64
2001	2,068	682	33%	2,914	4.27
2002	2,171	683	31%	2,835	4.15

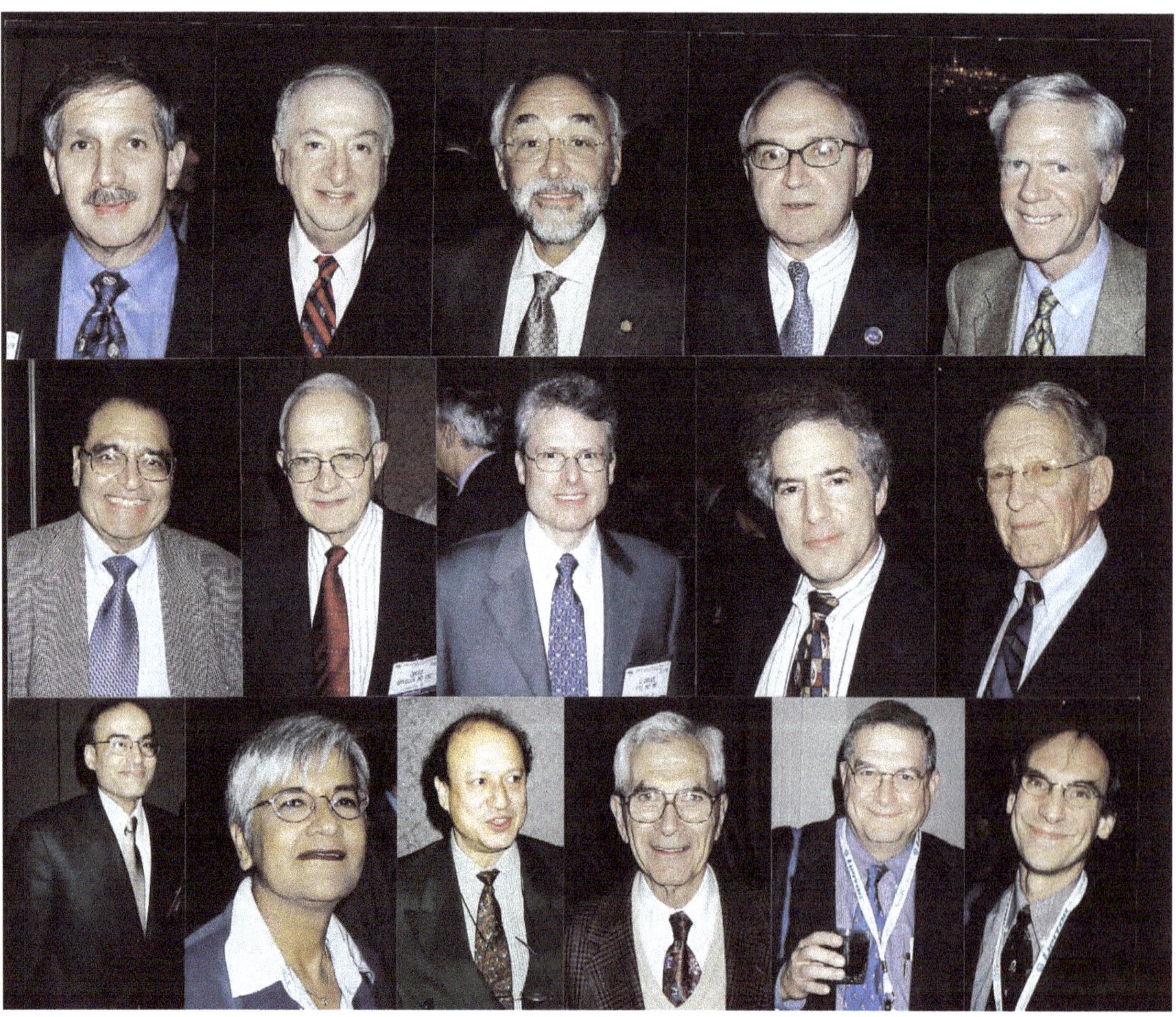

TABLE 7 Symposia in *The American Journal of Cardiology* in 2002

	Date of Publication	Subject of Symposium	Guest Editor(s)	Sponsor of Symposium	Articles	Pages	Discussion	Dates of Syposium	Interval (months) Symposium & Publication
A	January 24	Ramipril and telmisartan	Michael A. Weber Salim Yusuf	Boehringer Ingelheim GmbH	5	33	+	March 17, 2001	10
B	February 21	Techniques to measure plaques	Donald M. Black	Astra Zeneca	7	41	+	April 26, 2001	10
C	March 7	National cholesterol guidelines	Michael H. Davidson	Astra Zeneca	7	57	+	September 10, 2001	6
D	March 21	Cyclooxygenase-2 inhibition	Garret A. FitzGerald	Merck	6	48	0	—	—
E	June 20	Hormone replacement therapy	Daniel R. Mishell, Jr. Michael E. Mendelsohn	Ortho-McNeil	7	66	+	June 21, 2001	12
F	July 3	Hormone replacement therapy	Richard H. Karas Lori Mosca	Pharmacia	10	58	0	May 5, 2001	14
G	September 5	Diabetes mellitus	Barry J. Goldstein	Glaxo Smith Klein	7	50	0	July 11, 2001	14
H	September 24	Transcatheter cardiovascular therapeutics	Martin B. Leon Gregg W. Stone	Medtronic	Abstracts	217	0	September 24–28, 2002	—
I	October 17	Lipoprotein-modulated disease	Peter O. Kwiterovich, Jr.	LipoScience	9	84	0	October 13, 2001	12
J	November 18	Contrast echocardiography	Mani A. Vannan Sanjiv Kaul	Bracco Diagnostics	13	80	0	July 25–27, 2001	16
K	November 20	Combination therapy for dyslipidemia	Michael H. Davidson	Kos Pharmaceuticals Merck	7	60	0	March 2002	8
L	November 21	Atherosclerotic imaging	Paolo Raggi	Pfizer	12	64	0	May 31–June 2, 2002	6
12					90	858			(mean 11)

TABLE 8 Numbers of Symposia and the Numbers of Articles and Pages in Symposia in *The American Journal of Cardiology*, 1983–2002

Year	No. of Symposia	No. of Articles	No. of Pages
1983	5	60	341
1984	9	126	567
1985	15	192	1,161
1986	13	143	823
1987	19	279	1,576
1988	19	252	1,393
1989	20	232	1,240
1990	20	226	1,169
1991	9	99	631
1992	15	165	979
1993	13	167	1,076
1994	5	47	278
1995	11	156	872
1996	11	105	620
1997	17	166	1,119
1998	22	254	1,502
1999	18	172	1,133
2000	13	132	888
2001	14	108	703
2002	12	90	858
20 years	280	3,171	18,929

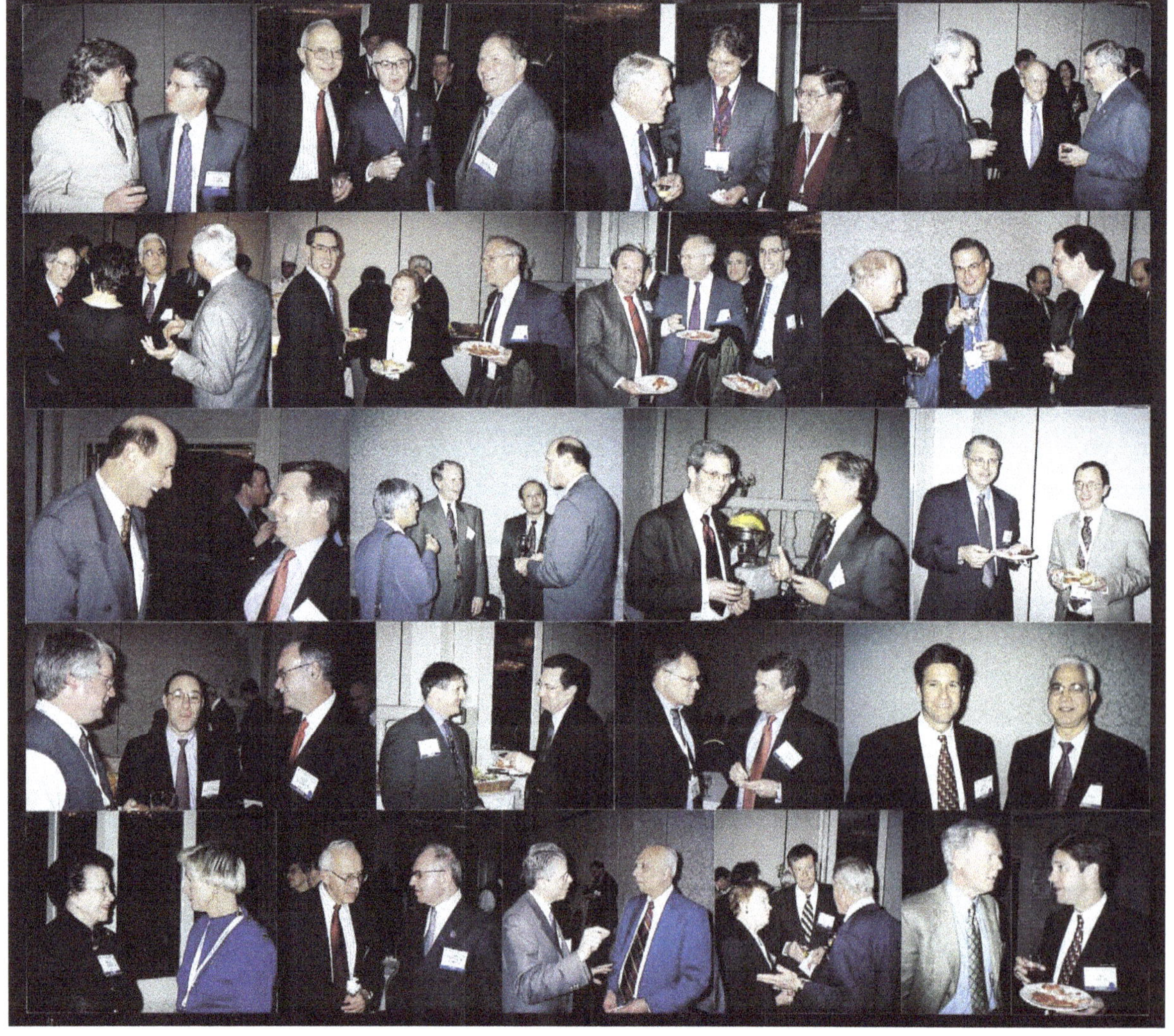

also listed in Table 6; that average is close to 4.0. The average pages per article, of course, would be smaller if so many figures and tables were not included.

9. *Sources of manuscripts submitted to the* AJC *in 2002:* Of the 2,171 manuscripts submitted in 2002, 881 (41%) came from the United States, and 422 (48%) were accepted; the remaining 1,290 manuscripts submitted in 2002 came from non-US countries and 261 (20%) were accepted.

10. *Number of manuscripts submitted to the* AJC *in 2002 with names of potential reviewers suggested by the authors:* The instructions to authors in the *AJC* urge submitting authors to suggest several potentially non-biased reviewers, located in cities other than those of the submitting author, who might provide non-biased reviews of their manuscripts. Of the 2,171 manuscripts submitted to the *AJC* in 2002, only 284 (13%) provided suggested reviewers. I would like to see that percentage increase considerably.

11. *Symposia published in the* AJC *in 2002:* A total of 12 supplements, including 90 articles occupying 858 editorial pages, were published in 2002 (Table 7). No advertisements, of course, appear in the supplement issues, which are published under a separate cover with a different color from that of the regular issues. The guest editors of these symposia are, for the most part, major leaders in cardiovascular disease around the world.

12. *Numbers of symposia and numbers of articles and pages in symposia in the* AJC *from 1983 through 2002:* These are listed in Table 8. During this 20-year period, 280 symposia were published and they included 3,171 articles occupying 18,929 pages.

The meeting produced several comments and suggestions from the editorial board members (see photographs) and was followed by a fine reception provided by the publisher.

William C. Roberts

William C. Roberts, MD
Editor in Chief
Baylor Heart and Vascular Institute
Baylor University Medical Center
Dallas, Texas 75246

Proceedings of the Editorial Board Meeting of *The American Journal of Cardiology* on 8 March 2004

The 2004 meeting of the Editorial Board of *The American Journal of Cardiology* (*AJC*) was held on 8 March at the time of the Annual Scientific Sessions of the American College of Cardiology. The meeting's purpose was to review the *AJC* publication results for 2003, to recognize particularly those *AJC* board members who reviewed the most manuscripts in 2003, and to receive criticisms and suggestions from the board members on how to improve the journal. The meeting went as follows:

1. *Ms. Christine B. Rullo, the publisher, introduced the Elsevier Science staff,* and described the *AJC*'s status relative to other cardiovascular journals, focusing particularly on the impact factor (see item 12 in this piece).

2. *Introduction of new* AJC *board members appointed in 2003*: These are listed in Table 1.

3. AJC *board members who reviewed the most manuscripts in 2003*: These are listed in Table 2.

4. *Number of manuscripts submitted and accepted for 2003*: These are shown in Table 3. Of the 2,190 manuscripts submitted in 2003, 783 (36%) were accepted. The percentage is higher than in some other cardiology journals because so many of the long reports are converted into brief reports. Otherwise, the percent would be much lower. The numbers of editorial pages available for articles in the *AJC* have been relatively constant over the past 21 years.

5. *Sources of manuscripts submitted to the* AJC *in 2003*: Of the 2,190 manuscripts submitted in 2003, 813 (37%) came from the USA, and 429 (53%) were accepted; the remaining 1,377 (63%) manuscripts submitted in 2003 came from non-USA countries and 354 (26%) were accepted.

6. *Number of manuscripts submitted to the* AJC *in 2003 with names of potential reviewers suggested by the investigators*: The instructions to authors in the *AJC* urge submitting investigators to suggest several potentially nonbiased reviewers, located in cities other than those of the submitting investigator, who might provide nonbiased reviews of their manuscripts. Of the 2,190 manuscripts submitted to the *AJC* in 2003, only 163 (7%) provided suggested reviewers. I would like to see that percent increase considerably.

7. *Number of editorial pages published and number of manuscripts published in the regular issues of the* AJC *in 2003*: A total of 3,358 editorial pages (nonadvertising pages) were published in the regular issues of the *AJC* in 2003 (Table 4). These included 2,982 pages for articles, 35 pages for Readers' Comments, and the remaining 341 pages (10%) for listings of the staff and editorial board, contents with abstracts, instructions to authors, and volume indexes. A total of 763 articles were published in the regular issues of the *AJC* in 2003, including 236 long reports (31%), 487 brief reports (64%), 16 editorials, 9 case reports, 7 interviews, and 8 from-the-editor columns. These numbers and percentages were virtually identical to those published in 2002. The brief reports, of course, allow the *AJC* to publish many more articles than would be possible if only long reports were published. Most of the published brief reports had been submitted originally as long reports.

8. *Number of pages for articles and Readers' Comments published and number of articles, Readers' Comments, and Brief Reports published in the* AJC *from 1983 to 2003 (during the present editor-in-chief's tenure)*: These are tabulated for each of the 21 years in Table 5.

9. *Interviews published in the* AJC: Table 6 lists the interviews published and 1 other scheduled for publication in 2004.

10. *Symposia published in the* AJC *in 2003*: A total of 14 supplements, including 95 articles occupying 620 editorial pages, were published in 2003 (Table 7). No advertisements, of course, appear in the supplement issues, which are published under separate cover with a different color from that of the regular issues. The guest editors of these symposia are, for the most part, major leaders in cardiovascular disease around the world.

11. *Numbers of symposia and numbers of articles and pages in symposia in the* AJC *from 1983 to 2003*: These are shown in Table 8. During this 21-year period, 294 symposia were published, and they included 3,266 articles occupying 19,549 pages.

12. *The impact factor and its significance*: Ms. Rullo indicated that the impact factor (IF) for the *AJC* in 2002, the latest year available, was 2.327. This number placed the *AJC* in 15th place among 66 cardiovascular journals published worldwide. This number was disturbing to me and stimulated me to study better what the IF was and how it was derived. The IF is a number derived by dividing the number of original research articles and reviews published in a particular journal during a specified period (2 years) into the number of citations to that journal in the year following the 2-year specified period.

Let's look at the derivation of the 2002 IF for the *AJC*. In 2000 and 2001 a total of 1,349 original research articles were published in the regular issues of the *AJC*, but no reviews were published during either of these 2 years. Also, during 2000 and 2001, a

TABLE 1 New Board Members Beginning 2003
William Gregory Hundley
Mark J. Eisenberg
Gregory Y.H. Lip
Ronald Gary Victor

TABLE 2 *The American Journal of Cardiology* Editorial Board Top Reviewers in 2003

Board Member	Number of Manuscripts
Sanjiv Kaul	7
Robert A. Kloner	7
Gary S. Mintz	7
David H. Spodick	7
James A. de Lemos	6
Gerald F. Fletcher	6
David R. Holmes, Jr.	6
Arthur Moss	6
Erik Magnus Ohman	6
Jonathan M. Tobis	6
Eric J. Topol	6
Barry L. Zaret	6

TABLE 3 Number of Manuscripts Submitted and Published in *The American Journal of Cardiology* 1983–2003

Year	Number of Manuscripts Submitted	Number of Manuscripts Published or Accepted	Percent Accepted
1983	1,234	643	52%
1984	1,605	747	46%
1985	1,707	645	38%
1986	1,574	616	39%
1987	1,525	695	46%
1988	1,496	636	42%
1989	1,740	699	40%
1990	1,717	662	38%
1991	1,615	680	42%
1992	1,873	664	35%
1993	1,997	619	31%
1994	1,783	604	34%
1995	1,844	668	36%
1996	1,930	701	36%
1997	1,898	768	40%
1998	1,992	631	31%
1999	2,170	703	32%
2000	2,226	630	28%
2001	2,068	682	33%
2002	2,171	683	31%
2003	2,190	783	36%

total of 240 articles were published in the 27 symposia issues during those 2 years. Thus, a total of 1,589 original research articles or reviews were published in those 2 years. Sixty of those articles, however, were editorials or interviews or Readers' Comments and they do not count as "original research articles" or "reviews" and that number had to be subtracted from the total number of articles in the denominator, leaving a total of 1,529 articles published in the 2-year period. During 2002, the year following the 2-year period (2000 and 2001), 3,558 *AJC* articles were cited. Dividing the number of articles (1,529) published in the 2 years into the number of citations (3,558) appearing the following year yielded an IF of 2.327.

How can the IF be increased in any journal? There are 3 ways: (1) by decreasing the numbers of articles published, (2) by increasing the numbers of citations, or (3) by the combination of 1 and 2.

TABLE 4 Number of Editorial Pages and Articles Published in *The American Journal of Cardiology in 2003* (Volumes 91 + 92) (non-Symposium issues)

Number of editorial pages–total	3,358 (100%)
Articles	2,982
Readers' Comments (number)[replies]	35(32)[5] (90%)
Staff & editorial board	48 (1%)
Contents with abstracts	125 (4%)
Instructions to Authors	44 (1%)
Volume indexes	124 (4%)
Number of articles—total	763 (100%)
Long reports	236 (31%)
Brief Reports	487 (64%)
Case Reports	9 (1%)
Interviews	7 (1%)
Editorials	16 (2%)
From-the-Editor columns	8 (1%)

Why is the IF of the AJC, a journal with nearly 30,000 paid readers, lower than it appears to deserve? In my view there are at least 4 reasons: (1) *the number of articles published in the* AJC *is large.* The 1,529 articles published in the AJC in the year 2000 and 2001 are well over twice the number published by 12 of the 14 cardiovascular journals with higher IFs in 2002, and the smaller the number of articles published, the greater the probability of a higher IF. (2) *The number of reviews published in the* AJC *is essentially zero.* Reviews are usually highly referenced and not publishing reviews puts the *AJC* at a disadvantage in this regard. All 14 cardiovascular journals with higher IFs publish reviews and some of them publish numerous ones. (3) *The number of references in articles published in the* AJC *is limited and that restriction limits the number of citations to previously published articles in the AJC.* The number of references in "long reports" in the *AJC* is limited to 30 and in "brief reports," to 20. Limiting the number of citations in articles in the *AJC*, of course, limits the numbers of citations to the *AJC* (as well as to other journals). Self citations are probably much greater when numbers of references are not limited and no cardiovascular journals have reference limitations as strict as the *AJC*. Furthermore, self citations are probably much greater in *Circulation* and the *Journal of the American College of Cardiology* than in the *AJC* because more articles in the *AJC* are by investigators with far fewer publications than in the other 2 medical journals, and, as a consequence, there are fewer self citations in the *AJC*. (4) *It is likely that "brief reports" are not cited as frequently as "long reports,"* and now more "brief reports" are published in the *AJC* than are "long

TABLE 5 Number of Articles and Editorial Pages for Articles and Readers' Comments Published in the Regular Issues of *The American Journal of Cardiology* 1983–2003

Year	Pages for Articles	Pages for Readers' Comments	Total	Number of Articles	Average Pages per Article	Numbers of Readers' Comments	Brief Reports (% of articles)
1983	3,130	27	3,157	643	4.87	53	81 (13%)
1984	3,077	36	3,113	747	4.12	80	204 (27%)
1985	2,623	21	2,602	645	4.07	40	172 (27%)
1986	2,627	17	2,644	616	4.26	40	160 (26%)
1987	2,810	23	2,833	695	4.04	45	203 (29%)
1988	2,646	26	2,672	636	4.15	60	152 (24%)
1989	2,903	19	2,922	699	4.15	36	187 (27%)
1990	3,001	20	3,021	662	4.53	40	158 (24%)
1991	3,165	38	3,203	680	4.65	59	182 (27%)
1992	3,211	46	3,257	711	4.51	53	166 (23%)
1993	2,890	37	2,927	650	4.45	64	209 (32%)
1994	2,493	31	2,524	604	4.13	46	221 (32%)
1995	2,570	34	2,604	668	3.85	52	268 (40%)
1996	2,775	29	2,804	658	3.96	52	273 (41%)
1997	3,328	32	3,360	826	4.33	45	409 (49%)
1998	3,048	35	3,083	664	4.11	37	263 (40%)
1999	3,015	38	3,053	680	3.90	42	268 (39%)
2000	2,926	38	2,964	648	4.64	37	287 (42%)
2001	2,862	37	2,899	701	4.27	39	370 (53%)
2002	2,835	45	2,880	680	4.15	45	363 (53%)
2003	2,982	35	3,017	763	3.91	32	487 (64%)
Totals (21 Years)	60,917	664	61,539	14,276	4.27	997	5,083 (36%)

TABLE 6 Interviews Published in the *AJC*

Eric Jeffrey Topol	(July 1, 1996)	Francis Robicsek	(June 1, 2000)
W. Bruce Fye	(August 1, 1996)	Richard John Bing	(July 1, 2000)
James Thronton Willerson	(February 15, 1997)	Valentin Fuster	(July 15, 2000)
Michael Ellis DeBakey	(April 1, 1997)	Henry Arthur Solomon	(July 15, 2000)
Denton Arthur Cooley	(April 15, 1997)	Myrvin Harold Ellestad	(December 1, 2000)
Joseph Stephan Alpert	(May 1, 1997)	Melvin Mayer Scheinman	(March 1, 2001)
Jesse Efrem Edwards	(April 1, 1998)	James Stuart Forrester, III	(December 1, 2001)
John Webster Kirklin	(April 15, 1998)	Carl J. Pepine	(December 15, 2001)
Howard Bertram Burchell	(May 15, 1998)	Kenneth Hardy Cooper	(February 1, 2002)
William Howard Frishman	(June 1, 1998)	Watkins Proctor Harvey	(February 15, 2002)
Robert Ogdon Bonow	(June 15, 1998)	Joseph Kayle Perloff	(March 1, 2002)
Eugene Braunwald	(July 1, 1998)	Charles Richard Conti	(March 15, 2002)
Joseph Cholmondeley Greenfield	(July 15, 1998)	William Watts Parmley	(May 1, 2002)
David Coston Sabiston, Jr.	(August 1, 1998)	Dean Michael Ornish	(August 1, 2002)
Norman Mayer Kaplan	(August 15, 1998)	Dean Towle Mason	(December 15, 2002)
Robert McKinnon Califf	(September 1, 1998)	George Allan Beller	(January 15, 2003)
Bernard John Gersh	(November 1, 1998)	Leslie David Hillis	(February 1, 2003)
Dean James Kereiakes	(November 15, 1998)	Douglas P. Zipes	(April 1, 2003)
Jeffrey Michael Isner	(January 1, 1999)	Nanette Kass Wenger	(May 15, 2003)
Scott Montgomery Grundy	(January 15, 1999)	Andrew Peter Selwyn	(June 15, 2003)
Burton Elias Sobel	(February 1, 1999)	Arthur Garson, Jr.	(August 15, 2003)
Robert Anthony O'Rourke	(April 1, 1999)	Edward David Frolich	(September 1, 2003)
David Kempton Cartwright Cooper	(April 15, 1999)	Magdi Habib Yacoub	(January 15, 2004)
Spencer Bidwell King III	(May 1, 1999)	Robert A. Vogel	(April 1, 2004)
Robert Roberts	(May 15, 1999)	Steven E. Nissen	
Eugene Auston Stead, Jr.	(September 15, 1999)		
Bertram Pitt	(October 1, 1999)		
Christopher John Dillon Packard	(November 15, 1999)		
Terje Rolf Pedersen	(November 15, 1999)		

reports." In 2003, abstracts of the brief reports were moved to the beginning of the reports and printed in bold type. Previously, they had been at the article's end and in nonbold type. We believe that this change will produce more citations to the brief reports, but it will take another 2 years before this effect on the IF can be determined.

Thus, the IF has serious limitations as a measure of a journal's success. The number of subscribers to the *AJC* continues to increase and the number of manu-

	TABLE 7 Symposia in *The American Journal of Cardiology* in 2003						
	Date of Publication	Subject of Symposium	Guest Editor(s)	Sponsor of Symposium	Articles	Pages	Interval (months) Symposium to Publication
A	February 6	Biology of Atherosclerosis	Joseph A. Franciosa R. Wayne Alexander	AtheroGenics	9	53	11
B	February 20	Atorvastatin	Andrew P. Selwyn Jeffrey J. Popma	Pfizer	7	35	—
C	March 6	Rosuvastatin	Evan A. Stein	Astra Zeneca	6	28	12
D	March 20	Cardiac Resynchronization Therapy	Gerald V. Naccarelli	Pfizer	9	66	7
E	April 3	Rosuvastatin	H. Bryan Brewer, Jr.	Astra Zeneca	7	39	5
F	May 8	Biventricular Pacing–Defibrillation	Italo de Luca, Robert O. Bonow, Mihai Gheorghiade, Francesco Fedele	ERREKAPPA	11	94	13
G	May 22	Perindopril	Peter Sleight Thomas Unger	Boehringer Ingelheim GmbH	6	34	14–18
H	August 24	Management after Percutaneous Coronary Intervention	Andrew P. Selwyn	Pfizer	6	32	42–66
I	July 3	Simvastatin	Antonio M. Gotto, Jr.	Merck	6	50	—
J	August 18	Diabetes Mellitus, Insulin Resistance and Cardiovascaular Disease	Willa. A Hsueh	Glaxo Smith Kline	8	60	—
K	August 21	Rosuvastatin	H. Bryan Brewer	Astra Zeneca	5	29	9
L	September	Abstracts—Transcatheter Cardiovascular Therapeutics-2003	—	Metronic AVE	—	260	0
M	November 6	Tadalafil	Robert A. Kloner	Lilly ICOS LLC	8	65	27
N	November 7	Angiogenic Gene Therapy	Victor J. Dzau Berlex Joachim-Friedrich Kapp		7	35	11
14					95	620*	—

*Excludes abstracts of Symposium L.

TABLE 8 Number of Symposia and the Number of Articles and Pages in Symposia in *The American Journal of Cardiology* 1983–2003			
Year	Number of Symposia	Number of Articles	Number of Pages
1983	5	60	341
1984	9	126	567
1985	15	192	1,161
1986	13	143	823
1987	19	279	1,576
1988	19	252	1,393
1989	20	232	1,240
1990	20	226	1,169
1991	9	99	631
1992	15	165	979
1993	13	167	1,076
1994	5	47	278
1995	11	156	872
1996	11	105	620
1997	17	166	1,119
1998	22	254	1,502
1999	18	172	1,133
2000	13	132	888
2001	14	108	703
2002	12	90	858
2003	14	95	620
21 Years	294	3,266	19,549

scripts submitted each year continues to climb, albeit slightly. I believe the latter 2 measures are better indicators of how a journal is doing than is the IF. The editorial board members, after the above discussion, also appeared to agree that the *AJC* need not be concerned with the IF.

13. *Structured versus nonstructured abstracts*: Dr. Arthur Moss suggested that the abstracts for long reports in the *AJC* be structured like in so many other medical journals. I expressed my preference for nonstructured abstracts because they save space and the flow of words might be smoother. After a brief discussion, a vote was held and the nonstructured version of the abstract won decidedly over the structured abstract.

The meeting was followed by a fine reception provided by the publisher.

William C. Roberts

William Clifford Roberts, MD
Editor in Chief
Baylor Heart and Vascular Institute
Baylor University Medical Center
Dallas, Texas 75246

Proceedings of the Editorial Board Meeting of *The American Journal of Cardiology* on 7 March 2005

The 2005 meeting of the Editorial Board of *The American Journal of Cardiology* (AJC) was held on 7 March at the time of the Annual Scientific Sessions of the American College of Cardiology. The meeting's purpose was to review the AJC publication results for 2004, to recognize particularly those AJC board members who reviewed the most manuscripts in 2004, and to receive criticism and suggestions from the board members on how to improve the journal. Additionally, changes to be made in the Journal beginning in July 2005 were discussed. The meeting went as follows:

1. *Introduction of new board member:* The new board member for 2004 is Dr. Attilio Maseri.
2. *AJC Board members who reviewed the most manuscripts in 2004*: These are listed in Table 1.
3. *Number of manuscripts submitted and accepted in 2004*: Of the 2,109 manuscripts submitted, 842 (39%) were accepted: 820 (39%) came from the USA and 406 (49%) were accepted; 1,289 (61%) were submitted from non-USA countries and 436 (34%) were accepted. Were not so many of initially submitted long reports converted to brief reports, these acceptance rates would be much lower.
4. *Number of manuscripts submitted in 2004 with names of potential reviewers suggested by the authors:* The Instructions to Authors in the AJC urge submitting investigators to suggest several potential, non-biased reviewers, located in cities other than those of the submitting authors, who might provide non-biased reviews of their manuscript. Of the 2,109 manuscripts submitted to the AJC in 2004, 672 (32%) authors provided names for suggested reviewers. This percent in 2003, in contrast, was only 7%; so in 2004 there was a 4 times increase in names of potential reviewers. I am always grateful to authors who provide the names of the potential reviewers of their manuscripts.
5. *Number of editorial pages published and number of manuscripts published in the regular issues of the AJC in 2004*: A total of 3,523 editorial pages (non-advertising pages) were published in the regular issues of the AJC in 2004 (Table 2). These included 3,131 pages for articles and 39 pages for Readers' Comments, and the remaining 10% of the editorial pages were for listings of the staff and editorial board, contents with abstracts, Instructions to Authors, and volume indexes. A total of 808 articles were published in the regular issues of the AJC in 2004, including 247 (31%) long reports, 516 (64%) brief reports, 16 (2%) editorials, 13 case reports (2%), 5 interviews, 4 reviews, and 7 from-the-editor columns. The brief reports, of course, allow the AJC to publish many more articles than would be possible if only long reports were published. Most of the published

TABLE 1 *The American Journal of Cardiology* Editorial Board Top Reviewers in 2004

Board Member	Number of Manuscripts
James A. de Lemos	7
George A. Diamond	7
Gregory Y.H. Lip	7
Barry Maron	7
Robert J. Siegel	7
Monty M. Bodenheimer	6
Jeffrey S. Borer	6
Bernard R. Chaitman	6
Gerald F. Fletcher	6
Julius M. Gardin	6
David R. Holmes Jr.	6
Dean J. Kereiakes	6
Morton J. Kern	6
Gerald V. Naccarelli	6
Navin C. Nanda	6
David H. Spodick	6
David J. Sahn	6

TABLE 2 Number of Editorial Pages and Articles Published in *The American Journal of Cardiology* in 2004 (Volumes 93 + 94) (Non-Symposium Issues)

Number of editorial pages—total	3523 (100%)
Articles	3131 (90%)
Readers' Comments (number)[replies]	39(42)[4]
Staff & editorial board	48 (1%)
Contents with abstracts	130 (4%)
Instructions to Authors	48 (1%)
Volume indexes	127 (4%)
Number of articles—total	808 (100%)
Long reports	247 (31%)
Brief Reports	516 (64%)
Case Reports	13 (2%)
Interviews	5 (<1%)
Reviews	4 (<1%)
Editorials	16 (2%)
From-the-Editor columns	7 (<1%)

TABLE 3 Number of Articles and Editorial Pages for Articles and Readers' Comments Published in the Regular Issues of *The American Journal of Cardiology* 1983–2004

Year	Pages for Articles	Pages for Readers' Comments	Total	Number of Articles	Numbers of Readers' Comments	Brief Reports (% of Articles)
1983	3,130	27	3,157	643	53	81 (13%)
1984	3,077	36	3,113	747	80	204 (27%)
1985	2,623	21	2,602	645	40	172 (27%)
1986	2,627	17	2,644	616	40	160 (26%)
1987	2,810	23	2,833	695	45	203 (29%)
1988	2,646	26	2,672	636	60	152 (24%)
1989	2,903	19	2,922	699	36	187 (27%)
1990	3,001	20	3,021	662	40	158 (24%)
1991	3,165	38	3,203	680	59	182 (27%)
1992	3,211	46	3,257	711	53	166 (23%)
1993	2,890	37	2,927	650	64	209 (32%)
1994	2,493	31	2,524	604	46	221 (32%)
1995	2,570	34	2,604	668	52	268 (40%)
1996	2,775	29	2,804	658	52	273 (41%)
1997	3,328	32	3,360	826	45	409 (49%)
1998	3,048	35	3,083	664	37	263 (40%)
1999	3,015	38	3,053	680	42	268 (39%)
2000	2,926	38	2,964	648	37	287 (42%)
2001	2,862	37	2,899	701	39	370 (53%)
2002	2,835	45	2,880	680	45	363 (53%)
2003	2,982	35	3,017	763	32	487 (64%)
2004	3,131	39	3,170	808	42	516 (64%)
Totals (22 Years)	64,048	703	64,709	15,084	1,039	5,599 (37%)

TABLE 4 Numbers of Manuscripts Submitted and Published and Numbers of Editorial Pages Published in the *AJC* 1983–2004

Year	Number of Manuscripts Submitted	Number of Manuscripts Published or Accepted	Percent Accepted	Number of Editorial Pages for Articles	Average Pages Per Article
1983	1,234	643	52%	3,130	4.87
1984	1,605	747	46%	3,077	4.12
1985	1,707	645	38%	2,623	4.07
1986	1,574	616	39%	2,627	4.26
1987	1,525	695	46%	2,810	4.04
1988	1,496	636	42%	2,642	4.15
1989	1,740	699	40%	2,903	4.15
1990	1,717	662	38%	3,001	4.53
1991	1,615	680	42%	3,165	4.65
1992	1,873	664	35%	3,211	4.51
1993	1,997	619	31%	2,890	4.45
1994	1,783	604	34%	2,493	4.13
1995	1,844	668	36%	2,570	3.85
1996	1,930	701	36%	2,775	3.96
1997	1,898	768	40%	3,328	4.33
1998	1,992	631	31%	2,598	4.11
1999	2,170	703	32%	2,745	3.90
2000	2,226	630	28%	2,926	4.64
2001	2,068	682	33%	2,914	4.27
2002	2,171	683	31%	2,835	4.15
2003	2,190	783	36%	2,982	3.81
2004	2,109	842	39%	3,131	3.72
Totals (22 Years)	40,464	15,001	37%	63,376	4.22

Brief Reports had been submitted originally as long reports.

6. *Number of pages for articles, Readers' Comments, and Brief Reports published in the AJC from 1983 to 2004 (during the present editor-in-chief's tenure)*: These are tabulated for each of the 22 years in Table 3.
7. *Numbers of manuscripts submitted, numbers published, percent accepted, numbers of editorial pages published and average pages per article in the AJC 1983 to 2004*: These are listed in Table 4. During the 22 years of the present editorship, over 40,000 manuscripts were submitted and just over 15,000 were accepted (37%). The number of editorial pages for articles published during that period was 63,376 and the average pages per article was 4.22. In 2004, the average article length was 3.72 pages, the shortest of any in these

TABLE 5 Interviews Published in the *AJC*

Name	Date	Name	Date
Eric Jeffrey Topol	(July 1, 1996)	Francis Robicsek	(June 1, 2000)
W. Bruce Fye	(August 1, 1996)	Richard John Bing	(July 1, 2000)
James Thronton Willerson	(February 15, 1997)	Valentin Fuster	(July 15, 2000)
Michael Ellis DeBakey	(April 1, 1997)	Henry Arthur Solomon	(July 15, 2000)
Denton Arthur Cooley	(April 15, 1997)	Myrvin Harold Ellestad	(December 1, 2000)
Joseph Stephan Alpert	(May 1, 1997)	Melvin Mayer Scheinman	(March 1, 2001)
Jesse Efrem Edwards	(April 1, 1998)	James Stuart Forrester, III	(December 1, 2001)
John Webster Kirklin	(April 15, 1998)	Carl J. Pepine	(December 15, 2001)
Howard Bertram Burchell	(May 15, 1998)	Kenneth Hardy Cooper	(February 1, 2002)
William Howard Frishman	(June 1, 1998)	Watkins Proctor Harvey	(February 15, 2002)
Robert Ogdon Bonow	(June 15, 1998)	Joseph Kayle Perloff	(March 1, 2002)
Eugene Braunwald	(July 1, 1998)	Charles Richard Conti	(March 15, 2002)
Joseph Cholmondeley Greenfield	(July 15, 1998)	William Watts Parmley	(May 1, 2002)
David Coston Sabiston, Jr.	(August 1, 1998)	Dean Michael Ornish	(August 1, 2002)
Norman Mayer Kaplan	(August 15, 1998)	Dean Towle Mason	(December 15, 2002)
Robert McKinnon Califf	(September 1, 1998)	George Allan Beller	(January 15, 2003)
Bernard John Gersh	(November 1, 1998)	Leslie David Hillis	(February 1, 2003)
Dean James Kereiakes	(November 15, 1998)	Douglas P. Zipes	(April 1, 2003)
Jeffrey Michael Isner	(January 1, 1999)	Nanette Kass Wenger	(May 15, 2003)
Scott Montgomery Grundy	(January 15, 1999)	Andrew Peter Selwyn	(June 15, 2003)
Burton Elias Sobel	(February 1, 1999)	Arthur Garson, Jr.	(August 15, 2003)
Robert Anthony O'Rourke	(April 1, 1999)	Edward David Frolich	(September 1, 2003)
David Kempton Cartwright Cooper	(April 15, 1999)	Magdi Habib Yacoub	(January 15, 2004)
Spencer Bidwell King, III	(May 1, 1999)	Robert A. Vogel	(April 1, 2004)
Robert Roberts	(May 15, 1999)	Ferid Murad	(July 1, 2004)
Eugene Auston Stead, Jr.	(September 15, 1999)	Steven Evan Nissen	(August 1, 2004)
Bertram Pitt	(October 1, 1999)	William Peter Castelli	(September 1, 2004)
Christopher John Dillon Packard	(November 15, 1999)	William Bruce Fye, III	(January 1, 2005)
Terje Rolf Pedersen	(November 15, 1999)	Anthony Nicolas DeMaria	(January 15, 2005)
		Barry L. Zaret	(May 15, 2005)

TABLE 6 Symposia in *The American Journal of Cardiology* in 2004

	Date of Publication	Subject of Symposium	Guest Editor(s)	Sponsor of Symposium	Articles	Pages	Interval (months) Symposium to Publication
A	April 22	Nutritional supplements and aminoacids in cardiovascular disease and diabetes mellitus	Mihai Gheorghiade	Professional Dietetics SRL	11	46	16
B	May 6	Carvedilol	Mihai Gheorghiade Gregg C. Fonarow	GlaxoSmithKline	17	81	—
C	June 3	Atherosclerosis, diabetes, and the metabolic syndrome	Michael H. Davidson	AstraZeneca	7	52	8
D	July 22	Adenosine stress imaging	Manuel D. Cerqueira	Fujisawa Healthcare	6	42	6
E	September 30	Abstracts: Transcatheter Cardiovascular Therapeutics	—	—	—	260	—
F	November 4	Over-the-counter statins	Thomas A. Pearson	Johnson & Johnson/Merck	7	39	—
Total					48	520	

22 years. Some of the manuscripts accepted in any particular year were not published until the following year. The interval from acceptance to publication throughout these 22 years has averaged 4 months, an interval less than that for publication of abstracts for most national and international cardiologic meetings.

8. *Interviews published in the AJC*: These are listed in Table 5. Five were published in 2004.
9. *Symposia published in the AJC in 2004*: These are listed in Table 6. No advertisements, of course, appear in the supplement issues that are published under separate cover with a different color from that of the regular issues. The guest editors of these symposia are, for the most part, major leaders in cardiovascular disease around the world.
10. *Changes to be made in the AJC beginning July 2005*: The publisher, David Dionne, introduced his staff and summarized changes to be made in the AJC beginning with the July 2005 issue:
    1) There will no longer be a separate section for brief reports. The brief reports will be placed under the general headings with the long reports, such as coronary artery disease, systemic hypertension, heart failure, etc., along with the long reports. Additionally, each re-

port, whether long or brief, will start on a separate page. This change will allow more prominent placing for the brief reports and will allow the editor to place brief reports at times before long reports in the various subheadings. The length of a manuscript does not determine its significance!

2) The AJC's cover will be changed such that some of the contents will be displayed on the cover.
3) The listings of the contents of each issue in the volume index will be eliminated.
4) The issue's contents with abstracts will be eliminated.
5) Electronic submissions and electronic reviewing of manuscripts will begin in April 2005.

The meeting was followed by a fine reception provided by the publisher.

William C. Roberts

William Clifford Roberts, MD
Editor-in-chief
Baylor Heart and Vascular Institute Baylor University Medical Center
Dallas, Texas 75246

Proceedings of the Editorial Board Meeting of *The American Journal of Cardiology* on 13 March 2006

The 2006 meeting of the Editorial Board of *The American Journal of Cardiology* (*AJC*) was held on 13 March in Atlanta, Georgia, at the time of the Annual Scientific Sessions of The American College of Cardiology. The meeting's purpose was to review the *AJC* publication results for 2005, to recognize particularly those *AJC* board members who reviewed the most manuscripts in 2005, and to receive criticisms and suggestions from the board members on how to improve the journal. The year 2005 was a big year for the *AJC*, with major format changes beginning July 1, 2005, and conversion to full electronic submission and processing of manuscripts on April 18, 2005. The meeting went as follows.

1. *Introduction of new editorial board members*: These are listed in Table 1.

2. *AJC board members who reviewed the most manuscripts in 2005*: These names are listed in Table 2.

3. *Number of manuscripts submitted and accepted for 2005*: Of the 2,661 manuscripts submitted in 2005, 984 (37%) were accepted. This percentage is higher than in some other cardiology journals, because so many of the long reports are converted into brief reports. Otherwise, the percent would be much lower. The percent accepted in 2006 will be much lower, I suspect. The number of manuscripts submitted in 2005 was 552 more than in 2004 (Table 3), a 21% increase. Additionally, the number of manuscripts submitted in the 2 months of January and February 2006 was 613 compared with 335 submitted in the same 2 months in 2005, a 45% increase. The number of manuscripts submitted and published in the *AJC* 1983 to 2005, the period of the present editorship, is shown in Table 3.

Table 1
New Board Members in 2005

Jeroen J. Bax
David L. Brown
Mun K. Hong
Robert C. Kowal
Darren K. McGuire
Richard V. Milani
Don Poldermans
Teresa S.M. Tsang
Michael Emmett

Table 2
Top AJC Board Reviewers in 2005

Name	Number Reviewed
Stephen P. Glasser	14
Eric Bates	13
Joseph A. Franciosa	13
Charles E. Rackley	13
Myrvin H. Ellestad	12
K. Lance Gould	12
Carl J. Lavie	12
Joseph Lindsay, Jr.	12
Prediman K. Shah	12
Monty M. Bodenheimer	11
George A. Diamond	11
Jack Ferlinz	11
Frank I. Marcus	11
Alan B. Miller	11
Hector O. Ventura	11
Warren G. Guntheroth	11
Marc Cohen	10
Michael E. Cain	10
Toby R. Engel	10
Gerald F. Fletcher	10
Donald C. Harrison	10
Raymond G. McKay	10
David J. Schneider	10
Ross J. Simpson, Jr.	10
Steven N. Singh	10
Eric J. Topol	10
Robert A. Vogel	10

Table 3
Numbers of manuscripts submitted and published in *AJC* from 1983 to 2005

Year	Number of Manuscripts Submitted	Number of Manuscripts Published or Accepted	Percent Accepted
1983	1,234	643	52%
1984	1,605	747	46%
1985	1,707	645	38%
1986	1,574	616	39%
1987	1,525	695	46%
1988	1,496	636	42%
1989	1,740	699	40%
1990	1,717	662	38%
1991	1,615	680	42%
1992	1,873	664	35%
1993	1,997	619	31%
1994	1,783	604	34%
1995	1,844	668	36%
1996	1,930	701	36%
1997	1,898	768	40%
1998	1,992	631	31%
1999	2,170	703	32%
2000	2,226	630	28%
2001	2,068	682	33%
2002	2,171	683	31%
2003	2,190	783	36%
2004	2,109	842	39%
2005	2,661	984	37%

4. *Sources of manuscripts submitted to the AJC in 2005*: Of the 2,661 manuscripts submitted in 2005, 1,203 (45%) came from the USA, and 541 (45%) were accepted; the remaining 1,458 (55%) manuscripts submitted in 2005 came from non-USA countries, and 443 (30%) were accepted. The countries from which the manuscripts were submitted and the percent accepted are listed in Table 4.

5. *Number of manuscripts submitted to the AJC in 2005 with names of potential reviewers suggested by the investigators:* The Instructions to Authors in the *AJC* urge submitting investigators to suggest several potentially nonbiased reviewers, located in cities other than those of the submitting investigators, who might provide nonbiased reviews of their manuscripts. Of the 2,661 manuscripts submitted to the *AJC* in 2005, 894 (34%) provided names of suggested reviewers. I would like to see this percent increase considerably. *Circulation* now provides a similar option.

Table 4
Number of manuscripts received and accepted from non-USA countries April 18 to December 31, 2005

Country	Number Submitted	Number Accepted (%)
Italy	141	29 (21%)
Japan	121	25 (21%)
Germany	82	14 (17%)
Turkey	77	9 (12%)
The Netherlands	69	33 (48%)
Taiwan	51	5 (10%)
Spain	48	7 (15%)
Greece	46	6 (13%)
Israel	43	9 (21%)
Canada	38	13 (34%)
S. Korea	33	6 (18%)
China	26	2 (8%)
Brazil	23	3 (13%)
India	23	3 (9%)
Sweden	23	5 (22%)
Australia	19	5 (26%)
Belgium	16	7 (44%)
Poland	14	2 (14%)
Austria	13	3 (23%)
Denmark	10	5 (50%)
Switzerland	10	3 (30%)
Twenty-eight other countries each <10	98	11 (11%)
Total (non-USA)	1,024	204 (20%)
Total (USA)	1,203	541 (45%)

6. *Number of editorial pages published and number of manuscripts published in the regular issues of the AJC in 2005*: A total of 3,542 editorial pages (nonadvertising pages) were published in the regular issues of the *AJC* in 2005 (Table 5). These included 3,242 pages for articles, 43 pages for Readers' Comments, and the remaining 257 pages (8%) for listings of the staff and editorial board, table of contents, instructions to authors, and volume indexes. A total of 736 articles were published in the regular issues of the *AJC* in 2005, including 259 long reports (35%), 442 brief reports (60%), 8 case reports, 4 interviews, 12 editorials, 4 reviews, 6 from-the-editor columns, and 1 editor's roundtable. The brief reports, of course, allow the *AJC* to publish many more articles than would be possible if only long reports were published. Most of the brief reports had been submitted originally as long reports.

7. *Comparison of numbers of editorial pages and numbers of articles published in Volume 95 (January to June 2005) versus Volume 96 (July to December 2005)*: The design of the *AJC* changed with the July 1, 2005, issue. Table 5 shows the numbers of editorial pages and numbers of articles in each of these 2 half years. Compared with volume 95, volume 96 had more editorial pages (1,874 vs 1,668 [11%]) but 6% less articles: the numbers of long reports increased from 104 to 155 (33% ↑), and the number of brief reports decreased from 259 to 183 (29% ↓). The contents with abstracts were eliminated beginning with the July 1 issue, and as a consequence the number of pages for tables of contents decreased from 61 to 36 (41% ↓). The

Table 5
Number of editorial pages and articles published in *The AJC* in 2005 (volumes 95 and 95) (non-symposium issues)

	Totals	Volume 95 Jan–June	Volume 96 July–Dec	Change
Number of editorial pages–total	3,542	1668	1,874	11% ↑
Articles	3,242	1,513 (91%)	1,729 (92%)	13% ↑
Readers' Comment (numbers)[replies]	43 (49) [6]	19 (23) [4]		21% ↑
Staff editorial board	48	24 (1%)	24 (26) [2]	0
Contents	97	61 (4%)	24 (1%)	41% ↓
Instructions to Authors	40	18 (1%)	36 (2%)	18% ↑
Volume indexes	72	33 (2%)	22 (1%)	15% ↑
			39 (2%)	
Number of articles–total	736	379		6% ↓
Long reports	259	104 (27%)	357	33% ↑
Brief reports	442	259 (68%)	155 (43%)	29% ↓
Case reports	8	3 (1%)	183 (51%)	
Interviews	4	3 (1%)	5 (1%)	
Editor's Roundtable	1	0	1	
Editorials	12	8 (2%)	1	
Reviews	4	0	4 (1%)	
From the Editor columns	6	2	4 (1%)	
			4 (1%)	

Table 6
Number of articles and editorial pages for articles and Readers' Comments published in the regular issues of *The AJC* 1983 to 2005

Year	Pages for Articles	Pages for Readers' Comments	Total	Number of Articles	Number of Readers' Comments	Number of Brief Reports (% of articles)
1983	3,130	27	3,157	643	53	81 (13%)
1984	3,007	36	3,113	747	80	204 (27%)
1985	2,623	21	2,602	645	40	172 (27%)
1986	2,627	17	2,644	616	40	160 (26%)
1987	2,810	23	2,833	695	45	203 (29%)
1988	2,646	26	2,672	636	60	152 (24%)
1989	2,903	19	2,922	699	36	187 (27%)
1990	3,001	20	3,021	662	40	158 (24%)
1991	3,165	38	3,203	680	59	182 (27%)
1992	3,211	46	3,257	711	53	166 (23%)
1993	2,890	37	2,927	650	64	209 (32%)
1994	2,493	31	2,524	604	46	221 (32%)
1995	2,570	34	2,604	668	52	268 (40%)
1996	2,775	29	2,804	658	52	273 (41%)
1997	3,328	32	3,360	826	45	409 (49%)
1998	3,048	35	3,083	664	37	263 (40%)
1999	3,015	38	3,053	680	42	268 (39%)
2000	2,926	38	2,964	648	37	287 (42%)
2001	2,862	37	2,899	701	39	370 (53%)
2002	2,835	45	2,880	680	45	363 (53%)
2003	2,982	35	3,017	763	32	487 (64%)
2004	3,131	39	3,170	808	42	516 (64%)
2005	3,242	43	3,285	736	49	442 (60%)
Totals (23 years)	67,290	746	67,994	15,820	1,088	6,041 (38%)

Table 7
Interviews published in *The AJC* (1996 to 2006)

Name	Date
Eric Jeffrey Topol	July 1, 1996
Wallace Bruce Fye	August 1, 1996
James Thornton Willerson	February 15, 1997
Michael Ellis DeBakey	April 1, 1997
Denton Arthur Cooley	April 15, 1997
Joseph Stephan Alpert	May 1, 1007
John Willis Hurst	February 15, 1998
Jesse Efrem Edwards	April 1, 1998
John Webster Kirklin	April 15, 1998
Howard Bertram Burchell	May 15, 1998
William Howard Frishman	June 1, 1998
Robert Ogdon Bonow	June 15, 1998
Eugene Braunwald	July 1, 1998
Joseph Cholmondeley Greenfield	July 15, 1998
David Coston Sabiston, Jr.	August 1, 1998
Norman Mayer Kaplan	August 15, 1998
Robert McKinnon Califf	September 1, 1998
Bernard John Gersh	November 1, 1998
Dean James Kereiakes	November 15, 1998
Jeffrey Michael Isner	January 1, 1999
Scott Montgomery Grundy	January 15, 1999
Burton Elias Sobel	February 1, 1999
Robert Anthony O'Rourke	April 1, 1999
David Kempton Cartwright Cooper	April 15, 1999
Spencer Bidwell King, III	May 1, 1999
Robert Roberts	May 15, 1999
Eugene Auston Stead, Jr.	September 15, 1999
Bertram Pitt	October 1, 1999
Christopher John Dillon Packard	November 15, 1999
Terje Rolf Pedersen	November 15, 1999
Francis Robicsek	June 1, 2000
Richard John Bing	July 1, 2000
Valentin Fuster	July 15, 2000
Henry Arthur Solomon	July 15, 2000
Harvey Stanley Hecht	November 1, 2000
Myrvin Harold Ellestad	December 1, 2000
Melvin Mayer Scheinman	March 1, 2001
James Stuart Forrester III	December 1, 2001
Carl John Pepine	December 15, 2001
Kenneth Hardy Cooper	February 1, 2002
Watkins Proctor Harvey	February 15, 2002
Joseph Kayle Perloff	March 1, 2002
Charles Richard Conti	March 15, 2002
William Watts Parmley	May 1, 2002
Dean Michael Ornish	August 1, 2002
Dean Towle Mason	December 15, 2002
George Allan Beller	January 15, 2003
Leslie David Hillis	February 1, 2003
Douglas P. Zipes	April 1, 2003
Nanette Kass Wenger	May 15, 2003
Andrew Peter Selwyn	June 15, 2003
Arthur Garson, Jr.	August 15, 2003
Edward David Frolich	September 1, 2003
Magdi Habib Yacoub	January 15, 2004
Robert A. Vogel	April 1, 2004
Ferid Murad	July 1, 2004
Steven Evan Nissen	August 1, 2004
William Peter Castelli	September 1, 2004
Wallace Bruce Fye, III	January 1, 2005
Anthony Nicolas DeMaria	January 15, 2005
Barry L. Zaret	May 15, 2005
Lawrence Harvey Cohn	March 15, 2006
Joseph Loscalzo	April 1, 2006
Donald Carey Harrison	May 1, 2006
Hollis Bryan Brewer	June 15, 2006

pages for volume indexes increased from 33 to 39 (15% ↑). No reviews were published in the first half of 2005 and 4 were published in the second half.

The reasons for the decrease in numbers in articles published in the second half of 2005 compared to the first half have to do with changes in the journal's format. Beginning with the July 1 issue, each article, whether a brief report or a long report or case report, etc., started on a separate page, whereas in the first half of 2005, brief reports, which constituted 68% of the manuscripts published in the first half of 2005, were placed back to back. The starting of each article on a separate page results in space lost at the end of most articles. Additionally, the numbers of lines per page decreased with the new change in appearance of the journal beginning July 1. Previously, there were a maximum of 62 lines per column (2 columns/page), the type was relatively large, and there was little space between lines. Beginning with the July 1 issue, the maximum number of lines per column dropped to 56 (10% ↓) despite smaller type, and there was more space between lines. Losing 12 lines per page in a 150-page issue theoretically adds up to a loss of 1,800 lines or 11 editorial pages. Figures and tables, of course, prevent using these calculations with assured accuracy. The publisher is now changing the format slightly to make each page more compact in an attempt to produce maximum information per page.

8. *Number of pages for articles and Readers' Comments published and number of articles, Readers' Comments, and brief reports published in the AJC from 1983 through 2005 (during the present editor in chief's tenure)*: These are tabulated for each of the 23 full years in Table 6.

9. *Interviews published in the AJC*: Table 7 lists the interviews published and the 4 scheduled for publication in 2006.

10. *Symposia published in the AJC in 2005*: A total of 13 supplements, including 105 articles, occupying 696 editorial pages plus abstracts for 2 international meetings, occupying 310 editorial pages, were published in 2005 (Table 8). The interval from the occurrence of the symposium from which the manuscripts for the supplements were obtained preceded publication of the supplement from 9 to 31 months (mean 15). Obviously, it is most desirable to have the interval between the occurrence of the symposium and publication of the supplement to be as short as possible.

11. *Number of symposia and numbers of articles and pages in symposia in the AJC from 1983 through 2005*: These are shown in Table 9. During this 23-year period, 313 symposia were published, and they included 3,419 articles occupying 21,085 pages.

12. *Major changes in the AJC in 2005*: The most striking change, of course, was the change in its format beginning July 1, 2005. The new look decreased the size of the name of the journal, which previously occupied two thirds of the journal's cover, to a reduction where it occupies no more than 25% of the journal's cover. Parts of the table of contents now are listed on the cover, and the full table of contents is listed just inside the cover. Abstracts were eliminated from the table of contents. Both the publisher and the editor have received favorable comments from readers regarding the changes. These changes were initiated after the publisher had 3 focus groups in 3 different US cities seeking opinions from 8 practicing cardiologists in each focus group.

The other major change was the initiation of online submission and processing of manuscripts beginning April 18, 2005. This innovation makes the processing of manuscripts more efficient. For editing, however, I have manuscripts that appear desirable for acceptance printed out so I can insert my editing suggestions.

13. *The impact factor and its significance*: The impact factor (IF) for the *AJC* has risen to above 3.0 (Table 10). The impact factor is a number derived by dividing the number of original research articles and reviews published in a particular journal during a specified period (2 years) into the number of citations to that journal in the year following the 2-year specified period. The IF increases when reviews are published in a journal and as a consequence, we now do publish some reviews. Articles published in the symposia issues count with those published in the regular issues, and this number adds to the denominator. The IF can be improved in any journal by 3 means: (1) by decreasing the number of articles published (the denominator), (2) by increasing the number of citations (the numerator), or (3) by a combination of 1 and 2.

The IF of the *AJC*, a journal received by over 30,000 readers, could be increased by doing the following: (1) by decreasing the number of articles (about 880/year) published in the *AJC*, a means of decreasing the denominator. (The smaller the number of articles published, the greater the probability of a higher IF.) 2) By publishing reviews, which we started doing in 2005 (The cardiovascular journals with higher IFs than the *AJC* publish reviews and some of them publish numerous ones.) (3) By increasing the number of references in articles published in the *AJC*. (This restriction will continue in the *AJC* except for reviews.) The number of references in long reports in the *AJC* is limited to 30 and in brief reports, to 20. Limiting the number of citations in articles in the *AJC*, of course, limits the number of citations to the *AJC* (as well as to other journals). Self citations are probably greater when numbers of references are not limited and no cardiovascular journals have reference limitations as strict as those in the *AJC*. (4) It is likely that brief reports are not cited as frequently as long reports and now more brief reports are published in the *AJC* than are long reports. Starting each article on a separate page, a change beginning July 1, 2005, will probably increase the references to brief reports.

Although the IF of the *AJC* is not as high as I think it should be, the number of citations to the AJC articles is third highest among the world's cardiologic journals. The *AJC* had 29,703 citations in 2004, the latest year these data are available.

14. *Consequence of the large increase in manuscripts submitted*: The sharp increase in manuscripts submitted in 2005 (552 more than in 2004) and the even greater increase in the first 2 months of 2006 compared with the first 2 months of 2005 (613 manuscripts vs 335 manuscripts, a

Table 8
Symposia in the *AJC* in 2005

Number	Date of Publication	Subject of Symposium	Guest Editor	Sponsor of Symposium	Number of Articles	Number of Pages	Interval (months) Symposium to Publication
A	April 28–30	Angioplasty Summit 2005 TCT Asia Pacific-ABSTRACTS	—	Cardiovascular Research Foundation Asia and Asian Medical Center (Seoul)	—	84	—
B	May 2	Hyponatremia in heart failure	Kenu Chatterjee	Astellas Pharma US	4	34	—
C	June 6	Immune activation and inflammation in heart failure	Craig M. Pratt Guillermo Torrc-Amione	Vasogen	6	40	31
D	July 4	Role of plant stanol esters in cholesterol management	Gilbert R. Thompson Scott M. Grundy	McNeil Nutritionals	10	54	22
E	August 22	Preventing obesity, the metabolic syndrome, and diabetes mellitus	Alan A. Brown	AstraZeneca	14	69	10
F	September 5	Time to benefit in lipid-lowering trials	Eugene Braunwald Antonio M. Gotto	Pfizer	10	75	9
G	September 19	Acute heart failure syndromes	Mihai Gheorghiade Alaxandre Mebazaa	Abbott	13	99	—
H	October 17–21	Transcatheter cardiovascular therapeutics-ABSTRACTS	—	Medtronic	—	236	—
I	October 10	Nitric oxide-enhancing therapy in heart failure	Anne L. Taylor Clyde W. Yancy	NitroMed	6	48	13
J	October 17	Noninvasive testing in preventive cardiology	Noel Bairey Merz	Astellas Pharma US	6	41	9
K	November 7	Combination therapy for dyslipidemia in the metabolic syndrome	Michael H. Davidson	Abbott Laboratories	10	70	13
L	December 19	Proceedings of IX International Meeting in Ostuni, Italy	Halo de Luca Mihai Gheorghiade Robert O. Bonow	AstraZeneca, Bayer, Guidant, Merck Sharp & Dhome, Novartis, Pfizer	11	75	14
M	December 26	Sexual dysfunction and cardiac risk	John B. Kostis Raymond C. Rosen	Pfizer, Lilly/ICOS, Bayer/Glaxo Smith Kliein, Vivus, Solvay, Sanofi-Aventis	19	91	18
13					105	1,016	Mean 15

Table 9
Number of Symposia and the number of articles and pages in symposia in *The AJC* 1983 to 2005

Year	Number of Symposia	Number of Articles	Number of Pages
1983	5	60	341
1984	9	126	567
1985	15	192	1,161
1986	13	143	823
1987	19	279	1,576
1988	19	252	1,393
1989	20	232	1,240
1990	20	226	1,169
1991	9	99	631
1992	15	165	979
1993	13	167	1076
1994	5	47	278
1995	11	156	872
1996	11	105	620
1997	17	166	1,119
1998	22	254	1,502
1999	18	172	1,133
2000	13	132	888
2001	14	108	703
2002	12	90	858
2003	14	95	620
2004	6	48	520
2005	13	105	1,016
23 years	313	3,419	21,085

45% increase) has, of course, put an added, but nevertheless, welcomed burden on the editorial office. As a consequence, the interval between acceptance of a manuscript and its publication has increased from 3.5 to 6 months in recent times. We are making every effort now to shorten that lag time to a more acceptable 4 months. To do so, more good manuscripts will have to be declined than in the past, and our acceptance rate will drop.

Table 10
Journal article cites and impact factor in 2004

Journal	Cites	Impact Factor
New England Journal of Medicine	159,498	38.57
Journal of America Medical Association	88,864	24.83
Lancet	126,002	21.71
Annals of Internal Medicine	36,932	13.11
Archives of Internal Medicine	26,525	7.51
American Journal of Medicine	21,000	4.18
Circulation	115,133	12.56
Journal of the American College of Cardiology	40,841	9.1
American Heart Journal	14,243	3.68
American Journal of Cardiology	29,703	3.14
European Heart Journal	10,890	6.25
Heart	6,023	3.27

The publisher, David Dionne, followed my presentation with additional *AJC* data. The journal's circulation remains good. On-line printouts of *AJC* articles are huge. The publisher is to be congratulated for improving the *AJC's* format and for initiating the on-line processing system for manuscripts.

We appreciate the support of readers and authors, and we will all continue to strive to produce the most clinically useful cardiologic journal possible.

Thank you all for your help.

The meeting was followed by a fine reception provided by the publisher.

William Clifford Roberts, MD
Editor in Chief
Baylor Heart and Vascular Institute
Baylor University Medical Center
Dallas, Texas 75246

Proceedings of the Editorial Board Meeting of *The American Journal of Cardiology* on 26 March 2007

The 2007 meeting of the editorial board of *The American Journal of Cardiology (AJC)*was held on 26 March 2007 in New Orleans, Louisiana, at the time of the Annual Scientific Sessions of The American College of Cardiology. The meeting's purpose was to review the AJC publication results for 2006, to recognize particularly those *AJC* board members who reviewed the most manuscripts in 2006, and to receive criticisms and suggestions from board members on how to improve the journal. The meeting went as follows:

1. *Introduction of new editorial board members:*These are listed in Table 1.
2. *AJC board members reviewing the most manuscripts in 2006:*Their names are listed in Table 2. It is not the editor's intention to send any board member 16 manuscripts to review a year. We owe Dr. Jeroen J. Bax hearty thanks, and we promise to go easy on him in 2007.
3. *Number of manuscripts submitted and accepted in 2006:* Of the 3,082 manuscripts received in 2006 (these do not include Readers' Comments submitted), 653 (21%) were accepted, 2,408 (>78%) were declined, and 21 (<1%) were withdrawn (Table 3). Probably, the 21 withdrawn would not have been accepted.

Table 1
New board members 2006

Antonio Abbatte
J. Dawn Abbott
Yuling Hong
Vincent E. Friedewald
Charles Maynard
Darren K. McGuire
Sebastian T. Palmeri
Maurice E. Sarano
Ron Waksman

Table 2
Top *AJC* board reviewers in 2006

Name	Number Reviewed
Jeroen J. Bax	16
Martin A. Alpert	11
Don Poldermans	11
George A. Diamond	10
Charles Landau	10
Gregory Y. H. Lip	10
Hector O. Ventura	10

The numbers of manuscripts submitted and published in the *AJC* 1983 to 2006, the period of the present editorship, is shown in Table 4.

There has been a considerable increase in the number of manuscripts submitted in the past 2 years. From 1992 to 2004 (12 years) the number of manuscripts submitted to the regular issues of the *AJC* (excluding those submitted to the Supplement issues) ranged from about 1,800 to 2,200 (Table 4). In 2005, the number rose to 2,661 manuscripts, a 21% increase compared with the 2109 submitted in 2004. The 3,061 manuscripts submitted in 2006 represents a 13% increase compared with the 2,661 submitted in

Table 3
Manuscripts submitted to *The AJC* in 2006

Total	3,082 (100%)
Withdrawn	21
Accepted	653 (21%)
Declined	2,408 (79%)

Table 4
Numbers of manuscripts submitted and published in *The American Journal of Cardiology* 1983–2006

Year	Number of Manuscripts Submitted	Number of Manuscripts Published or Accepted	Percent Accepted
1983	1,234	643	52%
1984	1,605	747	46%
1985	1,707	645	38%
1986	1,574	616	39%
1987	1,525	695	46%
1988	1,496	636	42%
1989	1,740	699	40%
1990	1,717	662	38%
1991	1,615	680	42%
1992	1,873	664	35%
1993	1,997	619	31%
1994	1,783	604	34%
1995	1,844	668	36%
1996	1,930	701	36%
1997	1,898	768	40%
1998	1,992	631	31%
1999	2,170	703	32%
2000	2,226	630	28%
2001	2,068	682	33%
2002	2,171	683	31%
2003	2,190	783	36%
2004	2,109	842	39%
2005	2,661	984	37%
2006	3,061	653	21%

Table 5
Number of manuscripts received and accepted from non-USA countries January 1 to December 31, 2006

Country	Number Submitted	Number Accepted (%)
Italy	236	37 (16%)
Japan	232	26 (11%)
Turkey	142	8 (6%)
The Netherlands	117	27 (23%)
Germany	116	14 (12%)
United Kingdom	90	10 (11%)
China	85	5 (6%)
Spain	85	12 (14%)
Korea	84	10 (12%)
Canada	82	16 (20%)
Greece	80	13 (16%)
Taiwan	76	7 (9%)
France	73	8 (11%)
Israel	62	13 (21%)
Brazil	46	5 (11%)
Poland	37	4 (11%)
Australia	31	5 (16%)
Switzerland	28	4 (14%)
Austria	26	1 (4%)
Finland	23	4 (17%)
Norway	21	4 (19%)
Belgium	20	5 (25%)
Sweden	20	2 (10%)
Denmark	17	6 (35%)
Iran	17	1 (6%)
Argentina	16	5 (31%)
Hungary	16	0 (0%)
India	12	0 (0%)
29 other countries with under 10 submissions	86	4 (5%)

Table 6
Number of editorial pages and articles published in *The American Journal of Cardiology* in 2006 (volumes 97 & 98) (non-Symposium issues)

	Jan 1–Dec 15 Volumes 97 & 98
Editorial pages—Total	3,602
Articles	3,406
Readers' Comments (numbers) [replies]	65 (70) [1]
Staff and editorial board	48
Contents	69
Instructions to Authors	14
Volume indexes	0
Articles—Total	695
Multipatient studies	640
Case reports	10
Reviews	16
Editorials	11
Editor's Roundtable	1
Interviews	4
From-the-Editor columns	4
Non-patient studies	9
Topics of articles	695
Coronary artery disease	313 (45%)
Preventive cardiology	69 (10%)
Arrhythmias and conduction disturbances	55 (8%)
Heart failure	60 (9%)
Valvular heart disease	32 (5%)
Cardiomyopathy	27 (4%)
Congenital heart disease	30 (4%)
Methods	16 (2%)
Miscellaneous	78 (11%)
Historical studies	3 (<1%)
Cardiovascular pharmacology	1 (<1%)
Systemic hypertension	7 (1%)
Interviews	4 (<1%)

2005. Thus, in the past 2 years (2005 and 2006), there has been a 25% increase in the numbers of manuscripts submitted compared with 2003 and 2004, when 2,190 and 2,109, respectively, were submitted. As a consequence, the numbers of manuscripts accepted in 2006, namely 21%, is a considerable drop from the percent in previous years.

The reason for the sharp increase in numbers of manuscripts submitted during the past 2 years is probably due to several factors, including: (1) a change in the journal's format, such that every manuscript starts on a separate page; (2) the move to online submission and processing of manuscripts, and; (3) the decrease in the numbers of clinically relevant manuscripts accepted in competing US cardiologic journals.

4. *Sources of manuscripts submitted to the AJC in 2006:*Of the 3,061 manuscripts submitted in 2006, 1,085 (35%) came from the USA, and 397 (37%) of them were accepted; 1,976 (65%) came from non-USA countries, and 256 (13%) were accepted. The non-USA sources of the manuscripts submitted in 2006 are listed in Table 5.
5. *Numbers of manuscripts submitted to the AJC in 2006 with names of potential reviewers suggested by the manuscript's authors*: Of the 3,061 manuscripts submitted in 2006, 1,194 (39%) provided names of potential reviewers, a much higher percentage than in previous years. Other journals, e.g., *Circulation,*also encourage this option.

The *Instructions to Authors*in the *AJC* urge submitting authors to suggest several potentially nonbiased reviewers located in cities other than those of the authors, or, in the case of non-USA countries, potential reviewers residing in countries other than their own.

6. *Number of editorial pages published, types of articles, and topics of articles published in the regular issues of the AJC in 2006:*A total of 3,602 editorial pages (non-advertising pages) were published in the regular issues of the *AJC* in 2006 (Table 6), including 3,406 pages for articles, 65 pages for Reader's Comments, and 131 pages (4%) for listings of staff and editorial board, issue contents, and Instructions to Authors. The volume indexes no longer are listed in the journal but are available online.

Of the 695 articles published in 2006, 640 (92%) were multipatient studies, 10 (1%) case reports, 16 reviews, 15

Table 7
Interviews published in *The American Journal of Cardiology*

Eric Jeffrey Topol	July 1, 1996	Harvey Stanley Hecht	November 1, 2000
Wallace Bruce Fye III	August 1, 1996	Myrvin Harold Ellestad	December 1, 2000
James Thornton Willerson	February 15, 1997	Melvin Mayer Scheinman	March 1, 2001
Michael Ellis DeBakey	April 1, 1997	James Stuart Forrester III	December 1, 2001
Denton Arthur Cooley	April 15, 1997	Carl John Pepine	December 15, 2001
Joseph Stephan Alpert	May 1, 1997	Kenneth Hardy Cooper	February 1, 2001
John Willis Hurst	February 15, 1998	Watkins Proctor Harvey	February 15, 2001
Jesse Efrem Edwards	April 1, 1998	Joseph Kayle Perloff	March 1, 2002
John Webster Kirklin	April 15, 1998	Charles Richard Conti	March 15, 2002
Howard Bertram Burchell	May 15, 1998	William Watts Parmley	May 1, 2002
William Howard Frishman	June 1, 1998	Dean Michael Ornish	August 1, 2002
Robert Ogdon Bonow	June 15, 1998	Dean Towle Mason	December 15, 2002
Eugene Braunwald	July 1, 1998	George Allan Beller	January 15, 2003
Joseph Cholmondeley Greenfield	July 15, 1998	Leslie David Hillis	February 1, 2003
David Coston Sabiston, Jr.	August 1, 1998	Douglas P. Zipes	April 1, 2003
Norman Mayer Kaplan	August 15, 1998	Nanette Kass Wenger	May 15, 2003
Robert McKinnon Califf	September 1, 1998	Andrew Peter Selwyn	June 15, 2003
Bernard John Gersh	November 1, 1998	Arthur Garson, Jr.	August 15, 2003
Dean James Kerlakes	November 15, 1998	Edward David Frolich	September 1, 2003
Jeffrey Michael Isner	January 1, 1999	Magdi Habib Yacoub	January 15, 2003
Scott Montgomery Grundy	January 15, 1999	Robert A. Vogel	April 1, 2004
Burton Elias Sobel	February 1, 1999	Ferid Murad	July 1, 2004
Robert Anothomy O'Rourke	April 1, 1999	Steven Evan Nissen	August 1, 2004
David Kempton Cartwright Cooper	April 15, 1999	William Peter Castelli	September 1, 2004
Spencer Bidwell King III	May 1, 1999	Wallace Bruce Fye III	January 1, 2005
Robert Roberts	May 15, 1999	Anthony Nicolas DeMaria	January 15, 2005
Eugene Austin Stead, Jr.	September 15, 1999	Barry L. Zaret	May 15, 2005
Bertram Pitt	October 1, 1999	Lawrence Harvey Cohn	March 15, 2006
Christopher John Dillon Packard	November 15, 1999	Joseph Loscalzo	April 1, 2006
Terje Rolf Pedersen	November 15, 1999	Donald Carey Harrison	May 1, 2006
Francis Robicsek	June 1, 2000	Hollis Bryan Brewer	June 15, 2006
Richard John Bing	July 1, 2000	Barry Joel Maron	May 1, 2007
Valentin Fuster	July 15, 2000	Lawrence Sorrell Cohen	2007
Henry Arthur Solomon	July 15, 2000		

Table 8
Number of articles and editorial pages for articles and Readers' Comments published in the Regular Issues of *The AJC* 1983 to 2006

Year	Pages for Articles	Pages for Readers' Comments	Total	Number of Articles	Number of Readers' Comments
1983	3,130	27	3,157	643	53
1984	3,007	36	3,113	747	80
1985	2,623	21	2,602	645	40
1986	2,627	17	2,644	616	40
1987	2,810	23	2,833	695	45
1988	2,646	26	2,672	636	60
1989	2,903	19	2,922	699	36
1990	3,001	20	3,021	662	40
1991	3,165	38	3,203	680	59
1992	3,211	46	3,257	711	53
1993	2,890	37	2,927	650	64
1994	2,493	31	2,524	604	46
1995	2,570	34	2,604	668	52
1996	2,775	29	2,804	658	52
1997	3,328	32	3,360	826	45
1998	3,048	35	3,083	664	37
1999	3,015	38	3,053	680	42
2000	2,962	38	2,964	648	37
2001	3,862	37	2,899	701	39
2002	2,835	45	2,880	680	45
2003	2,982	35	3,017	763	32
2004	3,131	39	3,170	808	42
2005	3,242	43	3,285	736	49
2006	3,406	65	3,471 (5% ↑)	695 (6% ↓)	70 (30% ↑)
Totals (24 years)	70,696	811	71,465	16,515	1,158

Table 9
Symposia in *The American Journal of Cardiology* in 2006

No.	Date of Publication	Topic	Sponsor	Symposium Guest Editors	Number of Articles	Number of Pages	Interval (months) Symposium to Publication
A	January 16	Dyslipidemia and inflammation	AstraZeneca	Paul M. Ridker		41	14
C	April 17	Statin safety	Abbott, AstraZeneca, Kos, Merck/Schering-Plough, Sanyko	James M. McKenney	14	97	9
D	April 26–28	Angioplasty summit 2006 TCT Asia Pacific	Cardiovascular Research Foundation, Korea	Seung-Jung Park Gary S. Mintz	0 (abstracts)	106	0
E	May 8	Nonopioid analgesia	McNeil	J. Michael Gaziano C. Michael Gibson	5	40	25
F	May 22	Heart failure after myocardial infarction and Aldosterone blockage	Pfizer, Vascular Biology Working Group	Carl J. Pepine Arthur M. Feldman	5	40	—
G	June 19	Bypass-vs-angioplasty in type 2 diabetes mellitus	NHLBI+NIDDK + 7 pharmaceutical companies	Katherine M. Detre Robert L. Frye Saul Genuth	8	65	—
H	July 17	Vulnerable plaque + patient (SHAPE)	Pfizer	Morteza Naghavi Valentin Fuster Prediman K. Shah Erling Falk	3	16	—
I	August 21	Omega-3 fatty acids	Reliant	Michael H. Davidson	9	76	—
J	September 4	Trimetazidine	Servier	William C. Stanley	6	33	12
K	September 18	Contrast-induced nephropathy	GE Healthcare	William Laskey	9	77	12
L	October 2	Carvedilol-controlled release version	GlaxoSmithKline	Domenic A. Sica	10	69	—
M	October 22–27	Transcatheter Cardiovascular Therapeutics	Abbott Vascular	Martin B. Leon Gregg W. Stone	0 (abstracts)	275	0
N	November 20	Platelet monitoring	Accumetrics	Christopher P. Cannon	7	38	—
P	December 4	Pleotrophic effects of statins	Pfizer	Peter Libby	6	41	
Q	December 18	Preventing myocardial infarction	Bristol-Myers Squibb Sarofi-Aventis	Christopher P. Cannon Deepak L. Bhatt	6	48	13
15					94 Excludes abstract issues	1062	9–25 (15) Excludes abstract issues

Table 10
Number of symposia and the number of articles and pages in symposia in *The AJC* 1983 to 2006

Year	Number of Symposia	Number of Articles	Number of Pages
1983	5	60	341
1984	9	126	567
1985	15	192	1,161
1986	13	143	823
1987	19	279	1,576
1988	19	252	1,393
1989	20	232	1,240
1990	20	226	1,169
1991	9	99	631
1992	15	165	979
1993	13	167	1,076
1994	5	47	278
1995	11	156	872
1996	11	105	620
1997	17	166	1,119
1998	22	254	1,502
1999	18	172	1,133
2000	13	132	888
2001	14	108	703
2002	12	90	858
2003	14	95	620
2004	6	48	520
2005	13	105	1,016
2006	15	94*	1,062
24 years	328	3,513	22,147

* Excludes abstracts

editorials, 4 interviews, and 9 non-patient studies. The Editor's Roundtable—discussions by experts—were initiated in 2006, and 1 was published that year. Probably 15 or so will be published in 2007. The names of the interviewees since this feature was initiated in 1996 are shown in Table 7.

The topics of the articles published in 2006 are listed in Table 6. Articles on coronary artery disease, of course, continue to dominate, numbering 313 (45%). There has been a considerable increase in articles concerning preventive cardiology, numbering 69 (10%) in 2006. Only 7 articles (1%) on systemic hypertension were published in the *AJC* in 2006, and yet about 65 million Americans have it.

7. *Number of pages for articles and Readers' Comments published and number of articles and Readers' Comments published in the AJC from 1983 through 2006 (during the present editor-in chief's tenure):* These are listed in Table 8. Although there was a 5% increase in 2006 compared to 2005 in the numbers of pages available for articles and Readers' Comments (from 3,285 → 3,471), there was a 6% decrease in numbers of articles published (736 to 695) and a 30% increase in the numbers of Readers' Comments published (49 → 70).

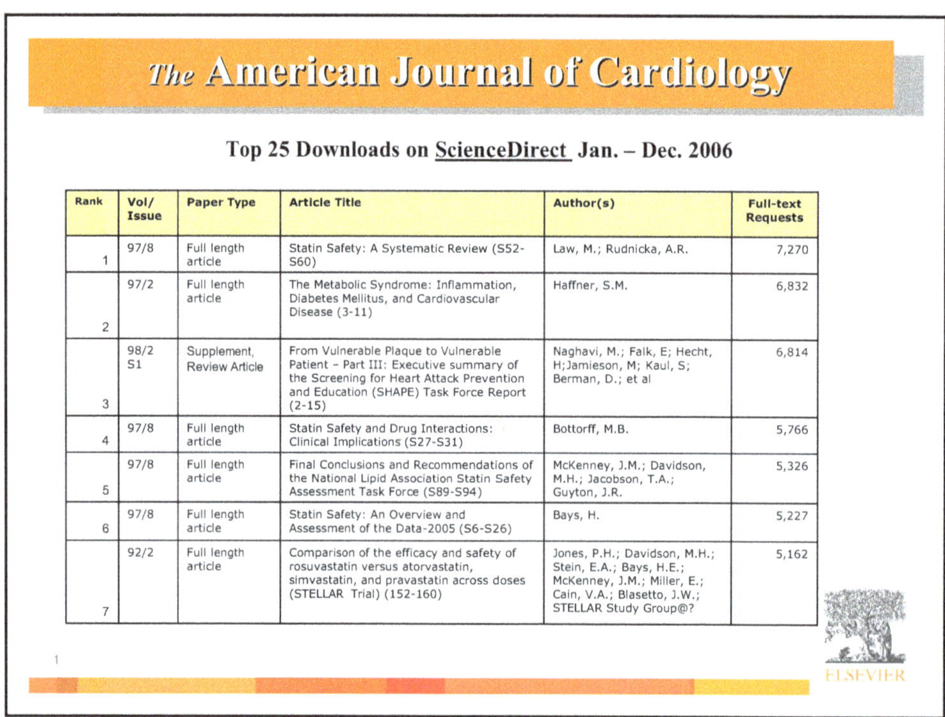

Rank	Vol/ Issue	Paper Type	Article Title	Author(s)	Full-text Requests
1	97/8	Full length article	Statin Safety: A Systematic Review (S52-S60)	Law, M.; Rudnicka, A.R.	7,270
2	97/2	Full length article	The Metabolic Syndrome: Inflammation, Diabetes Mellitus, and Cardiovascular Disease (3-11)	Haffner, S.M.	6,832
3	98/2 S1	Supplement, Review Article	From Vulnerable Plaque to Vulnerable Patient – Part III: Executive summary of the Screening for Heart Attack Prevention and Education (SHAPE) Task Force Report (2-15)	Naghavi, M.; Falk, E; Hecht, H;Jamieson, M; Kaul, S; Berman, D.; et al	6,814
4	97/8	Full length article	Statin Safety and Drug Interactions: Clinical Implications (S27-S31)	Bottorff, M.B.	5,766
5	97/8	Full length article	Final Conclusions and Recommendations of the National Lipid Association Statin Safety Assessment Task Force (S89-S94)	McKenney, J.M.; Davidson, M.H.; Jacobson, T.A.; Guyton, J.R.	5,326
6	97/8	Full length article	Statin Safety: An Overview and Assessment of the Data-2005 (S6-S26)	Bays, H.	5,227
7	92/2	Full length article	Comparison of the efficacy and safety of rosuvastatin versus atorvastatin, simvastatin, and pravastatin across doses (STELLAR Trial) (152-160)	Jones, P.H.; Davidson, M.H.; Stein, E.A.; Bays, H.E.; McKenney, J.M.; Miller, E.; Cain, V.A.; Blasetto, J.W.; STELLAR Study Group@?	5,162

Figure 1. Top 25 downloads on ScienceDirect.

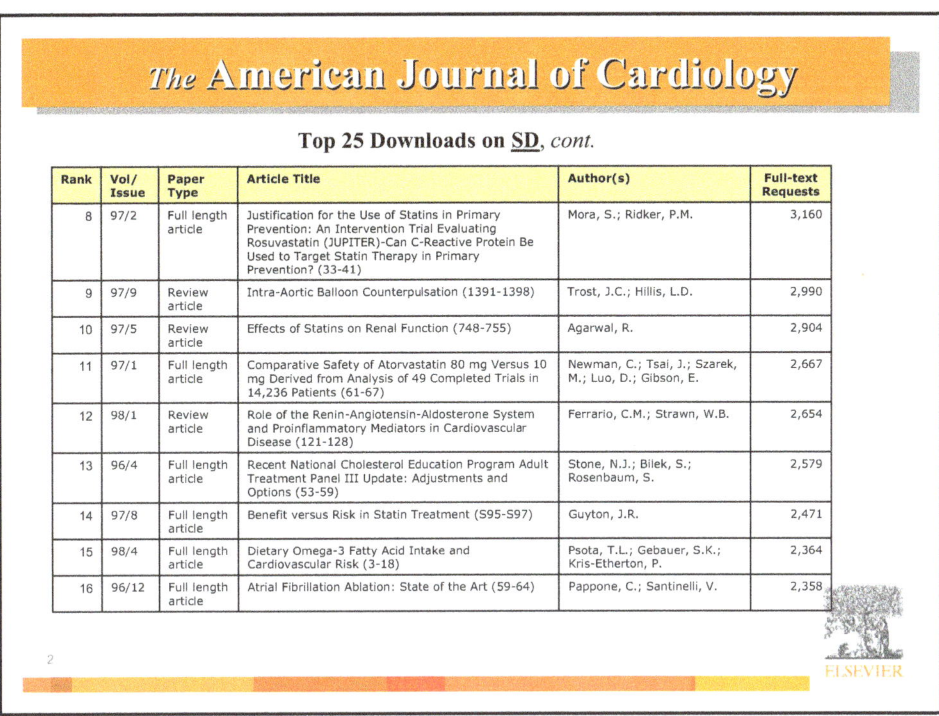

The American Journal of Cardiology

Top 25 Downloads on SD, *cont.*

Rank	Vol/ Issue	Paper Type	Article Title	Author(s)	Full-text Requests
8	97/2	Full length article	Justification for the Use of Statins in Primary Prevention: An Intervention Trial Evaluating Rosuvastatin (JUPITER)-Can C-Reactive Protein Be Used to Target Statin Therapy in Primary Prevention? (33-41)	Mora, S.; Ridker, P.M.	3,160
9	97/9	Review article	Intra-Aortic Balloon Counterpulsation (1391-1398)	Trost, J.C.; Hillis, L.D.	2,990
10	97/5	Review article	Effects of Statins on Renal Function (748-755)	Agarwal, R.	2,904
11	97/1	Full length article	Comparative Safety of Atorvastatin 80 mg Versus 10 mg Derived from Analysis of 49 Completed Trials in 14,236 Patients (61-67)	Newman, C.; Tsai, J.; Szarek, M.; Luo, D.; Gibson, E.	2,667
12	98/1	Review article	Role of the Renin-Angiotensin-Aldosterone System and Proinflammatory Mediators in Cardiovascular Disease (121-128)	Ferrario, C.M.; Strawn, W.B.	2,654
13	96/4	Full length article	Recent National Cholesterol Education Program Adult Treatment Panel III Update: Adjustments and Options (53-59)	Stone, N.J.; Bilek, S.; Rosenbaum, S.	2,579
14	97/8	Full length article	Benefit versus Risk in Statin Treatment (S95-S97)	Guyton, J.R.	2,471
15	98/4	Full length article	Dietary Omega-3 Fatty Acid Intake and Cardiovascular Risk (3-18)	Psota, T.L.; Gebauer, S.K.; Kris-Etherton, P.	2,364
16	96/12	Full length article	Atrial Fibrillation Ablation: State of the Art (59-64)	Pappone, C.; Santinelli, V.	2,358

2

ELSEVIER

Figure 2. Top 25 downloads on ScienceDirect *(continued).*

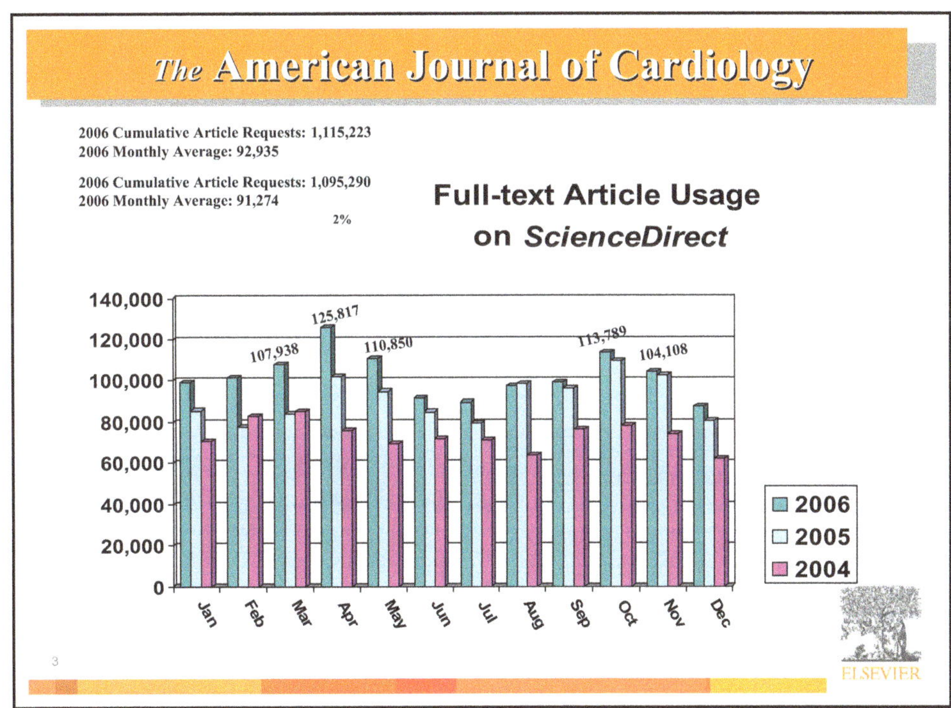

Figure 3. Full text usage on ScienceDirect.

8. *Symposia published in the AJC in 2006*: A total of 13 symposia and 2 abstract issues were published in 2006 (Table 9).
9. *Number of symposia and numbers of articles and pages in symposia in the AJC from 1983 through 2006 (during the present editor's tenure):* These are shown in Table 10. During this 24-year tenure, 328 symposia, including 3,513 articles occupying 22,147 pages have been published.

Following my comments, the publisher, David Dionne, of the *AJC* reviewed some other developments in the *AJC* in 2006. He showed a few power point slides detailing the Top 25 Article Downloads (January to December 2006) (Figures

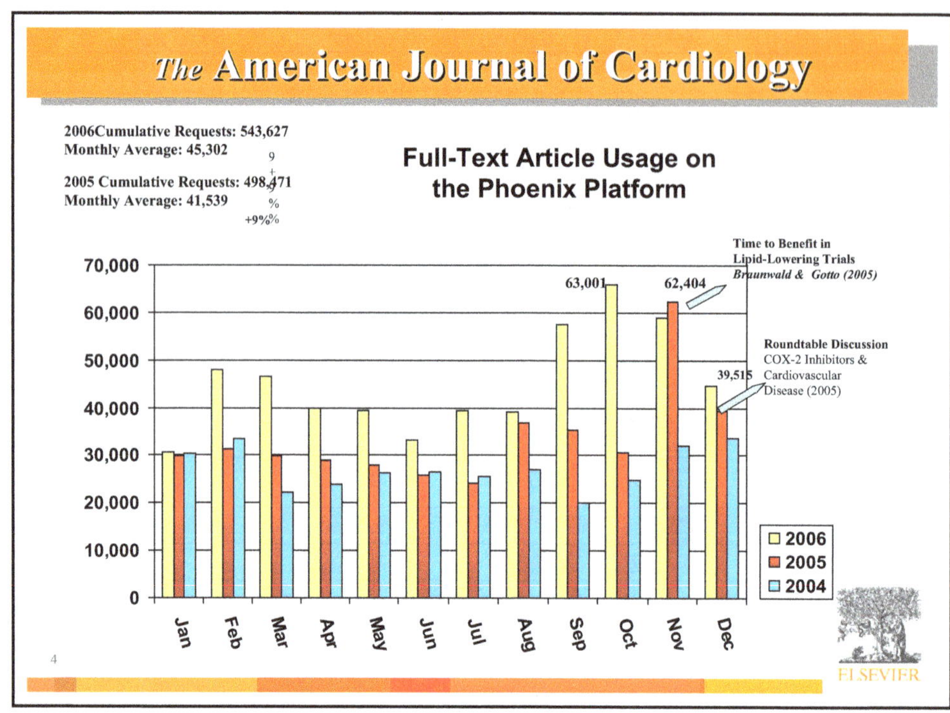

Figure 4. Full text usage on the Phoenix Platform.

The American Journal of Cardiology
Congratulations Bill !
25 Years as Editor-in-Chief
The
American Journal
of Cardiology
ELSEVIER

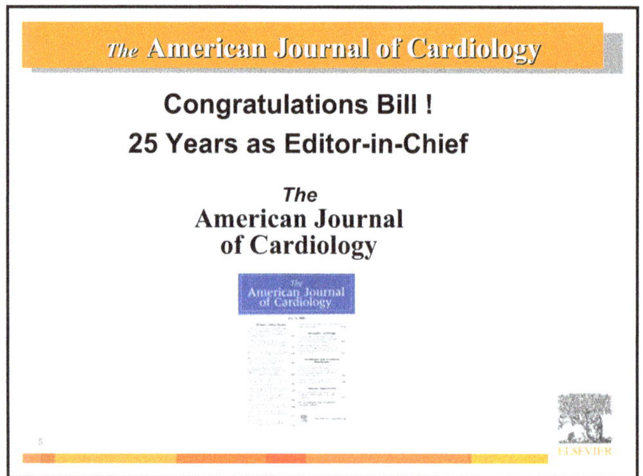

Figure 5. Congratulations for 25 years as Editor in Chief.

1 and 2) by individuals at institutions that have license agreements with ScienceDirect. Sixty-eight percent of the 25 articles focused on statins (risks and benefits), safety recommendations and large population statin studies, comparisons of various statin drugs, and cholesterol-lowering and lipid-lowering guidelines.

In addition, David showed the group 2 slides pertaining to full-text article usage during that same period on Science Direct and on the journal's Phoenix Platform, a platform where individual print subscribers access the full-text of the journal at www.AJConline.org. The slides showed that "usage" activity on both Platforms was considerable with a 2% increase in cumulative article requests (1,095,290 in 2005 to 1,115, 223 in 2006) on ScienceDirect (Figure 3) and a 9% increase in activity on the Phoenix Platform (Figure 4) from 498,471 article requests in 2005 to 543,627 requests in 2006.

David also detailed for the editorial board members some of the new features of the print journal as well as some enhancements to the full-text website. A new, irregular section with free CME was added to the journal by Dr. Vince Friedewald, now an Assistant Editor of the *AJC*, and me toward the end of 2006, entitled, *The Editor's Roundtable Discussion*. In this section, the *AJC* gathers together a group of experts, who discuss and debate a specific relevant clinical topic in cardiovascular disease, transcribes the meeting, and finally prints the Roundtable Discussion with references in the AJC. David pointed out at the meeting that a "navigational button" had been created at the journal's full-text website to collect all the Roundtable Discussions in one place and conveniently offer them to subscribers with free CME online. Six Roundtable Discussions have already appeared in the *AJC* with an additional 12 to 14 scheduled during the next 10 months.

I have interviewed close to 70 well-known cardiologists and cardiovascular surgeons since 1996 and have had them printed in the *AJC* as a permanent archival record. The Publisher has created an "Interviews Collection" button at the website with all 70 interviews collected there; it is a very convenient location to keep these valuable interviews.

The Articles in Press navigational button on the full-text web site has been posting articles for >2 years now—the articles are posted more than 4 to 6 weeks before the print version appears. The *AJC* has been receiving more and more video clips from authors on submission of their manuscripts to the editorial office. Because of the growing number of

The American Journal of Cardiology
Presented To
William C. Roberts, MD
In Recognition and Appreciation of Your Outstanding Service for
25 Years as Editor in Chief
The American Journal of Cardiology
From David, Dori, Judy, Greg, Donna, the Editorial Board and Your Friends at Elsevier
ELSEVIER

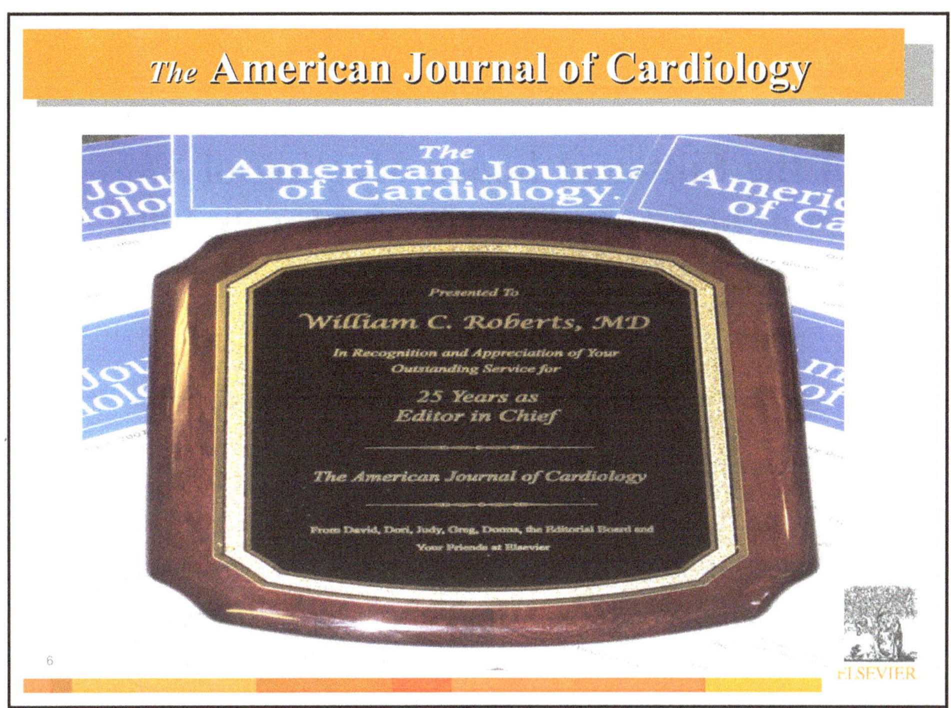

Figure 6. The plaque received from David Dionne and Elsevier.

video clips, 3-dimensional images, and animations, the *AJC* has been receiving with manuscripts during the past 10 months, the Publisher has created a "Multimedia Library Collection." All accepted manuscripts with multimedia components will not only appear embedded online with the article, but will also be extracted and posted with other multimedia in the site's Multimedia Library Collection.

Much to my surprise, David and his colleagues at Elsevier presented me with a plaque acknowledging their appreciation of my directing the AJC as Editor in Chief for the past 25 years (Figures 5 and 6). Dori Birch, the Sr. Journal Manager, who has been with the *AJC* for the past 11 years, presented me with an engraved, Tiffany's sterling silver pen. I am most grateful for the wonderful surprise and our subsequent reception following the editorial board meeting.

William Clifford Roberts, MD
Editor in Chief
Baylor Heart and Vascular Institute
Baylor University Medical Center
Dallas, Texas 75246

Proceedings of the Editorial Board Meeting of *The American Journal of Cardiology* on 30 March 2008

The 2008 meeting of the Editorial Board of *The American Journal of Cardiology* (*AJC*) was held on March 30 in Chicago, Illinois, at the time of the Annual Scientific Sessions of the American College of Cardiology. The meeting's purpose was to review the *AJC*'s publication results for 2007, to recognize particularly those *AJC* members who reviewed the most manuscripts in 2007, and to receive criticisms and suggestions from the board members on how to improve the journal. The meeting went as follows.

1. *Introduction of new board members* (Table 1).
2. AJC *board members who reviewed the most manuscripts in 2007* (Table 2).
3. *Number of manuscripts submitted and accepted for 2007* (Table 3). Of the 3,208 manuscripts submitted in 2007, 24 were eventually withdrawn, leaving 3,184, of which 710 (22%) were accepted and 2,474 (78%) were declined. Of these 3,184 manuscripts, 2,125 were received from countries other than the United States, of which 322 (15%) were accepted; of the 1,059 manuscripts received from the United States, 388 (37%) were accepted. During 2007, manuscripts were received from 53 different countries. The countries submitting the most manuscripts were Italy (42), Japan (36), The Netherlands (33), Australia (16), the United Kingdom (15), and Israel (13).
4. *Number of manuscripts submitted and published or accepted from 1983 through 2007,* during the 25 years of the present editorship (Table 4). The acceptance rate has decreased considerably during the past 2 years, mainly because of a marked increase in the number of manuscripts submitted without a major increase in the number of editorial pages available.
5. *Number of editorial pages published, number of manuscripts published, and topics of manuscripts published in the regular issues of the AJC in 2007* (Table 5). A total of 3,715 editorial pages (non-revenue-producing pages) were published in 2007: 3,540 (95%) were used for articles, and another 50 (1%) were used for readers' comments. A total of 695 articles were published in the AJC in 2007. Of the 695 articles published during 2007, 321 (46%) concerned coronary artery disease, and 80 (12%) concerned preventive cardiology.
6. *Number of articles and editorial pages for articles and readers' comments published in the regular issues of the AJC from 1983 to 2007* (Table 6). A total of 77,951 pages for articles were published during the 25 years of the present editorship, and 861 pages were used for readers' comments. A total of 17,210 articles and 1,217 readers' comments were published during this 25-year period.
7. *Interviews published in the* AJC (Table 7).
8. *Symposia published in the* AJC *in 2007* (Table 8). A total of 15 supplements, including 101 articles occupying 1,149 editorial pages, plus abstracts from 2 international meetings occupying 361 editorial pages, were published in the *AJC* in 2007. The occurrence of the symposia from which the manuscripts for the supplements were obtained preceded publication of the supplements by 12 to 42 months (mean 20) for the 7 supplements for which this information was available. Obviously, it is most desirable to have a short interval between the occurrence of a symposium and its publication.
9. *Number of symposia and number of articles and pages in symposia in the* AJC *from 1983 to 2007,* during the 25 years of the present editorship (Table 9). Three hundred forty-three symposia were published, including 3,614 articles occupying 23,296 editorial pages.
10. *Changes expected to affect the* AJC *in 2008.* Dr. Clyde W. Yancy has been selected to be the Overview Editor for the symposia to be published in 2008 and thereafter. Up to this point, the guest editors of the symposia have been in charge of reviewing the manuscripts submitted. Some of them have swapped manuscripts around among symposia members to review one another's manuscripts. An occasional symposium through the years has been reviewed by an outside editor selected by either the guest editor of the symposium or the editor of the *AJC*. Dr. Yancy will work in conjunction with the guest editor to make sure that the articles appearing in the symposia are of high quality.
11. *New managing editor in New York.* John Porter is his name, and the journal is in good hands with him.

In summary, 2007 was a good year for the *AJC*. The number of manuscripts submitted was >3,000, and the percentage accepted was near 20%. The roundtables appear to be popular, as do the interviews, particularly for those individuals being interviewed. Subscriptions are staying up.

We appreciate, of course, the readers and authors, and we will continue to strive to produce a most useful clinical cardiologic journal. I thank the Editorial Board members for their good help through the year.

The meeting was followed by a fine reception provided by the publisher, Mr. David Dionne, with who I have a fine working relationship.

Table 1
New Editorial Board members, 2007

George S. Abela
Pablo Avanzas
Martin S. Maron
Bernhard Meier
Wayne L. Miller
Seung-Jung Park
Jeffrey M. Schussler
Patrick W. Serruys

Table 2
Top *American Journal of Cardiology* Editorial Board reviewers, 2007

Name	No. of Manuscripts Reviewed
Monty M. Bodenheimer	11
Antonio Abbate	10
Eric Bates	10
James A. de Lemos	10
Joseph Lindsay, Jr.	10
David Waters	10

Table 3
Sources of manuscripts submitted to *The American Journal of Cardiology*, 2007

Source	Submitted	Accepted
Non–United States	2,125	322 (15%)
United States	1,059	388 (37%)
Total	3,184	710 (22%)

Table 4
Numbers of manuscripts submitted to and published in *The American Journal of Cardiology*, 1983 to 2007

Year	No. of Manuscripts Submitted	No. of Manuscripts Published or Accepted	Percentage Accepted
1983	1,234	643	52%
1984	1,605	747	46%
1985	1,707	645	38%
1986	1,574	616	39%
1987	1,525	695	46%
1988	1,496	636	42%
1989	1,740	699	40%
1990	1,717	662	38%
1991	1,615	680	42%
1992	1,873	664	35%
1993	1,997	619	31%
1994	1,783	604	34%
1995	1,844	668	36%
1996	1,930	701	36%
1997	1,898	768	40%
1998	1,992	631	31%
1999	2,170	703	32%
2000	2,226	630	28%
2001	2,068	682	33%
2002	2,171	683	31%
2003	2,190	783	36%
2004	2,109	842	39%
2005	2,661	984	37%
2006	3,061	653	21%
2007	3,184	710	22%

Table 5
Number of editorial pages and articles published in *The American Journal of Cardiology*, 2007 (Volumes 99 and 100, nonsymposium issues)

Category	January 1 to December 15 (Volumes 99 and 100)
Total editorial pages	3,715
Articles	3,540 (95%)
Readers' comments (no. of comments [no. of replies])	50 (59 [5]) (1%)
Staff and editorial board	48 (1%)
Tables of contents	69 (2%)
Instructions to authors	8 (0.2%)
Volume indexes	0 (0)
No. of articles	695
Multipatient studies	617 (89%)
Case reports	19 (3%)
Reviews	12 (2%)
Editorials	26 (4%)
Editor's Roundtables	15 (2%)
Interviews	2 (<1%)
Nonpatient studies	2 (<1%)
From the Editor columns	2 (<1%)
Topics of articles	695
Coronary artery disease	321 (46%)
Preventive cardiology	80 (12%)
Arrhythmias and conduction disturbances	35 (5%)
Systemic hypertension	10 (1%)
Heart failure	61 (9%)
Valvular heart disease	24 (3%)
Cardiomyopathy	30 (4%)
Congenital heart disease	29 (4%)
Miscellaneous	81 (12%)
Methods	16 (2%)
Cardiovascular pharmacology	3 (0.4%)
Historical studies	3 (0.4%)
Interviews	2 (0.3%)

Table 6
Number of articles and editorial pages for articles and readers' comments published in the regular issues of *The American Journal of Cardiology*, 1983 to 2007

Year	Pages for Articles	Pages for Readers' Comments	Total	Number of Articles	Number of Readers' Comments
1983	3,130	27	3,157	643	53
1984	3,007	36	3,113	747	80
1985	2,623	21	2,602	645	40
1986	2,627	17	2,644	616	40
1987	2,810	23	2,833	695	45
1988	2,646	26	2,672	636	60
1989	2,903	19	2,922	699	36
1990	3,001	20	3,021	662	40
1991	3,165	38	3,203	680	59
1992	3,211	46	3,257	711	53
1993	2,890	37	2,927	650	64
1994	2,493	31	2,524	604	46
1995	2,570	34	2,604	668	52
1996	2,775	29	2,804	658	52
1997	3,328	32	3,360	826	45
1998	3,048	35	3,083	664	37
1999	3,015	38	3,053	680	42
2000	2,962	38	2,964	648	37
2001	3,862	37	2,899	701	39
2002	2,835	45	2,880	680	45
2003	2,982	35	3,017	763	32
2004	3,131	39	3,170	808	42
2005	3,242	43	3,285	736	49
2006	3,406	65	3,471	695	70
2007	3,540	50	3,590	695	59
Total (25 years)	77,951	861	75,055	17,210	1,217

Table 7
Interviews published in *The American Journal of Cardiology*

Interviewee	Date	Interviewee	Date
Eric Jeffrey Topol	July 1, 1996	Harvey Stanley Hecht	November 1, 2000
Wallace Bruce	August 1, 1996	Myrvin Harold Ellestad	December 1, 2000
James Thornton Willerson	February 15, 1997	Melvin Mayer Scheinman	March 1, 2001
Michael Ellis DeBakey	April 1, 1997	James Stuart Forrester, III	December 1, 2001
Denton Arthur Cooley	April 15, 1997	Carl John Pepine	December 15, 2001
Joseph Stephan Alpert	May 1, 1997	Kenneth Hardy Cooper	February 1, 2001
John Willis Hurst	February 15, 1998	Watkins Proctor Harvey	February 15, 2001
Jesse Efrem Edwards	April 1, 1998	Joseph Kayle Perloff	March 1, 2002
John Webster Kirklin	April 15, 1998	Charles Richard Conti	March 15, 2002
Howard Bertram Burchell	May 15, 1998	William Watts Parmley	May 1, 2002
William Howard Frishman	June 1, 1998	Dean Michael Ornish	August 1, 2002
Robert Ogdon Bonow	June 15, 1998	Dean Towle Mason	December 15, 2002
Eugene Braunwald	July 1, 1998	George Allan Beller	January 15, 2003
Joseph Cholmondeley Greenfield	July 15, 1998	Leslie David Hillis	February 1, 2003
David Coston Sabiston, Jr.	August 1, 1998	Douglas P. Zipes	April 1, 2003
Norman Mayer Kaplan	August 15, 1998	Nanette Kass Wenger	May 15, 2003
Robert McKinnon Califf	September 1, 1998	Andrew Peter Selwyn	June 15, 2003
Bernard John Gersh	November 1, 1998	Arthur Garson, Jr.	August 15, 2003
Dean James Keriakes	November 15, 1998	Edward David Frolich	September 1, 2003
Jeffrey Michael Isner	January 1, 1999	Magdi Habib Yacoub	January 15, 2003
Scott Montgomery Grundy	January 15, 1999	Robert A. Vogel	April 1, 2004
Burton Elias Sobel	February 1, 1999	Ferid Murad	July 1, 2004
Robert Anthony O'Rourke	April 1, 1999	Steven Evan Nissen	August 1, 2004
David Kempton Cartwright Cooper	April 15, 1999	William Peter Castelli	September 1, 2004
Spencer Bidwell King, III	May 1, 1999	Wallace Bruce Fye, III	January 1, 2005
Robert Roberts	May 15, 1999	Anthony Nicolas DeMaria	January 15, 2005
Eugene Austin Stead, Jr.	September 15, 1999	Barry L. Zaret	May 15, 2005
Bertram Pitt	October 1, 1999	Lawrence Harvey Cohn	March 15, 2006
Christopher John Dillon Packard	November 15, 1999	Joseph Loscalzo	April 1, 2006
Terje Rolf Pedersen	November 15, 1999	Donald Carey Harrison	May 1, 2006
Francis Robicsek	June 1, 2000	Hollis Bryan Brewer	June 15, 2006
Richard John Bing	July 1, 2000	Barry Joel Maron	May 1, 2007
Valentin Fuster	July 15, 2000	Robert William (Bobby) Brown	March 1, 2008
Henry Arthur Solomon	July 15, 2000	Lawrence Cohen	March 15, 2008

Table 8
Symposia published in *The American Journal of Cardiology*, 2007

No.	Date of Publication	Topic	Sponsor	Symposium Guest Editors	No. of Articles	No. of Pages	Interval (mo) from Symposium to Publication
A	January 22	Istaroxime for heart failure	Sigma-Tau Pharmaceuticals	Mihai Gheorghiade, Hani N. Sabbah	6	56	—
B	February 19	Glucose control in diabetes mellitus	Abbott Laboratories, AstraZeneca, Sanofi-Aventis, Takeda Pharmaceuticals	Michael H. Davidson	14	140	—
C	March 19	Safety of fibrates, niacin, omega-3 fatty acids, ezetimibe, cholestyramine, colestipol, colesevelam	Abbott Laboratories, AstraZeneca, Kos Pharmaceuticals, Merck/ Schering-Plough, Daiichi Sankyo	James M. McKenney	9	58	13
D	March 26	Heart failure	Nitromed	Elizabeth Ofili	7	37	32
E	March 27	Drugs for secondary prevention	Sanofi-Aventis	Gerald F. Fletcher	1	35	—
F	April 25–27	Abstracts, Angioplasty Summit–TCT Asia Pacific	Cardiovascular Research Foundation, Korea	—	—	103	—
G	May 21	OptiVol fluid status monitoring in heart failure	Medtronic	W.H. Wilson Tang	8	44	13
H	June 4	Controlling hyperglycemia	Sanofi-Aventis	Christopher P. Cannon	3	18	15
I	June 18	Controlling cardiovascular risk in diabetes mellitus	National Heart, Lung, and Blood Institute; National Institute of Diabetes and Digestive and Kidney Diseases; National Eye Institute; National Institute of Aging; Centers for Disease Control and Prevention	Robert P. Byington, Saul Genuth, William T. Friedewald, Denise G. Simons-Morton	11	122	—
J	August 6	Antihypertensive therapy	Boehringer Ingelheim	Toshiro Fujita, Giuseppe Mancia	9	60	15
K	September 3	Coronary restenosis prevention	Otsuka America Pharmaceutical	John S. Douglas, Jr., Spencer B. King, III	5	31	42
L	October 20–25	Abstracts, 19th TCT Symposium, Washington, District of Columbia	Abbott Vascular	Cardiovascular Research Foundation, Columbia University Medical Center	—	258	—
M	October 22	Drug-eluting stents	Medtronic Vascular	Ron Waksman	11	83	—
N	December 3	High-density lipoprotein therapy	Pfizer	Michael H. Davidson, Peter P. Toth	11	67	12
P	December 17	Endocannabinoid system	Sanofi-Aventis	Carl J. Pepine, Jorge Plutzky	6	37	—
15					101	1,149	Mean 20

TCT = Transcatheter Cardiovascular Therapeutics.

Table 9
Number of symposia and number of articles and pages in symposia in *The American Journal of Cardiology*, 1983 to 2007

Year	No. of Symposia	No. of Articles	No. of Pages
1983	5	60	341
1984	9	126	567
1985	15	192	1,161
1986	13	143	823
1987	19	279	1,576
1988	19	252	1,393
1989	20	232	1,240
1990	20	226	1,169
1991	9	99	631
1992	15	165	979
1993	13	167	1,076
1994	5	47	278
1995	11	156	872
1996	11	105	620
1997	17	166	1,119
1998	22	254	1,502
1999	18	172	1,133
2000	13	132	888
2001	14	108	703
2002	12	90	858
2003	14	95	620
2004	6	48	520
2005	13	105	1,016
2006	15	94*	1,062
2007	15	101*	1,149
Total (25 years)	343	3,614	23,296

* Excludes abstracts.

William C. Roberts, MD
Editor in Chief
Baylor Heart and Vascular Institute
Baylor University Medical Center
Dallas, Texas

From the Publisher

Remarks by the publisher at the Editorial Board Meeting of 2008

The editor's presentation was followed by a presentation by the publisher, Mr. David Dionne:

1. *Top downloads on Science Direct of* The American Journal of Cardiology, *January–December 2007* (Figure 1); 2. *Top 10 ELS medical journal downloads in 2007 from Science Direct* (Figure 2); 3. *New features @ AJConline.org in 2007–2008:* Articles in Press–S200s are forwarded to MEDLINE; The Editor's Roundtable (14 published to date–6 in 2008 with free CME); "Interviews" Collection; Indexes ONLINE only; Multimedia Component Library, and FOCUS-Interactive Gateway; 4. *E-article requests stats: Science Direct and Phoenix platforms* (Figures 3 and 4); 5. *Circulation: Demographics and distribution* (Figures 5 and 6); 6. *Article sources:* (Figures 7 and 8).

Top 25 Downloads on ScienceDirect Jan. – Dec. 2007

Rank	Vol/ Iss	Cover Date	Article Title	Author(s)	Full-text Requests
1	99/4	01-Feb-2007	Inflammation in Diabetes Mellitus: Role of Peroxisome Proliferator-Activated Receptor-@a and Peroxisome Proliferator-Activated Receptor-@c Agonists (27-40)	Libby, P.; Plutzky, J.	3,356
2	99/1	01-Jan-2007	Risk of Cardiovascular Events in Patients Receiving Celecoxib: A Meta-Analysis of Randomized Clinical Trials (91-98)	White, W.B.; West, C.R.; Borer, J.S.; Gorelick, P.B.; Lavange, et al.	3,060
3	98/12	01-Dec-2006	Atherosclerosis: Disease Biology Affecting the Coronary Vasculature (S3-S9)	Libby, P.	3,031
4	99/5	01-Mar-2007	Efficacy and Safety of Rosuvastatin 40 mg Alone or in Combination With Ezetimibe in Patients at High Risk of Cardiovascular Disease (Results from the EXPLORER Study) (673-680)	EXPLORER Study Investigators; Ballantyne, C.M.; Weiss, R.; Moccetti, T.; Vogt, et al.	2,875
5	92/2	01-Jul-2003	Comparison of the efficacy and safety of rosuvastatin versus atorvastatin, simvastatin, and pravastatin across doses (STELLAR Trial) 152-160)	Jones, P.H.; Davidson, M.H.; Stein, E.A.; Bays, H.E.; McKenney, J.M.; et al.	2,778
6	99/2	01-Jan-2007	Review of Current and Investigational Pharmacologic Agents for Acute Heart Failure Syndromes (S4-S23)	Shin, D.D.; Brandimarte, F.; De Luca, L.; Sabbah, H.N.; Fonarow, G.C.; et al.	2,774
7	97/8	01-Apr-2006	Statin Safety: A Systematic Review (S52-S60)	Law, M.; Rudnicka, A.R.	2,529
8	98/12	01-Dec-2006	Evolving Management of ST-Segment Elevation Myocardial Infarction: Update on Recent Data (S10-S21)	Cannon, C.P.	2,468
9	98/4	01-Aug-2006	Dietary Omega-3 Fatty Acid Intake and Cardiovascular Risk (3-18)	Psota, T.L.; Gebauer, S.K.; Kris-Etherton, P.	2,229
10	99/5	01-Mar-2007	The Inflammation Hypothesis and Its Potential Relevance to Statin Therapy (732-738)	Forrester, J.S.; Libby, P.	2,223
11	98/2 S1	7/17/2006	Screening For Heart Attack Prevention and Education (SHAPE) Task Force Report: Executive Summary (2-16)	Morteza Naghavi	2,204
12	99/4	01-Feb-2007	Weight Management for Type 2 Diabetes Mellitus: Global Cardiovascular Risk Reduction (68-79)	Lee, M.; Aronne, L.J.	2,177
13	99/5	01-Mar-2007	Comparison of the Effects of High Doses of Rosuvastatin Versus Atorvastatin on the Subpopulations of High-Density Lipoproteins (681-685)	Asztalos, B.F.; Le Maulf, F.; Dallal, G.E.; Stein, E.; Jones, P.H.; et al.	2,092
14	99/6	01-Mar-2007	Acute Decompensated Heart Failure: Pathophysiology and Treatment (S25-S30)	Onwuanyi, A.; Taylor, M.	2,090
15	99/4	01-Feb-2007	Role of Insulin Resistance and Hyperglycemia in the Development of Atherosclerosis (6-14)	Bansilal, S.; Farkouh, M.E.; Fuster, V.	2,085
16	99/12	01-Jun-2007	Comparison of Effects of Ezetimibe/Simvastatin Versus Simvastatin Versus Atorvastatin in Reducing C-Reactive Protein and Low-Density Lipoprotein Cholesterol Levels (1706-1713.e1)	Pearson, T.; Ballantyne, C.; Sisk, C.; Shah, A.; Veltri, E.; Maccubbin, D.	2,073
17	99/2	01-Jan-2007	The Evolving Pattern of Symptomatic Coronary Artery Disease in the United States and Canada: Baseline Characteristics of the Clinical Outcomes Utilizing Revascularization and Aggressive DruG Evaluation (COURAGE) Trial (208-212)	COURAGE Trial Co-Principal Investigators and Study Coordinators; Boden, W.E.; O'Rourke, R.A.; Teo, K.K.; Hartigan, P.M.; Maron, D.J.; et al.	2,000

Figure 1. Top 25 downloads on ScienceDirect, Jan.–Dec. 2007.

18	99/10	01-May-2007	Effect of Coenzyme Q10 on Myopathic Symptoms in Patients Treated With Statins (1409-1412)	Caso, G.; Kelly, P.; McNurlan, M.A.; Lawson, W.E.	1,915
19	98/11	01-Dec-2006	Oxidative Biomarkers in the Diagnosis and Prognosis of Cardiovascular Disease (S9-S17)	Tsimikas, S.	1,844
20	98/11	01-Dec-2006	Emerging Strategies for Increasing High-Density Lipoprotein (1542-1549)	Forrester, J.S.; Shah, P.K.	1,839
21	100/3	01-Aug-2007	Angiotensin Receptor Blockers versus Angiotensin-Converting Enzyme Inhibitors: Where Do We Stand Now? (s38-S44)	Bohm, M.	1,695
22	98/10	01-Nov-2006	Current Options in Platelet Function Testing (S4-S10)	Michelson, A.D.; Frelinger, A.L.; Furman, M.I.	1,621
23	97/8	01-Apr-2006	Statin Safety and Drug Interactions: Clinical Implications (S27-S31)	Bottorff, M.B.	1,602
24	99/6	01-Mar-2007	Safety Considerations with Fibrate Therapy (S3-S18)	Davidson, M.H.; Armani, A.; McKenney, J.M.; Jacobson, T.A.	1,573
25	99/6	01-Mar-2007	Efficacy of Drug Therapy in the Secondary Prevention of Cardiovascular Disease and Stroke (S1-S35)	Fletcher, G.F.; Bufalino, V.; Costa, F.; Goldstein, L.B.; Jones, D.; et al.	1,571

Figure 1. *(continued).*

Science Direct in 2007

Top 10 Medical Journal Downloads

(Only Elsevier Medical Journals)

Journal	Total	Articles Online
Journal of the American College of Cardiology	**1,803,507**	**28,263**
Biological Psychiatry	**1,221,296**	**13,601**
The American Journal of Cardiology	**1,155,974**	**33,590**
Journal of Allergy and Clinical Immunology	**977,296**	**26,371**
International Journal of Radiation Oncology*Biology*Physics	**939,509**	**19,001**
American Journal of Obstetrics and Gynecology	**919,262**	**15,231**
Gastroenterology	**842,825**	**28,423**
Annals of Thoracic Surgery, The	**817,231**	**16,279**
American Journal of Medicine, The	**783,967**	**25,392**
Fertility and Sterility	**765,324**	**17,719**

Figure 2. Top 10 ELS medical journal downloads in 2007 from ScienceDirect.

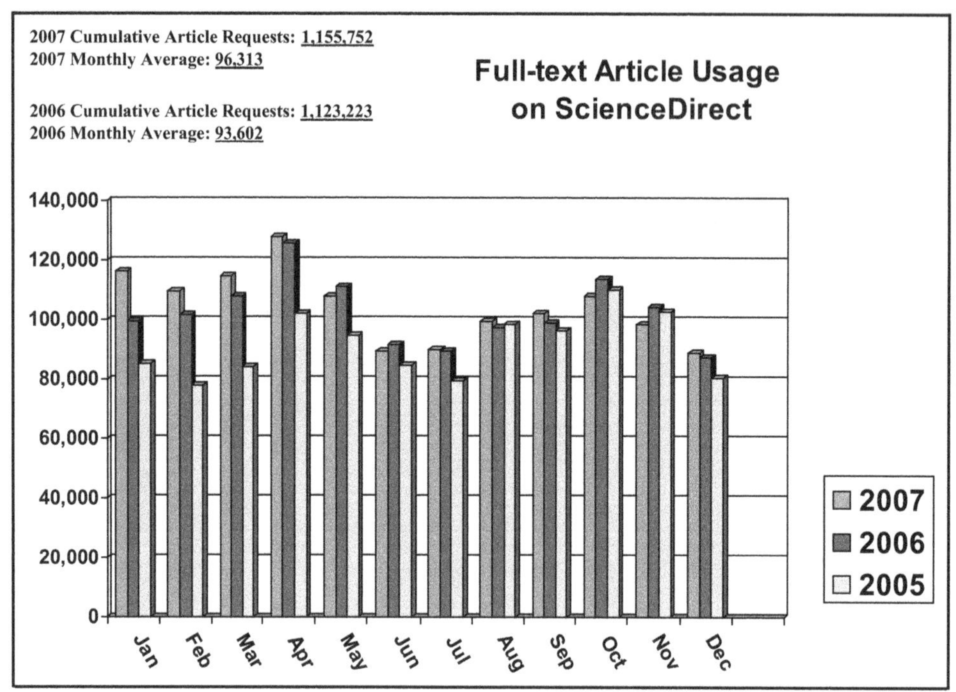

Figure 3. E-article requests stats: ScienceDirect platform.

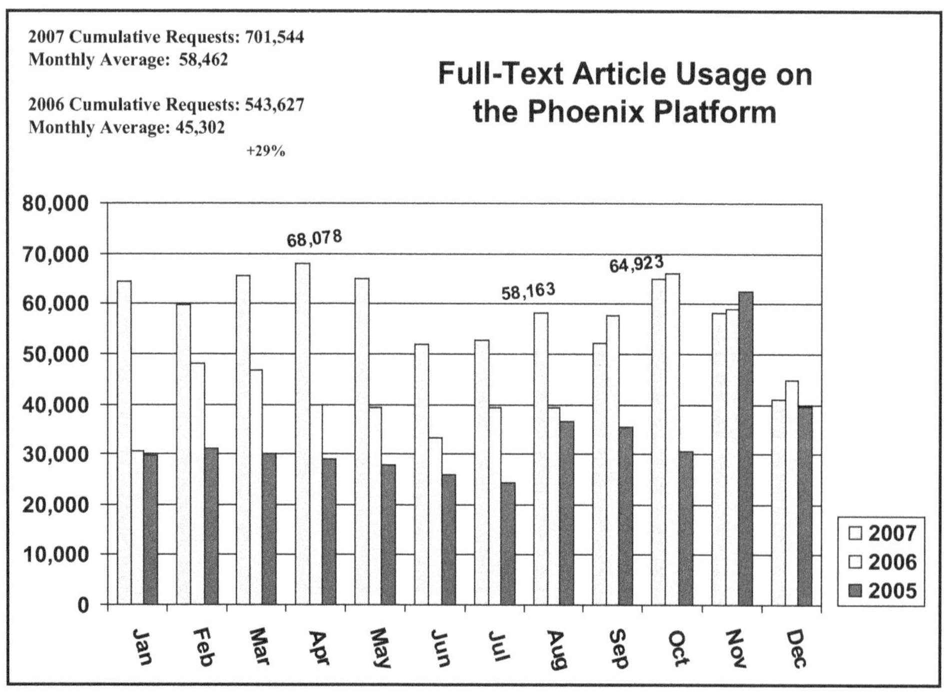

Figure 4. E-article requests stats: Phoenix platform.

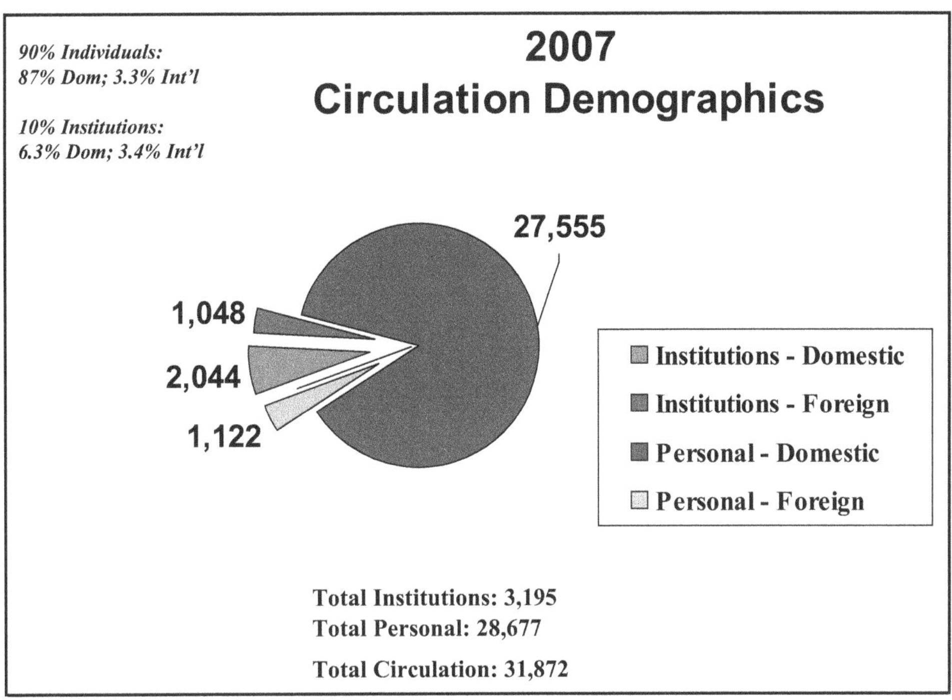

Figure 5. Circulation: Demographics and distribution.

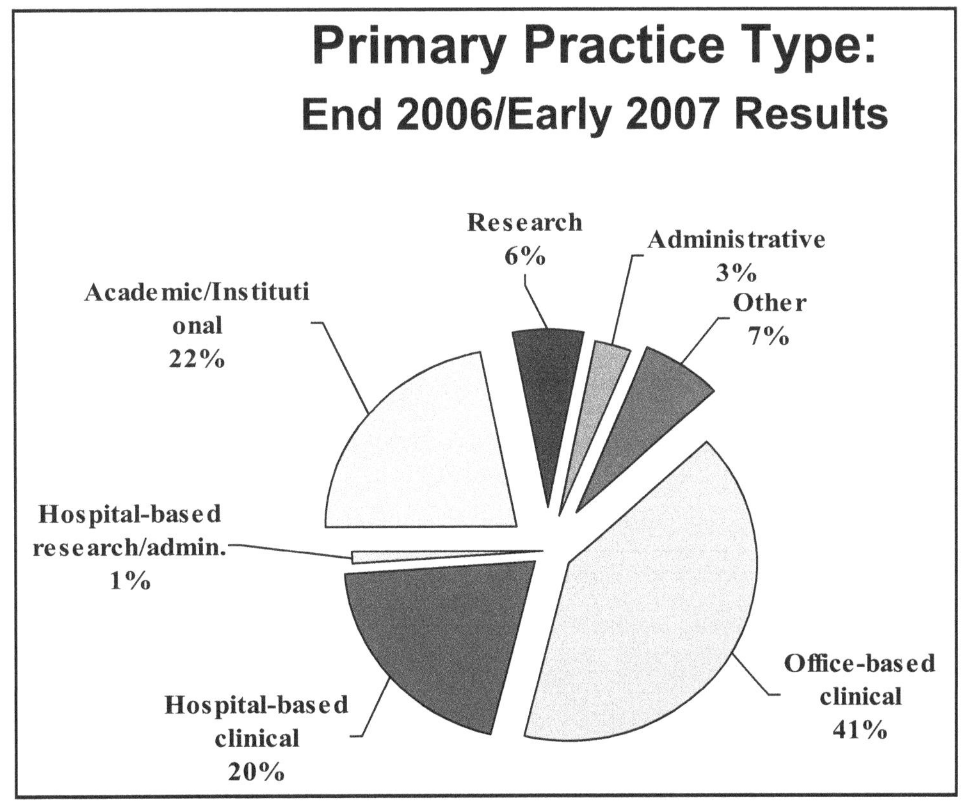

Figure 6. Circulation: Demographics and distribution.

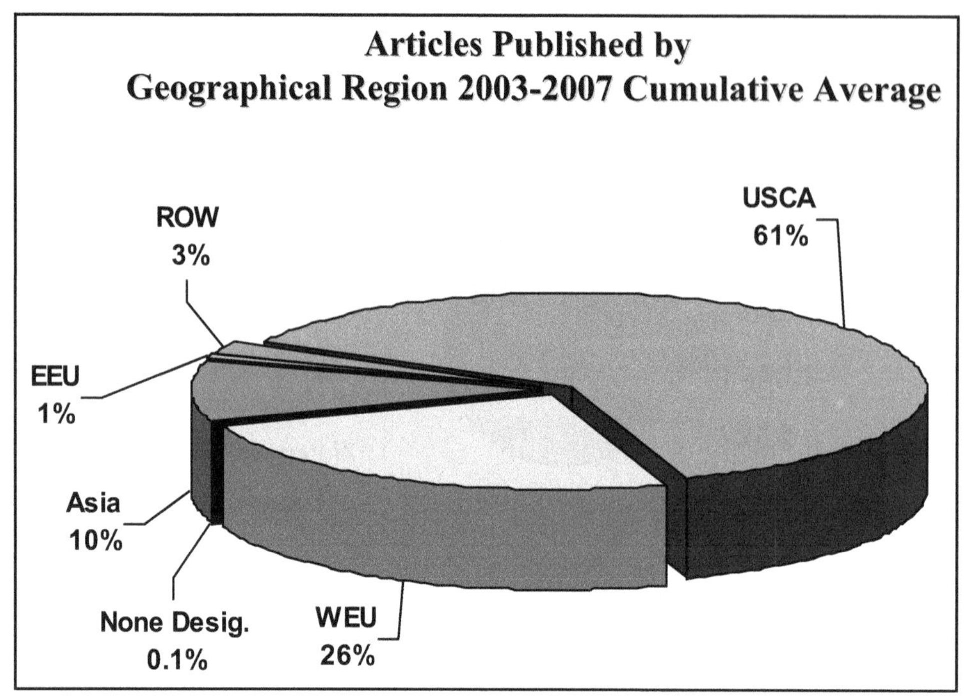

Figure 7. Article sources.

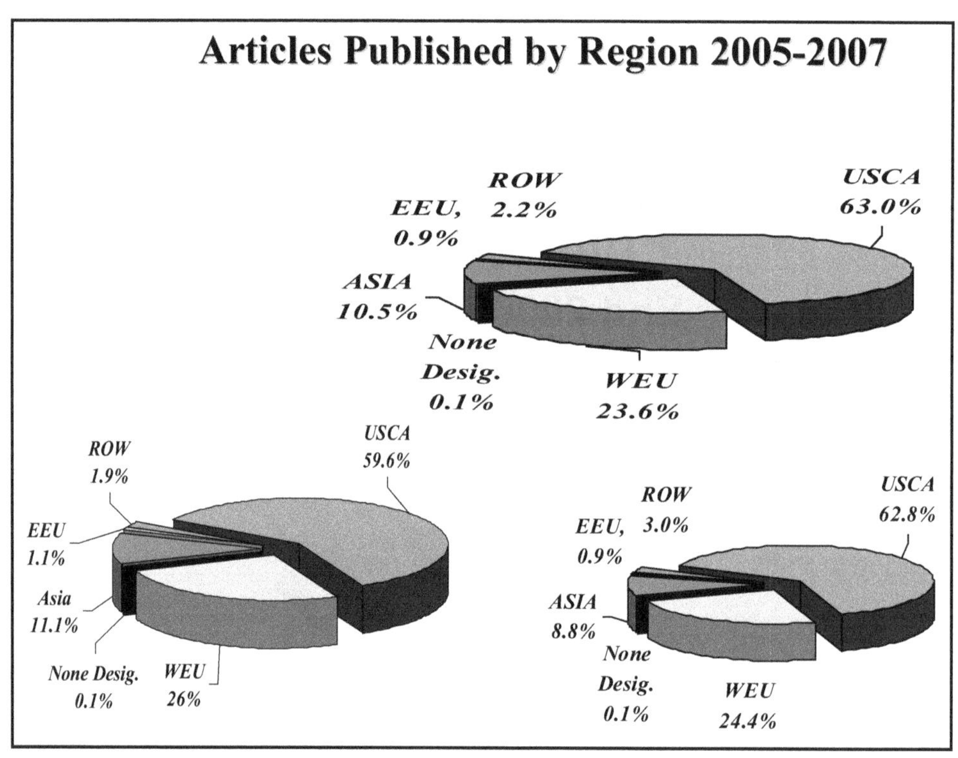

Figure 8. Article sources.

David Dionne
Publisher
Elsevier Inc.
New York, New York

Proceedings of the Editorial Board Meeting of *The American Journal of Cardiology* on March 29, 2009

The 2009 meeting of the editorial board of *The American Journal of Cardiology* (*AJC*) was held on March 29, 2009, in Orlando, Florida, at the time of the Annual Scientific Sessions of the American College of Cardiology. The meetings purpose was to review the *AJC*'s publication results for 2008, to recognize particularly those *AJC* board members who reviewed the most manuscripts in 2008, and to receive criticisms and suggestions from board members on how to improve the journal. The meeting went as follows.

1. Introduction of new editorial board members: these are listed in Table 1.
2. *AJC* board members reviewing the most manuscripts in 2008: their names are listed in Table 2.
3. Numbers of manuscripts submitted, withdrawn, accepted, and declined in 2008: a total of 2,912 manuscripts were received in 2008 (excluding readers' comments): 709 (25%) were accepted, 2,179 (75%) were declined, and 24 (<1%) were withdrawn (Table 3).
4. Numbers of manuscripts submitted and published or accepted (excluding readers' comments) in the *AJC*, 1983 through 2008, the period of the present editorship (Table 4): the number of manuscripts submitted in 2008 was 9% less than in 2007, whereas the number of manuscripts published or accepted was virtually identical to the previous year. The major reason the acceptance rate is in the midtwenties is because most of the manuscripts that are published are shortened considerably, and that allows space for more reports.
5. Sources of manuscripts submitted to the *AJC* in 2008: of the 1,912 manuscripts submitted from outside the United States, 307 (16%) were accepted; of the 976 submitted from the United States, 402 (41%) were accepted. Thus, of the total of 2,912 submitted in 2008, 709 (24%) were accepted.
6. Numbers of manuscripts received and accepted from countries other than the United States in 2008: these are listed in Table 5.
7. Numbers of editorial pages, types of reports, and topics of reports published in the *AJC* in 2008: these are summarized in Table 6. Of the 3,642 editorial pages published in 2008, 97% were used for reports and/or readers' comments. Of the 647 reports published, 591 (91%) involved multiple patients, and 11 involved studies of single patients. Three reviews, 3 interviews, and 9 Editor's Roundtables were published in 2008. Apparently, these roundtables are quite popular. The topics of the 647 reports are also listed in Table 6. Reports having to do with coronary artery disease of course led the list (at 39%), and those dealing with preventive cardiology, heart failure, and miscellaneous subjects each represented 11% of the reports. Although there are apparently 65 million Americans with systemic hypertension, only 8 reports were published on this topic in the *AJC* in 2008.
8. Numbers of reports and editorial pages for reports and readers' comments published in the regular issues of the *AJC* from 1983 through 2008: these are listed in Table 7. These include the 26 full years of the present editorship. The total pages for reports and readers' comments in 2008 numbered 3,522, a 2% reduction from the previous year.
9. Interviews published in the *AJC* from 1996 through 2008: these are listed in Table 8. Three interviews were published in 2008.
10. Supplements published in the *AJC* in 2008: these are listed in Table 9. Supplements are published separately from the regular issues, which have blue and white covers and contain advertisements. The supplements, which are underwritten by ≥1 pharmaceutical or device company, have white covers and do not contain advertisements.

Comments

The year 2008 was a very successful one for the *AJC* despite the appearance of 6 new cardiology journals in that year. Four of the new journals are published by the American Heart Association and the other 2 by the American College of Cardiology. The number of manuscripts submitted to the *AJC* in 2008 represented a 9% reduction from 2007; nevertheless, the number submitted in 2008 represents a 27% increase over the number submitted in 2004, only 4 years earlier. The percentage of manuscripts submitted from outside the United States in 2008 was similar to that in 2007.

Table 1
New board members in 2008

Jamil Aboulhosn
Bruce T. Liang
Francisco Lopez-Jimenez
Jennifer G. Robinson
Gregory W. Stone

Table 2
Top *American Journal of Cardiology* board reviewers in 2008

Name	Manuscripts Reviewed
David D. Waters	11
Antonio Abbate	10
Stephen P. Glasser	10
Ami E. Iskandrian	10
Pablo Avanzas	9
K. Lance Gould	9
Don Poldermans	9
George S. Abela	8
Monty M. Bodenheimer	8
Jeffrey S. Borer	8
Michael E. Cain	8
Marc Cohen	8
James A. de Lemos	8
N.A. Mark Estes	8
David R. Holmes, Jr.	8
Carl J. Lavie	8
Arthur J. Moss	8
Charles E. Rackley	8
John C. Somberg	8

Table 3
Manuscripts submitted to *The American Journal of Cardiology* in 2008

Total	2,912 (100%)
Withdrawn	24 (1%)
Accepted	709 (24%)
Declined	2,179 (75%)

Table 4
Numbers of manuscripts submitted and published in *The American Journal of Cardiology*, 1983 to 2008

Year	Manuscripts Submitted	Manuscripts Published or Accepted	Percentage Accepted
1983	1,234	643	52%
1984	1,605	747	46%
1985	1,707	645	38%
1986	1,574	616	39%
1987	1,525	695	46%
1988	1,496	636	42%
1989	1,740	699	40%
1990	1,717	662	38%
1991	1,615	680	42%
1992	1,873	664	35%
1993	1,997	619	31%
1994	1,783	604	34%
1995	1,844	668	36%
1996	1,930	701	36%
1997	1,898	768	40%
1998	1,992	631	31%
1999	2,170	703	32%
2000	2,226	630	28%
2001	2,068	682	33%
2002	2,171	683	31%
2003	2,190	783	36%
2004	2,109	842	39%
2005	2,661	984	37%
2006	3,061	653	21%
2007	3,184	710	22%
2008	2,912	709	24%

Table 5
Number of manuscripts received and accepted from countries other than the United States in 2008

Country	Submitted	Accepted
Italy	253	43 (17%)
Japan	233	21 (9%)
The Netherlands	140	35 (25%)
China	125	11 (9%)
Germany	104	13 (13%)
Turkey	97	4 (4%)
Korea	96	15 (16%)
Canada	82	22 (27%)
France	78	13 (17%)
Taiwan	70	5 (7%)
United Kingdom	70	16 (23%)
Spain	64	15 (23%)
Israel	61	18 (30%)
Greece	55	6 (11%)
Australia	49	13 (27%)
Brazil	46	5 (11%)
Switzerland	30	7 (23%)
Poland	28	3 (11%)
Denmark	24	5 (21%)
India	21	0 (0%)
Iran	21	1 (5%)
Belgium	19	3 (16%)
Norway	17	6 (35%)
Sweden	16	6 (38%)
Austria	15	3 (20%)
Finland	13	6 (46%)
Hong Kong	12	4 (33%)
34 countries with ≤10 submissions	73	8 (11%)
Total	1,912	307 (16%)

Table 6
Number of editorial pages and reports published in *The American Journal of Cardiology* in 2008 (Volumes 101 and 102) (nonsymposium issues)

Total editorial pages	3,642
Reports	3,474 (95%)
Readers' comments (numbers) [replys] (percentage)	48 (59) [7] (1%)
Staff and editorial board	48 (1%)
Contents	68 (2%)
Instructions to authors	4 (<1%)
Volume indexes	0
Types of reports	647
Multipatient studies	591 (91%)
Case reports	11 (2%)
Reviews	3 (<1%)
Editorials	18 (3%)
Editor's Roundtables	9 (1%)
Interviews	3 (<1%)
Nonpatient studies	10 (2%)
Topics of reports	647
Coronary artery disease	255 (39%)
Preventive cardiology	74 (11%)
Arrhythmias or conduction defects	51 (8%)
Heart failure	68 (11%)
Valvular heart disease	31 (5%)
Cardiomyopathy	30 (5%)
Congenital heart disease	32 (5%)
Methods	16 (2%)
Miscellaneous	71 (11%)
Historical studies	4 (<1%)
Systemic hypertension	8 (1%)
Cardiovascular pharmacology	4 (<1%)
Interviews	3 (<1%)

Table 7
Number of reports and editorial pages for reports and readers' comments published in *The American Journal of Cardiology*, 1983 to 2008

Year	Pages for Reports	Pages for Readers' Comments	Total	Number of Reports	Number of Readers' Comments
1983	3,130	27	3,157	643	53
1984	3,007	36	3,043	747	80
1985	2,623	21	2,644	645	40
1986	2,627	17	2,644	616	40
1987	2,810	23	2,833	695	45
1988	2,646	26	2,672	636	60
1989	2,903	19	2,922	699	36
1990	3,001	20	3,021	662	40
1991	3,165	38	3,203	680	59
1992	3,211	46	3,257	711	53
1993	2,890	37	2,927	650	64
1994	2,493	31	2,524	604	46
1995	2,570	34	2,604	668	52
1996	2,775	29	2,804	658	52
1997	3,328	32	3,360	826	45
1998	3,048	35	3,083	664	37
1999	3,015	38	3,053	680	42
2000	2,962	38	3,000	648	37
2001	3,862	37	3,899	701	39
2002	2,835	45	2,880	680	45
2003	2,982	35	3,017	763	32
2004	3,131	39	3,170	808	42
2005	3,242	43	3,285	736	49
2006	3,406	65	3,471	695	70
2007	3,540	50	3,590	695	59
2008	3,474	48	3,522	647	59
Total	78,676	909	79,585	17,857	1,276

Table 8
Interviews published in *The American Journal of Cardiology*

Subject	Date	Subject	Date
Eric Jeffrey Topol	July 1, 1996	Melvin Mayer Scheinman	March 1, 2001
Wallace Bruce	August 1, 1996	James Stuart Forrester III	December 1, 2001
James Thoraton Willerson	February 15, 1997	Carl John Pepine	December 15, 2001
Michael Ellis DeBakey	April 1, 1997	Kenneth Hardy Cooper	February 1, 2001
Denton Arthur Cooley	April 15, 1997	Watkins Proctor Harvey	February 15, 2001
Joseph Stephan Alpert	May 1, 1997	Joseph Kayle Perloff	March 1, 2002
John Willis Hurst	February 15, 1998	Charles Richard Conti	March 15, 2002
Jesse Efrem Edwards	April 1, 1998	William Watts Parmley	May 1, 2002
John Webster Kirklin	April 15, 1998	Dean Michael Ornish	August 1, 2002
Howard Bertram Burchell	May 15, 1998	Dean Towle Mason	December 15, 2002
William Howard Frishman	June 1, 1998	George Allan Beller	January 15, 2003
Robert Ogdon Bonow	June 15, 1998	Leslie David Hillis	February 1, 2003
Eugene Braunwald	July 1, 1998	Douglas P. Zipes	April 1, 2003
Joseph Cholmondeley Greenfield	July 15, 1998	Nanette Kass Wenger	May 15, 2003
David Coston Sabiston, Jr.	August 1, 1998	Andrew Peter Selwyn	June 15, 2003
Norman Mayer Kaplan	August 15, 1998	Arthur Garson, Jr.	August 15, 2003
Robert McKinnon Califf	September 1, 1998	Edward David Frolich	September 1, 2003
Bernard John Gersh	November 1, 1998	Magdi Habib Yacoub	January 15, 2003
Dean James Keriakes	November 15, 1998	Robert A. Vogel	April 1, 2004
Jeffrey Michael Isner	January 1, 1999	Ferid Murad	July 1, 2004
Scott Montgomery Grundy	January 15, 1999	Steven Evan Nissen	August 1, 2004
Burton Elias Sobel	February 1, 1999	William Peter Castelli	September 1, 2004
Robert Anthony O'Rourke	April 1, 1999	Wallace Bruce Fye III	January 1, 2005
David Kempton Cartwright Cooper	April 15, 1999	Anthony Nicolas DeMaria	January 15, 2005
Spencer Bidwell King III	May 1, 1999	Barry L. Zaret	May 15, 2005
Robert Roberts	May 15, 1999	Lawrence Harvey Cohn	March 15, 2006
Eugene Austin Stead, Jr.	September 15, 1999	Joseph Loscalzo	April 1, 2006
Bertram Pitt	October 1, 1999	Donald Carey Harrison	May 1, 2006
Christopher John Dillon Packard	November 15, 1999	Hollis Bryan Brewer	June 15, 2006
Terje Rolf Pedersen	November 15, 1999	Barry Joel Maron	May 1, 2007
Francis Robicsek	June 1, 2000	William Clifford Roberts	July 15, 2007
Richard John Bing	July 1, 2000	Jean Schlatter Kan	January 1, 2008
Valentin Fuster	July 15, 2000	Robert William (Bobby) Brown	March 1, 2008
Henry Arthur Solomon	July 15, 2000	Lawrence Sorel Cohen	March 15, 2008
Myrvin Harold Ellestad	December 1, 2000		

Table 9
Supplements published in the 2008 *American Journal of Cardiology* supplement issues

Topic of Supplement	Date of Publication	Guest Editor(s)	No. of Articles	No. of Pages	Interval from Symposium to Publication (mos)	Sponsor(s)
A. Consensus on N-terminal–pro-brain natriuretic peptide	February 4	James L. Januzzi, Jr., and A. Mark Richards	17	94	15	Roche, Dade-Behring, and Ortho Diagnostics
B. Niacin for mixed dyslipidemia	April 17	Michael H. Davidson and Christie M. Ballantyne	10	62	0	Abbott Laboratories
C. Abstracts, Summit 2008 Transcatheter Cardiovascular Therapeutics Asia Pacific	April 23–25		0	107	0	CardioVascular Research Foundation, Korea
D. Oxidative stress and heart disease	May 22	Deepak L. Bhatt and Frederic J. Pashkow	12	86	16	Cardax
E. Amino acids in cardiovascular and metabolic diseases	June 2	Mihai Gheorghiade, Gerasimos S. Filippatos, Gregg C. Fonarow, and Stefan D. Anker	18	115	0	Professional Dietetics
F. Ruptured plaque and phospholipase A_2	June 16	Michael H. Davidson	7	57	0	diaDexus
G. Left ventricular function after myocardial infarction	September 8	Mihai Gheorghiade, James D. Flaherty, and Gregg C. Fonarow	9	67	21	GlaxoSmithKline and Medtronic
H. Rate vs rhythm in atrial fibrillation	September 22	James A. Reiffel	4	30	16	Astellas Pharma
I. Abstracts, Transcatheter Cardiovascular Therapeutics in 2008	October 12–17		0	270	0	CardioVascular Research Foundation
J. Coronary stenting: drug-eluting vs bare-metal stents	November 3	David G. Rizik	6	37	12	Cordis
K. Metabolic syndrome, diabetes mellitus, and fenofibrate	November 17	Jean-Charles Fruchart, Frank M. Sacks, and Michel P. Hermans	1	34	0	Solvay
L. Reducing risk for dyslipidemia	December 22	Frank M. Sacks	8	47	0	Abbott Laboratories

William Clifford Roberts, MD
Baylor Heart and Vascular Institute
Baylor University Medical Center
Dallas, Texas
March 24, 2009

Proceedings of the Editorial Board Meeting of *The American Journal of Cardiology* on March 14, 2010

The 2010 meeting of the editorial board of *The American Journal of Cardiology* (AJC) was held on March 14, 2010, in Atlanta, Georgia, at the time of the Annual Scientific Sessions of the American College of Cardiology. The meeting's purpose was to review the AJC's publication results for 2009, to recognize, in particular, those AJC board members who had reviewed the most manuscripts in 2009, and to receive criticisms and suggestions from board members on how to improve the journal. The meeting went as follows:

1. Introduction of new editorial board members: these are listed in Table 1.
2. AJC board members reviewing the most manuscripts in 2009: their names are listed in Table 2.
3. Numbers of manuscripts submitted, withdrawn, accepted, and refused in 2009: 2,878 manuscripts were received in 2009 (excluding readers' comments); 728 (25%) were accepted, 2,136 (75%) were refused, and 14 (<1%) were withdrawn. The number of manuscripts received in 2009 represented a 1% decrease from the number received in 2008.
4. Numbers of manuscripts submitted and published or accepted (excluding readers' comments) in the AJC for 1983 to 2009, the period of the present editorship (Table 3): the major reason the acceptance rate was in the mid-20s was that most of the manuscripts published were shortened considerably, allowing space for more reports.
5. Sources of manuscripts submitted to the AJC in 2009: of the 1,916 manuscripts submitted from non-United States countries, 341 (18%) were accepted. Of the 948 submitted from the United States, 387 (41%) were accepted.
6. Numbers of editorial pages, types of reports, and topics of reports published in the AJC in 2009: these are summarized in Table 4. Of the 3,641 editorial pages published in 2009, 3,491 were used for articles and 32 for readers' comments, such that 97% were used for the publication of manuscripts. Of the 632 reports published, 577 (91%) involved multiple patients and 8 (1%), single patients. Twelve reviews, 22 editorials, 5 editor's roundtables and 8 from-the-editor columns were published in 2009. The topics of the articles published in 2009 are also listed in Table 4. Articles having to do with coronary artery disease led the list (45%), and preventive cardiology articles increased to 12%.
7. Numbers of reports and editorial pages for reports and readers' comments published in the regular issues of the AJC from 1983 to 2009: these are

Table 1
New Board Members in 2009

Jack P. Chen
Jean-Pierre Després
Allen L. Dollar
S. David Gertz
Greg L. Kaluza
Ellen C. Keeley
Lynda E. Rosenfeld

Table 2
Top *American Journal of Cardiology* board reviewers in 2009

Name	No. Reviewed
Toby R. Engel	10
Antonio Abbate	9
Ami E. Iskandrian	9
Gregory Y. H. Lip	9
Myrvin H. Ellestad	8
Stephen P. Glasser	8
Monty M. Bodenheimer	8
Carl J. Lavie	8

Table 3
Numbers of manuscripts submitted and published, 1983 to 2009

Year	No. of Manuscripts Submitted	No. of Manuscripts Published or Accepted	Percentage Accepted
1983	1,234	643	52%
1984	1,605	747	46%
1985	1,707	645	38%
1986	1,574	616	39%
1987	1,525	695	46%
1988	1,496	636	42%
1989	1,740	699	40%
1990	1,717	662	38%
1991	1,615	680	42%
1992	1,873	664	35%
1993	1,997	619	31%
1994	1,783	604	34%
1995	1,844	668	36%
1996	1,930	701	36%
1997	1,898	768	40%
1998	1,992	631	31%
1999	2,170	703	32%
2000	2,226	630	28%
2001	2,068	682	33%
2002	2,171	683	31%
2003	2,190	783	36%
2004	2,109	842	39%
2005	2,661	984	37%
2006	3,061	653	21%
2007	3,184	710	22%
2008	2,888	709	25%
2009	2,864	728	25%

Table 4
Number of editorial pages and types of articles published in the *American Journal of Cardiology* in 2009 (volumes 103 and 104; nonsymposium issues)

	2009, January 1 to December 15, Volumes 103 and 104
Editorial pages	
Total	3,641
Articles	3,491 (96%)
Readers' comments, total, replies	32, 46, 5 (1%)
Staff and editorial board	48
Contents	66
Instructions to authors	4
Types of articles	632
Multipatient studies	577 (91%)
Case reports	8 (1%)
Reviews	12 (2%)
Editorials	22 (3%)
Editor's roundtable (consensus)	5 (1%)
Interviews	0
From-the-editor columns	8 (1%)
Topics of articles	
Total	632
Coronary artery disease	287 (45%)
Preventive cardiology	78 (12%)
Arrhythmias and conduction disturbances	33 (5%)
Heart failure	56 (10%)
Valvular heart disease	23 (4%)
Cardiomyopathy	32 (5%)
Congenital heart disease	34 (5%)
Methods	8 (1%)
Miscellaneous	61 (10%)
Historical studies	2 (<1%)
Cardiovascular pharmacology	2 (<1%)
Systemic hypertension	8 (1%)
Nonpatient studies	8 (1%)

Table 5
Number of articles and editorial pages for articles and Readers' comments published in 1983 to 2009

Year	Pages for Reports	Pages for Readers' Comments	Total	No. of Reports	No. of Readers' Comments
1983	3,130	27	3,157	643	53
1984	3,007	36	3,043	747	80
1985	2,623	21	2,644	645	40
1986	2,627	17	2,644	616	40
1987	2,810	23	2,833	695	45
1988	2,646	26	2,672	636	60
1989	2,903	19	2,922	699	36
1990	3,001	20	3,021	662	40
1991	3,165	38	3,203	680	59
1992	3,211	46	3,257	711	53
1993	2,890	37	2,927	650	64
1994	2,493	31	2,524	604	46
1995	2,570	34	2,604	668	52
1996	2,775	29	2,804	658	52
1997	3,328	32	3,360	826	45
1998	3,048	35	3,083	664	37
1999	3,015	38	3,053	680	42
2000	2,962	38	3,000	648	37
2001	3,862	37	3,899	701	39
2002	2,835	45	2,880	680	45
2003	2,982	35	3,017	763	32
2004	3,131	39	3,170	808	42
2005	3,242	43	3,285	736	49
2006	3,406	65	3,471	695	70
2007	3,540	50	3,590	695	59
2008	3,474	48	3,522	647	59
2009	3,491	32	3,523	632	46

Table 6
Supplements published in the 2009 American Journal of Cardiology supplement issues

Topic of Supplement	Publication Date	Guest Editors	No. of Articles	No. of Pages	Sponsor
Antiplatelet therapy	February 2	Dominick J. Angiolillo	7	51	Daiichi Sankyo, Eli Lilly
Abstracts: Angioplasty Summit TCT Asia Pacific 2009	April 22			128	Cardiovascular Research Foundation
Antiplatelet therapy in coronary syndromes and its safety	September 7	Steven V. Manoukian	12	63	Sanofi-Aventis
Abstracts: transcatheter cardiovascular	Sept 21			242	Cardiovascular Research Foundation
High-density lipoprotein as a therapeutic target	Nov 19	Michael H. Davidson	9	57	Roche Pharmaceuticals
Total (n = 5)			28	541	

listed in Table 5. These include the 27 full years of the present editorship.

8. Supplements published in the AJC in 2009: these are listed in Table 6. Supplements are published separately from the regular issues, which have blue and white covers and contain advertisements. The supplements, which are underwritten by one or more pharmaceutical or device companies, have white covers and do not contain advertisements.
9. Reviewers of articles published in the AJC in 2009: this supplementary data can be found, in the online version, at doi:10.1016/j.amjcard.2010.03.054.

The 2009 year was a very successful one for the AJC. My presentation was followed by a report by Jane Grochowski, the publisher, and her discussion, as was mine, was followed by a brief question and comment session. The meeting adjourned to a splendid reception provided by the publisher.

William Clifford Roberts, MD
Baylor Heart and Vascular Institute
Baylor University Medical Center
Dallas, Texas
March 26, 2010

Proceedings of the Editorial Board Meeting of *The American Journal of Cardiology* on April 3, 2011

The 2011 meeting of the Editorial Board of *The American Journal of Cardiology* (*AJC*) was held on April 3, 2011, in New Orleans, Louisiana, at the time of the Annual Scientific Sessions of the American College of Cardiology. The meeting's purpose was to review the *AJC*'s publication results in 2010, to recognize particularly those *AJC* board members who reviewed the most manuscripts in 2010, and to receive suggestions and criticisms from board members on ways to improve the journal. The meeting went as follows:

1. *Introduction of new editorial board members* (Table 1).
2. AJC *board members reviewing the most manuscripts in 2010*. The publisher provided plaques to each of the 7 top *AJC* reviewers for 2010 (Table 2), and they read as follows:

   In appreciation to
   NAME
   Top Reviewer
   The American Journal of Cardiology
   2010
3. *Number of manuscripts submitted, withdrawn, accepted, and declined in 2010* (Table 3).
4. *Sources of manuscripts submitted to the* AJC *in 2010* (Table 4).
5. *Number of editorial pages, types and topics of articles published in the* AJC *in 2010* (Table 5).
6. *Number of manuscripts submitted and published and/or accepted in the* AJC *in 1983 through 2010, the 28 full years of the present editorship* (Table 6).
7. *Number of articles and Readers' Comments published and number of editorial pages utilized in the* AJC *from 1983 through 2010, the 28 full years of the present editorship* (Table 7).

Manuscript received April 8, 2011; revised manuscript received and accepted April 8, 2011.

Comments

The year 2010 was a good one for the *AJC*. The number of manuscripts submitted remained high (nearly 3,000), the number of manuscripts accepted remained high (nearly 700), and the manuscript quality remained good. The number of editorial pages provided by the publisher for articles and Readers' Comments was outstanding (3,650).

Some changes have occurred. The supplement issues sponsored by 1 or more pharmaceutical or device companies have virtually disappeared for the print issues. Some style changes initiated in 2009 were apparent in all issues in 2010. These included the elimination of all subheadings in the reports except for "Methods," "Results," and "Discussion." Their elimination allows a more attractive presentation of each report, and much space is preserved for text, tables, and figures. I believe that more tables and figures are published in the *AJC* than in any other cardiology journal.

We think 2011 will also be a good year for the *AJC*. Already in the first 3 months of 2011, just over 800 manuscripts have been submitted, and many are superb. The publisher, Ms. Jane Grochowski, working with Dr. Vincent E. Friedewald, 1 of the 3 associate editors of the *AJC*, and Mr. Brian Jenkins, are expanding the online version of the print *AJC*, and the innovations will appear in 2011. Ms. Grochowski and Mr. Jenkins presented some of these innovations to the *AJC* Editorial Board.

The meeting was adjourned to a splendid reception provided by the publisher.

Supplementary data

Supplementary data associated with this article can be found, in the online version, at doi:10.1016/j.amjcard.2011.04.002.

William Clifford Roberts, MD
Baylor Heart and Vascular InstituteBaylor University Medical Center, Dallas, Texas

Table 1
New Editorial Board members for 2010

Evan Applebaum
James P. Daubert
Giovanni Filardo
Hani Jneid
Lori Jean Mosca
Hartzell V. Schaff

Table 2
Top *American Journal of Cardiology* Editorial Board reviewers in 2010

Name	Manuscripts Reviewed
Antonio Abbate	10
Pablo Avanzas	9
Monty M. Bodenheimer	9
Marc Cohen	9
Toby R. Engel	9
Gregory Y.H. Lip	9
Don Poldermans	9

Table 3
Manuscripts submitted to *The American Journal of Cardiology* in 2010

Total	2,917 (100%)
Withdrawn	24
Accepted	684 (24%)
Declined	2,209 (76%)

Table 4
Sources of manuscripts submitted to *The American Journal of Cardiology* in 2010

Source	Submitted	Accepted
Outside the United States	1,915	344 (18%)
United States	978	340 (35%)
Total	2,893	684 (24%)

Table 5
Number of editorial pages and types and topics of reports published in *The American Journal of Cardiology* in 2010 (Volumes 105 and 106, January 1 to December 15; nonsymposium issues)

Editorial pages—Total	3,769
Reports	3,585
Readers' Comments (number of comments/number of replies)	65 (68/10)
Staff and Editorial Board	48 (1%)
Contents	67 (2%)
Instructions to authors	4 (0.001%)
Types of articles	626
Multipatient studies	562 (90%)
Case reports	8 (1%)
Reviews	22 (4%)
Editorials	12 (2%)
Editor's Roundtables (consensus statements)	5 (1%)
Interviews	0
From the Editor columns	4 (1%)
Nonpatient studies	5 (1%)
Historical studies	8 (1%)
Topics of articles	626
Coronary artery disease	252 (40%)
Preventive cardiology	66 (11%)
Arrhythmias and conduction disturbances	41 (7%)
Heart failure	49 (8%)
Valvular heart disease	35 (6%)
Cardiomyopathy	33 (5%)
Congenital heart disease	49 (8%)
Methods	14 (2%)
Systemic hypertension	11 (11%)
Miscellaneous	68 (1%)
Historical studies	8 (2%)

Table 6
Number of manuscripts submitted and published in *The American Journal of Cardiology* (1983 to 2010)

Year	Number Submitted	Published or Accepted	Percentage Accepted
1983	1,234	643	52%
1984	1,605	747	46%
1985	1,707	645	38%
1986	1,574	616	39%
1987	1,525	695	46%
1988	1,496	636	42%
1989	1,740	699	40%
1990	1,717	662	38%
1991	1,615	680	42%
1992	1,873	664	35%
1993	1,997	619	31%
1994	1,783	604	34%
1995	1,844	668	36%
1996	1,930	701	36%
1997	1,898	768	40%
1998	1,992	631	31%
1999	2,170	703	32%
2000	2,226	630	28%
2001	2,068	682	33%
2002	2,171	683	31%
2003	2,190	783	36%
2004	2,109	842	39%
2005	2,661	984	37%
2006	3,061	653	21%
2007	3,184	710	22%
2008	2,888	709	25%
2009	2,864	728	25%
2010	2,893	684	24%
Total	58,015	19,469	

Table 7
Number of reports and editorial pages for reports and Readers' Comments published in *The American Journal of Cardiology* (1983 to 2010)

Year	Pages for Reports	Pages for Readers' Comments	Total	Number of Reports	Number of Readers' Comments
1983	3,130	27	3,157	643	53
1984	3,007	36	3,043	747	80
1985	2,623	21	2,644	645	40
1986	2,627	17	2,644	616	40
1987	2,810	23	2,833	695	45
1988	2,646	26	2,672	636	60
1989	2,903	19	2,922	699	36
1990	3,001	20	3,021	662	40
1991	3,165	38	3,203	680	59
1992	3,211	46	3,257	711	53
1993	2,890	37	2,927	650	64
1994	2,493	31	2,524	604	46
1995	2,570	34	2,604	668	52
1996	2,775	29	2,804	658	52
1997	3,328	32	3,360	826	45
1998	3,048	35	3,083	664	37
1999	3,015	38	3,053	680	42
2000	2,962	38	3,000	648	37
2001	3,862	37	3,899	701	39
2002	2,835	45	2,880	680	45
2003	2,982	35	3,017	763	32
2004	3,131	39	3,170	808	42
2005	3,242	43	3,285	736	49
2006	3,406	65	3,471	695	70
2007	3,540	50	3,590	695	59
2008	3,474	48	3,522	647	59
2009	3,491	32	3,523	632	46
2010	3,585	65	3,650	626	68
Total	85,752	1,006	86,758	19,115	1,390

Proceedings of the Editorial Board Meeting of *The American Journal of Cardiology* on March 25, 2012

The 2012 meeting of the editorial board of *The American Journal of Cardiology* (*AJC*) was held on March 25, 2012, in Chicago, Illinois, at the time of the Annual Scientific Sessions of the American College of Cardiology. The meeting's purpose was to review the *AJC*'s publication results for 2011, to recognize in particular those *AJC* board members who had reviewed the most manuscripts in 2011, and to receive criticisms and suggestions from board members on how to improve the journal. The meeting went as follows:

1. *The publisher of the* AJC, *Jane Grochowski, presented information on how the* AJC *stands compared with other cardiology journals.*
2. *Introduction of new editorial board members* (Table 1).
3. AJC *board members reviewing the most manuscripts in 2011* (Table 2): Jane Grochowski provided plaques to each of these 9 top reviewers who during 2011 reviewed 8 or 9 manuscripts.
4. *Numbers of manuscripts submitted, withdrawn, accepted, and declined in 2011*: A total of 2,965 manuscripts were received in 2011; 14 were withdrawn by the authors, 702 (24%) were accepted, and 2,249 (76%) were declined. Of the 982 manuscripts submitted from the USA in 2011, 356 (35%) were accepted; of the 1,969 manuscripts submitted from non-USA countries, 346 (18%) were accepted.
5. *Numbers of editorial pages, types and topics of reports published in the* AJC *in 2011* (Table 3): Of the 3,820 editorial pages published, 3,637 (95%) were used for articles and an additional 32, for Readers' Comments, such that 97% of the editorial pages published in 2011 were used for publication of manuscripts. Of the 612 reports published, 555 (91%) involved multiple patients and 11 (2%), single patients. Eighteen reviews, 9 editorials, 7 Editor's Roundtables, and 5 From-the-Editor columns were published in 2011. The topics of the articles published in 2011 are also listed in Table 3.
6. *Numbers of manuscripts submitted and published in* AJC *1983 through 2011* (Table 4): In 1983, the first full year of the present editorship, 1,234 manuscripts were submitted and 643 were accepted. In 2011, 2,951 were submitted and 702 were accepted. During these 29 full years of the present editorship

Manuscript received and accepted April 13, 2012.

Table 1
New board members 2011

Eloisa Arbustini
Cristina Basso
Johnson Francis
Joseph A. Hill
Bradley A. Maron
Peter A. McCullough
Frank Pelosi

Table 2
Top *AJC* board reviewers in 2011

Monty M. Bodenheimer (9)
Steven P. Glasser (9)
Gregory Y.H. Lip (9)
Eugene R. Passamani (9)
David D. Waters (8)
Martin A. Alpert (8)
Eric R. Bates (8)
Mun K. Hong (8)
Charles Maynard (8)

Table 3
Number of editorial pages and types and topics of articles in *The American Journal of Cardiology* (regular issues) in 2011

	Volumes 107 and 108 January to December 2011
Editorial pages—total	3,820
Articles	3,637 (95%)
Readers' Comments (number) [replies]	62 (60) [10] (2%)
Staff and editorial board	48 (1%)
Table of contents	72 (2%)
Instructions to authors	1
Types of Articles	612
Multipatient studies	555 (91%)
Case reports	11 (2%)
Reviews	18 (3%)
Editorials	9 (1%)
Editor's Roundtables	7 (1%)
Historical	7 (1%)
Nonpatient studies	0
From-the-Editor columns	5 (1%)
Topics of articles	612
Coronary artery disease	241 (39%)
Preventive cardiology	44 (7%)
Arrhythmias and conduction disturbances	43 (7%)
Heart failure	66 (11%)
Valvular heart disease	50 (8%)
Cardiomyopathy	29 (5%)
Congenital heart disease	41 (7%)
Methods	9 (1%)
Systemic hypertension	13 (2%)
Historical studies	6 (1%)
Miscellaneous	69 (11%)
Interviews	1

Table 4
Numbers of manuscripts submitted and published in *The American Journal of Cardiology* 1983 to 2011

Year	Number of Manuscripts Submitted	Number of Manuscripts Published or Accepted	Percentage Accepted
1983	1,234	643	52%
1984	1,605	747	46%
1985	1,707	645	38%
1986	1,574	616	39%
1987	1,525	695	46%
1988	1,496	636	42%
1989	1,740	699	40%
1990	1,717	662	38%
1991	1,615	680	42%
1992	1,873	664	35%
1993	1,997	619	31%
1994	1,783	604	34%
1995	1,844	668	36%
1996	1,930	701	36%
1997	1,898	768	40%
1998	1,992	631	31%
1999	2,170	703	32%
2000	2,226	630	28%
2001	2,068	682	33%
2002	2,171	683	31%
2003	2,190	783	36%
2004	2,109	842	39%
2005	2,661	984	37%
2006	3,061	653	21%
2007	3,184	710	22%
2008	2,888	709	25%
2009	2,864	728	25%
2010	2,893	684	24%
2011	2,951	702	24%
Total	60,966	20,171	33%

Table 5
Number of editorial pages for articles and Readers' Comments published in *The American Journal of Cardiology* 1983 to 2011

Year	Pages for Articles	Pages for Readers' Comments	Total	Number of Articles	Number of Readers' Comments
1983	3,130	27	3,157	643	53
1984	3,007	36	3,043	747	80
1985	2,623	21	2,644	645	40
1986	2,627	17	2,644	616	40
1987	2,810	23	2,833	695	45
1988	2,646	26	2,672	636	60
1989	2,903	19	2,922	699	36
1990	3,001	20	3,021	662	40
1991	3,165	38	3,203	680	59
1992	3,211	46	3,257	711	53
1993	2,890	37	2,927	650	64
1994	2,493	31	2,524	604	46
1995	2,570	34	2,604	668	52
1996	2,775	29	2,804	658	52
1997	3,328	32	3,360	826	45
1998	3,048	35	3,083	664	37
1999	3,015	38	3,053	680	42
2000	2,962	38	3,000	648	37
2001	3,862	37	3,899	701	39
2002	2,835	45	2,880	680	45
2003	2,982	35	3,017	763	32
2004	3,131	39	3,170	808	42
2005	3,242	43	3,285	736	49
2006	3,406	65	3,471	695	70
2007	3,540	50	3,590	695	59
2008	3,474	48	3,522	647	59
2009	3,491	32	3,523	632	46
2010	3,585	65	3,650	626	68
2011	3,637	62	3,699	612	70
Total	89,389	1,068	90,457	19,727	1,460

a total of 60,966 manuscripts were submitted and 20,171 (33%) were accepted. The acceptance rate continues to drop despite the publisher's providing more editorial pages and the manuscript length continues to decline.

7. *Number of editorial pages for articles and Readers' Comments published in the* AJC *1983 through 2011* (Table 5): During the 29 full years of the present editorship, 89,389 editorial pages have been used for articles and 1,068, for Readers' Comments, totaling 90,457 pages. The number of articles published during these 29 years in the *AJC* totaled 19,727 and the number of Readers' Comments, 1,460.

Following discussion of the above items, the impact factor and the Eigenfactor® were discussed. These later items are discussed more fully in an upcoming article.[1]

The meeting produced a number of questions and answers and was followed by a lovely reception provided by the publisher.

Supplementary data

Supplementary data associated with this article can be found, in the online version, at http:/dx.doi.org/10.1016/j.amjcard.2012.04.013.

William Clifford Roberts, MD
Baylor Heart and Vascular Institute
Baylor University Medical Center
Dallas, Texas

1. Roberts WC. Formulating an answerable question, displaying data, illustrating, writing, reviewing, and editing manuscripts for publication in medical journals. *Am J Cardiol* 2012;110:290–306.

Proceedings of the Editorial Board Meeting of *The American Journal of Cardiology* on March 10, 2013

The 2013 meeting of the editorial board of *The American Journal of Cardiology* (*AJC*) was held on March 10, 2013, in San Francisco, California, at the time of the Annual Scientific Sessions of the American College of Cardiology Foundation. The meeting's purpose was to review the *AJC*'s publication results for 2012, to recognize in particular those *AJC* board members who had reviewed the most manuscripts in 2012, and to receive criticisms and suggestions from board members on how to improve the journal. The meeting went as follows:

1. *The publisher of the AJC, Jane Grochowski, presented information on how the AJC stands compared with other cardiology journals.* She emphasized that *AJC* article downloads continue with an upward trend, that the ScienceDirect and HealthAdvance platforms were upgraded, and that paper to electronic migration continues. She pointed out that the redesign of the cover now allows the entire table of contents to fit on the cover, and I am very pleased by that move. She also presented the top cited articles published in the *AJC* in 2012. *AJC* article downloads in 2012 numbered 1,261,223, essentially no change from downloads in 2011. She provided a list of the top downloaded articles on the *AJC* Web site in 2012. Interesting (to me) is the fact that none of the top 10 concerned percutaneous coronary intervention studies. Grochowski also showed on-line usage by country and, the United States was first followed by Great Britain, Japan, India, Italy, Canada, and so on. Grochowski also discussed Elsevier's clinical key, which is an on-line clinical reference product designed for clinicians in the hospital setting. It includes 500 journals, 800 books, and 1,000s of videos, images, clinical guidelines, point-of-care clinical summaries, patient education content, and clinical trial information. She also discussed developments in mobile access provided by ScienceDirect apps. The access through smart phones and iPad tablets provides search, retrieval of full text, and bookmark for later use. User log-in is required. She indicated that the average print circulation in 2012 was just under 24,000 and 97% of that was in the United States. Readership among cardiologists in the American Medical Association registry indicated that only 2 journals were ahead of the *AJC* in readership and they were the *Journal of the American College of Cardiology* and *Clinical Cardiology*. She also described how Elsevier continues to market actively their journals. During my editorship, the *AJC* has been published by several different companies. In my view, Elsevier is the absolute tops and is truly an editorial content-oriented company. They want the best articles available in their journals.
2. *Introduction of new editorial board members:* We welcomed Drs. Subhash Banerjee and H. Vernon Anderson.
3. *AJC board members reviewing the most manuscripts in 2012* (Table 1): Jane Grochowski provided plaques to each of these 5 top reviewers, who during 2012, reviewed 8 or 9 manuscripts.
4. *Numbers of manuscripts submitted, withdrawn, accepted, and declined in 2012:* A total of 2,720 manuscripts were received in 2012: 7 were withdrawn by the authors, 685 (25%) were accepted, and 2,028 (75%) were declined. Of the 910 submitted from the United States in 2012, 363 (40%) were accepted; of the 1,803 manuscripts submitted from non-United States countries, 322 (18%) were accepted.
5. *Numbers of editorial pages, types and topics of reports published in the AJC in 2012* (Table 2): Of the 3,779 editorial pages published, 3,605 were used for articles and an additional 52 for Readers' Comments, such that 96% of the editorial pages published in 2012 were used for publication of manuscripts. Of the 597 articles published, 557 (93%) involved multiple patients and 5 (1%), single patients. Thirteen reviews, 7 editorials, 2 Editor's Roundtables, and 4 From-the-Editor columns were published in 2012. The topics of the articles published in 2012 are also listed in Table 2.
6. *Numbers of manuscripts submitted and published in the AJC, 1983 through 2012* (Table 3): In 1983, the first full year of the present editorship, 1,234 manuscripts were submitted and 643 were accepted. In 2012, a total of 2,713 were submitted and 685 were accepted. During these 30 full years of the present editorship, a total of 63,679 manuscripts were submitted and 20,856 (33%) were accepted. The acceptance rate has remained the same in recent

Manuscript received April 10, 2013; accepted April 10, 2013.

Table 1
Top *American Journal of Cardiology* Board reviewers in 2012

Antonio Abbate
Monty M. Bodenheimer
Marc Cohen
Johnson Francis
Donald C. Harrison
Charles E. Rackley

Table 2
Number of pages, types of articles and topics of articles published in *The American Journal Cardiology* in 2012

	Volumes 109 and 110 January 2012 to December 2012		
Editorial pages	3,779		
Articles		3,605	(95%)
Staff and editorial board		48	
Table of contents		72	
Readers' Comments (Page No.) [Replies]		52(53)[11](1%)	
Types of articles (excludes Readers' Comments)	597		
Multipatient studies		557	(93%)
Case reports		5	(1%)
Reviews		13	(2%)
Editorials		7	22 (4%)
Editor's Roundtables		2	
Historical		4	
Nonpatient studies		3	
Interviews		2	
From-the-editor columns		4	
Topics of articles (excludes Readers' Comments)	597		
Coronary artery disease		238	(40%)
Preventive cardiology		54	(9%)
Arrhythmias and conduction disturbances		55	(9%)
Heart failure		45	(8%)
Valvular heart disease		38	(6%)
Cardiomyopathy		29	(5%)
Congenital heart disease		29	(5%)
Methods		9	(1%)
Systemic hypertension		10	(1%)
Historical studies		4	(1%)
Miscellaneous		86	(14%)
Interviews		2	

years despite the publisher providing more editorial pages. The *AJC* publishes more tables and figures than other cardiology journals and if we were to decrease that number, as some other journals have done, we would be publishing more manuscripts, but I favor publication of multiple tables and figures. Our acceptance rate would be lower if submitted manuscripts were not shortened considerably before acceptance.

Table 3
Numbers of manuscripts submitted and published in *The American Journal of Cardiology* (1983 to 2012)

Year	Number of Manuscripts Submitted	Number of Manuscripts Published or Accepted	Percentage Accepted
1983	1,234	643	52
1984	1,605	747	46
1985	1,707	645	38
1986	1,574	616	39
1987	1,525	695	46
1988	1,496	636	42
1989	1,740	699	40
1990	1,717	662	38
1991	1,615	680	42
1992	1,873	664	35
1993	1,997	619	31
1994	1,783	604	34
1995	1,844	668	36
1996	1,930	701	36
1997	1,898	768	40
1998	1,992	631	31
1999	2,170	703	32
2000	2,226	630	28
2001	2,068	682	33
2002	2,171	683	31
2003	2,190	783	36
2004	2,109	842	39
2005	2,661	984	37
2006	3,061	653	21
2007	3,184	710	22
2008	2,888	709	25
2009	2,864	728	25
2010	2,893	684	24
2011	2,951	702	24
2012	2,713	685	25
Total	63,679	20,856	33

7. *Number of editorial pages for articles and Readers' Comments published in the AJC, 1983 through 2012* (Table 4). During the 30 full years of the present editorship, 92,994 editorial pages have been used for articles and 1,120 for Readers' Comments, totaling 94,114. The number of articles published during these 30 years in the *AJC* totaled 20,324 and the number of Readers' Comments, 1,513.
8. *Report from Brian Jenkins, Elsevier Multimedia Editor, Elsevier Multimedia Publishing:* Jenkins discussed endeavors by Elsevier to increase usage of continuing medical education activities as a part of the *AJC*. He also oversees the symposia, 3 of which were published in 2012 (Table 5).

My presentation followed Jane Grochowski's report and mine was followed by Brian Jenkens' report. Thereafter, the floor was open to board members for questions and comments. I detected good vibes about the journal from board members. The meeting was followed by a warm reception provided by the publisher.

Table 4
Number of editorial pages for articles and Readers' Comments published in *The American Journal of Cardiology* (1983 to 2012)

Year	Pages for Articles	Pages for Readers' Comments	Total	Number of Articles	Number of Readers' Comments
1983	3,130	27	3,157	643	53
1984	3,007	36	3,043	747	80
1985	2,623	21	2,644	645	40
1986	2,627	17	2,644	616	40
1987	2,810	23	2,833	695	45
1988	2,646	26	2,672	636	60
1989	2,903	19	2,922	699	36
1990	3,001	20	3,021	662	40
1991	3,165	38	3,203	680	59
1992	3,211	46	3,257	711	53
1993	2,890	37	2,927	650	64
1994	2,493	31	2,524	604	46
1995	2,570	34	2,604	668	52
1996	2,775	29	2,804	658	52
1997	3,328	32	3,360	826	45
1998	3,048	35	3,083	664	37
1999	3,015	38	3,053	680	42
2000	2,962	38	3,000	648	37
2001	3,862	37	3,899	701	39
2002	2,835	45	2,880	680	45
2003	2,982	35	3,017	763	32
2004	3,131	39	3,170	808	42
2005	3,242	43	3,285	736	49
2006	3,406	65	3,471	695	70
2007	3,540	50	3,590	695	59
2008	3,474	48	3,522	647	59
2009	3,491	32	3,523	632	46
2010	3,585	65	3,650	626	68
2011	3,637	62	3,699	612	70
2012	3,605	52	3,657	597	53
Total	92,994	1,120	94,114	20,324	1,513

Table 5
Symposia published in *The American Journal of Cardiology* (separate from the regular issues) in 2012

Number	Publication Date	Guest Editor(s)	Topic	Number of Articles	Number of Pages
1S	July 1	Antonio M. Gotto, Jr	Evaluation and management of cardiovascular risk	3	26
6S	September 15	Marc Humbert, Vallerie McLaughlin	Right ventricle in pulmonary hypertension	8	51
9S	November 6	Michael H. Davidson	Diabetes and cardiovascular disease	8	68
3				19	145

Supplementary Data

Supplementary data associated with this article can be found, in the online version, at http://dx.doi.org/10.1016/j.amjcard.2013.04.005.

William Clifford Roberts, MD
Baylor Heart and Vascular Institute
Baylor University Medical Center
Dallas, Texas

Proceedings of the Editorial Board Meeting of *The American Journal of Cardiology* on March 30, 2014

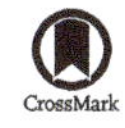

The annual *American Journal of Cardiology* (*AJC*) editorial board meeting was held on March 30, 2014, at the time of the Annual Scientific Sessions of the American College of Cardiology. A major purpose of the meeting is to bring the board members up to date on activities during the previous year and to thank them for reviewing manuscripts during the year. The meeting began with a discussion by the publisher, Ms. Jane M. Grochowski, who described several exciting initiatives that Elsevier has innovated during the past year for many of their journals, including the *AJC*. Ms. Grochowski provided a number of additional editorial pages for the *AJC* during the later months of 2013 and those additional pages allowed us to decrease the lag time from acceptance of a manuscript to its publication from approximately 5 months to its present 3 months. The following editorial matters then were discussed:

1. *Introduction of new 2013 editorial board members* (Table 1).
2. *AJC board members reviewing the most manuscripts in 2013* (Table 2).
3. *Top non-board reviewers for the AJC in 2013* (Table 3). The proven non-board reviewers are the obvious ones to replace "resting" present board members.
4. *Manuscripts submitted to the AJC in 2013* (Table 4). A total of 2,904 manuscripts were submitted in 2013 and 665 (23%) were accepted.
5. *Sources of manuscripts submitted to the AJC in 2013* (Table 5). Of the 2,881 manuscripts submitted (excludes the 23 withdrawn), 1,922 came from non-USA countries and 332 (17%) were accepted; 959 came from the USA and 333 (35%) were accepted.
6. *Numbers of manuscripts submitted and published in the AJC 1983–2013 (31 years) during the present editorship* (Table 6). During these 31 full years, 66,583 manuscripts were submitted, and 21,521 were accepted. The acceptance rate has declined significantly in recent years. The reason the acceptance rate is as high as it is is because most manuscripts are shortened considerably and therefore space exists to publish more manuscripts. The *AJC* publishes more manuscripts each year than any other cardiology journal in the world.
7. *Numbers of editorial pages, types and topics of reports published in the AJC in 2013* (Table 7). A total of 622 articles were published in the *AJC* in 2013 and they occupied 3,749 pages. Additionally, 48 readers' comments were published, occupying 55 editorial pages. Coronary artery disease topics comprised 40% of all articles published.
8. *Numbers of editorial pages for articles and readers' comments published in the AJC, 1983–2013 (31 years)* (Table 8). During my 31 years of editorship more editorial pages were provided by the publisher in 2013 than in any previous year, a total of 3,804 editorial pages: 3,749 were used for articles and 55, for readers' comments. During the entire 31 years of the present editorship a total of 96,743 editorial pages have been published for articles and 1,175 for readers' comments. The number of articles published during the 31 years was 20,946 and the numbers of readers' comments, 1,561.

After an informative question-and-answer period all enjoyed a wonderful reception provided by the publisher.

Table 1
New 2013 editorial board members

Lars Berglund
James C. Blankenship
Todd M. Brown
Gaetano M. De Ferrari
Ian C. Gilchrist
Christopher Hansen
Elizabeth M. Holper
Paul Muntner
Alexander Opotowsky
Charles S. Roberts
James L. Vacek

Table 2
Top *AJC* Board Reviewers in 2013

9 Manuscripts Reviewed	*8 Manuscripts Reviewed*
Marc Cohen	Hugh D. Allen
Lars Berglund	Stephen P. Glasser
James C. Blankenship	Monty M. Bodenheimer
	Toby Ross Engel
	Eric R. Bates
	Antonio Abbate
7 Manuscripts Reviewed	
Martin A. Alpert	Christopher Hansen
David L. Brown	Joseph A. Franciosa
H. Vernon Anderson	Donald Carey Harrison
J. Dawn Abbott	Charles E. Rackley
Jeffrey A. Brinker	Jeroen J. Bax
Johnson Francis	Joseph A. Hill
Richard L. Page	Pablo Avanzas
Steven N. Singh	Gerald V. Naccarelli
Ted E. Feldman	

Table 3
Top *AJC* non-board reviewers in 2013

9 Manuscripts Reviewed	*8 Manuscripts Reviewed*
Neil Filipchuk	Luigi Fiocca
Robert John Mentz	Matthew E. Harinstein
	Roger M. Mills
7 Manuscripts Reviewed	
Olivier François Bertrand	Gülmisal Güder
Danny Chu	Thomas Kahan
Eugene H. Chung	Tomoko Sugiyama Kato
Fabrizio D'Ascenzo	Malte Kelm
Roberto Elosua	Miklos David Kertai
Dmitriy N. Feldman	Alexander Mazur
Tamas Forster	Gjin Ndrepepa
Akira Fujiki	Giampaolo Niccoli
Philip Green	Parin J. Patel

Table 4
Manuscripts submitted to the *AJC* in 2013

Total	2,904 (100%)
Withdrawn	−23
Accepted	665 (23%)
Declined	2,216 (77%)

Table 5
Sources of manuscripts submitted to the *AJC* in 2013

Source	Submitted	Accepted
Non-USA	1,922	332 (17%)
USA	959	333 (35%)
Total	2,881	665 (23%)

Table 6
Number of manuscripts submitted and published in the *AJC* (1983−2013) (31 Years)

Year	Number of Manuscripts Submitted	Number of Manuscripts Published or Accepted	Percentage Accepted
1983	1,234	643	52%
1984	1,605	747	46%
1985	1,707	645	38%
1986	1,574	616	39%
1987	1,525	695	46%
1988	1,496	636	42%
1989	1,740	699	40%
1990	1,717	662	38%
1991	1,615	680	42%
1992	1,873	664	35%
1993	1,997	619	31%
1994	1,783	604	34%
1995	1,844	668	36%
1996	1,930	701	36%
1997	1,898	768	40%
1998	1,992	631	31%
1999	2,170	703	32%
2000	2,226	630	28%
2001	2,068	682	33%
2002	2,171	683	31%
2003	2,190	783	36%
2004	2,109	842	39%
2005	2,661	984	37%
2006	3,061	653	21%
2007	3,184	710	22%
2008	2,888	709	25%
2009	2,864	728	25%
2010	2,893	684	24%
2011	2,951	702	24%
2012	2,713	685	25%
2013	2,904	665	23%
Total	66,583	21,521	32%

Table 7
Number of editorial pages, types, and topics of articles published in the *AJC* in 2013 (Volumes 111 and 112) (Non-symposium Issues)

Editorial pages	3,925	
Articles		3,749 (96%)
Staff and editorial board		48
Table of Contents		73
Readers' comments (total) [replies]		55 (48) [8]
Types of Articles − Total	622	
Multipatient studies		573
Case reports		11
Reviews		20
Editorials		8
Editor's Roundtables		2
Interviews		1
From-the-editor columns		2
Non-patient reports		5
Topics of articles − Total	622	
Coronary artery disease		247 (40%)
Miscellaneous		77
Arrhythmias and conduction disturbances		62
Valvular heart disease		58
Preventive cardiology		49
Heart failure		42
Cardiomyopathy		36
Congenital heart disease		36
Systemic Hypertension		8
Historical studies		5
Methods		2

Table 8
Number of editorial pages for articles and readers' comments published in the *AJC* (1983–2013) (31 Years)

Year	Pages for Articles	Pages for Readers' Comments	Total	Number of Articles	Number of Readers' Comments
1983	3,130	27	3,157	643	53
1984	3,007	36	3,043	747	80
1985	2,623	21	2,644	645	40
1986	2,627	17	2,644	616	40
1987	2,810	23	2,833	695	45
1988	2,646	26	2,672	636	60
1989	2,903	19	2,922	699	36
1990	3,001	20	3,021	662	40
1991	3,165	38	3,203	680	59
1992	3,211	46	3,257	711	53
1993	2,890	37	2,927	650	64
1994	2,493	31	2,524	604	46
1995	2,570	34	2,604	668	52
1996	2,775	29	2,804	658	52
1997	3,328	32	3,360	826	45
1998	3,048	35	3,083	664	37
1999	3,015	38	3,053	680	42
2000	2,962	38	3,000	648	37
2001	3,862	37	3,899	701	39
2002	2,835	45	2,880	680	45
2003	2,982	35	3,017	763	32
2004	3,131	39	3,170	808	42
2005	3,242	43	3,285	736	49
2006	3,406	65	3,471	695	70
2007	3,540	50	3,590	695	59
2008	3,474	48	3,522	647	59
2009	3,491	32	3,523	632	46
2010	3,585	65	3,650	626	68
2011	3,637	62	3,699	612	70
2012	3,605	52	3,657	597	53
2013	3,749	55	3,804	622	48
Total	96,743	1,175	97,918	20,946	1,561

Supplementary Data

Supplementary data associated with this article can be found, in the online version, at http://dx.doi.org/10.1016/j.amjcard.2014.04.020.

William Clifford Roberts, MD
Baylor Heart and Vascular Institute
Baylor University Medical Center
Dallas, Texas

Proceedings of the Editorial Board Meeting of *The American Journal of Cardiology* on March 15, 2015

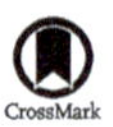

The annual *American Journal of Cardiology* (*AJC*) editorial board meeting was held on March 15, 2015, at the time of the Annual Scientific Sessions of the American College of Cardiology in San Diego, California. The major purposes of the meeting are to bring the board members up to date on activities during the previous year and to thank them for reviewing manuscripts. The meeting began with a discussion by the new publisher, Ms. Joan Anuels, who described several initiatives that Elsevier has introduced during the past year for many of the journals, including the *AJC*. Mr. Brian Jenkins, also of Elsevier, discussed some upcoming supplements planned for 2015. The following editorial matters were then discussed:

1) *Introduction of new 2014 editorial board members* (Table 1). These new board members, most of whom I do not know personally, have been appointed to the board because of supplying excellent and timely reviews for the journal during recent times. We are always looking for good prompt reviewers so suggestions are always welcomed. The proven non-board reviewers are the obvious ones to replace "resting" board members, a number of whom were replaced in 2014.
2) *AJC* board *members reviewing the most manuscripts in 2014* (Table 2). These board members will receive a certificate from the publisher indicating their top performance during 2014.
3) *Manuscripts submitted to the AJC in 2014*. A total of 3,057 manuscripts were submitted in 2014: 14 were withdrawn and a total of 670 (22%) were accepted. Of the 3,036 submitted and not withdrawn, 930 came from the USA and 356 (38%) were accepted; 2,106 were submitted from non-USA countries and 314 (15%) were accepted. The non-USA countries submitting the most manuscripts in 2014 were China (382), Japan (258), Italy (251), Turkey (113), Korea (107), Spain (86), Canada (76), France (72), Germany

Table 1
New board members 2014

Olivier François Bertrand	Danny Chu
Eugene H. Chung	Fabrizio D'Ascenzo
Roberto Elosua	Dmitriy N. Feldman
Gemma Figtree	Akira Fujiki
Philip Green	Matthew E. Harinstein
Thomas Kahan	Tomoko Sugiyama Kato
Malte Kelm	Miklos David Kertai
Alexander Mazur	Robert John Mentz
Roger M. Mills	Gjin Ndrepepa
Giampaolo Niccoli	Parin J. Patel
Augusto Pichard	Fadi N. Salloum

Table 2
Top *AJC* Board Reviewers in 2014

Monty M. Bodenheimer	James C. Blankenship
Akira Fujiki	Matthew E. Harinstein
Malte Kelm	Lars Berglund
Danny Chu	Eugene H. Chung
Marc Cohen	Fabrizio D'Ascenzo
Stephen P. Glasser	Donald Carey Harrison
Tomoko Sugiyama Kato	Roger M. Mills
Gjin Ndrepepa	

Table 3
Number of manuscripts submitted and published in the *AJC* (1983-2014) (32 Years)

Year	Number of Manuscripts Submitted	Number of Manuscripts Published or Accepted	Percentage Accepted
1983	1,234	643	52%
1984	1,605	747	46%
1985	1,707	645	38%
1986	1,574	616	39%
1987	1,525	695	46%
1988	1,496	636	42%
1989	1,740	699	40%
1990	1,717	662	38%
1991	1,615	680	42%
1992	1,873	664	35%
1993	1,997	619	31%
1994	1,783	604	34%
1995	1,844	668	36%
1996	1,930	701	36%
1997	1,898	768	40%
1998	1,992	631	31%
1999	2,170	703	32%
2000	2,226	630	28%
2001	2,068	682	33%
2002	2,171	683	31%
2003	2,190	783	36%
2004	2,109	842	39%
2005	2,661	984	37%
2006	3,061	653	21%
2007	3,184	710	22%
2008	2,888	709	25%
2009	2,864	728	25%
2010	2,893	684	24%
2011	2,951	702	24%
2012	2,713	685	25%
2013	2,904	665	23%
2014	3,057 (5%↑)	670	22%
Total	69,640	22,191	32%

Manuscript received March 19, 2015; revised manuscript received and accepted March 20, 2015.

Table 4
Number of editorial pages, types and topics of articles published in the *AJC* in 2014

	Volumes 113 & 114 Jan – Dec 2014	
Editorial pages	4139	
Articles	3976	(96%)
Staff and editorial board	48	(1%)
Table of contents	71	(2%)
Readers' comments (total) [replies]	44(41) [8]	(1%)
Types of articles – Total	649	
Multi-patient studies	598	
Case reports	8	
Reviews	27	
Editorials	8	
Interviews	3	
Non-patient reports	2	
From-the-editor columns	3	
Topics of articles – Total	649	
Coronary artery disease	251	
Arrhythmias & conduction disturbances	65	
Preventive cardiology	39	
Heart failure	57	
Valvular heart disease	58	
Cardiomyopathy	44	
Congenital heart disease	29	
Systemic hypertension	11	
Miscellaneous	77	
Historical studies	4	
Interviews	3	
Methods	10	

(70), United Kingdom (62), Israel (59), and The Netherlands (59). Fifty-one other countries submitted a total of 511 manuscripts. The acceptance rate among them ranged from 0% to 45%.

4) *Numbers of manuscripts submitted and published in the AJC 1983-2014 (32 years) during the present editorship* (Table 3). During these 32 full years 69,640 manuscripts were submitted and 22,191 were accepted. The acceptance rate has declined significantly in recent years. The reason the acceptance rate is as high as it is is because most manuscripts are shortened considerably and therefore space exists to publish more manuscripts. Subheadings, for example, are not used in the methods, results and discussion portions, and that saves space, and references, except in reviews, are limited to no more than 30. The *AJC* publishes more manuscripts each year than any other cardiology journal in the world.

5) *Numbers of editorial pages, types and topics of reports published in the AJC in 2014* (Table 4). A total of 649 articles were published in the *AJC* in 2014, a 4% increase from the previous year. Additionally, 44 readers' comments were published in 2014. The articles occupied 3,976 pages and the readers' comments, 44 pages. Only 3% of the pages were used for listings of the staff and editorial board, and for the table of contents. Thus, 97% of the editorial pages included articles and readers' comments. Most articles were multi-patient studies. Only 8 case reports and 27 reviews were published in

Table 5
Number of editorial pages for Articles and Readers' Comments published in the *AJC* (1983 to 2012)

Year	Pages for Articles	Pages for Readers' Comments	Total	Number of Articles	Number of Readers' Comments
1983	3,130	27	3,157	643	53
1984	3,007	36	3,043	747	80
1985	2,623	21	2,644	645	40
1986	2,627	17	2,644	616	40
1987	2,810	23	2,833	695	45
1988	2,646	26	2,672	636	60
1989	2,903	19	2,922	699	36
1990	3,001	20	3,021	662	40
1991	3,165	38	3,203	680	59
1992	3,211	46	3,257	711	53
1993	2,890	37	2,927	650	64
1994	2,493	31	2,524	604	46
1995	2,570	34	2,604	668	52
1996	2,775	29	2,804	658	52
1997	3,328	32	3,360	826	45
1998	3,048	35	3,083	664	37
1999	3,015	38	3,053	680	42
2000	2,962	38	3,000	648	37
2001	3,862	37	3,899	701	39
2002	2,835	45	2,880	680	45
2003	2,982	35	3,017	763	32
2004	3,131	39	3,170	808	42
2005	3,242	43	3,285	736	49
2006	3,406	65	3,471	695	70
2007	3,540	50	3,590	695	59
2008	3,474	48	3,522	647	59
2009	3,491	32	3,523	632	46
2010	3,585	65	3,650	626	68
2011	3,637	62	3,699	612	70
2012	3,605	52	3,657	597	53
2013	3,749	55	3,804	622	48
2014	3,976	44	4,020	649	41
Total	100,719	1,219	101,938	21,595	1,602

2014. Coronary artery disease, of course, continues to be the most popular topic published in most cardiology journals. Miscellaneous topics include conditions such as those affecting peripheral arteries, pulmonary arteries, aorta, and the heart in various system diseases. The number of articles having to do with preventive cardiology continues to rise.

6) *Number of editorial pages for articles and readers' comments published in the AJC, 1983-2014 (32 years)* (Table 5). During my 32+ years of editorship, more editorial pages were provided by the publisher in 2014 than any previous year, a total of 4,020: 3,976 were used for articles and 44, for readers' comments. During these 32 years, 100,719 total pages have been provided by the publisher for articles and an additional 1,219 for readers' comments. The number of articles published during the 32 full years was 21,595 and the number of readers' comments, 1,602.

7) *Interviews published in the AJC 1996-2014* (Table 6): During this 19-year period, 77 interviews of prominent cardiologists and cardiovascular surgeons have been published in the *AJC*. It is now time to put all these

Table 6
Interviews published in *The American Journal of Cardiology*

Eric Jeffrey Topol	July 1, 1996	Eugene Austin Stead, Jr.	September 15, 1999	Edward David Frolich	September 1, 2003
Wallace Bruce	August 1, 1996	Bertram Pitt	October 1, 1999	Magdi Habib Yacoub	January 15, 2003
James Thornton Willerson	February 15, 1997	Christopher John Dillon Packard	November 15, 1999	Robert A. Vogel	April 1, 2004
Michael Ellis DeBakey	April 1, 1997	Terje Rolf Pedersen	November 15, 1999	Ferid Murad	July 1, 2004
Denton Arthur Cooley	April 15, 1997	Francis Robicsek	June 1, 2000	Steven Evan Nissen	August 1, 2004
Joseph Stephan Alpert	May 1, 1997	Richard John Bing	July 1, 2000	William Peter Castelli	September 1, 2004
John Willis Hurst	February 15, 1998	Valentin Fuster	July 15, 2000	Wallace Bruce Fye III	January 1, 2005
Jesse Efrem Edwards	April 1, 1998	Henry Arthur Solomon	July 15, 2000	Anthony Nicolas DeMaria	January 15, 2005
John Webster Kirklin	April 15, 1998	Harvey Stanley Hecht	November 1, 2000	Barry L. Zaret	May 15, 2005
Howard Bertram Burchell	May 15, 1998	Myrvin Harold Ellestad	December 1, 2000	Lawrence Harvey Cohn	March 15, 2006
William Howard Frishman	June 1, 1998	Melvin Mayer Scheinman	March 1, 2001	Joseph Loscalzo	April 1, 2006
Robert Ogdon Bonow	June 15, 1998	James Stuart Forrester III	December 1, 2001	Donald Carey Harrison	May 1, 2006
Eugene Braunwald	July 1, 1998	Carl John Pepine	December 15, 2001	Hollis Bryan Brewer	June 15, 2006
Joseph Cholmondeley Greenfield	July 15, 1998	Kenneth Hardy Cooper	February 1, 2001	Barry Joel Maron	May 1, 2007
David Coston Sabiston, Jr.	August 1, 1998	Watkins Proctor Harvey	February 15, 2001	William Clifford Roberts	July 15, 2007
Norman Mayer Kaplan	August 15, 1998	Joseph Kayle Perloff	March 1, 2002	Jean Schlatter Kan	January 1, 2008
Robert McKinnon Califf	September 1, 1998	Charles Richard Conti	March 15, 2002	Robert William (Bobby) Brown	March 1, 2008
Bernard John Gersh	November 1, 1998	William Watts Parmley	May 1, 2002	Lawrence Cohen	March 15, 2008
Dean James Keriakes	November 15, 1998	Dean Michael Ornish	August 1, 2002	Paul Alan Grayburn	July 15, 2011
Jeffrey Michael Isner	January 1, 1999	Dean Towle Mason	December 15, 2002	William Edward Boden	July 1, 2012
Scott Montgomery Grundy	January 15, 1999	George Allan Beller	January 15, 2003	Peter Libby	September 1, 2012
Burton Elias Sobel	February 1, 1999	Leslie David Hillis	February 1, 2003	Lazar John Greenfield	November 1, 2013
Robert Anthony O'Rourke	April 1, 1999	Douglas P. Zipes	April 1, 2003	Peter Russell Kowey	June 1, 2014
David Kempton Cartwright Cooper	April 15, 1999	Nanette Kass Wenger	May 15, 2003	Jagat Narula	June 15, 2014
Spencer Bidwell King III	May 1, 1999	Andrew Peter Selwyn	June 15, 2003	Peter Andrew McCullough	December 1, 2014
Robert Roberts	May 15, 1999	Arthur Garson, Jr.	August 15, 2003		

interviews together in a book and I am trying to find a publisher desirous of doing so.

After an informative question-and-answer period all enjoyed a wonderful reception provided by the publisher.

William C. Roberts, MD
Baylor Heart and Vascular Institute
Baylor University Medical Center
Dallas, Texas

www.ingramcontent.com/pod-product-compliance
Lightning Source LLC
Chambersburg PA
CBHW082010150426
42814CB00005BA/278

* 9 7 8 0 9 8 4 5 2 3 7 6 4 *